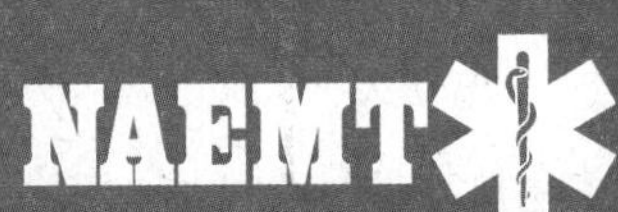

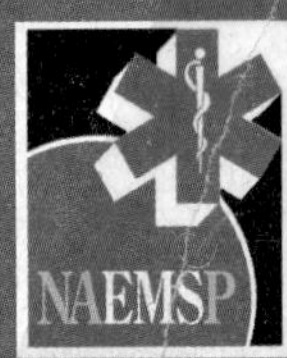

FOUR

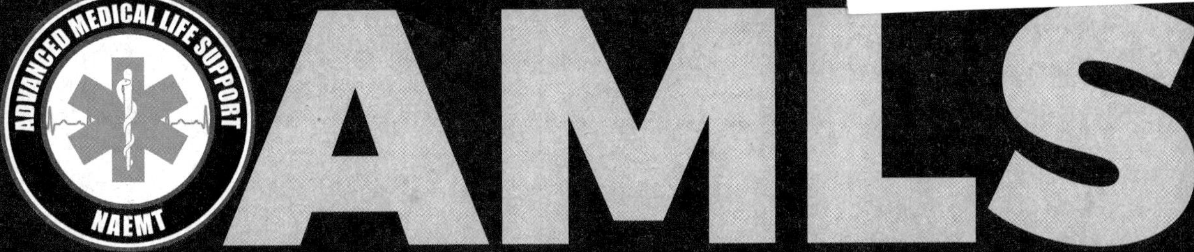

Advanced Medical Life Support

AN ASSESSMENT-BASED APPROACH

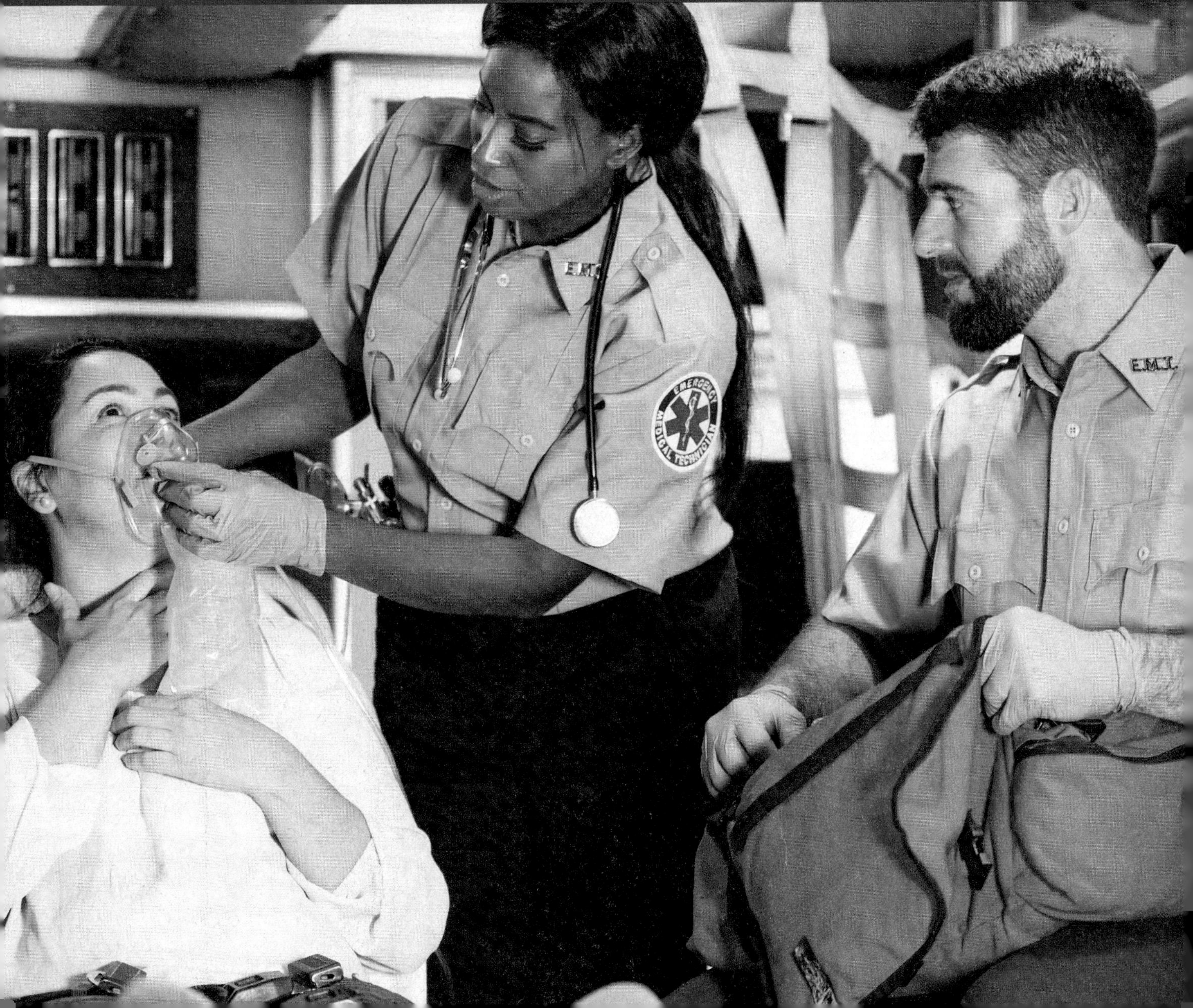

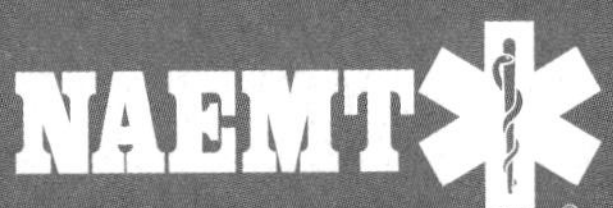
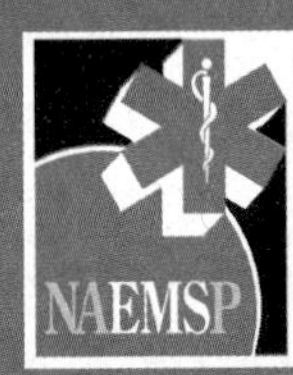

FOURTH EDITION

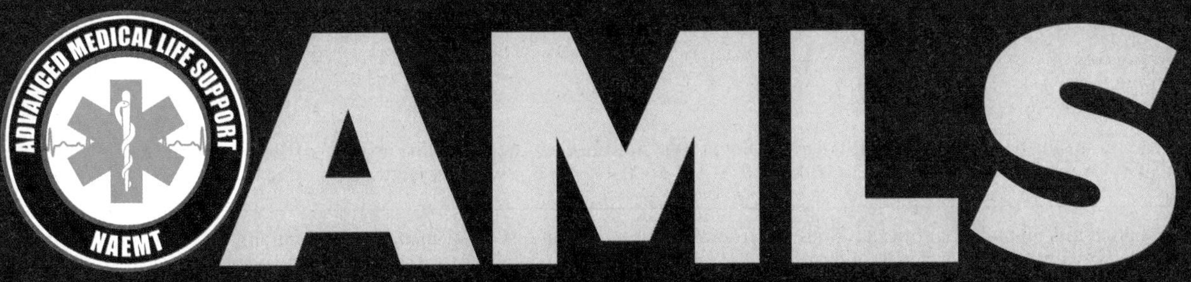

Advanced Medical Life Support

AN ASSESSMENT-BASED APPROACH

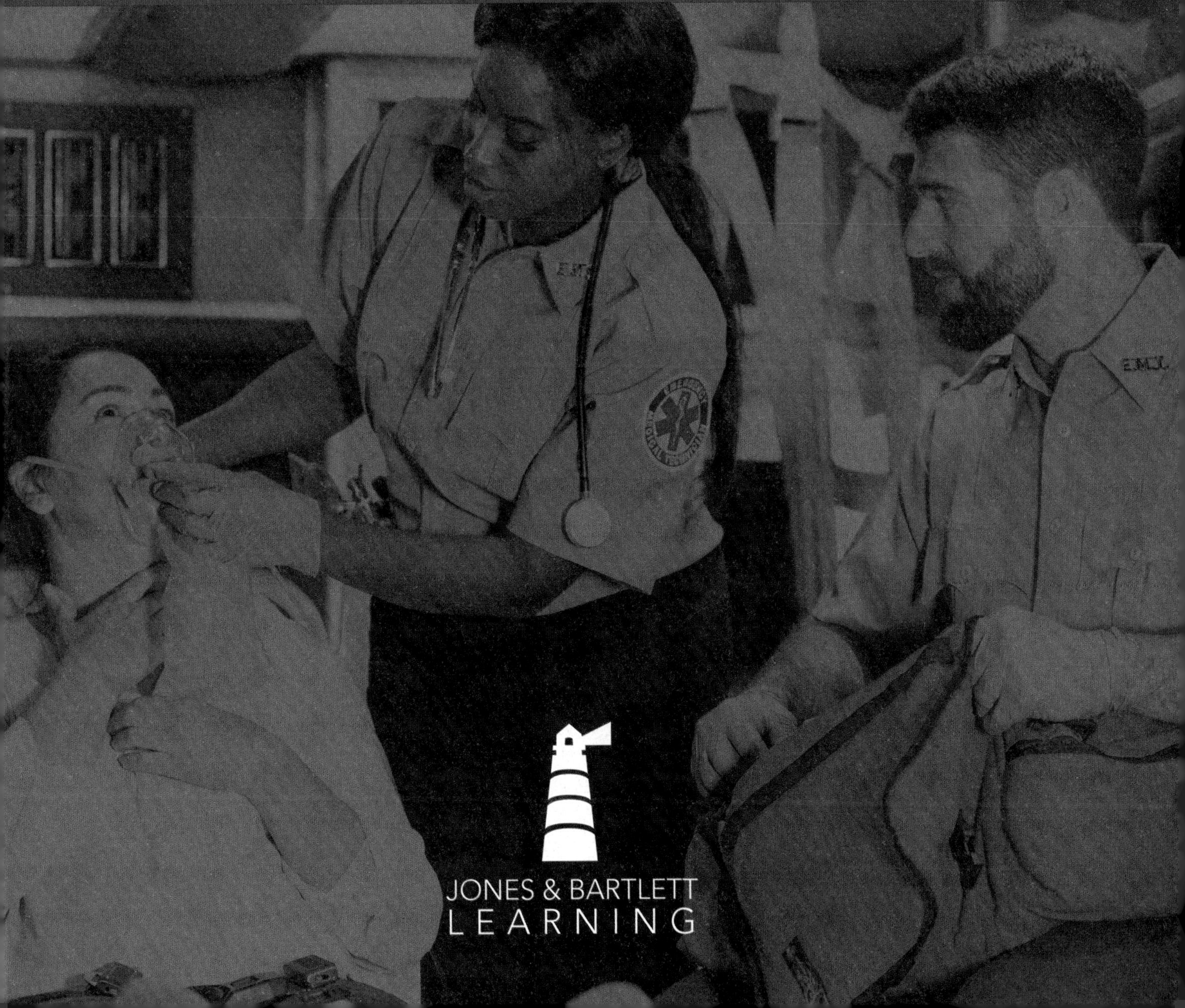

JONES & BARTLETT
LEARNING

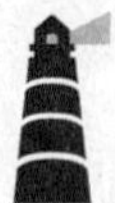

World Headquarters
Jones & Bartlett Learning
25 Mall Road
Burlington, MA 01803
978-443-5000
info@jblearning.com
www.jblearning.com
www.psglearning.com

Jones & Bartlett Learning books and products are available through most bookstores and online booksellers. To contact the Jones & Bartlett Learning Public Safety Group directly, call 800-832-0034, fax 978-443-8000, or visit our website, www.psglearning.com.

Substantial discounts on bulk quantities of Jones & Bartlett Learning publications are available to corporations, professional associations, and other qualified organizations. For details and specific discount information, contact the special sales department at Jones & Bartlett Learning via the above contact information or send an email to specialsales@jblearning.com.

29269-5

Production Credits
Vice President, Product Management: Marisa R. Urbano
Vice President, Content Strategy and Implementation: Christine Emerton
Director, Product Management: Cathy Esperti
Director, Content Management: Donna Gridley
Manager, Content Strategy: Tiffany Sliter
Content Strategist: ABP
Content Coordinator: Michaela MacQuarrie
Development Editor: Heather Ehlers
Director, Project Management and Content Services: Karen Scott
Manager, Project Management: Jackie Reynen
Project Manager: Erin Bosco
Senior Digital Project Specialist: Angela Dooley
Senior Product Marketing Manager: Elaine Riordan
Content Services Manager: Colleen Lamy
Senior Director of Supply Chain: Ed Schneider
Procurement Manager: Wendy Kilborn
Composition: S4Carlisle Publishing Services
Cover/Text Design: Scott Moden
Senior Media Development Editors: Troy Liston, Faith Brosnan
Rights & Permissions Manager: John Rusk
Rights Specialists: Liz Kincaid, Robin Silverman
Cover Image (Title Page): © kali9/E+/Getty images
Printing and Binding: Lakeside Book Company

Library of Congress Cataloging-in-Publication Data
Names: National Association of Emergency Medical Technicians (U.S.), issuing body.
Title: Advanced medical life support / National Association of Emergency Medical Technicians (NAEMT).
Other titles: AMLS.
Description: Fourth edition. | Burlington, MA : Jones & Bartlett Learning, [2025] | Preceded by AMLS : advanced medical life support : an assessment-based approach / Advanced Medical Life Support Committee of the National Association of Emergency Medical Technicians. Third edition. [2021]. | Includes bibliographical references and index.
Identifiers: LCCN 2023049747 | ISBN 9781284292695 (paperback)
Subjects: MESH: Advanced Trauma Life Support Care--methods | Emergency Treatment--methods | Emergency Medical Services | Needs Assessment | Emergency Medical Technicians
Classification: LCC RA645.5 | NLM WX 162 | DDC 362.18--dc23/eng/20231220
LC record available at https://lccn.loc.gov/2023049747

6048

Printed in the United States of America
28 27 26 25 24 10 9 8 7 6 5 4 3 2 1

Brief Contents

Table of Contents

Chapter 7 Infectious Diseases 225

Chapter 8 Neurologic Disorders 283

Acknowledgments

The NAEMT Advanced Medical Life Support Committee and AMLS textbook medical editors offer their gratitude to the many individuals who devoted countless hours of their time in the development of the fourth edition of *Advanced Medical Life Support* (AMLS). An exemplary group of subject matter experts composed of physicians, EMS clinicians, and educators served as chapter editors, authors, and reviewers. This collaboration has resulted in a textbook that reflects the diversity of thought leadership in prehospital medicine and is consistent with NAEMT's education mission and philosophy. We also wish to recognize the NAEMT editorial staff for their expertise and continuous attention to detail.

The National Association of EMS Physicians (NAEMSP) has supported the participation of its members as medical editors and chapter authors. Our gratitude is extended to NAEMSP for its ongoing support for this important prehospital program.

We also extend our appreciation to the many AMLS instructors and students who provided their feedback and suggestions for improvement to the fourth edition of AMLS. Their feedback has been incorporated into the chapters, the course slides, and the patient simulations.

Finally, we thank the EMS clinicians who serve in this profession, who positively impact patient outcomes through thoughtful assessments and evidence-based out-of-hospital health care. Your tireless commitment inspires us.

It has been our great pleasure and a true honor to work with everyone involved in bringing the Fourth Edition to publication. It is our hope this latest edition continues to make AMLS the premier source of education for advanced assessment and clinical decision-making while treating out-of-hospital patients with medical conditions.

Douglas F. Kupas, MD, EMT-P, FACEP, FAEMS
Vincent N. Mosesso, Jr., MD, FACEP, FAEMS
Jon R. Krohmer, MD, FACEP, FAEMS

Contributors

© Ralf Hiemisch/fStop/Getty Images

Medical Editor

Douglas F. Kupas, MD, EMT-P, FAEMS, FACEP
Medical Editor, *Advanced Medical Life Support, 4th Edition*
NAEMT Medical Director
Professor of Emergency Medicine
Medical Director, Geisinger EMS
Director, Resuscitation Program, Geisinger Medical Center
Danville, Pennsylvania

Associate Medical Editors

Vincent N. Mosesso, Jr., MD, FACEP, FAEMS
Associate Medical Editor, *Advanced Medical Life Support, 4th Edition*
Medical Director, NAEMT Advanced Medical Life Support Committee
Professor of Emergency Medicine
Associate Chief, Division of EMS
University of Pittsburgh School of Medicine
Medical Director, UPMC Prehospital Care
Pittsburgh, Pennsylvania

Jon R. Krohmer, MD, FACEP, FAEMS
Associate Medical Editor, *Advanced Medical Life Support, 4th Edition*
Adjunct Professor of Emergency Medicine
Michigan State University College of Human Medicine
East Lansing, Michigan

Editorial Director

Nancy Hoffmann, MSW
Senior Director, Education Publishing
National Association of Emergency Medical Technicians

Chapter Editors

Priyanka Amin, MD
Assistant Professor of Psychiatry
University of Pittsburgh
Medical Director, Patient Safety
UPMC Western Psychiatric Hospital
Pittsburgh, Pennsylvania

E. Stein Bronsky, MD
Co-Chief Medical Director
Colorado Springs Fire Department
Co-Chief Medical Director, American Medical Response
Medical Director, El Paso-Teller 911 Authority
Emergency Department Physician, Centura Health
Colorado Springs, Colorado

Erica Carney, MD, FAEMS
Medical Director
Kansas City, Missouri

Rommie L. Duckworth, MPA, LP, EFO, FO
Director, New England Center for Rescue and Emergency Medicine
Captain, Ridgefield Fire Department
Ridgefield, Connecticut

B. Craig Ellis, MBChB, Dip IMC (RCSEd), FACEM
Medical Director
St John, New Zealand

Bryan A. Everitt, MD, NRP, FAAEM
Assistant Clinical Professor
EMS Physician/Medical Director
University of Texas Health San Antonio
Department of Emergency Medicine
San Antonio, Texas

Raymond L. Fowler, MD, FACEP, FAEMS
Professor of Emergency Medicine and Emergency Medical Services
James M. Atkins MD Distinguished Professor of Emergency Medical Services
Department of Emergency Medicine
University of Texas Southwestern Medical Center
Dallas, Texas

David M. French, MD, FACEP, FAEMS
EMS Medical Director
Charleston, South Carolina

Joshua B. Gaither, MD, FACEP, FAEMS
Director, EMS Fellowship
Director, BS in Emergency Medical Services
Medical Director, Tucson Fire Department
Professor of Emergency Medicine
University of Arizona College of Medicine
Tucson, Arizona

Austin W. Gay, MD
Academic Chief Resident
Emergency Medicine
University of Texas Health—San Antonio
San Antonio, Texas

W. Scott Gilmore, MD, FACEP, FAEMS
Medical Director
St. Louis Fire Department
St. Louis, Missouri

Jonathan Jui, MD, MPH
Professor of Emergency Medicine
Oregon Health and Sciences University
Medical Director, Multnomah County EMS
Portland, Oregon

Dustin P. LeBlanc, MD
Assistant Professor of Emergency Medicine
Medical University of South Carolina
Charleston, South Carolina

Michael Levy, MD, FAEMS, FACEP, FACP
Medical Director for Anchorage Fire Department and Areawide EMS
Medical Director for EMS Kenai Peninsula Borough Alaska
Medical Director for Emergency Programs State of Alaska
Affiliate Associate Professor, College of Health
University of Alaska, Anchorage
Anchorage, Alaska

Melanie Lippmann, MD
Associate Professor of Emergency Medicine
Brown University, Alpert Medical School
Rhode Island Hospital and The Miriam Hospital
Providence, Rhode Island

Ratna M. Malkan, DO
EMS Physician, Emergency Medicine
University of Texas Health San Antonio
Department of Emergency Medicine
San Antonio, Texas

Christian Martin-Gill, MD, MPH
Chief, Division of EMS
Associate Professor of Emergency Medicine
University of Pittsburgh School of Medicine
Pittsburgh, Pennsylvania

Karin H. Molander, MD, FACEP
Emergency Medicine, Mills Peninsula Medical Center
Burlingame, California
Board of Directors, Sepsis Alliance
San Diego, California

Matthew R. Neth, MD
Assistant Professor, OHSU Department of Emergency Medicine
Associate Medical Director, Multnomah County EMS
Portland, Oregon

Emily Nichols, MD
Attending Physician, Department of Emergency Medicine
Ochsner Medical Center
Deputy Medical Director, New Orleans EMS
New Orleans, Louisiana

Cecilio Padrón, MD
EMS Fellow
Department of Emergency Medicine
University of North Carolina
Chapel Hill, North Carolina

Carolina C. Pereira, MD, FACEP, FAEMS
Fort Myers, Florida

Benjamin D. Pilkey, MD
2022–2023 Academic Chief Resident
2023–2024 Emergency Medical Services Fellow
University of Texas Health San Antonio
San Antonio, Texas

Stephen J. Rahm, NRP, FcEHS
Chief, Office of Clinical Direction
Co-Chair, Centre for Emergency Health Sciences
Spring Branch, Texas

Benjamin Smith, MD
Medical Director, Carolina Air Care
Medical Director, Air Life NC
Clinical Assistant Professor
Department of Emergency Medicine, University of North Carolina
Chapel Hill, North Carolina

Rickquel Tripp, MD, MPH, Commander United States Navy
Vice Chair of Diversity, Equity, and Inclusion for UPMC Medical Education
Vice Chair of Diversity, Inclusion, and Health Equity for Department of Emergency Medicine
Assistant Professor, Department of Emergency Medicine
EMS Medical Director, UPMC Prehospital
Pittsburgh, Pennsylvania

Shawn M. Varney, MD, FACEP, FAACT, FACMT
Professor, Department of Emergency Medicine
University of Texas Health San Antonio
Medical Director
South Texas Poison Center
San Antonio, Texas

Mark Warth, BHS, NRP
Medical Program Coordinator
Colorado Springs Fire Department
Colorado Springs, Colorado

Lauren Young Work, MSW, LCSW
Medical Social Work/MIH Coordinator
Palm Beach County Fire Rescue
Palm Beach County, Florida

Scott T. Youngquist, MD, MSc
Professor of Emergency Medicine
University of Utah School of Medicine
Medical Director, Salt Lake City Fire Department and 911 Dispatch
Salt Lake City, Utah

National Association of Emergency Medical Technicians 2024 Board of Directors

Officers

President: Susan Bailey
President-Elect: Chris Way
Immediate Past President: Bruce Evans
Secretary: Troy Tuke
Treasurer: Robert Luckritz
Medical Director: Douglas F. Kupas, MD

Directors

Rommie Duckworth, Director, Region I
Steven Kroll, Director, Region I
Juan C. Cardona, Director, Region II
Melissa McNally, Director, Region II
David Edgar, Director, Region III
Shannon Watson, Director, Region III
Tim Dienst, Director, Region IV
Karen Larsen, Director, Region IV
Maria Beermann-Foat, At-Large Director
Matt Zavadsky, At-Large Director

AMLS Committee

Cory S. Richter, BA, NRP
Chair, AMLS Committee
NAEMT Region II Education Coordinator
IT Director
Indian River Shores Public Safety Department
Indian River County, Florida

Vincent N. Mosesso, Jr., MD, FACEP, FAEMS
Medical Director, AMLS Committee

Jeffrey L. Jarvis, MD, MS, EMT-P
Associate Medical Director, AMLS Committee
Chief Medical Officer and System Medical Director
Metropolitan Area EMS Authority, MedStar
Fort Worth, Texas

R. Zachary Louderback, MD
Associate Medical Director, AMLS Committee
Emergency Medicine Physician
EMS Director, US Acute Care Solutions
Medical Director, West Metro Fire Rescue
Denver, Colorado

Douglas F. Kupas, MD, EMT-P, FAEMS, FACEP
Medical Editor, AMLS Committee

Jon R. Krohmer, MD, FACEP, FAEMS
Associate Medical Editor, AMLS Committee

Anne Austin Ellerbee, AAS, AF, NRP
Member, AMLS Committee
EMS Coordinator
Lamar County Fire & Rescue
Barnesville, Georgia

Bengt Eriksson, MD, PhD
Member, AMLS Committee
Consultant Anesthetist
Anesthesiology Department, Mora Iasaretti
Medical Director Prehospital Care Region Dalama
National CMD PHTLS and AMLS
Sweden

Michael Kaduce, MPS, NRP
Member, AMLS Committee
EMT Program Director
UCLA David Geffen School of Medicine
UCLA Center for Prehospital Care
Los Angeles, California

Kelly Kohler, MS, CCP-C, CHSE, NCEE
Member, AMLS Committee
Assistant Professor of Emergency Medical Services
Touro College of Osteopathic Medicine
Simulation Specialist
Middletown, New York

Jeff J. Messerole, EMT-P
Member, AMLS Committee
EMS Continuing Education Programmer
Iowa Lakes Community College
Spirit Lake, Iowa

Alex Protzman, Paramedic
Member, AMLS Committee
Major of Clinical Operations
Riley County EMS
Manhattan, Kansas

Reviewers

Fourth Edition Reviewers

Lisa Aiken, NRP
Central Virginia Community College
Lynchburg, Virginia

Jamie J. Barton, EMT-P, CCEMT-P, NYS CIC
Wilton Emergency Squad, Inc.
Saratoga Springs, New York

Ryan Batenhorst, EdD(c), MEd, NRP
Creighton University
Omaha, Nebraska

Patricia Binion, SEI
Skagit Valley College
Mount Vernon, Washington

Stephen Blackburn, BS, NR-P, CP-C
Cape Fear Community College
Wilmington, North Carolina

Graeme Bockrath, NREMT-P
Apollo Career Center
Lima, Ohio

Mark A. Boisclair, MPA, NRP
EMS Program Director
Chattahoochee Valley Community College
Phenix City, Alabama

Gary Bonewald, MEd, LP
Wharton County Junior College
Wharton, Texas

Leslie W. Brock Jr., CCT-P, ABA, EMSI
SafeTec Training Education Services
Bensalem, Pennsylvania

Fred D. Chambers, LP, BS, EMS-C$_{\text{(Advanced)}}$
Houston Community College–Northeast
Houston, Texas

John C Cook, EdD, MBA, NRP
Radford University
Roanoke, Virginia

Kevin Curry, AS, CCEMTP, NRP
Waldoboro EMS
Waldoboro, Maine

Julia Cusimano, EMT-P, EMSI, BS
Clark State College
Springfield, Ohio

Sylvia Davis, BS, NREMT-P, Paramedic, IC, FF
AHA BLS, ACLS, PALS Instructor
Educational Program Manager
Critical Care Transfer, Inc.
Ulysses, Kansas
Adjunct Faculty Fire and EMS Education
Butler Community College
Andover, Kansas

Brandy DeBarge, Paramedic
Patriot Ambulance
Chelmsford, Massachusetts

Melissa M. Doak, NRP, Battalion Chief of EMS
York County Fire and Life Safety
York County, Virginia

Ronald B. Estanislao, BA, NRP, NCEE, FP-C
Cambridge College
Boston, Massachusetts

William Faust, MPA, Paramedic
Western Carolina University
School of Health Sciences, Emergency Medical Care Program
Cullowhee, North Carolina

Darrell W. Fixler, AAS, RRT, CC-NRP
Parris Island Fire & EMS
Beaufort, South Carolina

Daniel R. Gerard, MS, RN, NRP

Lee Gillum, MPH, LIC-P, EMS-CC
Montgomery County Hospital District EMS
Conroe, Texas

Kevin M. Gurney, MS, CCEMT-P, I/C
Delta Ambulance
Waterville, Maine

Rick Hilinski, BA, EMT-P, CCP
CCAC Public Safety Institute
Pittsburgh, Pennsylvania

Mikka House-Moore, NRP, MEd
Tulsa Technology Center
Tulsa, Oklahoma

Joseph L. Hurlburt, BS, NREMT
Paramedic/Instructor Coordinator
Northwest Wexford Emergency Authority
Mesick, Michigan

Sandra Hultz, NRP, EMS Faculty
Holmes Community College
Ridgeland, Mississippi

Joseph Itzkowitz, AS, CCEMTP, NRP
Emergency Care Programs
Brooklyn, New York

Dorothy Jensen, AEMT

Peter D. Johnson, NREMT-P, EMSI
EMS Training Coordinator
Bridgewater Fire Department
Bridgewater, Connecticut

Bill Kane, BA, NREMT, AEMT
EMS Incident Commander
New Hampshire and Maine
Owner/Director
The Kane Schools, Wild & Rescue Medicine
Former Chief, VP BOD
Fryeburg Rescue
Fryeburg, Maine

Michael Kaduce, MPS, NRP
UCLA David Geffen School of Medicine
Los Angeles, California

Blake Klingle, MS, RN, CEN, CCEMT-P
Waukesha County Technical College
Pewaukee, Wisconsin

Lawrence Linder, MA, MS, NRP
Hillsborough Community College
Ruskin, Florida

Lt. Scott McCormack, EMT-P, EMS-EC, AAS
Richlands Fire Rescue
Richlands, Virginia

John R. McFarland, MS, EMT-P, NCEE, PI
Jay County EMS
Portland, Indiana

Terry Mendez, EdM, Paramedic
Western Nevada College
Carson City, Nevada

Nicholas J. Montelauro, MBA-HM, NRP, FP-C, NCEE, CHSE
Indiana University Health
Indianapolis, Indiana

Gregory S. Neiman, MS, NRP, NCEE
VCU Health
Richmond, Virginia

Jim O'Connor, Paramedic
Ohio Fire Academy
Reynoldsburg, Ohio

George Olschewski, BSN, RN, CFRN, CTRN, TCRN, CEN, MICN
Hackensack UMC Specialty Care Transport Unit
Hackensack, New Jersey

Keito Ortiz, Paramedic CIC, NCEE NAEMSE Level II
Continued Education Specialist
American Medical Response Metro NY
Bayshore, New York

Melissa Osborne, BA, CCEMT-P, NRP, EMS-I
Ambulance Service of Manchester
Manchester, Connecticut

Leo T. Pernesky Jr., Paramedic, EMS Instructor
Jefferson County EMS
Punxsutawney, Pennsylvania
Penn Highlands Healthcare
Du Bois, Pennsylvania

Jared K. Priddy, NRP
Frederick County Fire and Rescue
Frederick County, Virginia

Stephanie Scheib, MS, Paramedic, I/C
Great Lakes Bay Consortium for EMS Education
Saginaw, Michigan

Jeb Sheidler, DMSc, PA-C, NRP, TP-C, WP-C
Associate Director, Center of Operational Medicine
Director, EMS Academy
Medical College of Georgia at Augusta University
Augusta, Georgia

Craig Spector
EMS Instructor
CPR Heart Starters Safety Training
Warrington, Pennsylvania

Josh Steele, MBA, FP-C, NRP, CMTE
Hospital Wing
Memphis, Tennessee

Michael E. Tanner
Ritchie County Ambulance Authority
Harrisville, West Virginia
WVPST Mid-Ohio Valley Region
Parkersburg, West Virginia

Gilberto Torres, L-P, BA
Willacy County EMS
Raymondville, Texas

Adam Voydik, NRP, FP-C
VAMS, EMskillz LLC
Clarksville, Tennessee

Benjamin Vu, EMT-P, BS
Mt. San Antonio College
Walnut, California

Amy Wasko, Paramedic, Lead Instructor, NAEMSE Level II Instructor
College of DuPage
Glen Ellyn, Illinois

Joseph Welsh, NREMT
Life-Savers, Inc.
Louisville, Kentucky

R. Greg West
North Shore Community College
Danvers, Massachusetts

Crystal Campbell Youmans
Saint Matthews, South Carolina

Third Edition Reviewers

J. Adam Alford, NRP
Piedmont Virginia Community College
Charlottesville, Virginia

Ryan Batenhorst, MEd, NRP, EMSI
Southeast Community College
Lincoln, Nebraska

Dana Baumgartner, NRP, BS
Nicolet College
Eagle River, Wisconsin

Mark A. Boisclair, MPA, NRP USA (ret)
Chattahoochee Valley Community College
Phenix City, Alabama

John C. Cook, EdD, MBA, NRP, NCEE
Jefferson College of Health Sciences
Roanoke, Virginia

Mark Cromer, PhD, MS, MBA, NRP
Carilion Clinic
Salem, Virginia

Kevin Curry, AS, NRP, CCEMTP
United Training Center
Lewiston, Maine

William Faust, MPA, NRP
Western Carolina University
Cullowhee, North Carolina

Darrell W. Fixler Jr., RRT, NRP, FP-C
Parris Island Fire & Rescue
Beaufort, South Carolina

Lori Gallian, BS, EMT-P
Summit Sciences
Citrus Heights, California

Scott A. Gano, BS, NRP, FP-C, CCEMT-P
Columbus State Community College
Columbus, Ohio

Kevin M. Gurney, MS, CCEMT-P, I/C
Delta Ambulance
Waterville, Maine

Bradley R. Hughes, AAS, CP-C, NRP, NCEE
Putnam County EMS
Winfield, West Virginia

Sandra Hultz, NRP
Holmes Community College
Ridgeland, Mississippi

Joseph Hurlburt, BS, NRP
North Flight EMS
Manton, Michigan

Jared Kimball, NRP
Tulane Trauma Education
New Orleans, Louisiana

Timothy M. Kimble, BA, AAS, CEM, NRP
Craig County Office of Emergency Services
New Castle, Virginia

Blake E. Klingle, MS, RN, CCEMT-P
Waukesha County Technical College
Pewaukee, Wisconsin

Keri Wydner Krause
Lakeshore Technical College
Cleveland, Wisconsin

Michael K. Matheny, BS, NRP, NCEE, PI
Community Health Network, EMS Education
Indianapolis, Indiana

Nicholas Montelauro, BS, NRP, FP-C, NCEE, CHSE
Indianapolis, Indiana

Gregory S. Neiman, MS, NRP, NCEE
EMS Community Liaison, VCU Health
Richmond, Virginia

Jim O'Connor, Paramedic
Ohio Fire Academy
Logan, Ohio

Keito Ortiz, Paramedic, NAEMSE II
Jamaica Hospital Medical Center
Jamaica, New York

Matthew Ozanich, MHHS, NRP
Trumbull Regional Medical Center
Warren, Ohio

Debbie Petty
St. Charles County Ambulance District
St. Peters, Missouri

Tim Petreit, MBA, NRP
Montgomery Fire/Rescue
Montgomery, Alabama

Deborah Richeal, NRP
MedAire
Phoenix, Arizona

Captain Bruce J. Stark, NRP
Fairfax County Fire and Rescue Department
Fairfax, Virginia

Josh Steele, MBA-HA, BS, AAS, NRP, FP-C, CMTE
Hospital Wing Memphis
Memphis, Tennessee

Nerina J. Stepanovsky, PhD, MSN, CTRN, Paramedic
Caduceus Educational Consulting LLC
Parrish, Florida

Richard Stump, NRP
Central Carolina Community College
Sanford, North Carolina

William Torres Jr., NRP
Marcus Daly Memorial Hospital
Hamilton, Montana

Gary S. Walter, MS, BA, NRP
Eugene, Oregon

Rekeisha A. Watson-Love, AAS, NRP
Paramedic/Instructor Coordinator
Las Vegas, Nevada

Foreword

EMS education, like EMS care itself, has evolved dramatically. Early EMS education focused heavily on the most basic priority of emergency care: resuscitation. Education courses addressed the important resuscitative roles that EMS clinicians perform for critical patients. However, as prehospital clinicians—and EMS itself—matured and anchored their place in the patient care continuum, it became readily apparent that much of EMS care is not life or death resuscitation, but rather the care of acutely ill and injured patients. EMS clinicians and medical directors grew to understand that there was a need for education on the "nuts and bolts" of prehospital patient care—that is, talking to patients; identifying their physical, psychological, and social needs; differentiating between emergent and nonemergent patient presentations; and communicating with other health care providers to optimize patient care. This foundational understanding led to the development of Advanced Medical Life Support (AMLS).

The foundation for the AMLS textbook and course is based on a simple, but not easy, premise: that, although EMS clinicians do perform critical resuscitative skills, the most important roles of the EMS clinician are "less sexy" and focus on talking to and understanding patients; collecting and interpreting the patient's chief complaint and medical history; assessing the impact of the environment on patient care; providing empathy and comfort; and integrating all of these pieces to create a patient management plan based on the best information available at the time. These components of prehospital care require training (technical skills), education (ability to integrate varied and sometimes contradictory information), critical thinking, and affective skills (understanding and empathy to manage patients with a variety of emotional, cognitive, and even drug- or alcohol-impacted issues). Further, it requires that the clinician communicate all the necessary information calmly, clearly, and nonjudgmentally—in essence, making EMS care human. By comparison, running a cardiac arrest is a "walk in the park."

AMLS is structured to help EMS clinicians learn to better address this complex milieu. It begins by addressing the foundational skills of communication, understanding patients, scene assessment, information gathering, and assessing the patient's capacity to accept or refuse care. It then moves forward to address undifferentiated complaints that are varied, may be life threatening, or are just serious enough to require timely intervention to prevent bad outcomes. Increasingly, patients and clinicians will assess whether emergency care is required, or whether patients will receive transport to alternative facilities; a telemedicine consultation with a physician, advanced practice provider, or triage nurse; or be treated in place by EMS; all in a timely and cost-effective manner. All of these components are what comprise the practice of prehospital medical care.

To optimize the learning of this EMS practice, AMLS is supported and endorsed by the National Association of EMS Physicians, the course medical directors, and a host of accomplished authors. The goal of this support is to provide medical direction, to make certain that the direction of EMS care is *medical*, and, importantly, is focused on ensuring that all EMS care is patient centered and driven by optimal patient outcomes.

While I address the role that medical direction plays in this program, I would be remiss if I didn't recognize the impact that Dr. Craig Manifold has had on prehospital care. Dr. Manifold served as the medical director of the National Association of Emergency Medical Technicians, as the medical editor of the 3rd edition AMLS textbook, and as a visionary force in improving EMS patient care. Sadly, Dr. Manifold has passed away far too soon. We miss his kind and thoughtful presence, but the AMLS program is part of a rich legacy that has improved EMS care to all of our patients.

Robert Swor, DO, FACEP, FAEMS
Professor, Department of Emergency Medicine
Oakland University William Beaumont
School of Medicine
Auburn Hills, Michigan

Preface

AMLS Course Education Philosophy

First published in 1999, *Advanced Medical Life Support* (AMLS) was the first EMS education program that fully addressed how to best evaluate and manage patients in medical crises. AMLS is now globally recognized as the leading course for the assessment and treatment of medical conditions in the prehospital/out-of-hospital environments.

This latest edition of the AMLS textbook serves as the medical foundation of the AMLS fourth edition course and as a key reference for paramedics and other out-of-hospital clinicians around the world. AMLS serves an expanding audience of clinicians who seek high-quality, evidence-based education focusing on critical thinking, history taking, and a physical assessment to develop a list of potential differential diagnoses in the medical patient. The AMLS Assessment Pathway, one of the core features of the AMLS course and upon which the course lessons are built, has been demonstrated to be a highly reliable tool to assist out-of-hospital clinicians in identifying a differential diagnosis that will guide patient treatment.

The fourth edition of the AMLS course remains true to the AMLS philosophy of using critical thinking when assessing patients and formulating treatment plans. The case-based lesson presentations provide students with the opportunity for interactive discussion. Patient simulations throughout the course challenge students to apply their knowledge to a variety of realistic situations, including both high- and low-acuity patients; some may require emergent care and transport, whereas others may benefit from alternate destination transport or additional patient navigation.

AMLS is endorsed by the National Association of EMS Physicians (NAEMSP), and this support is reflected in the many NAEMSP members who lent their time and expertise as chapter editors to revise and update the textbook. The AMLS approach emphasizes early identification of a patient's cardinal presentation or chief complaint. In addition to the AMLS Assessment Pathway, AMLS provides (1) a foundation of anatomy, physiology, and pathophysiology and (2) an efficient yet thorough presentation of pertinent historical, physical exam, and diagnostic findings, which enhances students' ability to narrow the patient's differential diagnoses. All prehospital and out-of-hospital clinicians—whether paramedics, advanced EMTs, EMTs, nurses, or other advanced practice providers and physicians—as well as in-hospital clinicians assessing emergent patients, require expertise in clinical reasoning and decision making to accurately determine probable diagnoses and initiate treatment. All aspects of AMLS are focused on an assessment-based approach to reduce morbidity and mortality and improve positive patient outcomes.

Although the AMLS textbook and course are written with advanced clinicians in mind, NAEMT encourages all prehospital and out-of-hospital clinicians to take AMLS, recognizing that critical thinking is important at all licensure levels. Whether taught as continuing or initial education, AMLS prepares and enhances the prehospital clinician's ability to care for the majority of their patients.

Features

For the fourth edition, figures, tables, Rapid Recall boxes, and Tip boxes have been updated and included throughout the textbook, lessons, and course manual to serve as learning tools. Each chapter opens with a case-based scenario with critical-thinking questions to assist the student in formulating a differential diagnosis. New features to the fourth edition include:

- Revised table of contents
- Updates to all chapters, with a focus on current literature-based evidence
- New chapter on *Women's Health Emergencies*
- New or updated case-based lesson presentations
- Revised and new patient simulations.

We, the medical editors, along with the AMLS Committee and NAEMT, hope you find that the information contained in the fourth edition AMLS textbook, lessons, patient simulations, and course manual enhances your knowledge about the variety of medical emergencies to which you respond, better preparing you to serve your patients and communities with compassionate, competent, and up-to-date medical care.

Douglas F. Kupas, MD, EMT-P, FACEP, FAEMS
Vincent N. Mosesso, Jr., MD, FACEP, FAEMS
Jon R. Krohmer, MD, FACEP, FAEMS

National Association of Emergency Medical Technicians

Founded in 1975, NAEMT is the only national organization in the United States that represents and serves the professional interests of EMS practitioners, including paramedics, emergency medical technicians, emergency medical responders, and other professionals providing prehospital and out-of-hospital emergent, urgent, or preventive medical care. NAEMT members work in all sectors of EMS, including government service agencies, fire departments, hospital-based ambulance services, private companies, industrial and special operations settings, and the military.

NAEMT serves its members by advocating on issues that impact their ability to provide quality patient care, providing high-quality education that improves the knowledge and skills of practitioners, and supporting EMS research and innovation.

One of NAEMT's principal activities is EMS education. The mission of NAEMT education programs is to improve patient care through high-quality, cost-effective, evidence-based education that strengthens and enhances the knowledge and skills of EMS practitioners.

NAEMT strives to provide the highest quality education programs. All NAEMT education programs are developed by highly experienced EMS educators, clinicians, and medical directors. Course content incorporates the latest research, newest techniques, and innovative approaches in EMS learning. All NAEMT education programs promote critical thinking as the foundation for providing quality care. This is based on the belief that EMS practitioners make the best decisions on behalf of their patients when given a sound foundation of evidence-based knowledge and key principles.

Once developed, education programs are tested and refined to ensure that course materials are clear, accurate, and relevant to the needs of EMS practitioners. Finally, all education programs are reviewed and updated every 4 years or as needed to ensure that the content reflects the most up-to-date research and practices.

NAEMT provides ongoing support to its instructors and the EMS training centers that hold its courses. Over 2,500 training centers, including colleges, EMS agencies, fire departments, hospitals, and other medical training facilities located in the United States and more than 80 other countries, offer NAEMT education programs. NAEMT headquarters staff work with the network of education program faculty engaged as committee members; authors; national, regional, and state coordinators; and affiliate faculty to provide administrative and educational support.

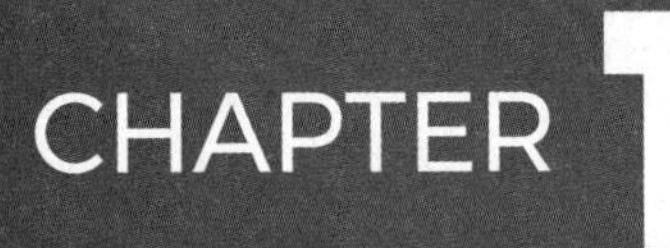

Advanced Medical Life Support Assessment for the Medical Patient

Chapter Editors

Vincent N. Mosesso, Jr., MD, FACEP, FAEMS
Jon R. Krohmer, MD, FACEP, FAEMS
Douglas F. Kupas, MD, EMT-P, FAEMS, FACEP
Rickquel Tripp, MD, MPH, CDR USN

In this chapter, clinicians will apply their knowledge of anatomy, physiology, pathophysiology, and epidemiology to the comprehensive, efficient Advanced Medical Life Support (AMLS) assessment process using their clinical reasoning to list differential diagnoses and formulate management strategies for a variety of medical emergencies.

LEARNING OBJECTIVES

At the conclusion of this chapter, you will be able to:

- Identify situations that compromise the safety of prehospital clinicians and patients.
- Apply the AMLS Assessment Pathway to identify nonemergent, emergent, and potentially life-threatening patient presentations.
- Identify the components of the first impression and the elements of the primary survey for patients with a variety of medical emergencies.
- Apply the AMLS Assessment Pathway to rule in or out differential diagnoses, based on a patient's initial presentation, assessment, and diagnostic findings.
- Integrate the patient's history (OPQRST and SAMPLER), pain assessment, physical examination, and diagnostic findings to determine working diagnoses and treatment interventions.
- Select appropriate diagnostic assessment tools, from basic to advanced, for a variety of medical emergencies.
- Correlate the symptoms of a patient's cardinal presentation to the appropriate body system to assess various potential diagnoses.
- Discuss how cultural awareness can help counter any unconscious prejudices that might impede the assessment process.
- Compare and contrast the assessment concepts of clinical decision making and clinical reasoning.
- Understand the potential impact of cognitive and unconscious biases on clinical decision making.
- Understand how basic life support (BLS) assessment and treatment combined with advanced life support (ALS) assessment and treatment supports an integrated team approach to patient care.

SCENARIO

EMS responds to a residence to care for an 86-year-old man. Dispatch indicates the patient is experiencing fatigue and feels faint when standing. This patient was transported twice last week by EMS to the local hospital for vague, but similar, complaints. On examination, the patient responds to verbal stimuli. He remains seated

(continues)

SCENARIO (CONTINUED)

in a chair during the assessment and says he is unusually tired and agitated. He is not feeling any better after several days. His body positioning is not concerning, but you notice a walker beside the chair. No difficulty in breathing is noted. He slowly answers questions regarding his current symptoms but is unsure if he took his medications today. His daughter provides his medications for hypertension and constipation. She tells you that "he takes some sort of blood thinner for an irregular heartbeat." When obtaining vital signs, the EMT and paramedic notice that the patient's skin is pale and clammy. The patient's respirations are 22 breaths/min and regular, his blood pressure is 110/84 mm Hg, and his pulse rate is 126 beats/min and irregular. The clinicians consider various differential diagnoses and begin the focused assessment.

- What conditions are you going to consider as possible diagnoses based on the information gathered thus far in your assessment?
- Which additional assessments will you perform based on this patient's chief complaint and the history you have obtained?
- What issues might you encounter as a result of the patient's age?

This chapter provides guidance for all levels of health care clinicians on how to apply their knowledge of anatomy, physiology, pathophysiology, and epidemiology to the Advanced Medical Life Support (AMLS) assessment process. An accurate patient assessment relies not only on a clinician's foundational knowledge and experience, but also on therapeutic communication techniques, clinical reasoning, and clinical decision-making skills.

An organized, systematic evaluation of the patient's initial presentation, medical history, physical exam findings, and diagnostic test results is essential. These findings help determine the criticality of the patient's condition, working diagnoses, and management strategies. The ability of the health care clinician to communicate effectively and use clinical reasoning enables the clinician to consider all possible etiologies related to the presenting symptoms. A thorough patient assessment ensures appropriate interventions and better patient outcomes.

It is important to understand that the foundation of the AMLS Assessment Pathway is based on effective therapeutic communication skills, keen clinical-reasoning abilities, and expert clinical decision making. BLS and ALS clinicians working efficiently as a team enhance the timeliness and quality of care of the patient.

Therapeutic Communication

Therapeutic communication uses various communication techniques and strategies, both verbal and nonverbal, to encourage patients to express how they are feeling and to achieve a positive, empathetic relationship with the patient. Obtaining a comprehensive medical history and being able to perform a thorough physical examination depend on good therapeutic interpersonal communication techniques. To obtain critical information about the patient's condition, BLS and ALS clinicians need to effectively communicate with the patient, family, bystanders, and the entire health care team. The information obtained can often provide clues to help identify the specific injuries sustained or point toward a particular diagnosis.

Effective Verbal and Nonverbal Communication

Effective verbal communication is a dynamic process. According to the Bayer Institute for Health Care Communication, health care clinicians carry out four principal communication tasks called the four Es: engagement, empathy, education, and enlistment.

- *Engagement* is the connection between you and your patients. You must establish a comfortable rapport with patients to help them stay calm and elicit a thorough, accurate history. Your words *and actions* convey your genuine concern. Failing to introduce yourself; grilling patients with aggressive, rapid-fire questions; and interrupting them when they are talking undermine the bond you need to develop and may cause the patient to disengage. During initial contact with patients and bystanders, be sure to introduce yourself and your title or role. Developing a rapport with patients also facilitates open communication. Be mindful in the moment, hear what the patient is saying to you, and observe the patient's reactions and body language. If you portray a calm deliberateness, you will quickly gain your patient's trust and confidence in your abilities. Make a positive first impression.

- *Empathy* refers to your sincere identification with the patient's feelings of anxiety, pain, suffering, fear, panic, or loss. Empathy is rooted in a sense of compassion for what the patient is going through. It is not about trying to convince the patient that you know exactly what they are feeling. Acknowledge to the patient what you hear and understand by summarizing or paraphrasing the information the patient has shared. Accept what the patient tells you, regardless of the circumstances surrounding the call. Empathy is especially important in situations such as suicide attempts and other behavioral health presentations, accidental drug overdoses, and cases of domestic assault. It is a skill that should be matured and improved upon throughout one's career.
- *Education* of your patients fortifies your bond by letting them know what is happening and what you are doing. Begin by asking what the patient already knows and follow up with questions until you have all the information you need. Keep patients informed during the entire call. Describe tests and procedures in simple, straightforward terms, which will help minimize the patient's anxiety.
- *Enlistment* involves encouraging patients to participate in their own care and treatment decisions. When you ask for a patient's consent for treatment, be sure to explain fully any possible side effects or potential adverse outcomes associated with the intervention. For example, before starting an IV, ask the patient if they have a preference for which arm is used. Give the patient choices in their care when possible, and ask for their help in making your examination easier and more thorough.

Nonverbal communication, which includes facial expressions, body language, and eye contact, is a powerful form of communication. It is important that you are aware of the body language of both you and your patients. Your gestures, body movements, and attitude toward the patient are critically important in gaining the trust of each patient and that of any family or caregivers present (**Figure 1-1**). Look for nonverbal behaviors (cues), such as facial affect and body positioning, indicating whether the

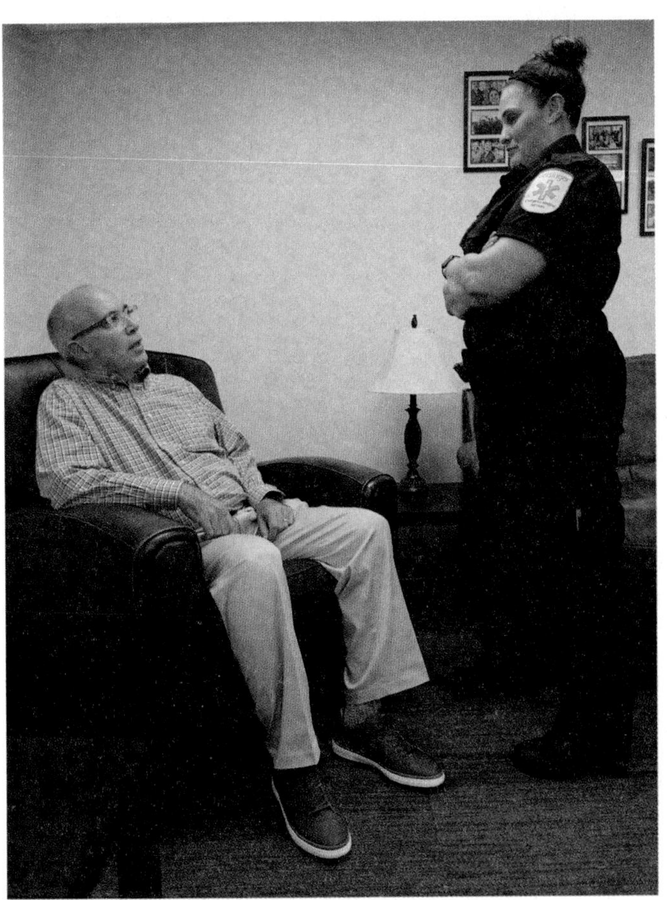

A

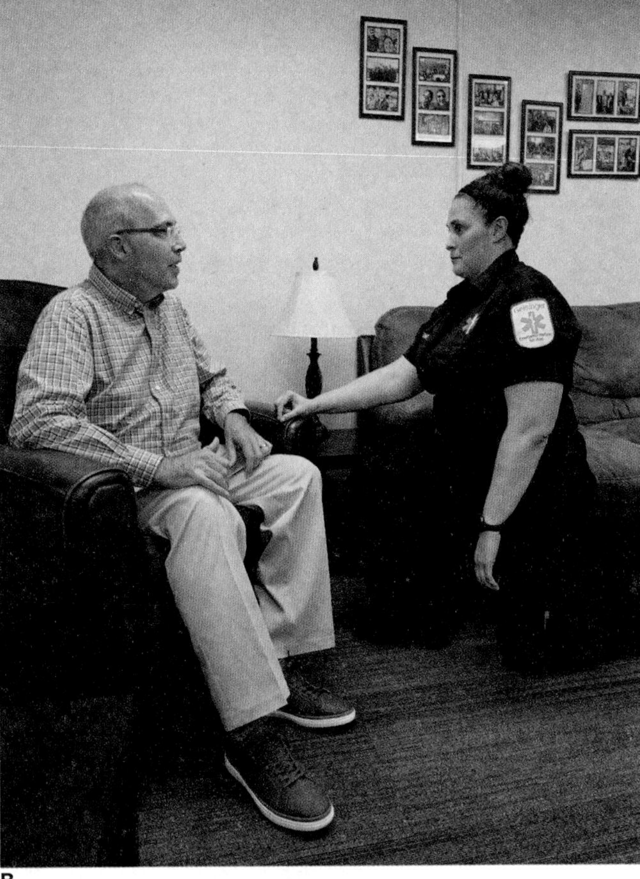

B

Figure 1-1 Watch your body language, because patients may misinterpret your gestures, movements, and attitude. Figure **A** shows an EMT with an imposing stance over a patient with arms crossed. Figure **B** shows an open and comfortable interaction with an EMT who is at eye-level to the patient with hands open and inviting.

patient feels at ease (**Figure 1-2**). These findings can be key indicators of the levels of discomfort, pain, or fear. Keep in mind that patients may present with comorbid conditions that can complicate assessment and delay implementation of appropriate management strategies. Patience is essential when such a complex assessment must be made.

Therapeutic communication is a skill developed over time. To assist in developing these skills, the following verbal and nonverbal communication techniques are important to incorporate into your daily interactions:

- Unless there are issues of safety or a critically ill patient, greet the patient in a friendly yet professional manner and introduce yourself and your role. Ask the patient their name, and ask how they want to be addressed. It is better to start more formally and only address the patient by a first or informal name if they request it.
- Talk with the patient at the patient's eye level and maintain good eye contact while talking. Some studies indicate that patients perceive longer interaction times with clinicians when the clinician is seated versus standing. This is especially important with patients who are frightened, hard of hearing, or elderly.
- Speak clearly and slowly. Even if the patient has a hearing impairment, only raise your voice if the patient asks.
- Maintain an open, attentive body position during the interview. Try not to appear rushed or flustered.
- Acknowledge your understanding of what the patient is saying by nodding and paraphrasing the patient's words.
- Avoid distracting mannerisms such as writing while the patient is talking, tapping or clicking a pen, or fidgeting with keys or coins in your pocket.
- Your nonverbal language should reassure patients you are there to help.
- Inform patients of what you and your colleagues are doing and why. Tell them where they are being transported and what to expect when they arrive.
- Avoid questions that may be taken as accusatory.
- Sometimes, you must ask a closed "yes-or-no" question to get specific information, but start with open-ended questions to get the broadest understanding of what happened.
- Show empathy by acknowledging the patient's pain, distress, anger, and other feelings. Answer the patient's questions to assist in decreasing anxiety and fear. Your patient won't care how much you know until they know how much you care.
- Respond to and reinforce empathetic and caring behavior.
- Respect the patient's right to confidentiality by keeping your voice down as much as possible in

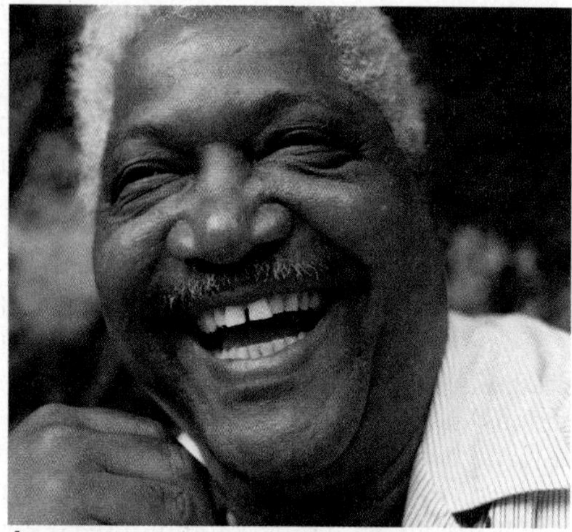

A

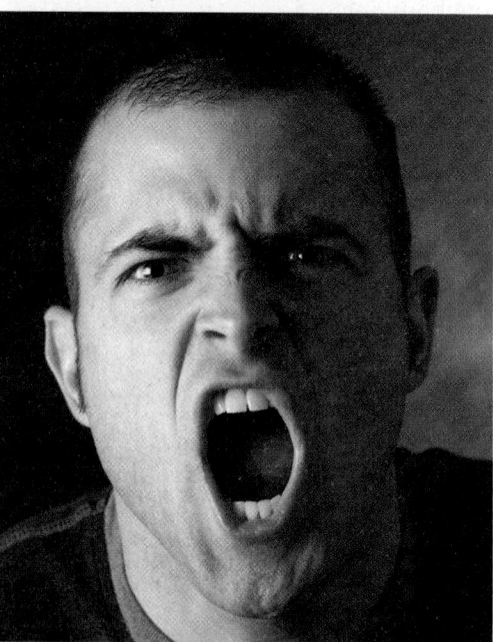

B

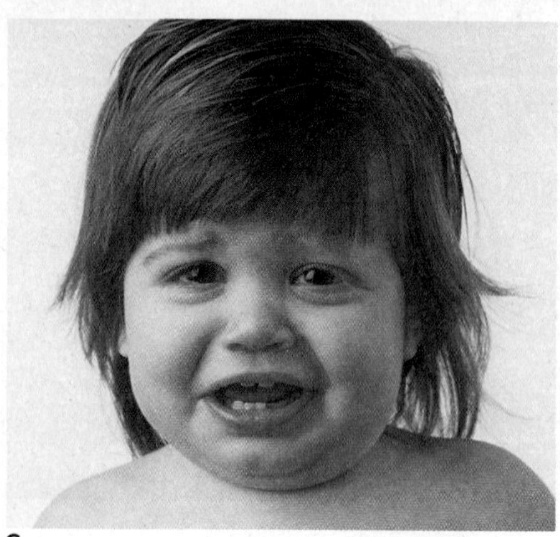

C

Figure 1-2 The effectiveness of body language. **A.** Happy. **B.** Angry. **C.** Sad.

public or semiprivate settings, such as at the scene and in the receiving facility.
- Protect the patient's modesty by keeping the patient covered as much as possible during the physical examination. Doing so will increase the patient's level of trust in the care you are providing and make the patient more willing to share pertinent health information.
- If you suspect a patient may become violent, interact with the patient in a calm, reassuring manner and call for additional resources. Do not try to handle a violent patient alone.

Communicating in Special Situations

You may need to adjust your communication technique or ask for assistance in special situations, such as when sign language is necessary for a hearing-impaired patient.

As a general rule, communicate with patients using terminology that matches their knowledge and understanding. For example, it may be more appropriate to ask the patient about a history of heart problems rather than asking about previous episodes of myocardial infarction.

Language Barriers and Hearing-Impaired Patients

In many areas, particularly large urban centers, segments of the population may not speak English. It would be beneficial for you to learn some common words and phrases in the language(s) spoken. Bilingual family members or bystanders may be able to offer assistance and interpret for you, but this is not ideal because it may violate a patient's privacy. In some cases, you may need to access interpreter translation services. Increasingly, EMS agencies have access to mobile electronic applications or resources that can connect the patient and clinician through a live interpreter.

People who are hearing impaired may communicate through sign language, gestures, writing, or lip reading—any or all of which may be difficult to do when they are ill or injured. Some people with deafness have partial speech or hearing. You may also be able to exchange written questions and answers with the patient. The patient's family members or friends may be able to help. In addition, learning how to ask a few basic questions in sign language, and interpret the answers, can be helpful.

Try to determine what the patient's abilities and preferences are to communicate as effectively as possible.

Cultural Differences

All health care clinicians encounter patients from diverse cultural backgrounds, including ethnicity, race, religion, ability, or sexual orientation. This diversity is reflected in how patients and clinicians interact. For example, some cultures encourage people to express their emotions, whereas others perceive emotional expressiveness as a sign of weakness. Physical proximity can indicate acceptance and familiarity to some people, whereas others may be offended or intimidated by close contact. Some clinicians may consciously or subconsciously apply their cultural values onto patient encounters, either believing their values are better (implicit bias) or assuming theirs is the "cultural norm." This attitude can bias your approach to treatment; for example, studies have shown significant variations in pain management for various age groups and cultural backgrounds or for those with a history of substance abuse or mental illness. Clinician attitudes can also impair developing a rapport with the patient and family, resulting in ineffective communication or even miscommunication and poor treatment.

When encountering a patient from another culture, clinicians must be careful to be considerate of other norms. For example, some cultures prohibit female patients from being examined by a male clinician, or they have expectations that some body parts may not be directly seen or examined. Some patients may have cultural or religious reasons for insisting that head coverings remain in place, even during physician examination. EMS clinicians should do their best to understand and respect their patients' cultural norms and expectations.

Clinical Reasoning

Most health care clinicians would agree that procedural skills proficiency alone cannot ensure quality care. **Clinical reasoning** skills are also essential. Clinical reasoning involves good judgment combined with a knowledge of anatomy, physiology, and pathophysiology seasoned by clinical experience to direct questioning about the patient's complaints. An understanding of the epidemiology of human disease processes is essential for early diagnosis, particularly when the patient's signs and symptoms do not point to an obvious cause. The following elements contribute to clinical reasoning:

- Knowledge in medical sciences
- Ability to gather and organize data
- Ability to focus on specific and multiple data
- Ability to identify medical ambiguity
- Ability to understand relevant/irrelevant data
- Ability to analyze and compare situations
- Ability to explain reasoning

As the patient responds to your interview questions, you begin to analyze their answers based on your underlying medical knowledge. Once the chief complaint, history of the present illness, past medical history, and review of body systems have been completed, you can begin to formulate a list of **differential diagnoses**, which are working hypotheses of the nature of the problem. As historical information, assessment findings, and test results are evaluated, a number of illnesses or conditions can be ruled out. The differential diagnoses therefore become narrowed until the clinician formulates a **working diagnosis**—the presumed cause of the patient's condition. The working diagnosis becomes a definitive diagnosis pending confirmation by further diagnostic tests, usually performed at the receiving facility. Early in patient care, the clinician may not be able to identify a single working diagnosis and may need to broadly treat the patient's symptoms until the differential diagnoses are narrowed down. When several plausible diagnoses are considered, it is important to include the most life-threatening working diagnosis in the patient care plan.

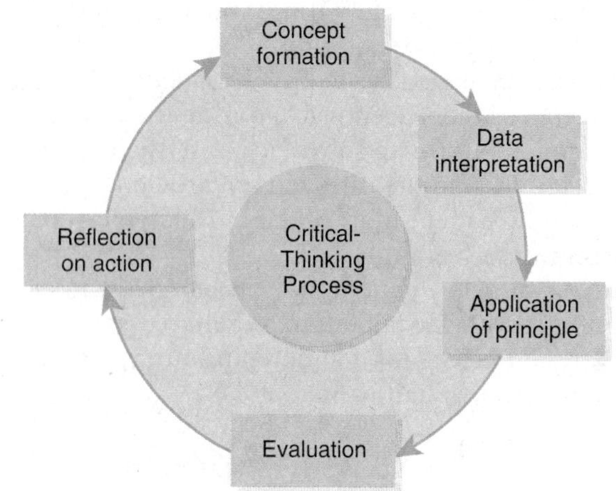

Figure 1-3 Critical-thinking process.

Reproduced from Sanders MJ. *Mosby's Paramedic Textbook*. Revised reprint. 3rd ed. Mosby; 2007.

Scope of Clinical Reasoning

Creating a mental list of differential diagnoses is not a static process. Vital signs, lung sounds, neurologic examination findings, oxygen saturation measurements, responses to interventions, laboratory and radiographic test results, and other information are used to evaluate potential diagnoses. When you are developing differential diagnoses, start with broad possibilities—that is, which body systems might be contributing to the patient's complaint. For example, chest pain could involve the cardiac, respiratory, or gastrointestinal systems. This approach will help you to avoid tunnel vision, which is defined as locking into a diagnosis early before considering all the possibilities. Because chest pain could involve multiple systems, it is important for clinicians to consider all the possible diagnoses and rule each one out systematically in order to determine a working diagnosis.

You should begin by considering the patient's chief complaint. A significant number of illnesses or injuries can be ruled out quickly by just determining the chief complaint. For example, suppose your patient reports chest pain. Your knowledge gives insight into the potential problems causing chest pain. Your list of differential diagnoses might include acute coronary syndrome, gastroesophageal reflux, pulmonary embolism, or aortic dissection. A patient reporting chest pain is not likely to have gastrointestinal bleeding; therefore, you can use the chief complaint to immediately narrow the diagnosis. In addition to the chief complaint, the associated signs and symptoms along with the history will narrow the possible causes even further.

The physical exam (discussed in detail later in the chapter) is another important aspect of clinical reasoning. Tenderness or other specific exam findings that point you toward specific anatomic locations can help refine your diagnostic possibilities. Once you are able to identify the possible organ systems involved, you can use your knowledge of pathophysiology to determine the most likely diagnosis.

Of course, clinical reasoning is not an exact science. Just like a scientist, however, you can test your differential diagnosis to determine whether it holds true. This is accomplished through further assessment and testing. The process evolves as different questions are asked based on the patient's answers. You may use various diagnostics to test these theories, such as a glucose check or a 12-lead electrocardiogram (ECG). The additional information is combined with the existing knowledge, and your differential diagnosis can be confirmed or modified.

To provide the best quality care for the patient, every clinician must possess the core knowledge required at the level to which they have been trained (**Figure 1-3**). This knowledge should be enhanced with experience and common sense to develop reliable clinical reasoning skills. A clinician must be able to think and perform quickly and effectively under extreme pressure using critical reasoning to determine an accurate working diagnosis and treatment plan based on patient care protocols or standing orders.

Clinical Decision Making

Clinical decision making is a process in which decisions are made about a patient's health care problems and appropriate therapeutic interventions are considered and implemented to improve the patient's outcome. Like clinical reasoning, clinical decision making is an ongoing process that takes place at every stage of care, beginning with the creation of the differential diagnosis. Both require a sufficient knowledge of anatomy, physiology, and pathophysiology; an ability to perform specific assessment skills; and the resourcefulness to apply complex diagnostic tools to a broad range of medical emergencies. Though we are not always conscious of the process, clinical decision-making approaches include the following:

- **Pattern recognition**: A process of recognizing and classifying data (patterns) based on past knowledge and experience. The clinician compares the patient's presentation with similar, previously encountered patient presentations. Analyzing similar diagnoses and which strategies were effective and which were not is a useful foundation for clinical decision making.
- *Hypothesis generation*: This can be described as utilizing the scientific method by starting with the patient's chief complaint, generating possible explanations (i.e., the hypotheses), collecting and synthesizing information, and ultimately accepting or rejecting one or more hypotheses.
- *Likelihood and probability estimates*: These influence our processing of the information we collect during patient assessments. For example, we might rule out tropical causes of a chief complaint if we can confidently determine our patient has neither traveled out of the country nor come in contact with anyone who has.
- *Differential diagnoses*: These are integral to the orderly application of the AMLS Assessment Pathway. We begin by generating an initial list of differential diagnoses—a list of potential causes for the patient's condition. It is structured with the most likely cause at the top of the list. The differential diagnoses are then refined or reorganized as we obtain additional information from the patient's history, physical exam, and diagnostic testing. Although we may not be able to completely refine our differential down to a single diagnosis, the process of creating, revising, and refining is very helpful to clinical decision making and helps to avoid overlooking a diagnostic possibility.

The combination of well-honed therapeutic communication techniques, the ability to recognize patterns, generation of likely differential diagnoses as hypotheses, assessment of the likelihood of particular diagnoses, and dependable clinical-reasoning skills enables prudent clinical decision making, allowing clinicians to gauge the severity of the patient's illness or injury and initiate appropriate, timely interventions. One's clinical decision-making skills become more reliable with experience. However, other processes can interfere with clinical decision making.

Biases

Bias is a tendency, preference, or inclination (either known or unknown) toward or against something or someone that prevents objectivity. If a person recognizes, or is conscious, of bias, it is considered *explicit*. If a person is unaware, or is unconscious, of bias, it is considered *implicit*. Implicit biases are automatic mental associations created as a product of our environment, exposure to specific ideas, and societal and cultural conditioning that begins at an early age; these biases are altered over time by personal experiences. Implicit bias may run counter to our stated beliefs or values. Explicit and implicit bias are not mutually exclusive; both influence behavior and may reinforce each other, leading to further bias, discrimination, and increased inequity. Bias may lead to preconceived, unfavorable, and unreasonable (even hostile) feelings, attitudes, and/or opinions about a certain group of people, referred to as prejudice.

Cognitive Biases

Who has not heard an instructor, supervisor, or partner caution you not to "tunnel" on a particular cause or diagnosis? So-called tunnel vision can be attributed to the well-known **cognitive bias** constructs of anchoring bias, confirmation bias, and premature closure (Table 1-1). Cognitive scientists have defined two systems that manage our processing of information: intuitive and analytic. The interaction of these two systems of information management can result in cognitive bias. Our intuitive system

Table 1-1 Common Cognitive Errors

Type of Cognitive Bias	Description
Anchoring bias	The tendency to perceptually lock onto salient features in the patient's initial presentation too early in the diagnostic process, and then failing to adjust this initial impression in the light of later information.
Confirmation bias	The tendency to rely upon confirming evidence to support a diagnosis rather than the disconfirming evidence to refute it, despite the latter often being more persuasive and definitive.
Premature closure	The tendency to apply premature closure to the decision-making process, accepting a diagnosis before it has been fully verified.

Modified from Saposnik G, Redelmeier D, Ruff CC, Tobler PN. Cognitive biases associated with medical decisions: a systematic review. *BMC Med Inform Decis Mak*. 2016;16(1):138. doi:10.1186/s12911-016-0377-1 quickly processes information, connecting and integrating facts, feelings, and observations, often subconsciously, but not necessarily or always leading to objectively correct conclusions. "Trusting your gut" relies on this intuitive system, and the result can be uncanny accuracy or dismaying error. Our slower analytic system is typically conscious and deliberate, processing stored facts. In an AMLS context, our intuitive system will quickly generate initial diagnoses of varying real-world accuracy, whereas our analytic system more deliberately processes the information gathered through patient assessment and diagnostic testing. The interplay of the systems leads us to a treatment path for a particular patient. Hasty action, prompted by our intuitive system, without confirmation by our analytic system, can lead us to suboptimal approaches to patient care. The AMLS Assessment Pathway provides a framework for careful, systematic processing of patient information, building on insights gained over time through the assessment and treatment of numerous patients.

Cognitive science has also validated the notion that our analytic system can falter under pressure. Using the six Rs can help the clinician put it all together and make better judgments under pressure (**Rapid Recall Box 1-1**). The AMLS Assessment Pathway gives you an efficient process to apply your clinical reasoning and clinical decision-making skills to effectively manage your patients.

RAPID RECALL BOX 1-1

The Six Rs

1. **R**ead the scene. Observe environmental conditions, safety hazards, and likely mechanisms of injury.
2. **R**ead the patient. Assess the patient's condition, take their vital signs, treat life threats, review the chief complaint, and record your general impression.
3. **R**eact. Manage life threats (ABCs) in the order in which they are discovered, and treat the patient based on their cardinal presentation.
4. **R**eevaluate. Reassess vital signs, and reconsider the patient's initial medical management
5. **R**evise the management plan. On the basis of your reevaluation and additional historical data, physical examination findings, diagnostic test results, and the patient's response to early interventions, revise your management plan to accord with the patient's new clinical picture.
6. **R**eview performance. Critiquing the call or patient encounter gives you a chance to reflect on your clinical decision making and target areas in which more advanced skills or a deeper level of knowledge is needed.

Gender Considerations in Health Care

Medical research has shown that women are assessed, diagnosed, referred, and treated differently, with a lower quality of care, compared to the standard of care given to men with comparable health problems. Physicians are more likely to interpret men's symptoms as organic, with physical causes, and women's as psychosocial and/or stemming from emotional causes. They are also more likely to give nonspecific diagnoses to women and prescribe them more psychoactive medications. Gender bias in health care includes disbelief or minimizing of the symptoms or concerns of women and gender-diverse patients by clinicians, causing delayed diagnoses, inadequate care management, and worse health disparities (i.e., higher complication rates, higher morbidity, and higher mortality). Gender bias also fosters distrust by these patients for the medical community and has resulted in gaps in medical research and knowledge about female, intersex, and transgender health. The global impact of gender bias in health care is such that the United Nations Department of Economic and Social Affairs has included gender equality as one of its 17 Sustainable Development Goals. These biases are obviously in addition to conscious and unconscious biases based on race, color, nationality, age, religion, socioeconomic status, geography, physical attributes or physical conditions, and many others.

Addressing Biases in Health Care

The first step in addressing gender, racial, or other bias is acknowledging and understanding that it exists and influences decision making by all health care clinicians, whether intentionally or unintentionally. In EMS, we have the ability and awareness to monitor ourselves and others in everyday practice to mitigate implicit bias and ensure equal opportunity for improved equitable patient care. One strategy is to implement evidence-based protocols and guidelines that have objective indices that must be met, decreasing the ability to deviate based on subjective elements such as gender bias. Just as with a medication error, when gender or racial bias is identified, an investigation should occur within a just culture framework to analyze the systemic/institutional and individual causes leading to the incorrect or biased management of a patient, develop tools to prevent any reoccurrence, and promote education throughout the department/agency. Thus, clinicians will have improved knowledge and behavior to recognize and mitigate bias, leading to our collective goal of equitable care and better health outcomes for all patients.

Educating clinicians on situations associated with biased processes, reactions, and treatments, along with addressing attitudes and preconceptions about gender, race, and other biases, would help prevent these biases in health care. Evaluations of clinicians with patients should be performed to determine the effect that gender perspective has on gender-biased assessments. Likewise, similar approaches related to racial and other forms of bias may improve these. Understanding one's interpretations and bias may lead to improved clinical reasoning and decision making, conduct in patient care, and health outcomes.

AMLS Assessment Pathway ▸▸▸▸

The **Advanced Medical Life Support (AMLS) Assessment Pathway** is a reliable process for reducing patient morbidity and mortality by identifying a broad range of medical emergencies early and managing them effectively. Determination of an accurate field or in-hospital diagnosis and initiation of a timely, effective management plan hinge on a reliable patient assessment process.

The success of the AMLS Assessment Pathway depends on the integration of BLS patient assessment and interventions and the early integration of ALS assessment and interventions. Taken together, the patient's initial presentation, history, chief complaint, physical exam findings, and diagnostic results should begin to suggest possible diagnoses. For example, if the chief complaint is low back pain, the clinician should pursue that lead by asking patients follow-up questions, such as the following:

- Have you recently had any injuries?
- Are you having weakness or numbness in your arms, legs, or groin?
- Are you having any problems with bowel movements or urination?
- Have you had a fever?
- Does the pain seem to move around or does it stay in one place?
- What makes it better or worse?
- Is the pain constant or does it come and go?
- Have you experienced these symptoms before?

The presence or absence of pertinent signs and symptoms associated with the initial presentation is equally important. Information gleaned from the patient's answers will help clinicians prioritize various differential diagnoses by using clinical decision-making skills. When clinicians have repeatedly seen how a condition presents in multiple patients, they can identify similarities to past cases almost immediately based on experience. Active listening, generating differential diagnoses, identifying distinguishing signs and symptoms, and recalling past success with specific treatment approaches and considerations provide the basis for evaluation of the current patient's presentation. A health care clinician's knowledge of pathophysiology combined with the knowledge gained from patient care experience enhances the effectiveness of this clinical decision-making approach.

As clinicians talk to the patient to obtain a history and perform a physical exam, they are looking for life-threatening, emergent, and nonemergent problems that must be managed within their scope of practice and adherence to medical protocols and guidelines. They are also forming a general impression of the patient's condition. Of course, all findings should be thoroughly documented and clearly communicated to the receiving facility.

The AMLS Assessment Pathway supports **assessment-based patient management**. This process is not driven by rote performance skills. Instead, the AMLS Assessment Pathway recognizes that although all components of the assessment process (**Figure 1-4**) are important to patient care, they are conducted based on the patient's unique presentation. For example, if you have a high index of suspicion the patient has sustained an injury, performing a rapid head-to-toe physical exam based on a trauma-focused secondary assessment may be a higher priority than obtaining a past medical history. The history is not omitted, however; it is merely given a lower priority during the assessment process. The opposite is also true. With a medically ill patient, it may be more appropriate to immediately obtain a history of the patient's present illness and a past medical history and then perform a focused physical exam based upon their history. The physical exam and present and past medical history are not segregated entities. They are typically evaluated in tandem.

During the secondary survey, the health care clinician should follow a dynamic, flexible approach to the patient assessment process. The process should be systematic, but it must remain dynamic and adaptable in order to confirm or eliminate diagnoses as more findings are noted and the patient's therapeutic response is observed.

Although the AMLS Assessment Pathway supports flexibility in deciding when to obtain specific details of a patient's history and physical exam, one important principle is that initial observations at the scene must be made to ensure that the scene is safe before the **primary survey** is performed so any life-threatening medical emergencies can be identified and managed without delay. The discussion of the AMLS Assessment Pathway that follows reflects the algorithm in Figure 1-4.

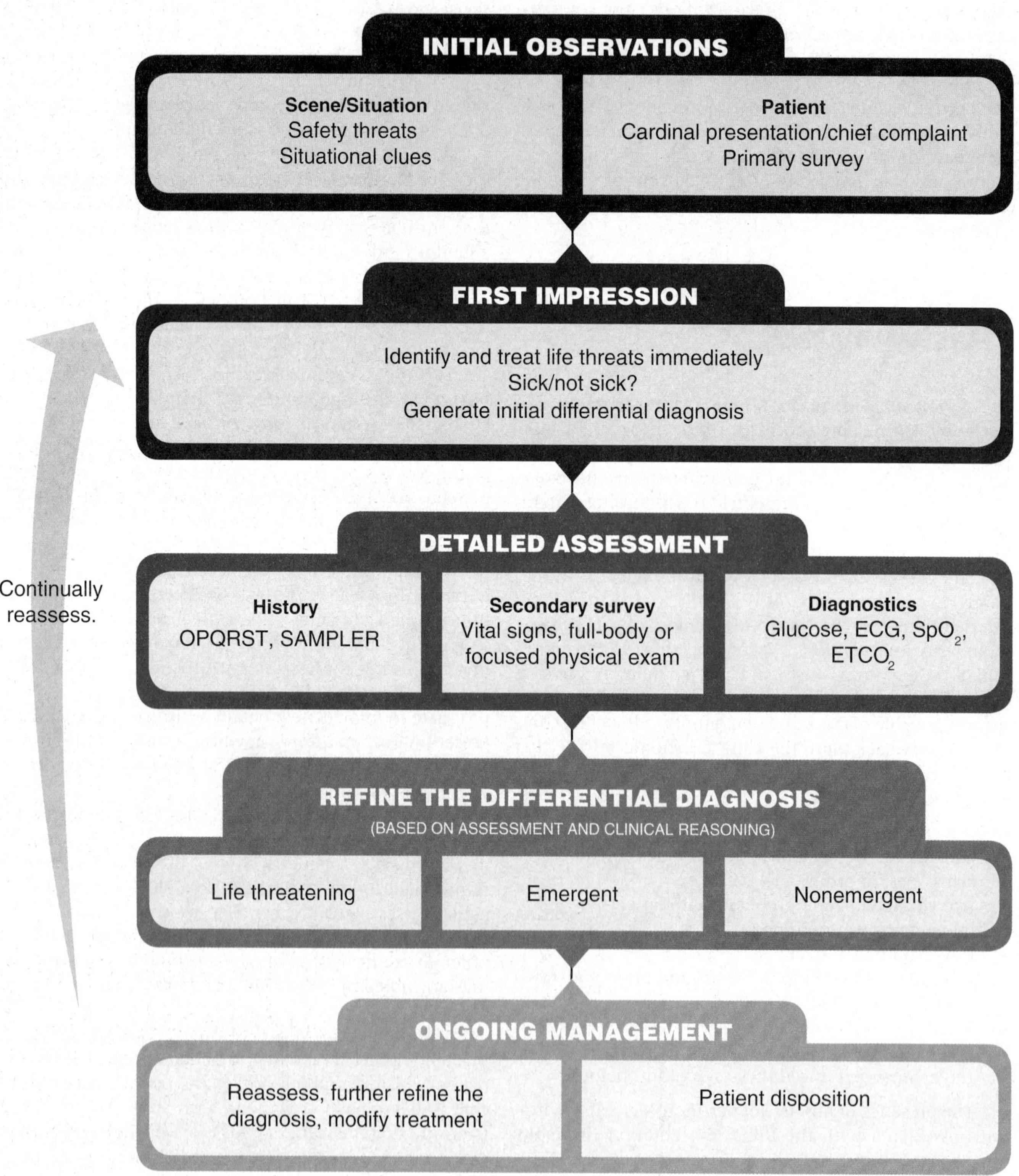

Figure 1-4 Algorithm for the AMLS Assessment Pathway.

Initial Observations

Scene Considerations

Safety and Situational Clues

Prehospital clinicians reach the scene or situation before they reach the patient. For prehospital personnel, this gives them a moment to integrate what the dispatcher has stated with their own judicious observation of the scene. The scene and the potential for safety hazards or threats are continually evaluated until patient care has been transferred (**Figure 1-5**). In-hospital environments may also place patients in an unsafe set of circumstances, such as when side rails are left down and the patient has an altered level of consciousness.

Prehospital clinicians enter the patient's environment, which may be a home, office, or vehicle. Anger or anxiety may be part of the environment, particularly when a stressful event such as an injury or assault has just occurred. The presence of EMS, law enforcement, or fire department personnel may make a violent person feel threatened. Behavioral red flags may precede an angry outburst or assault. Staying alert to potential or real threats of violence is equally as important in any health care institution, even if there are security personnel on site. All health care personnel must be aware of a gradual acceleration of emotion or concerning behavioral clues, such as pacing, gesturing, and hostile words that indicate an escalation of a dangerous situation.

Before approaching the patient, survey the environment and the patient's affect. This vigilance is essential in both prehospital and in-hospital situations. Determine the number of patients, family members, or bystanders present and whether any additional resources are needed, such as more ambulances, law enforcement, and fire or hazardous materials (hazmat) assistance. Evidence of weapons, alcohol, or drug paraphernalia can be an early indicator that the situation is unsafe and law enforcement backup is needed. In the prehospital setting, ominous background noise such as people arguing should cause enough concern for you to contact law enforcement to assist at the scene. Less-menacing distractions such as televisions should be turned off or otherwise eliminated.

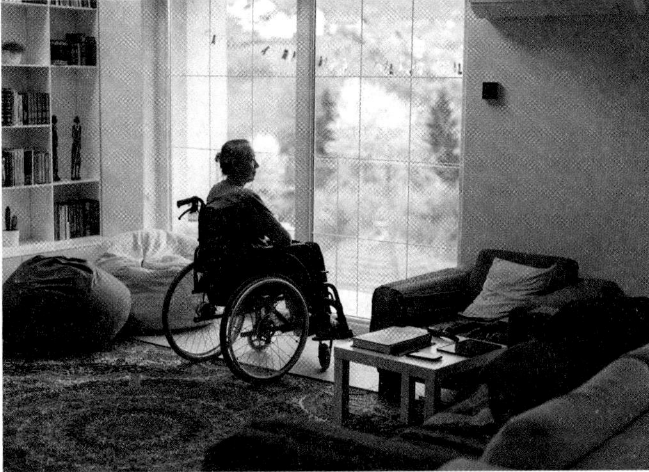

Figure 1-5 Throw rugs are a hazard; it is important to evaluate the safety of the patient's residence.

It is important to protect the integrity of a crime scene and the preservation of associated evidence, as well as the safety of the victim. Work with your colleagues to keep the scene safe. Designate one person to have contact with the patient while the other remains alert for problems, a practice followed in law enforcement. Keep your communication equipment with you. On calls involving overdose, violent crime, or potential hazardous materials exposure, stage at a reasonable distance and wait for law enforcement to advise you the scene is safe. Listen to your instincts—if the situation does not feel right, leave, if appropriate, and call for help. Always follow local or institutional protocols for such situations. Ensure that documentation is timely and is an accurate reflection of the situation.

All personnel should evaluate each scene and patient situation as a potential threat to safety. Close observation of nonverbal behavior and communication with family members can lead to clues of a possibly unstable environment.

In addition to clues related to safety or violence, many medical clues can be observed at the scene before engaging the patient. Assess the situation for assistive devices, such as canes, wheelchairs, and oxygen concentrators, which indicate chronic conditions with the potential for poor perfusion presentations.

Standard Precautions

Standard precautions and personal protective equipment (PPE) need to be considered and adapted to the task at hand. PPE includes gloves, protective eyewear, gowns, face masks, and respirators (e.g., N-95) (**Figure 1-6**). If weapons of mass destruction have been used or other hazardous materials have been dispersed, a higher level of PPE may be necessary to prevent contamination by potentially lethal materials. The COVID-19 pandemic demonstrated the importance of vigilance for possible infectious diseases and the importance of understanding modes of transmission for viral diseases and appropriate PPE and other protective actions.

The Centers for Disease Control and Prevention (CDC) recommends following standard precautions to prevent transmission of infectious diseases. These precautions apply to all patients in every health care setting, regardless of whether the patient is known to be infected

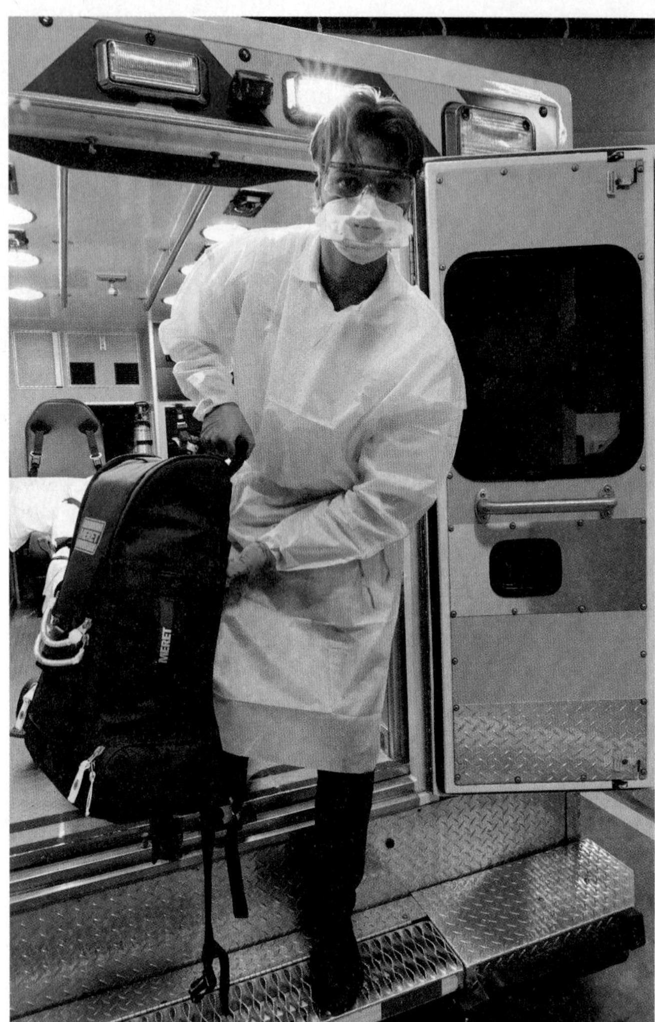

Figure 1-6 Proper personal protective equipment (PPE) is vital when you are called to a scene in which you may be exposed to blood or other body fluids.

Courtesy of Douglas F. Kupas, MD.

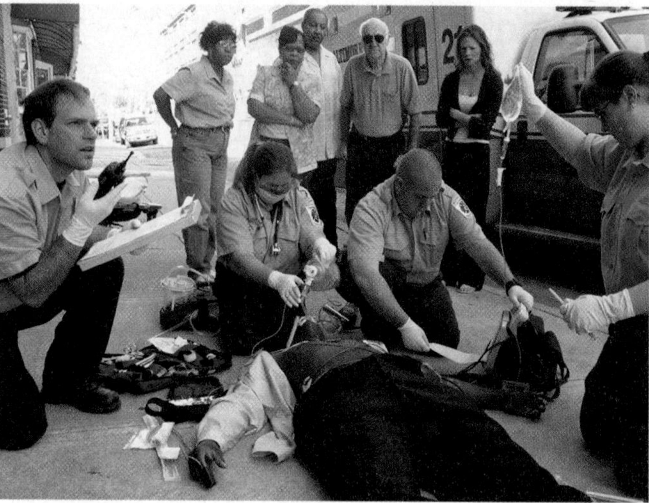

Figure 1-7 Standard precautions require that health care personnel do not carry infectious agents on their hands. Gloves are essential.

© Jones & Bartlett Learning. Courtesy of MIEMSS.

or only suspected of having an infection. Standard precautions include the following:

- Use of proper hand hygiene techniques, including hand washing and/or use of hand sanitizer before and after every patient encounter and after removal of gloves and disinfection of equipment
- Use of gloves, gown, mask (surgical or N-95), and eye protection/face shield, depending on the anticipated exposure
- Safe injection and disposal practices
- Proper cleaning and disposal of equipment and items in the patient's environment likely to have been contaminated with infectious body fluids

Standard precautions protect not only health care clinicians, but also patients by ensuring that health care personnel do not carry infectious agents from patient to patient on their hands or transmit them via equipment used during patient care (**Figure 1-7**). An exposure can occur by contact with blood or through inhalation or ingestion of respiratory secretions, airborne droplets, or saliva. Occupational Safety and Health Administration (OSHA) regulations specify training requirements, mandatory vaccinations, exposure control plans, and PPE.

Other Hazards

Assess the scene for other hazards such as downed electrical lines, fires, imminent structural collapse, and the presence of hazardous materials. Animals should be secured in advance of your entry. If you do receive an animal bite, contact local animal control authorities so the animal can be confined and tested for diseases. If toxic substances are present or you cannot rule out the possibility, call in the hazardous materials (hazmat) team.

Patient Considerations

Patient Cardinal Presentation/Chief Complaint

The chief complaint is what the patient, family member, friend, or bystander reports to you as the primary concern. The chief complaint answers the question, "Why did you call for help?" The **cardinal presentation** is the condition or complaint recognized by medical clinicians as a key concern. Usually this will be based on the chief complaint, but sometimes it will reflect your recognition of what is the most critical condition to be evaluated.

With a responsive medical patient, you must first identify the chief complaint. In most cases, some type of pain, discomfort, or body dysfunction prompts the call for help. In some cases, the complaint may be vague. Vague complaints also challenge you to ask the right questions and be a patient listener as you obtain the information you need to make appropriate care decisions.

Primary Survey

The primary survey identifies life-threatening presentations and establishes immediate management strategies. If no life threats are found, continue to formulate an initial impression of the patient's condition and determine whether the patient's condition is emergent (the patient is injured or ill and in need of immediate medical attention) or nonemergent (the patient is not in need of immediate medical attention).

To determine the patient's status, clinicians must evaluate the patient's level of consciousness and identify any airway, breathing, circulation, or hemorrhage problems. If a life threat is identified, immediate interventions must be initiated before further assessment is performed. The remaining history taking and physical exam can be performed en route to the receiving facility.

If the primary survey reveals immediately life-threatening conditions (e.g., obstructed airway, inadequate respiration, or uncontrolled bleeding), the EMS clinician should address the immediate life threats before continuing with the assessment. If the patient's condition continues to be life threatening, the prehospital emergency medical team must then make transport decisions. Is the patient to be transported by ground or air? What are the implications of either mode of transportation? Which is the closest, most appropriate medical center? At each step, the transport crew or type of vehicle can be upgraded based on additional information.

If the assessment does not reveal an immediate life threat, the patient should be evaluated for emergent conditions. An emergent patient has a poor general impression or decreased level of consciousness; is unresponsive; shows signs and symptoms of shock; complains of severe pain; has sustained multiple injuries; or is having trouble breathing, has symptoms of acute coronary syndrome, or has internal uncontrolled bleeding.

At this point in the assessment process, clinicians may not be able to pinpoint a working diagnosis, but differential diagnoses should begin to be formulated. Keep in mind the various possible causes of the patient's signs and symptoms as further assessment data become available and are interpreted.

Level of Consciousness

Assessment of the patient's mental status, or level of consciousness, involves evaluation of brain function. As clinicians approach the patient, they need to carefully observe the patient's level of consciousness to immediately determine any potential life-threatening presentations. For example, if the patient is conscious, note the patient's responsiveness. A patient with a limited attention span or a patient who seems to be daydreaming should be assessed for hypoglycemia, dehydration, cardiovascular compromise, stroke, or head trauma.

Level of consciousness is associated with the function of the reticular activating system (RAS) and the cerebral hemispheres. The RAS is located in the upper brainstem and is responsible for maintenance of consciousness, specifically a person's level of arousal. The cerebral hemispheres are responsible for awareness and understanding. Reacting to the environment occurs through the cerebral hemispheres. The RAS alerts the cerebral hemispheres so they activate a response to the stimulus, such as an emotional or physical reaction. Coma can be caused by dysfunction of the RAS or both cerebral hemispheres.

The quickest and simplest way to assess the patient's level of consciousness is to use the AVPU process (Table 1-2).

When you are classifying the response to stimuli, grade the patient according to the best response you can elicit. For example, a patient passed out on the street who moans in response to a loud shout from the clinician would score a V on the AVPU scale. Response to painful tactile stimuli, such as pinching a nail bed, would be graded a P. No response to verbal or tactile stimuli would be classified as U.

Awareness is a high-level neurologic function and demonstrates an orientation to person, place, time, and situation. Note that wakefulness and awareness (orientation) are two separate functions. A patient can be awake but disoriented (not aware), indicating adequate RAS function but cerebral hemisphere dysfunction, or can be not awake but still aware of what is being said or done to them.

The Glasgow Coma Scale (GCS), used to assess victims of trauma or critical medical illness, is a tool for assessing neurologic function and is particularly important in establishing the patient's baseline level of

Table 1-2 Mental Status and AVPU

AVPU Level	Assessment Findings
Alert	Responds and eyes open spontaneously, patient tracks examiner/environment, follows commands
Verbal	Responds to verbal stimuli
Pain	Responds only to painful stimuli applied by the examiner
Unresponsive	Does not respond to stimuli

consciousness (Table 1-3). The score is also helpful in providing additional information on patients with changes in mental status. Documented changes in the GCS score that indicate diminishing neurologic function guide in-hospital diagnostic testing and inpatient placement.

The GCS includes the patient's eye-opening response and the best verbal and motor responses. The score for each of these responses should be documented (e.g., E = 3, V = 4, M = 4, for a total GCS score of 11). A score of 8 or less often indicates the need for aggressive airway management. Although 15 is the highest score possible, a patient with a GCS of 15 may still have some subtle deficits in mental status. Definitive care should not be based on the GCS findings alone but in conjunction with other diagnostic and historical data obtained. It is also important to consider the presence of any medications you have given the patient when relaying the GCS; for example, ketamine can result in a GCS of 3, but this has far different implications than a GCS of 3 without ketamine. EMS clinicians should be aware that the GCS is frequently miscalculated by EMS and in-hospital clinicians. Do not guess or estimate the level of GCS. Each component should be assessed and accurately calculated. The GCS is utilized in the prehospital field and is a common examination question.

Recent studies have shown that a simple distinction of brain function based on only the motor component of the GCS is strongly predictive of patient outcome in trauma patients. A simple assessment of whether a patient follows commands (GCS motor = 6) or not (GCS motor ≤ 5) differentiates between function and communication among various parts of the brain. In addition to AVPU, it is good practice for EMS clinicians to simply determine and report whether the patient follows commands or does not follow commands.

Assessment of level of consciousness helps determine whether the patient's neurologic and perfusion status are stable and allows life-threatening conditions to be identified and managed early. Patients with difficulties in mentation should receive a complete neurologic examination.

If the patient is unresponsive and flaccid with no signs of life, you should immediately check for the presence of a pulse. If you cannot detect a pulse within 10 seconds or if uncertain, begin chest compressions immediately and proceed with cardiopulmonary resuscitation (CPR).

Airway and Breathing

After assessing level of consciousness and ensuring that the patient has a pulse, the patient's airway status must be rapidly evaluated. Airway patency must be established and maintained. A patent airway allows good airflow and is free of fluids, secretions, teeth, and other types of foreign bodies (such as food or dentures) obstructing airflow. A patient's inability to maintain a patent airway is a life-threatening emergency and necessitates emergency interventions and immediate transport to an appropriate medical facility. Assessment of a patient's airway is completed in the same way regardless of the patient's age. In responsive patients of any age, talking or crying will give clues about the adequacy of the airway. For all unresponsive patients, you must establish responsiveness and assess breathing. Open the airway and observe the mouth and upper airway for air movement. Performing

Table 1-3 Glasgow Coma Scale

Eye Opening	Score	Best Verbal Response	Score	Best Motor Response	Score
Spontaneous	4	Oriented and converses	5	Follows commands	6
To verbal command	3	Disoriented conversation	4	Localizes pain	5
To pain	2	Speaking but nonsensical	3	Withdraws to pain	4
No response	1	Moans or makes unintelligible sounds	2	Decorticate flexion	3
		No response	1	Decerebrate extension	2
				No response	1

Scores:
15: Normal GCS
13–14: Mild dysfunction
9–12: Moderate to severe dysfunction
8 or less: Severe dysfunction (The lowest possible score is 3.)

a jaw-thrust maneuver without head tilt on a trauma patient is appropriate if the potential for head, neck, or spine injury is noted. In cases of suspected trauma, manually protect the cervical spine from movement by positioning the patient in a neutral, in-line position. Look for evidence of upper airway problems, such as facial trauma, and check for the presence of vomitus and blood.

During the assessment of a patient's airway, observe the patient's position or posture. Is the patient lying in an unnatural position on the ground or in bed? Does the patient seem to favor an upright position or the tripod position? Certain positions maximize airflow and indicate increased work of breathing and respiratory fatigue, distress, and imminent failure.

A compromised airway may require suctioning or removal of a foreign object. In the case of obstruction, such as by food, BLS procedures to clear the obstruction require no equipment and can be done quickly. Suctioning, however, may be necessary to clear the airway. Suctioning takes longer (because of the need to set up and use the equipment) and is a more complicated procedure than positioning a patient to improve airflow. If you suction the patient for too long, you may create new problems, such as hypoxia and bradycardia secondary to vagal stimulation.

If there is a foreign body obstruction, use appropriate techniques to remove the object. This might include direct visualization and the use of Magill forceps by advanced clinicians.

If a mechanical means is required to keep the airway patent, you must choose an airway adjunct. If you decide to place an oropharyngeal or nasopharyngeal airway, you must measure and choose the right size for the specific patient and then properly insert the airway. If you determine the patient cannot maintain a patent airway and you cannot maintain it by any other means, you need to use a more invasive technique, such as endotracheal intubation. BLS and ALS adjuncts include the following:

- BLS adjuncts
  - Suction
  - Manual maneuvers
  - Oropharyngeal/nasopharyngeal device
- ALS adjuncts
  - Supraglottic or blindly inserted airway devices (BIADs), including various laryngeal tube airways and laryngeal mask airways (**Rapid Recall Box 1-2**)
  - Endotracheal intubation (oral, nasal)
  - Chest decompression
  - Needle or surgical cricothyrotomy

Initially, BLS interventions can be used and, when appropriate, progress to definitive ALS interventions. A thorough assessment will determine the urgency of airway management and suggest which devices are most likely to be effective.

RAPID RECALL BOX 1-2

Blindly Inserted Airway Devices (BIADs)

Supraglottic, or extraglottic, airway devices refer to a variety of products such as laryngeal tube airways and laryngeal mask airways that may be placed in the hypopharynx as an alternative to endotracheal intubation. These are also referred to as blindly inserted airway devices (BIADs) because they can be placed without visualization of the glottis. These devices provide some protection from aspiration when compared with bag-valve mask (BVM) ventilation, but the risk of aspiration may be higher than with endotracheal intubation, as they do not occlude the trachea. Also, they cannot be used if there is significant upper airway/oropharyngeal trauma or severe swelling of the glottis/upper airway.

A person's breathing status is directly related to airway adequacy. Breathing rate, rhythm, and effort are evaluated in the primary survey. A normal respiratory rate varies widely in adults, ranging from 12 to 20 breaths/min. Children breathe at even faster rates, 15 to 30 breaths/min. The clinician assesses the patient's rate of breathing. With practice, you will be able to estimate the rate and determine whether it is too fast or too slow. When vital signs are taken during the secondary survey, it is important to specifically measure the respiratory rate, but during the primary survey, the clinician should be making a general interpretation of adequate breathing by subjectively estimating rate, rhythm, and depth of respiratory effort. Lung sounds may be auscultated in the primary survey if labored respirations are noted. The patient's respiratory rhythm should be easy, regular, and without distress. Inadequate respiratory rates or irregular breathing patterns should be noted as they may affect adequacy of ventilation and oxygenation. Painful or irregular breaths may indicate a medical or trauma-related emergency and should be evaluated further to determine the cause of the abnormal breathing pattern (Table 1-4). Symmetry of the chest rise and utilization of accessory muscles should be noted. Nasal flaring, agitation, and the ability to speak only two or three words without stopping for a breath are indications of distress and compromised air exchange.

Conditions and injuries causing a life-threatening compromise of the patient's ability to breathe include tension pneumothorax, flail chest, cardiac tamponade, pulmonary embolus, or any other condition diminishing tidal and minute volume and increasing the work and effort of breathing.

Table 1-4 Breathing Patterns

Pattern	Description	Cause	Comments
Normal (eupnea)	Regular, comfortable, and quiet respirations (12–20 breaths/min).	N/A	
Agonal	Slow and gasping respirations immediately preceding or during early cardiac arrest.	Poor or no perfusion to the brainstem, where breathing is controlled	Agonal respirations in patients with cardiac arrest are often confused with normal breathing and can delay the initiation of CPR. EMS clinicians and dispatchers should recognize agonal respirations and intervene immediately.
Apneustic	A long, gasping inspiration followed by a very short expiration in which the breath is not completely expelled. The result is chest hyperinflation.	Brain lesion	Causes severe hypoxemia
Ataxic	Significant disorganization with irregular and varying depths of respiration.	Stroke Trauma Neurologic disorder	
Biot respiration	Irregularly interspersed periods of apnea in a disorganized sequence of breaths; similar to Cheyne-Stokes but with an irregular pattern instead of a repeating pattern.	Meningitis Increased intracranial pressure Neurologic emergency	Think of it as the atrial fibrillation of the respiratory system (irregularly irregular).
Bradypnea	Slower-than-normal respiratory rate (< 12 breaths/min).	Narcotic/sedative drugs, including alcohol Metabolic disorders Hypoperfusion Fatigue Brain injury	In addition to bradypnea, the patient may have episodes of apnea. The patient may require both oxygen and ventilatory assistance.
Central neurogenic hyperventilation	A very deep, rapid respiratory rate (> 25 breaths/min).	Tumor or lesion of the brainstem that causes increased intracranial pressure or direct injury to the brainstem Stroke	Central nervous system acidosis triggers rapid, deep breathing, leading to systemic alkalosis.

Pattern	Description	Cause	Comments
Cheyne-Stokes respiration	A respiratory pattern with alternating periods of increasing and decreasing rate and depth with brief periods of apnea.	Increased intracranial pressure Congestive heart failure Renal failure Toxin Acidosis	May indicate spinal cord injury or brain dysfunction.
Kussmaul respiration	Deep and fast breaths lacking any apneic periods.	Metabolic acidosis Renal failure Diabetic ketoacidosis	Deep, labored breathing that indicates severe acidosis. Kussmaul respirations are a type of tachypnea and are often related to diabetic ketoacidosis.
Tachypnea	Increased respiratory rate (> 20 breaths/min).	Fever Respiratory distress Toxins Hypoperfusion Brain lesion Metabolic acidosis Anxiety	One of the body's coping mechanisms, but it can have a harmful effect by promoting respiratory alkalosis. The patient may require supplemental oxygen.

Respiratory distress can result from hypoxia, a condition in which too little oxygen is available to the body's tissues. Hypoxia can be caused by any of the aforementioned conditions or by asthma; chronic obstructive pulmonary disease (COPD); airway obstruction; or any condition that restricts normal gas exchange by the alveoli, such as pneumonia, pulmonary edema, or abnormal mucus secretions.

When the patient's chief complaint is respiratory distress, another possible syndrome is hyperventilation, which will lead to respiratory alkalosis. Hyperventilation may be compensating for metabolic acidosis, anxiety, fear, or central nervous system (CNS) insult. Working diagnoses may include possible causes such as stroke and diabetic ketoacidosis.

An elevated level of carbon dioxide in the blood caused by hypoventilation is called hypercapnia (hypercarbia). Hypercapnia occurs when the body cannot rid itself of carbon dioxide, causing it to build up in the bloodstream, leading to respiratory failure. Hypercapnia should be considered in every patient with decreased mental status, especially if the patient appears somnolent or very fatigued.

In the primary survey, midaxillary lung sounds are auscultated if the patient presents with a diminished level of consciousness, difficulty in breathing, or poor perfusion. Audible respiratory sounds such as wheezing are an important clinical finding. Gurgling and stridor are upper airway sounds (above the carina), and the other abnormal breath sounds are lower airway sounds. Abnormal breath sounds are as follows:

- *Gurgling.* A hollow bubbling sound; an upper airway condition.
- *Stridor.* A harsh, high-pitched sound heard during inhalation; indicates narrowing, usually as a result of swelling or foreign body in the upper airway. Stridor is best heard over the anterior neck.
- *Wheezing.* High-pitched, whistling sounds generated in bronchioles by air being forced through narrowed airways. Despite low flow, the high velocity makes them vibrate, much like the reed in a musical instrument; wheezing suggests small airways are swollen and/or constricted, such as in patients with asthma. Wheezing occurs during expiration or both inspiration and expiration, but never inspiration alone.
- *Crackles (rales).* These are discrete, primarily inspiratory sounds caused by the abrupt opening of small airways. Very small airways lead to high-pitched sounds often called fine crackles, and larger bronchioles cause lower-pitched sounds

known as coarse crackles. Crackles can be simulated by rolling hair between your fingers.
- *Rhonchi.* Low-pitched, coarse loud sounds caused by secretions in the larger airways; rhonchi can be a sign of chronic obstructive pulmonary disease or an infectious process such as bronchitis. Rhonchi, like wheezing, occurs in expiration, or both inspiration and expiration, but never inspiration alone.

Accessory muscle use and retraction can be seen at the suprasternal notch, beneath and between the ribs. If the work of breathing is increased, or the patient's breathing becomes progressively more difficult, the patient should be monitored for respiratory distress and imminent collapse. The combination of abnormal breath sounds and accessory muscle use or retraction is a more ominous sign than abnormal breath sounds alone. When you are assessing breathing, you must obtain the following information:

- Respiratory rate
- Rhythm: regular or irregular
- Quality/character of breathing
- Depth of breathing

As you assess the patient's breathing, ask yourself the following questions:

- Does the patient appear to be choking?
- Is the respiratory rate too fast or too slow?
- Are the patient's respirations shallow or deep?
- Is the patient cyanotic?
- Do you hear abnormal sounds when listening to the lungs?
- Is the patient moving air into and out of the lungs on both sides equally?
- Can the patient speak a full sentence without pausing for breath?

Other important questions the patient may be able to answer include:

- Did the difficulty breathing come on suddenly or get worse over several days?
- Is this problem chronic?
- Do you have any associated symptoms, such as a productive cough, chest pain, or a fever?
- Did you try to treat the condition on your own? If so, how?

Compromising breathing patterns should be identified and managed in the primary survey. Intervention for immediate life threats in airway or ventilation can include opening the airway, clearing an obstruction, assisting ventilation with BVM, administering supplemental oxygen, initiating positive-pressure ventilation, or decompressing a suspected tension pneumothorax. If a patient seems to experience difficulty breathing after your primary assessment, you should immediately reevaluate the airway. Remember: Air exchange is the critical issue, not the number of breaths.

Circulation/Perfusion

Assessing circulation helps you to evaluate how well blood is perfusing the major organs, including the brain, lungs, heart, kidneys, and the rest of the body. The patient's pulse rate, quality, and regularity should be obtained. Palpating the radial, carotid, or femoral artery is essential. An apical pulse can be palpated at the apex of the heart near the fifth intercostal space, a landmark known as the point of maximum impulse (PMI), but this does not allow assessment of pulse strength. The normal resting pulse rate for an adult is between 60 and 100 beats/min, with rates closer to 100 beats/min being normal for geriatric patients. In pediatric patients, the younger the patient, the faster the pulse will be.

Pulse quality is described as absent, weak, thready, bounding, or strong. A bounding pulse may indicate increased pulse pressures, such as with aortic regurgitation or elevated systolic blood pressure. A weak pulse may indicate poor perfusion. A weak and rapid pulse is often referred to as "thready" pulse. Factors that can decrease myocardial contractility include hypoxia, hyperkalemia, and hypercapnia. Early identification of irregular, weak, or thready pulses in the primary survey indicates poor perfusion and may prompt urgent application and interpretation of ECG findings.

The pulse should also be evaluated to determine whether it is regular or irregular. A normal rhythm is regular, like the ticking of a clock. If some beats come early or late or are skipped, the pulse is considered irregular. An irregular heartbeat may have a cardiac or respiratory cause, or it may be brought on by toxic substances or drugs.

If a patient has inadequate circulation, you must take immediate action to restore or improve circulation, control severe bleeding, and improve oxygen delivery to the tissues. At this point, perform a rapid exam to identify any major external bleeding. External severe uncontrolled bleeding is an immediate life threat that should be addressed before moving to a secondary assessment.

Once the pulse rate, quality, and regularity have been assessed, the skin needs to be assessed for color, temperature, moisture, and **capillary refill**. Capillary refill time can be evaluated to determine the status of the cardiovascular system. To perform this test, pressure is applied to the nail bed until it turns white. The clinician then measures the time it takes for normal color to return. A blanching time of more than 2 seconds is considered an indicator that capillary blood is being inappropriately shunted. This test can be unreliable in adult patients for several reasons. Older adults, especially those who take many medications and those with diabetes or immune system or renal disease, tend to have poor distal circulation. The temperature of the environment can also reduce the accuracy of the capillary refill test; cooler environments cause vasoconstriction as a compensatory mechanism and may give a false impression of poor perfusion status.

Pulse pressure is calculated by subtracting diastolic blood pressure from systolic blood pressure (e.g., 110 [systolic] − 70 [diastolic] = 40 [pulse pressure]). Normal pulse pressure is 30 to 40 mm Hg. If pulse pressure is low (< 25% of systolic blood pressure), the cause may be low stroke volume or increased peripheral resistance. *A narrowing pulse pressure may indicate shock or cardiac tamponade.* Identification of pulse pressure changes is also used to identify increased intracranial pressure (ICP). Observation of hypertension with a widening pulse pressure, bradycardia, and an irregular breathing pattern is a key indicator of increased ICP and is identified as Cushing's triad.

Information from dispatch, the initial observations of the scene and the patient, the patient's chief complaint, level of consciousness, patency of the airway and breathing, and circulation/perfusion status should suggest potential underlying diagnoses and initiate appropriate initial treatment interventions. Immediate life threats should be managed during the primary assessment. Diagnoses and patient management are dynamic throughout the call. They are continually reevaluated and modified as additional patient history, physical exam findings, and diagnostic results are obtained. The patient's response to treatment is used in modifying ongoing treatment.

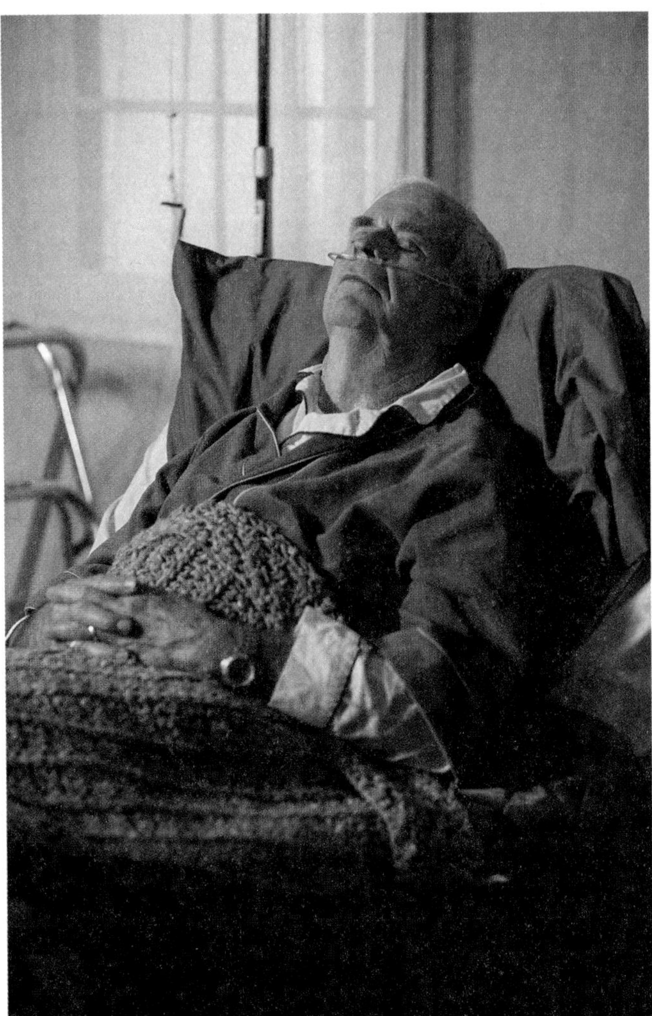

Figure 1-8 A person on home oxygen indicates a chronic disease process.

▼ First Impression

The first impression is formed based on all the initial information available when first contact is made with the patient. More often than not, you will form the first impression of your patient based on the initial patient presentation and chief complaint. Visual, olfactory, auditory, and tactile observations at the scene will add valuable information to your patient assessment process to help determine the patient's differential diagnoses.

Visual Observation

You should think of your initial impression of the patient as a visual assessment. Extrinsic clues can include body positioning, expressions of pain, and abnormal respiratory effort, which are all cause for concern. In patients with respiratory distress, the tripod position can be a sign of impending respiratory failure. Visual indications of extreme distress, such as a patient guarding their chest or abdomen or a chest pain patient holding a fist on the chest, known as Levine sign, help to formulate a first impression.

Look around for assistive devices indicating a chronic disease process. Walkers, canes, wheelchairs, oxygen concentrators, portable nebulizer devices, and hospital beds in private residences (**Figure 1-8**) are examples. Prosthetic and mobility devices indicate possible mobility problems associated with chronic respiratory, cardiovascular, musculoskeletal, or neurologic deficits.

Oxygen in the home can be stored as compressed gas or liquid oxygen or may be generated with an oxygen concentrator. Oxygen may be delivered by nasal cannula, oxygen mask, tracheostomy, ventilator, continuous positive airway pressure (CPAP), or biphasic positive airway pressure (BiPAP; **Figure 1-9**).

The care of patients who are dependent on technology such as ventilators can be complicated by chronic illness and medical devices. Some patients will require automatic transport ventilators. These ventilators should be identified on arrival. Patients are placed on these ventilators to provide extended positive-pressure ventilation.

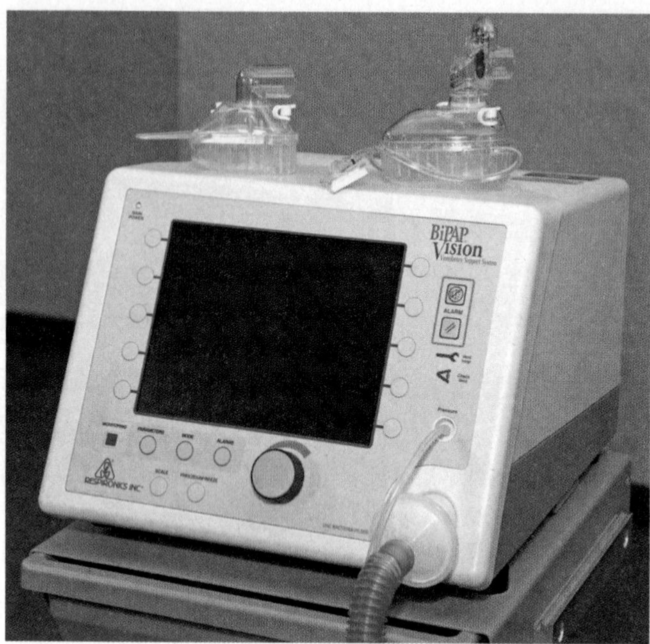

Figure 1-9 Home BiPAP machine.

To ensure quality continuity of care, prehospital clinicians should disclose information on patients who are dependent on technology to the receiving facility as soon as it is identified. Typically, patients and their family members are well-versed in the operations of the machines they use. They can provide tremendous assistance if you are unfamiliar with the devices.

Auditory Observation

Your sense of hearing can provide valuable information regarding your patient's condition. Severe wheezing or stridor can sometimes be heard from across the room without a stethoscope. Irregular and slow gasping may indicate agonal respirations in a patient in cardiac arrest, and gurgling respirations may lead one to suspect aspiration of fluids into the respiratory tract. These audible cues can help to narrow the first impression and identify patients with significant respiratory issues.

Olfactory Observation

Odors can also serve as warning signs of an unsafe environment even before patient contact is established. Evidence of gas fumes, especially with multiple patients complaining of similar distressing symptoms, indicates the need for immediate evacuation. Odors associated with spoiled food, mold, or insect or rodent infiltration may indicate an unhealthy environment for the patient and family members. This type of environment may indicate failure to thrive or may be evidence of neglect or domestic abuse. This observation should be reported to the proper authorities per local protocols and statutory requirements.

Also note unusual patient odors. Certain smells are associated with various acute or chronic disease processes, such as a fruity acetone breath odor with diabetic ketoacidosis. Observation of any excreted patient fluids such as blood, vomitus, urine, or feces may indicate dysfunction of the CNS. Other odors, such as a musty breath odor, can point toward chronic liver dysfunction. Significant body odor and uncleanliness may be evidence that the patient can no longer perform the activities of daily living without assistance.

Tactile Observation

The sense of touch also gives clues to the patient's condition. Patients may have skin that feels cool, cold, warm, hot, or sweaty. Excessively warm or hot skin may indicate an elevated core body temperature. A hot day with high humidity can lead to hyperthermia. Intrinsic causes of hot skin include stroke, fever, and heatstroke.

Likewise, an extremely cold environment may cause hypothermia. However, in older adult patients, hypothermia can occur even in a warm environment. Immobility, compromised cardiovascular and neurologic systems, endocrine disease, inappropriate clothing, drug toxicities, and comorbid conditions cause poor perfusion and diminished compensatory mechanisms. Cool, clammy skin can also be the result of shock or compensatory mechanisms such as vasoconstriction.

Moist or wet skin is typically found in patients with heat exhaustion, exertion, or drug toxicity. Patients with cardiovascular compromise leading to poor perfusion can also present with moist skin. Patients who are dehydrated will have dry skin. Deterioration of thirst and taste mechanisms often accompany advancing age, so it is especially important to evaluate older adult patients for dry skin and dehydration.

Touch also provides essential assessment information by allowing you to feel the patient's pulse and determine the rate—too fast or too slow, weak, thready, or bounding. Touch can help identify an irregular pulse, which may indicate cardiovascular compromise.

Building on dispatch information, initial observations, the patient's chief complaint, the primary survey, and information gained by what the clinician sees, hears, smells, and touches, EMS clinicians can form a first impression and can develop a plan to focus patient care through a more detailed assessment.

Sick or Not Sick

One component of the AMLS Assessment Pathway is the conceptual determination of whether the patient has an emergent condition and is acutely ill, or not. During the initial assessment this is based on System 1 thinking, essentially your gut instinct, which becomes more accurate with education and experience. The reason this is included in AMLS is to encourage clinicians to be highly vigilant for patients who are "sick" so that time-sensitive treatments are not delayed.

Throughout your encounter with a patient, you should continually consider whether there are indications that the patient is "sick." This is particularly true in the out-of-hospital setting where there are limitations to patient information and diagnostic testing. However, ultimately, clinicians should rely on the comprehensive assessment of history, exam, and diagnostic testing to use deductive reasoning to determine the patient's clinical status.

Detailed Assessment

History Taking

For patients with medical emergencies, historical information can be obtained before the physical exam is performed. Modifying the approach to obtaining historical information before performing a physical exam is dependent on the patient's initial presentation. Many diagnostic assessments are ordered on the basis of additional information obtained during the patient interview. An efficient, systematic, comprehensive interview, then, can help clinicians eliminate differential diagnoses, establish a working diagnosis, and determine treatment interventions.

History of the Present Illness

The history of the present illness can be obtained by using the mnemonic OPQRST (**Rapid Recall Box 1-3**). This tool helps analyze the patient's complaint by focusing on obtaining a clear, chronologic account of the symptoms the patient is experiencing.

Onset

First, determine the time of onset and origin of the symptom or condition. Find out what the patient was doing when symptoms began. Ask about any similar episodes the patient may have had. Obtaining the following information will assist you in determining a differential diagnosis:

- What the patient was doing when symptoms began.
- Whether the onset of symptoms was gradual or sudden.
- Any associated complaints, which may help to further refine the differential diagnoses and indicate whether multiple body systems are involved. Associated symptoms of importance include the following:
    - Trouble breathing
    - Shortness of breath
    - Chest pain or pressure
    - Palpitations
    - Nausea or vomiting
    - Syncope (fainting)
    - Lightheadedness or dizziness
    - Numbness or tingling
    - Indigestion (epigastric pain, abdominal pain, or bloating)
    - Confusion or disorientation
    - Fatigue
    - General feeling of illness or being out of sorts
- Any information offered by bystanders.
- Whether the patient has experienced similar symptoms before. Ask whether the patient is under a doctor's care, and, if so, when the last visit was. Inquire about medications prescribed and other treatments given.

RAPID RECALL BOX 1-3

History of the Present Illness: OPQRST

To assess the cause of a patient's injury or illness, clinicians need to collect details about the chief complaint. Errors in care can be made when all patients with similar chief complaints are treated the same without looking for important differences. For example, "chest pain" is a common complaint, but the cause (and subsequent treatment) may vary widely; retrosternal chest pain that started with exertion and radiates to the jaw may be caused by acute coronary syndrome, but chest pain in the unilateral chest that is sharp and worsens with each breath may be from a pulmonary embolus or pneumothorax. The OPQRST mnemonic will help you remember which questions to ask in order to elicit the most pertinent answers from the patient:

- **O**nset—What were you doing when the symptom started? Did it start suddenly, or did it develop gradually over time?
- **P**alliation/**P**rovocation—Does anything make the symptom go away or feel better or feel worse?
- **Q**uality—Describe the symptom or nature of the pain (burning, sharp, dull, ache, stabbing) or attributes of the condition.
- **R**egion/**R**adiation/**R**eferral—Can you point to the place where it hurts? Does the symptom move from its initial location or extend beyond the location of origin?
- **S**everity—On a scale of 1 to 10, with 1 being very minor and 10 the most severe you have ever felt, how would you rate this?
- **T**ime/duration—How long have you had this symptom/condition? What is the time course since onset—constant, worsening, improving, or waxing and waning?

Palliation/Provocation

Palliation and provocation refer to factors that make the patient's symptoms better (palliate them) or worse (provoke them). A patient whose chief complaint is dizziness, for example, might say the symptoms are better when lying down (palliation) and worse with movement, such as suddenly trying to get out of bed (provocation). A patient with chest pain may state that it is worse with inspiration, also known as pleuritic chest pain. A patient with chest pain from angina may state that it occurs during the exertion of climbing steps or walking uphill.

Quality

The patient's perception of the quality of the pain or discomfort can be an important diagnostic clue. Ask for a description of the type of pain or discomfort. Some common descriptions include terms such as *sharp, dull, tearing, ripping, crushing, pressure,* and *stabbing*. The patient's description can suggest whether the pain is of visceral or somatic origin, which will help in determining the differential diagnosis. Visceral pain is from internal organs and is often vague and difficult to localize, whereas somatic pain (typically caused by skin, tissues, or muscle) can be precisely located and is more likely to be sharp or stabbing in nature. Assessing whether the discomfort is constant or occurs only intermittently, either randomly or with certain breathing patterns or movements, can be a key indicator of the body system involved and the severity of the etiology. Along with palliation and provocation, how a patient describes the quality of the pain or discomfort can also indicate the underlying body system affected. Use quotation marks to document exactly how patients describe their symptoms (e.g., "my stomach feels like it's on fire").

Region/Radiation/Referral

Region, radiation, and referral are all associated with the location of the pain or discomfort. Ask the patient to point to where it hurts or indicate whether the pain seems to radiate or move anywhere else (Table 1-5). Try to ascertain whether the pain is referred, such as abdominal distention with pain in the shoulder (Kehr sign).

Table 1-5 Regions of Referred Pain

Location	Organ
Left shoulder pain	Diaphragm irritation (colon; blood or debris from rupture of abdominal structures such as bowel, ovaries, or spleen; heart due to myocardial infarction or pericarditis)
Right shoulder pain	Diaphragm irritation (liver or gallbladder, rupture of abdominal structures such as bowel, ovaries, or spleen)
Right scapular pain	Liver and gallbladder
Epigastric	Stomach, pancreas, lung, cardiac
Umbilical	Small intestine, appendix
Back	Aorta, stomach, pancreas
Flanks to groin	Kidney, ureter
Perineal	Bladder
Suprapubic	Bladder, colon

Severity

The majority of patients seen by health care clinicians have experienced either acute or chronic pain or discomfort. Pain and discomfort can result from infection, inflammation, trauma, and neurologic dysfunction. Injury and overuse of muscles and the skeletal system can generate acute or chronic pain. Organs in every body system can elicit pain and discomfort. Activation of nociceptive pain fibers is the root cause of both chronic and acute pain. When the fibers are stimulated, the pain impulse will travel via nerve fibers to the spinal cord to the brain.

Pain or discomfort can present with very vague signs and symptoms, especially in patients who are poor historians, as in the elderly. Oftentimes, patients are taking over-the-counter (OTC) medications, self-remedies, or multiple medications. Whether medications are OTC or prescribed, their effects may mask the quality and severity of pain. Historical information regarding pain may present differently based on the patient's cultural background and religious belief systems, making assessment and management challenging.

Any and all complaints of pain or discomfort must be taken seriously. Exercise patience in determining the location, severity, and quality of pain. Precise patient descriptions of the pain can help you differentiate pain associated with a life-threatening medical emergency from less-critical pain and allow you to provide appropriate pain management.

Ask the patient to rate the level of the pain or discomfort on a scale from 1 to 10, with 1 being the least discomfort or pain and 10 the highest. This numeric scale is commonly used by both EMS and hospital personnel. Not only will the patient's report of the severity of the pain help narrow down its source, but it might also set a useful baseline by which to gauge whether the patient's condition is improving or worsening. The Wong-Baker

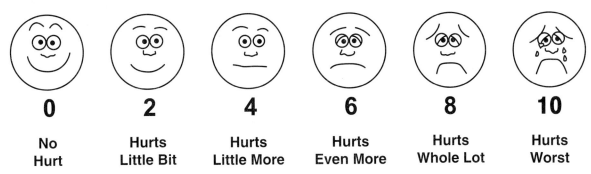

Figure 1-10 Wong-Baker FACES Pain Rating Scale. To use this scale, point to each face and use the words to describe the pain intensity. Ask the patient to choose the face that best describes the pain, and document the number.

FACES Pain Rating Scale is a useful alternative for children or patients who may not be able to communicate verbally (**Figure 1-10**).

Time/Duration

Finally, ask patients how long (time/duration) they have had the pain or discomfort. If the patient cannot respond or is not sure, ask a family member or a bystander to tell you exactly how long ago the patient last seemed to be feeling normal. Narrowing down the time frame of the discomfort may become crucial for sound medical decision making about certain conditions, such as deciding whether to administer fibrinolytic agents to a stroke patient or whether to catheterize a patient with suspected myocardial infarction.

Past Medical History

The past medical history gives the clinician an opportunity to learn about any pertinent or chronic underlying medical conditions the patient may have. Whereas not all aspects of the past history may seem important at the present time, a careful and thorough history will help paint a clear picture of the patient's overall health status. The SAMPLER mnemonic can also be useful in the interviewing process (**Rapid Recall Box 1-4**).

Signs and Symptoms

Symptoms are the subjective perceptions of what the patient feels, such as nausea, or has experienced, such as a sensation of seeing flashing lights. **Signs** are objective data you or another health care professional have observed, felt, seen, heard, smelled, or measured, such as data indicating tachycardia. A symptom reported by the patient, such as diarrhea, becomes a sign as well when observed by a health care clinician. All signs and symptoms should be well documented (**Figure 1-11**).

In awake and alert patients with no cognitive deficits, it is appropriate to use open-ended questions when asking how they are feeling. Such patients are able to process the question and give a reply. Patients with speech, hearing, or cognitive difficulties may respond more easily to yes-or-no questions. Often a simple head nod or shake can communicate effectively enough to help you complete the history. Be sure to exercise patience with older

RAPID RECALL BOX 1-4

The SAMPLER Approach to Past Medical History

The SAMPLER mnemonic represents a sensible approach to inquiring about a patient's medical conditions:

- **S**igns/symptoms
- **A**llergies
- **M**edications
- **P**ertinent past medical history
- **L**ast known well/**L**ast oral intake
- **E**vents preceding the current illness or injury
- **R**isk factors

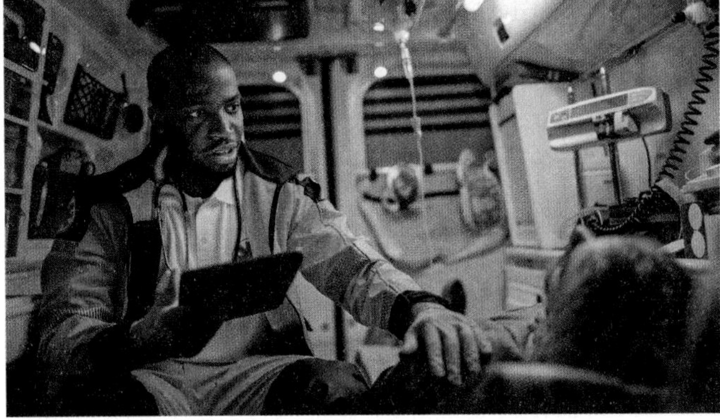

Figure 1-11 Be especially patient when you are obtaining information about a patient's symptoms.

and frail adults and persons with speech, hearing, or cognitive disabilities. Allowing enough time for the patient to answer the question can often be challenging. Rushing a verbal response, however, will inhibit rapport, might be frustrating or intimidating, and could impede the patient's willingness to share information. Use of therapeutic communication techniques will help you obtain more complete and accurate information.

Allergies

Many patients have allergies to prescribed or OTC medications, animals, food, or environmental conditions. Ask the patient about any known causes of allergic reactions and which symptoms are normally experienced, such as hives or trouble breathing. Find out how quickly the symptoms tend to develop.

Some symptoms are more worrisome than others. A patient who breaks out in a slight rash when around cats raises fewer concerns than a patient who develops stridor when a particular food is eaten. Some untoward responses are adverse reactions rather than true allergic responses. Many patients may misinterpret hypersensitivity to a food, animal, or medication as an allergy, so it becomes important to evaluate exactly how the patient responds to contact with the reported allergen or irritant. This information will help distinguish a hypersensitivity response from an allergic or anaphylactic reaction.

Medications

In written documentation, include a record of all medications the patient takes regularly—OTC drugs and medications prescribed by all the patient's doctors. Health care clinicians may or may not know what the patient's physician has prescribed. Drug interactions and adverse reactions must be considered in the overall medication profile. When listing medications, patients often forget to include inhalers, eye drops, and herbal medications. It is important to identify medications that the patient only takes on occasion, such as albuterol for exercise-induced asthma or the use of medication for erectile dysfunction that can have catastrophic consequences if not known and an EMS clinician administers nitroglycerin to the patient.

Some patients also take OTC drugs or dietary supplements that are considered to be holistic, herbal, homeopathic, or alternative medications. Trends in the legalization of cannabis indicate the inclusion of additional patient questioning regarding the use of cannabis for recreational or medicinal use. Remember to ask about liquid OTC drinks and herbal teas having a high content of caffeine, vitamins, or other ingredients that could cause the patient's signs and symptoms. Hypertensive patients who take OTC medications that contain dextromethorphan or guaifenesin, such as cough suppressants or antitussive agents, in conjunction with monoamine oxidase inhibitors or selective serotonin reuptake inhibitors can experience elevations in blood pressure.

A variety of pain remedies may be encountered. Acetaminophen and nonsteroidal anti-inflammatory drugs (NSAIDs) such as ibuprofen and naproxen are nonopioid OTC medications. Opioid analgesics, such as morphine, hydrocodone, and oxycodone, are prescribed for acute and chronic pain.

Obtain as much information as possible on which pain medications the patient has been taking, including amount, frequency, and time of last dose. Based on the additional information gathered in the history of present illness, diagnoses and possible treatments can evaluated and modified.

Pertinent Past Medical History

Try to discern which medical history is pertinent to the presenting complaint. If the patient is having chest pain and had a stent recently placed, for example, that information is pertinent. A femur fracture occurring 2 years ago is most likely not essential information.

A description of past surgeries, especially recent ones, is important historical information to obtain. The risk of an embolus can be identified, for example, if the patient has recently undergone a cesarean section, hip or knee replacement, or gallbladder removal. Gastric bypass surgical interventions should be identified for patients with unstable vital signs or history of gastrointestinal upset with fever, vomiting, constipation, or diarrhea.

In a premenopausal woman, the menstrual history should be obtained when the presentation includes abdominal or pelvic symptoms or when gynecologic/obstetric conditions are part of the differential diagnoses.

Last Known Well/Last Oral Intake

Time-sensitive illnesses have time-dependent treatments. The time "last known well" is important in the definitive treatment of ST-elevation myocardial infarction (STEMI) and stroke. Often the witness who has this information may not be directly available to the hospital staff, and therefore it is critical for EMS clinicians to obtain this information.

For STEMI patients, the time last known well is the time of onset of continuous chest pain or symptoms of acute coronary syndrome. For stroke patients, the time last known well may be the time that the stroke symptoms are definitively known to have started, or it may be the time that the patient was last seen by a witness to be well. For example, patients who awaken with stroke symptoms were last known well when someone last saw them without symptoms. In situations where time last known well is important, this pertinent information should be specifically provided as part of the SAMPLER history.

Time of last oral intake has traditionally been used in trauma patients who may require surgery, because unconsciousness or sedation may carry risk of aspiration of stomach contents into the lungs if the patient vomits. Recent evidence no longer supports avoiding sedation or anesthesia in patients who have recently eaten when the patient requires surgery or sedation for an emergent procedure. It is still reasonable to obtain this information, but it is of less utility than in the past. It is also helpful to obtain information about the last oral intake and what was consumed in patients with certain medical conditions, such as hypoglycemia. Ask patients when and what they last ate and drank.

Events Preceding the Current Illness or Injury

Find out which events led to the decision to request an ambulance or go to the hospital. Ask the patient, bystanders, and family the following questions: What happened today? Why did you call EMS? What has made the discomfort better or worse? This last question is appropriate when the events elapsed slowly, such as when a patient has trouble breathing for a couple days but does not call EMS or obtain medical care until symptoms begin to worsen.

Risk Factors

Risk factors for a patient's given condition can be environmental, social, psychological, or familial, or they may involve other medical and physiologic conditions. Is the patient living alone and at risk for falls? Does the residence contain any fall-related hazards? Is the patient confined to bed and dependent on someone else for meals and care? Other significant risk factors for medical problems include recent travel, surgeries, diabetes, hypertension, sex, race, age, smoking, and obesity.

Some risk factors are permanent, such as a chronic medical disease, whereas others are temporary. Consider that a recent fracture with temporary immobilization may predispose to a venous thrombus for several weeks, and postpartum status is associated with some clinical conditions for up to a year.

EMS clinicians should focus on risk factors that alter the list of differential diagnoses that they are building during the history and secondary survey.

Current Health Status

The personal habits of patients relevant to their overall health history can be important in determining the acuity of the current complaint. Frequent visits to their physician or the emergency department for similar complaints may indicate the need for evaluation of a chronic condition, change in treatment regimens, or further patient education.

Alcohol or Substance Abuse and Tobacco Use

Asking patients about their use of drugs (licit or illicit, including the use of prescription drugs not prescribed to them), tobacco products, and alcohol and other recreational substances may elicit important information about the potential for multiple underlying etiologies. Assure the patient of confidentiality when making such inquiries. The CAGE questionnaire can be used to help identify alcohol abuse patterns of behavior (**Rapid Recall Box 1-5**). Such an evaluation can indicate a chronic versus acute condition with the potential for traumatic injury. For example, a patient with chronic alcoholic use disorder is at increased risk for bleeding, particularly subdural bleeding following a fall.

RAPID RECALL BOX 1-5

CAGE Questionnaire

- **C:** Have you ever been concerned about your own drinking? Have you ever found the need to cut down on drinking?
- **A:** Have you ever felt annoyed by criticism of your drinking?
- **G:** Have you ever felt guilty about your drinking? Have you ever felt guilty about something you said or did while you were drinking?
- **E:** Have you ever felt the need for a morning "eye-opener" drink?

Modified from Ewing JA. Detecting alcoholism: the CAGE questionnaire. *JAMA*. 1984;252:1905.

Immunizations

Information about recent screening tests performed and an immunization record help identify patients at risk for communicable diseases. Recent travel history outside the country or immigration status is also helpful in identifying conditions that should be included in the differential diagnosis.

Family History

Family history may be important if the differential diagnosis includes inherited conditions such as sickle cell disease or contagious diseases such as tuberculosis. Once the patient's historical information is obtained, additional underlying etiologies and diagnoses should be modified and either disregarded or considered.

Secondary Survey

The **secondary survey** consists of two elements: obtaining vital signs and performing a head-to-toe examination evaluating the specific body organ systems. The assessment is done in a sequential manner, starting with the head and moving down to the toes, ensuring that every aspect of the body's function is evaluated. Of course, the conditions in the prehospital setting may determine precisely how the secondary survey is performed.

Sometimes, it may be condensed. For example, for an unresponsive medical patient or a trauma patient with a significant mechanism of injury, there may only be time to perform a rapid exam. The amount of time spent on this exam and its thoroughness will be directly related to your scope of practice as a health care clinician, the patient's status, transport time to definitive care, and the diagnostic assessment tools available.

In medical patients, vital signs are taken and a history is often obtained before a physical exam is performed. Depending on the severity of the patient's condition, the availability of other health care personnel, and the estimated transport time to the appropriate health care facility, the physical exam may be performed either at the scene or en route to the receiving facility.

Confirming or ruling out whether life threats and emergent or nonemergent conditions exist are core considerations for initiating care at the scene, prior to packaging for transport. Modifying or establishing a care regimen will be based on continued information gathering during the secondary survey.

Vital Signs

When several clinicians are available, vital signs and the secondary survey can be done simultaneously. In this case, the clinicians must ensure that the patient is paying full attention to the parts of the exam that require patient input. Vital signs are generally the first component of the secondary survey. Vital signs traditionally include pulse rate, regularity, and quality; respiratory rate, regularity, and depth; pulse oximetry; blood pressure; and body temperature. You should measure and document these parameters frequently and repeatedly. Monitors allow for continuous reading of heart rate, respiratory rate, and oxygen saturation. Even if the patient's initial presentation does not suggest an immediate life threat, the patient's condition may deteriorate. Establishing baseline vital signs and being alert for trends during ongoing monitoring can aid in early identification of any adverse change. Even if the patient's condition remains stable and nonemergent, vital signs are indispensable to sound medical decision making. They guide clinicians in establishing a specific diagnosis and formulating a treatment plan likely to be effective.

Pulse

Patients with suspected medical emergencies should be assessed for both central and peripheral pulses. The rate, regularity, and quality should be reevaluated, as previously discussed. Abnormal findings can lead to early application of ECG monitoring.

Respiration

In addition to depth, rate, and regularity, the work of breathing and symmetry of breath sounds should be assessed. For a detailed discussion of breathing, see the earlier section. Pulse oximetry (discussed later) provides additional information on the patient's oxygenation status.

Blood Pressure

Evaluation of blood pressure provides an estimate of the patient's perfusion status and can identify pulsus paradoxus and pulse pressure. **Blood pressure** is the tension exerted by blood on the arterial walls. Blood pressure is calculated using the following equation:

$$\textbf{Blood pressure} = \textbf{Flow} \times \textbf{Resistance}$$

If flow or resistance is altered, blood pressure will increase or decrease. Resistance is altered when vessels narrow, increasing resistance and raising pressure, and when vessels dilate, decreasing resistance and lowering pressure.

In patients with a life-threatening cardiac or pulmonary condition, such as cardiac tamponade or tension pneumothorax, pulsus paradoxus may be present. Pulsus paradoxus is defined as a fall in systolic blood pressure of more than 10 mm Hg during inspiration compared to expiration. Normally the difference is less than 10 mm Hg. This can only be detected when taking blood pressure by auscultation. It is caused by the decrease in intrathoracic pressure with inspiration leading to decreased left ventricular filling and stroke volume. Although classically a sign of cardiac tamponade, pulsus paradoxus also occurs in the setting of right ventricular myocardial infarction, restrictive cardiomyopathy (e.g., amyloidosis), severe COPD and asthma, tension pneumothorax, large bilateral pleural effusion, pulmonary embolism, and severe hypovolemic shock.

A baseline blood pressure should be taken during initial contact with the patient. Measure blood pressure a minimum of two times while treating the patient in the prehospital environment. Ideally, the second blood pressure reading is obtained once the patient has been secured in the ambulance or other transport vehicle. Depending on the status of the patient and transport time, a third measurement is taken en route to the receiving facility. An initial blood pressure should be taken manually, and reassessment of blood pressure can be done using an automated device. Generally, vital signs for patients in stable condition are obtained twice and then every 15 minutes thereafter. Vital signs for patients in unstable condition are obtained every 5 minutes.

Temperature

Oral, rectal, esophageal, tympanic, temporal (forehead), or axillary temperature measurements may be taken, depending on the patient's injuries, age, and level of consciousness (**Tip Box 1-1**). Some patients with a decreased level of consciousness may be too agitated for an oral

TIP BOX 1-1

Obtaining Temperature

Obtaining an accurate temperature is a challenge for EMS clinicians. Reliance on skin temperature devices and axillary measurements do not help you in identifying patients with alterations in temperature regulation, and tympanic thermometers are less accurate than core temperatures. A core temperature is preferred in patients who are ill, but rectal and esophageal temperatures are not always feasible in a prehospital setting, and these are often limited to critical care out-of-hospital practice. Work with your agency to ensure your ability to obtain an accurate temperature in the field.

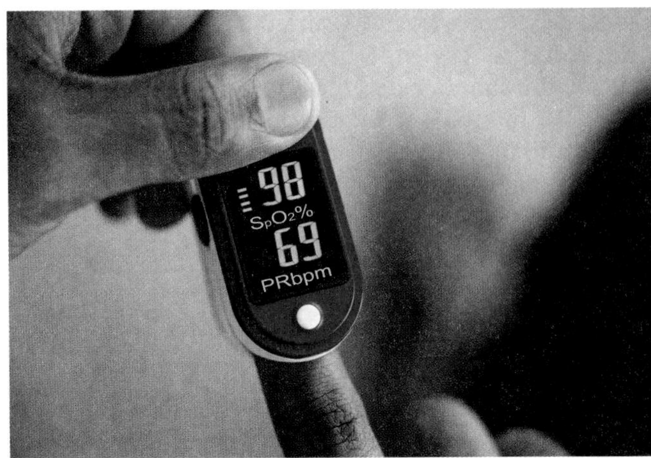

Figure 1-12 A pulse oximeter.

measurement. Facial or other injuries may also preclude use of an oral thermometer.

Hyperthermia can be caused by sepsis (infection) and heat illness (particularly heatstroke). Other causes include autoimmune/inflammatory conditions, medications, sympathomimetic substances, and hyperthyroidism. Hypothermia can be caused by exposure, shock, alcohol or other drug use, and hypothyroidism, and it can occur in patients who are severely burned and unable to regulate their body temperature. The environment, whether too warm, cold, or humid, may affect the patient's skin temperature and should be considered when evaluating skin vital signs. Keep in mind that, under certain conditions (exposure to wind/cold water, very young or old patients, certain medications, etc.), hypothermia can be present even if environmental temperatures are above freezing.

Pulse Oximetry

A pulse oximeter takes advantage of hemoglobin's propensity to absorb light, which results in an indirect measurement of oxygen saturation when a pulse oximetry probe is placed on a finger or toe (without nail polish) or earlobe (**Figure 1-12**). Oxygen saturation is an indication of, on average, how many of the oxygen-binding sites in each molecule of hemoglobin are occupied by (saturated with) oxygen molecules. This measurement is expressed as a percentage. Healthy people have an oxygen saturation of 97% to 99%. In a patient with a normal hemoglobin level, a saturation of 90% is minimally acceptable, although some patients with severe COPD, pulmonary hypertension, or other chronic pulmonary conditions may have lower baseline saturations (between 80% and 90%). Oxygen should be administered to patients with breathlessness, signs of heart failure or shock, and those with acute illness and an oxygen saturation of less than 94%. Another indication for oxygen therapy is suspected carbon monoxide poisoning. In this instance, oxygen should be delivered at the highest concentration available because carboxyhemoglobin is measured as oxygen by pulse oximetry, and a normal oxygen saturation on pulse oximeter will be deceivingly elevated.

In some patients, it may be difficult to obtain an accurate pulse oximetry reading when the patient has poor perfusion or the measurement of light waves are inhibited by other factors. These limitations include patients with cold extremities (distal vasoconstriction), significant history of smoking, advanced peripheral vascular disease, nail polish, fake nails, and variations in patient skin pigmentation. In addition to carbon monoxide poisoning, pulse oximetry may give false or inaccurate readings in patients with methemoglobinemia.

A patient with medical complaints and whose oxygen saturation is less than 94% should be administered supplemental oxygen by a nasal cannula or nonrebreather mask. The percentage of supplemental oxygen administered will depend on assessment findings. Oxygen saturation findings are helpful if assessed before and after application of supplemental oxygen.

Other Vital Signs

The vital signs offer important information to help you formulate a more in-depth impression about the patient's health status and treatment needs. In patients with alterations in mentation, also assess the pupils and perform an abbreviated neurologic exam during the assessment of vital signs. Motor and sensory function, distal pulses, and capillary refill should be evaluated as well. In addition, blood glucose levels should be obtained.

Physical Exam

The physical examination of a patient in the prehospital setting is the most important skill a health care clinician can master. This ability is first developed as an EMT and should be refined as an advanced clinician. The goal of this process is to identify hidden injuries or conditions and identify abnormalities that may not have been found during the primary survey. The goal is also to further develop the list of differential diagnoses by ruling in or ruling out conditions suspected during the initial patient history. The exam can be a full-body head-to-toe exam or a focused exam. The health care clinician must determine, based on the acuity of the patient, which exam is most appropriate. In most emergency response situations, a focused exam is appropriate in conscious patients. A full-body head-to-toe exam is necessary in patients who are unconscious or have a diminished level of consciousness and in those whose presentation indicates possible substance abuse or toxicity. Detailed physical exams may be more practical in the hospital, although a detailed exam may be performed by prehospital personnel as transport time allows.

The physical exam findings should augment the historical data and diagnostic assessment information already obtained to rule in or rule out certain differential diagnoses. As information is gathered and critically evaluated, an appropriate treatment pathway will be identified and implemented.

Inspection, auscultation, palpation, and percussion are critical components of the assessment process. Stethoscopes, otoscopes, and ophthalmoscopes are common equipment used to gather valuable information when performing a physical exam, but the tools are only as good as the examiner's scope of practice and observation skills. The physical examination will help identify life threats in the primary or secondary survey. In an unconscious patient, the physical exam may be the only way to obtain clues to identify the problem.

In many medical patients, historical information is typically obtained before the physical exam is performed. Altering the order of the components of the assessment is dependent on the severity of symptoms, the criticality of the patient's status, and the initial presentation. The physical exam during the primary survey may be performed prior to obtaining the history or simultaneously with obtaining the history if enough personnel are present. The opposite may be true of traumatic injuries: in trauma patients, a rapid physical exam may be carried out before medical information is obtained.

Examination Techniques

Inspection

Inspection is the visual assessment of the patient to look for abnormalities. You begin observing visual clues to the patient's condition during the initial observation period. This preliminary inspection can reveal the implications of the environment and the severity of the patient's condition before the history is taken or the physical exam is performed. Other aspects readily apparent and worth noting include dress, hygiene, expression, overall size, posture, and overall state of health.

Significant injury should be identified during your visual exam. Bruising, abrasions, surgical scars (particularly evidence of previous surgeries such as cardiac surgery or lung removal, because they may be pertinent to dyspnea or other respiratory distress), and rashes should be noted. Note whether a stoma is present. Read and document any medical alert tags.

The trachea should be observed and potentially palpated to be midline. The shape of the patient's chest can offer the first clue to chronic lung disease. A barrel chest can indicate underlying COPD such as emphysema or chronic bronchitis.

A patient in a supine position with flattened neck veins may have hypovolemia. Look for any unusual neck masses, jugular venous distention (JVD), and swelling (**Figure 1-13**). JVD with diminished or absent breath sounds may indicate tension pneumothorax and cardiac tamponade. JVD increasing with palpation of the liver (hepatojugular reflex) may indicate fluid overload, as seen in congestive heart failure.

Assess the patient for vascular access devices, such as a peripherally inserted central catheter (PICC) line, centrally inserted central line, and subcutaneous ports, that indicate chronic disease processes and the need for nutritional support or long-term vascular access, as in the case of chemotherapy regimens or frequent blood samples.

Tracheal tugging and use of intercostal and neck muscles are signs of distress. Asymmetry, grunting, and deep or shallow respiratory movement are abnormal. Immediate intervention should be initiated to improve

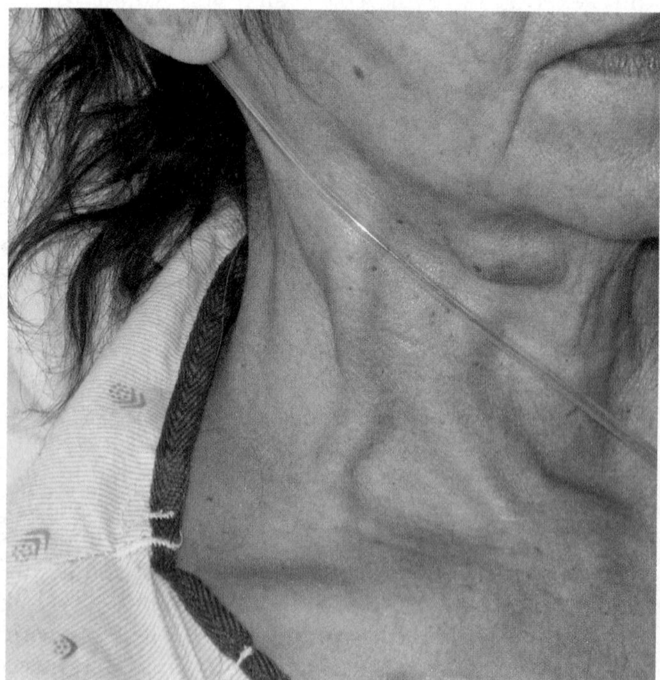

Figure 1-13 Jugular venous distention (JVD).

oxygenation and ventilation, stabilize the work of breathing, and promote adequate perfusion.

In patients with chronic renal failure, especially those on dialysis, you may note grafts or fistulae. Patients who receive peritoneal dialysis at home will have an abdominal catheter. In addition, a gastric tube may be used in the home setting to remove fluids and gas, instill irrigation solutions or medications, or administer enteral feedings. Be alert for the possibility the patient has aspirated gastric contents, and make sure the device is working properly.

With keen observation, clinicians will note kyphosis (spinal curvature), pressure ulcers, moles, abrasions, rashes, ecchymosis or hematoma, bleeding, needle or track marks, and discoloration. Observe the patient's chest and breathing efforts. Ask the patient to take a deep breath. Patients having acute asthma attacks tend to have more trouble exhaling than inhaling. If deep breathing causes pain or discomfort, the patient may have underlying pleurisy or a pulmonary embolism.

Auscultation

Auscultation is the use of a stethoscope or your ears to evaluate the sounds the body makes, such as the flow of blood against the brachial artery with the head of the stethoscope. Lung sounds, heart sounds, and bowel sounds can be evaluated using auscultation. Patency of dialysis grafts can be determined by listening for a bruit (sound of high-flow blood through the graft).

The lungs initially should be auscultated in the upper and lower lung fields, both anteriorly and posteriorly. When the differential diagnosis includes pneumothorax or when assuring that ventilation to the lungs is equal, it is essential to compare breath sounds on both sides in the midaxillary line. It is common for breath sounds to be transmitted from one side to the other, so comparing equality from the midaxillary line helps to reduce misinterpretation due to transmitted sounds. Performing auscultation early in the assessment can reveal life-threatening respiratory compromise attributable to tension pneumothorax, acute asthma, or pulmonary edema.

Lung sounds vary based on the part of the airway over which you are auscultating and the presence of abnormal conditions (**Figure 1-14**):

- Vesicular lung sounds are auscultated over the anterior and posterior part of the chest. Normally these sounds are soft, low-pitched sounds heard over healthy lung tissue.
- Bronchovesicular sounds are auscultated over the main bronchi. These sounds are lower than the vesicular sounds and have a medium pitch.
- Bronchial sounds are heard over the trachea, near the manubrium of the sternum. They are loud, harsh, and high pitched.
- A sandpaper-like sound is an indication that the visceral and parietal pleura are rubbing together. This sign is called a friction rub and is associated with pulmonary diseases such as pleurisy.
- Adventitious lung sounds are abnormal sounds, such as crackles, rhonchi, and wheezing, each of which reveals valuable clues about lower airway disease.

Abnormal lung sounds can also result from cardiovascular compromise affecting both the cardiovascular and respiratory systems. For example, crackles can signal pulmonary congestion from heart failure. Using the proper assessment tools will help you confirm or eliminate differential diagnoses related to the respiratory system. The findings of such supplemental assessments will aid your clinical reasoning and ensure that your medical decision making is well informed and accurate.

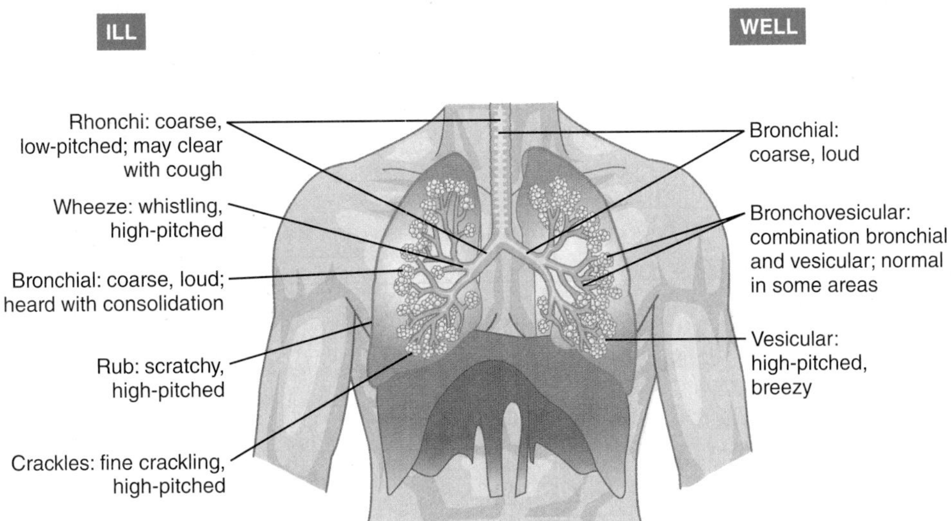

Figure 1-14 Abnormal (left) and normal (right) breath sounds.

Heart tones are auscultated for loudness (intensity), length (duration), pitch (frequency), and timing of the cardiac cycle. When listening at the fifth intercostal space, toward the apex of the heart, the normal heart sounds of S_1 and S_2 can be heard. These sounds are caused by heart valves closing and are best heard if the patient is leaning forward, sitting up, or in a left lateral recumbent position.

Abnormal heart sounds, such as murmurs, indicate a problem with the blood flow in and out of the heart. Bruits are abnormal sounds sometimes heard when the carotid arteries are auscultated; they produce high-pitched sounds indicating blood flow obstruction in those vessels. In the case of an aneurysm, a fine tremor or vibration that can identify a blockage can be felt; these are commonly called thrills. Murmurs, bruits, and thrills can be benign or life threatening.

In patients with a history of heart failure, additional heart sounds can be heard. Additional heart sounds occur in the presence of ventricular disease and are often identified as S_3 and S_4. The S_3 sound, identified as a third heart sound, is an early clue to a diagnosis of left heart failure. Difficult to detect, it can be referred to as a gallop, which would sound similar to a horse's gallop. It appears approximately 0.12 to 0.16 second after the second heart sound and results from rapid expansion of the ventricles as they fill with blood. The S_4 sound occurs during the second phase of ventricular filling, when the atrium contracts. This sound is thought to be caused by valvular and ventricular wall vibration. It is typically heard when there is increased resistance to ventricular filling.

Auscultation of bowel sounds, although not often performed during the prehospital evaluation, can help identify bowel obstruction. Bowel sounds should be auscultated for 30 to 60 seconds before palpation. A normal bowel makes a gurgling noise and sounds fairly similar in each quadrant. Hypoactive or hyperactive bowel sounds, particularly with high-pitched tinkles, in the presence of a distended abdomen may indicate a bowel obstruction. An obstruction or accumulation of gases can lead to a rupture of the intestinal wall. When examining the abdomen, auscultation should precede palpation to ensure that the intestinal activity is not altered by the palpation.

Palpation

Palpation is physical touching for the purpose of obtaining information, such as when you feel for a pulse. Some patients may feel palpation is a form of invasion of their personal space, so be sure to ask the patient for permission before you use this technique. Palpation should be gentle and respectful.

When traumatic injury is suspected, palpate the chest wall. Feel the torso for instability of bony structures. Palpate the chest for subcutaneous emphysema. Palpate the trachea for proper midline positioning; deviation can be a late sign of pneumothorax.

The abdomen should be palpated in all four quadrants. It should be soft and nontender, with no tension, swelling, or masses. The quadrant with the most reported discomfort should be palpated last. Palpation should be used to evaluate pain when gentle pressure is applied. It is also a means of identifying an increase in pain on removal of gentle pressure, known as rebound tenderness. This sign is a red flag for peritonitis. Guarding, or involuntarily tensing the abdominal muscles in response to tenderness, is an abnormal finding that indicates pain and possible underlying injury. Abdominal rigidity (firmness or contraction of the abdominal wall) can be a sign of internal bleeding or other potential life threats. Upper right quadrant tenderness that worsens with inspiration, known as Murphy's sign, is an indication of gallbladder inflammation from the presence of gallstones or cholecystitis (**Figure 1-15**).

McBurney's point is the name of the area over the right side of the abdomen, one-third of the distance from the anterior superior iliac spine to the umbilicus. Localized tenderness in this area is a sign of acute appendicitis. Referred tenderness, palpation of the left lower quadrant eliciting pain in the right lower quadrant, called Rovsing sign, can also be an indicator of appendicitis. Abdominal pain that cannot be elicited on palpation can be caused by renal calculi or a urinary tract infection. Flank and back pain often accompany both of these diagnoses.

In addition to auscultation, the skin over a dialysis graft can be palpated for a thrill (vibration felt from high flow) to confirm that the graft is patent.

Percussion

Percussion entails gently striking the surface of the body, typically where it overlies various body cavities. Sound waves are heard as percussion tones, which change according to the density of the tissue.

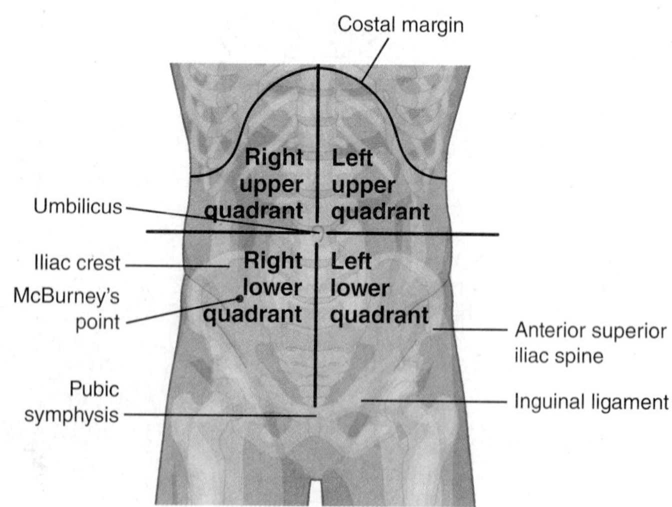

Figure 1-15 The four quadrants.

RAPID RECALL BOX 1-6

DCAP-BTLS

D Deformities
C Contusions
A Abrasions
P Punctures/Penetrations
B Burns
T Tenderness
L Lacerations
S Swelling

Percussion is not typically performed in the prehospital environment, particularly because ambient noise may make it difficult to hear subtle differences. However, this assessment provides important information regarding the abdominal cavity. If a dullness is heard during percussion, an abundance of fluid may be accumulating in this cavity (ascites or hemorrhage), as occurs in liver failure. A hyperresonant sound may indicate air, as opposed to fluid, is abundant.

The Full-Body Physical Exam

The full-body physical exam is a systematic head-to-toe physical examination. The full-body exam includes looking, listening where appropriate, and palpating. Any patient who has sustained a significant mechanism of injury, is unresponsive, or is in critical condition should receive this type of examination. DCAP-BTLS (**Rapid Recall Box 1-6**) is a helpful mnemonic when examining parts of the body for injury, but these findings can also be helpful in assessing medical etiologies. To perform this physical exam of a patient with no suspected spinal injuries, follow the steps listed:

1. Look at the face for obvious swelling, lacerations, bruises, fluids, and deformities.
2. Inspect the area around the eyes and eyelids.
3. Examine the eyes for redness, contact lenses, and yellow or reddened sclera. Assess the pupils using a penlight.
4. Use the penlight to look for drainage of spinal fluid or blood from the ears.
5. Look for bruising and lacerations about the head. Palpate for tenderness, depressions of the skull, and deformities.
6. Palpate the zygomas for tenderness, symmetry, and instability.
7. Palpate the stability of the maxilla.
8. Check the nose for blood, drainage, or nasal flaring.
9. Palpate the stability of the mandible.
10. Assess the mouth for cyanosis, foreign bodies (including loose or broken teeth or dentures), bleeding, lacerations, and deformities.
11. Check for unusual odors on the patient's breath.
12. Look at the neck for obvious lacerations, bruises, and deformities. Observe for JVD and/or tracheal deviation and thyroid gland enlargement.
13. Palpate the front and the back of the neck for tenderness and deformity. Auscultate for bruits if perfusion is compromised.
14. Look at the chest for obvious signs of injury before you begin palpation. Be sure to watch for movement of the chest with respirations. Assess for neck chains, bruising, and scars as evidence of a previous surgery. Observe placement of central line catheters, such as a Hickman, Broviac, or Groshong catheter. Assess the work of breathing.
15. Gently palpate over the ribs to assess structural integrity and elicit tenderness. Avoid pressing over obvious bruises and fractures.
16. Listen for breath sounds over the midaxillary and midclavicular lines—a minimum of four fields.
17. Lung assessment must include the bases and apices of the lungs. At this point, also assess the back for tenderness and deformities. Logroll the patient only once. Remember, if a spinal cord injury is suspected, use spinal precautions as you logroll the patient.
18. Look at the abdomen and pelvis for obvious lacerations, bruises, and deformities. Gently palpate the abdomen for pain on pressure or rebound tenderness. Observe for tenderness, guarding, rigidity, and pulsating masses.
19. Gently compress the pelvis and iliac crest from the sides to assess for tenderness, instability, and/or crepitus.
20. Inspect all four extremities for lacerations, bruises, swelling, tenderness, deformities, ports or fistulae, and medical alert anklets or bracelets. Also assess distal pulses and motor and sensory function in all extremities. Compare the right and left sides to determine strength and weakness variances.

The Focused Physical Assessment

A focused physical assessment is generally performed on responsive medical patients and patients who have sustained nonsignificant mechanisms of injury. This type of examination is based on the cardinal presentation/chief complaint. For example, in a person reporting a headache, you should carefully and systematically assess the head and neurologic system. A person with an isolated laceration on the arm may need to have only the arm evaluated. The focused assessment concentrates on the immediate problem.

Mental Status

Evaluation of a patient's mental status involves assessing cognitive function (the patient's ability to use reasoning). At a minimum, evaluate the patient's degree of alertness. Use the AVPU mnemonic as described in the *Primary Survey* section to help identify the patient's level of consciousness. You can further assess mental status by considering whether the patient is oriented in four areas (O × 4): person, place, day of the week, and the event itself. A standard method of assessing mental status and neurologic function is the GCS, which was described earlier. The GCS assigns a point value (score) for eye-opening, verbal response, and motor response; these values are added together for a total score. The GCS score provides insight into the patient's overall neurologic function.

Skin, Hair, and Nails

The skin, which is the largest organ system in the body, serves three major functions: temperature regulation, sensation of the environment, and protection from the environment. Examination of the skin involves both inspection and palpation. Pay careful attention to the skin color, moisture, temperature, texture, turgor, and any significant lesions. Look for evidence of diminished perfusion and evaluate for pallor, cyanosis, and diaphoresis. Flushed skin is usually apparent in patients with fever, and it may be seen in patients who are experiencing an allergic reaction.

Be sure to assess the color of the skin and nail beds. The skin should be dry to the touch and feel neither cool nor hot. If the patient has anything but skin that is warm, dry, and of normal coloration, you should look for the cause of the altered perfusion. Assessing perfusion or cyanosis via skin color can be challenging in patients with altered or darker skin color. In those situations, the color of the patient's mucous membranes may help with the assessment.

Examination of the hair is done by inspection and palpation. In this survey, note the quantity, distribution, and texture of the hair. Recent changes in the growth or loss of hair can indicate an underlying endocrine disorder, such as diabetes, or may result from treatment modalities, such as chemotherapy or radiation.

The examination of the fingernails and toenails can reveal many subtle findings. The color, shape, texture, and presence or absence of lesions should all be assessed. Normal changes to the nails with aging include the development of striation and a change in color (yellowish tint) related to the reduction in body calcium. Overly thick nails or nails that have lines running parallel to the finger often suggest a fungal infection.

Head, Eyes, Ears, Nose, and Throat

Physical exam of the head, eyes, ears, nose, and throat consists of a comprehensive evaluation of the head and related structures. The eyes are a nervous system structure involving both motor pathways (lids, extraocular muscles, pupillary constrictors, corneal blink reflex) and sensory pathways. The ears provide for both hearing and balance control. The nose is a sensory organ involved with the senses of smell and taste. It also plays an important role in assisting with breathing. The throat consists of the mouth and posterior pharynx and all the structures intrinsic to them. This complicated structure simultaneously coordinates many motor and sensory functions, as well as the initial activities of both the respiratory and digestive systems.

When you are examining the head, you should both feel it and inspect it visually. This step is important in the management of potential trauma patients and patients who have altered mental status or are unresponsive. Inspect and feel the entire cranium for signs of deformity or asymmetry, being careful not to palpate any depressions because you do not want to push bone fragments into the cranial vault or the brain. If you find evidence of external bleeding, attempt to separate the hair manually and apply direct pressure. When you are evaluating the face, observe the color and moisture of the skin, as well as expression, symmetry, and contour of the face itself. Asymmetry of the face could suggest an underlying nervous system problem such as a stroke or facial nerve palsy. Take the following steps to examine the head:

1. Visually inspect the head, looking for any obvious DCAP-BTLS.
2. Palpate the top and back of the head to locate any subtle abnormalities. Use a systematic approach, going from front to back, to ensure that nothing is missed.
3. Part the hair in several places to examine the condition of the scalp. Identify any lesions under the hair.
4. Note any pain or discomfort during the process. This exam should not cause the patient any pain.
5. Palpate the structure of the face, noting any DCAP-BTLS.

The eyes are a tremendously complex sensory organ and are a critical link to the CNS—they provide a useful glimpse into the patient's neurologic status. Retinal receptor cells process light stimuli for the brain so that the brain can decode light impulses entering the eyes and form a visual image. Assess the eyes for a conjugate gaze. In an awake and alert patient, the eyes should be open, should look in the same direction, and should move in tandem. Eyes that are focusing in two different directions are dysconjugate (**Figure 1-16**).

Normal pupils are equal, round, and briskly reactive to light. Pinpoint pupils suggest opioid use or injury to the pons region of the brain. Pupil dilation indicates toxicity or diminished neurologic function. Shining a light into the patient's eyes should cause the pupils to constrict quickly. Be sure to assess for this response in both eyes. Unilateral dilatation in an unconscious patient may be a sign of brain herniation. Some patients may present with anisocoria, a condition characterized by pupils that are noticeably unequal in size. Pupils appearing unequal in shape and size may be normal in some patients but may also suggest glaucoma or other serious conditions.

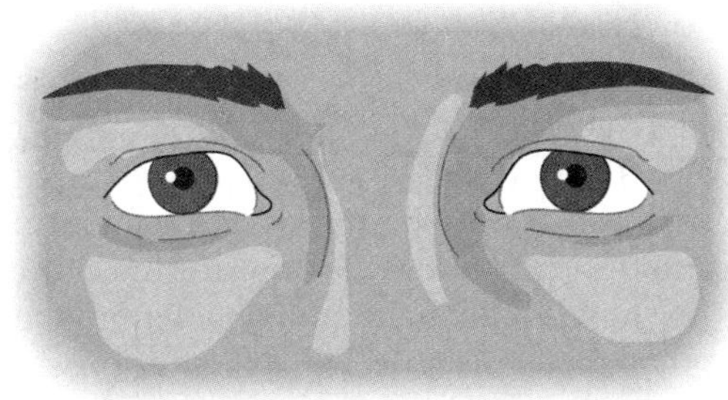

A

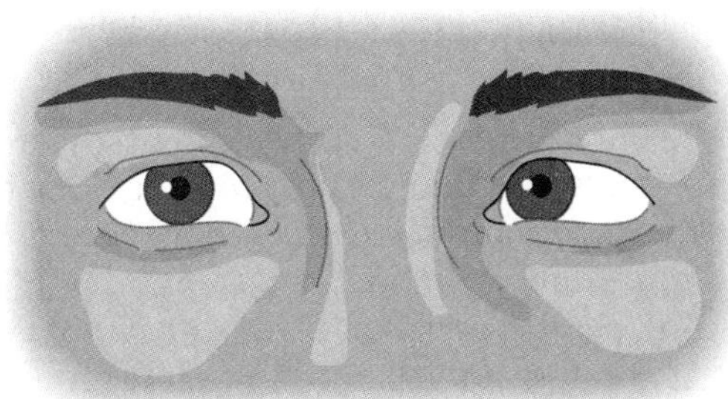

B

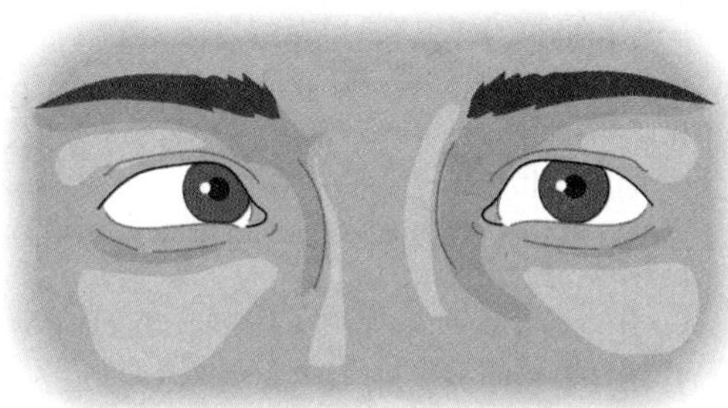

C

Figure 1-16 **A.** Baseline eye and lid position in central position. **B.** Right gaze with impaired abduction (away from the nose) of the right eye. **C.** Left gaze with impaired abduction of the left eye.

Irregular pupils can be seen after cataract or other surgery. Take the following steps to examine the eyes:

1. Examine the exterior portion of the eye. Look for any obvious trauma or deformity.
2. Ask the patient about any pain, altered vision (blurred or double vision), discharge, or sensitivity to light. If the patient has double vision, determine if it is vertical (two objects on top of each other) or horizontal (two objects side by side), and if only present with both eyes open.
3. Check for visual field defects by checking if the patient can see your moving finger in each of the four quadrants (top, bottom, right, left). Perform this exam on each eye independently of the other by testing one eye while the other eye is covered.
4. Examine the pupils for size, shape, and symmetry. They should be equal and round.
5. Test the pupils for their reaction to light. Both pupils should constrict when exposed to light, and they should be equal in their response.
6. Inspect the eyelids, lashes, and tear ducts for evidence of trauma, foreign bodies, or discharge.

Assessing the ears involves checking for new changes in hearing plus inspecting and palpating for wounds, swelling, or drainage (blood, pus, cerebrospinal fluid). Abnormalities of the external auditory canal and tympanic membrane are visualized by use of an otoscope. Take the following steps to examine the middle ears with the otoscope if allowed:

1. Select an appropriately sized speculum. Dim the lights in the room as much as possible.
2. Ensure that the ear is free of foreign bodies.
3. Place your hand firmly against the patient's head and gently grasp the patient's auricle. Move the ear to best visualize the canal, usually upward and back in the adult patient.
4. Ask the patient not to move during the exam to avoid damaging the ear.
5. Turn on the otoscope, and insert the speculum into the ear. Insertion toward the patient's nose usually provides the best view. Do not insert the speculum deeply into the canal.
6. Inspect the canal for any lesions or discharge. A small amount of ear wax is normal.
7. Visualize the tympanic membrane (eardrum) and inspect it for integrity and color. Note any signs of inflammation.

Using an otoscope is rarely performed in the prehospital setting; however, it may be a useful skill for community paramedics.

When you are checking the nose, assess it both anteriorly and inferiorly. Look for evidence of asymmetry, deformity, wounds, foreign bodies, discharge or bleeding, and tenderness. Assessment of the throat should include an evaluation of the mouth, the pharynx, and sometimes the neck. The throat is a conduit for both respiration and digestion, and it is in close proximity to numerous vital neurovascular structures. Take the following steps to examine the nose and throat:

1. Inspect the exterior of the nose, looking for color changes and structural abnormalities.
2. Examine the external column of the nose; it should be midline with the face.
3. Inspect the septum for any deviation from midline or for a hematoma.
4. Note gross abnormalities and any drainage or discharge. Small amounts of mucosal discharge are normal, but large amounts of mucus and any blood or cerebrospinal fluid are serious findings.
5. Ask the patient to open their mouth, and inspect the tongue, mucosal tissue, and teeth.
6. Examine the throat, or pharynx, with a light. If needed, a tongue depressor can be used to improve the view. Look for signs of inflammation and white pus or exudate.

As part of the assessment of overall hydration status, pay close attention to the lips, oral mucosa, and tongue. In patients who present with a markedly altered mental status, you will need to rapidly determine upper airway status. Prompt assessment of the throat and upper airway structures is mandatory. Always be ready to assist with clearing the pharynx using manual techniques and suction.

Take the following steps to examine the neck:

1. If trauma is suspected, take precautions to protect the cervical spine.
2. Assess for usage of accessory muscles during respiration.
3. Palpate the neck to find any structural abnormalities or subcutaneous air, and ensure that the trachea is midline. Begin at the suprasternal notch and work your way toward the head. Be careful about applying pressure to the area of the carotid arteries because it may stimulate a vagal response.
4. Assess the lymph nodes and note any swelling, which may indicate infection.
5. Assess for JVD; this may indicate a problem with blood returning to the heart and is associated with conditions such as heart failure, cardiac tamponade, or pneumothorax. Ideally, JVD should be evaluated with the patient sitting at about 45 degrees. Any JVD should be reported in centimeters above the level of the sternal notch.

Cervical Spine

The cervical spine is the pathway by which the spinal cord makes its way out of the brain and into the torso, enabling the spinal nerves to emanate to and innervate the rest of the body. Be aware that the most common mechanism for spinal cord injury in older persons is falling. Evaluate the patient first for the mechanism of injury and then for the presence of pain.

When you are examining the cervical spine, inspect and palpate it, looking for evidence of tenderness and deformity. Pain is the single most reliable indicator of a spine injury or spinal cord injury. Any manipulations resulting in pain, tenderness, or tingling should prompt you to stop the exam immediately and provide spinal motion restriction. Continued assessment of a patient's range of motion should take place only when there is no potential for cervical spine injury.

Chest

Typically, the chest exam proceeds in three phases: The chest wall is checked, a pulmonary evaluation is conducted, and finally the cardiovascular assessment is performed. The chest must be inspected for deformities as well as to look for external clues of respiratory distress. Expose the chest, while maintaining patient modesty and ensuring that the clinician is not exposed to risks of impropriety, and then begin the assessment, using the techniques of inspection, palpation, and auscultation. The examination of the posterior chest is the same as the examination of the anterior chest. Take the following steps to examine the chest:

1. Ensure the patient's privacy as best you can.
2. Inspect the patient's breathing, looking for suprasternal, subcostal, or intercostal muscle retractions with breathing.
3. Inspect the chest for any obvious DCAP-BTLS.
4. If you find any open wounds, dress them appropriately.
5. Note the shape of the patient's chest—it can give you clues to many underlying medical conditions, such as emphysema.
6. Look for any surgical scars or catheter ports indicating previous cardiac surgery and chronic illness.
7. Auscultate lung fields, noting any abnormal lung sounds.
8. Observe and palpate for subcutaneous emphysema.
9. Auscultate for heart tones.
10. Repeat the appropriate portions of the examination for the posterior aspect of the thorax.

Cardiovascular System

When you are examining a patient's cardiovascular system, pay attention to distal pulses, noting their location, rate, rhythm, and quality. Are the pulses fast or slow? Regular or irregular? Is the quality weak and thready or strong and bounding? Obtain an accurate blood pressure reading and repeat this measurement periodically to assess the patient's hemodynamic stability. Note if the patient has a history of hypertension. Auscultate the carotid arteries with the bell of the stethoscope to assess for any bruits. While inspecting and palpating the chest, listen for heart sounds. Feel the chest wall to locate the point of maximum impulse and appreciate the apical pulse.

For a suspected heart problem, assess the pulse for regularity and strength, and examine the skin for signs of hypoperfusion (pallor, cool, wet) or oxygen desaturation (cyanosis). If the pulse feels irregular or slow, assess it over 1 minute, rather than 30 seconds, in order to obtain a more accurate rate. Hypotension with sustained or progressive tachycardia is common in cardiogenic shock; stay alert for this condition because its mortality rate is more than 80%. Examine the extremities for signs of peripheral edema that may result from right-sided heart failure.

Abdomen

One of the most challenging complaints for you to assess in the field setting is abdominal pain because it can result from multiple causes and often presents with few or no external signs. Always proceed with abdominal assessment in a systematic fashion, routinely performing inspection, auscultation, and palpation, quadrant by quadrant. Take the following steps to examine the abdomen:

1. Inspect the abdomen for any DCAP-BTLS.
2. Note any surgical scars; they may be clues to an underlying illness.
3. Look for symmetry and the presence of distention.
4. Auscultate the abdomen for bowel sounds.
5. Palpate the four quadrants of the abdomen utilizing a systematic approach, beginning with the quadrant farthest from the patient's complaint of pain.
6. Note any tenderness or rigidity and pay special attention to the patient's expressions; they may yield valuable information.

Female and Male Genitalia and Anus

In general, assessment of female genitalia is performed in a limited and discreet fashion and only when needed for the immediate treatment of an emergent condition. Reasons to examine the genitalia include concern over life-threatening hemorrhage or imminent delivery in childbirth (checking for crowning). Assessment of the female genitalia can be performed while you are assessing the abdomen. Palpate both the bilateral inguinal regions and the hypogastric region. If the decision is made to inspect the genitalia specifically, limit the examination to inspection only. Note the amount and quality of any bleeding, as well as the presence of injury, inflammation, discharge, swelling, or lesions of the genitalia.

When you are examining male genitalia, make certain the exam is performed in a limited and discreet fashion and only when needed to treat an emergent condition. Always assess the entire abdomen and note any pertinent findings because occasionally pain from lower abdominal problems is referred to the genitalia. Testicular torsion and inguinal hernia sometimes present with a complaint of lower abdominal pain but minimal abdominal tenderness. In the case of a trauma patient, assess for the possibility of significant genital bleeding, bleeding from the urethra, and other injury.

The anus is often evaluated at the same time as the genitalia. It is examined in only a limited number of circumstances. Examine the sacrococcygeal and perineal areas, noting obvious bleeding trauma, lumps, ulcers, inflammation, rash, abrasions, or evidence of fecal incontinence.

Examinations of the genitalia and anus should be performed with a partner or a witness present. This may not be practical in all scenarios, and your local policy should be followed.

Musculoskeletal System

When you are examining the skeleton and joints, pay attention to their structure and function. Consider how the joint and associated extremity look and how well they work. Does the extremity look normal, and does it move in a normal range of motion? In particular, note any limitation of range of motion, pain with range of motion, or bony crepitus. When you are assessing the joints and extremities, look for evidence of inflammation or injury, such as swelling, tenderness, warmth, redness, ecchymosis, or decreased function. Also evaluate the joint or extremity for obvious deformity, diminished strength, atrophy, or asymmetry from one side to the other. The examination of the musculoskeletal system should not cause the patient any pain. If any pain occurs, it should be considered an abnormal finding. Take the following steps to examine the musculoskeletal system:

1. Beginning with the upper extremities, inspect the skin overlying the muscles, bones, and joints for soft-tissue damage.
2. Note any deformities or abnormal structure.
3. Check for adequate distal pulse, motor, and sensation to each extremity.
4. Inspect and palpate hands and wrists, noting any DCAP-BTLS.
5. Ask the patient to flex and extend the joints of fingers, hands, and wrist, noting any abnormalities in range of motion. If the patient experiences any discomfort, stop that portion of the exam.

6. Inspect and palpate the elbows, noting any abnormalities. Ask the patient to flex and extend the elbow to determine range of motion.
7. Ask the patient to turn the hand from palm-down position to palm-up position and back again, noting any pain or abnormalities.
8. Inspect and palpate the shoulders. Ask the patient to shrug the shoulders and raise and extend both arms.
9. Inspect the skin overlying the lower extremities.
10. Ask the patient to point and bend the toes to establish the range of motion.
11. Ask the patient to rotate the ankle, checking for pain or restricted range of motion.
12. Inspect and palpate the knee joints and patella. Ask the patient to bend and straighten both to establish the range of motion.
13. Check for structural integrity of the pelvis by applying gentle pressure to the iliac crests and pushing in and then down.
14. Ask the patient to lift both legs by bending at the hip and then turning legs inward and outward. Note any abnormalities.

Peripheral Vascular System

When you are assessing the peripheral vascular system, pay attention to both the upper and lower extremities. Look for signs indicative of either acute or chronic vascular problems. A wide range of disorders can affect the peripheral vascular system—from chronic venous stasis and lymphedema to intermittent claudication (crampy pain in the lower legs during ambulation due to poor circulation) and acute arterial occlusion. Peripheral vascular disease can manifest in many forms, depending on the point in the vasculature where the abnormality is located. Carotid artery disease can manifest as a stroke. Obstruction of the mesenteric vessels can result in bowel ischemia and necrosis. Take the following steps to examine the peripheral vascular system:

1. When you are examining the upper extremities, note any abnormalities in the radial pulse, skin color, and warmth. Always compare one extremity to the opposing extremity.
2. If abnormalities are noted in the distal pulse, work your way proximally, checking pulse points and noting your findings.
3. Examine the lower extremities, noting any abnormalities in the size and symmetry of the legs.
4. Inspect the skin color and warmth, noting any abnormal venous patterns or enlargement.
5. Check distal pulses, noting any abnormalities.
6. Palpate the inguinal nodes for swelling and tenderness.
7. Evaluate the temperature of each leg relative to the rest of the body and to each other.
8. Evaluate for pitting edema in the legs and feet.

Spine

Assessment of the cervical spine was introduced after the section on examination of the throat and neck. This section lists the complete assessment steps for the examination of the spine:

1. Inspect the cervical, thoracic, and lumbar curves for any abnormalities.
2. Evaluate the heights of the shoulders and the iliac crests. Differences from one side to the other may indicate abnormal curvature of the spine.
3. Palpate the posterior portion of the cervical spine, noting any point tenderness or structural abnormalities.
4. In the nontrauma patient and in the absence of reported pain, ask the patient to move the head forward, backward, and from side to side.
5. Move down the spine, palpating each vertebra with the thumbs to note any tenderness or instability.
6. In the absence of pain or trauma, ask the patient to bend at the waist in each direction to establish the range of motion.

Nervous System

The nervous system includes two portions: the central nervous system, which consists of the brain and spinal cord, and the peripheral nervous system, which includes the remaining motor and sensory nerves. Motor and sensory function should be evaluated in all patients whether they are conscious, unconscious, or have altered mental status. If the patient is conscious, gently touch the hands and feet to determine the ability to feel light touch, indicating that distal perfusion is adequate and sensory nerve tracts are functioning properly. Movement confirms intact motor function. Withdrawal of an extremity may indicate pain or discomfort. Assessing for sensation will determine the function of the afferent sensory nerve tracts in the posterior spinal column. Thorough assessment of the nervous system is one of the most time-consuming elements of the physical exam.

The 12 cranial nerves originate in the brain and brainstem rather than from the spinal cord. Although it is not necessary for EMS clinicians to examine all of these cranial nerves, EMS clinicians frequently check some of them when looking for pupil reaction, extraocular eye movement, and facial muscle symmetry.

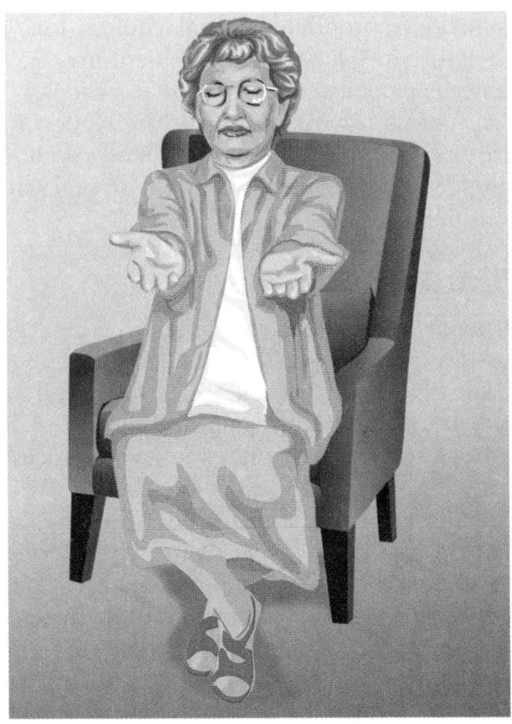

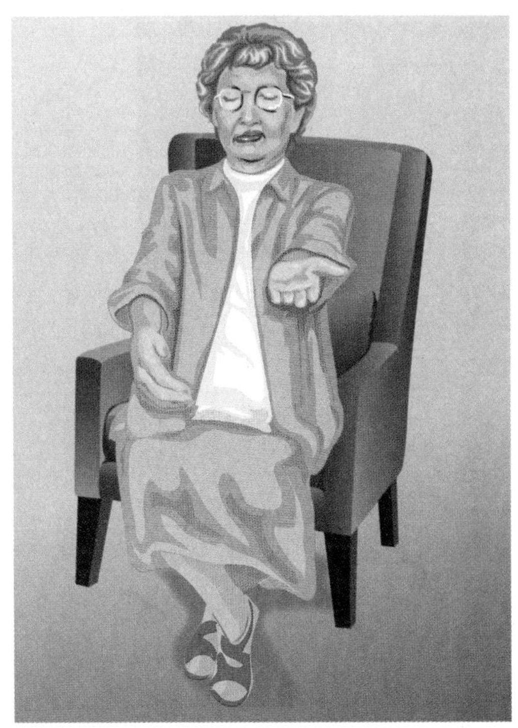

A B

Figure 1-17 Demonstration of assessment of arm drift to identify subtle muscle weakness that may be seen acutely in a stroke. **A.** Normal exam and normal strength. **B.** Right upper extremity drift seen with upper extremity weakness.

Motor function in all extremities should be evaluated for bilateral equality and strength. Unequal responses of left and right limbs should be considered a sign of hemiparesis (unilateral paralysis) or hemiplegia (unilateral weakness), which can be caused by stroke, meningitis, brain tumors, or seizure activity. Bilateral upper or lower extremity weakness should raise concern for a spinal cord lesion.

Cerebellar function can be evaluated by how a patient stands and walks. Ataxia (unsteady gait) may indicate damage from toxicity or chronic neurologic dysfunction. A shuffling gait may indicate neurologic damage caused by Huntington disease or Parkinson disease. Tremors, muscle rigidity, and repetitive motion may indicate degeneration of the nervous system attributable to Alzheimer disease or Parkinson disease.

Patients with a variety of psychological or behavioral disorders may take antipsychotic medications that have spasmodic muscle movement as a side effect. These medications may also induce muscle dystonia, expressed as contortion of the extremities or facial tics.

The arm drift (**Figure 1-17**) is used to evaluate motor and proprioception function in a suspected stroke patient. Patients are asked to extend their arms with palms up and then close their eyes. Note any downward drift or drop or any inward rotation of either arm.

The Babinski test may be used to check for neurologic function in conscious patients and in patients with altered mental status. To perform this exam, take a pen or similar dull object and run it along the lateral length of the sole of the foot from heel to toes. Normal reaction to this stimulation is for the toes to curl downward, a response known as plantar flexion. An abnormal Babinski test is indicated by extension of the great toe and fanning of the remaining toes. This movement suggests neurologic dysfunction (**Figure 1-18**).

Periodic reevaluation of the patient's response to questions about pain, discomfort, and difficulty breathing is important in gauging the effectiveness of interventions. The patient's physical exam should also be reevaluated, as appropriate, for diminished pain and discomfort, bleeding, and edema. Capillary refill time; distal pulses; and skin color, temperature, and moisture should also be reevaluated. CNS function should be reassessed for improvement in GCS scores and motor, sensory, and pupil response.

Take the following steps to examine the nervous system:

1. Assess the patient's mental status by using the AVPU mnemonic. If the patient is alert or responsive verbally, determine orientation (to person, place, time, and situation).
2. Note the patient's posture.
3. Assess the patient's pupils for equality, shape, and reactivity to light. Normal is often

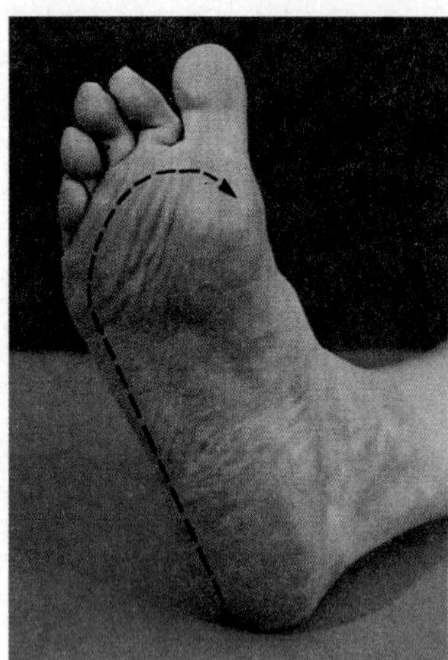

Figure 1-18 Check to determine the presence or absence of the Babinski sign.

described as "pupils equal, round, and reactive to light," or PERRL. Check extraocular muscle strength by assessing the patient's gaze in the four corners of a square in front of the patient.

4. Evaluate the patient's neuromuscular status by checking muscle strength against resistance.
5. Evaluate the patient's coordination by performing the finger-to-nose test using alternating hands.
6. If appropriate, check the patient's gait and balance by having the patient walk heel to toe or perform the heel-to-shin stance.
7. Perform the arm drift test. There should be no difference in movement on either side.
8. Evaluate the patient's sensory function by checking the responses to both gross and light touch.

Trauma Patients

Any trauma patient who is unresponsive or has altered mentation should be considered a high-risk, priority patient and requires immediate transport to a trauma center. An unresponsive patient may have a traumatic brain injury, stroke, hypoglycemia, or alcohol or drug intoxication. All are serious and potentially lethal events.

Mentally piece together all you know about your patient, including the chief complaint, the history of the present event, the medical history, and any information about the patient's current health status. Combine that knowledge with the other information and insights you have gained from your various assessments, along with the information obtained from your diagnostics (discussed next), and you should have enough information to make appropriate clinical choices for your patient. Keep in mind that a trauma patient may have also experienced a medical event and that a medical patient may also have a traumatic injury. The clinician must prioritize the most urgent complaint and condition for treatment. Some cases may involve both medical and trauma considerations.

Diagnostics

Whereas the history taking and secondary survey process are the best methods for determining a differential diagnosis in the patient, the use of certain diagnostic and monitoring devices in addition to performing laboratory tests aids in the assessment process. These devices are designed to assist the clinician with diagnostic assessment and monitoring of patients. Keep in mind that though these devices are helpful, they cannot replace a good history and physical exam. Patient history, physical exam, and diagnostic tools can be targeted to a specific body system. Each body system presents a set of unique assessment options to rule in or rule out differential diagnoses. Using clinical reasoning, the clinician can integrate new information pertinent to the current patient with previous assessment and treatment knowledge.

Diagnostic tools can help identify a broad range of medical conditions and can provide valuable information and prompt early, lifesaving intervention.

Laboratory Studies

A variety of elements found in the blood can aid you in determining a differential diagnosis. Measuring the blood glucose level of every patient who has altered mentation is required. Point-of-care testing (POCT) is becoming more available in prehospital settings, particularly in critical care and air medical systems. These include tests for hemoglobin, electrolytes, creatinine, and blood gases. EMS agencies may be required to obtain a specific laboratory license to use some POCTs. Clinicians should strive to be knowledgeable in their interpretation.

Capnography

Capnography (**Table 1-6**) is used to monitor carbon dioxide levels in exhaled gases, or end-tidal carbon dioxide ($ETCO_2$). This diagnostic assessment can give you a better understanding of the patient's ventilatory status. Capnography is projected as a waveform and a numeric value. The normal value of arterial CO_2 in the blood is between 35 and 45 mm Hg. Typically, the $ETCO_2$ will be slightly lower (3 to 5 mm Hg) than the pCO_2 level obtained through a blood gas.

Capnography is a waveform tracing showing the level of exhaled carbon dioxide and the characteristics

Table 1-6 Capnography-Related Terms

Term	Description
Capnograph	A device that provides a numeric reading of exhaled CO_2 concentrations and a waveform (tracing).
Capnography	Continuous analysis and recording of CO_2 concentrations in respiratory gases. Output is displayed as a waveform. Graphic display of the CO_2 concentration versus time during a respiratory cycle. CO_2 concentration may also be plotted versus expiratory volume.
Capnometer	Device used to measure the concentration of CO_2 at the end of exhalation.
Capnometry	A numeric reading of exhaled CO_2 concentrations without a continuous written record or waveform. Output is a numeric value. Numeric display of CO_2 on a monitor.
Colorimetric $ETCO_2$ detector	A device that recognizes the presence of CO_2 by chemical reaction on pH-sensitive litmus paper housed in the detector. The presence of CO_2 (evidenced by a color change on the colorimetric device) suggests tracheal placement. False readings are common with these devices, and in cardiac arrest or low perfusion states, they are less accurate than simple auscultation. They do not provide a quantitative reading of $ETCO_2$ level.

$ETCO_2$, End-tidal carbon dioxide.
Data from Aehlert BJ. *Paramedic Practice Today: Above and Beyond*. MosbyJems; 2010.

of the breath during exhalation. A capnograph allows for continual monitoring of $ETCO_2$, respiratory rate, and respiratory patterns. Abnormalities in inhalation or exhalation will alter the pattern of the waveforms and can indicate specific airway issues. Capnography is the gold standard for verifying and monitoring the correct placement and ventilation through an advanced airway. During spontaneous respiration, the $ETCO_2$ is inversely proportional to the minute ventilation (respiratory rate × tidal volume), but in poor perfusion states such as cardiac arrest, the $ETCO_2$ is directly proportional to pulmonary blood flow or perfusion. The quantitative values of $ETCO_2$ can be helpful in ensuring maximal perfusion during CPR.

Capnometry is the quantitative measurement of CO_2 without the waveform.

A colorimetric CO_2 detector provides semiquantitative information. Colorimetric devices use litmus paper to assess for CO_2 in exhaled air. They are less accurate than auscultation, and therefore they may lead to inaccurate information about tube location. In addition to having a high rate of false negatives in poor perfusion states such as cardiac arrest, if the litmus paper is exposed to stomach contents, it will present as a false positive due to the acidity. After a period of time, the litmus paper becomes less sensitive and may falsely suggest proper advanced airway placement. Importantly, because colorimetric devices do not provide a level of $ETCO_2$, they are not valuable in predicting perfusion during CPR or other physiologic conditions related to the $ETCO_2$ value. For these reasons, waveform capnography is overwhelmingly preferred.

Hypoventilation causes retention of CO_2, leading to respiratory acidosis. Increasing the percentage of supplemental oxygen, checking proper tracheal tube placement, and assisting ventilation with a bag-mask device are essential in addressing this issue.

Electrocardiography

An ECG records the electrical activity of the atrial and ventricular cells of the heart and represents this activity as specific waveforms and complexes. The ECG continuously detects and measures electrical flow on the patient's skin. Electrocardiographic testing is used to detect acute myocardial ischemia and to monitor a patient's heart rate and rhythm, evaluate the effects of disease or injury on heart function, analyze pacemaker function, and assess response to medications. The ECG does not provide information about the heart's contractile (mechanical) function.

Whether using a 3-, 12-, 15-, or 18-lead ECG, reviewing various views of the frontal surface, horizontal axis, and left ventricle of the heart provides key information about ischemia and infarction. The standard 12-lead ECG visualizes the heart in the frontal and horizontal planes and views the surfaces of the left ventricle from 12 different angles. Having multiple views of the heart makes possible the recognition of bundle branch blocks; the identification of ST-segment changes such as ischemia, injury, or infarct; and the analysis of ECG changes associated with medications. Extended lead placement, as in the 15- and 18-lead devices, allows additional anterior and posterior views to further demonstrate possible areas of injury.

ECG monitoring is typically performed in patients who are having difficulty breathing or who have chest or epigastric discomfort or pain. ST-segment elevation may indicate an acute, evolving myocardial infarction or STEMI. Non–ST-segment elevation myocardial infarction (NSTEMI) may show up on an ECG as ST-segment depression and T-wave inversion also demonstrating cardiac muscle injury. When reviewing 12-lead ECGs, several patterns may mimic ST elevation, including left bundle branch block (LBBB) and pericarditis.

Continuing advances in electronics and miniaturization of previously large diagnostic tools are making more diagnostic resources available to the prehospital environment. Devices such as point-of-care ultrasound, laboratory chemical testing, and bioassays are now available for field use. These devices may provide valuable feedback and allow for rapid interventions of patient care. EMS agencies and their medical directors must assess the training requirements and balance the potential advantages with the potential false negatives that are associated with each device.

Refine the Differential Diagnosis

Throughout the assessment process, the clinician will be distinguishing one disease from another based on accumulated data and clinical reasoning. The clues obtained from the patient's symptoms, history, physical examination, and diagnostic testing help narrow the possible diagnoses. Refining the differential diagnosis, which is the process of the elimination of potential diagnoses, eventually leads to one or more of the most likely diagnoses. In the prehospital setting it is usually not possible to determine an absolute diagnosis.

The patient's differential diagnosis also helps you decide whether the patient's condition is life threatening, emergent, or nonemergent. At any moment your patient's condition may deteriorate from being emergent to life threatening, and appropriate management and transport must begin without delay.

Ongoing Management

Reassess the Patient

After the primary survey, reassessment is the single most important process you will perform. When performing reassessment, you must evaluate the patient's airway, breathing, and circulation/perfusion (ABCs); make certain you have adequately addressed the chief complaint; obtain another set of vital signs; and reassess pertinent examination findings after treatment interventions (e.g., lung sounds after receiving albuterol for an asthma exacerbation). Reassessment represents a continuous, yet cyclical, process you perform throughout transport, right up to the time you transfer patient care to the receiving facility. For patients in stable condition, you should do a reassessment every 15 minutes. For patients in unstable condition, a goal is to reassess vital signs and pertinent exam and diagnostics every 5 minutes while providing appropriate interventions.

Reassessment combines repetition of the primary survey, repeated taking of vital signs and breath sounds, and repetition of the secondary survey. During the reassessment, you continue to reevaluate the patient's status and any condition changes from treatments already administered. Trends in the patient's current condition may give clues about the effectiveness of treatments. Compare vital signs. Have interventions improved the patient's condition?

Further Refine the Differential Diagnosis

As you perform your reassessment, you will continually be able to rule in or rule out certain conditions from your differential diagnosis. Keep an open mind as you gather patient information and modify your differential diagnosis based on new findings.

Modify Treatment

After reassessing the patient, think about your present care plan. Have you addressed all life threats? On the basis of what you know now, do you need to revise your priority list? If so, make the change and continue with patient care. In contrast, if your plan is working well and you have addressed the patient's complaints, there is no need to revise the care plan.

Patient Disposition

As you are reevaluating your patient care priorities, you should also reassess the transport plan. Should routine transport be stepped up to priority? Is the patient's condition worsening to the point you need to consider diverting to a closer facility? Do you need to set up a rendezvous with an air ambulance and fly the patient to the health care facility? If your patient's condition has improved and stabilized, you should decrease the priority and consider canceling critical care resources or transporting to a lower-level facility.

Population-Specific Considerations

Older Adult Patients

In the United States, approximately 40% of all EMS calls involve an older adult patient. Many older adults lead healthy, active lives, but others have chronic health problems. Assessment of the geriatric patient is more challenging than that of a younger adult for a variety of reasons.

Geriatric patients lack appropriate compensatory mechanisms and therefore may not show signs of deterioration as their conditions become unstable. In addition, many of these patients have underlying diseases or take medications that may mask true assessment findings. Orthostatic hypotension attributable to diminished baroreceptor function can be a concern during the physical exam. Take care to have older patients move slowly to better accommodate blood volume changes.

Medications

Polypharmacy refers to taking more than one prescription medication, but definitions vary and some consider polypharmacy to be taking more than five different medications simultaneously for one or more medical conditions. Either way, most older adults take multiple medications for several chronic conditions. **Pharmacokinetics**—the absorption, distribution, metabolism, and excretion of medications—differs in older adults compared to younger patients. As a result of pharmacokinetic differences and polypharmacy, older adults tend to have adverse drug reactions more often, especially when they are also taking OTC medications or dietary supplements such as herbal preparations or nutritional drinks. Common adverse reactions to medications include confusion, sedation, loss of balance, nausea, and electrolyte abnormalities.

Communication

Communication may be difficult if the patient has a hearing or speech–language impairment. However, many older adults are able to hear normally. If a patient does have hearing aids, make sure they are set at the proper volume.

Patience is vital when taking a history. Older adults sometimes cannot recall the names of medications or the conditions for which they have been prescribed. In addition, they may process questions slowly and feel obligated to share information they believe is important before answering the question directly. Such extra information may prove helpful when trying to work through the differential diagnosis.

Pulmonary System Changes

The pulmonary system undergoes changes in the older adult. The kyphosis (curvature) of the thoracic spine that often occurs with advancing age can make expanding the lungs more difficult. The respiratory muscles weaken, causing respiratory fatigue and failure earlier than in younger adults. In addition, the elasticity of the lungs and chest wall decreases with age, diminishing tidal volume. Pulmonary problems may also occur from lifelong exposure to smoking or environmental pollutants or due to repeated lung infections over the years. Because of these changes, the respiratory rate normally increases to compensate and maintain an adequate minute volume.

Cardiovascular System Changes

Many changes occur in the cardiovascular system of an older adult patient. Large arteries become less elastic, creating more pressure in the arteriole system during systole. This raises systolic blood pressure, leading, in turn, to a widened pulse pressure (the difference between systolic and diastolic blood pressure). Isolated systolic hypertension is the most common form of hypertension in the elderly. Many elderly patients rely on this elevated pressure, and overtreatment to "normal" pressures may lead to dizziness, syncope, and falls. Common cardiac problems among older adults include myocardial infarction, heart failure, dysrhythmias, aneurysms, and hypertension.

When obtaining a history from the older adult patient complaining of chest pain or discomfort, try to ascertain level of cardiovascular fitness. Older people who regularly engage in physical activity are able to maintain more efficient cardiac function.

Nervous System Changes

Assessment of the older adult for cognitive changes can be difficult without family members or friends to whom you can direct questions about the patient's history. If possible, determine the patient's baseline mental status, and then assess for any changes in behavior, thought processes, and mood. Ask family or friends about any recent changes in the patient's hygiene and food preparation habits.

Patients at End of Life

Hospice services include supportive social, emotional, and spiritual care for patients and their families at the end of life. Patients who are terminally ill or who have end-stage disease, such as those with advanced cancer, end-stage congestive heart failure, or advanced dementia, often receive palliative care (comfort care). Medical needs vary depending on the disease but typically center on pain and symptom management.

Patients who are terminally ill may have medical and legal documents such as advance directives or do-not-resuscitate (DNR) orders. The Physician Orders for Life Sustaining Treatment (POLST) document is particularly helpful for delineating specific parameters of care that should or should not be provided based on the patient's goals for care and discussion between the patient (or surrogate) and physician. Some states have specific DNR paperwork, thus health care clinicians should be familiar with specific policies, procedures, and regulations that apply to their patients and them.

Bariatric Patients

Obesity is related to many diseases and health risks, and obese patients can present challenges in care and transportation for EMS agencies and clinicians. Obesity is when a person has an excessive amount of weight relative to height. The CDC defines obesity in terms of body mass index (BMI), a height–weight ratio calculated as follows:

$$\textbf{BMI} = \textbf{Weight (kg)/[Height (m)]}^2$$

Overweight is defined as a BMI of 25 to 29.9 kg/m^2. A BMI over 30 kg/m^2 is classified as obese, and individuals with a BMI over 39 kg/m^2 are considered morbidly obese. Note that the use of BMI to measure obesity has become increasingly controversial, with many questioning labeling patients by these cutoffs and the application of BMI to taller individuals. In addition, it is an overly simplistic determination that does not correlate perfectly with health risks or obesity.

Obesity is a chronic disease and is a leading factor in preventable death in the United States (behind tobacco use). Patients with obesity are referred to as bariatric patients. Bariatric patients are at increased risk of diabetes, hypertension, coronary heart disease, dyslipidemia, stroke, liver disease, gallbladder disease, sleep apnea, respiratory disorders, osteoarthritis, and certain types of cancer; obese women are also at increased risk of infertility. Morbidly obese people may develop pulmonary hypertension and right-sided heart failure, known as cor pulmonale.

Moving a Bariatric Patient

Health care personnel must have policies and specialized equipment for moving and lifting bariatric patients because of the additional risk they pose to clinicians and the extra demands they place on staff and resources. Scene and situational assessment is especially important because a specially equipped bariatric ambulance and additional clinicians may be necessary (**Figure 1-19**). Ask the patient's weight, and call for assistance if necessary.

Both clinician and patient are at particularly high risk as the obese patient is being moved. Clinicians are subject to lifting-related injuries. Patients can be dropped or may roll off surfaces not designed to accommodate them, such as standard-sized backboards and some stretchers. High-capacity carrying sheets made of plastic with built-in side handles may be a good alternative to moving the patient on a stretcher.

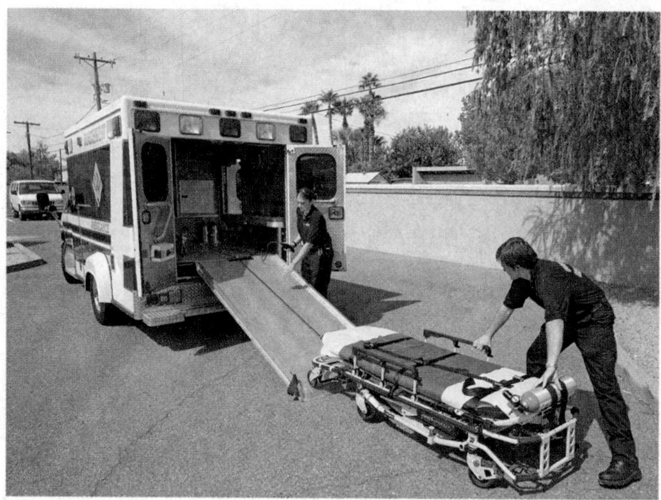

Figure 1-19 Some EMS systems have specialized equipment and vehicles to care for bariatric patients.

Specialized Equipment, Medical Devices, and Supplies

All EMS agencies and health care institutions must have the proper bariatric equipment and supplies needed to care for obese patients, such as extra-large blood pressure cuffs; long-length needles for intramuscular injections or needle decompression; large cervical collars; extra-long straps and taping supplies; and large gowns, sheets, and blankets.

Understanding Sex versus Gender

Gender is defined as an internal sense of how someone identifies and refers to the constant ongoing social construction of what is considered "feminine" and "masculine" based on sociocultural norms about women and men and the interactions between them. Specifically, **gender identity** refers to a person's internal sense of being a man, a woman, or something else; **gender expression** refers to the way a person communicates gender identity to the outside world through behavior/mannerisms, clothing, hairstyles, voice, and/or body characteristics. **Sex** refers to the biological characteristics a person was born with or assigned at birth, such as anatomy and physiology with reproductive organs, chromosomes, and hormones. Thus, sex is a biological construct, and gender is a social construct based on societal and cultural-bound

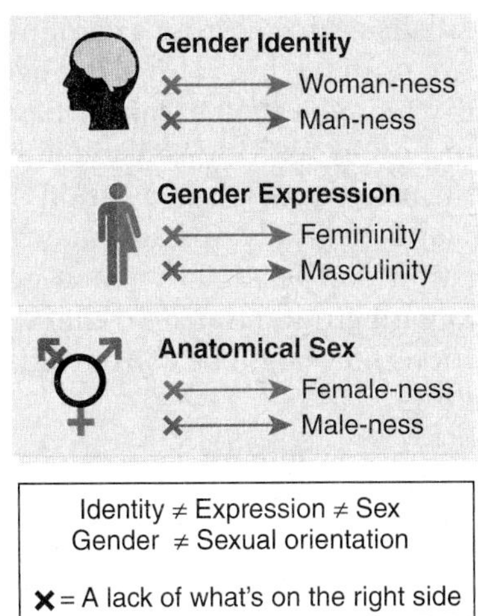

Figure 1-20 Sex is a biological construct. Gender is a social construct based on societal and cultural roles of men and women.

conventions, roles, and behaviors for, as well as relations between and among, women and men and boys and girls (**Figure 1-20**).

Biases can be generated based on both sex and gender and often occur simultaneously. They arise from either assuming sameness and/or equity between the sexes when there are genuine differences in anatomy, physiology, pathophysiology, course, or response to treatment, or from assuming that differences exist when they actually do not. It is important to understand, however, that both sex and gender exist on spectrums. Human sex development is naturally diverse with many variations of possible genitalia, hormones, internal anatomy, and/or chromosomes. The umbrella term *intersex* is used to describe a variety of naturally occurring clinical situations in which a person is born with reproductive anatomy or sex traits that do not fit binary medical definitions of "female" or "male." For example, some intersex people may be born with both ovarian and testicular tissues along with having combinations of chromosomes. Traditionally, a child born with two X chromosomes is determined to be female and a child born with one X and one Y chromosome is determined to be male. Some patients, however, may be born an extra copy of the X chromosome (XXY), as in those with Klinefelter syndrome, and will not have a traditional male or female physical appearance. It is estimated that about 1.7% of the U.S. population has an intersex trait and approximately 0.5% have clinically identifiable sexual or reproductive variations.

Transgender, or "trans," is an umbrella term for persons whose gender identity, gender expression, or behavior does not conform to that typically associated with the sex to which they were assigned at birth. When caring for a transgender patient, ask if they have undergone any gender-affirming treatments (e.g., hormone therapy, surgery, and/or other means to make their bodies as congruent as possible with their gender identities), as these changes affect medical decision making regarding certain diagnoses and treatments. It is also essential to inquire about and use the patient's preferred pronouns to help build rapport.

The dichotomy (or division) of sex and gender may lead to issues when addressing patients because both sex and gender are vital to understanding a patient's health concerns. For example, in the prehospital setting, a clinician may be dispatched to a male with severe abdominal pain. However, the patient could be a transman who still has female reproductive organs that could lead to life-threatening conditions such as a ruptured ectopic pregnancy. Thus, a gender-inclusive perspective in medicine consists of life conditions, lifestyles, and positions in society of men and women; societal expectations about "femininity" and "masculinity"; and biological concepts. In addition, aspects of gender may differ across various cultures. This perspective is important in professional encounters and relationships as well as when theorizing about women and men.

Clinical Assessment Considerations

To date, extensive literature demonstrates gender differences in medicine and medical emergencies. To ensure optimal effectiveness, EMS clinicians should understand the implications of sex and gender differences on health, societal roles, lifestyle, and well-being.

When caring for persons in the prehospital setting, clinicians should recognize the intrinsic power differential between the clinician and patient. This structural imbalance is often compounded by the effects of gender diversity and gender expression. It is best overcome by a clinician's early actions to build trust and rapport with the patient. When speaking to patients, particularly when the sex and/or gender of the patient is discordant from the clinician's, one can display sensitivity through the use of language that minimizes gender stereotypes. Clinicians can also maintain patient dignity by explaining their role and actions in appropriate terms as often as able and utilizing gowns and sheets to keep patients covered when performing procedures. Additionally, utilizing effective communication and validating patient experiences with empathy and self-disclosure facilitates both the patient and clinician experience.

Clinicians must be able to perform a sex-specific and gender-appropriate history and physical examination. This includes asking patients their name and preferred pronouns in addition to asking "What sex were you assigned at birth?" and "How would you describe your gender identity?" These questions should be asked as naturally as "Are you sexually active?" However, one should not request details of the patient's sexual history or sexual preferences when it is not clinically indicated.

In addition to obtaining a history of present illness, clinicians should place similar emphasis on reviewing a patient's medication list, recent EMS encounters, and inquiring about recent changes in health or recent medical procedures. For example, hormonal use as contraception or as therapy during perimenopause affects an individual's risk for thromboembolic disease—this treatment may not be disclosed as a medication unless it is directly asked. Similarly, when caring for transgender patients, it is important to consider whether an individual is taking exogenous hormones to help align their body with their identity. Obtaining a thorough history could include inquiring about gender-affirming surgery, but this information will rarely impact the prehospital examination and assessment. However, a history of nonsurgical practices such as tucking (manually displacing the testes and penis) and chest binding have clinical implications and may impact the differential diagnosis of acute disease in transgender individuals. Clinicians should be prepared to educate patients and explain why they are obtaining this information when patients express concern about "irrelevant" or "intrusive" questions.

When caring for a transgender individual and considering a clinical impression and treatment plan, clinicians should consider the following questions:

- How would this presentation be different if the patient's sex/gender were different?
- How would the treatment be different if the patient were male/female?
- How would the evaluation be different if the clinician were male/female?
- How would the outcome be different if the patient's sex/gender were different?

When developing a treatment plan and preparing for clinician handoff at the receiving facility, clinicians must consider their own gender bias and the differential impact of gender on care within health care systems. The latter is especially pertinent when caring for transgender and gender-diverse patients. Utilizing a patient's preferred name and pronouns during report and patient handoff helps to build rapport and establish trust for not only the prehospital clinician but also the receiving clinician.

Special Transport Considerations

Air Transport

Depending on the patient's location and condition and proximity to the appropriate receiving facility, some patients might be best transported directly by air. Interfacility transfers, such as from a community hospital to a tertiary care hospital, may also occur by air. Helicopters and fixed-wing aircraft (airplanes) have been used for patient transport by both civilian and military medical systems almost since the dawn of aviation. Patients who are critically ill and medically unstable may be considered for helicopter transport, especially when definitive care will be delayed with ground transport times. Examples of medical conditions that might be considered for air transport are as follows:

- Bleeding from or imminent rupture of an aortic aneurysm
- Intracranial bleeding
- Acute (time-dependent for treatment) ischemic stroke
- Severe hypothermia and hyperthermia
- STEMI and other cardiac conditions requiring immediate intervention
- Status asthmaticus
- Status epilepticus
- Major trauma

Some patients may have time-dependent transport needs or require more advanced care that can be delivered by an air team. Therefore, each EMS clinician should be familiar with local ground and air transport options. The decision to transport a patient by air has both advantages and drawbacks (Table 1-7). Air transport allows the patient to be rescued in a remote area if necessary, transported quickly, and transferred rapidly to a specialty unit. In addition, specialized personnel (critical care) or supplies (e.g., antivenin, blood products) can often be delivered more quickly via aircraft. However, flying may be restricted by bad weather, and aircraft have load restrictions limiting the number and weight of patients who can be transported. These factors will be taken into consideration when consulting the air medical program. EMS clinicians should know local helicopter and fixed-wing safety requirements and communication procedures.

Flight Physiology

The prehospital clinician—in many instances the paramedic—must select the most suitable mode of transportation for patients based on their condition; the specialty care offered at the receiving facility; and the safest, most efficient means available by which to move them. Likewise, in-hospital clinicians use similar criteria to determine whether to transfer a patient by air or ground.

If air medical transport is thought to be in the best clinical interest of the patient, you must prepare the patient for transport. Although the transport crew is responsible for the patient's safety during the flight, proper preflight preparation is the responsibility of the prehospital or in-hospital clinician, who must be aware of factors that affect the patient during flight. For example, you

Table 1-7 Advantages and Disadvantages of Air Medical Transport

Advantages
▪ Can provide critical care equipment, medications, and clinician expertise that are not otherwise available to the patient during transport ▪ May provide quicker access to time-sensitive treatments and interventions ▪ Can provide access to and enable extrication of patients from austere environments that may not be accessible by ground EMS agencies
Disadvantages
▪ Weather restrictions ▪ Maximum weight capacity ▪ Fuel limitations ▪ Agitated or combative patients present safety risks ▪ Must provide care in confined space ▪ "Helicopter shopping" ▪ Higher cost of operation than ambulance

Data from Lyng JW, Braithwaite S, Abraham H, et al. Appropriate air medical services utilization and recommendations for integration of air medical services resources into the EMS system of care: a joint position statement and resource document of NAEMSP, ACEP, and AMPA. Prehosp Emerg Care. 2021;25(6):854-873.

should understand how factors such as vertigo (dizziness), changes in temperature and barometric pressure, gravity, and spatial disorientation might affect the patient.

Putting It All Together

A systematic, thorough, efficient patient assessment process is the backbone of effectively managing patients with medical or traumatic emergencies. The AMLS Assessment Pathway is built on the assumption that clinicians already have a broad understanding of human anatomy, physiology, pathophysiology, and epidemiology to complement the assessment and clinical management processes. Most AMLS clinicians also have an understanding of primary and secondary surveys used in patient assessment by EMS clinicians, but the AMLS Assessment Pathway seeks to expand a learner's clinical reasoning, therapeutic communication, and clinical decision-making skills. This allows clinicians to integrate historical information, physical exam findings, and the results of diagnostic assessments to develop and refine differential diagnoses and arrive at a working diagnosis or diagnoses. Implementation of appropriate treatment modalities hinges on the accuracy of this assessment information.

Initial patient presentations are often subtle—your judgment is the key to timely, effective intervention. Most of the assessment information, especially in patients with emergent presentations, is obtained during history taking. When patients are poor historians, you must use your senses and let your experience guide your decisions.

Initial observations begin with the dispatch information or a prehospital radio report. A scene or situation assessment gives you a preview of the patient's condition even before any direct interaction takes place. All scenes or situations, whether prehospital or in-hospital, should be evaluated for safety. Home environments should be assessed for medical devices, environmental issues, and indications of chronic disease processes. Once the area is deemed safe, clinicians should note the patient's affect and body position, breath sounds and respiratory pattern, color, odor, and other physical characteristics. Any life threats must be addressed immediately. Proceed to the primary survey to identify and manage life threats relevant to airway, breathing, circulation, or perfusion. This assessment, while finished in a matter of seconds, should be systematic and thorough to identify any emergent conditions for which intervention is needed. Determine an initial impression, including how sick the patient is and whether the patient is likely to deteriorate. If deterioration seems imminent, determine which body systems might be affected and addressed.

History taking is then performed. Historical information is obtained by soliciting information about the present illness (OPQRST) and past medical history (SAMPLER). During the secondary survey, the clinician applies clinical reasoning to the patient's initial presentation. Vital signs, pain assessment, and a physical exam help rule in or rule out differential diagnoses to determine a working diagnosis. Diagnostic information is obtained and interpreted from pulse oximetry devices, blood glucose meters, laboratory tests as available, 3- or 12-lead ECG monitoring, and capnography to eliminate or confirm diagnoses.

A focused physical exam should be performed on patients with localized complaints or nonemergent presentations. A full-body (head-to-toe) physical exam is performed on patients with altered mental status or potential trauma if on-scene and transport time allow.

Communication, assessment, and management barriers can be encountered in patients with special challenges, such as bariatric patients, older adults, and obstetric patients. Transport decisions take into consideration the patient's condition but must also include factors such as weather, maximum aircraft load capacity, capabilities of the receiving hospital, and distance of the most appropriate facility.

Health care clinicians at all levels and scopes of practice work as a team to apply the AMLS Assessment Pathway to provide comprehensive assessment and management of patients experiencing medical emergencies. The AMLS Assessment Pathway is a dynamic and ongoing assessment process in which conclusions are continually revised as more information about the patient's history and current status becomes available. The process promotes teamwork for efficient and accurate patient assessment and care from dispatch to delivery at the receiving facility.

SCENARIO SOLUTION

- The clinicians should investigate for congestive heart failure, bowel impaction, stroke, dehydration and nutrition concerns, head injury or bruising from falls or abuse, and STEMI or cardiac rhythm changes.
- Assessment should include a thorough OPQRST and SAMPLER exam to note current status and any changes since last week's complaints, as well as a neurologic exam to include motor/sensory and pupil status. A focused physical exam should evaluate pulmonary or systemic edema. Auscultation of breath, heart, and bowel sounds should be performed. Diagnostic evaluation of blood glucose, pulse oximetry, ECG, and waveform capnography should be performed.
- Reassessment en route to the receiving facility is essential to determine if the patient's condition is stable or deteriorating, despite interventions.
- Several communication barriers may inhibit an efficient assessment. The patient may have hearing deficits or a short attention span due to fatigue and feelings of frustration. This requires the clinicians to use closed-ended questions and actively listen to what the patient and daughter state. Assistive devices may indicate inability to care for self. This patient may not be an accurate historian, so an efficient and thorough history and physical assessment are necessary to determine if this patient's presentation is life threatening. At this time, the patient's condition appears to be a potential life threat.

The clinicians should be concerned about the patient's condition rapidly deteriorating; therefore, an organized, systematic approach to assessment and management is essential. Multiple underlying diagnoses in this patient are a concern due to the decrease in efficiency of all body systems in the elderly. Changes in metabolic rates, reduction in blood vessel elasticity, osteoarthritis, slowed reflexes, and diminished neurotransmitter activity all contribute to diminished efficiency of body systems in the elderly. Respiratory, cardiovascular, and neurologic assessments are key to determining differential diagnoses and ultimately a working diagnosis. The AMLS Assessment Pathway, although dynamic and flexible, can provide a tool for systematic and comprehensive assessments in patients with challenging medical presentations.

SUMMARY

- The AMLS Assessment Pathway is a dependable framework that allows for early recognition and management of a variety of medical emergencies with a goal of improved patient outcome.
- The patient's history, physical exam, risk factors, chief complaint, and cardinal presentation help suggest possible differential diagnoses.
- Therapeutic communication skills, keen clinical reasoning abilities, and expert clinical decision making are the foundation for the AMLS assessment.
- Clinicians more accurately diagnose and care for patients when they recognize and attempt to eliminate the effect of their extrinsic and intrinsic biases in caring for patients related to gender, race, socioeconomic status, and other biases.
- Patient assessment and management can be hindered by social, language, behavioral, or psychological barriers.
- Effective clinical reasoning requires gathering and organizing relevant historical and diagnostic information, filtering out irrelevant or extraneous information, and reflecting on similar experiences to efficiently determine working diagnoses and management priorities.
- Clinical reasoning is a bridge between historical information and diagnostic test results, allowing the provider to draw inferences about

underlying etiologies to formulate differential diagnoses.
- Barriers for efficient assessment and management of patient presentations involve the level of medical knowledge and experience and scope of practice of the health care provider.
- The primary survey consists of identifying and managing life-threatening medical emergencies related to the patient's level of consciousness, as well as hemorrhage, airway, breathing, circulatory, and perfusion status.
- An emergent patient is one who is hemodynamically unstable and "sick," with a decreased level of consciousness, signs and symptoms of shock, severe pain, and difficulty breathing.
- The clinician's senses can contribute and enhance information obtained from observation of the scene and the initial presentation of the patient.
- The physical exam can be a focused exam related to the chief complaint or initial presentation or a full-body head-to-toe exam.
- All health care clinicians should be familiar with the benefits and risks in transportation options for patients.

Key Terms

Advanced Medical Life Support (AMLS) Assessment Pathway A dependable framework to support the reduction of morbidity and mortality by using an assessment-based approach to determine a differential diagnosis and effectively manage a broad range of medical emergencies.

assessment-based patient management Utilizing the patient's cardinal presentation; historical, diagnostic, and physical exam findings; and one's own critical-thinking skills as a health care professional to diagnose and treat a patient.

bias A tendency, preference, or inclination (either known or unknown) toward or against something or someone that prevents objectivity.

blood pressure The tension exerted by blood on the arterial walls. Blood pressure is calculated using the following equation: Blood pressure = Flow × Resistance.

capillary refill Time for tissues to reperfuse after compression (e.g., nail beds, fingers, toes).

cardinal presentation The patient's primary presenting sign or symptom from the clinician's perspective; often this is similar to the patient's chief complaint, but it may be an objective finding such as unconsciousness or choking.

clinical decision making The ability to integrate assessment findings and test data with experience and evidence-based guidelines to make decisions regarding the most appropriate treatment.

clinical reasoning The combination of good judgment with clinical experience to make accurate diagnoses and initiate proper treatment. This process assumes the clinician has a strong foundation of clinical knowledge.

cognitive bias A systematic error in thinking that impacts how one interprets information from the environment and distorts judgment in favor of or against certain ideas, actions, or people.

differential diagnoses The possible causes of the patient's clinical condition.

gender The internal sense of how someone identifies in relation to the socially constructed roles and characteristics of men and women, rather than biological characteristics.

gender expression The way a person communicates gender identity to the outside world.

gender identity The personal sense of one's own gender.

pattern recognition A process of recognizing and classifying data based on past knowledge and experience.

pharmacokinetics The absorption, distribution, metabolism, and excretion of medications.

primary survey The process of initially assessing the airway, breathing, circulation, and disability status to identify and manage life-threatening conditions and establish priorities for further assessment, treatment, and transport.

pulse pressure The difference between the systolic and diastolic blood pressures; normal pulse pressure is 30 to 40 mm Hg.

secondary survey An in-depth systematic head-to-toe physical examination, including vital signs.

sex The biological characteristics a person was born with or assigned at birth, such as anatomy and physiology with reproductive organs, chromosomes, and hormones.

signs Objective evidence that a health care professional observes, feels, sees, hears, touches, or smells.

symptoms Subjective perceptions by patients indicating what they feel, such as nausea, or have experienced, such as a sensation of seeing flashing lights.

therapeutic communication A communication process in which the health care clinician uses effective communication skills to obtain information about the patient's condition, including the use of the four Es: engagement, empathy, education, and enlistment.

transgender Persons whose gender identity or gender expression does not conform to that typically associated with the sex to which they were assigned at birth.

working diagnosis The presumed cause of the patient's condition, arrived at by evaluating all assessment information thus far obtained while conducting further diagnostic testing to definitively diagnose the illness.

Bibliography

Aehlert B. *Paramedic Practice Today: Above and Beyond.* Mosby; 2009.

American Academy of Orthopaedic Surgeons, American College of Emergency Physicians, University of Maryland, Baltimore County. *Critical Care Transport*, 2nd ed. Jones & Bartlett Learning; 2018.

American Academy of Orthopaedic Surgeons. *Emergency Care and Transportation of the Sick and Injured*, 11th ed. Jones & Bartlett Learning; 2017.

American Academy of Orthopaedic Surgeons. *Nancy Caroline's Emergency Care in the Streets*, 8th ed. Jones & Bartlett Learning; 2018.

American Psychological Association. Answers to your questions about transgender people, gender identity, and gender expression. March 9, 2023. Updated June 6, 2023. https://www.apa.org/topics/lgbtq/transgender-people-gender-identity-gender-expression

Assessing your assessment. *JEMS.* January 23, 2008. https://www.jems.com/patient-care/assessing-your-assessment/

Centers for Disease Control and Prevention. III. *Precautions to Prevent Transmission of Infectious Agents: Guideline for Isolation Precautions: Preventing Transmission of Infectious Agents in Healthcare Settings.* 2007. https://www.cdc.gov/infectioncontrol/guidelines/isolation/precautions.html

Centers for Disease Control and Prevention and Healthcare Infection Control Practices Advisory Committee. *Guide to Infection Prevention for Outpatient Settings: Minimum Expectations for Safe Care.* Version 2.3. September 2016. Accessed October 19, 2023. https://www.cdc.gov/infectioncontrol/pdf/outpatient/guide.pdf

Colameco S, Becker LA, Simpson M. Sex bias in the assessment of patient complaints. *J Fam Pract.* 1983;16:1117–1121.

Croskerry P. From mindless to mindful practice—cognitive bias and clinical decision making. *N Engl J Med.* 2013; 368(26):2445–2448. doi:10.1056/NEJMp1303712

Donohue D. Medical triage for WMD incidents: An adaptation of daily triage. *JEMS.* 2008;33(5). http://www.jems.com/article/major-incidents/medical-triage-wmd-incidents-i

Gladwell M. *Blink: The Power of Thinking Without Thinking.* Little, Brown and Co; 2005.

Graveris D. How common is intersex: 2023 intersex population figures & facts. *SexualAlpha.* February 8, 2023. https://sexualalpha.com/how-common-is-intersex/

Hamilton G, Sanders A, Strange G, et al. *Emergency Medicine: An Approach to Clinical Problem-Solving*, 2nd ed. Saunders; 2003.

Healey C, Osler TM, Rogers FB, et al. Improving the Glasgow Coma Scale score: motor score alone is a better predictor. *J Trauma.* 2003;54(4):671–678.

Johnson RL, Sadosty AT, Weaver AL, Goyal DG. To sit or not to sit? *Ann Emerg Med.* 2008;51(2):188–193.e2. doi:10.1016/j.annemergmed.2007.04.024

Kahneman D. *Thinking Fast and Slow.* Farrar, Straus and Giroux; 2011.

Krieger N. Genders, sexes, and health: what are the connections—and why does it matter? *Int J Epidemiol.* 2003;32(4):652–657.

Kupas DF, Melnychuk EM, Young AJ. Glasgow Coma Scale motor component ("patient does not follow commands") performs similarly to total Glasgow Coma Scale in predicting severe injury in predicting severe injury in trauma patients. *Ann Emerg Med.* 2016;68(6):744–750.

Lyng JW, Braithwaite S, Abraham H, et al. Appropriate air medical services utilization and recommendations for integration of air medical services resources into the EMS system of care: a joint position statement and resource document of NAEMSP, ACEP, and AMPA. *Prehosp Emerg Care.* 2021;25(6):854–873.

Marx J, Hockberger R, Walls R, eds. *Rosen's Emergency Medicine: Concepts and Clinical Practice*, 5th ed. Mosby; 2002.

Mock K. Effective clinician–patient communication. *Physician's News Digest.* 2001. https://physiciansnews.com/2001/02/14/effective-clinician-patient-communication/

National EMS Information System (NEMSIS). 2021 NEMSIS National EMS Data Report. November 4, 2022. https://nemsis.org/2021-nemsis-national-ems-data-report/

National Highway Traffic Safety Administration. Drug and Human Performance Fact Sheets. July 2005. https://www.nhtsa.gov/sites/nhtsa.gov/files/809725-drugshumanperformfs.pdf

Occupational Safety and Health Administration. *General description and discussion of the levels of protection and protective gear, Standard 1910.120, App B.* https://www.osha.gov/laws-regs/regulations/standardnumber/1910/1910.120AppB

Occupational Safety and Health Administration. *Toxic and hazardous substances: Bloodborne pathogens, Standard 1910.1030.* https://www.osha.gov/laws-regs/regulations/standardnumber/1910/1910.1030

Ogden CL, Carroll MD, Kit BK, et al. Prevalence of childhood and adult obesity in the United States, 2011–2012. *JAMA.* 2014;311(8):806–814. doi:10.1001/jama.2014.732

O'Neill LB, Bhansali P, Bost JE, Chamberlain JM, Ottolini MC. "Sick or not sick?" A mixed methods study evaluating the rapid determination of illness severity in a pediatric emergency department. *Diagnosis (Berl).* 2021;9(2):207–215. doi:10.1515/dx-2021-0093

Pagana K, Pagana T. *Mosby's Diagnostic and Laboratory Test Reference.* Mosby; 1997.

Paramedic Association of Canada. *National Occupational Competency Profile for Paramedic Practitioners.* Paramedic Association of Canada; 2001.

Reisner SL, Keuroghlian AS, Potter J. Gender identity: terminology, demographics, and epidemiology. In: Keuroghlian AS, Potter J, Reisner SL. eds. *Transgender and Gender Diverse Health Care: The Fenway Guide.* McGraw Hill; 2022.

Risberg G, Johansson EE, Hamber K. A theoretical model for analyzing gender bias in medicine. *Int J Equity Health.* 2009;8:28.

Saposnik G, Redelmeier D, Ruff CC, et al. Cognitive biases associated with medical decisions: a systematic review. *BMC Med Inform Decis Mak.* 2016;16(1):138. doi:10.1186/s12911-016-0377-1

Segal ES. Maintaining communication in a time of uncertainty. *Arch Fam Med.* 1995;4(12):1066–1067.

Smith RC, Gardiner JC, Lyles JS, et al. Exploration of DSM-IV criteria in primary care patients with medically unexplained symptoms. *Psychosom Med.* 2005;67:123–129.

Swayden KJ, Anderson KK, Connelly LM, Moran JS, McMahon JK, Arnold PM. Effect of sitting vs. standing on perception of provider time at bedside: a pilot study. *Patient Ed Counsel.* 2012;86(2):166–171. doi:10.1016/j.pec.2011.05.024

United Nations. The 17 goals. https://sdgs.un.org/goals.

Urden L. *Priorities in Critical Care Nursing,* 2nd ed. Mosby; 1996.

U.S. Department of Transportation National Highway Traffic Safety Administration. *EMT-Paramedic National Standard Curriculum.* U.S. Department of Transportation National Highway Traffic Safety Administration; 1998.

U.S. Department of Transportation National Highway Traffic Safety Administration. *National EMS Education Standards, Draft 3.0.* U.S. Department of Transportation National Highway Traffic Safety Administration; 2008.

Villinez Z. What to know about gender bias in healthcare. Medical News Today. October 25, 2021. https://www.medicalnewstoday.com/articles/gender-bias-in-healthcare

Wiswell J, Tsao K, Bellolio MF, Hess EP, Cabrera D. "Sick" or "not-sick": accuracy of System 1 diagnostic reasoning for the prediction of disposition and acuity in patients presenting to an academic ED. *Am J Emerg Med.* 2013;31(10):1448–1452. doi:10.1016/j.ajem.2013.07.018

Woolever D. The art and science of clinical decision making. *Fam Prac Manag.* 2008;15(5):31.

CHAPTER 2

Clinical Approach to Pharmacology

Chapter Editors
Mark Warth, BHS, NRP
E. Stein Bronsky, MD

Pharmacology is the study of interactions between substances and living organisms. The etymology of pharmacy, *pharmikeia*, predates the Greek and is loosely translated as the use of drugs or potions. This term was later adapted in the late 1600s to *pharmaco*, or pharmacology in modern verbiage. Around the 17th century, King James I created an independent pharmacist association in England, leading to the development of apothecaries, where specially trained individuals both dispensed remedies and offered advice, paving the way for modern-day pharmacists. In the 19th century, organic synthetic chemistry was created by a scientist named Friedrich Wohler, laying a foundation for the practice of pharmacology.

What does all this mean in the world of emergency medical services (EMS) medicine? Simply put, the understanding and use of medications have been described throughout history to improve pharmacologic sciences, advance scientific research, and develop new drugs in medicine, all in an effort to positively influence the health of patients. In this chapter, we discuss several foundational terms and principles that the health care clinician should appreciate for the successful understanding, management, and administration of medications. The framework of this chapter is not intended to be a traditional annex listing of medications, dosages, and side effects, but rather is organized with the goal of offering EMS clinicians a vantage point from which to critically process key concepts related to what medications are, how they interact with the human body, when and how to appropriately administer them, and how to do so with a safe and realistic approach. After reading this chapter, EMS clinicians should be able to juxtapose job-specific medications against the general concepts discussed here.

LEARNING OBJECTIVES

At the conclusion of this chapter, you will be able to:

- Identify the benefits of medication safety practice.
- Recognize the impact of medication errors.
- Describe a culture of safety.
- Define pharmacokinetics and pharmacodynamics.
- Discuss special considerations related to controlled substances, pregnancy, geriatrics, and weight-based dosing.
- Identify priorities in the face of medication shortages.

Philosophy

Pharmacology

Traditionally, an introduction to **pharmacology** lists specific definitions of key terms and analyzes each component of the pharmacologic process in detail. In this chapter, however, we will first discuss the philosophical framework encompassing medication administration. This can be summed up by four main ideologies: clinical decision making, benefit–risk analysis, cost-feasibility analysis, and professional responsibility. Medications are like words: When used in the right situation or environment, they can prove beneficial, but if administered in the wrong situation, they can be harmful. Either way, it is important to consider that drugs can have lasting effects and, most of the time, are best delivered in moderation. EMS systems must also consider the cost and feasibility of adding medications to their formulary. Such costs include not only the price of the medication, but also the costs to train EMS clinicians, properly store and carry medications, and replace expired medications if used infrequently. For many EMS medications, an agency has no way to directly charge for medications used on a patient. *Primum non nocere* is a Latin expression that means "first, do no harm." It is the *professional responsibility* of the health care clinician to be grounded in beneficence and to have a sound foundational understanding of the environment, history of the present illness, and available medications.

Using this information helps with clinical reasoning, judgment, and overall clinical decision making. In the end, it is simply about benefit–risk analysis. To administer the appropriate medication, a clinician has to weigh the potential benefits and harms, including any potential downstream effects. This is where terms such as **indications**, contraindications, untoward effects, relative precautions, adverse reactions, and special considerations come into play. Regarding pharmacologic philosophy, it is crucial for the clinician to have a working knowledge of these terms to ensure the safety and appropriateness of any medication administered.

Culture of Safety

For years, the medical community at all levels has been trying to adopt or utilize rules to prevent medication errors. These rules quickly morphed into the 6 Rights, which refer to the right patient, right drug, right dose, right route, right time, and right documentation as key components of safe medication administration (**Rapid Recall Box 2-1**). Over time, the 6 Rights have been extended to include three more "rights": right reason, right drug formulation, and right line attachment.

RAPID RECALL BOX 2-1

The 6 Rights

- Right patient
- Right drug
- Right dose
- Right route
- Right time
- Right documentation

Plus 3

- Right reason
- Right drug formulation
- Right line attachment

Unfortunately, the 6 Rights do not mitigate all of the issues faced by EMS clinicians and may actually play into the hands of poor professional practice enhanced by **normalization of deviance**. Normalization of deviance occurs when improper practice or standards gradually become tolerable and accepted, resulting in repeated deviant behavior (as long as disastrous results do not occur) that then becomes the procedural norm. In short, the 6 Rights focus on the individual's practice instead of human factors or system-related flaws. According to the vice president of the Institute for Safe Medication Practices, Judy Smetzer, the "rights" are general goals of medication safety practice that do not offer practical guidance on how to achieve them and thus inadequately safeguard against errors. To mitigate medication errors as much as possible, it may be more constructive to discover the common pitfalls and pathways to these errors by evaluating human imperfections and system-related operational flaws that set clinicians up for failure. No clinician intentionally sets out to make errors in medication administration, yet it is a universal constant that these errors occur. Solely blaming the clinician for the errors may lead to overlooking potential system flaws that can be changed to set up clinicians for greater success.

The administration of medications might seem simple, but in actuality it is a fairly complex process. It is the professional responsibility of the clinician to evaluate the situation to ensure overall safe delivery of a beneficial, yet still potentially dangerous, administration of a medication. EMS clinicians have limited available space to carry medications, and every additional medication carried adds to the risk of medication error due to accidentally selecting the wrong medication. The administration procedure itself can range from 10 to 20 steps, depending on the drug. If managing all of these elements were not difficult enough, the clinician must be aware of basic human nature, which can include bias, amplification of distractions, and the creation of shortcuts, all of which can lead to critical errors. In the hospital or prehospital environment, this same human nature can create other challenges adding to the difficulty of safe administrative practice, including, but not limited to, poor lighting, poor communication, difficult environment, inadequate staffing, long hours, ever-changing **medication concentrations**, a technology-enriched environment contributing to alarm/alert fatigue, frequent distractions, carrying multiple medications in a relatively small EMS response bag, and ambiguous drug labels. Combine those factors with normalization of deviance, and one can easily see the potential for disaster. In other words, this is where the mantras "to err is human" and "no harm, no foul" collide, creating poor professional practice, which can be the springboard for sustained errors.

In the United States, more than 1.5 million annual medication errors occur per year, leading to between

7,000 and 9,000 deaths and more than $3 billion of additional health care costs. If the average health care clinician was asked to define "medication error," undoubtedly the majority of responses would revolve around a failure involving one of the 6 Rights. The U.S. Food and Drug Administration (FDA) defines a medication error as "any preventable event that may cause or lead to inappropriate medication use or patient harm while the medication is in the control of a healthcare professional, patient, or consumer." Another way to state this definition is that a medication error is the possible preventable harm occurring from the misadministration of a medication. Two words in these definitions that should be emphasized are *may* and *possible*. It is important to remember that completed medication administration itself does not have to cause harm to be deemed a medication error; near misses are just as critical to identify.

Look-alike or sound-alike medication names are one factor that increases the risk of medication errors. The Institute for Safe Medical Practices (ISMP) has a goal of reducing medication errors in all settings and maintains a list of mixed case (sometimes called "Tall Man") lettering recommendations for medication names. The capitalization of parts of the medication name in the mixed case scheme places emphasis on certain parts of the name to avoid mix-ups with similarly spelled medications. Some of the medications used in the EMS setting can be confused when read in protocols. Examples of these medication names include DOBUTamine and DOPamine. To emphasize the mixed case recommendations, they will be used throughout this text in tables, charts, and lists when referencing applicable medication names. Table 2-1 is a selected list of commonly used medications for which mixed case lettering recommendations have been made.

Table 2-1 Selected Commonly Used EMS Medications with Look-Alike Names and Recommended Mixed Case (Tall Man) Lettering

acetaZOLAMIDE
BUPivacaine
carBAMazepine
ceFAZolin
cloNIDine
dexAMETHasone
diazePAM
dilTIAZem
diphenhydrAMINE
DOBUTamine
DOPamine
droPERidol
EPINEPHrine
fentaNYL
hydrALAZINE
hydroCLOROthiazide
HYDROmorphone
levETIRAcetam
LORazepam
methylPREDNISolone
niCARdipine
OLANZapine
oxyCODONE
PHYSostigmine
prednisoLONE
predniSONE
raNITIdine
risperiDONE
SUMAtriptan

Data from Institute for Safe Medication Practices. List of confused drug names. July 26, 2023. https://www.ismp.org/recommendations/confused-drug-names-list

How do health care professionals improve the safety of medication administration? They must buy into a **culture of safety**—a concept defined by the American Nurses Association as the "core values and behaviors resulting from a collective and continuous commitment by organizational leadership, managers, and health care workers to emphasize safety over competing goals." In a sense, a culture of safety is the attitude that "we are all in it together to ensure patient safety." Leadership must then work to establish a system of just culture; this approach to workplace safety assumes that humans, despite their best intentions to do the right thing, will inevitably make errors. The just culture ideology, when combined with a robust quality improvement program promoting accurate, honest reporting, can limit errors and should focus on identifying any errors' root causes. Clinicians must feel safe when reporting an error, which will in turn increase their personal responsibility to report a completed error or near miss. Overall, a culture of safety makes it easier to instill the "duty to report" ideology in all personnel so that individual and/or system failures are found and alleviated much sooner.

Another aspect of laying the groundwork for a culture of safety is self-reporting. Self-reporting is critical to system improvements and ought to be highly encouraged; it should *not* be used as a pathway to punitive measures. Unfortunately, health care clinicians who commit errors often fear potential malpractice lawsuits, discipline, career-ending repercussions, embarrassment, and/or lack of institutional support, all of which contribute to a culture of blame and punishment. This perception of personal risk, combined with an inadequate definition of medication errors, can lead individuals to commit acts of omission—that is, concealing an error rather than disclosing it. Through the development of a safe self-reporting environment, it becomes easier for organizational leaders to gather constructive information for the continued safe administration of medications—not just for mistakes already identified, but for the many more near misses that might have previously gone unidentified due to clinicians' fears about self-reporting.

When an error is identified or reported, a question that always comes up shortly afterward is, "Does the patient have a moral, ethical, and/or legal right to know?" This question is very difficult to answer, as it depends on the system in which the clinician operates. EMS agencies should develop processes to guide how errors should be disclosed to leadership; how the agency leadership and medical director will investigate the error; and the process for how, who, and when any errors are disclosed to the patient. The creation or implementation of error disclosure policies emphasizing honest, open communication without blaming tends to benefit everyone through the reduction of unscripted individual responses (or lack thereof), promoting an open disclosure culture that is, once again, an organizational culture and responsibility.

An additional component of a culture of safety revolves around the physical ability to administer a medication. If adhering to the 6 Rights fails to produce the desired outcomes, is there a better way? The short answer is yes. Because mnemonics help individuals learn, one possibility is the use of the mnemonic *SAD*, because that is how we feel afterward if a mistake occurs (**Rapid Recall Box 2-2**). First, **S**low down; never rush toward an error. By slowing down, the clinician can engage in critical thinking rather than relying on muscle memory, thereby avoiding the autopilot mentality. This forces the clinician to maintain an elevated situational awareness, looking for potential errors. Next, **A**void distractions, which include anything that disrupts, disturbs, or diverts the clinician's focus from the task at hand. Several studies have revealed distractions, especially early in a task, can substantially increase mistakes. Focusing on the immediate task, while always maintaining situational awareness, will help clinicians avoid potential errors. Lastly, institute an independent **D**ouble-check system. This might seem counterproductive in a world of hospital and prehospital clinicians, but it helps assist with the first element of SAD, which is to slow down. Double-checking involves two clinicians separately checking each component of the administration process, from dose to route to appropriateness of the drug. Performing these checks independently highlights the reality that two people are unlikely to make the same mistake, and it also avoids any bias. Studies have demonstrated that when performed properly, double-checking can diminish errors by as much as 99%. The key of any double-check system is to be consistent, utilize standardized resources and protocols, and fight the potential for the process to become mundane. If logistics prevent the independent double-check, then use of other resources such as quick-reference guides can be beneficial.

RAPID RECALL BOX 2-2

SAD

Slow down.
Avoid distractions.
Institute an independent **D**ouble-check system.

The last factor to help develop a culture of safety is proper education, stressing designated roles. Taking a professional approach to dedicated, regular, and environmentally realistic simulations including built-in errors can help improve health care clinician education, test the system, and potentially identify any early weaknesses. Taking a page from the airline industry, the health care industry has adapted simulated patient care from the idea of flight simulation, and has introduced crew resource management (CRM) as a means to reduce medical errors, including adverse drug events. CRM emphasizes closed-loop communication, defined roles, checklists, and organized decision making. Through a well-operated and -designed simulation incorporating the human element and highlighting assigned roles, medication errors can be reduced. Patient safety profits when CRM and simulation are a part of clinicians' regular practice and education.

Another teamwork-based approach to patient safety was developed jointly by the Agency for Research in Healthcare Quality (ARHQ) and the U.S. Department of Defense. TeamSTEPPS (Team Strategies and Tools to Enhance Performance and Patient Safety) teaches health care clinicians to use tools related to team leadership, communication, situation monitoring, and mutual support to change team knowledge, dynamics, and performance. The AHRQ provides a publicly available curriculum and training for instructors who deliver courses.

In the end, safety is the ultimate responsibility of all individuals involved with patient care. Having a clear and concise definition of medication errors, developing a culture of safety emphasizing the practice of a just culture, encouraging self-reporting, and implementing a standardized independent double-check system can prevent potential medication errors.

Foundational Knowledge

It is important not only to understand the philosophy behind why and how we medicate patients, but also to have a fundamental appreciation for how drugs interact with the human body. Two equally important concepts—pharmacokinetics and pharmacodynamics—must be understood to have the necessary appreciation of rudimentary human–drug interactions.

Pharmacokinetics

Pharmacokinetics refers to *what the body does to a drug*. It is an important concept to understand to customize a medication and dose for a patient. The principles of pharmacokinetics include drug absorption, distribution, metabolism, and elimination from the body. This is a very broad and nuanced topic, so for the purposes of this chapter we will focus on elements that are most important to the health care clinician.

Absorption, or how the body takes the specific drug into the circulation, includes elements at the discretion of the clinician, such as various formulations (e.g., immediate versus extended release) and route of administration (e.g., oral, sublingual, inhaled, parenteral, topical, intranasal [IN], or rectal). Parenteral refers to administration of a medication by a route that is outside of the enteral (or gastrointestinal [GI]) tract. In other words, parenteral describes medications that are given by the intramuscular (IM), subcutaneous, intravenous (IV), and intraosseous (IO) routes. For medications given orally, another factor in absorption is GI motility. Medications that slow down the GI tract, such as anticholinergic drugs (e.g., diphenhydramine) and opioids, can delay the absorption of drugs, especially in the setting of an overdose. Selecting the appropriate formulation and route to deliver the medication based on the patient's needs and the access routes available (e.g., IM versus IV) helps the clinician elicit the desired response in a timely manner.

Distribution of a medication has multiple components. It can be affected by a patient's perfusion to the site of action: Can the medication be transported to where it needs to act? Also, it is affected by body composition (e.g., patients with more adipose tissue can have accumulation of lipophilic medications in their fatty tissues), body and/or tissue pH compared to a drug's pH, and permeability of cellular membranes, which can create easy access or obstacles for a medication to reach the intended **receptors**. Knowledge of absorption and distribution properties will help a clinician predict the onset of action and magnitude of effect of a medication after its administration.

The body's **metabolism** breaks down a drug into either inactive components or active **metabolites**; the latter can cause an effect on the body. Many of the enzymes involved with drug metabolism are located in the liver and can be affected by liver disease or poor perfusion to the liver. In addition, metabolism can be affected by a patient's genetics or other medications, which can interact with the intended medication and can inhibit, induce, and/or accelerate its actions. Being aware of medication interactions and how one medication may influence the activity of another is an important consideration for clinicians.

The kidneys primarily carry out **elimination**—removal of the medication from the body. Because the kidneys excrete water-soluble drugs, metabolites, or other dispersible by-products broken down by the liver, this process can be affected by acute and chronic kidney disease. To a lesser extent, drugs can be eliminated through feces, and to an even lesser extent, alternative routes such as exhalation through the lungs, sweat, or tears. Knowledge of medication- and patient-specific factors affecting metabolism and elimination can help predict a drug's duration of action and whether the dose needs to be adjusted prior to administration. Applying these principles of pharmacokinetics helps the clinician select the most optimal medication, route, and dosage based on properties of the drug and factors unique to the clinician and the patient's circumstances.

Pharmacodynamics

Pharmacodynamics refers to *what the drug does to the body*. It is based on where and which receptors, enzymes, or other proteins a drug binds to and how the drug is modified in the body. A thorough understanding of a drug's mechanism of action and site of activity helps the clinician understand both the expected therapeutic response and potential adverse effects. A drug's pharmacodynamics can be modulated by a variety of factors, including genetics as well as certain physiologic disorders and medical conditions (e.g., hypo/hyperthyroidism, elderly patients, acidosis). For example, vasopressors such as EPINEPHrine can have decreased receptor binding (and thus decreased efficacy) in the setting of profound acidosis during a prolonged cardiac arrest. Again, it is important to keep the potential for drug interactions in mind. Knowing if and how the medications already in the body might alter the binding sites or the body's response to a medication enables the clinician to avoid compounding therapeutic effects, such as oversedation, and prevent adverse reactions. In conjunction with knowledge of pharmacokinetics, a clinician can incorporate the pharmacodynamics of a drug to predict a patient's response to a particular medication and dose.

Special Considerations

Many other considerations concerning medication categorization and administration are worthy of discussion: how controlled substances are categorized and managed; how and if medications may need to be modified in specific patient populations, including in pregnancy and in elderly patients; how to determine the best method of dosing medications using weight-based versus standardized dosing; issues of drug compatibility and mixing; and how to assess and manage potential drug shortages.

Controlled Substance Schedules

The Controlled Substances Act created the first list of federally controlled medications in 1970. Since then, this

Table 2-2 Medication Classifications: U.S. Drug Enforcement Agency Schedule

Schedule	Definition	Example Drugs
I	High abuse potential; most have no currently accepted medical use	Ecstasy, heroin, lysergic acid diethylamide (LSD), marijuana, methaqualone, and peyote
II	High abuse potential, including severe psychological or physical dependence	Amphetamines (e.g., methamphetamine, dextroamphetamine, methylphenidate) cocaine, fentaNYL, HYDROmorphone, methadone, morphine, oxyCODONE
III	Low to moderate potential for physical and psychological dependence	Codeine (< 90 mg per dose), ketamine, testosterone
IV	Low potential for abuse or dependence	ALPRAZolam, diazePAM, LORazepam, traMADol, zolpidem
V	Lowest potential for abuse or dependence	Atropine/diphenoxylate, cough preparations with < 200 mg codeine per 100 mL (e.g., Robitussin AC), pregabalin

Modified from United States Drug Enforcement Agency. Drug scheduling. July 10, 2018. Accessed September 28, 2023. https://www.dea.gov/drug-scheduling

list has been repeatedly modified and updated as additional medications have been determined to have abuse potential or dependence risk. Controlled substances encompass an array of medications having varying degrees of abuse or dependence potential for the user; they are also classified based on whether they have a currently acceptable medicinal use. The manufacture, distribution, and dispensing of controlled substances are regulated and enforced by the U.S. Drug Enforcement Agency. Drugs are categorized into schedules ranging from I to V, with a higher number indicating a lower risk of inducing dependence in the user (Table 2-2). Category I is unique in that it includes substances that do not currently have a medically approved use in the United States, although an increasing number of states now have medical marijuana programs for the clinical treatment of some diseases.

Clinicians in the prehospital and emergency settings need to have a firm understanding of the controlled medications to which they have access, as well as the rules and regulations for prescribing, dispensing, storing, and administering these medications, and documentation of their administration and waste. Health care professionals should remain vigilant for diversion of controlled substances by both patients and colleagues. In particular, EMS clinicians are at a disadvantage for monitoring for diversion. The original Controlled Substances Act did not specifically provide guidance on how EMS teams should handle, document, and monitor these drugs.

Some crews have to rely on rudimentary paper documentation to account for medication administration and waste. Fortunately, most electronic patient care records (ePCRs) facilitate record keeping for controlled substances. In a high-stress environment such as the prehospital and emergency scene, there is a risk for clinicians to divert either to self-medicate or for profit. Such diversion not only violates federal law, but also turns the individual into a liability and creates risks in terms of patient safety, their team members, and the individual's own health. A variety of publications and resources have recommended best practices for controlled substance monitoring in the prehospital and hospital settings. It is ultimately the responsibility of the individual agency to regularly evaluate and maintain the chain of custody, distribution, and protection of all scheduled medications.

Pregnancy

In 2015, the FDA created new drug labeling regulations for medication use in pregnancy through the Pregnancy and Lactation Labeling Rule. This initiative creates a narrative summary of the risks of medications in pregnancy and the supporting data, rather than relying on a strict letter category system. Drugs approved after June 2015 are required to use this new system, and drugs approved after June 30, 2001, are required to submit updated labeling. The FDA determined that the previous letter system (A, B, C, D, and X) did not accurately communicate the risk–benefit evidence and often was perceived as confusing or misinterpreted by clinicians. For reference, the previous labeling ranged from A, indicating no evidence of fetal risk from the drug in well-controlled animal and human studies, to X, indicating clear evidence of teratogenic harm from the drug that outweighed any possible benefit. Category C in the previous labeling indicated either there was no information on use in pregnancy or there were reported adverse effects in animal studies but no information in human studies. This ambiguity sometimes led clinicians to avoid this category of medications even when a Category C medication might have benefited a patient with a particular disease/condition if the suboptimal management of the disease/condition was a detriment to the patient or to fetal development. Table 2-3 shows the information that is now included under the *Pregnancy* subsection of a drug label.

This new labeling system is intended to help clinicians make more informed decisions based on the currently available research and reports. Pregnancy is a complex condition, and the clinician must weigh the complications from untreated disease or progression of a condition against the potential risk of an adverse outcome for fetal development, taking advantage of the available information on a medication to benefit patients as much as possible.

Many medications have limited adverse effects with one-time or short-term exposures. Other than drugs that have well-established teratogenicity, most medications in an emergency setting will have more benefit in improving a pregnant patient's condition than potential harm to the fetus. For example, a seizing pregnant patient may benefit from administration of a benzodiazepine, which will help halt the seizures and restore proper oxygenation to mother and fetus. However, benzodiazepines also carry a risk of premature birth and low birth weight, as well as the development of neonatal withdrawal symptoms (typically with frequent or continuous exposures). The clinician must quickly weigh the benefits of terminating the seizures with the potential risk of detrimental effects on the fetus from both the continuation of the seizures and the administration of a benzodiazepine.

Table 2-4 lists resources that provide quick but comprehensive summaries of medications and exposures and their associated fetal risks. Many are available as applications that can be downloaded to your mobile device for easy access.

Table 2-3 Medication Classifications for Pregnant Patients

Pregnancy Exposure Registry	If a registry for a pregnant person currently taking the drug is available, contact information for enrollment is included. Registry data are tracked for adverse outcomes with a particular medication, though submitting such data is a voluntary process.
Risk Summary	Includes a summary of available human, animal, and research data that describe the risk of adverse effects on fetal development when a drug is used during pregnancy. It also states if there are no risk data, and provides birth defect rates in the United States when no drug exposure occurred for comparison.
Clinical Considerations	If data are available, includes disease versus drug benefit–risk analysis, dose adjustments in pregnancy, maternal and fetal/neonatal reported adverse reactions, and effects on labor and delivery. It also can include effects of specific dosing, timing during pregnancy stages, and duration of exposure (e.g., one-time doses versus long-term use).
Data	Summarizes available human data and animal data.

Geriatric Considerations

Geriatric patients, typically defined as those 65 years of age and older, are at a higher risk for developing medication-related **side effects** and drug–drug interactions due to an increased number of comorbidities, which can lead to changes in their pharmacokinetics, and incidence of polypharmacy (taking multiple medications at a time). Additionally, this patient population tends to have decreased renal function, which places them at risk for drug accumulation if the doses of renally eliminated medications are not adjusted. Members of this already vulnerable population are at a higher risk for functional decline and readmission to the hospital and have a higher mortality risk following an emergency department admission. Older adult patients also have a lower threshold for tolerating medication errors or adverse effects if one occurs.

Table 2-4 Medication Risks to Fetuses

Resource[a]	How to Access	Fee/Availability	Features
Infant Risk Center	Call 1-806-352-2519 or www.infantrisk.com Applications: Professional: Infant Risk Center Health Care Mobile Consumer: MommyMeds	Call center: Free M–F, 0800–1700 CST	Texas Tech University Health Sciences Center with director Thomas Hale, PhD, RPh, a leading expert in pregnancy and lactation Based on information found in *Medications and Mothers' Milk* publication Accurate, up-to-date information on drugs and exposures
MotherToBaby	Call 1-866-626-6847 or text 1-855-999-3525	Free; varies by state but typically M–F, 0800–1700	Organization of teratology information specialists National call center routes to state-based center Evidence-based information on drugs and other exposures
REPROTOX	www.reprotox.org Application: Reprotox	Fee-based subscription, either individual, group, or institutional. Free for trainees	Nonprofit Toxicologists, geneticists, and reproductive specialists Quick overview of literature and animal/human studies Includes more than 5,000 drugs and exposures
LactMed	https://www.ncbi.nlm.nih.gov/books/NBK501922/ Application: LactMed	Free	Peer-reviewed, maintained by National Library of Medicine Focused on medications in lactation, risk, and alternatives
Lexi-Drugs[b]	https://www.wolterskluwercdi.com/lexicomp-online/ Application: Lexicomp	Fee-based subscription, either individual, group, or institutional	Short summaries within drug database on pregnancy risk factor and pregnancy considerations
Drug labels	Provided in medication box/container Database for drug labels: https://dailymed.nlm.nih.gov/dailymed	Free	FDA-labeled pregnancy summaries or pregnancy categories

[a]Modified from Temming LA, Cahill AG, Riley LE. Clinical management of medications in pregnancy and lactation. *Am J Obstet Gynecol.* 2016;214(6):698–702, Table 1. doi:10.1016/j.ajog.2016.01.187

[b]*Up-to-Date* (another clinical reference) and Lexicomp have merged. Lexi-Drugs can now be accessed through *Up-to-Date* by typing in the drug name either online or in the mobile application.

To help mitigate these risks, health care clinicians need to be cognizant of both potential medication-related adverse effects that might cause elderly patients to require care and treatment medications in the clinician's arsenal that might need to be adjusted or avoided in this population. For example, geriatric patients are at increased risk for medication-induced delirium caused by polypharmacy, overmedication (especially with

resulting in widespread and long-lasting drug shortages in the United States. The COVID-19 pandemic in 2020 is another example of how medication supply can drastically be affected. During the early days of the pandemic there was a fear that drug manufacturing would be severely impacted by China's shutdown of its facilities that produced raw materials used in such manufacturing. Surprisingly, the temporary halt of raw material manufacturing from China did not cause as large a disruption as initially feared. However, the worldwide ripples of the pandemic, along with associated multinational economic freezes, temporary as well as permanent production facility closures, workforce shortages, and ubiquitous multilevel supply chain disruptions, did (and continue to) play a large part in downstream drug supply shortages. Even in 2023, as the world was emerging from the pandemic, health care systems were experiencing the largest drug supply shortages ever seen.

Thus, it has never been as important for medical providers to look at alternatives when dealing with pharmacologic therapy as it is today. Shortages can adversely affect patient care by forcing substitution of safe and effective therapies with alternative treatments, compromising or delaying medical procedures, and causing medication errors. To effectively deliver patient care in this dynamic situation, health care clinicians must become comfortable in their understanding and utilization of drugs as an unstable variable in medical treatment and must adapt to this changing environment to provide some level of consistency in patient care. To best mitigate the untoward ramifications of ever-increasing drug shortages, it is paramount that educational emphasis is placed on the global understanding of why, how, and when specific types of drugs (and classifications) are used for various pathologies, rather than concentrating on the traditional model of learning about a specific drug for a specific indication. It is also critical that, when medication shortages occur, protocol modifications and appropriate education are implemented to allow for those alternative medications.

Establishing and Institutionalizing a Suite of Contingencies for Clinical Care

In 2012, the Institute of Medicine (IOM) of the National Academies (now called the National Academy of Medicine) created a framework called *Crisis Standards of Care: A Systems Framework for Catastrophic Disaster Response*. Among many other issues, the framework identifies a host of strategies to address medication shortages:

- Prepare: planning and training for emergency patient care and responses; anticipating potential resource shortfalls and possible adaptive strategies
- Substitute: using functionally equivalent equipment and supplies
- Conserve: placing restrictions on the use of therapies and interventions to preserve supplies
- Reuse: reusing equipment with appropriate cleaning, disinfection, or sterilization
- Reallocate: prioritizing of therapy to those patients who have the best chance of having a favorable outcome, who are most likely to benefit, or who require the least resource investment

EMS and other health care professionals must be prepared with alternative strategy plans should they face a drug shortage. This plan should serve as a reliable decision-support tool by clearly articulating the various options, indicating priorities, laying out the conditions under which they will be executed, and identifying other operational considerations (appropriate education and protocol modifications). One illustration of how this framework is translated to a real-world application can be extracted from the Association of State and Territorial Health Officials' Drug Shortage Mitigation Algorithm, shown in Table 2-5. This tool is designed to facilitate a structured approach to drug shortages. It illustrates one way to facilitate structured and informed decision making and action when a drug-shortage intervention needs to be initiated. The tool has been modified by adding the last column, "Strategy," to link the various decision points to the IOM's Crisis Standards of Care framework.

As mentioned previously, there are several potential avenues to help alleviate the burden created by drug shortages. Expanding expiration dates, utilizing compounded medications, shared resourcing, tiered utilization (priority given to selected patients with medical necessity), discontinued use of medical interventions with questionable utility, adjusting the dosage concentration and/or route of delivery, drug substitution, and medication sparing are all options as part of an organized action plan when faced with drug shortages. Each of these pathways has its distinct benefits, as well as potential disadvantages and challenges. All of these options must be accompanied by appropriate clinician education and agency and medical director approval.

Expanded Expiration Dates

There is a strong opinion that under proper conditions and if clinical circumstances dictated, using out-of-date drugs would be one potentially viable option for mitigating drug shortages, taking into account the effectiveness of the drug and the seriousness of the patient's condition, especially if the health care clinician was faced with the decision of using an expired drug versus no drug at all. Favorable data exist for many classes of drugs regarding stability and efficacy beyond expiration. This option can provide dosing consistency; provide assurance the drug would be readily available, thus avoiding delays in administration; and aid in reducing unnecessary waste of a limited resource.

Table 2-5 Medication Shortage Strategies

Drug Shortage Mitigation Algorithm (Prioritized by Patient Safety) Decision Point	Comment	Contingency	Strategy
1	Baseline SOP	None: Continue with current policies/procedures	Plan and prepare
2a	Does not require medication changes	Utilize expired medications	Adapt
2b	Does not require medication changes	Utilize compounded medications	Adapt
2c	Does not require medication changes	Discontinue use of medication for interventions with questionable utility	Conserve
3	Requires new dose calculations and training	Utilize the same drug with a different concentration	Substitute
4	Requires new dose calculations and training	Utilize the same drug given via a different route (oral versus IV)	Substitute
5	Requires new dose calculations and training	Utilize a different drug from the same class (midazolam versus diazePAM)	Substitute
6	Requires new dose calculations and training	Utilize a different drug from a different class (droPERidol versus ondansetron)	Substitute
7	Does not require medication changes	Stay in service without the medication (failed mitigation)	Transition to crisis care

IV, intravenous; SOP, standard operating procedure.

Traditionally, the FDA had no control over the factors leading to drug shortages and has had limited authority to assist in managing shortages. The FDA's role in the management of drug shortages has changed in recent years. The Food and Drug Administration Safety and Innovation Act (FDASIA), which was passed by Congress in 2012, provides the FDA with the authority to address the challenges posed by an increasingly global drug supply chain. Prior to FDASIA, manufacturers were not always required to notify the FDA of a potential drug shortage or disruption in supply. FDASIA broadens the scope of mandatory early notifications, which greatly improves the FDA's ability to help manage shortages. Recently, the FDA has been working closely with drug manufacturers to extend the expiration dates for many critical medications. Based on stability data provided by manufacturers and reviewed by the FDA, extended use dates are supported for specific drugs, allowing these medications to be used for longer periods to help mitigate supply issues. As more data become available, the lists of the drugs eligible for extended use dates can continue to expand.

However, if the FDA has not specifically made formal notification of expiration date extensions for specific drugs and manufacturing lots (control number), the original expiration date continues to apply. Use of expired medications should occur only with agency and medical director approval. In addition, if replacement products become available during the extension period, then the FDA expects the expired drugs to be replaced and properly disposed of as soon as possible. Some states and pharmacy boards specifically prohibit the extension of expiration dates, and some consider it to be a felony. Always be aware of your local jurisdiction's policies and procedures.

Shared Resourcing

Whenever possible, collaborative arrangements among health care entities should be established to create a system of medication sharing. Large health systems and EMS agency coalitions can often address drug shortages by shifting drug inventory among their sites and can operationally afford to shift medications to other agencies. Information regarding possible alternative therapies should also be shared among health care entities. There are some downsides to shared resourcing, including the added difficulty of tracking responsibility for and management of medications and supplies. Appropriate record keeping of medication tracking must occur.

Using Compounded Medications

Compounding refers to the practice of a licensed pharmacist making a particular medication by mixing together different ingredients when a specific dose or form of a medication is not being manufactured already or is not commercially available. The use of compounding pharmacies has potential benefits in offsetting drug shortages and is another means to increase drug availability. Compounding can create immediate availability of a product that is not commercially accessible. It is especially useful in meeting the individual medical needs of certain unique patient populations.

The regulations for compounding medications differ from those governing mass production of drugs, and usually result in fewer barriers and time constraints on drug accessibility while ensuring appropriate manufacturing, storage, and efficacy of the medication. Potential disadvantages of compounding medications include product safety and efficacy secondary to poorly compounded drug recipes or human errors in the compounding process (unlikely in appropriately licensed facilities); greater expense; a shorter shelf life, leading to potential wastage; and lack of local and governmental oversight. Health care clinicians can investigate the utilization of 503b-classified pharmacies (compounding pharmacies) to assist in alleviating medication shortages; hospital pharmacies may also have this capability.

Conservation

Conservation is an alternative option that addresses medication utilization, allowing for prudent management of a scarce resource with the goal of preserving preferred treatment for life-threatening situations or specific medical indications where treatment alternatives are limited or unavailable. Conservation can be accomplished by tiered utilization (priority given to selected patients with medical necessity), discontinuing use of medical treatments with debatable utility, adjusting drug dosage concentrations by titrating to effect, and changing the route of administration. Potential areas of concern associated with this approach include perceived treatment inequity, potentially subtherapeutic treatments, and the need to create a sound operational framework to support treatment decisions.

Substitution

Substitution is the act of identifying alternative in-class drugs or therapeutic equivalents from a different drug class. This option provides an alternative path for treatment when the preferred drug is not readily available or is being reserved for high-priority situations. It potentially allows for timely treatment and may also reduce inappropriate hoarding of first-choice medications during a shortage. Same-class drug substitution is preferable to using drugs from a different class because it minimizes differences in side-effect profiles and clinician education requirements. Drawbacks that must be seriously considered are a possible lack of health care clinician familiarity and professional competence with rarely or never before administered drugs, increasing the likelihood of medical errors and subsequent patient safety concerns. In addition, alternative drugs may not have obtained FDA approval for some indications (off-label use) or special patient populations. Medication substitution is a commonly used tool for mitigating drug shortages; therefore, it is imperative to create viable operational and clinical training in anticipation of this need.

Sparing

Sparing refers to the use of multidose vials of drugs to treat multiple patients. When faced with a shortage of a drug that comes in a single-use vial, consideration may be given to splitting the medication in multidose vials among multiple patients. Like some of the other options, this will result in a more robust drug-of-choice inventory and reduce medication wasting. Some of the challenges associated with this practice are the potential for product contamination and dosing errors, issues with medication tracking and diversion, and the need to establish guidelines and documentation for proper vial storage and usage once opened. In addition to EMS clinicians using multidose vials for multiple drug administrations (to be discouraged for multiple patients), hospital pharmacies and compounding pharmacies may be able to produce multiple unit-dose syringes or vials for single patient use from a single multidose vial.

Putting It All Together

Pharmacology is a complex subject and is a subspecialty unto itself. A basic understanding of pharmacology is essential for any health care clinician, and it plays a central role in medical care. Knowledge of pharmacology encompasses more than just memorizing a list of drugs, their indications, and dosages: It also includes the philosophy behind why, when, and how medications are administered; drug pharmacodynamics and pharmacokinetics; considerations for special patient populations; options for dosing and administration; concerns about drug–drug compatibility and interactions; and ways to adapt and safely overcome increasing drug shortages. All of these elements need to be taken into account as treatment decisions are made. Medication administration is a complex task that can be fraught with potential errors. It is best to nurture a system and culture that account for human error, promote disclosure of errors, and establish paradigms promoting system improvement and positioning clinicians for successful patient treatment.

Reinforcement of Learning

Case studies are a great way to apply text material to real-life patient encounters. As you read through the following case studies, try to imagine yourself as the clinician, immerse yourself in the scene, and navigate through the case with the goal of identifying the best pharmacologic approach to your patient care, while at the same time recognizing potential pitfalls and dangers related to medication administration.

Case Study: Pain Management

Prehospital: Dispatch for Abdominal Pain

Upon arrival at a single-story residence, you find a 36-year-old female in the front living room clutching her abdomen. She has a previous medical history of gestational diabetes and is currently 38 weeks pregnant with her third child. The patient states that she was in a car accident earlier today: She was the passenger in a small sedan that was rear-ended at approximately 30 mph. The chief complaint is 9/10 severe, nonradiating lower abdominal pain associated with nausea. She describes the pain as different from previous contractions; it is sharp and constant in nature. She denies vaginal bleeding or other discharge, and denies any other history or complaint.

Physical Findings

A gravid female is alert and oriented with slight anxiousness. The airway is open and patent, and the patient is able to answer all questions without distress. Her skin is pale and nondiaphoretic; she is able to ambulate without assistance or staggering gait and has full movement of extremities with good range of motion without restriction. The heart rate is in the 90s. Upon inspection of the abdomen, you see positive guarding and bruising just below the umbilicus, approximately 7 cm in width and 30 cm in length. No noted contractions, rigidity, or other trauma is found. Bowel sounds are present and active. Fetal heart tones are present at 160 beats per minute. No vaginal bleeding is described.

Vital Signs

- BP: 136/88
- HR: 95, regular
- SpO_2: 92% on room air
- RR: 18, shallow
- Lungs: Clear
- Mental status: Alert and oriented
- Temp: 36°C (96.8°F)

Discussion

The etiology of abdominal pain in any patient can be elusive. The addition of trauma and pregnancy makes the differential diagnosis even more extensive in this case. The history and physical examination can help narrow possible etiologies, but specific diagnostic testing, which can take time, may be needed to identify the exact pathology. Pain is an important consideration in patient assessment. In general, pain can easily be brushed aside or underprioritized, leading to undertreatment, especially in the presence of trauma. In fact, one study identified that trauma patients experienced more pain initially compared with medical patients. This knowledge can be applied to abdominal complaints of pain, as well as pregnancies. As a health care professional, it is important to realize that pain, no matter what the history or cause, is important to address and manage. Utilize the current history and presentation of the patient as a compass when choosing the most appropriate medication for pain management and try to avoid using these elements as an excuse to avoid pain management.

Medication Considerations

Various types of medications are used to treat pain acutely. Each medication has unique aspects of pharmacokinetics and pharmacodynamics. Each drug also has a unique set of adverse reactions. Several factors should be taken into account when choosing the right pain medication for any specific situation, including drug availability, drug class, mechanism of action, pharmacokinetics, pharmacodynamics, hemodynamic stability, and route of administration. Following are common therapies for pain management:

- **Acetaminophen (APAP**, from *N*-acetyl-para-aminophenol**):** This is a nonopioid analgesia option. Although its mechanism of action is not fully understood, APAP may provide pain relief through inhibition of the perception of pain through the central nervous system (CNS). It is available orally, rectally, and IV as a 15-minute infusion. The IV formulation may be beneficial in nauseated patients, may be used by EMS clinicians at intermediate scopes of practice who do not carry controlled substances, and may reduce the use of opioid analgesics in some systems. The oral formulation can start to have effects in less than 1 hour, while the IV formulation can start to have an effect as quickly as 10 minutes, with peak pain relief within 1 hour. Attention should be given to the total amount of APAP given to a patient, as high doses (> 4 g/day in healthy patients and > 2–3 g/day in patients with hepatic disease/cirrhosis) can create a toxic metabolite. Acetaminophen is safe for use in pregnancy and does not have any effects on the patient's hemodynamics.
- **Nonsteroidal anti-inflammatory drugs (NSAIDs):** NSAIDs are a nonopioid analgesia option that also possess anti-inflammatory properties. These agents act by decreasing the production of prostaglandins, which cause pain, fever, and inflammation; however, prostaglandins are also beneficial, as they protect the stomach from the effects of acid and support the clotting function of platelets. Therefore, some of the side effects of NSAIDs include platelet dysfunction and GI ulcers and/or bleeding. NSAIDs are available orally (e.g., ibuprofen, naproxen) as well as IV/IM (e.g., ketorolac). IV ketorolac has a more rapid effect in the ureteral spasms of biliary colic, but for other conditions, several studies have shown no difference between the use of oral NSAIDs and parenteral ketorolac. NSAIDs should be used with caution and/or in lower doses in patients with renal disease or decreased renal function (e.g., older patients), as they can cause kidney failure. These medications should generally be avoided in pregnancy due to the increased risk of miscarriage early in pregnancy and premature closure of the ductus arteriosus in the later stages of pregnancy. They do not have any effects on the patient's hemodynamics.
- **Opioids:** This group of analgesics works on a variety of receptors, including opioid and mu receptors, within the CNS to increase a patient's pain threshold, inhibit neural pain pathways, and decrease the perception of pain. All opioids are controlled substances, and run the risk of creating dependence or re-activating previous addictive tendencies in patients. One of their biggest side effects is respiratory depression, which occurs even in opioid-tolerant patients. Caution should be used with dosing to avoid oversedation and respiratory depression, especially in older patients. One-time doses are not known to confer a high risk of birth defects in pregnancy and should be considered if the benefits outweigh the risks. Some opioids (e.g., morphine) have metabolites that accumulate in patients with renal dysfunction and increase the risk of respiratory depression due to the prolongation of effects. Synthetic (e.g., fentaNYL and traMADol), semi-synthetic (e.g., oxyCODONE, HYDROcodone, and HYDROmorphone), and natural (e.g., morphine and codeine) opioids are available. Natural opioids have the greatest risk of causing hypotension due to their more profound release of histamine (causes vasodilation similar to the effects of an allergic reaction) compared to synthetic opioids, which have a much smaller degree of decreasing the blood pressure.

  Opioids are available for administration through a variety of routes, including oral (both immediate- and extended-release formulations), IN, IM, IO, and IV, as well as less common forms such as patches, lozenges, buccal films, sublingual sprays and tablets, and subcutaneous. Administration via the IV and IO routes generally has an instantaneous effect, the IN and IM routes typically have an onset of less than 10 minutes, and administration by the oral route takes effect in approximately 30 minutes. There are some differences in onset and duration of action among individual opioids, with fentaNYL having the shortest time to onset (instant) but the shortest duration (30 minutes to 1 hour), and HYDROmorphone having an effect in less than 5 minutes but lasting 3 to 4 hours. It is important to recognize these differences in individual drugs to select the best option for a patient, based on how long the pain relief is required and the hemodynamic effects.
- **Ketamine:** This unique agent has recently gained acceptance for various medical conditions. It works by a variety of mechanisms (primarily inhibition of glutamate, an excitatory neurotransmitter) that, in addition to producing analgesic effects, can decrease sensitization to opioids (hyperalgesia), reduce opioid tolerance, and cause dissociative effects. Ketamine, a controlled substance, and carries a lower risk of respiratory depression compared to opioids, but can cause a brief apneic period if

administered too quickly (IV bolus) in higher and/or concentrated doses. Its dissociative properties have benefits for pain management, including assisting with the posttraumatic stress of an event. Potential undesired effects of disassociation can occur with higher doses, rapid administration, and/or closer dosing intervals. In addition, ketamine can potentially induce a temporary emergence reaction or emergence psychosis, causing auditory and visual hallucinations, agitation, disorientation, and erratic behavior. When treating pain, the psychomimetic side effects of ketamine can be decreased by using lower doses (0.3 mg/kg) mixed in 50 to 100 mL of normal saline solution and administering by infusion over 15 minutes rather than by direct IV bolus. Some clinicians also mitigate this risk by administering benzodiazepines, but mixing medications leads to less predictability of side effects. No dose adjustments are required for patients with renal or hepatic impairment, but the lowest effective dose should be used in older adults due to this drug's CNS effects. There is a risk of ketamine increasing uterine contractions in a dose-dependent manner, but it has been utilized as an anesthetic and adjunctive analgesic during childbirth. Therefore, the risks versus benefits of a one-time dose should be considered on a case-by-case basis in pregnancy.

Ketamine can be delivered IN, IM, and IV. Typically, the IV formulation has an instantaneous onset of action, while the IN and IM versions can take up to 10 minutes to have an effect. However, delivery by the IN and IM routes produces a longer duration of effect (up to 1 hour) and a lower risk of apnea due to the delayed absorption compared to the IV route. There is also a recovery period that typically occurs with higher doses and causes the patient to continue to be in a confused state after the analgesic and/or dissociative effects have worn off. Because it can cause the release of endogenous catecholamines (naturally occurring epinephrine, norepinephrine, dopamine, and other substances in the body), ketamine is the only analgesic medication that increases blood pressure and pulse. Preliminary military data regarding the administration of ketamine early in the posttrauma phase have shown a decrease in posttraumatic stress disorder symptoms associated with its use.

- **DroPERidol:** Like haloperidol, droPERidol is a butyrophenone. These medications have analgesic properties but use different receptors than the opioid receptors or the mechanisms of NSAIDs and acetaminophen. DroPERidol is also a potent antiemetic, and it may have particular benefits in treating painful conditions that also are associated with nausea—such as migraine headaches and nonspecific abdominal pain with nausea. The usual dosing is 1.25 mg IV or IM for adults.
- **Ketorolac:** Ketorolac, an NSAID, has traditionally been given in doses that are higher than currently needed (e.g., 60 mg IM and 30 mg IV). Ketorolac 10 mg IV/IM essentially provides the same analgesic effect as 800 mg of ibuprofen. The lower dosing minimizes adverse effects. In addition to parenteral ketorolac being equivalent to oral ibuprofen in its level of pain reduction, it works just as quickly as ibuprofen for most pain: Even when given parenterally, it must pass through liver metabolism before it is active. Ketorolac does appear to have a special effect on the peristaltic ureteral pain in renal colic from kidney stones (or cholelithiasis).

Table 2-6 summarizes a collection of Cochrane reviews comparing the number of people who need to be treated for one person to get 50% pain relief for severe pain. Other studies have demonstrated that *nonopioid options performed favorably when compared to opioid options,* even more significantly when used in combination.

Other Considerations

Developing a strong pain management guideline can help the clinician navigate through the complexities some patients might exhibit and lead to better pain management compliance. For health care clinicians, there are several concepts to keep in mind with the administration of pain medications. First is the patient's potential for opioid tolerance from chronic use of various medications. This factor can alter the efficacy of medications used for general or acute pain management or require alternative nonopioid options. Second is the potential for addiction, both for the patient and for the clinician. Having a strong tracking system, a defined policy for regulation, and addiction risk assessment education can help deter diversion. Lastly is the human bias element when judging whether to administer an analgesic medication based on the clinician's perception of the patient's pain and history. This issue ties into the ongoing battle of clinician compassion fatigue and does not have a clearly defined solution.

The lack of formal teaching of pain management in medical programs for physicians, nurses, and prehospital clinicians can contribute to the misunderstanding of pain and its priority in overall treatment. The improvement of current practice patterns can occur through the implementation of regular, robust, scientifically supported education.

Several recent studies have demonstrated the possibility of bias within the realm of pain management. These biases can be attributed to race, socioeconomic status, gender, ethnicity, religion, and age. It is difficult to provide comprehensive examples of bias because they vary by cultural, local, regional, national, and international

Table 2-6 Cochrane Reviews of Pain Relief Studies

Study	Population	Interventions	Outcomes	Comments
Chang A, et al. *JAMA* 2017	RCT; ED patients with moderate-severe acute leg/arm pain ($n = 416$)	Single doses of: ibuprofen 400 mg + 1,000 mg APAP vs. oxyCODONE 5 mg + 325 mg APAP vs. HYDROcodone 5 mg + 300 mg APAP vs. codeine 30 mg + 300 mg APAP	Primary outcome: No statistically significant differences between groups in pain decline at 2 hours after ingestion using an 11-point NRS. Mean declines of 4.3, 4.4, 3.5, and 3.9, respectively, from baseline mean of 8.7.	1 in 5 patients required additional medication to control pain. Limited to pain control at 2 hours post ingestion. Nonopioids may be equally efficacious in strain, sprain, or fracture of extremities.
Bronsky ES, et al. *Prehosp Emerg Care* 2019	Retrospective, cohort, matched study; prehospital with severe pain of NRS 7–10 ($n = 79$ matched pairs)	Low-dose ketamine IV (mean 0.3 mg/kg) vs. fentaNYL IV	Primary outcome: Change in pain score from baseline after treatment. Larger mean decrease in pain after treatment with ketamine (–5.5 vs. –2.5, $p < 0.001$). 50% pain reduction in greater proportion of patients (67% vs. 19%, $p < 0.001$). Only AEs in fentaNYL-treated patients (2 respiratory depression, 2 hemodynamic instability).	Limited due to retrospective, observational nature of small study. Significant pain reduction in both groups, but significantly greater response to low- dose ketamine. Relative cardiovascular and respiratory safety of ketamine compared to opioid option.
Masoumi B, et al. *Adv Biomed Res* 2017	RCT; ED patients with long bone fractures ($n = 88$)	Ketorolac 10 mg IV followed by 5 mg IV every 5–20 min PRN vs. morphine 5 mg IV followed by 2.5 mg every 5–20 min PRN	Primary outcome: Pain reduction 1 hour after administration was reduced to means of 1.41 and 1.61, respectively, with no significant differences from mean baselines of 7.59 and 7.93. Patients received 31.8% additional dose of ketorolac vs. 18.2% for morphine, but not statistically significant.	Significantly more nausea associated with morphine. Comparable pain relief efficacy between ketorolac and opioid options with fewer adverse effects.

AEs, adverse effects; APAP, acetaminophen; ED, emergency department; IV, intravenous; *n*, number of patients enrolled in each study; NRS, Numerical Rating Scale; PRN, as needed; RCT, randomized controlled trial.

characteristics, but it is important to understand that these implicit biases exist within clinicians and have been shown to affect the overall assessment and medical management of patients. Remember that all patients—regardless of their age, appearance, socioeconomic status, gender, religious practice, and ethnicity—warrant compassion and equitable medical treatment.

Questions

- This patient is pregnant. Are there any adjustments to the use of pain medications because of the pregnancy?
- What would you do if a colleague with whom you are working does not want to treat the patient's pain because they are concerned it will mask the etiology and make it more difficult for caregivers to identify the patient's diagnosis?
- What would you do if the patient is hypotensive? Are there certain drugs to avoid or, conversely, to preferably use in a hypotensive patient? Remember to consider why the patient may be hypotensive. Is relative hypotension a normal pregnancy state, or would hypotension be secondary to internal bleeding? How can you tell?
- You witness a coworker exchange normal saline for an opioid, pocket the opioid, and then inject the patient with the swapped saline. What would you do?

Case Study Wrap-Up

Pain is easily managed. Human bias does exist in regard to pain, however, and can influence the decision of when and how to treat pain appropriately. Try to avoid the undertreatment pitfalls stemming from lack of proper assessment and acknowledgment, cultural biases, and/or not understanding that acute pain is a true emergency and deserves treatment as such. This situation of undertreating pain is complicated by the current opioid crisis: Clinicians should remain cognizant of the crisis but find a suitable balance between inappropriate overuse and judicious appropriate opioid use.

Case Study: Anaphylaxis

Prehospital: Dispatch for an Allergic Reaction

You arrive at a local construction site where you see a 25-year-old male surrounded by his coworkers, who are holding him up. They state he was stung by a bee and became very anxious, short of breath, and flushed. They were getting ready to place him in their truck and drive him to the emergency department, but before they could do so, he became difficult to keep awake and his breathing become more labored. They called 911. Currently, the patient is unable to speak and additional history is difficult to obtain from his coworkers.

Physical Findings

You see a male, approximately 80 kg (176 lb), who is extremely anxious and in obvious respiratory distress. You lay the patient down. Upon inspection of his airway, you hear audible stridor and wheezes with secretions that are easily controlled with suction. Physical examination shows swelling of the lips, with urticaria around the right cheek, with a raised area where it appears he was stung. Distal pulses are weak with no apparent movement of extremities, but you do notice the skin is flushed with hives that appear widespread.

Vital Signs

- BP: 88/50
- HR: 118, regular
- SpO_2: 89% on room air
- RR: 28, labored
- Lungs: Stridor and wheezes
- Mental status: Alert, but extremely anxious
- Temp: 36°C (96.8°F)

Discussion

Anaphylaxis is a potentially deadly allergic reaction to some form of antigen and represents one of the most critical emergencies health care clinicians face. It can progress in just a few minutes to respiratory or cardiovascular failure and death. Incidence of anaphylaxis in allergic reactions is approximately 2%, with an overall low mortality rate of less than 1%. There could be several reasons for the low mortality rate, which include better education and awareness of common food and venom allergies, increased speed to medical care, and improved access to epinephrine. Because death can occur quickly and symptoms can be unpredictable, the health care clinician must be diligent and prompt with their assessment. This will help in the delivery of lifesaving medications and prevent progression of symptoms.

Medication Considerations

Overall, the pharmacologic treatments of anaphylaxis have not changed much in the past few decades. The mnemonic EASII assists clinicians in the treatment regimen; it stands for **e**pinephrine, **a**ntihistamines, **s**teroids, **i**nhaled beta-2 agonists, and **i**sotonic fluids.

- **EPINEPHrine:** This very well-studied medication has been shown to be critical in preventing death in patients with anaphylaxis. In fact, to prevent further advancement of severe symptoms, systemic anaphylactic reactions are best treated immediately with EPINEPHrine. It works through activation of both alpha- and beta-adrenergic receptors, which counteracts the primary pathology of anaphylaxis by causing vasoconstriction, decreasing vascular permeability, and increasing the force of cardiac contractions, thereby improving a patient's hemodynamic stability. This medication also provides a beneficial respiratory effect through bronchodilation. EPINEPHrine works immediately. In patients not in cardiac arrest, it is recommended to administer (0.1 mg/mL concentration) the drug via the IM route to the outer upper thigh due to its rapid IM absorption. This dose can be repeated every 5 to 10 minutes if there is insufficient response to the initial dose. Subcutaneous administration is not recommended due to erratic absorption by that route, which can delay the effects of the drug. Patients requiring resuscitation or those refractory to IM EPINEPHrine can be given IV EPINEPHrine as a bolus or infusion in a diluted concentration (compared to the IM route); however, due to the more potent effects, this route has a higher arrhythmogenic risk and elevates cardiac oxygen consumption, potentially leading to chest pain and/or myocardial infarction. For these reasons, many protocols include diluted (0.01 mg/mL or 10 mcg/mL) push-dose EPINEPHrine in titrated smaller amounts until the drug has the appropriate effect on blood pressure. In high-quality observational studies, prompt IM injection of EPINEPHrine was found to reduce hospital admissions, and the IM route has been found to be 10-fold safer than the IV injection due to its lower risk of cardiac side effects.

- **Antihistamines:** H_1 histamine receptor blockers (H_1 blockers) such as diphenhydrAMINE work well in relieving itching and urticaria but should not be relied upon to reverse any airway obstruction or hypotension. Unfortunately, antihistamines have a slow peak onset and rarely provide any immediate benefit; thus, they should never replace EPINEPHrine as first-line treatment in the patient with potential anaphylaxis. H_2 receptor histamine blockers such as famotine or raNITidine can also be given for additional histamine antagonism and assist in the relief of hives, but also have a slower onset; little evidence supports their administration as having a significant immediate benefit. Both classes of histamine blockers have no major side effects, so in the majority of cases the potential benefit far outweighs the risk. For anaphylactic reactions, both should be preferably given IV, but they can also be administered orally for mild allergic reactions.
- **Steroids:** Glucocorticoids such as methylPREDNISolone are commonly administered and are continually being studied to determine their role in anaphylactic reaction therapy. They have a slower onset of action (hours) in decreasing the inflammatory and immunologic response to anaphylaxis, but may be effective in helping mitigate prolonged or two-phase anaphylactic reactions. Generally, due to the patient's respiratory difficulties in an anaphylactic reaction, steroids should be preferably administered IV.
- **Inhaled beta-2 agonists:** Medications such as albuterol have been shown to safely and effectively reverse bronchospasm in patients with anaphylaxis through beta-2 agonism, which causes dilation of the bronchioles. These agents can be administered as a nebulized solution or an aerosol spray. They should be considered lower-priority medications when administered in the acute treatment of anaphylaxis, because EPINEPHrine is the drug of choice and provides the beta-2 bronchodilation as well as the important alpha-1 vasoconstriction.
- **Isotonic fluid administration:** Third spacing can rapidly occur in patients experiencing anaphylaxis. For this reason, large amounts of isotonic fluid resuscitation should be initiated early, in addition to epinephrine, in the treatment regimen to treat distributive shock and hypotension.
- Other considerations include administering glucagon for patients who routinely take beta blockers and are refractory to EPINEPHrine administration. Glucagon can improve patients' cardiac symptoms and hemodynamics, but will not affect the respiratory system. Inhaled ipratropium bromide can be considered to help relieve bronchospasm and excessive secretions, but little evidence supports its routine use in anaphylaxis. In those patients who are truly refractory to any treatment, the clinician can also consider a vasopressor, including DOPamine, norepinephrine, or vasopressin.

Other Considerations

Always be vigilant for the rapid decline of a patient suspected of having anaphylaxis. Constant monitoring and aggressive pharmacologic interventions are necessary to avoid respiratory and/or circulatory collapse.

Questions

- What would you do if a patient is hypotensive?
- What should you consider if the patient does not respond to the initial treatment? What is the best route to administer EPINEPHrine initially?

- When should you consider IV administration of EPINEPHrine?
- What is the concentration difference when using IV versus IM EPINEPHrine?
- What dysrhythmias should you be prepared for after IV administration of EPINEPHrine?

Case Wrap-Up

Anaphylaxis is a multisystem disease process in which symptoms can vary and be unpredictable; sometimes, it presents with only hypotension. This creates difficulty in recognition, delaying lifesaving interventions. The clinician should always have a high index of suspicion when dealing with this type of patient to avoid a delay in care and prevent a potential poor outcome.

Case Study: Pharmacologic Treatment for Delirium with Agitated Behavior

Prehospital: Dispatch for General Illness

You are dispatched to a "disturbance" at a downtown apartment at 2300 hours. You arrive to find a large group of young adults having a party where there are obvious signs of alcohol and drug use. You are guided into an upstairs bedroom, where four people have cornered a mid-20s male in a closet and are trying to calm him down. Bystanders report the patient has been using drugs, including synthetic marijuana, and a minimal amount of alcohol. The patient is reported to be extremely violent and delirious; he has already caused physical harm to a bystander who was attempting to calm him.

Physical Findings

You find a well-developed, young adult male standing in a closet, naked, and screaming for everyone to move out of the way so he can jump out of the third-story bedroom window. His verbal responses to questions are nonsense statements. He is diaphoretic, flushed in color, and extremely agitated. His pupils are equal and normal size, as best you can see. He is tachypneic, but in no obvious respiratory distress. There is no gross evidence of trauma. He will not follow commands. You are unable to get him to cooperate so that you can touch or approach him or for obtaining vital signs.

Vital Signs

- BP: Unknown
- HR: Unknown
- SpO_2: Unknown
- RR: Rapid
- Lungs: Unknown
- Mental status: Not following commands, delirium
- Temp: Unknown

Discussion

Administration of medications by EMS clinicians to sedate delirious and often violent patients in the prehospital environment is sometimes necessary if it is not possible to gain the patient's cooperation through verbal de-escalation or simple physical restraints. Safety is the primary consideration for the use of sedative or calming medications. Patients who are violent due to psychiatric disorders and/or substance use often become delirious and do not have the ability to respond to verbal calming techniques. As a result, they present a significant health and safety risk to themselves and to those around them. Death may result from severe metabolic abnormalities that are worsened by uncontrolled agitation and struggling.

If possible, stepwise management of violent patient situations begins with implementation of verbal calming and de-escalation techniques. If this method does not achieve the desired results, physical containment and/or sedation may be required. The goal is to safeguard the patient while also reducing the risk of violence directed against health care clinicians or others. Coordination with law enforcement is critical to the safe management of violent patients. This partnership between EMS and law enforcement is intentional and preplanned and is the result of a national effort to decrease the risk of in-custody death. Appropriate uses of physical containment and restraints, as well as sedation with pharmacologic agents, are critical tools for the safety of both the patients and the responders who are called to care for them.

Allowing delirious and agitated patients to struggle against physical restraints is medically dangerous and increases the risk of injury or death. Appropriate physical restraint, when needed, is mandatory. All people in this condition require constant monitoring and safe transport by EMS to an emergency department for further evaluation. It should not be assumed that this is purely a psychiatric issue; they are clearly medical patients until their condition is fully diagnosed, treated, and stabilized.

Medication Considerations

A variety of medications are currently considered appropriate options for sedation in this setting. Benzodiazepines, butyrophenones/antipsychotic agents, and ketamine are widely accepted drugs to be used for sedation in the field. Each type of medication has specific characteristics that need to be considered when a health care clinician is determining which drug, or combination of drugs, should be used in a particular situation.

Benzodiazepines (e.g., LORazepam, DiazePAM, Midazolam)

One of the safest options in patients with unknown intoxications and unknown histories is the benzodiazepines, which lack the significant cardiac side effects seen with alternative sedating medications. This class of drugs binds to and inhibits gamma-amino butyric acid (GABA) receptors in the CNS and causes sedation by decreasing neuronal excitability. In addition to producing sedation, this GABA binding is beneficial in treatment of alcohol withdrawal as well as treatment of seizures in at-risk patients (especially those who have ingested seizure threshold–lowering substances). Although benzodiazepines may cause respiratory depression, this effect typically occurs at very high doses or in combination with other respiratory-depressant medications already ingested by the patient. Hypotension may also be seen in patients, particularly with rapid administration. These medications are helpful in combative patients as they can be administered IM as well as IV, and midazolam and LORazepam can even be given IN. For more cooperative patients who do not require immediate sedation, all of the agents are available orally. Administration by the IV route typically has the quickest onset, within minutes, followed by the IN route of within 5 minutes; administration by the IM route typically has an effect within 5 to 10 minutes, but may take up to 15 to 20 minutes. Doses can be rapidly escalated or repeated until the desired sedation level is achieved.

Antipsychotic Agents (e.g., DroPERidol, Haloperidol, Ziprasidone, OLANZapine)

Antipsychotic agents work on various neurotransmitters in the brain, but their mechanism of action is not entirely known. All of these agents may help treat an underlying psychiatric disorder in combative patients more effectively than alternative options. Butyrophenones such as droPERidol and haloperidol are commonly used for pharmacologic treatment of delirium with agitated behavior.

First-generation antipsychotics (e.g., haloperidol) especially have anticholinergic/antihistamine effects. These agents should be utilized with caution in patients with cardiac disorders and in patients with co-ingestions known to cause cardiac dysrhythmias, as they can prolong QTc, with ziprasidone having the greatest potentiation of this effect. Higher doses of all first-generation antipsychotics increase the risk of QTc prolongation and subsequent risk of progression to torsades de pointes, although this is not a significant risk with the doses used in this setting. Because of this risk, ziprasidone can only be given IM. The other agents can be given IM or IV, with the oral route available for more cooperative patients. Antipsychotic agents may also potentiate the anticholinergic effects of agents already ingested and can potentially result in extrapyramidal side effects. Haloperidol has an immediate onset when given IV and can be repeated within 5 minutes if the initial dose is ineffective. Ziprasidone and OLANZapine can take up to 15 minutes for maximum effect when given IM; it is recommended to wait longer before repeating a dose of these medications. For health care clinicians, it is important to know the maximum effective doses of each of these first-generation agents and the threshold beyond which the significantly increased risk of adverse effects outweighs their benefits. OLANZapine has the advantage of being available in an oral dissolving tablet formulation, which works well in cooperative patients.

Alcohol potentiates the sedative effects of these medications, which may progress to ventilatory failure. These patients require continuous monitoring of vital signs, including continuous pulse oximetry. Continuous end-tidal carbon dioxide capnography can be helpful in monitoring patients receiving sedation because it can be the earliest indicator of apnea.

One medication that has been gaining increased popularity within the EMS community for behavioral emergencies is droPERidol, a butyrophenone. An equivalent of haloperidol, it has high potency and substantial antidopaminergic action. The increased prehospital use of droPERidol can be attributed to its rapid onset of sedation—3 to 10 minutes IM—and its high efficacy of sedation as compared to other medications such as midazolam or haloperidol. In a prospective before and after study of droPERidol for acute out-of-hospital behavioral emergencies, the results showed that it had fewer adverse events, quicker time to sedation, and less need for additional sedation as compared to midazolam. The benefits and safety are not only demonstrated in the adult population but in the pediatric population as well.

In patients with behavioral emergencies, it can be very difficult to determine their underlying diseases/conditions, ascertain their history, or obtain a baseline vital signs assessment. Also, with medications that can cause sedation, decreased respiratory drive, QT prolongation, and dysrhythmia, there is a higher risk for rapid decline in patient stability. Therefore, it is critical for clinicians to monitor vital signs such as blood pressure, blood glucose, electrocardiogram, oxygen saturations, and capnography as soon as it is safe to do so.

Ketamine

Ketamine is often utilized in the prehospital and emergency settings due to its low risk of respiratory depressant effects (especially with the IM route) and rapid onset. At higher doses, it provides rapid dissociative effects in acutely agitated patients—something that is needed when patient and clinician safety is at stake. Studies report that very few patients who receive ketamine for delirium with agitated behavior require repeat doses. While it can affect patients' hemodynamics, ketamine has a low risk of triggering cardiac arrhythmias compared to antipsychotic agents. Due to its potential for emergence reactions, it is recommended to avoid use of this agent in patients with known history of schizophrenia due to its ability to exacerbate these psychotic symptoms.

Note the differences in ketamine dosing when this drug is administered for analgesic versus sedation effects. While low-dose ketamine is given by an infusion for painful conditions, higher doses given by IM or IV bolus are used to achieve quicker results and sedation in patients with delirium and agitated behavior. All patients receiving ketamine (or any of the listed agents for agitation) must be constantly monitored (all vital signs, including continuous pulse oximetry and, if available, capnography) and appropriately stabilized for transport. Refer to the previous pain management scenario for more specific details.

Other Considerations

During a behavioral emergency, you are treating an undiagnosed patient and may have only a limited medical history available to you. Remember that there are many causes of behavioral agitation, such as mental illness or intoxication, closed head injury, hypoglycemia, hypoxia, infection, stroke, and a postictal phase of a seizure disorder. The health care clinician should perform a thorough medical examination and look for the patient's specific cause.

Questions

- What should you do if your patient goes into cardiac arrest after administration of a behavioral control medication?
- What should you do if your patient starts hypersalivating after administration of ketamine?
- What should you do if you are accidently punctured with a used needle while trying to subdue a patient?

Case Wrap-Up

Properly treating the delirious and potentially violent patient with pharmacologic measures ensures a safe and effective medical evaluation to help identify the potential root cause of the patient's behavior. Always remember that the choice to apply behavioral sedation should be a medical decision; it should never be used for retribution or punishment. When the clinician administers medications to sedate a patient, it should be because they have the best interests of the patient at heart.

Key Terms

absorption How the body takes in a specific drug.

culture of safety An organizational culture in which organizational leaders, directors, and staff emphasize safety over opposing goals.

distribution The distribution of a medication throughout the body (between the plasma and the other body components).

elimination The process by which a drug is excreted from the body. In humans, this is typically via the kidneys or the liver. Physiologic effects on these organs can affect how fast or how much of a medication is removed from the body

ideal body weight (IBW) A measure used for medication dosing. IBW (kg) = 50 (males) or 45.5 (females) + 2.3 kg × each inch over 5 feet.

indications Conditions or circumstances for which a medication is administered.

medication concentration The amount of a drug in the body related to the concentration of the drug measured in a biologic fluid (blood).

metabolism The process by which a drug is broken down (degraded) into inactive components or to active metabolites causing an effect on the body.

metabolites Breakdown products of a drug, Inactive metabolites no longer exert a pharmacologic effect; active metabolites continue to exert a metabolic effect (which may be the same or different from the parent drug's effect).

normalization of deviance Occurs when an improper practice or standard gradually becomes tolerable and accepted, resulting in repeated deviant behavior (without disastrous results) that then becomes the procedural norm.

pharmacodynamics The effect that a drug exerts on the body. It is based on where and which receptors, enzymes, or other proteins a drug binds to in the body.

pharmacokinetics What the body does to a drug; how the drug is absorbed, metabolized, and excreted.

pharmacology The study of interactions between substances and living organisms.

receptors Chemical structures that receive or interact with a drug or hormone and transduce signals, which may be integrated into a biologic system. Receptors typically relay, amplify, or integrate a chemical or electrical signal.

side effects Unexpected or untoward effects caused by a drug that occur in addition to the desired therapeutic effect of a medication.

Bibliography

Academy of Managed Care Pharmacy. Medication errors. Published July 18, 2019. Accessed September 24, 2023. https://www.amcp.org/about/managed-care-pharmacy-101/concepts-managed-care-pharmacy/medication-errors

Acetaminophen. In *Lexi-drugs*. Wolters Kluwer Clinical Drug Information; 2018.

Agency for Healthcare Research and Quality. TeamSTEPPS. Accessed September 24, 2023. https://www.ahrq.gov/teamstepps-program/index.html

Albrecht E. Undertreatment of acute pain (oligoanalgesia) and medical practice variation in prehospital analgesia of adult trauma patients: a 10 yr retrospective study. *Br J Anaesth*. 2013;110(1):96-106.

Alvarez-Perea A, Tanno LK, Baeza ML. How to manage anaphylaxis in primary care. *Clin Transl Allergy*. 2017;7:45. doi:10.1186/s13601-017-0182-7

American Geriatrics Society 2015 Beers Criteria Update Expert Panel. American Geriatrics Society 2015 updated Beers criteria for potentially inappropriate medication use in older adults. *J Am Geriatr Soc*. 2015;63(11):2227-2246.

American Nurses Association. 2016 culture of safety. Accessed September 24, 2023. https://community.ana.org/pages/cultureofsafety?ssopc=1

Arora S, Wagner JG, Herbert M. Myth: parenteral ketorolac provides more effective analgesia than oral ibuprofen. *CJEM*. 2007;9(1):30-32. doi:10.1017/s1481803500014718

Azithromycin. In: *Lexi-drugs*. Wolters Kluwer Clinical Drug Information; 2018.

Axelband J, Malka A, Jacoby J, Reed J. Can emergency personnel accurately estimate adult patient weights? *Ann Emerg Med*. 2004;44(4)(suppl):S81.

Bakkelund KE, Sundland E, Moen S, et al. Undertreatment of pain in the prehospital setting: a comparison between trauma patients and patients with chest pain. *Eur J Emerg Med*. 2013;20(6):428-430.

Banja J. The normalization of deviance in healthcare delivery. *Bus Horiz*. 2010;53(2):139-148.

Bentley J, Heard K, Collins G, Chung C. Mixing medicines: how to ensure patient safety. *Pharmaceut J*. 2015;294(7859). doi:10.1211/PJ.2015.20068289

Bonhomme L, Benhamou D, Comoy E, Preaux N. Stability of epinephrine in alkalinized solutions. *Ann Emerg Med*. 1990;19(11):1242-1244.

British Columbia Institute of Technology. 6.2 safe medication administration: clinical procedures for safer patient care. Published August 31, 2018. Accessed September 24, 2023. https://opentextbc.ca/clinicalskills/chapter/6-1-safe-medication-adminstration

Bronsky ES, Koola C, Orlando A, et al. Intravenous low-dose ketamine provides greater pain control compared to fentanyl in a civilian prehospital trauma system: a propensity matched analysis. *Prehosp Emerg Care*. 2019;23(1):1-8.

Burdette SD, Trotman R, Cmar J. Mobile infectious disease references: from the bedside to the beach. *Clin Infect Dis*. 2012;55(1):114-125.

Campbell RL. Anaphylaxis: emergency treatment. *UpToDate*. Last updated June 24, 2023. Accessed September 24, 2023. https://www.uptodate.com/contents/anaphylaxis-emergency-treatment

Centers for Disease Control and Prevention. Opioid data analysis and resources. Last reviewed June 1, 2022. Accessed September 24, 2023. https://www.cdc.gov/opioids/data/analysis-resources.html

Centers for Medicare and Medicaid Services, Department of Health and Human Services. Partners in integrity: what is a prescriber's role in preventing the diversion of prescription drugs? Published March 2015. Accessed September 24, 2023. https://www.cms.gov/files/document/prescriber-role-drugdiversion-033115pdf

Chang AK, Bijur PE, Esses D, et al. Effect of a single dose of oral opioid and nonopioid analgesics on acute extremity pain in the emergency department. *JAMA*. 2017;318(17):1661-1667.

Cronshaw HL, Daniels R, Bleetman, et al. Impact of Surviving Sepsis campaign on the recognition and management of severe sepsis in the emergency department: are we failing? *Emerg Med J*. 2011;28(8):670-675.

Derry C, Derry S. Single dose oral naproxen and naproxen sodium for acute postoperative pain in adults. *Cochrane Database Syst Rev*. 2009;2009(1):CD004234. doi:10.1002/14651858.CD004234.pub3

Derry C, Derry S, Moore R. Single dose oral ibuprofen plus paracetamol (acetaminophen) for acute postoperative pain (review). *Cochrane Database Syst Rev*. 2013;2013(6):CD010210. doi:10.1002/14651858.CD010210.pub2

Diazepam. In: *Lexi-drugs*. Wolters Kluwer Clinical Drug Information; 2018.

Diphenhydramine. In: *Lexi-drugs*. Wolters Kluwer Clinical Drug Information; 2018.

Duffull SB, Wright DFB, Marra CA, et al. A philosophical framework for pharmacy in the 21st century guided by ethical principles. *Res Social Administr Pharmacy*. 2018;14(3):309-316.

Eagles EMS Medical Directors Consortium. *Sedation of Prehospital Patients* [Position statement]. June 2018.

Farinde A. Overview of pharmacodynamics. *Merck Manual*. Reviewed/revised June 2021. Modified September 2022. Accessed September 24, 2023. https://www.merckmanuals.com/professional/clinical-pharmacology/pharmacodynamics/overview-of-pharmacodynamics

Fentanyl. In: *Lexi-drugs*. Wolters Kluwer Clinical Drug Information; 2018.

Fox E, Birt A, James K, et al. ASHP guidelines on managing drug product shortages in hospitals and health systems. *Am J Health Syst Pharm*. 2009;66:1399-1406.

Gaskell H, Derry S, Moore R, McQuay HJ. Single dose oral oxycodone and oxycodone plus paracetamol (acetaminophen) for acute postoperative pain in adults. *Cochrane Database Syst Rev*. 2009;2009(3):CD002763. doi:10.1002/14651858.CD002763.pub2

Gleason W, Richmond N. Best practices for controlled substance monitoring. *J Emerg Med Serv*. Published November 1, 2017. Accessed September 24, 2023. https://www.jems.com/operations/best-practices-for-controlled-substance-monitoring

Guthrie K. Behavioural emergency management. *Life in the Fast Lane*. Published September 12, 2019. https://litfl.com/behavioural-emergency-management

Haloperidol. In: *Lexi-drugs*. Wolters Kluwer Clinical Drug Information; 2018.

Hughes RG, Blegen MA. Medication administration safety. In: RG Hughes, ed. *Patient Safety and Quality: An Evidence-Based Handbook for Nurses*. Agency for Healthcare Research and Quality; 2008. Accessed September 24, 2023. https://www.ncbi.nlm.nih.gov/books/NBK2656

Hydromorphone. In: *Lexi-drugs*. Wolters Kluwer Clinical Drug Information; 2018.

Ibuprofen. In: *Lexi-drugs*. Wolters Kluwer Clinical Drug Information; 2018.

Institute for Safe Medication Practices. Independent double checks: undervalued and misused: selective use of this strategy can play an important role in medication safety. Published June 13, 2013. Accessed September 24, 2023. https://www.ismp.org/resources/independent-double-checks-undervalued-and-misused-selective-use-strategy-can-play

Institute for Safe Medication Practices. Look-alike drug names with recommended tall-man (mixed case) letters. Published January 26, 2023. Accessed September 24, 2023. https://www.ismp.org/recommendations/tall-man-letters-list

Institute for Safe Medication Practices. Side tracks on the safety express: interruptions lead to errors and unfinished ... wait, what was I doing? Published November 29, 2012. Accessed September 24, 2023. https://www.ismp.org/resources/side-tracks-safety-express-interruptions-lead-errors-and-unfinished-wait-what-was-i-doing

Institute of Medicine. *Crisis Standards of Care: A Systems Framework for Catastrophic Disaster Response*. National Academies Press; 2012.

Kalil AC, Metersky ML, Klompas M, et al.. Management of adults with hospital-acquired and ventilator-associated pneumonia: 2016 clinical practice guidelines by the Infectious Diseases Society of America and the American Thoracic Society. *Clin Infect Dis*. 2016;63(5):e61-e111.

Kapusta D. Drug excretion. In: *xPharm: The Comprehensive Pharmacology Reference*. Elsevier; 2007:1-2.

Ketamine. In: *Lexi-drugs*. Wolters Kluwer Clinical Drug Information; 2018.

Ketorolac. In: *Lexi-drugs*. Wolters Kluwer Clinical Drug Information; 2018.

Kim M, Mitchell SH, Gatewood M,, et al. Older adults and high-risk medication administration in the emergency department. *Drug Health Patient Saf*. 2017;8;9:105-112.

Kupas DF, Shayhorn M, Payton TF, Green P. Structured inspection of medications carried and stored by emergency medical services agencies identifies practices that may lead to medication errors. *Prehosp Emerg Care*. 2012;16(1):67-75.

Kupas DF, Wydro GC, Tan DK, et al. Clinical care and restraint of agitated or combative patients by emergency medical services practitioners, *Prehosp Emerg Care*. 2021;25:5:721-723. doi:10.1080/10903127.2021.1917736

Lavonas EJ, Drennan IR, Gabrielli A, et al. Part 10: special circumstances of resuscitation: 2015 American Heart Association guidelines update for cardiopulmonary resuscitation and emergency cardiovascular care. *Circulation*. 2015;132(18 suppl):S501-S518.

Le J. Overview of pharmacokinetics. *Merck Manual*. Reviewed/revised June 2022. Modified September 2022. Accessed September 24, 2023. https://www.merckmanuals.com/professional/clinical-pharmacology/pharmacokinetics/overview-of-pharmacokinetics

Levofloxacin. In: *Lexi-drugs*. Wolters Kluwer Clinical Drug Information; 2018.

Leykin Y, Pellis T, Lucca M, et al. The pharmacodynamics effects of rocuronium when dosed according to real body weight or ideal body weight in morbidly obese patients. *Anesth Analg*. 2004;99:1086-1089.

Lieberman P, Nicklas RA, Randolph C, et al. Anaphylaxis: a practice parameter update 2015. *Ann Allergy Asthma Immunol*. 2015;115:341-384.

Linder LM, Ross Ca, Weant KA. Ketamine for the acute management of excited delirium and agitation in the prehospital setting. *Pharmacotherapy*. 2018;38(1):139-151.

Lorazepam. In: *Lexi-drugs*. Wolters Kluwer Clinical Drug Information; 2018.

Mandell LA, Wunderink RG, Anzueto A, et al. Infectious Diseases Society of America/American Thoracic Society Consensus guidelines on the management of community-acquired pneumonia in adults. *Clin Infect Dis*. 2007;44:S27-S72.

Masoumi B, Farzaneh B, Ahmadi O, et al. Effect of intravenous morphine and ketorolac on pain control in long bone fractures. *Adv Biomed Res*. 2017;6:91.

McCabe JJ, Kennelly SP. Acute care of older patients in the emergency department: strategies to improve patient outcomes. *Open Access Emerg Med*. 2015;4;7:45-54.

Midazolam. In: *Lexi-drugs*. Wolters Kluwer Clinical Drug Information; 2018.

Minnesota Department of Health, Office of Emergency Preparedness, Minnesota Healthcare System Preparedness

Program. Patient care: strategies for scarce resource situations. Revised August 2021. https://www.health.state.mn.us/communities/ep/surge/crisis/standards.pdf

Morphine. In: *Lexi-drugs*. Wolters Kluwer Clinical Drug Information; 2018.

Motov SM, Khan AN. Problems and barriers of pain management in the emergency department: are we ever going to get better? *J Pain Res*. 2008;2:5-11.

Murney P. To mix or not to mix: compatibilities of parenteral drug solutions. *Aust Prescr.* 2008;31:98-191. Accessed September 24, 2023. https://www.nps.org.au/australian-prescriber/articles/to-mix-or-not-to-mix-compatibilities-of-parenteral-drug-solutions

Naproxen. In: *Lexi-drugs*. Wolters Kluwer Clinical Drug Information; 2018.

National Library of Medicine. About DailyMed. Accessed September 24, 2023. https://dailymed.nlm.nih.gov/dailymed/about-dailymed.cfm

Olanzapine. In: *Lexi-drugs*. Wolters Kluwer Clinical Drug Information; 2018.

Olasveengen TM, Mancini ME, Perkins GD, et al. Adult basic life support: 2020 international consensus on cardiopulmonary resuscitation and emergency cardiovascular care science with treatment recommendations. *Circulation.* 2020;142(16 suppl):S41-S91.

O'Mahony D, O'Sullivan D, Byrne S, et al. STOPP/START criteria for potentially inappropriate prescribing in older people: version 2. *Age Ageing*. 2015;44(2):213-218.

Overgaard CB, Dzavik V. Inotropes and vasopressors: review of physiology and clinical use in cardiovascular disease. *Circulation*. 2008;118:1047-1056. https://www.ahajournals.org/doi/pdf/10.1161/CIRCULATIONAHA.107.728840

Page CB, Parker LE, Rashford SJ, et al. A prospective before and after study of droperidol for prehospital acute behavioral disturbance. *Prehosp Emerg Care*. 2018;22(6):713-721. https://doi.org/10.1080/10903127.2018.1445329

Page CB, Parker LE, Rashford SJ, et al. A prospective study of the safety and effectiveness of droperidol in children for prehospital acute behavioral disturbance. *Prehosp Emerg Care*. 2018;23(4):519-526. https://doi.org/10.1080/10903127.2018.1542473

Pan S, Zhu L, Chen M, et al. Weight-based dosing in medication use: what should we know? *Patient Prefer Adher*. 2016;10:549-560.

Reber LL, Hernandez JD, Galli SJ. The pathophysiology of anaphylaxis. *J Allergy Clin Immunol*. 2017;140(2):335-348.

Ring J, Beyer K, Biedermann T, et al. Guideline for acute therapy and management of anaphylaxis. *Allergo J Int*. 2014;23(3):96-112.

Roberts JR. Physical and chemical restraint. In: *Roberts and Hedges' Clinical Procedures in Emergency Medicine and Acute Care*. 7th ed. Elsevier; 2017.

Sarfati L, Ranchone F, Vantard N, et al. Human-simulation-based learning to prevent medication error: a systematic review. *J Eval Clin Pract*. 2019;(1):11-20.

Scaggs TR, Glass DM, Hutchcraft MG, et al. Prehospital ketamine is a safe and effective treatment for excited delirium in a community hospital based EMS system. *Prehosp Disaster Med*. 2016;31(5):563-569.

Scheindlin S. A brief history of pharmacology. *Modern Drug Discovery*. Published January 2001. Accessed September 24, 2023. http://pubs.acs.org/subscribe/archive/mdd/v04/i05/html/05timeline.html

Schroers G, Ross JG, Moriarty H. Nurses' perceived causes of medication administration errors: a qualitative systematic review. *Jt Comm J Qual Patient Saf.* 2021;41(1):38-53.

Sherman R. Normalization of deviance: a nursing leadership challenge. *Emerging RN Leader.* Published March 13, 2014. Accessed September 24, 2023. https://www.emergingrnleader.com/normalization-deviance-nursing-leadership-challenge

Stark R. Drug diversion legal brief for EMS leaders. *EMS1*. Published November 10, 2016. Accessed September 24, 2023. https://www.ems1.com/opioids/articles/142756048-Drug-diversion-legal-brief-for-EMS-leaders

Tariq RA, Vashisht R, Sinha A, Scherbak Y. Medication dispensing errors and prevention. *StatPearls*. Last updated May 2, 2023. Accessed September 24, 2023. https://www.ncbi.nlm.nih.gov/books/NBK519065

Teater D. *Evidence for the efficacy of pain medications*. Accessed September 24, 2023. https://www.nsc.org/Portals/0/Documents/RxDrugOverdoseDocuments/Evidence-Efficacy-Pain-Medications.pdf

Temming LA. Cahill AG, Riley LE. Clinical management of medications in pregnancy and lactation. *Am J Obstet Gynecol.* 2016;214(6):698-702.

Thompson C. Senator proposes drug shortage law. *Am J Health Syst Pharm*. 2011;68:461.

Trissel's I.V. compatibility databases in facts and comparisons. In: *Lexicomp*. Wolters Kluwer Clinical Drug Information; 2018. Accessed September 24, 2023. https://www.wolterskluwer.com/en/solutions/lexicomp/resources/facts-comparisons-user-academy/trissels-iv-compatibility-databases.

Turner PJ, Jerschow E, Umasunthar T, et al. Fatal anaphylaxis: mortality rate and risk factors. *J Allergy Clin Immunol Pract.* 2017;5(5):1169-1178.

Umhoefer S, Finnefrock M. 6 steps for hospitals to take to prevent prescription drug abuse, diversion. *Hospitals & Health Networks*. Published May 31, 2016. Accessed September 24, 2023.

U.S. Department of Health and Human Services. FDA pregnancy categories. Last updated November 16, 2022. Accessed September 24, 2023. https://chemm.hhs.gov/pregnancycategories.htm

U.S. Drug Enforcement Administration. Drug scheduling. Accessed September 24, 2023. https://www.dea.gov/drug-scheduling

U.S. Food and Drug Administration. Content and format of labeling for human prescription drug and biological products, requirements for pregnancy and lactation *labeling,* Final Rule (79 FR 72063, December 4, 2014).

U.S. Food and Drug Administration. Transcript: managing drug shortages. Published September 4, 2015. Accessed September 24, 2023. https://www.fda.gov/drugs/fda-drug-info-rounds-video/transcript-managing-drug-shortages

U.S. Food and Drug Administration. Working to reduce medication errors. Accessed September 24, 2023. https://www.fda.gov/drugs/information-consumers-and-patients-drugs/working-reduce-medication-errors

U.S. Food and Drug Administration, Risk Communication Advisory Committee Meeting. FDA Briefing Document: Communicating information about risks in pregnancy in product labeling for patients and providers to make informed decisions about the use of drugs during pregnancy. March 5–6, 2018. Accessed September 24, 2023. https://www.fda.gov/downloads/AdvisoryCommittees/CommitteesMeetingMaterials/RiskCommunicationAdvisory Committee/UCM597309.pdf

Ventola CL. The drug shortage crisis in the United States: causes, impact, and management strategies. *PT*. 2011;36(11):740-757.

Weant KA, Bailey AM, Baker SN. Strategies for reducing medication errors in the emergency department. *Open Access Emerg Med*. 2014;6:45-55.

Weaver SJ, Lubomksi LH, Wilson RF, et al. Promoting a culture of safety as a patient safety strategy: a systematic review. *Ann Intern Med*. 2013;158(5 pt 2):369-374.

Wilson MP, Pepper D, Currier GW, et al. The psychopharmacology of agitation: consensus statement of the American Association for Emergency Psychiatry Project BETA Psychopharmacology Workgroup. *West J Emerg Med*. 2012;13(1):26-34.

Wolf ZR, Hughes RG. Error reporting and disclosure. In: RG Hughes, ed. *Patient Safety and Quality: An Evidence-Based Handbook for Nurses*. Agency for Healthcare Research and Quality; 2008. Accessed September 24, 2023. https://www.ncbi.nlm.nih.gov/books/NBK2652

Yu JE, Lin RY: The epidemiology of anaphylaxis. *Clin Rev Allergy Immunol*. 2018;54(3):366-374.

Zebroski R. A brief history of pharmacy: Humanity's search for wellness. Published 2003. Accessed September 24, 2023. https://handoutset.com/wp-content/uploads/2022/04/A-Brief-History-of-Pharmacy-Humanitys-Search-for-Wellness-by-Bob-Zebroski.pdf

Ziprasidone. In: *Lexi-drugs*. Wolters Kluwer Clinical Drug Information; 2018.

CHAPTER 3

Respiratory Disorders

Chapter Editors
David M. French, MD, FACEP, FAEMS
Dustin P. LeBlanc, MD

In this chapter, the anatomy and function of the respiratory system are discussed, and common diseases and conditions that generate respiratory complaints are described. More importantly, clinicians will learn how to thoroughly assess patients, determine whether a pathologic condition is present, identify the cause of the condition from among several plausible diagnoses, and apply clinical reasoning to select the best treatment plan for the patient. In addition, several critical procedures for monitoring and treating patients with respiratory complaints are reviewed.

LEARNING OBJECTIVES

At the conclusion of this chapter, you will be able to:

- Explain the anatomy, physiology, and pathophysiology of diseases and conditions often accompanied by respiratory complaints, and describe their typical clinical presentations.
- Describe how to obtain a thorough history from the patient with a respiratory complaint.
- Demonstrate a comprehensive physical examination of a patient with a respiratory complaint using the Advanced Medical Life Support (AMLS) Assessment Pathway.
- Form an initial impression and generate a list of likely differential diagnoses based on a patient's history, signs, and symptoms.
- Order or recommend appropriate diagnostic tests and apply the results of those tests to aid in diagnosis.
- Identify critical procedures necessary to stabilize and treat patients with emergent respiratory conditions.
- Follow accepted evidence-based practice guidelines for the overall management of each condition.
- Provide an ongoing assessment of the patient, revising your clinical impression and treatment strategy based on the patient's response to interventions.

SCENARIO

A 57-year-old man complains of a sore throat. As you greet him, you note that he appears ill. His eyes are red, and he constantly dabs sputum from the corners of his mouth. With a muffled voice, he explains that his symptoms began today. He says he feels achy, has had chills, and is experiencing pain in his ear and lower teeth. His medical history includes type 2 diabetes and hypertension. Initial vital signs include blood pressure, 104/72 mm Hg; pulse rate, 124 beats/min; respirations, 20 breaths/min; and temperature, 39.4°C (103°F). As you continue examining the patient, he becomes more anxious and restless. You note a high-pitched noise as he breathes in.

- Which diagnoses are you considering based on the information you have now?
- Which additional information will you need to narrow your differential diagnosis?
- What are your initial treatment priorities as you continue your patient care?

The function of the respiratory system is to bring in oxygen, eliminate carbon dioxide from the body, and protect the airway by keeping out secretions. If this process is interrupted, vital organs of the body will not function properly. Clinicians must understand the importance of early detection of airway problems, provide rapid and effective interventions, and continually reassess patients with compromised airway or inadequate breathing.

The Respiratory System: Anatomy

The respiratory system is composed of structures that facilitate air exchange through breathing. The two primary functions of breathing are intake of air for oxygenation of blood cells and exhalation of carbon dioxide (CO_2). This process, which is crucial to life, involves a series of conduits designed to warm, filter, humidify, and transfer inhaled air to the lungs during inspiration, followed by rapid elimination during exhalation.

The respiratory system can be divided into the upper and lower airways (**Figure 3-1**). The upper airway comprises all structures above the vocal cords (the nose, mouth, jaw, oral cavity, and pharynx), and the lower airway comprises the structures below the vocal cords (externally, from the thyroid cartilage to the xiphoid process; internally, from the glottis to the pulmonary capillary membrane). Most of the respiratory system and its structures lie within the thorax, sharing space with the cardiovascular and gastrointestinal structures. The patient who complains of chest pain, cough, shortness of breath, or a choking sensation may be experiencing symptoms from any of these structures, making diagnosis and treatment of the patient's condition more complicated.

The Upper Airway

The major functions of the upper airway are to warm, filter, and humidify air as it enters the body through the nose and mouth. Humidification occurs as the air picks up moisture from the soft tissues of the airway. The pharynx extends from the nose and mouth to the level of the esophagus and trachea. Air passing through the mouth to the posterior pharynx does not become as moist as air passing through the nasal cavity.

Nasal Cavity

The nasal cavity includes the following structures:

- Nares (nostrils)
- The nasal cavity, which contains the nasal turbinates (curved bony plates, or shelves, that extend from the lateral wall of the nasal cavity; they increase the surface area of the nasal mucosa, thereby facilitating the warming, filtering, and humidification of inhaled air)
- The nasopharynx, formed by the union of the facial bones

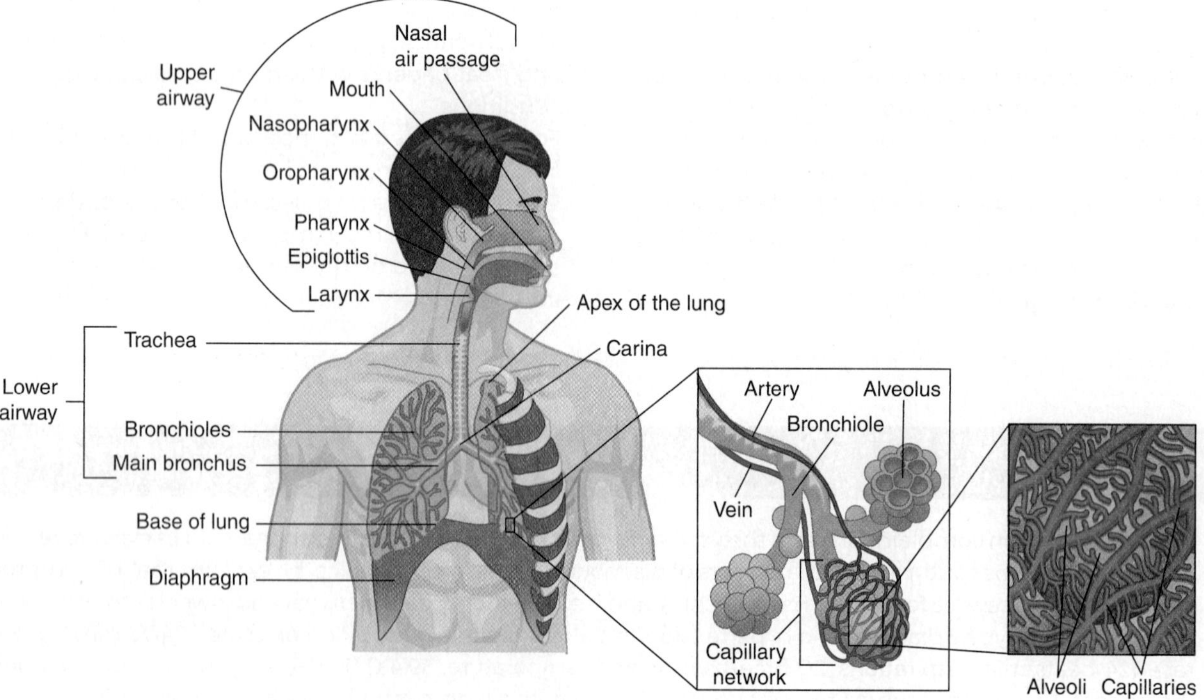

Figure 3-1 The upper and lower airways contain the structures in the body that help us breathe.

The nasal cavity serves several important purposes. First, it humidifies and warms inhaled air, protecting the lower mucosa. In addition, hair and mucus-producing cells line the nasopharynx and capture large airborne particles, preventing lower respiratory tract infections. Finally, the nasopharynx functions as a resonating chamber, giving the voice its timbre and pitch.

The extensive vascularization of the nasal cavity and the vulnerable position of the nose make a nosebleed, or epistaxis, a common occurrence. This bleeding generally involves vessels of the mucosa covering the cartilaginous portion of the septum. Possible causes include trauma, drying, infections, allergies, and clotting disorders. Hypertension can bring on a nosebleed by rupturing small vessels of the lamina propria.

Pharynx and Oral Cavity

Some structures of the mouth—the lips, teeth, gums, tongue, and salivary glands—are not dedicated to ventilation. Instead, they play roles in mastication and speech creation.

Inhaled air passes through the oral cavity, reaches the pharynx and then the hypopharynx, which is located immediately behind the base of the tongue (**Figure 3-2**). This area also contains the tonsils, lymph tissue that helps fight infection. Directly below the hypopharynx is the epiglottis, a cartilaginous flap covering the trachea during swallowing. This flap, which normally remains open, protects the airway from aspiration by closing involuntarily during swallowing when a bolus of liquid or

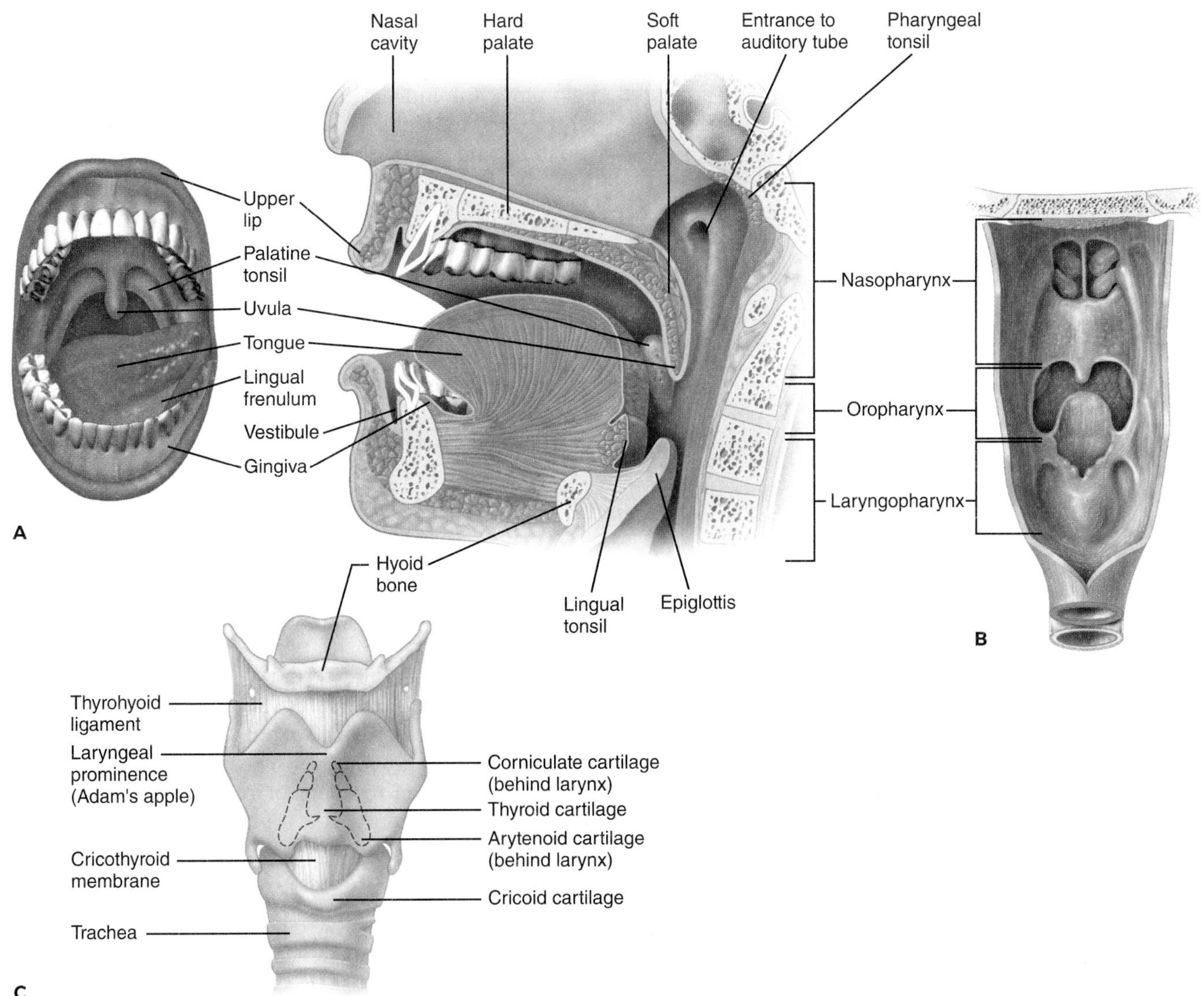

Figure 3-2 **A.** The oral cavity. **B.** The larynx. **C.** The pharynx.

food passes over it. In unconscious patients, this reflex is often absent, putting them at risk of aspirating food or liquid. Such aspiration can be a life-threatening event because of the volume and acidity of the stomach contents and the risk of subsequent infection.

Below the epiglottis lie three glottic structures:

1. The thyroid cartilage.
2. The arytenoid cartilages, which help support the vocal cords.
3. The false vocal cords and true vocal cords—mobile structures partially covering the glottis that move back and forth to create basic sounds, which are then tuned by the oropharynx and nasopharynx. The false vocal cords are made up of fibrous connective tissue and are attached to the true vocal cords. The true vocal cords are composed of fine ligamentous tissues. The space between the two true vocal cords, which is the narrowest portion of the adult airway, is referred to as the glottis.

The Lower Airway

The function of the lower airway is to exchange oxygen and carbon dioxide. When air enters the lower airway (**Figure 3-3**), it passes through the trachea and bronchi to the lungs, where it sweeps through the bronchioles and finally reaches the alveoli, the tiny sacs in which gas exchange takes place.

Trachea

The trachea, or windpipe, is the conduit for air entry into the lungs. This membranous tube is supported by a series of C-shaped cartilaginous rings. The trachea begins immediately below the cricoid cartilage, the only ring with a circumferential cartilage framework. Below the cricoid cartilage is a series of incomplete rings connected posteriorly by small muscles that help determine the diameter of the trachea as they relax and contract. This structure keeps the trachea from collapsing during vigorous coughing or in case of bronchial constriction.

At the level of the carina, the trachea divides into the right and left mainstem bronchi. The bronchi are the only source of ventilation for each lung. The right mainstem bronchus is straighter and larger in diameter than the left mainstem bronchus, making it more susceptible to aspiration and inadvertent unilateral intubation. Thus, an endotracheal tube inserted too far will often terminate in the right mainstem bronchus. This severely limits the ability of the left lung to participate in respiration and decreases capacity. These bronchi are also composed of C-shaped rings, which are connected in the back by a small muscle. The trachea and mainstem bronchi are lined with columnar epithelium, which provides humidification and secretes mucus to protect the lower airway against harmful particulates. Microscopic hairs called cilia help move the mucus and trapped particles up the respiratory tract, where this material is eventually expelled by coughing and expectoration.

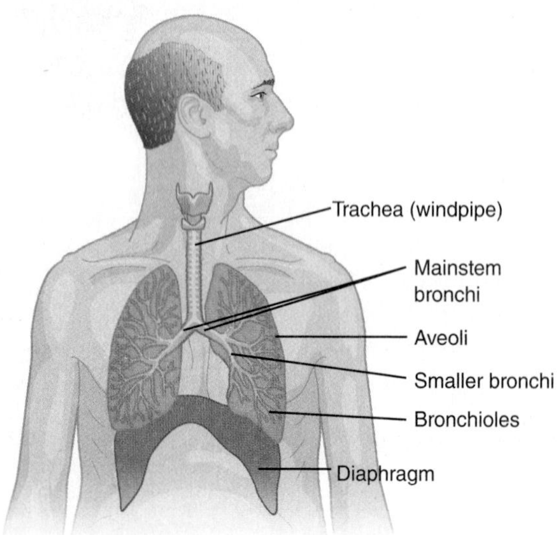

Figure 3-3 The trachea and lungs (lower airway structures).

Lungs

After the mainstem bronchi, there is further branching of the lower airway into a series of smaller bronchi, followed by bronchioles, and, at the smallest level, alveoli. Collectively, these structures form the lungs. The right lung has three main lobes: upper, middle, and lower. The left lung shares its side of the intrathoracic space with the heart and has only two lobes—upper and lower. These lobes are covered with a thin, slippery outer membrane called the visceral pleura. The parietal pleura lines the inside of the thoracic cavity. A small amount of fluid is found between the two pleurae, which decreases the friction between them during breathing.

On entering the lungs, each bronchus divides into increasingly smaller bronchi, which in turn subdivide into primary, secondary, and tertiary bronchioles. These increasingly smaller bronchioles distribute inhaled air to all areas of the lung for effective ventilation. The bronchiole walls are composed of muscle and connective tissue, which enable them to dilate or constrict in response to various stimuli. The smaller bronchioles eventually terminate in alveoli, small sacs with walls only a single cell thick, to allow gas exchange (respiration) to occur. Millions of alveoli exist in a healthy lung, forming grapelike clusters. **Gas exchange** takes place across the few layers of cells separating the alveoli from the pulmonary capillaries. This reciprocal passage of oxygen into the blood and carbon dioxide into the alveoli is called **respiration**. As it leaves the alveoli, oxygen passes through the single layer of cells of the alveolar wall, through a thin layer of interstitial tissue, and finally through the single layer of cells of the capillary wall. Any increase in the thickness of this cell layer can profoundly jeopardize respiration.

Alveoli are held open and in position by connective tissue in the interstitial tissues surrounding the alveoli. A chemical called *surfactant* coats the inner walls of the alveoli, helping to keep these tiny pouches open. Surfactant reduces surface tension in the alveoli walls and prevents the alveoli from collapsing on exhalation. Premature infants can have a deficiency of surfactant, which leads to serious respiratory problems; however, regardless of age, even normal amounts of surfactant and adequate connective-tissue support cannot completely prevent alveolar collapse, called atelectasis. Atelectasis can occur secondary to shallow breathing, infection, trauma, or inflammation, and can be reversed with a sigh or yawn. Atelectasis is a major risk factor for pneumonia.

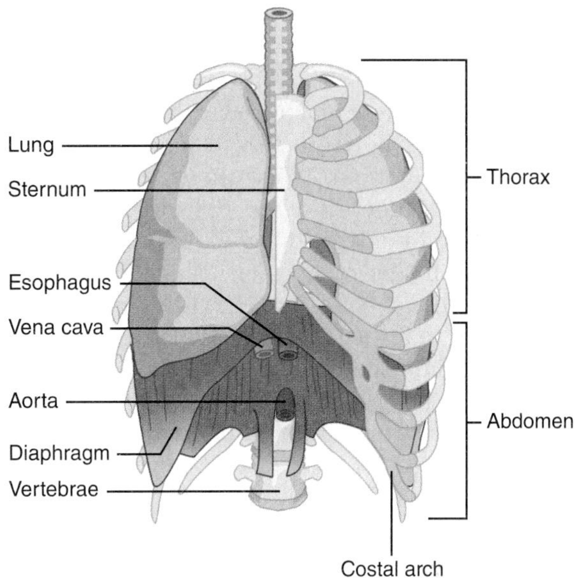

Figure 3-4 The thoracic cage. The dome-shaped diaphragm divides the thorax from the abdomen. It is pierced by the great vessels and the esophagus.

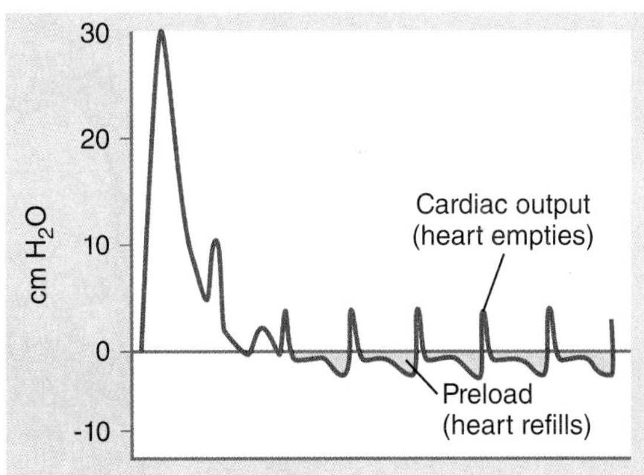

Figure 3-5 Negative intrathoracic pressure enhances venous blood return to the heart and increases stroke volume during systole.

Musculoskeletal Support of Respiration

The bones, muscles, and connective tissues serve an integral function in ventilation. Without the support of these structures, effective ventilation would be impossible. Structural support ranges from the cartilaginous trachea to the bony vault of the thorax, which maintains the pressure necessary for ventilation.

The main muscle of ventilation is the diaphragm, a thick muscle separating the thorax from the abdomen. Contraction of the diaphragm, along with the chest wall muscles, enlarges the thoracic cavity, leading to decreased intrathoracic pressure and drawing air into the lungs. The diaphragm is under both voluntary and involuntary control. It acts like a voluntary muscle when you take a deep breath, cough, or hold your breath; that is, you can control these variations in the way you breathe. However, unlike other skeletal or voluntary muscles, the diaphragm also performs an automatic function. Breathing continues during sleep and at all other times. Even though you can hold your breath or temporarily breathe faster or slower, you cannot continue these variations in breathing patterns indefinitely. When the concentration of carbon dioxide becomes too high, automatic regulation of breathing resumes. Therefore, although the diaphragm appears to be a voluntary skeletal muscle attached to the bony thorax, it behaves, for the most part, like an involuntary muscle. The diaphragm is innervated by the phrenic nerve, which signals the diaphragm to contract and relax. The phrenic nerve originates in the brainstem and exits from the cervical spine at levels C3, C4, and C5. Injury to the cervical spine at or above these levels, particularly from trauma, may cause fatal apnea.

The thoracic cage is the truss that supports and shelters the structures within the thoracic cavity, including the lungs (**Figure 3-4**). Its architecture facilitates the intrathoracic pressure changes necessary for ventilation. The ribs, sternum, and thoracic spine form a protective framework for the thoracic cavity. In addition to shielding the intrathoracic organs, the ribs help create the intrathoracic pressure changes that are necessary for inspiration and expiration (**Figure 3-5**). The anatomic structures that support ventilation and respiration share the intrathoracic space with several other important structures, including the heart, venae cavae, aorta, pulmonary trunk, and thoracic duct. The vascular structures circulate oxygenated blood to tissues and return deoxygenated blood to the lungs for removal of carbon dioxide.

The intercostal muscles run between the ribs and are considered accessory muscles to respiration, assisting the diaphragm in creating the pressure changes necessary for ventilation. Other accessory muscles include the abdominal and pectoral muscles. The muscles of the chest wall are innervated by the intercostal nerves. When the diaphragm contracts, it moves down slightly, enlarging the thoracic cage from top to bottom. When the external intercostal muscles contract, they move the ribs up and out. These actions combine to enlarge the chest cavity in all dimensions. Pressure in the cavity then falls, making it lower than atmospheric pressure, and air rushes into the lungs. This is referred to as negative-pressure breathing because air is "sucked" into the lungs. The inhalation part of the cycle is an active process, requiring the muscles to contract.

During exhalation or expiration, the diaphragm and the intercostal muscles relax. Unlike inhalation, exhalation does not normally require muscular effort. As these muscles relax, all dimensions of the thorax decrease, and the ribs and muscles assume a normal resting position. When the volume of the chest cavity decreases, air in the lungs is compressed into a smaller space, and pressure becomes greater than atmospheric pressure. Intrapulmonic pressure, which is the pressure within the lungs and airways, is increased, and air is pushed out through the trachea. This phase of the cycle is passive. Exhalation ends when the intrapleural pressure is equal to the atmospheric pressure, at which point air stops flowing from the lungs to the outside.

The process of breathing is typically easy and requires little muscular effort. If a patient is using accessory muscles to breathe, respiratory compromise or impending **respiratory failure** should be included in the differential diagnosis.

The heart is the pump of the cardiorespiratory system, and its proper functioning is critical for the distribution of blood, and therefore oxygen, throughout the body (**Figure 3-6**). Deoxygenated blood returns to the heart via

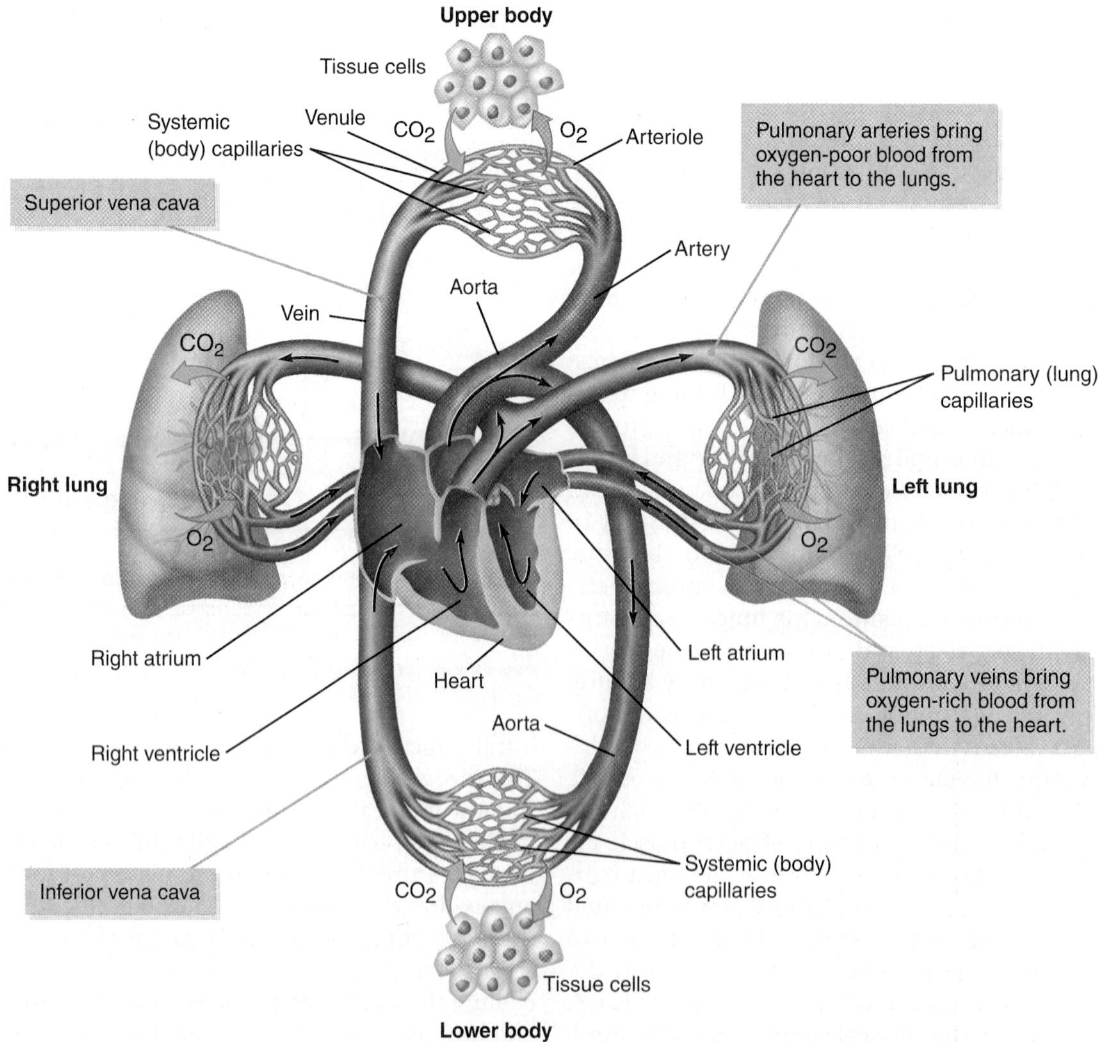

Figure 3-6 The circulatory system includes the heart, arteries, veins, and interconnecting capillaries. The capillaries are the smallest vessels and connect venules and arterioles. At the center of the system, and providing its driving force, is the heart.

the superior and inferior venae cavae. The superior vena cava returns the blood from the head, arms, and upper body, and the inferior vena cava returns blood from the lower body. Deoxygenated blood passes from the venae cavae into the right atrium and is pumped first into the right ventricle, then into the pulmonary trunk. The pulmonary trunk branches into the right and left pulmonary arteries, which flow into the lungs. Oxygenated blood returns to the heart and left atrium through the pulmonary veins. This is the only place in the body where the arteries carry deoxygenated blood, and the veins carry oxygenated blood.

The **thoracic duct**, located in the left upper thorax, is the largest lymph vessel in the body. The thoracic duct returns to the venae cavae any excess fluid from the lower extremities and abdomen that is not collected by the veins. The amount of lymph fluid returned is small compared with the blood volume that flows through the veins, but its evacuation is important because the fluid would otherwise pool in the lower extremities.

The Respiratory System: Physiology

The primary function of the respiratory system is respiration, the exchange of gases at the alveolocapillary membrane. Respiration and ventilation are regulated by a complex series of interactions involving nerves, sensors, and hormones. The level of CO_2 in the body is the primary modulator of ventilation. CO_2 is the chief waste product of metabolism. Metabolism is the process of breaking down sugars and other nutrients into energy for use by the cells of the body, and a high CO_2 level damages the cellular machinery responsible for this metabolism. **Aerobic metabolism**, in which glucose is converted into energy in the presence of oxygen, is the basic process of life. This process is efficient but relies on a steady supply of both oxygen and glucose because the cells cannot stockpile either resource.

When denied oxygen, the cells resort to **anaerobic metabolism**, which allows the cells to generate small amounts of energy but releases excessive acids as by-products, especially lactic and carbonic acids. This excess of acid must be removed by the carbonic acid–bicarbonate buffer system, or acidosis will result. Often, though, the same problem that impaired oxygen delivery also compromises the circulation so that levels of acids build up, causing cellular injury or tissue death.

When air from the environment enters the respiratory tract, the potential for infection is always present, but the body is quite efficient in responding to this threat. The respiratory system has several strategies for preventing disease-causing organisms (pathogens) from entering from the upper respiratory tract and reaching the alveoli.

If a pathogen bypasses the skin (which acts as the primary barrier against injury and infection) and enters the body through the respiratory tract, the lining of epithelial cells in the trachea acts as a secondary barrier against infection. The epithelium is made up of mucus-secreting goblet cells. The sticky mucus intercepts would-be invaders. Other cells contain microscopic hairs (cilia) that help move the mucus to the upper respiratory tract, where it can be expectorated (coughed). Mucus also contains an antibody called immunoglobulin A (IgA). IgA is secreted into body fluids and binds to pathogenic organisms, allowing white blood cells to recognize and destroy them.

In the lower respiratory tract, white cells can physically enter the alveoli and bronchioles by squeezing between the cell borders. White cells attack pathogens and engulf any small particles not carried away in the mucus of the upper airway. These white cells are often expectorated in mucus and account for the yellow-green color of sputum in patients with certain kinds of respiratory infections.

Respiration

Each time a person takes a breath, the alveoli receive a supply of oxygen-rich air. The oxygen then passes into a fine network of pulmonary capillaries, which are in close contact with the alveoli. The capillaries in the lungs are located in the walls of the alveoli. The walls of both the capillaries and the alveoli are extremely thin. Thus, air in the alveoli and blood in the capillaries are separated by two very thin layers of tissue.

Oxygen and carbon dioxide pass rapidly across these thin tissue layers by diffusion. Diffusion is a passive process in which molecules move from an area with a higher concentration of molecules to an area of lower concentration. There are more oxygen molecules in the alveoli than in the blood, so the oxygen molecules move from the alveoli into the blood. Conversely, because there are more carbon dioxide molecules in the blood than in the inhaled air, carbon dioxide moves from the blood into the alveoli.

The Chemical Control of Breathing

The brain—or more specifically, the respiratory center in the brainstem—controls breathing. This area is in one of the most highly protected parts of the nervous system, located deep within the skull. The nerves in the respiratory center act as sensors monitoring the level of carbon dioxide in the blood and subsequently the spinal fluid. The brain automatically controls breathing if the level of carbon dioxide or oxygen in the arterial blood is too high or too low. In fact, adjustments can be made in one breath.

Breathing is triggered by a buildup of carbon dioxide, which causes the pH to decrease in the cerebrospinal fluid. The cells are constantly working to eliminate carbon dioxide to regulate the acid–base balance of the body. When the level of carbon dioxide becomes too high, a slight change occurs in the pH (the measure of acidity) of the cerebrospinal fluid. The medulla oblongata (a portion of the brainstem), which is sensitive to pH changes, stimulates the phrenic nerve, sending a signal to the diaphragm to initiate a breath. The person then exhales to reduce the level of carbon dioxide in the body.

Chemical receptors, or **chemoreceptors**, sense changes in the composition of blood and body fluids. The primary chemical changes registered by chemoreceptors include levels of hydrogen (H^+), carbon dioxide (CO_2), and oxygen (O_2):

- *H^+*. The chemoreceptors sense an increase in the hydrogen level in the fluid surrounding the cells of the medulla, which stimulates an increase in the rate of ventilation. The opposite occurs when H^+ levels fall. This change can be detected in the bloodstream by measuring pH, which is inversely proportional to H^+—that is, the pH level goes down when the H^+ level goes up, and vice versa. Normal pH in the human body is 7.35 to 7.45.
- *CO_2*. The CO_2 level in the blood will rise if respiration is too slow or shallow, causing **hypercapnia** (also known as hypercarbia or CO_2 retention), or if the blood becomes too acidic. The excess CO_2 spills over into the cerebrospinal fluid, triggering an increase in H^+ and in turn precipitating an increase in the respiratory rate. This level can be measured in the blood by measuring the partial arterial pressure of CO_2 ($PaCO_2$). Normal $PaCO_2$ is 35 to 45 millimeters of mercury (mm Hg). The CO_2 level is the principal regulator of respiration.
- *O_2*. When peripheral chemoreceptors sense an excessive drop in the oxygen level, the respiratory rate increases. The normal partial arterial pressure of O_2 (PaO_2) is 75 to 100 mm Hg.

Normal respiration is controlled by the hypercapnic (high CO_2 level) drive, whereby respiration increases when CO_2 becomes even slightly elevated. The body also has a backup system, called the hypoxic drive, to control respiration. When the oxygen level falls, this system will stimulate breathing. Areas in the brain, the walls of the aorta, and the carotid arteries act as oxygen sensors. These sensors are easily satisfied by minimal levels of oxygen in the arterial blood. As a result, the backup system—that is, the hypoxic drive—is much less sensitive and less powerful than the carbon dioxide sensors in the brainstem.

Chemoreceptors undergo a change when chronic lung disease causes a perpetual elevation of the CO_2 level. Patients with chronically elevated levels of CO_2, including some patients with lung diseases like chronic obstructive pulmonary disease (COPD), may rely on the hypoxic drive to regulate their respiration. Such patients are dependent on low levels of oxygen to stimulate a rise in respiratory rate or depth. Patients with chronic lung disease should not be given excessive amounts of oxygen over the long term. However, in the initial management of patients with chronic lung disease, if marked hypoxemia is present and administering a high percentage of oxygen is necessary, patients should not be deprived of oxygen treatment for fear of causing respiratory arrest.

Buffer Systems

A buffer is a substance that absorbs or donates hydrogen ions (H^+). Buffers absorb H^+ when these ions are in excess and donate H^+ when these ions are depleted. Through this mechanism, buffer systems act as rapid defenses when acid–base changes affect the H^+ concentration in the extracellular fluid. The respiratory system and the renal system work in conjunction with the bicarbonate buffer to maintain homeostasis. The fastest way for the body to get rid of excess acid is through the respiratory system. Excess acid can be expelled as CO_2 and water from the lungs. Conversely, slowing respirations will increase CO_2 if the body is in an alkalotic state. The renal system regulates pH by filtering out more H^+ and retaining bicarbonate if the body is in an acidotic state, and by doing the reverse if it is in an alkalotic state. This is a slow process, however, and it may take days for enough H^+ to be eliminated to achieve acid–base balance.

The kidneys can sense decreased oxygen levels in the blood. When sensors in the renal artery detect hypoxia, they release erythropoietin, a hormone that stimulates the creation of red blood cells. When the sensors register chronically low levels of oxygen, more red blood cells are created. Patients with chronic bronchitis, for example, often have an elevated number of red blood cells, a condition called polycythemia. This disorder increases the risk of forming blood clots.

The Nervous System Control of Breathing

The dorsal respiratory group (DRG) in the medulla is the main pacemaker for breathing and is responsible for initiating inspiration. It sets the base pattern for respirations. The pons, another area within the brainstem, helps regulate the DRG's activities. The pons includes two areas that help regulate respiration. The **pneumotaxic center**, located in the superior portion of the pons, helps shut off the DRG, resulting in shorter, faster respirations. The **apneustic center**, located in the inferior portion of the pons, stimulates the DRG, resulting in longer, slower respirations. Both areas of the pons can help augment respirations during emotional or physical stress. Thus, the two areas of the medulla and the two areas of the pons work together to help regulate breathing.

Ventilation

A substantial amount of air can be moved within the respiratory system. An adult male has a total lung capacity of 6,000 mL, with females having about one-third less total capacity. The tidal volume is the amount of air moved into or out of the lungs during a single breath. The amount of air movement with each breath during rest is approximately 500 mL. The precise volume can be affected by many variables, including lung disease, body size, physical fitness, and less obvious factors such as elevation above sea level. Residual volume is the amount of air that remains in the lungs after maximum expiration; this air maintains partial inflation of the lungs. Vital capacity is the total amount of air moved in and out of the lungs with maximum inspiration and expiration.

There are two kinds of reserve capacity: expiratory and inspiratory. Expiratory reserve capacity is the difference between a normal exhalation and a maximal exhalation. You can demonstrate this concept by forcing as much air out of your lungs as possible after a normal exhalation—this volume of air is the expiratory reserve capacity. Likewise, inhaling as deeply as possible after a normal inhalation allows you to take in an additional volume of air, the inspiratory reserve capacity. This continued inhalation occurs through negative pressure created in the thoracic cavity. With assisted ventilations, the clinician actively moves air into the patient's lungs using positive pressure. The typical adult-size bag-valve mask (BVM) holds approximately 1,500 to 2,000 mL of air. Although the usual tidal volume is approximately 500 mL, some additional volume is required to compensate for dead space in the respiratory circuit. However, the full volume of air from the BVM should not be administered, to avoid hyperventilation and barotrauma from hyperinflation. Instead, the clinician should judge whether the volume administered is sufficient by assessing chest rise.

Dead space is the portion of the respiratory system having no alveoli and, therefore, where little or no exchange of gas between air and blood occurs. It includes the air in the upper airway and parts of the lower airway to the alveoli and is normally accepted to be about 150 mL. The mouth, trachea, bronchi, and bronchioles are all considered dead space. When a patient is ventilated with any device, more dead space is created. Gas must first fill the device before it can be moved into the patient. The amount of dead space can also increase when a disease process such as pulmonary embolism causes portions of the lung to have a loss of or decreased perfusion.

The depth or volume of each breath is critical information to know when assessing ventilation. Another measurement, called minute volume, provides a more accurate determination of effective ventilation. Minute volume, also referred to as minute ventilation, is the amount of air moving in and out of the lungs in 1 minute minus the dead space:

Minute Volume = Respiratory Rate × Tidal Volume

Dead space is an important factor to consider when determining whether the rate and depth of ventilation are adequate, as it must be subtracted from the tidal volume.

Survival requires an adequate amount of minute volume, not just an adequate respiratory rate. Consider a patient who is breathing at a rate of 20 breaths/min but has minimal chest rise and air movement. Even though the patient's respiratory rate seems adequate, the amount of air being moved is inadequate. The minute volume is too low, and the patient needs ventilatory assistance. Analysis of the volume of air involved in ventilation can help you understand the pathology of many respiratory diseases and evaluate how well a patient is responding to treatment (**Figure 3-7**).

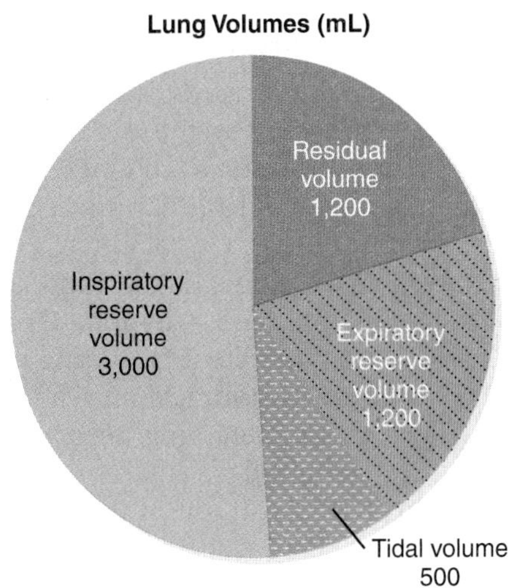

Figure 3-7 Lung volumes.

The AMLS Assessment Pathway ▸▸▸▸

▾ Initial Observations

Dyspnea (difficulty breathing) is both a sign and a symptom. An outward sign of dyspnea, for example, is the use of accessory muscles. The patient may complain of breathlessness or express an uncomfortable awareness of breathing difficulties, using terms such as *shortness of breath*, *chest tightness*, or *having trouble breathing*.

Scene Safety Considerations

Evaluating the scene for hazards is a key step in the AMLS Assessment Pathway. Patients with respiratory distress rarely pose a physical threat to emergency medical services (EMS) clinicians, but caution must be exercised when dealing with any hypoxic patient who is restless. In addition to restlessness, hypoxia can cause a patient to have altered mental status and agitation. These patients will resist being laid supine, because sitting upright has mechanical advantages for thoracic muscle and ribcage function and facilitates maintaining an open airway. It may be difficult to communicate with patients who are agitated due to hypoxia. Restraint of these patients may be necessary while quickly working to oxygenate them and reverse the hypoxia.

Standard Precautions

Perhaps the greatest safety concern when caring for a patient with a respiratory complaint is the risk of contagious diseases, particularly those spread by droplets and airborne transmission. Any combination of respiratory complaints with a history of fever warrants using barrier protection for your mucous membranes, especially while performing suctioning and airway procedures. Putting on a mask, gloves, gown, and eye protection seems so simple, but it is a precaution that is easy to forget when you are caring for a very sick patient. Be alert to situations requiring higher levels of respiratory protection, such as an N-95 respirator for patients with suspected COVID-19.

Other Hazards

When patients show evidence of mucous membrane irritation and increased work of breathing, especially when there is more than one patient with similar symptoms, paying special attention to the possible presence of toxic substances, such as carbon monoxide or chlorine gas, is warranted. Nontoxic substances such as natural gas (methane) may create a hypoxic environment. Hazardous materials (hazmat) equipment and teams may have to be dispatched before you enter the scene.

Evaluation of any scene should be done using all your senses. You should not normally see particulates suspended in the air or enter an area where the air is smoky, foggy, or dusty. If the patient is located in such an area, respiratory complications are likely. Look for chemical placards or pictograms within business settings. Obtain personal protection equipment and hazmat resources to gain safe entry to such scenes if you are trained to do so. Chemical odors may alert you to the presence of invisible chemicals in the air. The same protection and resources must be used if you detect this hazard.

Some patients with chronic respiratory diseases require airway and ventilatory support at home, ranging from oxygen therapy to mechanical ventilation. The presence of medical devices in the patient's environment should prompt you to ask if the devices are working properly and if the patient has been using them as prescribed. EMS clinicians are often called when a device malfunction leads to acute distress. Some fixes may be simple, such as unkinking oxygen tubing. In other cases, the problem may not be solvable on scene and the patient may require transport to the hospital.

Patient Cardinal Presentation/ Chief Complaint

Many patients with chronic respiratory diseases have some symptoms that are present all the time. A pertinent question for them is, "What changed that made you call for an ambulance?" Some common reasons for an acute change to a chronic respiratory problem include the following:

- Asthma with fever
- Running out of medicine, including medication for a nebulizer or metered-dose inhaler
- Travel-related problems after a lengthy journey
- Dyspnea triggers such as pets, perfume, or cigarette smoke
- Issues with allergens, bacteria, molds, and fungi
- Noncompliance with therapy
- Failure of technology, such as an oxygen tank regulator malfunction

Primary Survey

Level of Consciousness

As with all patients, rapidly assessing the level of consciousness is of primary importance when caring for a patient with a respiratory emergency. If the patient is awake, alert, and speaking, then the airway is obviously patent. When the patient is not fully awake and alert, then further evaluation of the airway is required. A decreased level of consciousness may be caused by respiratory failure, whether hypoxic or hypercapnic, so rapid assessment for these conditions must be done as part of your overall evaluation of patients with altered mental status. Recognizing and treating life threats are the priority in the primary survey and throughout care. Because many respiratory ailments are life threatening, the respiratory assessment is always an early step in patient assessment.

Airway and Breathing

In an unresponsive patient whose airway is being assessed, listen for abnormal breathing sounds such as snoring, gurgling, and stridor. Then open the airway with your gloved hands, using a jaw-thrust or head tilt–chin lift maneuver. The latter method should *not* be utilized if there is any possibility of a cervical spine injury. Look for signs of upper airway obstruction, such as secretions or blood inside the mouth. Suction should always be readily available for your use in the primary survey.

If you need to provide ongoing manual airway management, make an immediate plan for positioning or initiation of invasive techniques. Preoxygenation/ventilation is always the first step in the plan while you map out a safe, effective means of managing the airway based on your resources, the differential diagnosis, your location, and the patient's anatomy.

If the patient already has an airway device in place, evaluate its effectiveness and the patient's tolerance of the device. Confirm proper placement of the device before moving on to assess breathing.

Assessment of breathing begins upon your first encounter with the patient. Observe for labored breathing. Visualize the chest and observe for accessory muscle use, asymmetric chest rise, and abdominal breathing. Generally, any respiratory noises that are audible without a stethoscope are abnormal. Tactile (or vocal) fremitus is a vibration that is palpable when a person speaks; pneumonia will cause this vibration to be more prominent, whereas pneumothorax and pleural effusion lead to a decrease in fremitus. Listen to the patient speak. Is the patient hoarse, or does the patient complain of dysphagia (difficulty swallowing)? How many words can the patient speak in a sentence before taking a breath? The ability to speak only two to three words at a time is a sign of severe respiratory compromise.

Assessing the rate, volume, and quality of breathing is an obvious component of respiratory assessment, but rate and volume are often not determined accurately. The rate is a commonly assessed vital sign, but respiratory depth (volume) may be misjudged. A patient with an adequate rate but a low volume may still have an inadequate minute ventilation. The respiratory rate can vary significantly from minute to minute. Be sure to monitor trends in respiratory rate (whether it is decreasing or increasing) rather than solely focusing on the specific rate at the beginning of the assessment.

Distinguishing Respiratory Distress from Respiratory Failure

When a patient reports dyspnea or you observe increased work of breathing, you must pause and ask yourself a question: Is this patient in respiratory distress, or does the patient have signs of respiratory failure? If the patient's condition improves with simple resuscitative maneuvers, then respiratory distress is the answer. In contrast, if the patient's condition does not improve with basic interventions, or if any patient with respiratory distress has signs of fatigue or altered mental status, respiratory failure is imminent. Immediate interventions should be implemented to support the patient's airway and ventilation. Indicators of impending respiratory failure include the following findings:

- Respiratory rate > 30 or < 6 breaths/min
- Oxygen saturation $< 90\%$
- Use of multiple accessory muscle groups
- Inability to lie supine
- Tachycardia with a rate > 140 beats/min
- Mental status changes
- Inability to clear oral secretions/mucus
- Cyanosis of nail beds or lips

After the primary survey, you may have initiated some basic resuscitative maneuvers if warranted by the patient's condition. You may have supplied oxygen or continuous positive airway pressure (CPAP), or you may have administered positive-pressure ventilation with a BVM. Reevaluate how the patient is tolerating these interventions. Assess whether the patient is feeling better. Have the patient's vital signs improved? Is the patient's chest rising symmetrically with BVM ventilation? If these interventions fail to relieve the patient's distress, you may need to consider placement of a supraglottic (extraglottic) airway or endotracheal intubation and mechanical ventilation. Depending on the patient, pharmacologic sedation and/or paralysis may be appropriate to facilitate placement of an advanced airway.

Circulation/Perfusion

Assessing skin color is a fast way to begin forming an early impression of the patient's circulation and oxygenation. Although it is important to note the generalized cyanosis of oxygen desaturation or the profound pallor of shock, more subtle information can be gained by assessing the mucous membranes. The tissues inside the mouth, under the eyelids, and even under the nail beds are usually the same pink color in all healthy patients.

▼ First Impression

Your knowledge of anatomy, physiology, and pathophysiology is the first step in being able to perform a thorough physical exam and obtain an appropriate history from the patient to determine the cause of the breathing complaint. Chapter 1, *Advanced Medical Life Support Assessment for the Medical Patient*, outlines the process of forming that clinical impression.

Regardless of the setting, assess the patient's overall level of consciousness and work of breathing. In addition, do a quick check of their perfusion status.

All clinicians must be aware of the safety and environmental clues that can be assessed when first encountering the patient. Clues to a variety of pathologic conditions may be evident immediately, but keep in mind they are only clues. Avoid forming a hasty field impression based on minimal information. The patient's presentation may suggest a particular condition, but these suspicions must be confirmed by a thorough assessment.

Detailed Assessment

History Taking

Always ask the patient about a history of similar complaints, and compare the current episode's symptoms with those experienced previously—are they the same or different from the last time? A patient with a history of heart failure (HF) and an acute onset of dyspnea may relate that the symptoms today are the same as the last time pulmonary edema developed. Ask the patient what they think is wrong. Some patients are so familiar with their disorder that they can relate their current symptoms to how they felt on previous occasions and identify the cause. However, do not focus so intently on a particular diagnosis that you overlook alternative conditions.

History of Present Illness

The **history of present illness (HPI)** is perhaps the most important element of patient assessment. A common teaching in medicine is that the history is the most important contributor to making the correct diagnosis. The primary elements of the HPI are obtained through a systematic history. Identifying whether the patient has ever been intubated when experiencing similar symptoms can be a key indicator of the need for imminent airway management interventions and the likelihood of respiratory failure. If the dyspnea is present only with exertion, try to identify how much exertion is needed to provoke the dyspnea (walking to the mailbox versus walking across a room) and if this is different from the patient's baseline. Using the OPQRST and SAMPLER mnemonics, you can systematically obtain a basic HPI (see Chapter 1, *Advanced Medical Life Support Assessment for the Medical Patient*, for more information on the OPQRST and SAMPLER mnemonics).

Elicit information from the patient about aggravating or alleviating factors—what makes the symptoms worse, and what makes them better? A detailed HPI is required in developing an accurate differential diagnosis and formulating an effective treatment plan. Key findings in the patient with dyspnea are listed in Table 3-1. Important elements of a pulmonary history include the following:

- Fever or chills
- Ankle edema
- Calf swelling or tenderness
- Back, chest, or abdominal pain
- Orthopnea (shortness of breath when lying flat)
- Cough
- Dyspnea on exertion
- History of smoking or passive smoke exposure
- History of chronic lung disease
  - Asthma
  - COPD
- Blood in sputum
  - Color of sputum
  - History of sputum production
- Prior respiratory admissions
- Prior intubations
- Home nebulizer use

History taking should include an exploration of the patient's risk factors to help narrow the differential diagnosis. For example, the patient may have risk factors for the development of venous thrombosis and pulmonary embolus, such as use of oral contraceptives, obesity, smoking, recent surgery, long-distance travel, and a sedentary lifestyle.

Table 3-1 Key Findings in Patients with Dyspnea

Duration
■ Chronic or progressive dyspnea is usually related to cardiac disease, asthma, COPD, or neuromuscular disease (e.g., multiple sclerosis). ■ An acute dyspneic spell may be due to exacerbation of chronic lung condition; infection; pulmonary embolus; cardiac dysfunction; a psychogenic cause; or inhalation of a toxic substance, allergen, or foreign body.
Onset
■ Sudden onset of dyspnea should raise suspicion of pulmonary embolism or spontaneous pneumothorax. ■ Dyspnea developing slowly (hours to days) points toward pneumonia, HF, or exacerbation of asthma or COPD.
Patient Position
■ Orthopnea can be attributed to HF, COPD, or a neuromuscular disorder. ■ Paroxysmal nocturnal dyspnea (sudden onset of dyspnea while sleeping) is most common in patients with left-sided HF. ■ Exertional dyspnea is associated with COPD; myocardial ischemia; and the abdominal loading that occurs in obesity, ascites, and pregnancy.

COPD, chronic obstructive pulmonary disease; HF, heart failure.

Secondary Survey

Vital Signs

Obtain the patient's baseline vital signs—temperature, pulse, respiration, blood pressure, oxygen saturation, and, if an advanced airway is in place, end-tidal CO_2 ($ETCO_2$) measurements, and repeat these periodically, guided by the severity of the patient's condition. $ETCO_2$ monitoring is helpful in the safe monitoring of any patient who receives a sedating medication, and it provides some information about respiratory physiology in other selected situations as well. The patient's mental status should also be frequently reassessed for changes, especially in the presence of abnormal vital signs.

During the initial assessment of the patient, the work of breathing is assessed as being either quiet (normal) or increased, and the presence of respiratory distress determined. In the primary survey, you focus on attending to vital functions and addressing life threats. During the secondary survey, however, you should count the patient's breaths per minute to determine the respiratory rate and further assess the depth of breathing. An extremely high or low respiratory rate may alert you that a secondary organ system is responsible for the respiratory distress. For example, a patient who is breathing without difficulty, using no accessory muscles, but at a fast rate, is exhibiting tachypnea. This may be a clue to fever, anxiety, hypoxia, or metabolic acidosis (shock, diabetic ketoacidosis, and other causes). Tachypnea occurs when the chemoreceptors sense a rise in acidity (metabolic acidosis), stimulating the respiratory system to breathe faster to blow off excess CO_2. At the other end of the spectrum, a patient who is breathing slowly, with no accessory muscle use, is exhibiting bradypnea, which can be caused by a central nervous system (CNS) disturbance or by the action of respiratory depressant drugs.

When monitoring vital signs, it is especially important to keep a close eye on how respiration and perfusion are affecting the patient's mental status.

Physical Exam

By the time the patient's history has been elicited, some important information should be known about the patient's physical signs, such as their level of consciousness and degree of distress. This section presents the components of the focused physical exam in sequence, noting at each step the points of relevance to a patient with dyspnea.

Neurologic Exam

Assessing the level of consciousness is imperative in patients with dyspnea. Mental status is an indicator of adequate perfusion and oxygenation of the CNS. The brain is intolerant of prolonged interruption of its supply of oxygen or glucose. Mental status can deteriorate rapidly when either of these supplies is deficient for as little as a few minutes. Dysfunction of the pulmonary system can lead to hypoxia, hypercapnia, and decline of mental status even in the presence of a functioning circulatory system. The combination of new-onset altered mental status and respiratory distress is a hallmark of respiratory failure.

Neck Exam

In the neck, look for jugular venous distention (JVD) when the patient is in a semi-recumbent position. JVD is a condition in which the jugular veins become engorged with blood. When it is present, it can provide a rough measure of the pressure in the right atrium of the heart. Distended neck veins may implicate cardiac failure as the source of dyspnea. JVD may also indicate high pressure in the thorax, which keeps the blood from draining out of the head and neck. Cardiac tamponade, tension pneumothorax, HF, and COPD can all cause JVD.

Distention of the jugular veins must be interpreted in the context of the patient's position and other vital signs. Grossly distended jugular veins despite a blood pressure of 80/40 mm Hg in a trauma patient should cause considerable concern. In contrast, JVD in a healthy 20-year-old person while lying flat (but not while sitting) is of little concern.

While looking at the patient's neck, note the position of the trachea. Tracheal deviation may be seen or felt at the suprasternal notch and is a classic but late sign of a tension pneumothorax. The deviation occurs behind the sternum, so it may be difficult to assess. Consider palpating the trachea as part of your examination.

Hepatojugular reflux is specific to right-sided HF. When the right ventricle is not pumping effectively, the central venous pressure increases, making it difficult for the jugular veins and the large reservoir of blood in the liver to drain into the thorax. As a result, the combination of JVD and a distended liver may present in right-sided HF. Pressing gently on the liver will further engorge the jugular veins (hepatojugular reflux). You can elicit this sign of right-sided HF when a patient in respiratory distress is sitting up in a semi-Fowler's (45-degree) position.

Chest and Abdominal Exam

A key assessment for a patient with respiratory difficulty is auscultation of breath sounds. Evaluate the upper and lower lung fields, both anterior and posterior, during both inspiration and expiration. Assess whether breath sounds are diminished and if they are equal bilaterally. Best practices for performing auscultation are outlined here:

- Use the diaphragm of the stethoscope, placing the diaphragm directly on the patient's skin if possible.
- To eliminate outside interference, do not allow the stethoscope tubing to touch anything during auscultation.

- To avoid eliciting abnormal airway noises, ask the patient to breathe with the mouth open and the head in a neutral position or slightly extended.
- If you hear something unusual, stop, move the stethoscope to a new site, and listen again for comparison.

Breath sounds can be categorized simply as normal or abnormal (the latter are also referred to as adventitious breath sounds). You might hear normal sounds in one area and abnormal sounds in another. Sounds associated with particular respiratory disease processes are summarized in **Table 3-2**.

- Wheezing is the classic sound of lower airway narrowing or a reactive airway. Patients who exhibit this sign usually do not have trouble drawing air in, but they have difficulty letting air out, which causes expiration to be longer than inspiration. Wheezing is usually heard on expiration (although it can be heard on inhalation as well) and can have a musical quality or a harsh, discordant tone. The pitch varies with the size of the airway. Wheezing may be heard in many disease processes, especially asthma, bronchitis, and COPD, but can also be present with pneumonia and HF. Be wary of the silent or very quiet chest. To produce audible wheezing, sufficient air must move through the structures. A patient cannot wheeze if they are not moving enough air.
- The auscultation of crackles (also known as rales) on inspiration is associated with accumulated fluid in the alveoli. This sound has a fine, high-pitched, shrill quality and sometimes clears with coughing. If the sound clears after a few deep breaths, the patient probably has atelectasis. Pneumonia, HF, and pulmonary edema are the conditions most often associated with crackles, but this sound is also heard in patients with pulmonary fibrosis.
- The word *rhonchi* (the plural of rhonchus) derives from the Greek word *rhonkos*, meaning "snoring." Auscultation of rhonchi indicates narrowing or

Table 3-2 Breath Sounds Associated with Selected Conditions

Location	Sound	Phase	Disease Process
Upper airway	Stridor	Inspiration	Croup Epiglottitis Foreign body aspiration Deep-space neck infection Inhalation burn Swelling of upper airway
Lower airway	Rhonchi	Primarily expiration	Aspiration Bronchitis Cystic fibrosis
	Wheezing	Primarily expiration	Reactive airway disease Asthma Pulmonary edema Chronic bronchitis Emphysema Endobronchial obstruction
	Crackles (formerly rales)	End inspiration	Pneumonia Pulmonary edema Fibrosis
	Diminished breath sounds	Both	Emphysema Atelectasis Pneumothorax (simple or tension) Flail chest Neuromuscular disease Pleural effusion
Chest wall	Pleural rub	Either	Pleuritis Pleural effusion

obstruction, such as from secretions, in the larger airways. These loud, coarse, low-pitched sounds are often described as bubbly, rattling, or snoring, and are heard primarily on expiration. Acute bronchitis and chronic conditions such as bronchiectasis and cystic fibrosis are often accompanied by rhonchi.

- As noted earlier, the fluid present between the pleural layers reduces friction between them, helping the lungs expand and contract during normal respiration. When an area of the pleura becomes inflamed, the surface becomes roughened, and a pleural friction rub can be auscultated. This sign is associated with chest wall pain caused by pneumonia, pleurisy, and lung contusion. The friction rub may be heard in an area adjacent to the site of pain.
- Auscultation of diminished breath sounds is a classic sign of emphysema. Other disorders associated with diminished breath sounds include atelectasis, pneumothorax, pleural effusion, and neuromuscular disorders that limit inspiratory volume.
- Stridor is a sound produced by narrowing, such as from inflammation or a foreign body in the upper airway. It is heard only on inspiration and is described as a high-pitched musical sound. Viral croup and epiglottitis are two respiratory disorders accompanied by stridor. In addition, a foreign body airway obstruction, laryngitis, stenosis, or tumor of the airway may cause stridor and may be identified during history taking. Angioedema and trauma may also be associated with stridor.
- Whereas diminished breath sounds are associated with emphysema and other disorders, absent breath sounds (a quiet chest) is an ominous finding; the sounds listed here require sufficient air movement to produce them.

Examination of the Extremities

Does the patient have edema of the ankles or lower back? If so, does it pit when a finger is pushed into the edematous tissue? Is there peripheral cyanosis? Check the patient's pulse. The radial pulse is the point most commonly assessed in a stable patient, but you can gather additional information by evaluating the pulse at alternative arterial sites like the carotid, femoral, and dorsalis pedis. Proximal pulses correspond to larger arteries. The body can shift circulation to these larger vessels during times of stress or hemorrhage. When this occurs, the peripheral pulses may be weak or absent while central circulation is preserved. Does the patient have profound tachycardia (from exertion or hypoxia)? Also note the patient's skin temperature—whether an obvious fever is present or whether the patient's skin is cool and clammy from shock.

Diagnostics

Repeated vital signs, electrocardiography, and pulse oximetry readings are the data most commonly collected for patients with respiratory difficulty. In some situations, depending on the available equipment and the patient's condition, peak expiratory flow, waveform $ETCO_2$, and transcutaneous carbon monoxide levels might be recorded.

Pulse Oximeters

Under normal circumstances, a pulse oximeter is a noninvasive device that measures the percentage of a patient's hemoglobin saturated with oxygen. For example, an oxygen saturation (SpO_2) of 97% indicates that 97% of the patient's hemoglobin's oxygen receptors have oxygen attached to them. Although an $SpO_2 < 90\%$ is concerning clinically, many persons may not perceive shortness of breath until the saturation falls much lower. Thus, SpO_2 should be checked for all medically ill patients. Transcutaneous SpO_2 monitoring—also known as "pulse ox," "O_2 sat," and "sat monitoring"—has become an easy, commonplace way to assess blood oxygenation. Transcutaneous SpO_2 monitors are relatively inexpensive and can quickly approximate the level of oxygen in the blood without the need for an invasive procedure. This technology capitalizes on hemoglobin's ability to absorb infrared light to varying degrees, depending on the number of hemoglobin-binding sites occupied by (i.e., saturated by) oxygen molecules. The monitor calculates the amount of light absorption and translates it into a percentage that represents the SpO_2 level. This percentage is displayed on the monitor.

At rest, most healthy individuals have an SpO_2 of 95% to 100%. More accurate oxygen levels are assessed through invasive arterial blood gas (ABG) monitoring, which requires puncturing an artery to obtain a sample for testing. This test is valuable for patients experiencing respiratory distress/failure, for ventilated patients, and for the assessment of respiratory and metabolic acidosis. While this test is not typically performed in the prehospital environment, it is helpful during critical care transport.

Normal PaO_2 is 75 to 100 mm Hg. Generally, if the SpO_2 stays $> 90\%$, the PaO_2 will be > 60 mm Hg. As the oxygen level drops, the oxygen saturation monitor will show a declining reading. There is a slight lag during monitoring, so the patient's actual oxygen level may be lower before you see a change on the saturation monitor. Because of the relationship between the partial pressure of oxygen and the saturation percentage, the latter is not very sensitive to changes in $PaO_2 > 60$ mm Hg. When SpO_2 is 90%, PaO_2 is approximately 60 mm Hg. However, at an $SpO_2 < 90\%$, the saturation will decrease by a greater amount than the magnitude of decrease in the

PaO_2. For example, when intubating a severely hypoxic patient, if the patient initially shows a 70% saturation, the PaO_2 may be in the 40s. After intubation, the SpO_2 might improve to 80%, but the PaO_2 may improve only marginally, to about 50 mm Hg.

Other factors can compromise the reliability of SpO_2 monitoring. Nail polish, fake/false nails, paint, or stain/ink on the fingers; cool extremities or a cold environment; shock; poor sensor-to-skin contact; darkly pigmented skin; and low batteries can all cause inaccurate readings. The saturation monitor needs to sense a pulsatile flow in the digit and indicates this by a pulsating bar or flashing light. Make sure the saturation monitor is picking this flow up, as without it your readings may be unreliable. Nonfunctional hemoglobin, such as methemoglobin and carboxyhemoglobin (COHb, from carbon monoxide [CO] poisoning), can also cause false readings. In CO poisoning, the SpO_2 can be 100% but a significant amount of hemoglobin may be bound to CO; in methemoglobinemia, the SpO_2 can falsely approach 75%.

The bottom line on saturation monitoring is that the value you obtain indicates the amount of hemoglobin that is saturated with a gas. It does not verify effective ventilation, and it does not determine the amount of hemoglobin present. Thus, the saturation value can be high when, in fact, a patient is anemic, which can lead to hypoxia. Moreover, saturation monitoring does not indicate which gas is attached to the hemoglobin.

End-Tidal Carbon Dioxide Monitoring

Capnography, the measurement of **end-tidal carbon dioxide ($ETCO_2$)** displayed as a graphic and dynamic wave over time, is a reliable method of confirming proper initial placement of an endotracheal tube because the esophagus normally has a low level of CO_2 or none at all. It is also useful in detecting inadvertent extubation, effectiveness of chest compressions, and return of spontaneous circulation. Capnography employs a detector (mainstream) or a gas sampling device (sidestream) placed between the endotracheal tube and the ventilator or BVM. In addition to waveform capnography, other methods of measuring $ETCO_2$ are available, but are less useful and/or less reliable. These options include digital capnometry, which provides a numerical reading but not a dynamic graphic wave, and colorimetric detectors, which use color changes in pH-sensitive paper to detect $ETCO_2$. The gold standard is waveform capnography, which is the only method that is more reliable than physical examination for the detection of misplaced endotracheal tubes. (For additional discussion of $ETCO_2$ monitoring, see Chapter 1, *Advanced Medical Life Support Assessment for the Medical Patient*.)

Capnography takes CO_2 detection a step further by making the measurement graphic and dynamic, mapping the CO_2 level throughout the respiratory cycle and over time, providing information about the rate of airflow and quality of respiration. The resulting waveform can be broken down into the following phases representing metabolism in the body:

- Phase I is the initial exhalation, consisting of dead-space air that contains no significant amount of CO_2 and thus does not move the graph.
- Phase II is the exhalation of air from the lower airways, which contains escalating amounts of CO_2 owing to the increasing percentage of alveolar air.
- Phase III reflects all alveolar air; the CO_2 level eventually reaches a plateau, which is termed the end-tidal CO_2 level.
- Phase IV (sometimes called phase 0) is inspiration; in this phase, the CO_2 level decreases rapidly.

Figure 3-8 shows a typical waveform produced by capnography. Point A-B (phase I) shows the waveform at zero, or baseline, on the graph. This baseline occurs at the end of inspiration, just before exhalation. As exhalation begins, an upstroke appears on the waveform, represented by point B-C (phase II). This positive deflection occurs as the device immediately begins to detect CO_2. Point C-D (phase III) indicates a slowing of the velocity of the exhalation, with point D representing the peak of exhaled CO_2 at the end of exhalation. As the plateau

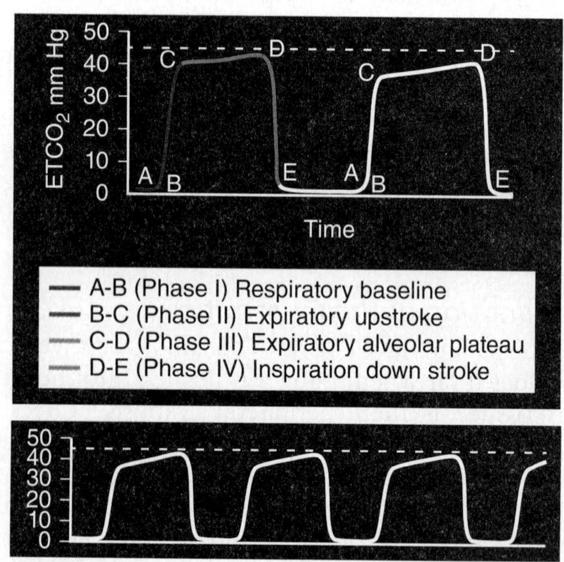

Figure 3-8 Four phases of a normal capnogram. **A-B.** Carbon dioxide–free portion of the respiratory cycle. **B-C.** Rapid upstroke of the curve, representing the transition from inspiration to expiration and the mixing of dead-space and alveolar gas. **C-D.** Alveolar plateau, representing alveolar gas rich in carbon dioxide and tending to slope gently upward with uneven emptying of alveoli. **D-E.** Respiratory downstroke, a nearly vertical drop to baseline.

of the wave is graphed, a negative deflection (dip), or cleft, may indicate the patient's spontaneous respiratory effort. This can be an early sign that neuromuscular paralysis is wearing off. Point D-E on the waveform reflects rapid inhalation as the next breath begins. This stroke is negatively deflected (moving in a downward direction) because little CO_2 is expelled during this part of the respiratory cycle.

Proper endotracheal tube placement should produce a regular, predictable waveform, as illustrated in Figure 3-8. Inadvertent placement of the endotracheal tube in the esophagus produces no regular waveform because there is no significant continuous production of CO_2. Placement of the tip of the endotracheal tube near the glottis may produce some irregular but measurable readings; however, they will not appear as a typical waveform. Any waveform that departs from the expected contours should prompt immediate reevaluation of the patient's intubation status.

As mentioned earlier, the waveform in the intubated patient is accompanied by a number. A normal $ETCO_2$ level is 30 to 40 mm Hg (usually 2 to 5 mm Hg less than in venous blood, but it can be lower) and is present when ventilation and perfusion are well matched. Conditions such as cardiac arrest, pulmonary embolism, and hypovolemic shock make it difficult to achieve normal $ETCO_2$ levels. These levels can also be used to monitor the status and anticipated course of patients with cardiac arrest who receive an advanced airway. An $ETCO_2 < 10$ mm Hg by waveform capnography after 20 minutes of cardiopulmonary resuscitation (CPR) is inconsistent with survival, and a sudden increase in the $ETCO_2$ may be a sign of return of spontaneous circulation.

Finally, the capnography waveform morphology can be used to assess ventilatory mechanics. In particular, a sloping and merging of the upstroke and plateau (phases II and III) indicates decreased airflow during expiration, typical of bronchospasm. This finding is often referred to as a "shark fin" configuration (**Figure 3-9**). With treatment and improvement in the obstructed outflow of air, this shape should normalize on repeated assessments.

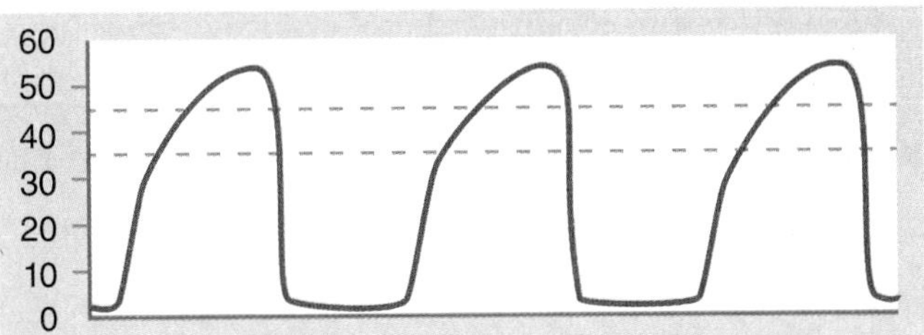

Figure 3-9 The "shark fin" appearance of the waveform indicates the patient is in bronchospasm: The bronchioles are spasming, causing prolonged expiration, and the patient is taking a longer time to blow off the carbon dioxide. The shark fin is a classic presentation for a patient with bronchospasm of any type.

Courtesy of Les R. Becker, PhD, MS.MedL, NRP, CHSE.

Waveform capnography is the "gold standard" assessment tool for verifying the initial and ongoing correct placement of an advanced airway or endotracheal tube. All advanced life support (ALS) agencies should have this technology available, and appropriate competencies in its use should be demonstrated by clinicians. Devices that display waveform capnography in intubated patients can be either mainstream or sidestream units, depending on whether the sensor is in a device attached to the airway or inside the monitor with small sampling line that draws expired air from the patient's airway.

Sidestream $ETCO_2$ Evaluation in the Nonintubated Patient

For patients who are breathing spontaneously without an advanced airway, the individual's CO_2 level at the end of exhalation is generally obtained through sidestream capnography, although this technology is less reliable than the methods used for intubated patients. A CO_2 sampling tube is placed within the patient's nose or mouth, and airway gas samples of the patient's exhalation are sent to a sensor in the machine. Monitoring of nonintubated patients can occur while simultaneously providing supplemental oxygen via cannula. Additionally, changes in respiratory status will be seen almost immediately, particularly in the respiratory rate, whereas it may take minutes for oxygen saturation to decrease, so capnography can be a useful tool when administering sedative medications or those that depress respiratory effort.

Carbon Monoxide Sensors

Carbon monoxide oximeters, also known as CO-oximeters, are indicators of the attachment of carbon monoxide molecules to hemoglobin. Hemoglobin has a higher affinity for carbon monoxide than for oxygen. When a patient has been exposed to carbon monoxide, it may be clinically useful to have a simple method of detecting the precise amount of carbon monoxide binding (measured as the percentage of **carboxyhemoglobin**) that has occurred. The sensor attaches to the patient the same way a traditional oximeter device does, but it relies on different wavelengths of light on the spectrum to detect carboxyhemoglobin in addition to oxyhemoglobin and deoxyhemoglobin. Comparing the results of carbon monoxide oximetry and standard carboxyhemoglobin detection using ABG analysis (an invasive laboratory test), the CO-oximetry method comes within 4.3% of the ABG result. Despite this information, controversy still exists regarding the accuracy and utility of carbon monoxide detection and monitoring in prehospital patients, and these results may not be of significant clinical utility in many patients.

For the earliest and most reliable diagnosis of carbon monoxide poisoning, environmental detectors that are carried by an EMS crew on their "first in" bag give an earlier warning, protect the patient and crew, and provide ongoing surveillance for a carbon monoxide threat even when this diagnosis has not been considered.

Chest Radiography

A chest radiograph is an important diagnostic test for assessing patients with chest pain and dyspnea. Although chest radiography and its interpretation are not part of the skill set required for EMS clinicians, and such imaging is not typically performed in the emergent out-of-hospital setting, critical care transport clinicians should have a basic understanding of chest radiograph interpretation.

Ultrasonography

Ultrasound examination, also called sonography or diagnostic medical sonography, is an imaging method that uses high-frequency sound waves to produce precise images of structures within the body. Such images often provide information that is useful in diagnosing and treating a variety of diseases and conditions.

Ultrasound imaging is a valuable assessment tool in emergency settings, where it is often referred to as POCUS (point-of-care ultrasound). It has many uses, including some that are valuable in assessing respiratory conditions. These applications include the detection of pleural effusion, pneumothorax, hemothorax, and even pneumonia. Ultrasound equipment is relatively expensive, however, and reliable ultrasound evaluation requires training and significant expertise. Such drawbacks tend to limit the availability of this diagnostic tool. Future research will delineate the role of ultrasound imaging in the prehospital environment.

Blood Tests: Arterial Blood Gases and Venous Blood Gases

Arterial blood gases (ABGs) and venous blood gases (VBGs) are used to evaluate both the oxygenation and the acid–base balance of the blood. ABGs are obtained by needle aspiration of arterial blood into a syringe. The blood is then analyzed rapidly and the findings used to direct clinical management of a patient in respiratory distress. A VBG analysis is an alternative method of estimating carbon dioxide and pH that does not require arterial blood sampling.

The pH reflects the acidic or alkalemic condition of the blood. Normal pH in the human body ranges between 7.35 and 7.45. A decreased pH level represents acidosis, whereas an elevated pH level represents alkalosis. Acidosis and alkalosis can be further divided into respiratory and metabolic components. Acidosis of a respiratory nature—that is, respiratory failure—can evolve rapidly. Metabolic conditions can also cause acidosis; diabetic ketoacidosis is a primary example, although shock is the most common cause of metabolic acidosis.

Measuring the PaO_2 is essential in evaluating the presence and degree of hypoxia. Normal values for patients who can breathe room air range from 75 to 100 mm Hg and typically are achieved while breathing 21% oxygen (room air). Hypoxia, defined as a PaO_2 ranging from 50 to 70 mm Hg, is not uncommon in patients with chronic lung disease such as COPD.

The bicarbonate (HCO_3) level reflects the body's acid–base status from a metabolic perspective. A low HCO_3 indicates a metabolic acidosis, and a high HCO_3 level indicates a metabolic alkalosis. The base excess (BE) or base deficit can also be used to evaluate the presence of a metabolic or respiratory condition. The BE normally ranges from –3 to +3. A negative value indicates metabolic acidosis; a positive value indicates metabolic alkalosis.

Arterial Blood Gas Interpretation

For EMS clinicians, it is important to have a basic understanding of ABG findings and their application. Proper mechanical ventilation of a patient is based on ABG findings interpreted in the specific clinical context. The ventilator settings should be guided by precise clinical findings, some of which include blood gases (Table 3-3).

Note that the change in the $PaCO_2$ is proportionately opposite to the pH and reflects a respiratory abnormality or adjustment. Also keep in mind that the BE and HCO_3 levels generally move in the same direction as the pH when a metabolic reason exists for the abnormality or body adjustment.

When you review blood gas results from the lab, a shortcut to guide you toward the correct interpretation is to place an arrow next to each result. Is the result from the patient higher than normal? If so, use an arrow pointing up. Is the result lower than the normal range? If so, use an arrow pointing down.

Table 3-3 Key Blood Gas Results

Parameter	Normal Range	Abnormal Findings	
		Acid	Alkali
pH	7.35–7.45	↓	↑
PCO_2, mm Hg	35–45	↑	↓
PaO_2, mm Hg	75–100	NA	NA
Base excess	−2 to +2	↓	↑
Bicarbonate, mEq/L	22–26	↓	↑

For example, suppose the patient's blood gas results read as follows:

- pH: 7.20
- $PaCO_2$: 78 mm Hg
- PaO_2: 60 mm Hg
- BE: –2
- HCO_3: 22 mEq/l

You note that the PaO_2 is low, indicating the delivery of oxygen is not sufficient. If the patient is breathing room air, you would consider administering oxygen. The pH is down, the $PaCO_2$ is up, and the BE and HCO_3 levels are normal. These findings, taken together, indicate acidosis—specifically, respiratory acidosis. All laboratory results must be correlated with the patient's clinical condition. In this case, you know the way to correct the acidosis is to increase the patient's minute volume. If you were providing mechanical ventilation to this patient, you could correct the minute volume by increasing the rate (frequency), the tidal volume, or both.

The body continually tries to recalibrate its balance, or homeostasis. The mechanisms by which the body adjusts for acid or alkali abnormalities are deployed first and most rapidly through the buffer system, second through the respiratory system, and third—over the course of several days—through the renal system.

The following blood gas results show successful compensation in a patient who is in early hemorrhagic shock:

- pH: 7.36
- $PaCO_2$: 25 mm Hg
- BE: –8
- HCO_3: 15 mEq/l

Clinically, this patient is demonstrating hyperventilation (an early sign of shock) and is blowing off CO_2 to minimize the availability of carbonic acid. In fact, the respiratory system has accomplished this so effectively that the patient's pH remains normal. This state is termed *complete compensation*. Alternatively, you could say the metabolic acidosis is fully compensated. However, this rarely occurs in the acute setting. An important clinical caveat is that patients with a severe metabolic acidosis require hyperventilation to reduce the acidosis, so be sure to provide sufficient ventilation if bagging or mechanically ventilating these patients. They should have a low $PaCO_2$.

Adjusting positive-pressure ventilation based on blood gas results is standard practice in the critical care arena. One way to do this from a practical standpoint is as follows:

1. $PaCO_2$ is largely a function of respiratory rate (rr) and tidal volume (TV).
   - For increased $PaCO_2$: Increase rr by 2 to 5 breaths/min or TV by 50 to 100 mL
   - For decreased $PaCO_2$: Decrease rr by 2 to 5 breaths/min or TV by 50 to 100 mL
2. Acute changes in SpO_2 as measured by pulse oximetry should be managed by adjusting the fraction of inspired oxygen (FiO_2) and the level of positive end-expiratory pressure (PEEP). PEEP increases the pressure within the alveoli and can open atelectatic or collapsed alveoli or drive oxygen into alveoli filled with fluid. Changes in PEEP must be undertaken with caution, especially when PEEP levels are > 7 to 10 cm H_2O.
   - For increases in $SpO_2 > 95\%$: Decrease FiO_2 in increments of 5% to maintain SpO_2 at $> 94\%$.

Venous Blood Gas Interpretation

Venous (rather than arterial) blood gases are often used in the emergency care setting. This practice has obvious clinical advantages: It reduces the number of high-risk arterial punctures required to obtain laboratory samples, it provides enough data for clinicians to determine the presence of most metabolic disorders, and it eliminates a painful experience for the patient. VBG values, except for the partial pressure of oxygen (PO_2), correlate closely with arterial values.

One disadvantage of VBG testing is that it does not measure the PaO_2 level. Pulse oximetry may be used as an adjunct to VBG sampling for this purpose. Table 3-4 demonstrates the differences in normal VBG and ABG values.

Pulmonary Function Tests

Pulmonary function tests (PFTs) are a group of tests often ordered by pulmonologists for patients with breathing difficulties to better characterize the nature and severity of their illness. PFTs measure how well the lungs take in and release air and how well they move gases such as oxygen from the atmosphere into the body's circulation.

Table 3-4 Comparison of Arterial and Venous Blood Gas Values in Healthy Volunteers

	Arterial Blood Gas Values	Venous Blood Gas Values
pH	7.38-7.42	7.35-7.38
PCO_2, mm Hg	38-42	44-48
PO_2, mm Hg	80-100	40
HCO_3, mEq/l	24	22-26

Reproduced from Sherman SC, Schindlbeck M. When is venous blood gas analysis enough? *Emerg Med.* 2006;38:44-48. Copyrighted 2015. IMNG. 119131:0815BN

In the field or emergency department (ED), you may measure a peak expiratory flow rate, or peak flow, in patients with bronchospasm. This rate is a measure of airflow and is evaluated against an expected norm based on age, height, and sex or against the patient's known baseline. Measurements can determine the effectiveness of your therapies or direct you to another cause of the patient's shortness of breath.

Refine the Differential Diagnosis

After you have obtained the patient's history and performed a physical exam and pertinent diagnostic tests based on the patient's chief complaint, you should develop a differential diagnosis. Differential diagnosis of dyspnea by body system is summarized in Table 3-5.

Table 3-5 Differential Diagnosis of Dyspnea by Body System

Life Threatening	Emergent	Nonemergent
	Pulmonary Diagnoses	
Airway obstruction	Spontaneous pneumothorax	Pleural effusion, stable or small
Pulmonary embolus	Asthma exacerbation	Neoplasm
Tension pneumothorax	COPD exacerbation	
Anaphylaxis	Aspiration pneumonia	COPD
	Noncardiogenic edema	
	Cardiac Diagnoses	
Pulmonary edema	Pericarditis	Coronary artery disease
Myocardial infarction/acute coronary syndrome (ACS)	Decompensated HF	Valvular heart disease
Cardiac tamponade		Cardiomyopathy
	Metabolic Diagnoses	
Diabetic ketoacidosis	Hyperglycemia, severe	
Thyroid storm	Hyperthyroidism	
	Infectious Diagnoses	
Sepsis	Pneumonia, viral (e.g., COVID-19, influenza)	Upper respiratory infection
Meningitis	Pneumonia, bacterial	Bronchitis
Epiglottitis	Pneumonia, fungal	Tuberculosis
Bacterial tracheitis	Empyema	
Retropharyngeal abscess	Large pleural effusion	
Foreign object aspiration	Lung abscess	
	Hematologic Diagnoses	
Severe anemia	Acute moderate anemia	Chronic anemia
Hemorrhage, gastrointestinal	Leukemia, acute complications	Lymphoma

Life Threatening	Emergent	Nonemergent
	Neurologic Diagnoses	
Intracerebral hemorrhage	Guillain-Barré syndrome	Neuromuscular degenerative disease (ALS)
		Myasthenia gravis
		Multiple sclerosis

ALS, amyotrophic lateral sclerosis; COPD, chronic obstructive pulmonary disease; HF, heart failure.

Ongoing Management

Before the treatments discussed in the following sections are administered, a variety of other standard interventions should have already been implemented. Supplemental oxygen to keep the oxygen saturation at > 94% and an intravenous line are typical interventions for any patient who needs advanced life support. Psychological support is also an important consideration for a patient with dyspnea. Your efforts to reduce the patient's anxiety with a calm, professional, and caring demeanor can help reduce the patient's heart rate and blood pressure and allow the patient to maximize breathing effectiveness.

Initial and Basic Management Techniques

Supplemental Oxygen

Supplemental oxygen is the easiest, quickest, and most efficient way to improve oxygenation in a breathing patient. Oxygen is usually delivered by nasal cannula, which can effectively provide a flow of 24% to 40% oxygen. Higher flow rates (i.e., > 6 L/min) can cause patient discomfort, especially when given over the long term. Specialized devices can safely deliver very high flow rates for neonatal, pediatric, and adult patients, which are effective for increasing oxygenation and lowering hypercapnia. Oxygen may be administered with humidification, reducing the drying effect of the inspired air.

Use of a face mask can increase the concentration of oxygen administered to as much as 60% when 15 L/min of oxygen is given. The Venturi (air entrainment) mask is a specialized face mask that gives the clinician more precise control over the amount of inspired oxygen, which can range from 28% to 40%. The Venturi mask and the standard face mask have one problem in common: Placing a device over both the nose and mouth of a dyspneic patient may increase the patient's anxiety and often results in the patient removing the mask.

The nonrebreather face mask adds an oxygen reservoir to the standard face mask, increasing the inspired oxygen level to 80% to 100% at 15 l/min of oxygen flow. The nonrebreather mask often functions as a bridging device to another modality because a patient who needs that much oxygen typically requires some other type of ventilatory support, such as **noninvasive positive-pressure ventilation (NIPPV)** or intubation. If aggressive care is successful, the patient can be weaned down to a lower FiO_2 instead of being intubated.

Positive-Pressure Ventilation

Patients with respiratory failure need positive-pressure ventilation to improve gas exchange and relieve their work of breathing. While some patients with chronic lung disease have chronically abnormal ABGs, acute respiratory failure is defined by the following criteria:

- $PaO_2 < 55$ mm Hg or $SpO_2 < 90\%$
- $PaCO_2 > 50$ mm Hg or $ETCO_2 > 55$ mm Hg
- pH < 7.32
- Decreasing mental status or severe fatigue in setting of labored breathing

You can provide this ventilatory support noninvasively through a BVM, CPAP, or bilevel positive airway pressure (BiPAP).

BVM

The BVM has become a standard respiratory resuscitation tool for patients of all ages. Certain considerations are typical regardless of which manual resuscitator system you purchase and use. You must stock and select the correct sizes of bags and masks for all patients.

Many newer BVMs have PEEP valve capability, especially in the hospital and interfacility transport settings. In addition, oxygenation is improved when a reservoir bag or tube is added *and* you administer ventilation slowly (over 1 to 2 seconds) with just enough TV to raise the chest. Standard adult bag devices are 1,500 to 2,000 mL in volume; note that TV should generally be approximately 400 to 500 mL. Newly designed BVM systems allow you to adjust PEEP and may limit the flow rate and provide metronome for timing of ventilations.

BVMs are the preferred initial choice for providing ventilation in a cardiac arrest scenario, but they can be

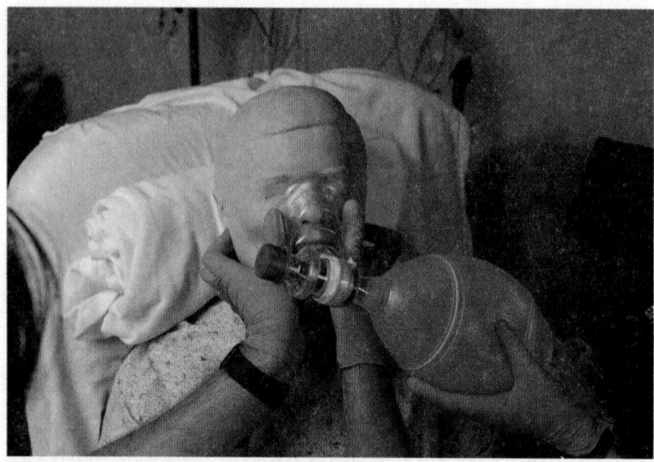

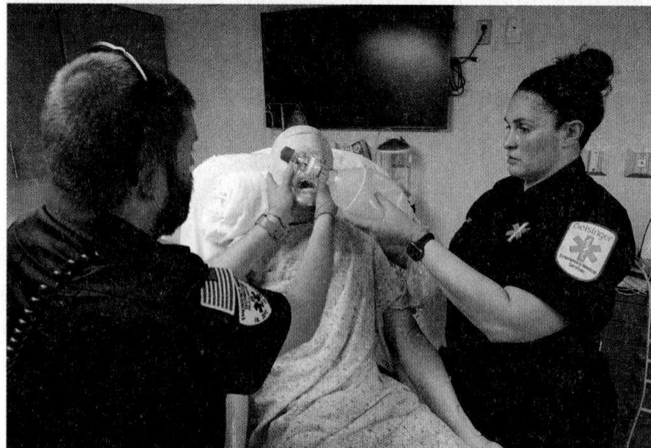

Figure 3-10 Demonstration of two-person, two-thumbs-up BVM ventilation in the sitting position.

beneficial in ventilating a conscious patient who is in acute respiratory distress as well. In the latter situation, the awake patient will have better respiratory dynamics if they remain sitting upright or in semi-Fowler's position (**Figure 3-10**) and the ventilating clinician approaches them from the front and applies the mask with a two-thumbs-up technique. The clinician's longest fingers can be used to add some jaw thrust, and PEEP can be added if available on the device. The BVM can also be used to ventilate and resuscitate a hypoxic patient with pulmonary edema or COPD.

A misconception about manual (self-inflating) BVM systems is that they all deliver 100% oxygen if you add 12 to 15 liters of oxygen to the reservoir. *If* you administer ventilation slowly, with moderate TV and a good mask seal, delivery can approach 100% oxygen using those devices—but it is difficult to do so. A more realistic estimate is 65% to 80% oxygenation. Non–self-inflating devices or anesthesia bags do deliver 100% oxygen to the patient. Clinicians in many critical care areas prefer these bags because they are sensitive to the patient's lung compliance while administering ventilation, although they are not easy to use in practice. The flow-control valve on an anesthesia bag gives it built-in PEEP capability.

BVM ventilation is an often underappreciated skill and one that is not always performed adequately. One-person BVM ventilation technique is notorious for difficult and less effective ventilation, and the value of two-person BVM ventilation with a two-thumbs-up approach has been increasingly favored when adequate resources are available. Education curricula should consider the importance and frequency of BVM utilization. Obtaining an effective seal and providing an appropriate TV and respiratory rate are critical to patient outcomes. Use of BVM ventilation is associated with high TVs and pressures. Clinicians must use great caution to avoid excessive TVs or respiratory rates. Some modern EMS monitors now include a respiratory sensor that can be attached to the BVM to provide real-time feedback on the TV and respiratory rate being delivered.

Continuous Positive Airway Pressure

CPAP is a ventilatory technique used to apply a modest amount of continuous positive pressure in the airway to an alert patient to keep smaller airways open, reduce the work of breathing, and improve alveolar oxygenation. CPAP devices can be beneficial for patients who are having moderate to severe respiratory difficulty, such as those with asthma, emphysema, and HF. This technique reduces left ventricular preload and afterload in patients with HF, and it has been shown to significantly decrease the need for intubation.

For the CPAP device to be effective, a good seal must be maintained between the mask and the patient's face. Various mask types may cover the nose and mouth, nose only, or full face, or use a nasal pillow. The mask is often secured to the face with adjustable straps, allowing the patient to relax rather than worry about holding the mask in place. CPAP is commonly utilized in the prehospital environment and is becoming recognized as a basic life support (BLS) skill in many geographic areas. It also has a substantial presence as a home therapy for patients with sleep apnea.

Bilevel Positive Airway Pressure

BiPAP (**Figure 3-11**) is a modality being used more frequently in the emergency setting, as it leverages the advantages of CPAP while adding more inspiratory support. This noninvasive technique can ease the work of breathing, improve ventilation, and greatly reduce the need for intubation.

BiPAP is a form of NIPPV, like CPAP, but it has two different levels of pressure support: one pressure during inspiration (inspiratory positive airway pressure) and a different pressure during exhalation (expiratory positive airway pressure). Ventilation is delivered through a mask that covers either the nose only or both the mouth and nose.

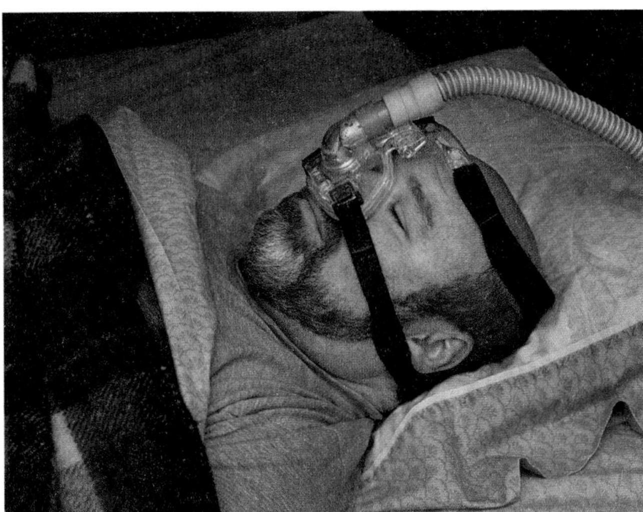

Figure 3-11 Patient with a bilevel positive airway pressure (BiPAP) mask applied.

Both CPAP and BiPAP are valuable noninvasive tools for supporting a patient's respiratory effort, but they are not without drawbacks. Some patients, especially those prone to claustrophobia, cannot tolerate having their nose and mouth covered—a factor that reduces compliance and can increase patients' sense of distress. The continuous positive pressure can impede venous return and thus reduce blood pressure; it may also contribute to gastric distention and raise the risk of aspiration. Finally, increased positive airway pressure carries the risk of barotrauma, specifically pneumothorax or tension pneumothorax (discussed later).

Intubation

Ultimately, patients who are in respiratory failure may need to be intubated and ventilated. Intubation can be lifesaving care, and many patients can be extubated within a day or two and have an excellent outcome. However, when you are deciding whether to intubate a patient, the following issues must be weighed along with the protocols, medical direction, and any expression of the patient's wishes:

- Intubation should be considered the last option for patients who have severe asthma. Patients with asthma are extremely difficult to ventilate and are prone to pneumothoraces and other complications of mechanical ventilation.
- Be proactive; ventilate patients before cardiac arrest occurs. When in doubt, attempt to ventilate. A patient who is combative may not be ready for intubation. If a patient allows you to apply positive-pressure ventilation, then this intervention was probably necessary. Patients who are conscious, yet still in respiratory distress, will require sedation and neuromuscular blocking medications (through rapid-sequence intubation) to facilitate intubation. Dissociative doses of ketamine are becoming popular for the sedation component due to their low risk of causing or worsening hypotension.
- Patients who are unresponsive may have little or no gag reflex, which poses a grave danger if the patient vomits. Consider intubating patients in these situations to protect the airway even if ventilation is adequate.
- Some patients who have diabetes or have overdosed present with an obvious need for intubation. However, if administration of dextrose or naloxone is likely to completely change the scenario, it might be better to use BVM ventilation for a few minutes to monitor the effect of the initial therapy. Ventilate slowly (over 1 second) and use only enough ventilation to produce visible chest rise.
- Evolving airway management strategies call for use of a high-flow nasal cannula for passive oxygenation (apneic oxygenation) during attempts at intubation. Sufficient sources of oxygen must be available.

Ventilator Management

Invasive Airway Ventilation

Emergent ventilatory management is always (or almost always) performed in response to a clinical presentation of respiratory distress and/or a declining level of consciousness. The initial goal of invasive airway ventilation is to ensure that the airway is secure and protected and that ventilation and oxygenation are adequate.

Invasive ventilation techniques for intubated patients include pressure-cycled and volume-cycled ventilators.

Pressure-Cycled Ventilation

In pressure-cycled ventilation, a breath is delivered using an operator-determined pressure level (rather than the TV). This predetermined level is, by definition, the peak inspiratory pressure. The operator must also set the respiratory rate and inspiratory time, which together with the set pressure and patient compliance determine the actual TV and minute volume.

Volume-Cycled Ventilation

In volume-cycled ventilation, a preset tidal volume is programmed into the device. Inhalation is terminated when the limit has been reached. A major advantage of this type of ventilator is that it delivers the tidal volume regardless of changes in lung compliance. Assist/control and intermittent mandatory ventilation are types of volume-cycled ventilators. This is the most commonly used type of ventilation in emergent settings.

Modes of Ventilatory Support

Four principal methods are used to deliver volume-cycled and pressure-cycled ventilation:

1. *Controlled mechanical ventilation (CMV)*. The ventilator delivers breaths at a preset interval, regardless of the patient's respiratory effort. This mode is appropriate only for apneic patients and for those who have been pharmacologically paralyzed. It is rarely used in the current setting of modern critical care medicine.
2. *Assist/controlled (A/C) ventilation*. The ventilator provides a set rate and TV. If the patient takes a breath, it triggers the ventilator to provide a full breath based on the set TV. This is a common ventilator setting during the early phase of ventilatory support.
3. *Intermittent mandatory ventilation (IMV)*. This mode combines CMV with the patient's spontaneous ventilation. The ventilator provides a set rate of mandatory breaths. If the patient puts forth a respiratory effort, the ventilator does not trigger a mechanical breath, although positive-pressure support can be provided. IMV in an alert patient requires less sedation and no paralysis, and it allows the patient to preserve muscle tone in the muscles of ventilation, which makes it easier to wean the patient from mechanical ventilation.
4. *Synchronous intermittent mandatory ventilation (SIMV)*. This mode is similar to IMV but delivers mandatory breaths in synchrony with patient breathing. Synchronous delivery prevents stacking of breaths (a mechanical breath being delivered at the same time as a spontaneous breath—a drawback of IMV), which may cause barotrauma from hyperinflation.

When choosing a mode, determine how the ventilator should respond to a patient's spontaneous respiration. Consider the patient's mental status, including whether the patient will be aware of the activity of the ventilator. Attempting to breathe and receiving no response from the ventilator can make even the calmest patient extremely anxious. Conscious patients can be placed on SIMV, and totally awake patients who are being prepared for extubation may be placed on pressure-support ventilation. A heavily sedated patient or one with severe brain injury, however, may put forth no respiratory effort. Such patients require near-total mechanical control and are candidates for A/C ventilation.

Mechanical Ventilator Settings

When initiating mechanical ventilation, you must select a ventilatory mode, TV or pressure support level, respiratory rate, and initial oxygenation concentration. Supplemental choices include PEEP. These parameters can be altered to meet specific clinical requirements, such as an anxious patient with respiratory failure and HF who prefers to breathe at a rate of 20 breaths/min but whose TV is less than that predicted on the basis of ideal body weight. Table 3-6 summarizes typical ventilator settings.

Minute Volume

Minute volume is the amount of air inspired per minute. Minute volume combines TV with the respiratory rate to ensure that enough air is inspired to support adequate ventilation.

Tidal Volume

The TV (ventilation volume) and respiratory rate should approximate the patient's own normal rate of respiration. Most adults draw a TV of between 5 and 10 milliliters per kilogram (mL/kg) of ideal body weight. Typical settings for an adult who is not in distress are a volume of 6 to 8 mL/kg of ideal body weight and a respiratory rate of 12 breaths/min. The ideal way to determine tidal volume is by using a height-based predicted body weight Table 3-7.

FiO_2

The FiO_2 is also chosen as an initial ventilator setting. Choices range from 100% down to 21%. A severely dyspneic patient who has a low PO_2 may benefit from an initial setting of 100% until their respiratory status has stabilized. Few patients who require emergent or urgent intubation will tolerate 21% oxygen, which is the same as room air. Virtually all patients requiring aggressive airway management will need some oxygen supplementation, but the precise degree will vary from patient to patient. Settings for FiO_2 typically fall between 40% and 80%.

Positive End-Expiratory Pressure

Most ventilators accommodate PEEP, a small amount of positive pressure that remains present even at the peak of expiration. Similar to CPAP in spontaneously breathing patients, this pressure opens small bronchioles and alveoli clogged with mucus, vomitus, infiltrate (in patients with pneumonia), and edema (in patients with HF), and helps keep them open. PEEP can help patients who have alveolar collapse, as is seen in pneumonia and pulmonary edema, and provides for stenting of the small airways that might otherwise collapse during exhalation. PEEP at approximately 5 cm H_2O reproduces the normal end-expiratory pressure observed in nonventilated patients. This level, called physiologic PEEP, should be

Table 3-6 Common Ventilator Settings

Setting	Description	Common Settings	Comments
Rate or frequency (f)	Number of breaths delivered per minute	6–20/min	
Tidal volume (TV)	Volume of gas delivered to the patient	6–8 mL/kg	
Oxygen (FiO_2)	Fraction of inspired oxygen delivered	21–100%	Blender required if $< 100\%$
Positive end-expiratory pressure (PEEP)	Positive pressure delivered at the end of exhalation	5–20 cm H_2O	This function improves oxygenation.
Pressure support (PS)	Pressure support to augment inspiratory effort	5–20 cm H_2O	
Inspiratory flow rate/time	Speed with which TV is delivered	40–80 l/min Time: 0.8–1.2 seconds	
Inspiration/expiration (I/E) ratio	Duration of inspiration to expiration	1:2	
Sensitivity	Determines the amount of effort the patient must generate to initiate a breath	0.5–1.5 cm H_2O below baseline pressure	
High pressure limit	Maximum pressure with which the ventilator can deliver the tidal volume	10–20 cm H_2O above peak inspiratory pressure	The ventilator will stop the breath and release the rest to the atmosphere when the limit is reached.

applied to nearly all ventilated patients. Higher PEEP is used therapeutically to improve oxygenation in patients with conditions such as those described earlier.

Complications of Mechanical Ventilation

Invasive mechanical ventilation is associated with several serious risks. Volutrauma is lung injury or alveolar rupture from overdistention of the alveoli. Barotrauma is lung injury from an excessively high airway pressure. These two terms are related and refer to similar types of lung injury. Pneumothorax and tension pneumothorax are the primary concerns in ventilator-induced barotrauma; pneumomediastinum and pneumoperitoneum are less-frequent complications. The risk of these complications is the driving force behind the use of lung-protective strategies.

Prolonged administration of high-concentration oxygen can damage cells and lead to atelectasis. Persistently high intrathoracic pressure can cause decreased cardiac return and low systolic blood pressure.

Another complication can arise when patients receive positive-pressure ventilation. As noted earlier, applying PEEP can help keep distal alveoli open and improve oxygenation. Ventilation of patients who have obstructive lung diseases such as asthma or COPD, however, may cause a complication called auto-PEEP. In this condition, too little time for exhalation leads to progressively increased air trapping. This phenomenon limits delivery of an effective TV and allows intrathoracic pressure to become so high that hemodynamic compromise occurs because of decreased venous return, which in turn

Table 3-7 Conversions for Determining Tidal Volume Based on Patient Height

Height	Predicted Body Weight (kg)	4 mL	5 mL	6 mL	7 mL	8 mL
			Women			
4'0" (48 in. [122 cm])	17.9	72	90	107	125	143
4'1" (49 in. [124.5 cm])	20.2	81	101	121	141	162
4'2" (50 in. [127 cm])	22.5	90	113	135	158	180
4'3" (51 in. [129.5 cm])	24.8	99	124	149	174	198
4'4" (52 in. [132 cm])	27.1	108	136	163	190	217
4'5" (53 in. [135 cm])	29.4	118	147	176	206	235
4'6" (54 in. [137 cm])	31.7	127	159	190	222	254
4'7" (55 in. [140 cm])	34	136	170	204	238	272
4'8" (56 in. [142 cm])	36.3	145	182	218	254	290
4'9" (57 in. [145 cm])	38.6	154	193	232	270	309
4'10" (58 in. [147 cm])	40.9	164	205	245	286	327
4'11" (59 in. [150 cm])	43.2	173	216	259	302	346
5'0" (60 in. [152 cm])	45.5	182	228	273	319	364
5'1" (61 in. [155 cm])	47.8	191	239	287	335	382
5'2" (62 in. [157.5 cm])	50.1	200	251	301	351	401
5'3" (63 in. [160 cm])	52.4	210	262	314	367	419
5'4" (64 in. [162.5 cm])	54.7	219	274	328	383	438
5'5" (65 in. [165 cm])	57	228	285	342	399	456
5'6" (66 in. [168 cm])	59.3	237	297	356	415	474
5'7" (67 in. [170 cm])	61.6	246	308	370	431	493
5'8" (68 in. [173 cm])	63.9	256	320	383	447	511
5'9" (69 in. [175 cm])	66.2	265	331	397	363	530
5'10" (70 in. [178 cm])	68.5	274	343	411	480	548
5'11" (71 in. [180 cm])	70.8	283	354	425	496	566
6'0" (72 in. [183 cm])	73.1	292	366	439	512	585
6'1" (73 in. [185 cm])	75.4	302	377	452	528	603
6'2" (74 in. [188 cm])	77.7	311	389	466	544	622
6'3" (75 in. [190.5 cm])	80	320	400	480	560	640
6'4" (76 in. [193 cm])	82.3	329	412	494	576	658

Height	Predicted Body Weight (kg)	4 mL	5 mL	6 mL	7 mL	8 mL
6'5" (77 in. [195.5 cm])	84.6	338	423	508	592	677
6'6" (78 in. [198 cm])	86.9	348	435	521	608	695
6'7" (79 in. [201 cm])	89.2	357	446	535	624	714
6'8" (80 in. [203 cm])	91.5	366	458	549	641	732
6'9" (81 in. [206 cm])	93.8	375	469	563	657	750
6'10" (82 in. [208 cm])	96.1	384	481	577	673	769
6'11" (83 in. [211 cm])	98.4	394	492	590	689	787
7'0" (84 in. [213 cm])	100.7	403	504	604	705	806
	Men					
4'0" (48 in. [122 cm])	22.4	90	112	134	157	179
4'1" (49 in. [124.5 cm])	24.7	99	124	148	173	198
4'2" (50 in. [127 cm])	27	108	135	162	189	216
4'3" (51 in. [129.5 cm])	29.3	117	147	176	205	234
4'4" (52 in. [132 cm])	31.6	126	158	190	221	253
4'5" (53 in. [135 cm])	33.9	136	170	203	237	271
4'6" (54 in. [137 cm])	36.2	145	181	217	253	290
4'7" (55 in. [140 cm])	38.5	154	193	231	270	308
4'8" (56 in. [142 cm])	40.8	163	204	245	286	326
4'9" (57 in. [145 cm])	43.1	172	216	259	302	345
4'10" (58 in. [147 cm])	45.4	182	227	272	318	363
4'11" (59 in. [150 cm])	47.7	191	239	286	334	382
5'0" (60 in. [152 cm])	50	200	250	300	350	400
5'1" (61 in. [155 cm])	52.3	209	262	314	366	418
5'2" (62 in. [157.5 cm])	54.6	218	273	328	382	437
5'3" (63 in. [160 cm])	56.9	228	285	341	398	455
5'4" (64 in. [162.5 cm])	59.2	237	296	355	414	474
5'5" (65 in. [165 cm])	61.5	246	308	369	431	492
5'6" (66 in. [168 cm])	63.8	255	319	383	447	510
5'7" (67 in. [170 cm])	66.1	264	331	397	463	529
5'8" (68 in. [173 cm])	68.4	274	342	410	479	547

(*continues*)

Table 3-7 Conversions for Determining Tidal Volume Based on Patient Height (*continued*)

Height	Predicted Body Weight (kg)	4 mL	5 mL	6 mL	7 mL	8 mL
5'9" (69 in. [175 cm])	70.7	283	354	424	495	566
5'10" (70 in. [178 cm])	73	292	365	438	511	584
5'11" (71 in. [180 cm])	75.3	301	377	452	527	602
6'0" (72 in. [183 cm])	77.6	310	388	466	543	621
6'1" (73 in. [185 cm])	79.9	320	400	479	559	639
6'2" (74 in. [188 cm])	82.2	329	411	493	575	658
6'3" (75 in. [190.5 cm])	84.5	338	423	507	592	676
6'4" (76 in. [193 cm])	86.8	347	434	521	608	694
6'5" (77 in. [195.5 cm])	89.1	356	446	535	624	713
6'6" (78 in. [198 cm])	91.4	366	457	548	640	731
6'7" (79 in. [201 cm])	93.7	375	469	562	656	750
6'8" (80 in. [203 cm])	96	384	480	576	672	768
6'9" (81 in. [206 cm])	98.3	393	492	590	688	786
6'10" (82 in. [208 cm])	100.6	402	503	604	704	805
6'11" (83 in. [211 cm])	102.9	412	515	617	720	823
7'0" (84 in. [213 cm])	105.2	421	526	631	736	842

Reproduced from Pennsylvania Department of Health Bureau of Emergency Medical Services. Pennsylvania Statewide Advanced Life Support Protocols. Pennsylvania Department of Health; 2020. https://www.health.pa.gov/topics/Documents/EMS/2020%20PA%20ALS%20Protocols%20Final.pdf

compromises cardiac output. Correction requires allowing longer expiratory times by altering the inspiratory to expiratory (I:E) ratio and/or decreasing the respiratory rate. External PEEP can help ameliorate auto-PEEP.

According to a consensus statement from the National Association of EMS Physicians, given the risk of lung injury and worse clinical outcomes associated with non-lung-protective ventilation in numerous clinical environments, it is reasonable to apply lung-protective strategies to the prehospital environment, even in the absence of direct studies demonstrating the benefit of this approach. These strategies include avoiding excessive pressure and volume during ventilation. The choices made during patients' prehospital management may also influence the settings that are subsequently used in the ED or inpatient units.

In an intubated patient, a rapidly declining condition may warrant a quick assessment of the most common causes of acute deterioration using the DOPE mnemonic (**Rapid Recall Box 3-1**).

Special Circumstances with Mechanical Ventilation

Closely monitoring the patient during intubation and subsequent mechanical ventilation is imperative because sedation that is adequate to allow mechanical ventilation can prevent the patient from communicating symptoms of an evolving complication. Immediately investigate and address any unexplained tachycardia, bradycardia, hypotension, or hypertension. Use waveform capnography and SpO_2 monitoring to direct your selection of ventilator settings. Reduce the FiO_2 as soon as possible, consistent with maintaining an adequate PO_2.

Patients with asthma or COPD may require a high inspiratory pressure, longer expiratory time, slower rate, and larger TV. These patients tend to retain air volume and have a high airway pressure, putting them at markedly increased risk of barotrauma. PEEP may help reduce air retention, for which these patients are at high risk.

The discussion of mechanical ventilation presented here is introductory in nature, and is included to stimulate

RAPID RECALL BOX 3-1

Assessing Causes of Acute Deterioration in the Intubated Patient

When you are evaluating an intubated patient for acute deterioration, begin by taking the patient off the ventilator and performing ventilation with a BVM during the assessment. Use the DOPE acronym to guide you.

- **D Displaced tube.** Has the tube been accidentally displaced? Auscultate for bilateral breath sounds and absence of epigastric sounds. Use capnography/capnometry. Gastric **D**istention is another potential cause of difficulty ventilating the patient.
- **O Obstructed tube.** Does the patient have thick secretions that have plugged the distal tube? Perform sterile suctioning. Is the patient biting on the tube to obstruct it? Insert a bite block.
- **P Pneumothorax.** Has pneumothorax occurred during positive-pressure ventilation? Listen for breath sounds. Sense lung compliance while ventilating with bag-valve device. Is it hard to squeeze the bag because of high intrathoracic pressure? If a tension pneumothorax is present, perform needle decompression until a chest tube can be inserted. When appropriate, adding **P**EEP can improve the patient's oxygenation.
- **E Equipment failure.** Has the ventilator run out of oxygen to drive the ventilatory pressure? Check the oxygen tank and ventilator for correct function. An endotracheal tube failure such as rupture of the balloon or a leak should be considered.

your lifelong learning motivation. Nevertheless, by itself, it does not provide you with adequate education, knowledge, or experience to care for mechanically ventilated patients. Formal education regarding mechanical ventilation and on the specific ventilator being used should be obtained before caring for these patients.

Upper Airway Conditions

The upper respiratory tract is vulnerable to many conditions that can obstruct the airway and consequently impair ventilation. Infection is the most common cause of such conditions, but allergic reactions and foreign bodies can also obstruct airflow. Patients with airway obstructions may have no obvious outward signs of illness (e.g., swelling and positional breathing) but may have difficulty swallowing (dysphagia) to the point of drooling. Abnormal sounds may be generated when they breathe or speak. The sound most commonly associated with upper airway obstruction is stridor, which is typically heard on inspiration.

Upper airway involvement may be minor, taking the form of rhinitis (inflammation and congestion of the nasal airway) or laryngitis (irritation of the larynx from overuse, irritation, or infection). Some upper airway diseases such as epiglottitis can become life threatening, and you must have a safe and smart plan for airway management in such cases that includes proper positioning of the patient. When you suspect the patient might have one of these conditions, avoid agitation and tongue depressor evaluations. These patients may also prefer to maintain an upright or "sniffing" position.

Upper Airway Obstruction

The most common cause of upper airway obstruction in a semiconscious or unconscious patient is the tongue relaxing posteriorly and obstructing the hypopharynx in a supine individual. Aspiration of foreign objects can be a source of upper airway obstruction as well.

Signs and Symptoms

Sudden onset of coughing, dyspnea, and signs of choking are the hallmarks of aspiration of a foreign object. Depending on the size and position of the object and the diameter of the airway, the patient may have either total or partial obstruction. Partial obstruction of the lower airway may cause air trapping, with a sudden change in thoracic pressure leading to pneumothorax or pneumomediastinum. Sudden onset of wheezing, especially in an infant or child and particularly in one lung, should raise suspicion that a foreign object has been aspirated.

In some cases, aspirated foreign objects may remain trapped in the airway for several days, weeks, or even months. Chronic blockage of a bronchus can cause bronchial collapse and obstructive pneumonia. Even obstructions in the esophagus can be responsible for airway compromise.

Treatment

Management of an aspirated foreign object should be dictated by the patient's ability to breathe or cough effectively. Supplemental oxygen may alleviate symptoms sufficiently to allow transport to the ED. Patients who exhibit severe stridor, low oxygen saturation, cyanosis, or signs of impending respiratory failure need immediate interventions. Management of such scenarios is challenging for even the most experienced clinician—not just the physical act of removing a foreign object from an anxious, dyspneic patient, but also calming the distressed caregivers.

For conscious adult patients with mild obstruction, provide supportive care and encourage coughing. For those with severe obstruction, administer abdominal thrusts. If the patient loses consciousness, initiation of chest compressions and ventilations is recommended, with the airway being checked for a visible foreign body before the first breath is administered. Administer oxygen if the patient is hypoxic. Suction should be on and available at the patient's side. Be ready to assist ventilations with a BVM. Direct laryngoscopy should be performed to look for a visible obstruction; if one is observed, attempt its removal with Magill forceps or other appropriate device. Consider intubation if the patient remains unresponsive. Preparing the family with a brief, simple description of the procedure before you attempt object removal can alleviate some of their anxiety.

An object visualized below the glottis may be difficult to grasp and not easily removed. In a case series, SLAT (simultaneous laryngoscopy and abdominal thrust) was successful in advancing the foreign body outward where it could be grasped with Magill forceps. Another technique shown to be successful is blindly passing an endotracheal tube into the trachea to move the object to a less-obstructive position, though this maneuver should be attempted only if you are a skilled, experienced clinician faced with a complete obstruction.

If you cannot clear the obstruction with BLS maneuvers and laryngoscopy, and you are unable to ventilate the patient, then it will be necessary to perform a cricothyrotomy. Attempt this procedure only if you are trained and it is allowed by local protocol.

After removal of a foreign object, intubation may still be indicated if the patient has a decreased level of consciousness, is intoxicated or bleeding, or requires oxygenation and respiratory support. Retain the object so it can be inspected at the receiving facility. The patient's post-transport condition or suspicion that portions of the aspirated object have been retained may warrant bronchoscopy in the hospital.

Anaphylactic Reactions

Anaphylaxis is an extreme systemic form of allergic reaction involving two or more body systems. Although the immune system is essential to life and health, sometimes it becomes overzealous in defending the body. The resulting problems may range in severity from hay fever to anaphylaxis, and may exist along a spectrum from a simple annoyance to a life-threatening crisis. During anaphylactic reactions, the immune system becomes hypersensitive to one or more substances. The body often has these reactions to substances that should not be identified as harmful by the immune system—substances such as ragweed, strawberries, and penicillin. The immune cells of a person with allergies are more sensitive than the immune cells of a person without allergies. Although these cells can recognize and react to dangerous invaders such as bacteria and viruses, they may also identify harmless substances as posing a threat.

Pathophysiology

When an invading substance enters the body, mast cells recognize it as potentially harmful and begin releasing chemical mediators. Histamine, one of the primary chemical weapons in this response, causes the blood vessels in the local area to dilate and the capillaries to leak. Leukotrienes, which are even more powerful, are released and cause additional dilation and leaking. White blood cells are called to the area to help engulf and destroy the enemy, and platelets begin to collect and clump together. In most cases, this overreaction to harmless invaders is usually restricted to the local area being invaded. The runny, itchy nose and swollen eyes associated with hay fever are examples of a local allergic reaction.

In the case of anaphylaxis, however, chemical mediators are released, and the effect involves more than one system throughout the body. The initial effect may reflect the release of histamine, which causes skin symptoms (hives), vomiting, and hypotension. Later responses involving the much more powerful leukotrienes compound the effects of histamine. The patient's respiratory status will deteriorate as these highly potent bronchoconstrictors are released.

Signs and Symptoms

Patients with anaphylaxis may present with CNS symptoms in response to decreased cerebral perfusion and hypoxia—for example, headache, dizziness, confusion, and anxiety. The most common complaints are usually respiratory symptoms, which often present as shortness of breath or dyspnea and tightness in the throat and chest. Stridor and/or hoarseness may also be noted. These signs and symptoms are often due to upper airway swelling in the laryngeal and epiglottic areas. Affected patients may report the sensation of a lump in the throat. The lower airway is often involved as well. Bronchoconstriction and increased secretions may result in wheezing and crackles. It is not uncommon for patients to cough or sneeze as the body tries to clear the airway. These symptoms may progress slowly or alarmingly fast. You may have only 1 to 3 minutes to halt this rapid, life-threatening process. Table 3-8 lists the signs and symptoms of anaphylaxis.

Differential Diagnosis

Determining a differential diagnosis in a patient having an anaphylactic reaction can be very challenging. You may

Table 3-8 Signs and Symptoms of Anaphylaxis*

System	Signs and Symptoms
Skin	▪ Warm ▪ Flushed ▪ Itching (pruritus) ▪ Swollen, red eyes ▪ **Swelling of the face and tongue** ▪ Swelling of the hands and feet ▪ **Hives (urticaria)**
Respiratory	▪ **Dyspnea** ▪ Tightness in the throat and chest ▪ Stridor ▪ Hoarseness ▪ Lump in throat ▪ **Wheezing** ▪ Coughing ▪ Sneezing
Cardiovascular	▪ Dysrhythmias ▪ **Hypotension** ▪ **Tachycardia**
Gastrointestinal	▪ Abdominal cramping ▪ Nausea ▪ Bloating ▪ Vomiting ▪ Abdominal distention ▪ Profuse, watery diarrhea
Central nervous system	▪ Headache ▪ Dizziness ▪ Confusion ▪ Anxiety and restlessness ▪ Sense of impending doom ▪ Altered mental status

*Key indicators are highlighted in bold type.

have to simultaneously assess the patient, identify the problem, and intervene within seconds of arriving on the scene to save the patient's life. Index of suspicion for anaphylaxis must be high on your list if any of the symptoms previously discussed are present. Studies have indicated that prehospital clinicians may recognize anaphylaxis only half of the time. Some clinicians may find this surprising, as it is easy to recognize a patient with hives and hypotension as having anaphylaxis. The difficulty lies in recognizing patients with other systemic involvement, such as CNS and gastrointestinal symptoms. The patient with nausea, vomiting, sweating, confusion, and hypotension may well be having an anaphylactic episode.

Treatment

Patients having allergic reactions are divided into two groups for management purposes. The first group includes patients who have signs of an allergic reaction—for example, hives—but no respiratory distress or dyspnea. The initial treatment of choice for such patients is antihistamines, including both rapid-acting H_1 blockers such as diphenhydramine and, if available, H_2 blockers such as famotidine. Continue to monitor for changes in the patient's condition, but recognize that most patients in this group will recover with no further problems. Depending on your protocols and the patient's disease severity, steroids and long-acting nonsedating antihistamines may also be administered.

The second group includes patients with signs of an allergic reaction and dyspnea, hypotension, or soft-tissue swelling affecting the airway. These patients require immediate treatment with EPINEPHrine. Oxygen should be administered for hypoxemia and an intravenous fluid (IVF) bolus for hypotension. Antihistamines may alleviate itching but do not otherwise treat anaphylaxis. Steroids may help stabilize the immune response but do not take effect immediately. Whenever dyspnea is present with signs of an allergic reaction, you should administer EPINEPHrine and monitor the patient for development of anaphylaxis. The administration of EPINEPHrine in patients with anaphylaxis is a crucial action and considered first-line treatment. Intramuscular (IM) EPINEPHrine may be administered by patients themselves, caregivers, bystanders, or EMS clinicians, via auto-injector or manual IM injection.

Psychological support is a crucial component of treatment. Anaphylaxis can progress rapidly and has the potential to be a life-threatening event. Patients and their families will need reassurance as you perform the necessary interventions. Many of the patients have experienced similar events and may recognize how serious their condition has become. For others, this may be a first-time event. You need to remain professional and reassuring and focus on early intervention and transport.

Pharyngitis and Tonsillitis

Pharyngitis and tonsillitis are both infections of the posterior pharynx. Although they share many of the same causes, *tonsillitis* specifically refers to infection of the tonsils, whereas *pharyngitis* refers to infection of the pharynx, which often includes some degree of tonsillitis.

Pathophysiology

The etiology of pharyngitis and tonsillitis is usually either viral or bacterial; about 40% to 60% of infections are viral, and 5% to 40% are bacterial. Most of these bacterial infections are caused by group A *Streptococcus*. A very small percentage of cases are due to trauma, cancer, allergy, or a toxic exposure.

Bacterial and viral infections cause inflammation of the local pharyngeal tissues. In addition, streptococcal infections release local toxins and proteins that may trigger additional inflammation. This inflammation and infection are usually self-limiting, but streptococcal infections have two important side effects. First, the bacterial surface carries antigens that are similar to proteins found normally in the heart. In the process of fighting off a streptococcal infection, the body's defenses can inadvertently attack the heart and heart valves, causing rheumatic fever. The likelihood of this complication is decreased by treatment with antibiotic. Second, the glomeruli in the kidneys can become damaged by the antibody–antigen combination, causing acute glomerulonephritis.

Signs and Symptoms

Signs and symptoms of pharyngitis and tonsillitis may include the following:

- Sore throat
- Fever
- Chills
- Muscle aches (myalgia)
- Abdominal pain
- Rhinorrhea
- Headache
- Earache

Physical exam will reveal a red and swollen posterior pharynx. Streptococcal infection is associated with enlarged and tender anterior cervical lymph nodes, and sometimes a fine red rash that feels like sandpaper. This rough-feeling rash, called scarlatina, begins on the torso and spreads to the entire body. In addition, whitish exudates (pockets of pus) on the tonsils may be seen. These exudates are more common with streptococcal infection, although their presence does not confirm a bacterial infection. Viral infections are more often associated with the presence of other upper respiratory infection (URI) signs and symptoms, such as cough and nasal congestion. A particular viral infection, mononucleosis, is associated with anterior and posterior cervical lymph node swelling and tenderness and should be precisely identified because of the potential for complications such as splenic rupture.

Treatment

Viral pharyngitis and tonsillitis are best treated symptomatically with fluids, antipyretic medications, and anti-inflammatory agents. In addition, bacterial infections are treated with antibiotics, usually penicillin or amoxicillin. Alternative antibiotics for patients who are allergic to penicillin include ceftriaxone, clindamycin, and erythromycin.

Peritonsillar Abscess

In **peritonsillar abscess**, a superficial soft-tissue infection progresses to create pockets of purulence in the submucosal space adjacent to the tonsils. This abscess and its accompanying inflammation may limit jaw opening (trismus), be accompanied by a hoarse voice (often described as a "hot potato voice"), and lead to uvular deviation to the opposite side (**Figure 3-12**).

Pathophysiology

Peritonsillar abscess is the most common infection of the peritonsillar region. The incidence of peritonsillar abscess in the United States is about 3 in 10,000 people annually. *Streptococcus* is often isolated in cultures of peritonsillar abscess, along with other bacteria such as *Peptostreptococcus*.

Signs and Symptoms

Signs and symptoms of peritonsillar abscess may include the following:

- Sore throat (especially unilaterally)
- Dysphagia
- Fever
- Chills
- Muscle aches
- Neck and anterior throat pain
- Hoarseness

Differential Diagnosis

The differential diagnosis for peritonsillar abscess includes other serious illnesses such as retropharyngeal

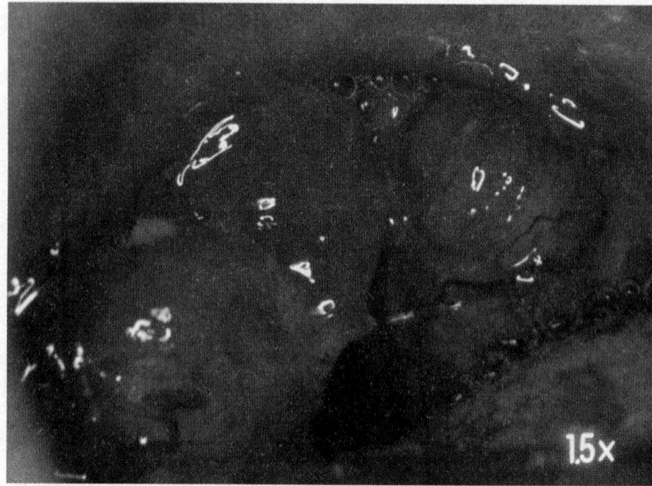

Figure 3-12 Peritonsillar abscess. Note the extensive swelling of the left tonsil and the deviation of the uvula.

and prevertebral abscess, epiglottitis, mononucleosis, herpes pharyngitis, carotid artery aneurysm, and cancer.

Treatment

Treatment includes hydration with intravenous (IV) fluids and administration of anti-inflammatory agents and antibiotics. If an abscess is present, drainage is indicated.

Epiglottitis

Epiglottitis is a life-threatening infection that causes inflammation of the epiglottis and often the supraglottic region. This swelling can lead to partial or complete obstruction of the trachea.

Once considered a disease of toddlers, the incidence of epiglottitis has changed dramatically since the United States began immunizing children against *Haemophilus influenzae* in 1985. Adults are now more likely to present with this illness in the emergency setting, with such patients having an average age of 45 years; men develop epiglottitis more often than women do. December is the most common month for cases to emerge. Mortality is estimated at 7% in adults and 1% in children.

Pathophysiology

Before a vaccine for *H. influenzae* type b (Hib) became available, epiglottitis occurred 2.6 times more often in children than in adults. *Streptococcus* species have now edged out *H. influenzae* as the pathogens most often responsible for causing epiglottitis.

Signs and Symptoms

Epiglottitis often begins with a sore throat and progresses to pain on swallowing and a muffled voice. Physical exam may reveal a patient in moderate or severe distress assuming a tripod position, with fever, heavy drooling, stridor, respiratory distress, tenderness when the larynx is palpated, tachycardia, and perhaps a low oxygen saturation. The stridor may be of a softer, lower pitch than that caused by croup.

Differential Diagnosis

The differential diagnosis for epiglottitis should include croup, retropharyngeal or prevertebral abscess, Ludwig angina, and peritonsillar abscess. A diagnosis of epiglottitis should be suspected based on clinical presentation and history, and can be confirmed with plain-film lateral neck radiographs. Computed tomography (CT) imaging may be performed but is often unnecessary because plain-film radiographs are usually sufficient. Fiber-optic laryngoscopy may provide direct information about the extent of airway edema and can assist in placement of an endotracheal tube.

Treatment

Emergency treatment for epiglottitis in the prehospital setting should be limited to maintaining adequate oxygenation and ventilation. Humidified oxygen can be of some relief to the patient, but the severity of this condition cannot be overstated. Avoid sticking anything in the patient's mouth. Limit suction to only those situations where secretions are obstructing the airway. If the patient is drooling heavily, have the patient sit up and lean forward to allow drooling. Intubation should be performed in the field only if absolutely necessary, such as for severe airway obstruction or respiratory arrest. Manipulating the epiglottis with a laryngoscope blade while the tissue is inflamed may irritate the airway and make further intubation attempts extremely difficult. Endotracheal intubation in this setting may best be achieved in the surgical suite. Antibiotics are indicated (often amoxicillin/sulbactam or clindamycin), as well as corticosteroids, inhaled beta-agonists, and nebulized epinephrine. If respiratory failure occurs with this condition, it is comforting to note that BVM ventilation is usually successful, even without endotracheal intubation.

Ludwig Angina

Named for the physician who first described it in the early 19th century, **Ludwig angina** refers not to chest pain but rather to a deep-space infection of the floor of the mouth and often extending into the anterior neck just below the mandible. Most patients with this condition report sensations of choking and suffocation.

Pathophysiology

Swelling, redness, and firmness of the soft tissue of the floor of the mouth and submandibular region are the most notable signs of Ludwig angina on clinical exam. This inflammation is caused by bacteria in the oral cavity, most often associated with dental infection. *Streptococcus* species are often cultured, but such infections are rarely due to a single organism and may contain anaerobic organisms.

Submental (beneath the chin) infection often migrates from dental caries in the incisors. Sublingual infection can usually be attributed to infection in the anterior mandibular teeth and can manifest as tongue elevation caused by swelling. Submandibular infection, which usually originates in the molars, is characterized by swelling in the angle of the jaw.

Since fluoridation of public drinking water became widespread in the 1970s, the prevalence of dental caries has decreased in developed countries. However, dental caries remain the most common chronic disease in the world.

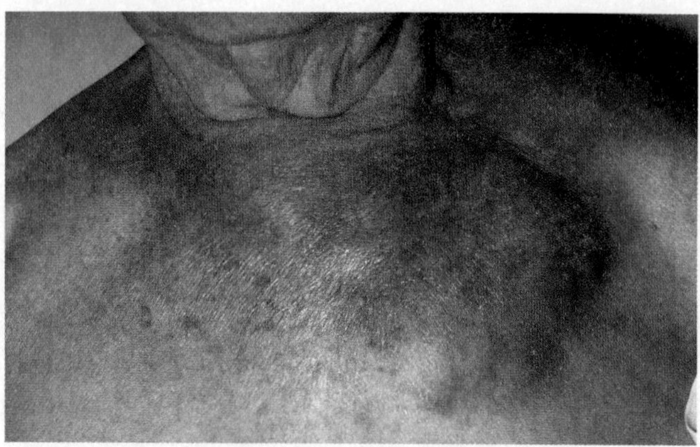

Figure 3-13 Ludwig angina. Rapid progression may compromise a patient's airway in a few hours.

Signs and Symptoms

Because it often arises from dental decay and subsequent infection, Ludwig angina is characterized by the following signs and symptoms:

- Severe gingivitis and cellulitis, with firm swelling and rapidly spreading infection in the submandibular, sublingual, and submental spaces (**Figure 3-13**)
- Swelling of the sublingual area and tongue
- Drooling
- Airway obstruction
- Elevation and posterior displacement of the tongue as a result of edema

Symptoms of Ludwig angina include sore throat, dysphagia, fever, chills, dental pain, and dyspnea. The patient tends to look anxious and toxic, with poor dentition and a firm, red, pronounced swelling in the anterior throat area. The location of caries may suggest which primary spaces are affected. The patient's tongue may be elevated, portending a difficult intubation should placement of a mechanical airway become necessary.

Differential Diagnosis

The differential diagnosis for Ludwig angina includes retropharyngeal and prevertebral abscess, as well as epiglottitis. Patients who have recently had chemotherapy or an organ transplant with immunosuppression are at increased risk of developing this infection, including abscess.

Treatment

A patient suspected of having Ludwig angina should be considered to have a life-threatening illness, perhaps accompanied by a compromised airway. Maintaining a patent airway is of paramount importance. In a rapidly progressing infection, prophylactic intubation may be performed electively in the ED or operating room. Stridor, dysphagia with difficulty controlling secretions, and dyspnea may prompt intubation. In the prehospital environment, supplemental humidified oxygen can make the patient more comfortable. Electrocardiographic monitoring and IV placement should be initiated. Antibiotics are initiated in the ED, and an ear, nose, and throat (ENT) surgeon may be consulted.

Retropharyngeal and Prevertebral Abscess

Retropharyngeal and prevertebral abscesses are both infections that develop behind the esophagus and in front of the cervical vertebrae. As noted earlier, an abscess is a localized collection of pus in a tissue or other confined space in the body. A retropharyngeal abscess may originate in the sinuses, teeth, or middle ear. As many as 67% of patients with such an abscess report having had a recent ENT infection. Retropharyngeal infections can be life threatening if they begin to cause airway obstruction. Infection that spreads to the mediastinum, called mediastinitis, is a grave complication that carries a startlingly high mortality rate of nearly 50%.

Pathophysiology

Common causal organisms in retropharyngeal abscess are *Staphylococcus* species, *Streptococcus* species, and *H. influenzae*, although the infection can be attributed to other organisms, especially anaerobes from the mouth. Retropharyngeal lesions can be seen in adults as well as in children, but usually affect persons who are 3 to 4 years old or younger.

Signs and Symptoms

Signs of retropharyngeal abscess include the following:

- Pharyngitis
- Dysphagia
- Dyspnea
- Fever
- Chills
- Neck pain, stiffness, swelling, or erythema
- Drooling

The following are worrisome signs of possible airway compromise:

- Difficulty opening the mouth (trismus)
- Vocal changes
- Inspiratory stridor

Differential Diagnosis

Early retropharyngeal abscess may be misdiagnosed as unspecified or streptococcal pharyngitis. If the patient's condition declines rapidly, you should consider more threatening illnesses such as epiglottitis and meningitis.

Treatment

Treatment includes ensuring a patent airway and providing supplemental oxygen. Be careful not to puncture the abscess during intubation, because aspiration of its purulent contents may be fatal. Initiate electrocardiographic monitoring and obtain IV access. Initiate appropriate fluid replenishment if the patient is dehydrated from decreased oral intake.

Definitive care often involves intubation in the operating suite (or under other controlled circumstances), surgical drainage of the lesion, and antibiotics. With aggressive management of retropharyngeal abscess before it progresses to mediastinitis, many patients recover promptly and can be extubated immediately following or a few days after the procedure.

Angioedema

Angioedema is a sudden swelling, usually of a head or neck structure such as the lip (especially the lower lip), earlobes, tongue, or uvula, though it has been described in other tissues, including the bowel. The pathophysiology of angioedema is not fully understood but is generally treated like an allergic reaction. Sometimes the cause is related to medications (such as angiotensin-converting enzyme [ACE] inhibitors and nonsteroidal anti-inflammatory drugs [NSAIDs]), but it may also be idiopathic (of unknown cause). A few cases are hereditary, referred to as hereditary angioedema.

As much as 15% of the general population experiences episodic idiopathic angioedema. No racial predominance exists. Females are more likely to have angioedema than are males, and the condition is most often seen in adults. Exposure to certain agents increases the risk of angioedema. Common triggers include the following:

- ACE inhibitors (captopril, enalapril, and others)
- Radiologic dyes
- Aspirin
- NSAIDs (ibuprofen, naproxen, and others)
- Hymenoptera insect stings (wasps, yellowjackets, and others)
- Food allergies
- Animal hair or dander (shed skin cells)
- Sunlight exposure
- Stress

Pathophysiology

In angioedema, some insult triggers leakage from the small-vessel circulation, prompting interstitial tissues to swell. Edema can originate in the epidermal and dermal tissues, in the subcutaneous tissues, or in both. This inflammation is a response to the actions of circulating hormones and histamines, serotonin, and bradykinins.

Signs and Symptoms

Signs of angioedema include clearly demarcated swelling with or without a rash, which is occasionally accompanied by dyspnea or anxiety. Stridor, wheezing on chest auscultation, or history of intubation should prompt careful observation for deterioration. Angioedema of the bowel may cause bowel obstruction with consequent nausea, vomiting, and abdominal pain.

Differential Diagnosis

Carefully assess the patient for other life-threatening illnesses, such as cellulitis or abscess, retropharyngeal abscess, and Ludwig angina. If the patient has hives, consider the possibility of anaphylaxis.

Treatment

Although extensive angioedema may threaten the airway, many cases are self-limiting or require only minimal treatment. Allow the patient to assume a comfortable position. If there are no signs of respiratory failure, the patient will be able to maintain a patent airway with simple positioning. Antihistamines are rarely beneficial, as angioedema is generally a bradykinin-mediated condition. Case reports demonstrate some beneficial effects from administering blood products (whole or packed red blood cells [PRBC]) in patients with hereditary angioedema. Additional pharmacologic agents are typically not available to prehospital personnel.

Emergent intubation can be extremely difficult in severe cases of angioedema because the swollen tissue may prevent adequate visualization of the vocal cords. In addition to normal intubation equipment, prepare rescue airway equipment before you attempt intubation. If time permits, intubation should be performed under controlled circumstances with adequate difficult-airway equipment. In nonemergent situations, it is prudent to initiate electrocardiographic monitoring, obtain IV access, and transport the patient to a nearby emergency facility.

Lower Airway Conditions

Obstructive lower airway diseases are characterized by diffuse obstruction of airflow within the lungs. The most commonly encountered obstructive airway diseases are emphysema, chronic bronchitis, and asthma; these three conditions collectively affect as many as 20% of adults in the United States.

Obstructive disease is characterized by constriction or blockage of small airways from the underlying disease. The positive intrathoracic pressure during exhalation causes the small airways to further collapse, trapping gas in the alveoli. The harder the patient tries to push air out, the more air that becomes trapped in the alveoli. Patients with obstructive disease may have large amounts of gas trapped in their lungs that they cannot effectively expel. Such individuals learn exhaling slowly at a low pressure is more effective than exhaling rapidly at high pressure.

Aspiration

The inhalation of anything other than breathable gases is called aspiration, and the resultant inflammatory response in the lungs is termed aspiration pneumonitis. Infection from aspirated bacteria or secondarily related to the inflammation is common. Patients can aspirate fresh or salt water, blood, vomitus, toxins, or food. Patients who receive tube feedings are at particular risk for aspiration if they are placed supine immediately after receiving a large feeding. A large percentage of geriatric patients have impaired swallowing from strokes or other neurologic impairments. Unresponsive patients are at risk for the aspiration of vomitus. The aspiration of stomach contents can be particularly irritating due to its acidity.

Pathophysiology

Aspiration of stomach contents into the lungs has a significantly high mortality rate. It is a common but profoundly dangerous complication in patients with trauma injuries and those who have overdosed. Aspiration of foreign bodies, such as nuts or broken teeth, may also occur. Most healthy adults are at risk of aspiration or choking only when they are intoxicated or traumatized or have a reduced gag reflex from aging. Chronic aspiration of food is also a common cause of pneumonia in older patients.

Signs and Symptoms

Consider the scenario surrounding the patient's sudden onset of dyspnea. Did it occur immediately after eating? Does the patient have a gastric feeding tube, and, if so, when was the last feeding and how large was it? Is the material suctioned from the patient's airway the same color as the tube feeding? Is there particulate matter in the suctioned material? A fever and cough may present several hours after an aspiration-prone event, such as a seizure or an episode of unresponsiveness. Some patients aspirate chronically and may have a history of aspiration pneumonia.

Treatment

Follow these guidelines when treating patients at risk for aspiration or who have aspirated:

- Reduce the risk of aspiration by avoiding gastric distention when ventilating and by decompressing the stomach with a nasogastric tube whenever appropriate.
- Monitor the patient's ability to protect and maintain a patent airway, and protect the patient's airway with an advanced airway when needed.
- Aggressively treat aspiration with suction and airway control if the other steps fail.

Asthma

Asthma is a very common disease, prompting millions of ED visits each year and accounting for 20% to 30% of all hospital admissions in the United States. Patients have a high relapse rate, with 10% to 20% returning within 2 weeks of treatment. In the United States, asthma prevalence is estimated at 7.8%. According to the Centers for Disease Control and Prevention, asthma is most prevalent in persons 20 to 24 years old (10.3%). It is more common in females (9.5%) than in males (6.1%); in persons of Black, American Indian/Alaska Native, and multiple non-Hispanic race/ethnicity; and in persons with lower economic status.

Children who have wheezing that begins before age 5 years and persists into adulthood have a greater likelihood of compromised lung function. Children who begin to wheeze after age 5 years have a lower incidence of pulmonary disease even if the wheezing persists into adulthood. As many as 90% of patients with asthma have their first symptoms before age 6 years. Some children present with nocturnal coughing as a symptom, without the typical wheezing.

Pathophysiology

Asthma is a chronic inflammation of the bronchi characterized by increased mucus production and contraction of the bronchial smooth muscles, resulting in narrowed bronchi and associated wheezing (**Figure 3-14**). The airways become overly sensitive to inhaled allergens, viruses, and other environmental irritants—even strong odors can precipitate an episode. This oversensitivity is

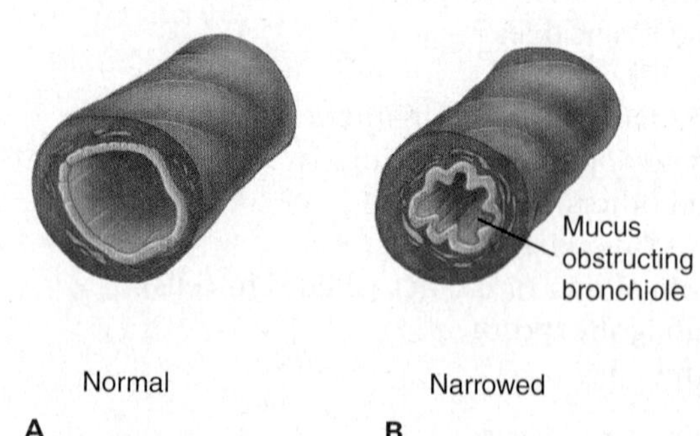

Figure 3-14 **A.** A normal bronchiole with no inflammation. **B.** A bronchiole in spasm, with contraction of the bronchial smooth muscle, resulting in narrowed bronchi, causing the associated wheezing of asthma.

responsible for the reactive airway component of the disease.

Inflammation and persistent bronchospasm are at the center of asthma symptoms such as dyspnea, wheezing, and coughing. Inflammation includes bronchial edema and tenacious mucus secretions that can cause bronchial plugging and atelectasis.

Signs and Symptoms

Patients with asthma are usually acutely aware of their symptoms, even if those symptoms are considered clinically mild. Early symptoms of asthma include some combination of the following:

- Wheezing
- Dyspnea
- Chest tightness
- Cough
- Signs of a recent URI, such as rhinorrhea, congestion, headache, pharyngitis, or myalgia
- Signs of exposure to allergens, such as rhinorrhea, pharyngitis, hoarseness, and cough
- Chest tightness, discomfort, or pain

The patient initially hyperventilates, causing a decrease in CO_2 levels (respiratory alkalosis). As the airways continue to narrow, complete exhalation becomes increasingly difficult; air trapping results and CO_2 levels begin to increase. The lungs become overinflated and stiff, increasing the work of breathing. Tachypnea, tachycardia, and pulsus paradoxus may occur, with accompanying agitation. Few retractions should be seen. Oxygen saturation should be near normal, even on room air.

Patients with moderate exacerbations may show increased tachycardia and tachypnea, with increased wheezing and decreased air movement. Oxygen saturation may dip, but should be easily restored with supplemental oxygen. Retractions may be seen, and the degree and types will increase with the severity of the episode. Recruitment of more muscle sets (e.g., intercostal, subcostal) indicates a worsening condition.

Certain factors in a carefully taken patient history may help predict the severity of an asthma episode: respiratory illness; exposure to potential allergens; compliance with home inhaled medications; and the frequency of ED visits, hospital admissions, prior intubation, and corticosteroid use.

Inhalation of allergens such as animal material and airborne ragweed and pollen particles frequently precipitates asthma episodes. Inhalation of smoke or cold, dry air may also touch off a flare-up. The following factors suggest that a patient is more likely to experience a severe asthma exacerbation:

- Presenting oxygen saturation < 92%
- Tachypnea
- Recent ED visit or hospitalization
- Frequent hospitalizations
- History of intubation for asthma
- Peak flows < 60% of predicted values
- Accessory muscle use and retraction
- Duration of symptoms > 2 days
- History of frequent corticosteroid use

Differential Diagnosis

When the clinician is gathering a history, new-onset wheezing is not enough to make a diagnosis of asthma. Instead, repeated bouts of this disease are usually necessary for a clinician to make a definitive diagnosis because many other conditions are also characterized by wheezing. Bacterial pneumonia, such as that caused by *Streptococcus* species, can cause wheezing, as can atypical infections from *Mycoplasma* and *Chlamydia*. Viral infections are also potential causes of wheezing, especially respiratory syncytial virus (RSV), an infection often seen among infants during the winter and early spring months.

What other diseases present with wheezing? The differential diagnosis should include both primary pulmonary and systemic diseases. What distinguishes asthma from COPD (chronic bronchitis and emphysema)? The reactive airway process in asthma, unlike in COPD, is largely reversible. Other primary pulmonary conditions include interstitial fibrosis, bronchiolitis, and bronchiectasis. Consider upper airway obstruction, such as that caused by croup, epiglottitis, or retropharyngeal infection, especially if stridor is present. Acute pulmonary edema and decompensated HF may present with acute wheezing, as can aspiration of a foreign object (see the earlier discussion) and pulmonary embolism (discussed later in the chapter). Chest pain may prompt evaluation for cardiac ischemia, especially if the quality of the pain is different from that experienced in previous asthma episodes. Potential systemic conditions include sarcoidosis and cystic fibrosis.

Treatment

Therapy should be scaled to the severity of the exacerbation. First-line treatment for actively wheezing patients includes inhaled rapid-onset beta-agonists such as albuterol and levalbuterol. Beta-2 agonists used early and aggressively in the course of disease can reduce the likelihood of hospitalization.

Parenteral beta-2 agonists may be a useful supplement for severe asthma episodes. Terbutaline, 0.25 mg, or 0.3 mg of 1:1,000 EPINEPHrine administered IM or subcutaneously, can facilitate the effects of inhaled beta-2 agonists. Because of their tendency to cause hypertension and increase myocardial workload and oxygen demand, however, these agents should be used with caution, especially in patients who have coexisting ischemic cardiac disease. IV or intraosseous (IO) administration of terbutaline or EPINEPHrine may also be indicated, but seek medical consultation first.

Ipratropium is an anticholinergic agent that treats bronchospasm by a different mechanism than beta-agonists do. It is delivered via a metered-dose inhaler (MDI) or nebulizer. Although this medication may be most effective in patients with COPD or a history of tobacco use, it can also be helpful for patients with asthma who do not respond to beta-agonists.

IV corticosteroids help slow down the inflammatory response, thereby reducing the edema that causes narrowing of the bronchial passageways. Although corticosteroids may take hours to work, their administration by EMS clinicians in the prehospital setting may decrease the patient's length of stay in the ED and need for hospital admission.

Magnesium sulfate given intravenously has shown promise in controlling severe exacerbations of asthma. This medication is typically given as a 2-gram dose over 30 to 60 minutes to help relax the smooth bronchial muscles. It is a third-line therapy, however, and its administration should not take priority over beta-agonists and steroids.

While not widely used, heliox—a gaseous mixture of helium and oxygen—is another inhaled agent showing promise for severe exacerbations. Given either in an 80:20 or a 70:30 mixture, helium acts as a lighter-than-air carrier to help distribute oxygen and nebulized agents and decrease the patient's work of breathing. Albuterol given with heliox requires twice the normal dose of albuterol at a flow rate of 8 to 10 l/min.

Despite aggressive pharmacologic therapy, some patients still face severe respiratory distress or respiratory failure from asthma episodes. In these patients, ketamine infusion may be useful as an adjunctive therapy. NIPPV should also be considered in these patients, particularly if the patient appears to be fatiguing.

Chronic Obstructive Pulmonary Disease

COPD is a collective term for chronic lung disease characterized by airflow obstruction caused by chronic bronchitis or loss of alveolar surface area associated with emphysema. Both forms are marked by wheezing and airway edema. In addition, even though their underlying mechanisms are slightly different from that associated with asthma, both are air-trapping diseases of the lungs. In asthma, airflow obstruction is completely reversible; in COPD, it is not. Chronic bronchitis is formally defined as a chronic productive cough for 3 months in each of 2 years, for which other causes of chronic cough have been excluded. Emphysema is defined by alveolar breakdown and loss of lung elasticity.

COPD is a chronic, devastating disease that is currently ranked as the third leading cause of death worldwide, albeit with the great majority of these deaths occurring in low- and middle-income countries. In the United States, it is the fourth-leading cause of death and affects more than 15 million people. The overall prevalence of COPD is approximately 6.0% of the U.S. population, with more females than males affected; its age-adjusted death rate is approximately 105 deaths per 100,000 population, and is higher in males than females.

The primary cause of COPD is cigarette smoking. Most patients with clinically significant COPD have smoked at least 1 pack per day for 20 years. An estimated 15% of all smokers develop clinically significant COPD. Many factors affect the rate at which COPD evolves, including the age at which the person began smoking, the number of packs smoked per day, the existence of other illnesses, the person's level of physical fitness, and the amount and duration of tobacco use. Secondhand smoke contributes to reduced pulmonary function, asthma exacerbations, and increased risk of upper respiratory tract infections. Other air pollutants can also lead to COPD. The only genetic risk factor known to cause COPD in nonsmokers is a deficiency of alpha$_1$-antitrypsin, a protein that inhibits neutrophil elastase, a lung enzyme.

Pathophysiology

Chronic exposure to inhaled toxic particles causes inflammation and injury to the airways. The body tries to repair this injury by remodeling the airways, a process that causes scarring and narrowing. Changes in the alveolar walls and connective tissue permanently enlarge the alveoli. On the other side of those alveoli, the important connection to the capillary membrane is remodeled with a thickened vessel wall, which impedes gas exchange. Mucus-secreting glands and goblet cells multiply, increasing mucus production. Cilia are destroyed, limiting the body's ability to clear this abundant mucus.

External changes in the body, such as a barrel-shaped chest (**Figure 3-15**), occur in response to the remodeled airways and chronic air trapping. Chronic shortness of breath and chronic cough are also manifestations of this remodeling. Because of chronic hypoxia, chemoreceptors fail to react to fluctuations in the blood's oxygen level. Unfortunately, these changes reflect a permanent adjustment of the body in response to chronic inhalation of irritants.

Over time, lung function gradually declines, sputum production increases, and the patient has retained secretions with a chronic cough. The classic air trapping is caused by the lungs' limited ability to move air out of the enlarged distal airspaces. The lungs become hyperinflated and decreased gas exchange occurs, which leads to hypoxia and high CO_2 levels. In patients with high levels of CO_2, the chronic hypercapnia blunts the body's normal chemoreceptor sensitivity, such that hypoxia becomes

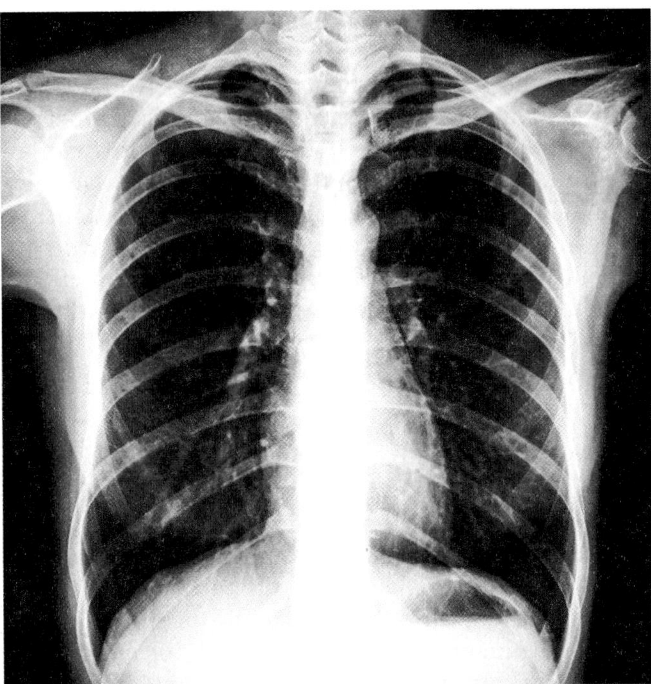

Figure 3-15 Common radiographic findings of a patient with COPD: elongated chest, hyperexpansion of the lungs, flattened diaphragm, and small heart.

the primary mechanism for ventilation control. At this stage, the patient is vulnerable to infection and intolerant of exercise. Any condition that increases the work of breathing may quickly lead to respiratory failure. To compensate for the CO_2 retention, the body must maintain a metabolic alkalosis.

Signs and Symptoms

Signs and symptoms of acute exacerbation of COPD may include the following findings:

- Dyspnea
- Cough
- Intolerance of exertion
- Wheezing
- Productive cough
- Chest pain or discomfort
- Diaphoresis
- Orthopnea

COPD is also associated with the following clinical signs:

- Wheezing
- Increased respiratory rate
- Decreased oxygen saturation
- Use of accessory muscles
- Elevated jugular pulse
- Peripheral edema
- Hyperinflated lungs
- Hyperresonance on percussion
- Coarse, scattered rhonchi

Critical episodes are indicated by the following signs and symptoms:

- Oxygen saturation below patient baseline
- Tachypnea (approximately 30 breaths/min)
- Peripheral or central cyanosis
- Mental status changes

Differential Diagnosis

The presentation of an apparent COPD exacerbation should prompt consideration of other serious diseases as potential causes, particularly because the chief complaint of dyspnea may be associated with chest pain. The differential diagnosis of COPD exacerbation should include asthma; acute bronchitis; pneumonia; pneumonitis; pulmonary fibrosis; pneumothorax; pulmonary hypertension; pulmonary embolus; and cardiac causes of dyspnea such as acute myocardial infarction, angina, and HF.

Treatment

Management of a COPD exacerbation hinges on maintaining oxygenation and ventilation. Emergency management includes supplemental oxygen delivered by either nasal cannula or Venturi mask and sufficient to maintain an oxygen saturation of 88% to 92%. Patients with COPD have adapted to a mildly hypoxic state, and their respiratory drive is based on these hypoxia receptors. In consequence, they have a risk of developing hypercarbia if a high oxygen concentration caused by administration of excessive supplemental oxygen decreases their stimulus to breathe at a necessary rate. If the patient remains hypoxic with low-flow oxygen, apply a nonrebreather mask with high-flow oxygen and prepare for aggressive airway and ventilation management. Evidence of inadequate ventilation or fatiguing, an SpO_2 that falls into the low 80s, and pale/ashen or cyanotic extremities indicate a need for aggressive intervention. Small studies have suggested that a trial of mask CPAP may be warranted before intubation attempts in an alert, acutely hypercapnic patient with COPD. Using CPAP has been shown to decrease the work of breathing, improve oxygenation and ventilation, and decrease the likelihood of intubation. Endotracheal intubation may be indicated in severe cases.

Bronchodilators, delivered by MDI or nebulization, should be administered initially, although these agents are not as effective in COPD as they are in asthma. Anticholinergic agents such as ipratropium bromide are beneficial, particularly in concert with beta-2 agonists. Although they do not act as quickly as the beta-2 agonists, the anticholinergics can provide an additional 20% to 40% bronchodilation when combined with beta-2 agonists.

Systemic corticosteroids are indicated for moderate to severe COPD exacerbations. While administration of these agents by the oral route is as effective as IV delivery, the latter route is typically used for severe exacerbations.

Patients with COPD who must be placed on invasive mechanical ventilation may prove difficult to wean and be vulnerable to ventilator-associated pneumonia. Mechanical ventilation is indicated when, despite aggressive therapy, the patient has mental status changes, acidosis, respiratory fatigue, and hypoxia. These patients may have discussed the use of long-term ventilatory support with family members or caregivers. Be sure to ask the family whether the patient has an advance directive and what the patient's wishes are regarding long-term mechanical ventilation.

Atelectasis

Atelectasis is the collapse of the alveolar air spaces of the lungs.

Pathophysiology

The alveoli are vulnerable to several disorders. They may collapse from obstruction somewhere in the proximal airways or from external pressures produced, for example, by pneumothorax or hemothorax. They may fill with pus in pneumonia, with blood in pulmonary contusion, or with fluid in near-drowning or HF. In addition, smoke or toxic gases may displace the fresh air that should be present in the alveoli.

The human body has billions of alveoli, and it is common for some of them to collapse from time to time. Humans periodically sigh, cough, sneeze, and change positions—all actions that are thought to help open closed alveoli and avoid decreased ventilation in any one part of the lung. When people do not use these actions—for example, because they are sedated or in a coma, or because deep breathing or moving causes pain—increasing numbers of alveoli may collapse and not reopen. Like balloons, alveoli are more difficult to open once they have completely collapsed. Eventually, entire lung segments collapse. This condition, which is termed atelectasis, increases the chance of pneumonia developing in the affected areas.

Signs and Symptoms

Although atelectasis can be a significant disorder by itself, the larger concern is that the affected areas become breeding grounds for pathogens, resulting in pneumonia. This possibility is a concern in any patient who has a fever in the days following chest or abdominal surgery, particularly if breath sounds are decreased or abnormally colored sputum is produced.

Treatment

Patients who sustained chest trauma and who are post surgery should be encouraged to cough, breathe deeply, and get out of bed, even though it is painful. Use of an incentive spirometer is helpful. EMS clinicians can reinforce the importance of deep breathing to these patients, and can be watchful for atelectasis in patients who are sedentary or who take medications with sedative effects, including some analgesics.

Pneumonia

Lung infection that causes fluid to collect in the alveoli is referred to as pneumonia. The resulting inflammation can cause dyspnea, fever, chills, chest pain, chest wall pain, and a productive cough. Three broad types of pneumonia are distinguished: community acquired, hospital acquired in nonventilated patients (nosocomial; begins 48 or more hours after hospital admission), and hospital acquired ventilator associated (begins 48 or more hours after intubation or within 48 hours of extubation). The cause may be viral, bacterial, fungal, or chemical (aspiration of gastric contents).

More than 3 million cases of pneumonia are diagnosed annually in the United States. Untreated pneumonia has a mortality rate approaching 30%. Even with appropriate and timely treatment, coexisting medical conditions (comorbidities) can drastically increase the likelihood of mortality. Advanced age increases susceptibility to pneumonia. In a 20-year study, overall mortality in pneumonia caused by *Streptococcus pneumoniae* was 20%, but in patients older than 80 years, mortality exceeded 37%.

Recovery may be complicated by comorbid conditions such as human immunodeficiency virus (HIV) infection or other causes of immunosuppression; HF; diabetes; leukemia; and pulmonary diseases such as asthma, COPD, and bronchitis. Development of pneumonia in an already compromised patient can touch off a downward spiral of dyspnea, destruction of lung tissue by infection, further infection, more dyspnea, and a worsening condition. Ravaged alveoli can be replaced by pus-filled saccules. This inflammatory material perpetuates the cycle, resulting in empyema or lung abscess, which can be difficult to treat without surgical intervention. Even in patients who recover, scarring from the infection can compromise respiratory gas exchange, reducing their pulmonary reserve capacity and increasing their susceptibility to another infection.

Pathophysiology

Pathogens causing community-acquired pneumonia include *S. pneumoniae*, *Legionella* species, *H. influenzae*,

Staphylococcus aureus, respiratory viruses, *Chlamydia*, and *Pseudomonas*. *Pseudomonas* is rarely the cause of community-acquired pneumonia, but is more likely to cause pneumonia in individuals with severe lung disease such as cystic fibrosis and COPD and persons recently discharged from the hospital. Hospital-acquired pneumonia can be caused by the same pathogens, along with *Klebsiella* and *Enterococcus* species. The two pathogens most commonly associated with ventilator-assisted pneumonia are *S. aureus* and *Pseudomonas aeruginosa*. Pneumonia most commonly develops because of a defect in the host's immune system or an overwhelming burden of strong pathogens.

Signs and Symptoms

Patients with pneumonia usually have the classic symptoms of shortness of breath, cough, and fever, but may also have more subtle signs, such as abdominal pain, low-grade fever, and weakness with accompanying tachycardia. An acute onset of symptoms and a rapid progression are more suggestive of a bacterial cause than a viral cause. Clinical signs and symptoms of pneumonia may include any of the following:

- Shortness of breath
- Fever
- Chills
- Cough
- Malaise
- Nausea and vomiting
- Diarrhea
- Myalgia
- Pleuritic chest pain
- Abdominal pain
- Anorexia
- Tachypnea
- Tachycardia
- Hypoxia
- Abnormal breath sounds, including crackles, rhonchi, and even wheezing

Altered mental status and cyanosis are signs of severe illness.

Differential Diagnosis

The differential diagnosis of pneumonia should include asthma, bronchitis, COPD exacerbation, tracheal or supraglottic foreign objects, epiglottitis, empyema, pulmonary abscess, HF, angina, and myocardial infarction.

Diagnosis can be made based on clinical presentation, a careful history of present illness, and a thorough physical exam. Radiologic evaluation, including anterior–posterior and lateral chest radiographs, shows fair to good sensitivity for presence of infiltrate, although normal findings do not rule out pneumonia. CT imaging is more sensitive to pneumonia but exposes the patient to higher radiation than plain films.

Treatment

Supplemental oxygen should be provided as needed for hypoxia or dyspnea, with the goal of maintaining oxygen saturation at $> 94\%$. Consider more aggressive airway maneuvers if this saturation cannot be achieved with supplemental oxygen alone. Use of a CPAP mask may alleviate the need for intubation in patients who are able to tolerate having the mask covering the face (see the earlier discussion).

Bronchodilators are indicated if wheezing or other evidence of bronchospasm is present. Antibiotics should be administered empirically as soon as possible. Studies have shown that administration of antibiotics within 6 hours of patients' arrival in the ED decreases morbidity and mortality in patients with pneumonia.

Patients with sepsis must be aggressively resuscitated. Sepsis is considered to be present when the patient has an identifiable infection and meets the clinical criteria for systemic inflammatory response syndrome (SIRS)—fever, tachycardia, tachypnea, and leukocytosis. If septic shock develops, vigorous fluid resuscitation and vasopressor therapy may be needed.

Acute Lung Injury/Acute Respiratory Distress Syndrome

Acute lung injury/acute respiratory distress syndrome (ALI/ARDS) is a syndrome of pulmonary inflammation and edema that can develop in association with other severe medical illness or trauma. When the lungs fail in ALI/ARDS, a noncardiogenic pulmonary edema develops, in which fluid from the blood plasma migrates into the lung parenchyma and fills the lung tissue and air spaces. This fluid shift is accompanied by respiratory distress, pulmonary edema, and respiratory failure. Ventilatory support may be required to treat the severe hypoxemia associated with this condition.

Pathophysiology

ARDS is seldom seen in the field, but EMS clinicians may have a vital role in preventing this devastating pathologic condition. This syndrome is caused by diffuse damage to the alveoli, perhaps because of shock, aspiration of gastric contents, pulmonary edema, or a hypoxic event. It seems to be worse when patients experience direct damage to the lungs—for example, in trauma patients who have severe pulmonary contusions. The onset of ALI/ARDS begins with a breakdown of the alveolar–capillary border, which allows fluid to seep into the alveoli, decreasing gas exchange in the lungs. In severe cases, high levels of oxygen are required to maintain adequate oxygenation.

Signs and Symptoms

Development of progressive dyspnea and hypoxemia within hours to days after an acute traumatic or medical event is the hallmark of ALI/ARDS; ARDS is most often seen in hospitalized patients, usually those being treated in the intensive care unit (ICU). The typical patient has recently undergone major surgery, seems to recover, and is in a non-ICU bed—and then phase 1 ALI/ARDS develops and the patient must be readmitted to the ICU. Physical signs of ALI/ARDS include the following:

- Dyspnea
- Hypoxemia, sometimes accompanied by cyanosis of the mucous membranes
- Tachypnea
- Tachycardia
- Increasing demand for supplemental oxygen to maintain adequate saturation
- Fever and hypotension in patients with sepsis
- Crackles/rales (may or may not be heard on auscultation)

Treatment

Supporting oxygenation and assisting ventilation are the cornerstones of ALI/ARDS treatment. Document SpO_2, breath sounds, and any sudden changes in the patient's condition. Patients with ARDS typically have "stiff" lungs (i.e., low compliance). No specific remedy exists other than aggressively managing the inciting medical or traumatic event. Intubation and mechanical ventilation, along with pressure support and suctioning as needed, are indicated. Once ventilatory support has been instituted, ventilation pressures should be monitored and care taken to not overventilate the lungs and cause further damage.

Severe Acute Respiratory Syndrome

Severe acute respiratory syndrome (SARS) is a disease that arose from the merger of two viruses, one from mammals and one from birds. The source of this unique coronavirus has been identified as bats found in Hong Kong. SARS was first reported in Asia in February 2003. Within a few months, the disease had spread to Canada, South America, and Europe. In the United States, there were eight confirmed cases (all mild) and no deaths; all the cases involved people who had traveled to areas where SARS cases had been reported. At this time, there has not been a case of SARS since 2004. However, a new strain of coronavirus caused coronavirus disease 2019 (COVID-19); it is covered in depth in Chapter 7, *Infectious Diseases*.

Pneumothorax

Pneumothorax is defined as air in the pleural space. As discussed earlier, normally the pleural space is occupied by only a small amount of fluid that lubricates the pleura to minimize friction. The vacuum (or negative intrathoracic pressure) between the pleural layers is essential for proper ventilatory functioning, assuring that as the chest wall expands, so will the lungs. When the outside surface of the lung is disrupted, however, air escapes into the pleural cavity (**Figure 3-16**), and the negative pressure is lost. The natural elasticity of the lung tissue causes the lung to collapse in proportion to the volume of pleural air. Although pneumothorax is most often caused by trauma, it also can be caused by some medical conditions or can be spontaneous, particularly in tall, thin males.

Pathophysiology

Primary spontaneous pneumothorax can occur without an obvious cause. Nearly all patients who experience primary spontaneous pneumothorax have bullae, or air pockets that rupture to cause the pneumothorax. Although this condition is seen predominantly in patients without a prior diagnosis of lung disease, more than 90% of persons who experience primary spontaneous pneumothorax are smokers. As noted earlier, the condition

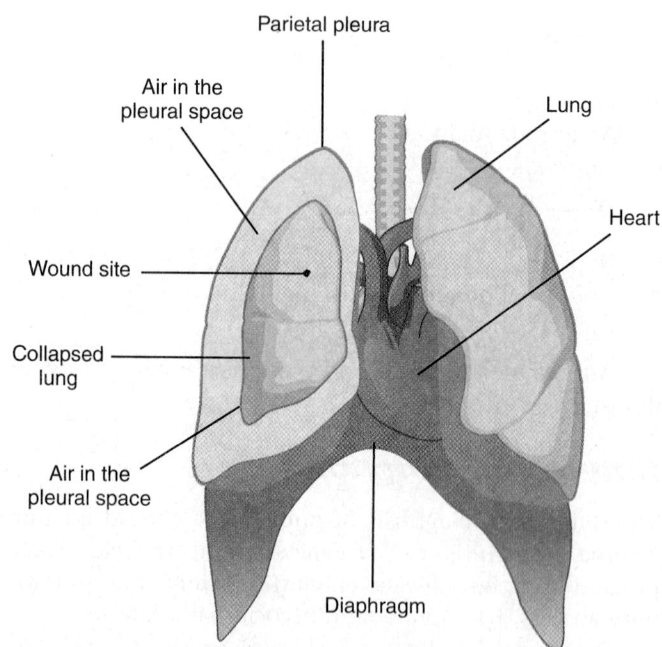

Figure 3-16 A pneumothorax occurs when air leaks into the pleural space from an opening in the chest wall or the surface of the lung. The lung collapses as air fills the pleural space and the two pleural surfaces are no longer in contact.

is also more common in tall, thin, young males. Developing evidence suggests that genetic factors may predispose patients to spontaneous pneumothorax. Huffing or inhaling recreational substances is also a risk factor for spontaneous pneumothorax.

Secondary spontaneous pneumothorax can be caused by a variety of lung diseases but occurs primarily in patients with asthma and COPD. Pulmonary fibrosis, sarcoidosis, tuberculosis, and infection with *Pneumocystis jirovecii* (almost exclusively in patients with acquired immunodeficiency syndrome [AIDS]) are other reported risk factors. Secondary spontaneous pneumothorax occurs more frequently in older patients.

Besides traumatic and spontaneous causes, pneumothorax may occur because of volutrauma or barotrauma from high intrathoracic pressure during positive-pressure ventilation.

Signs and Symptoms

The cardinal signs of spontaneous pneumothorax are chest pain and dyspnea. The chest pain is often described as having a sudden onset, sharp or stabbing, and made worse by breathing or other chest wall motion. Decreased lung reserve capacity, such as occurs in COPD, may make dyspnea more pronounced in patients with secondary spontaneous pneumothorax. Additional symptoms of pneumothorax may include diaphoresis, anxiety, back pain, cough, and malaise.

Look for the following clinical signs of spontaneous pneumothorax:

- Tachypnea
- Tachycardia
- Pulsus paradoxus
- Unilateral decreased breath sounds
- Subcutaneous emphysema
- Hyperresonance on percussion
- Hypoxia and altered mental status (in some patients)

The presence of breath sounds on the affected side does not rule out a pneumothorax because an estimated 25% of the lung would need to be collapsed before diminished breath sounds would be heard. Auscultating the midaxillary line may help you pick up on this indicator earlier. Hypotension, hypoxia, cyanosis, and increased JVD should prompt you to consider tension pneumothorax. In tension pneumothorax, a pneumothorax leads to significant hemodynamic compromise due to decreased venous return related to the increased intrathoracic pressure and, in some cases, kinking of the great vessels. The critical finding in persons with tension pneumothorax is hypotension in association with respiratory distress and the other signs and symptoms of pneumothorax.

Differential Diagnosis

In the differential diagnosis, the clinician should consider other causes of acute-onset respiratory distress and chest pain based on the clinical scenario. These possibilities include acute hemothorax, acute coronary syndrome, pulmonary embolism, aortic dissection, acute pericarditis, esophageal rupture, and acute cholecystitis.

Although a diagnosis can be made based on clinical exam findings, a chest radiograph can confirm the degree of pneumothorax. Performing a chest radiograph while the patient is exhaling will allow the practitioner to see the severity of the pneumothorax, although a regular chest radiograph is also acceptable. CT is a more sensitive imaging study and can be especially useful when the pneumothorax is small. Bedside ultrasound is also helpful in diagnosing pneumothorax.

In the diagnosis, a distinction should be made between spontaneous pneumothorax and tension pneumothorax (**Figure 3-17**). Accumulation of air in the pleural space on the affected side eventually forces the mediastinum to shift against the "good" lung and the vena cava. These changes cause worsening dyspnea, increased work of breathing, and a drop in cardiac output, leading to obstructive shock. The patient with unilateral diminished breath sounds who is clinically deteriorating and slipping into shock should be diagnosed with tension pneumothorax. Immediate lifesaving chest decompression must occur. When the patient is in severe respiratory distress, diagnosis of a tension pneumothorax must be clinical, not radiographic, and the condition must be treated immediately, as time does not allow for radiologic studies.

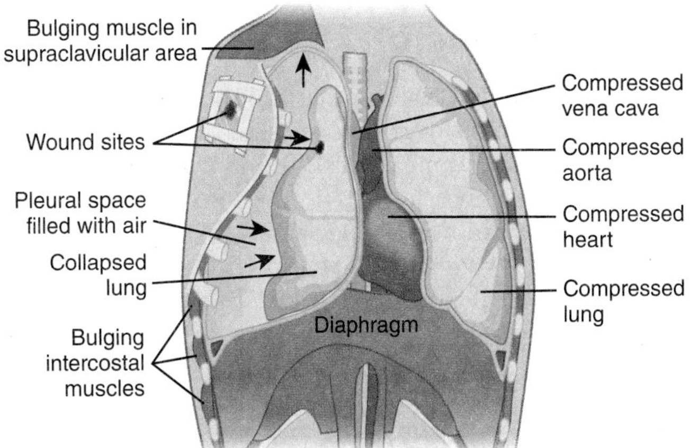

Figure 3-17 A tension pneumothorax can develop if a penetrating chest wound is bandaged tightly and air from a damaged lung cannot escape. The air then accumulates in the pleural space, eventually causing compression of the heart and great vessels.

Treatment

The goal when treating pneumothoraces is to restore an air-free pleural space. The treatment you select should be guided by the patient's medical history, comorbid conditions, and clinical status; the likelihood of resolution; and follow-up avenues. Most patients will not require acute intervention, such as needle chest decompression, but they must at least receive oxygen and have their respiratory status closely monitored en route to the hospital.

The least invasive management strategy is simple observation; this approach is ideal for stable patients with no comorbid conditions who have good oxygenation and reserve capacity and a small pneumothorax. These patients may be observed in the ED for a period of 6 hours. If a repeat chest radiograph shows no increase in the size of the pneumothorax, they can be discharged, provided they receive close follow-up in 24 to 96 hours.

Simple aspiration may be performed on certain patients whose condition is unlikely to resolve without intervention. Candidates include symptomatic but stable patients and those who have a small pneumothorax but comorbid conditions such as COPD. To perform this procedure, a needle is introduced into the pleural space under local anesthesia, and air is aspirated to induce reexpansion of the lung.

Patients who are significantly symptomatic often warrant tube **thoracostomy**. If time permits, local anesthesia and procedural sedation are provided. The tube may be connected to a Heimlich valve, a one-way valve that lets air escape but not enter the pleural space. Alternatively, the tube may be connected to continuous wall suction. Surgical intervention may be necessary in severe or prolonged cases, or in cases in which tube thoracostomy does not rectify the pneumothorax.

Pleural Effusion

Pleural effusion is a collection of fluid in the pleural cavity on one or both sides of the chest. It may compress the lung and cause dyspnea. This fluid may collect in large volumes in response to irritation, infection, HF, or cancer. Though it can build up gradually, over days or even weeks, patients often report that their dyspnea came on suddenly. Pleural effusions should be considered as a contributing diagnosis in any patient with lung cancer and shortness of breath (**Figure 3-18**).

Pathophysiology

When fluid collects between the visceral and parietal pleura, it produces a pleural effusion. Effusions can be caused by infections, tumors, or trauma.

Some pleural effusions can contain several liters of fluid. A large effusion decreases lung capacity and causes dyspnea.

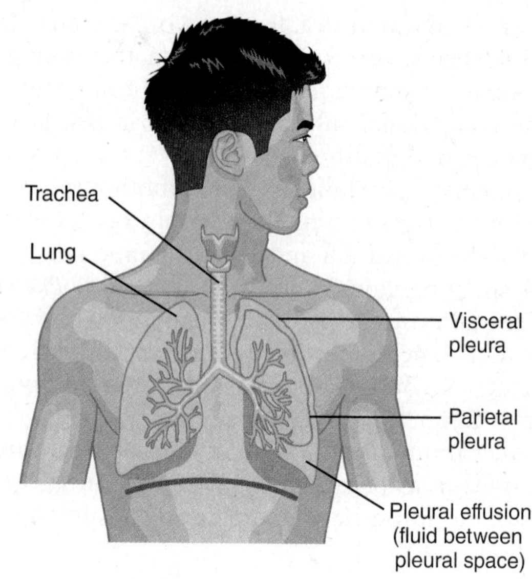

Figure 3-18 With a pleural effusion, fluid may accumulate in large volumes on one or both sides of the chest, compressing the lungs and causing dyspnea.

Signs and Symptoms

The most commonly noted symptom in patients with effusion is dyspnea. Chest pain (particularly pleuritic), cough, dyspnea on exertion, and orthopnea may also be present. The absence of a pleuritic component of chest pain does not rule out effusion. Certain etiologies of effusion may be associated with additional symptoms (e.g., pneumonia causing fever and productive cough), and systemic effects such as hypotension and hypoxia may suggest sepsis.

When you listen with a stethoscope to the chest of a patient with dyspnea resulting from pleural effusion, you will hear decreased breath sounds over the regions of the chest where fluid has moved the lung away from the chest wall. These patients frequently feel better if they are sitting upright. Nothing will really relieve their symptoms, however, except removal of the fluid (**thoracentesis**), which must be done by a physician in the hospital.

Differential Diagnosis

Effusions can be confirmed on chest radiograph, which can help guide treatment. Lateral decubitus films can help image smaller effusions but may be unnecessary with larger effusions. Approximately 200 mL of fluid is required to produce a layer of fluid throughout the lung when the patient is placed in the decubitus position. Supine films can help determine whether the fluid is loculated (within a cavity), which may suggest empyema.

Pneumonia, pulmonary abscess, empyema, pulmonary embolism, and hemothorax can have symptoms and physical findings similar to pleural effusion. Of these conditions, hemothorax often has a traumatic etiology, whereas the other causes are medical. Consider malignancy in patients who present with new pulmonary effusion. Consider tuberculosis in patients known to have been exposed to this infection.

HF should also be part of the differential diagnosis, as well as myocardial infarction and ischemia with accompanying HF. Collection of fluid in the pericardial space or in both the pericardial and pleural spaces after a recent myocardial infarction should prompt you to consider Dressler syndrome. In addition to the inflammation after a myocardial infarction, the pericarditis of Dressler syndrome can be caused by postsurgical changes or trauma.

Treatment

Allow patients to sit in a position of comfort, usually semi-erect or fully erect. Provide supportive care, including oxygen administration and analgesia, as needed.

In the hospital, fluid from significant effusions can be extracted by needle thoracentesis for both diagnostic purposes and symptomatic relief. Chemical and microscopic examination of the aspirated fluid can determine its etiology. Tube thoracostomy or surgery may be required to relieve very large effusions or to treat the cause of the effusion, as in the case of certain aggressive cancers. Imaging with CT may be performed in patients who have a new-onset effusion; this study can help diagnose lung cancer and tuberculosis that may be associated with the effusion.

Pulmonary Embolism

Pulmonary embolism is the sudden blockage of an artery in the lung by an embolus (plural, emboli), which could be a blood clot, an air bubble, a fatty plaque, or even a group of tumor cells that travel to the pulmonary circulation from elsewhere in the body. A clot that embolizes from a deep venous thrombosis (DVT) in an extremity is one of the most common causes of pulmonary embolism.

Pathophysiology

The pulmonary circulation may be compromised by a blood clot (embolism); a fat embolism from a broken bone; an amniotic fluid embolism during pregnancy; or an air embolism resulting from a large venous laceration, a central IV line, or barotrauma such as after scuba diving. A large embolus, of whatever type, will usually lodge in a major branch of the pulmonary artery and prevent blood flow through that branch; as a result, blood cannot perfuse the alveoli in the affected area.

Signs and Symptoms

Because some patients present with mild symptoms, and because the presentation may mimic more common conditions such as acute coronary syndrome, viral URIs, and COPD exacerbations, pulmonary embolism can be a very challenging diagnosis to make. Patients at risk of this condition include those who have recently had surgery or major trauma and those with indwelling catheters. Other risk factors include prolonged immobilization, including long travel; oral contraceptives; pregnancy; smoking; cancer; and prior history of DVT/pulmonary embolism. Signs and symptoms suggesting pulmonary embolism include the following:

- Chest pain, especially pleuritic
- Dyspnea
- Tachycardia
- Syncope
- Hemoptysis (blood-tinged sputum)
- New-onset wheezing
- Tachyarrhythmia

The classic triad of chest pain, hemoptysis, and dyspnea is seen in fewer than 20% of patients. Early symptoms of pulmonary embolism may be minimal, but massive pulmonary embolism evolves quickly and may rapidly become symptomatic, leading to cardiac arrest with pulseless electrical activity as the presenting rhythm.

Differential Diagnosis

Pulmonary embolism is one of the most frequently misdiagnosed conditions in emergency medicine because of its confusing presentation. The early presentation may reveal normal breath sounds with good peripheral aeration, diverting attention away from a pulmonary pathology. The classic presentation is sudden dyspnea and sharp pain in the chest. A hallmark of pulmonary embolism is that hypoxemia does not markedly improve with oxygen therapy.

On physical exam, massive pulmonary embolism can cause hypotension due to impaired venous return to the left atrium. New wheezing may be noted and can be deceptive, especially in patients with COPD or asthma. Lung sounds are often clear, as nothing prevents the air from moving in and out of the chest. Instead, the circulation is obstructed by the pulmonary embolism, leading to ventilation–perfusion mismatch.

Diagnostic Testing

A D-dimer test is very sensitive but cannot be fully relied upon in patients with moderate to high risk of pulmonary embolism. These patients will require a more definitive test such as CT angiography or a nuclear ventilation–perfusion scan to confirm the diagnosis. Chest radiographs are typically normal, unless the classic wedge-shaped pulmonary infarct has developed. Sinus tachycardia is the most common rhythm abnormality but is a nonspecific finding. Oxygen saturations show little improvement with oxygen administration.

Treatment

Treatment of suspected pulmonary embolism in the field includes supportive care with oxygen and NIPPV if necessary, and close monitoring including of pulse oximetry, blood pressure, and cardiac rhythm. Critical care teams may initiate or continue anticoagulation. In severe cases, thrombectomy may be performed.

Preventive measures include low-dose anticoagulation and compression stockings, and intermittent pneumatic compression devices; these are often used in hospitalized and bedridden patients to reduce the risk of blood clots forming in the legs. Especially for patients with a history of DVT, a Greenfield filter may be inserted by a physician. This device, which opens like a mesh umbrella in the inferior vena cava, is intended to catch clots that break loose and travel from the legs.

Pulmonary Arterial Hypertension

Pulmonary arterial hypertension (PAH), one of five types of pulmonary hypertension, is a rare chronic disease characterized by elevated pulmonary artery pressure. The high pressure in the pulmonary artery makes it difficult for the right side of the heart to pump enough blood to the lungs, and this decreased blood flow eventually affects both sides of the heart and the lungs.

Affecting only 5 to 15 people per 1 million population in the United States, the primary idiopathic and hereditary forms of the disease are clinically similar. Other causes of PAH include drugs and toxins, connective tissue disease, HIV, and congenital heart disease. The disease is most common among females of childbearing age and females in their 50s and 60s.

The four other types of pulmonary hypertension are related to severe chronic lung disease, left HF, chronic thromboembolism, and other chronic diseases.

Pathophysiology

Idiopathic or hereditary PAH begins with inflammation and changes in the cells lining the pulmonary arteries, leading to vasoconstriction, fibrotic changes, and micro-sized clots. These changes lead to an increased resistance to flow and elevated pressure in the pulmonary arteries, putting strain on the right ventricle. Many factors can contribute to the process that leads to the different types of pulmonary hypertension.

Signs and Symptoms

Signs and symptoms of PAH include the following:

- Dyspnea, especially on exertion (cardinal symptom)
- Weakness
- Fatigue
- Syncope
- Increased second heart sound (S_2)
- Tricuspid murmur
- Jugular venous pulsations
- Pitting edema

Lung sounds are often normal.

Differential Diagnosis

Many other heart and lung conditions that cause dyspnea and hypoxia must be considered. Echocardiography and blood tests can be performed to help confirm the diagnosis of PAH.

Treatment

Administering oxygen to dilate pulmonary vessels is an important part of treatment. The principal therapy for PAH is pulmonary vasodilation, using medications such as calcium-channel blockers, phoshopdiesterase-5 inhibitors, and endothelin receptor antagonists.

Other Conditions That Affect Respiratory Function

CNS Dysfunction

A wide range of CNS diseases can impair respiratory function, as shown in Table 3-9. In general, CNS disorders can be divided into three categories:

1. *Acute*. Illnesses lasting less than 1 week.
2. *Subacute*. Diseases and disorders lasting between 1 week and 2 months.
3. *Chronic*. Conditions lasting 2 months or longer.

Acute CNS Dysfunction

Acute CNS dysfunction can have numerous medical and traumatic causes. The focus here is on acute medical illnesses of the CNS that impair respiratory function. The primary concern in such cases is maintaining a patent airway. An occluded airway may lead to rapid deterioration and cerebral anoxia. Stroke, seizure, CNS infection, and other acute neuromuscular disorders may cause a decreased level of consciousness and place the patient at high risk for poor airway and ventilation control.

General changes in respiration such as hyperpnea, tachypnea, or both often accompany CNS dysfunction. Abnormal respiratory patterns sometimes suggest the etiology of the problem; they are presented in Chapter 1, *Advanced Medical Life Support Assessment for the Medical Patient*.

Table 3-9 CNS Conditions That Can Impair Respiration

Acute	Subacute	Chronic
Intoxication	Guillain-Barré syndrome	HIV/AIDS
Overdose	Encephalopathy	Neuromuscular degenerative disease (ALS)
Stroke/TIA	Meningitis	Dementia
Tick paralysis	Delirium	Myasthenia gravis paralysis
Myasthenia gravis paralysis	Myasthenia gravis paralysis	
Guillain-Barré syndrome		
Meningitis		
Encephalopathy		
Delirium		
Psychiatric illness		
Seizure		
Epidural abscess		

ALS, Amyotrophic lateral sclerosis; HIV/AIDS, human immunodeficiency virus/acquired immunodeficiency syndrome; TIA, transient ischemic attack.

Subacute CNS Dysfunction

Subacute CNS dysfunction can be responsible for prolonged respiratory compromise, including respiratory failure, atelectasis, pneumonia, lobar collapse, or infiltrate. An extended period of immobility can impair the ability to expel mucus, increase the risk of mucus plugging of the bronchi, and raise the risk of pneumonia as the alveoli lose their ability to expand. Persistent immobility can increase the threat of DVT and pulmonary embolism.

Chronic CNS Dysfunction

Chronic CNS dysfunction carries many of the same risks as subacute CNS dysfunction, such as an increased chance of DVT and pulmonary embolism. Prolonged respiratory compromise may necessitate a tracheostomy to maintain a secure airway. With this intervention, inspired air skirts the defenses of the upper airway, increasing the risk of a lower airway infection.

Furthermore, long-term care of CNS dysfunction is associated with exposure to hospitals and health care facilities, where serious infection with *Pseudomonas* species, health care–associated methicillin-resistant *S. aureus* (HA-MRSA), and vancomycin-resistant *Enterococcus* (VRE) is more likely.

Generalized Neurologic Disorders

Neuromuscular diseases such as myasthenia gravis and neuromuscular degenerative disease, often called amyotrophic lateral sclerosis (ALS) or Lou Gehrig's disease, are chronic diseases that have profound effects on the respiratory system. Respiratory muscle weakness or ineffective nervous system control can cause hypoventilation, resulting in atelectasis. Subsequent pneumonia can be life threatening in patients who are already debilitated by their neuromuscular disease. Acute respiratory failure can be superimposed on pneumonia or, conversely, pneumonia may precipitate respiratory failure.

A few chronic neuromuscular diseases bear mention individually. Guillain-Barré syndrome is an ascending paralysis believed to represent an overzealous response of the immune system to a viral infection. Patients with this disease may report having had a recent URI, with the ascending paralysis developing over the course of a few days. Respiratory compromise may be seen if the disorder progresses to involve the chest muscles and muscles of breathing.

Neuromuscular degenerative disease is a chronic muscle-wasting disease affecting the muscles of the extremities, some skeletal muscles, and the respiratory muscles. Respiratory muscle paralysis can be partial or complete and may make the patient permanently dependent on a ventilator.

A few final tips and cautions are in order:

- Do not use depolarizing neuromuscular blocking agents (i.e., succinylcholine) for medication-assisted intubation in patients with chronic neuromuscular diseases.
- Follow standard precautions because many nontraumatic respiratory complaints of CNS origin have an infectious origin.
- Provide supplemental oxygen and initiate appropriate airway management with any necessary sedation if you have any concern about the patient's ability to protect the airway.

Remember, all situations—acute, subacute, and chronic CNS dysfunction—should prompt meticulous attention to airway maintenance.

Medication Side Effects

Many medications have pulmonary side effects. Opioid medications induce sleep as well as respiratory depression. In a well patient, small to moderate doses of opioids induce pain relief and mild sedation. In larger doses, opioids induce respiratory depression and eventually respiratory arrest, to which almost all fatal opioid overdoses can be attributed. Both naloxone and naltrexone are effective in reversing opioid toxicity, although naloxone is more frequently given emergently because it is available in IV form. Naloxone can be administered to an adult by the IV, IM, or intranasal route, and its effects are both naloxone-dose and opioid-dose dependent. Alcohol has a synergistic effect with opioids, and acute intoxication with both substances increases the risk of respiratory depression.

Benzodiazepines such as diazepam, LORazepam, ALPRAZolam, and midazolam may also cause respiratory depression or, in significant quantities, respiratory failure, although they are much less likely to cause respiratory arrest compared to opioids. Like opioids, benzodiazepines have synergistic effects with alcohol, and combined ingestions increase the likelihood of an adverse outcome. Hypoventilation, respiratory depression, and respiratory failure can accompany major toxicity.

Use caution with any reversal agent in the setting of chronic use or abuse. Naloxone use may precipitate opioid withdrawal, which is rarely life threatening but almost always unwelcome. Withdrawal may make the patient less cooperative with clinicians, and some patients may threaten to leave against medical advice. Benzodiazepine withdrawal may precipitate seizures in severe cases. Treatment with flumazenil may complicate the management of withdrawal seizures and is not advised. Both naloxone and flumazenil have a variable duration, so monitor the patient carefully if airway compromise is suspected.

Cancer

Lung cancer is one of the most common forms of cancer, especially among people who smoke cigarettes and people who are exposed to occupational lung hazards, such as asbestos, coal dust, and secondhand smoke. Although lung cancer was traditionally considered predominantly a disease of men, today 45% of new cases of lung cancer occur in women, most likely because of the increased rate of smoking among women.

Signs and Symptoms

Lung cancer often is identified when tumors in the large airways bleed, causing hemoptysis (coughing up blood in the sputum) and uncontrollable coughing. It is frequently accompanied by COPD and impaired lung function. The lung is also a common site for the metastasis of cancer from other body sites.

Other cancers may invade the lymph nodes in the neck, producing tumors that threaten to occlude the upper airway. Patients with various types of cancer may have pulmonary complications from chemotherapy or radiation therapy. Lung irradiation, for example, may be associated with some degree of scarring or pulmonary edema. Tumors or treatment may also cause pleural effusion, which can present as rapidly progressing dyspnea.

Clinical symptoms mirror the extent of disease and metastasis but may include the following:

- Cough
- Dyspnea
- Dyspnea on exertion
- Wheezing
- Hemoptysis
- Chest wall pain from pleural irritation or pleural effusion (decreased breath sounds may not be noted until a significant pleural effusion develops)

Regional spread of the cancer can compress structures or destroy tissue, generating a broad range of symptoms. For example, superior vena cava obstruction can cause extensive central thrombus and emboli formation, paralysis of the recurrent laryngeal nerve can cause hoarseness, pressure on the esophagus can cause swallowing difficulties, and so on. The cancer may cause a markedly elevated calcium level, which then leads to muscle pain, renal problems, kidney stones, and mental status changes. A chest radiograph will often demonstrate the malignancy as well as any associated effusion.

Treatment

Treatment involves administering supplemental oxygen, assisting ventilation, ensuring a patent airway, and providing appropriate suctioning. Pneumothoraces are extremely rare with lung cancer, but consider this condition if the patient has had a recent lung biopsy. Pleural effusions, if present, are rarely drained emergently (see the earlier discussion).

Toxic Inhalations

Many potentially toxic substances can be inhaled into the lungs. The type of damage depends largely on the water solubility of the toxic gas.

Signs and Symptoms

Highly water-soluble gases like ammonia will react with the moist mucous membranes of the upper airway and cause swelling and irritation. If the substance gets in the patient's eyes, they will also burn and feel inflamed and irritated.

Less water-soluble gases may get deep into the lower airway, where they can do damage over time. Such toxic gases have been used in war to disable the enemy because they do not cause immediate distress, but rather cause pulmonary edema up to 24 hours later. The gases phosgene and nitrogen dioxide behave in this manner.

Some common gases—for example, chlorine—are moderately water soluble and cause problems somewhere between the extremes of irritation and pulmonary edema. Severe exposure may present with upper airway swelling, whereas lower-level exposure may present with the classic delayed onset and lower airway damage. A common household error is pouring drain cleaner and chlorine bleach into a drain to clear a clog, which may produce an irritant chlorine gas that sickens the person and everyone in the home or building. Industrial settings often use irritant gas–forming chemicals in large quantities and in higher concentrations than are available for home use, creating the potential for incidents that expose a larger number of people or involve a more toxic gas. EMS clinicians should note the industrial settings in their area that are at high risk for this type of incident.

Toxic gases can also affect people outside industrial settings. In particular, one common type of exposure is carbon monoxide. Natural gas has an odor because of a chemical additive, but carbon monoxide is colorless, odorless, and tasteless. Carbon monoxide is the leading cause of accidental poisoning deaths in the United States. People who survive carbon monoxide poisoning can have permanent brain damage.

Carbon monoxide is produced by household appliances such as gas water heaters, space heaters, grills, and generators, and it is even present in cigarette smoke. Many cases of carbon monoxide poisoning occur at the onset of cold weather, when people turn heaters on for the first time of the season. The combined effects of incomplete combustion and generally poor or no ventilation in a cold weather–sealed building result in the perfect scenario for producing toxic levels of carbon monoxide. Other sources of carbon monoxide poisoning include smoke from fires and motor vehicle exhaust. Some people attempt suicide by parking their car in their garage, turning the vehicle on, and inhaling the exhaust.

Table 3-10 Signs and Symptoms of Carbon Monoxide Poisoning

Severity	COHb Level	Signs and Symptoms
Mild	< 15–20%	Headache, nausea, vomiting, dizziness, blurred vision
Moderate	21–40%	Confusion, syncope, chest pain, dyspnea, weakness, tachycardia, tachypnea, rhabdomyolysis
Severe	41–59%	Palpitations, dysrhythmias, hypotension, myocardial ischemia, cardiac arrest, respiratory arrest, pulmonary edema, seizures, coma
Fatal	$> 60\%$	Death

COHb, carboxyhemoglobin.

People who are exposed to carbon monoxide may think they have the flu. They initially complain of headache, dizziness, fatigue, and nausea and vomiting. They may complain of dyspnea on exertion and chest pain, and display nervous system symptoms such as impaired judgment, confusion, or even hallucinations. The worst exposures may result in syncope or seizure. The signs and symptoms associated with carbon monoxide poisoning are listed in Table 3-10.

Differential Diagnosis

The relevant differential diagnosis will be based on the patient's actual signs and symptoms. For example, for upper airway irritation, a wide range of infections, allergy, and trauma should be considered in addition to toxic inhalation. For lower respiratory symptoms, a wide range of pulmonary and cardiac conditions as discussed in this chapter should be considered unless there is definitive evidence of a toxic exposure.

Treatment

A patient who has been exposed to a toxic gas must be removed from the environment immediately and provided with 100% supplemental oxygen or assisted ventilation if breathing is impaired (i.e., if there is reduced TV). If the upper airway is compromised, aggressive airway management (such as intubation or a cricothyrotomy) may be required.

Patients who have been exposed to slightly water-soluble gases may feel fine initially but develop acute dyspnea many hours later. When such an exposure is suspected, patients should strongly consider transport to the closest ED for observation and further assessment.

Special Populations

Older Adult Patients

The respiratory system of aging patients undergoes multiple changes, all of which ultimately impair the body's ability to oxygenate the blood. A wide range of physiologic changes can occur both within the respiratory tract and in the body structures that support ventilation. A summary of the physiologic changes associated with advancing age follows:

- Thinning of the epithelial linings
- Decreased mucus production
- Decreased motility of the respiratory cilia that clear mucus from the airways
- Reduced lung compliance due to calcification of cartilage in the trachea and bronchioles and calcification of interstitial tissues
- Decreasing respiratory surface area as the number of alveoli decreases
- Reduced intrathoracic volume secondary to fractures, slumping, or bone changes
- Less vigorous immune response, including fewer immunoglobulins and leukocytes
- Weakened muscles of respiration, including the diaphragm, intercostal muscles, and accessory muscles

Because these changes occur gradually, often over a period of years or even decades, the body has time to adapt to a significant decrease in function. A good example is the decrease in respiratory surface area that occurs as a person ages. The blood oxygen level (i.e., the partial pressure of oxygen) in a young adult normally averages 95 mm Hg. In an older adult, a value as low as 60 mm Hg is not uncommon. If the partial pressure of oxygen of 60 mm Hg is noted in a young, seemingly healthy individual, you should be quite concerned.

The likelihood of pathologic changes in the respiratory system and supporting structures increases as a patient ages. Some intrapleural diseases impair the lungs' ability to inspire and expire air. Others inhibit diffusion of oxygen into the blood and carbon dioxide out of the blood. In addition, tumors can occupy lung space, decreasing the area available for ventilation. Chronic smoking can damage alveoli, narrow bronchi and choke them with mucus, and displace functioning alveoli with large blebs, or air pockets. Circulatory changes can result in delivery of less or thinner blood to the lung capillaries, impairing oxygenation. Decreased hemoglobin levels can reduce the oxygen-carrying capacity of red blood cells.

All of these changes can combine to make it more difficult for an older adult to perform normal activities of daily living. In elderly patients, a relatively minor respiratory infection can pose a life threat. Pneumonia may cause an already marginally hypoxic elderly patient to become severely hypoxic, requiring respiratory support and mechanical ventilation.

Obstetric Patients

Pulmonary physiology changes in pregnancy. Upper airway mucosal edema, mucus secretion, nasal congestion, and rhinitis can create difficulties with BVM ventilation and endotracheal intubation. A pregnant patient has reduced respiratory reserve because of the elevated oxygen demand on their system. In a critical illness, rapid and severe respiratory decompensation may occur. A pregnant patient is also at greater risk of gastric aspiration.

The following conditions may cause respiratory disorders in a pregnant patient:

- Preeclampsia (hypertension and proteinuria occurring after the 20th week of gestation)
- Pulmonary embolism (may occur throughout pregnancy, but the highest incidence is in the immediate postpartum period)
- Respiratory infection (such as pneumonia and influenza)
- Asthma
- ARDS

Bariatric Patients

Increased body mass can impede or complicate many functions of the respiratory system:

- The larger body mass increases the amount of energy needed to carry out routine activities, with a consequent increase in the need for delivery of oxygen and removal of carbon dioxide and other waste products.
- The body's sheer physical mass limits the range of motion of the chest, reducing contraction of the diaphragm and subsequent expansion of the lungs. Obstructive sleep apnea is common, as are other respiratory conditions such as pulmonary embolism, COPD, HF, and pneumonia.

- When a person is lying supine, excessive weight in the anterior abdomen can shift to the upper abdomen, limiting expansion of the chest and perhaps decreasing TV, leading to hypercapnia and subsequent respiratory acidosis.

The lungs can expand somewhat in response to increased demand, but their size is limited by the abdomen and its contents. The chest can increase in diameter, a response often seen in patients who chronically use tobacco (an indicator of chronic bronchitis), but the size of the chest is also limited. The heart can become more efficient by pumping faster and harder, but these adjustments may have long-term cardiovascular side effects, including HF.

Putting It All Together

Disorders resulting in respiratory compromise are common in patients of all ages and are seen by all levels of health care clinicians. Respiratory complaints can result in significant oxygenation and ventilation compromise. A thorough patient history, physical exam, and evaluation of diagnostic findings will aid your early recognition of the underlying etiologies of respiratory distress and respiratory failure.

As a health care clinician, your understanding of the anatomy, physiology, and pathophysiology of the respiratory system and the diseases contributing to inadequate ventilation and oxygenation can be critical in evaluating your patient's level of distress and initiating proper care. Ineffective work of breathing may be due to a variety of dysfunctional processes. Be familiar with the differences and similarities of reactive airway diseases, bacterial versus viral infections, and the causes of airway occlusion—accidental, traumatic, and idiopathic. Maintain your skill levels at peak performance and be ready to initiate prompt BLS and ALS airway adjunct interventions. The expertise you bring to the work of responding to and attending patients with respiratory disorders can save lives.

SCENARIO SOLUTION

- Differential diagnoses may include pharyngitis, tonsillitis, peritonsillar abscess, epiglottitis, Ludwig angina, retropharyngeal abscess, and prevertebral abscess.
- To narrow your differential diagnosis, you will need to complete the history of present illness and obtain the past medical history as much as is possible. Perform a physical examination of the patient's mouth and throat. Do not insert anything into the mouth to examine the throat, as it could worsen airway swelling. Assess the patient's oxygen saturation. Palpate his submental area and his neck. This examination should not delay transport or transfer to an area where advanced airway management is possible.
- This patient has signs of impending airway obstruction. Airway management in patients with airway obstruction is best provided by emergency physicians, anesthesiology, or ENT surgeons when immediately available. Administer humidified oxygen. Prepare to suction his oropharynx (provide him with an emesis basin to spit secretions if he prefers). Establish vascular access and deliver IV fluids. Prepare to intubate. Select several tube sizes. Prepare equipment for cricothyrotomy if the airway cannot be secured by oral endotracheal intubation. Consider medication for fever, antibiotics, and pain once the airway is managed.

SUMMARY

- The upper and lower airways conduct air (ventilation) to the alveoli, the site of gas exchange (diffusion).
- Sensors within the body tell the respiratory system when and how to adjust ventilation to meet the body's needs for oxygen and carbon dioxide and maintain its acid-base balance.
- The interdependence of the respiratory anatomy on other thoracic structures helps it provide oxygen to all tissues and eliminate carbon dioxide.
- Diseases of the cardiovascular system, which shares intrathoracic space with the respiratory system, should be included in the differential diagnosis when the patient complains of

(continues)

SUMMARY (CONTINUED)

respiratory distress or failure, weakness, airway compromise, chest pain, altered mental status, cough, or fever.

- Specific disease processes that may compromise the upper airway include anatomic obstruction, aspiration, allergic reactions, and inflammation caused by infection.
- Specific disease processes characterized by lower airway dysfunction include asthma, COPD, pulmonary infections, pneumothorax, pleural effusion, pulmonary embolism, and pulmonary arterial hypertension.
- Other conditions that may potentially affect respiratory function include CNS dysfunction, generalized neurologic disorders, medication side effects, cancer, and toxic inhalations.
- Your assessment of the patient with respiratory complaints should include a standard emergency approach. Special monitoring and diagnostic clues can help you narrow the differential diagnoses.
- Patient management includes airway and ventilatory support, with ongoing assessment that reassures the patient that the treatment plan is being reassessed and carried out based on your findings.

Key Terms

acute lung injury/acute respiratory distress syndrome (ALI/ARDS) Syndrome that typically occurs in ill patients, which is characterized by alveolar and pulmonary capillary breakdown leading to edema and alveolar collapse; this leads to severe hypoxemia and difficult ventilation.

aerobic metabolism The normal metabolism that utilizes oxygen.

anaerobic metabolism The metabolism that takes place in the absence of oxygen; the principal by-product is lactic acid.

angioedema A vascular reaction that may have an allergic, hereditary, drug-induced, or other non-allergic cause and may result in profound swelling of the face, upper airway, and other regions of the body.

apneustic center A portion of the pons that assists in creating longer, slower respirations.

atelectasis The collapse of the alveolar air spaces of the lungs.

carboxyhemoglobin Hemoglobin bound to carbon monoxide.

chemoreceptors Chemical receptors that sense changes in the composition of blood and body fluids. The primary chemical changes registered by chemoreceptors are those involving levels of hydrogen (H^+), carbon dioxide (CO_2), and oxygen (O_2).

end-tidal carbon dioxide ($ETCO_2$) The CO_2 level in the expired air at the end of expiration.

gas exchange The process in which oxygen in the alveoli is taken up by circulating blood cells and carbon dioxide from the bloodstream is released to air in the alveoli.

history of present illness (HPI) Information about the patient's chief complaint and related symptoms. The primary elements of the HPI can be obtained by using the OPQRST and SAMPLER mnemonics. It is the most important element of patient assessment.

hypercapnia An abnormally elevated carbon dioxide level in the blood, caused by hypoventilation or lung disease. It may also be caused by exposure to environments containing abnormally high concentrations of carbon dioxide, or by rebreathing exhaled carbon dioxide. Usually defined as a carbon dioxide level > 45 mm Hg. This term is interchangeable with *hypercarbia*.

Ludwig angina A deep-space infection of the floor of the mouth and anterior neck just below the mandible.

noninvasive positive-pressure ventilation (NIPPV) A procedure in which positive pressure is provided through the upper airway by some type of mask or other noninvasive device.

peritonsillar abscess An abscess in the submucosal space adjacent to the tonsils. This abscess and its accompanying inflammation can cause the uvula to deviate to the opposing side.

pneumotaxic center Located in the pons, this center generally controls the rate and pattern of respiration.

respiration (1) Physiologically, the transfer of oxygen from the environment to the cells of the body and the reciprocal transfer of carbon dioxide from the body to the environment. (2) Biochemically, the generation of energy through the oxidation of nutrients.

respiratory failure A disorder in which the lungs become unable to perform their basic task of gas exchange—that is, the transfer of oxygen from inhaled air into the blood and the transfer of carbon dioxide from the blood into exhaled air.

thoracentesis A procedure to remove fluid or air from the pleural space.

thoracic duct Located in the left upper thorax; the largest lymph vessel in the body. It returns the excess fluid that is not collected by the veins from the lower extremities and abdomen to the venae cavae.

thoracostomy A procedure in which an opening is made through the skin into the pleural cavity; a tube is often placed through the opening to facilitate drainage of air, blood or other fluid.

ultrasound Also called *sonography* or *diagnostic medical sonography*; an imaging method that uses high-frequency sound waves to produce precise images of structures within the body.

Bibliography

Acerra JR. Pharyngitis. *Medscape.* Updated April 6, 2022. https://emedicine.medscape.com/article/764304-overview

Aceves SS, Wasserman SI. Evaluating and treating asthma, *Emerg Med.* 2005;37:20-29.

Akinbami LJ, Moorman JE, Bailey C, et al. *Trends in Asthma Prevalence, Health Care Use, and Mortality in the United States, 2001–2010.* NCHS Data Brief, No. 94. National Center for Health Statistics; 2012.

American Academy of Orthopaedic Surgeons. *Emergency Care and Transportation of the Sick and Injured.* 12th ed. Jones & Bartlett Learning; 2022.

American Academy of Orthopaedic Surgeons. *Nancy Caroline's Emergency Care in the Streets.* 9th ed. Jones & Bartlett Learning; 2022.

American Academy of Pediatrics. Prevention of choking among children. *Pediatrics.* 2010;125:601-607.

Amitai A. Ventilator management. *Medscape.* Updated April 7, 2020. https://emedicine.medscape.com/article/810126-overview

Asmussen J, Gellett S, Pilegaard H, et al. Conjunctival oxygen tension measurements for assessment of tissue oxygen tension during pulmonary surgery. *Eur Surg Res.* 1994;26:372-379.

Baez AA, Qasim Z, Wilcox S, et al. Prehospital mechanical ventilation: an NAEMSP position statement and resource document. *Prehosp Emerg Care.* 2022;26(suppl 1):88-95.

Benson BE. Stridor. *Medscape.* Updated April 7, 2022. https://emedicine.medscape.com/article/995267-overview

BMJ Best Practice. Acute exacerbation of chronic obstructive pulmonary disease. Updated June 8, 2023. https://bestpractice.bmj.com/topics/en-us/8

Boka K. Pleural effusion. *Medscape.* Updated October 15, 2021. https://emedicine.medscape.com/article/299959-overview.

Braud D, Dixon D, Torres M, et al. Brief research report: prehospital rapid sequence airway. *Prehosp Emerg Care.* 2021;25(4):583-587.

Centers for Disease Control and Prevention. Most recent national asthma data. Last reviewed May 10, 2023. https://www.cdc.gov/asthma/most_recent_national_asthma_data.htm

Centers for Disease Control and Prevention. National trends in COPD. Last reviewed July 20, 2022. https://www.cdc.gov/copd/data-and-statistics/national-trends.html

Daley BJ. Pneumothorax. *Medscape.* Updated May 9, 2022. https://emedicine.medscape.com/article/424547-overview.

Deitch K, Miner J, Chudnofsky CR, et al. Does end tidal CO_2 monitoring during emergency department procedural sedation and analgesia with propofol decrease the incidence of hypoxic events? A randomized, controlled trial. *Ann Emerg Med.* 2010;55(3):258-264.

Deitch K, Rowden A, Damiron K, et al. Unrecognized hypoxia and respiratory depression in emergency department patients sedated for psychomotor agitation: pilot study. *West J Emerg Med.* 2014;15(4):430-437.

Dumitru I. Heart failure. *Medscape.* Updated June 5, 2023. https://emedicine.medscape.com/article/163062-overview

Fink S, Abraham E, Ehrlich H. Postoperative monitoring of conjunctival oxygen tension and temperature. *Int J Clin Monit Comput.* 1988;5:37-43.

Flores J. Peritonsillar abscess in emergency medicine. *Medscape.* Updated October 13, 2022. https://emedicine.medscape.com/article/764188-overview

Gamache J. Bacterial pneumonia. *Medscape.* Updated September 30, 2020. https://emedicine.medscape.com/article/300157-overview

Gompf SG. Epiglottitis. *Medscape.* Updated April 5, 2022. https://emedicine.medscape.com/article/763612-overview

Green TE. Acute angioedema: overview of angioedema treatment. *Medscape.* Updated August 28, 2018. https://emedicine.medscape.com/article/756261-overview

Gresham C. Benzodiazepine toxicity. *Medscape.* Updated April 28, 2022. https://emedicine.medscape.com/article/813255-overview

Harman EM. Acute respiratory distress syndrome (ARDS). *Medscape.* Updated March 27, 2020. https://emedicine.medscape.com/article/165139-overview.

Howes DS. Encephalitis. *Medscape.* Updated August 7, 2018. https://emedicine.medscape.com/article/791896-overview

Hunter CL, Silvestri S, Ralls G, et al. A prehospital screening tool utilizing end-tidal carbon dioxide predicts sepsis and severe sepsis. *Am J Emerg Med.* 2016;34:813-819.

Jenkins W, Verdile VP, Paris PM. The syringe aspiration technique to verify endotracheal tube position. *Am J Emerg Med.* 1994;12(4):413-416.

Kaplan J. Barotrauma. *Medscape.* Updated April 27, 2022. https://emedicine.medscape.com/article/768618-overview

Khan JH. Retropharyngeal abscess. *Medscape.* Updated January 8, 2021. https://emedicine.medscape.com/article/764421-overview

Maffei FA, Lambert RL, Azar JM. Should the pediatric advanced life support DOPE mnemonic be revised? *Pediatr Emerg Care.* 2023;39(6):462. doi:10.1097/PEC.0000000000002957

Marx J, Walls R, Hockberger R. *Rosen's Emergency Medicine: Concepts and Clinical Practice.* 5th ed. Mosby; 2002.

Memon MA. Panic disorder. *Medscape.* Updated March 21, 2018. https://emedicine.medscape.com/article/287913-overview

Morris MJ. Asthma. *Medscape.* Updated January 12, 2023. https://emedicine.medscape.com/article/296301-overview

Mosenafir Z. Chronic obstructive pulmonary disease. *Medscape.* Updated June 3, 2022. https://emedicine.medscape.com/article/297664-overview

Murray AD. Deep neck infections. *Medscape.* Updated April 7, 2022. https://emedicine.medscape.com/article/837048-overview

Nadel JA, Murray JF, Mason RJ. *Murray & Nadel's Textbook pf Respiratory Medicine.* 4th ed. Elsevier Saunders; 2005.

National Highway Traffic Safety Administration. *National Emergency Medical Services Education Standards.* Published December 9, 2021. https://www.ems.gov/assets/EMS_Education-Standards_2021_FNL.pdf

Nguyen VQ. Dilated cardiomyopathy. *Medscape.* Updated March 2, 2021. https://emedicine.medscape.com/article/757668-overview.

Oudiz RJ. Idiopathic pulmonary arterial hypertension. *Medscape.* Updated February 6, 2023. https://emedicine.medscape.com/article/301450-overview

Ouellette DR. Pulmonary embolism (PE). *Medscape.* Updated September 18, 2020. https://emedicine.medscape.com/article/759765-overview.

Panchal AR, Bartos JA, Cabanas JG, et al. Part 3: adult basic and advanced life support: 2020 American Heart Association guidelines update for cardiopulmonary resuscitation and emergency cardiovascular care. *Circulation.* 2020;142(18 suppl 2):S366-S468.

Pappas DE, Hendley JO. Retropharyngeal abscess, lateral pharyngeal abscess and peritonsillar abscess. In: Kleigman RM, et al., eds. *Nelson Textbook of Pediatrics.* 18th ed. Saunders; 2007:1754-1755.

Paramedic Association of Canada. National occupational competency profile. Updated 2011. https://paramedic.ca/competencies/nocp

Paul M, Dueck M, Kampe S, et al. Intracranial placement of a nasotracheal tube after transnasal trans-sphenoidal surgery. *Br J Anaesth.* 2003;91:601-604.

Peng LF. Dental infections in emergency medicine. *Medscape.* Updated January 17, 2023. https://emedicine.medscape.com/article/763538-overview

Petrache I. Pleurodynia. *Medscape.* Updated December 8, 2020. https://emedicine.medscape.com/article/300049-overview

Qaseem A, Etxeandia-Ikobaltzeta I, Mustafa RA, et al. Appropriate use of point-of-care ultrasonography in patients with acute dyspnea in emergency department or inpatient settings: a clinical guideline from the American College of Physicians. *Ann Intern Med.* 2021;174(7):985-993.

Rackow E, O'Neil P, Astiz M, et al. Sublingual capnometry and indexes of tissue perfusion in patients with circulatory failure. *Chest.* 2001;120:1633-1638.

Ren X. Aortic stenosis. *Medscape.* Updated November 18, 2021. https://emedicine.medscape.com/article/150638-overview

Risavi BL, Wadas RJ, Thomas C, Kupas DF. A novel method for continuous environmental surveillance for carbon monoxide exposure to protect emergency medical services providers and patients. *J Emerg Med.* 2013;44(3):637-640.

Rubin J, Hopkins W. The epidemiology and pathogenesis of pulmonary arterial hypertension (Group 1). *UpToDate.* Updated November 28, 2022. https://www.uptodate.com/contents/the-epidemiology-and-pathogenesis-of-pulmonary-arterial-hypertension-group-1?search=pulmonary%20hypertension&topicRef=8249&source=see_link

Shah SN. Hypertrophic cardiomyopathy clinical presentation. *Medscape.* Updated April 29, 2022. https://emedicine.medscape.com/article/152913-clinical

Shapiro JM. Critical care of the obstetric patient. *J Intens Care Med.* 2006;21:278-286.

Shores C. Infections and disorders of the neck and upper airway. In: Tintinalli J, ed. *Emergency Medicine: A Comprehensive Study Guide.* McGraw-Hill Professional Publishing; 2004:1494-1501.

Snyder SR. Managing sepsis in the adult patient. *EMS World.* Published May 2012. https://www.hmpgloballearningnetwork.com/site/emsworld/article/10685110/managing-sepsis-adult-patient

Stephens E. Opioid toxicity. *Medscape.* Updated April 3, 2023. https://emedicine.medscape.com/article/815784-overview

Tan WW. Non-small cell lung cancer (NSCLC). *Medscape.* Updated June 7, 2023. https://emedicine.medscape.com/article/279960-overview

Tang WH. Myocarditis. *Medscape.* Updated December 28, 2021. https://emedicine.medscape.com/article/759212-overview

Tanigawa K, Takeda T, Goto E, et al. The efficacy of esophageal detector devices in verifying tracheal tube placement: a randomized cross-over study of out-of-hospital cardiac arrest patients. *Anesth Analg.* 2001;92:375-378.

Tatevossian RG, Wo CC, Velmahos GC, et al. Transcutaneous oxygen and CO_2 as early warning of tissue hypoxia and hemodynamic shock in critically ill emergency patients. *Crit Care Med.* 2000;28(7):2248-2253.

Urden L, Stacy K, Lough M. *Thelan's Critical Care Nursing: Diagnosis and Management.* 5th ed. Elsevier; 2006.

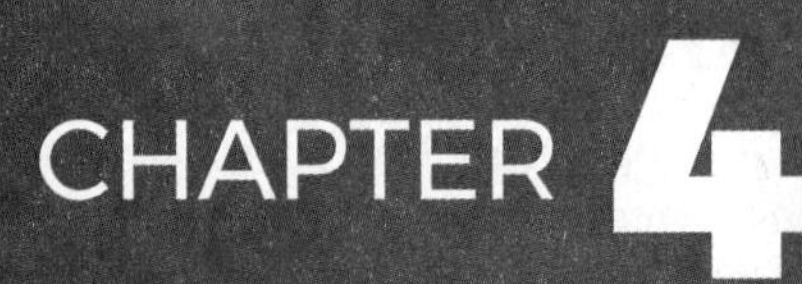

CHAPTER 4

Cardiovascular Disorders and Conditions Presenting as Chest Pain

Chapter Editors
Joshua B. Gaither, MD, FACEP, FAEMS
Michael Levy, MD, FACEP, FAEMS, FACP

Cardiovascular disorders are a common reason for adults to seek medical attention. Chest pain and chest discomfort are symptoms often described by patients, the causes of which may range from benign to life threatening. This chapter describes how to quickly assess the causes of chest pain and identify life-threatening causes by categorizing this common symptom based on the four possible systems affected: cardiovascular, pulmonary, gastrointestinal, or musculoskeletal. Additional descriptions will help you make an accurate field diagnosis, develop a treatment plan, and monitor the patient to adapt treatment as necessary.

LEARNING OBJECTIVES

At the conclusion of this chapter, you will be able to:

- Apply knowledge of anatomy, physiology, and pathophysiology to patients presenting with chest discomfort.
- Employ history collection and physical exam skills to direct the assessment for patients with chest discomfort.
- Apply knowledge of disease processes and the information obtained from the patient presentation, history, and physical exam to form a list of clinical impressions based on the degree of severity (life-threatening, emergent, and nonemergent diagnoses) using the AMLS Assessment Pathway.
- Manage patients with chest discomfort by making clinical decisions, performing diagnostic tests, and using the results to modify care as indicated. Decision making includes routing the patient to the correct resources and following accepted practice guidelines.
- Provide an ongoing assessment of a patient with chest discomfort and adapt treatment and management based on patient response and findings.

SCENARIO

A 37-year-old woman complains of dyspnea and chest pain. She has been feeling ill for about a week and vomited twice today. Her skin is flushed, and her heart rate is increased. She reports smoking two packs of cigarettes a day. Her only medications are birth control pills and insulin.

- Which differential diagnoses are you considering based on the information you have now?
- What additional information will you need to narrow your differential diagnosis?
- What are your initial treatment priorities as you continue your patient care?

Anatomy and Physiology

Chest pain can be caused by any of the structures in the chest, including the chest wall itself as well as intra-abdominal organs (**Figure 4-1**).

The Heart

The heart is a muscular organ composed of four chambers, divided into right and left sides, which are separated by a wall called the septum. The right side of the heart receives venous blood from the body and delivers it to the lungs for exchange of oxygen and carbon dioxide. The left side of the heart receives the oxygen-rich blood from the lungs and sends it to the rest of the body. The upper chambers (atria) and lower chambers (ventricles) on each side are separated by one-way valves that open and close, allowing for the blood to move in the intended direction. The heart is made of specialized muscle tissue called myocardium; its smooth inner surface is called the endocardium and its outer layer is called the epicardium. The epicardium, in turn, is the Innermost lining, or visceral pericardium, of the sac in which the heart resides, called the pericardium. The outer part of the sac, the parietal pericardium, is fibrous. Between these two layers there is a small amount of pericardial fluid.

A unique feature of myocardium is this muscle's ability to rhythmically contract. The contractions of the heart chambers are regulated by an electrical system within the heart that provides a pacemaker function. This electrical system controls the number of beats per minute and coordinates the contractions of all cardiac chambers through a specialized conduction system.

The Great Vessels

The great vessels include the aorta, superior and inferior venae cavae, pulmonary arteries, and pulmonary veins (**Figure 4-2**). The aorta exits from the top of the heart and arches to the left, down through the chest and into the abdomen, and then splits into the bilateral iliac arteries. A serious, life-threatening condition known as an aortic dissection occurs when the aorta becomes diseased or weakened and the innermost layer tears, allowing blood to dissect between the layers. The entire wall of the aorta can also become weak and bulge outward in an aortic aneurysm. A ruptured aortic aneurysm is a life-threatening emergency.

The Lungs and Pleurae

The anatomy and physiology of the respiratory system are briefly reviewed here; Chapter 3, *Respiratory Disorders*, covers the respiratory system in depth. The trachea, which conducts respiratory gases, divides into the bronchi, which further subdivide into the resistance airways that have muscle in addition to cartilage, allowing the small airways to constrict and expand. The lungs and airways bring in fresh oxygen-rich air and expel carbon dioxide, the product of cellular metabolism. During inhalation, the diaphragm and intercostal muscles contract and expand the chest. This expansion lowers the pressure in the chest below the outside air pressure. Air then flows in through the airways from an area of high pressure to low pressure and inflates the lungs. During exhalation, the diaphragm and intercostal muscles relax, and the weight of the chest wall along with the elasticity of the diaphragm and chest wall force the air out.

The lungs are enveloped with **pleurae** inside the chest cavity (**Figure 4-3**). The visceral pleura are directly

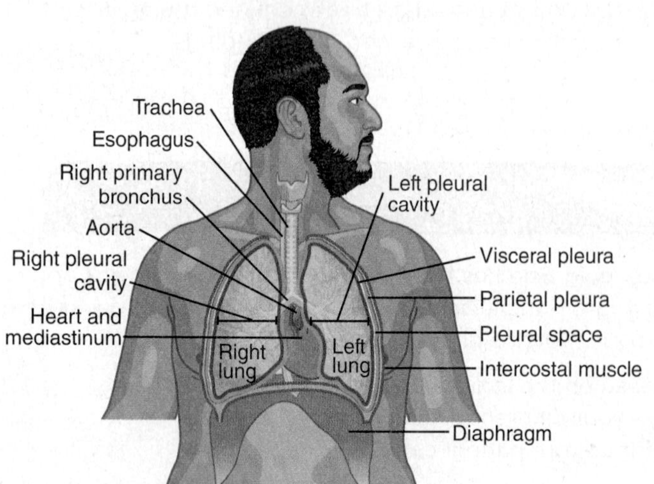

Figure 4-1 Thoracic cavity, including diaphragm, mediastinum, lungs, heart, bronchi, trachea, and esophagus.

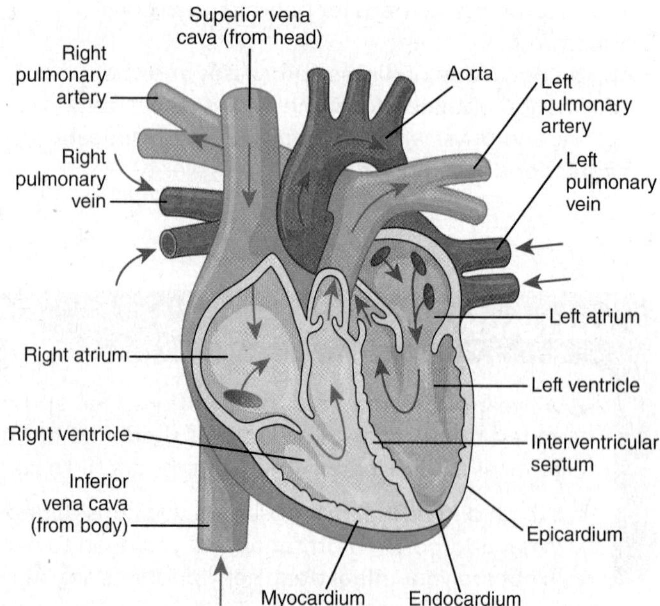

Figure 4-2 Pericardial reflections near the origins of the great vessels, shown after removal of the heart. Note that portions of the venae cavae lie within the pericardial space.

adherent to the lungs, and the parietal pleura to the chest wall. Between these two layers is a very small amount of pleural fluid that serves as lubricant, but there is no air. Therefore, when the chest wall and parietal pleurae expand, so do the visceral pleura and lungs. The pleurae have somatic sensory innervation, which may cause a patient to feel "sharp" pain—that is, somatic pain.

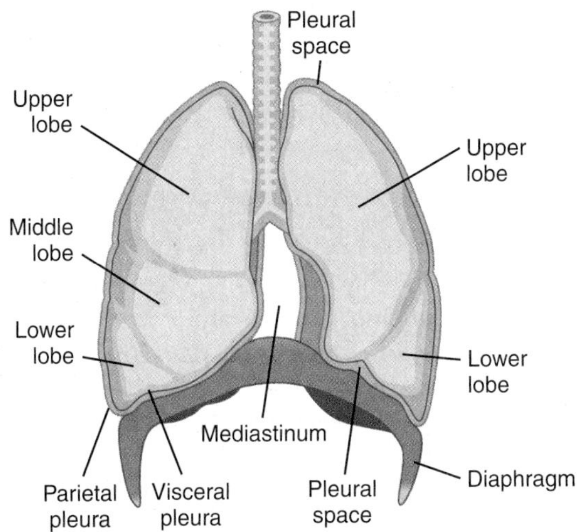

Figure 4-3 The pleurae lining the chest wall and covering the lungs are an essential part of the breathing mechanism.

The role of the lungs in the cardiovascular system is to transform the deoxygenated blood from the venous side of the circulation into the oxygen-rich blood needed to sustain life. Equally importantly, the lungs "exhaust" carbon dioxide (CO_2), the by-product of cellular energy production (**Figure 4-4**). Abnormalities of the lungs and chest wall can affect the function of the cardiovascular system, and abnormalities of the heart can affect the function of the lungs. This issue will be further explored elsewhere. Diseases and injuries of the lungs, pleurae, and chest wall are common causes of chest pain.

The Esophagus

The esophagus is a muscular tube lined with epithelial cells but lacking any fibrous outer layer. When food is swallowed, it passes from the pharynx into the esophagus, initiating rhythmic contractions (peristalsis) of the esophagus. This propels the food through the gastroesophageal (GE) sphincter into the stomach. Chest discomfort can occur if the muscular contractions are out of synchrony or spasm. Reflux of gastric contents back into the esophagus causes burning and pain (gastroesophageal reflux disease [GERD]). Forceful vomiting can tear the inside lining at the GE junction, causing pain and bleeding (Mallory-Weiss syndrome). A rare but catastrophic injury is a tear through the entire wall of the esophagus

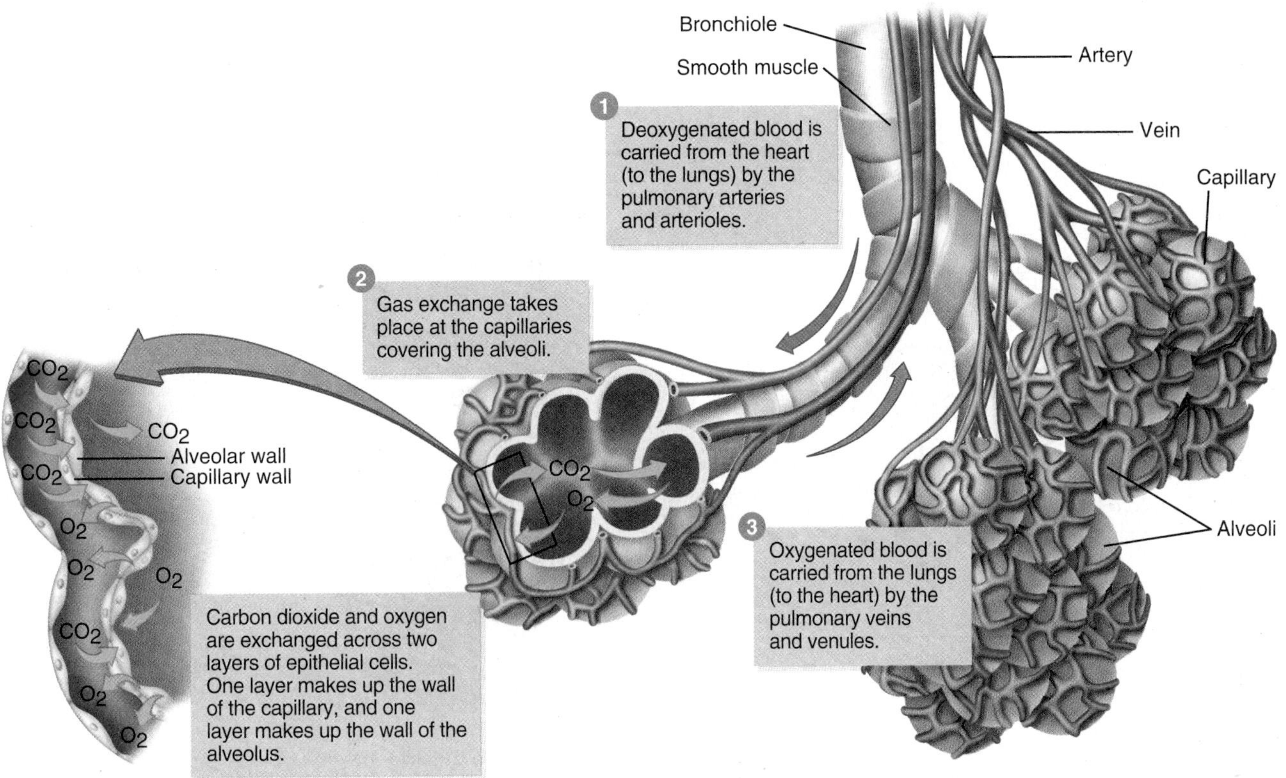

Figure 4-4 Exchange of gases in the lungs.

known as Boerhaave syndrome, which is usually associated with existing esophageal disease. In summary, chest pain can sometimes be caused by conditions involving the esophagus, but most of them are relatively benign. Because the symptoms of cardiac and esophageal causes of chest pain can be similar, it is always best to consider a cardiac etiology when unsure.

The Sensation of Chest Pain

The scientific and clinical definition of *pain* is an unpleasant sensory and emotional experience associated with actual or potential tissue damage. For the purposes of this chapter, *chest discomfort* includes not only pain, but also any feeling of discomfort to include burning, crushing, stabbing, pressure, heaviness, or squeezing sensations. Chest discomfort is the direct result of the stimulation of nerve fibers from potentially damaged tissues within the chest. This potential damage may be caused by mechanical obstruction, inflammation, infection, or **ischemia**. For example, with an **acute myocardial infarction (AMI)**, ischemic tissues send the brain sensory information that is interpreted as chest discomfort.

Many cardiovascular disorders cause chest discomfort. All complaints of chest discomfort should be taken seriously until potential life threats can be ruled out. At times, it may be difficult to distinguish chest discomfort from discomfort caused by organs or structures outside of the chest cavity (**Figure 4-5**). Although the boundaries of the chest cavity are well defined, organs or structures lying close to those boundaries may be served by similar nerve roots. A patient with gallbladder disease, for example, may complain of discomfort in the upper right side of the chest and shoulder because even though the gallbladder is located in the abdominal cavity, pain can be "referred" to the chest and shoulder. The converse may also be true: Pathophysiology inside the chest can be interpreted by the patient as symptoms outside the chest, such as in the abdomen, neck, and back. For example, AMI commonly presents with feelings of epigastric pain, nausea, and vomiting. **Tip Box 4-1** suggests ways to interpret and distinguish the pain patients may be feeling.

TIP BOX 4-1

Allow patients to tell you in their own words what they are experiencing. Pain coming from organs such as the heart may lead to unusual pain sensations, and if patients are offered terms to describe the pain, they may choose to use words that are potentially misleading. Although patients are not likely to use medical terminology, they will often describe the pain or discomfort they experience in terms of how it feels to them, using words such as "sharp," "burning," "tearing," or "squeezing."

To locate the cause of the discomfort, an understanding of somatic pain and visceral pain is important (**Table 4-1**).

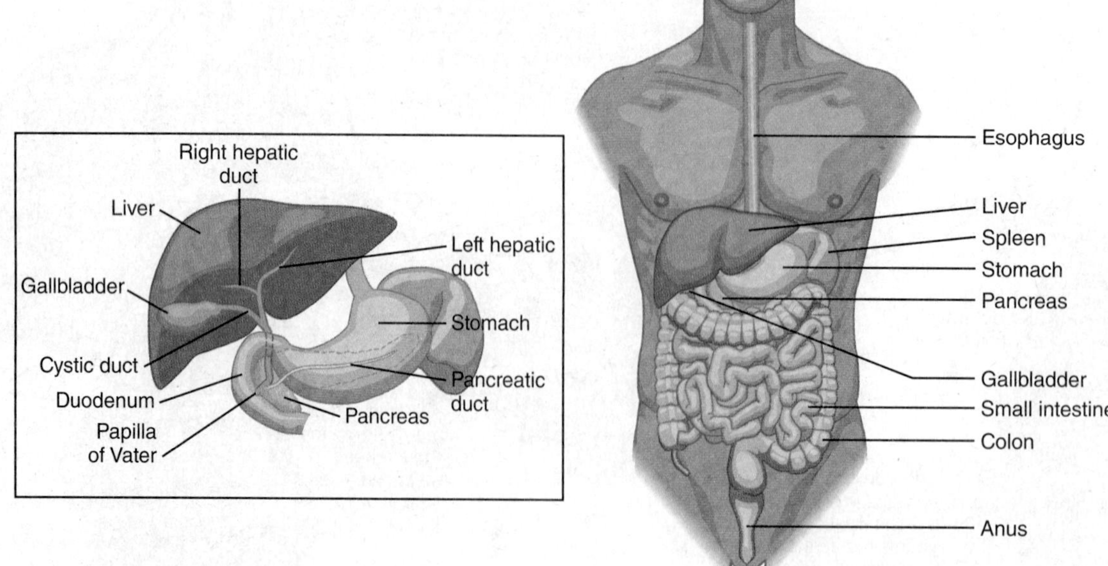

Figure 4-5 Structures causing chest discomfort or pain can be located outside the chest cavity, such as structures of the digestive system.

AMLS Assessment Pathway ▸▸▸▸

▾ Initial Observations

Patient Cardinal Presentation/ Chief Complaint

Patients may experience a wide range of symptoms when they have a cardiovascular problem. The most common complaints include chest pain, dyspnea, fainting, palpitations, nausea and vomiting, weakness, diaphoresis, and fatigue. Table 4-2 lists the common causes of chest pain.

Primary Survey

When first assessing a patient, the priority is looking for any life-threatening causes of chest discomfort. Should your primary survey reveal life-threatening signs, triage decisions must be made in both the prehospital and in-hospital settings, with the goal of moving the patient quickly toward a definitive intervention. Always begin your assessment by evaluating the patient's level of consciousness, airway, breathing, and circulation.

Level of Consciousness

The patient's level of consciousness is an excellent indicator of the adequacy of cerebral perfusion. If the patient is alert and oriented, the brain is receiving enough

Table 4-1 Somatic Pain versus Visceral Pain

	Description	Cause	Examples
Somatic pain	Well localized and often described as sharp.	Results from activation of nociceptors (sensory receptors that respond to pain) within the muscles, bones, and other soft tissues.	Rib fracture
Visceral pain	Often described as heaviness, pressure, aching, or burning that is not easy to pinpoint. May also radiate to other areas of the body and be accompanied by symptoms such as nausea and vomiting.	Results from activation of nociceptors within the organs of the chest and abdomen.	Acute coronary syndrome Pneumonia Pericarditis

Table 4-2 Critical Differential Diagnoses of Chest Discomfort

Cardiovascular Causes	Pulmonary Causes	Gastrointestinal Causes	Musculoskeletal Causes
Acute coronary syndrome	Pulmonary embolism	Esophageal rupture	Costochondritis
Acute decompensated heart failure	Tension/simple pneumothorax	Cholecystitis/biliary colic	Contusion
Aortic dissection	Respiratory infections (bacterial or viral)	Dyspepsia	Muscle spasm
Dysrhythmia	Pleurisy	Gastroesophageal reflux disease	Fracture
Myocarditis/pericarditis		Hiatal hernia	
		Pancreatitis	
		Peptic ulcer disease	

oxygen, which in turn means the heart is functioning adequately at that moment. Conversely, stupor or confusion may indicate poor cardiac output, which may indicate the presence of myocardial damage or dysfunction. The color and temperature of the patient's skin can provide you with valuable information about circulation; for example, cold, clammy skin suggests peripheral vasoconstriction.

Airway and Breathing

In some cases, the patient may be able to maintain an open airway. In other cases, depending on the patient's level of consciousness, you may need to clear an obstruction (e.g., debris, blood, or teeth) by properly positioning the head and/or placing an airway adjunct. If the patient can talk, the airway is patent. Note the rate, quality, depth, and work of breathing. Always listen to the lungs in patients who present with shortness of breath. If the patient's oxygen saturation (SpO_2) is $< 94\%$, consider administering supplemental oxygen (goal: SpO_2 95–99%). Remember, oxygen can be detrimental if administered in excess and has been shown to worsen outcomes in patients who are experiencing acute coronary syndrome (ACS) and stroke. Patients exhibiting signs and symptoms of myocardial ischemia should receive oxygen only if hypoxemic or demonstrating air hunger or rapid breathing.

Circulation/Perfusion

If the patient is conscious, check the radial pulse; if the patient is unconscious, first check the carotid pulse. Note the overall quality of the pulse and whether it is regular or irregular. Continue to assess the skin color and condition. Note any edema, poor turgor, or skin tenting.

▾ First Impression

When you respond to a call for a patient with a complaint of chest discomfort, your knowledge of anatomy, physiology, and pathophysiology will help guide you toward the common causes of chest pain.

By this point, you will have already made some observations when you first arrived and observed the patient, even before your primary assessment. What did you discern from across the room? Is the patient awake? What position is the patient in? Is the patient in a tripod position, indicating trouble breathing, or lying flat with minimal response to your presence? Is there increased work of breathing? Does the patient appear anxious? Is there an appearance of shock or poor perfusion? The patient's affect can also provide clues to the etiology or severity of the patient's condition. Your first impression of the patient may tell you whether the patient is "sick" or "not sick."

▾ Detailed Assessment

History Taking

Obtain the patient's history with the assistance of the patient, family members, or bystanders. A medication list may provide important clues to the patient's medical conditions.

OPQRST and SAMPLER

The OPQRST and SAMPLER mnemonics can be used to elaborate on the patient's chief complaint. Get the patient's description of the discomfort. Note the exact words the patient uses to describe symptoms and observe the patient's body language during your dialogue. Be sure to use open-ended questions to avoid leading the patient.

In patients with chest pain, the OPQRST and SAMPLER mnemonics are highly effective in documenting a description of the patient's pain. In addition, it can be helpful to specifically ask the following questions:

- How long have you had these signs and symptoms? Ask for a specific time of onset for the symptoms, as many facilities will request this information be relayed prior to the patient's arrival at the receiving facility (for instance, when patients are suspected to have ST-segment elevation myocardial infarction [STEMI]).
- What was the patient doing when the chest discomfort started? Ask about physical exertion or stress during the events leading to the onset of symptoms.
- Did the patient use any substances (stimulants or depressants) prior to onset of the pain?
- Did the pain gradually worsen or start at maximal intensity?
- What did the patient do to alleviate the symptoms?
- Did the patient use nitroglycerin to reduce the pain? Be careful about using nitroglycerin as a diagnostic tool—studies have shown that patients with noncardiac chest pain respond to treatment with nitroglycerin while some patients with ACS do not.
- Is there a position of comfort?
- Ask the patient to rate the pain on a scale of 0 to 10, with 0 being no discomfort and 10 being the worst pain ever felt.

Classic cardiac-related pain is accompanied by a sensation of moderate or severe pressure or squeezing ("there's an elephant on my chest") that starts fairly abruptly, escalates quickly in severity, and is associated with exertion. Unfortunately, this condition also has many nonclassical presentations, so the clinician must be very diligent and wary of misinterpreting these vague presentations. Such pain is sometimes described as indigestion. There may be radiation to the left or right arm or jaw. Severe chest pain that is described as a tearing pain in the upper back may indicate thoracic aortic dissection. Sometimes the only pain is felt in the arm or the jaw. It may manifest as sudden severe fatigue or breathlessness or as unexplained diaphoresis. Presentations may differ based on sex as well. Although the most common presentation for myocardial infarction (MI) in both sexes is chest discomfort, women are more likely to have atypical symptoms.

Knowledge of the patient's allergies to any medications is important because the patient may be given aspirin and other medications. All medications—including prescription, herbal, and over-the-counter products—are important to note. They may indicate a past medical history of coronary artery disease (CAD) or other heart condition. Medications such as nitroglycerin; aspirin; cholesterol-lowering medications; high blood pressure medications such as angiotensin-converting enzyme (ACE) inhibitors, beta blockers, and calcium-channel blockers; and oral hypoglycemics would all be pertinent when considering the possibility of CAD. Carefully ask about the use of phosphodiesterase inhibitors for erectile dysfunction. Patients taking these medications can have a life-threatening drop in blood pressure when given nitroglycerin, particularly within 24 hours of taking sildenafil or within 48 hours of taking tadalafil or vardenafil.

Does the patient have heart disease? Is there a family history of heart disease? Has the patient had an MI? Has the patient ever had a coronary artery bypass graft (CABG) or a percutaneous coronary intervention (PCI) with or without a stent to open a coronary vessel? Is there evidence of risk factors? These are all pertinent medical history questions to which you should attempt to gain answers. If the patient has undergone a prior PCI with stent, medication noncompliance could lead to stent closure.

You should also note whether a pacemaker or ventricular assist device is implanted in the patient's chest wall during your exam (**Figure 4-6**).

Determine the events associated with the patient's presentation. Were they engaged in physical activity or a high-stress situation, or did they wake up from sleep with discomfort? Has there been any use of cocaine or methamphetamines? Has there been a long period of inactivity such as an international flight or cross-country road trip (suggesting a pulmonary embolism [PE])?

In cases of dyspnea, explore the possibility of heart failure (HF). When did the dyspnea start? Did it awaken the patient from sleep? Can the patient lie flat and, if not, when did that start? If present previously, is it worse now? Does the patient awaken being unable to breathe? Paroxysmal nocturnal dyspnea is an acute episode of shortness of breath in which the patient suddenly awakens from sleep with a feeling of suffocation. It is a classic sign of left-sided HF (though rarely reported). Some patients will have such symptoms due to flash pulmonary edema, which can be due to a condition in which the heart does not relax normally (diastolic dysfunction).

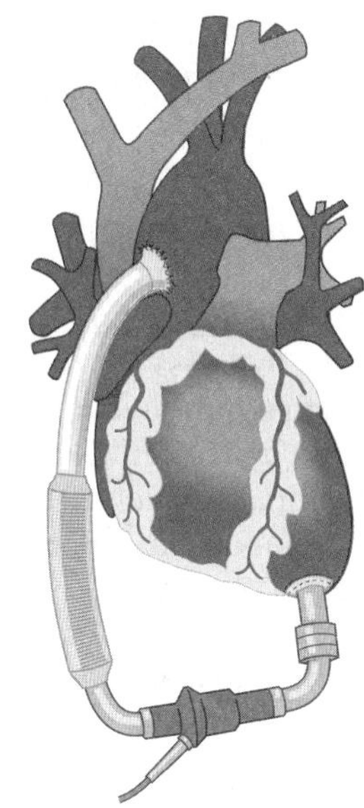

Figure 4-6 Left ventricular assist device. This device is a small, continuous-flow pump. The inflow cannula is connected to the cardiac apex, and the outflow graft is connected to the ascending aorta.

Fainting (syncope) occurs when cardiac output suddenly declines. Cardiac causes of syncope include dysrhythmias (either fast or slow heart rhythms), increased vagal tone (a situation known as vasovagal syncope, in which a decreased heart rate and dilatation of resistance blood vessels lead to a sudden drop in blood pressure), and structural problems with the heart such as those related to the heart valves. There are also numerous noncardiac causes of syncope (see Chapter 8, *Neurologic Disorders*). As part of the history taking from someone who has fainted, try to sort out whether the patient fainted from cardiac or noncardiac causes. Find out the circumstances under which the person fainted. A 25-year-old person who faints at the sight of blood is unlikely to have significant underlying heart disease. A 65-year-old person who faints after feeling some fluttering in the chest may have a dangerous cardiac dysrhythmia. Also, losing consciousness while sitting or lying down has more ominous implications than fainting while standing up.

Secondary Survey

Although the secondary survey for medical patients is often similar, when a patient presents with a cardiac problem, certain aspects warrant greater emphasis.

Vital Signs

The patient's pulse should be carefully examined. Although a rapid pulse may indicate anxiety, it may also occur secondary to severe pain, HF, or a cardiac dysrhythmia. If the pulse is weak and thready, cardiac output is compromised.

Abnormal vital signs findings include the following:

- *A pulse deficit.* This occurs when the palpated radial pulse rate is less than the apical pulse rate or monitored heart rate; it is reported as the difference between the two. To assess for a pulse deficit, check the peripheral radial pulse while listening to an apical pulse. Pulse deficit can occur during exercise or with simple premature ventricular complexes (PVCs), or it may involve more serious pathology such as dysrhythmias or cardiogenic shock.
- *Pulsus paradoxus.* This is an excessive drop (> 10 mm Hg) in systolic blood pressure during inspiration compared to during expiration. The finding is easiest to detect when the rhythm is regular. The affected pulse beats feel weaker than the others. Pulsus paradoxus can occur in patients with cardiac tamponade.
- *Pulsus alternans.* This occurs when the pulse alternates between strong and weak beats and typically is representative of left ventricular systolic damage.
- *Upper-extremity blood pressure discrepancies:* In patients with chest pain, particularly if it is felt largely in the back, obtaining blood pressures in both arms is advised. A significant difference in the systolic pressures could be an indication of thoracic aortic dissection.

Physical Exam

The focused cardiovascular physical exam starts with a general impression of the patient's overall status. Does the patient look "sick"? How is the patient's color? Is there obvious cyanosis around the mouth? Is there diaphoresis? Can the patient talk to you normally or only in bursts of a few words due to pain or dyspnea? After developing your first impression, look at the patient's neck, examine the chest wall, listen to lung sounds, and check pulses before examining the abdomen and extremities. Look at the neck and inspect for prominent neck veins when the patient is in an upright position if tolerated and, if not, in the supine position. Normally, these veins are collapsed when a person is sitting or standing. If the function of the right side of the heart is compromised, central venous pressure increases, causing jugular venous distention (JVD). Peripheral edema may be present as well.

Continue the assessment by inspecting and palpating the chest. Is chest pain replicated by pushing on the chest? If so, where? Surgical scars may indicate previous cardiac surgery. A bulge under the patient's skin may indicate a pacemaker or defibrillator (they look the same and often are present in the same device). These devices are usually implanted just below the right or left clavicle and are about the size of a half dollar.

Using your stethoscope, listen for crackles at the posterior bases of the lungs; their presence suggests excess fluid in the lungs, often due to heart failure, but they can be present in patients with chronic lung disease as well. Wheezing may also occur in both conditions. Many patients have both HF and chronic obstructive pulmonary disease (COPD), so caution is advised in interpreting lung sounds.

Palpate radial pulses and gauge the strength of each pulse such as weak, strong, thready, or bounding, for example.

Examine the abdomen. Fluid can accumulate in the abdomen with right-sided HF. Continuous gentle pressure on the liver (right upper quadrant) can cause engorgement of the neck veins when the patient is sitting upright; this so-called hepatojugular reflux is a sign of right-sided HF.

Examine the extremities and low back for edema; these may be signs of right-sided HF.

Diagnostics

Electrocardiography

In the prehospital setting, one of the most widely used diagnostic tools is the electrocardiogram (ECG). Cardiac rhythm monitoring can be performed using 3 leads or pacing/defibrillation pads. Rhythm monitoring is used in cardiac patients to monitor for dysrhythmias and to assess the effectiveness of treatments provided. Application of additional cardiac leads allows for rapid acquisition of a 12-lead ECG to diagnose **ST-elevation myocardial infarction (STEMI)**. Many agencies identify a key performance indicator for EMS clinicians as the ability to obtain a 12-lead ECG within 10 minutes of patient contact.

Rapid acquisition and transmission of a 12-lead ECG and diagnosis of STEMI in patients with chest pain allows prehospital clinicians to transport patients with STEMI to designated STEMI receiving facilities where cardiac catheterization and interventional services are available. EMS agencies should establish a system of care that ensures that patients with STEMI are quickly identified and then transported to centers capable of cardiac interventions. It is essential that EMS clinicians have a system to transmit or otherwise share 12-lead results with receiving facilities and activate in-hospital STEMI resources before patient arrival. The goal is to minimize the time from first patient contact to coronary intervention (or administration of thrombolytics in regions without interventional centers).

When you are obtaining the patient's vital signs, attach the cardiac monitor and pulse oximeter if indicated and if you have not already done so. Use the ECG and oxygen saturation measurement to guide your assessment and treatment. In patients who are unstable or have a clinical presentation that is concerning for STEMI, consider repeating the 12-lead ECG every 5 to 10 minutes. During the prehospital care interval, ECG findings can evolve from nonspecific changes to changes consistent with a STEMI.

Blood Tests: Troponins

Diagnosis of **non-ST-elevation myocardial infarction (NSTEMI)** is typically confirmed by measuring the serum levels of cardiac markers such as troponins. Elevated blood levels in the setting of cardiac chest pain usually confirm the diagnosis; however, the tests may not be positive for a few hours after onset of the condition. These tests can be done with a portable device for "point of care" evaluation, and some ground EMS systems utilize this test in the field (**Tip Box 4-2**). Such a capability is more commonly found in air ambulance and critical care transport services.

Cardiac Catheterization

Cardiac catheterization is the gold standard for diagnosing coronary blockages and provides the best means for treating most lesions. This procedure involves advancing a catheter via the femoral or radial artery through the aorta to the coronary arteries. Fluid (contrast dye) that can be seen by x-ray is then injected into the selected coronary artery, which allows visualization of any narrowing or obstructions in the vessel. Using the same port of access and the map produced by the injection of contrast, a physician can advance devices that can aspirate a clot, dilate the vessel, and apply a stent to forestall subsequent reclotting or collapse. This procedure is referred to as primary percutaneous coronary intervention (PPCI). The contraction of the heart can also be seen using the catheter and contrast, which can show when injured heart muscle does not move normally.

Echocardiography

Another commonly performed test is echocardiography. This modality employs ultrasound to show views of the heart in motion, demonstrating such aspects as the health of the valves and abnormalities of heart wall movement that may indicate MI or ischemia. Pericardial fluid and signs of tamponade can also be identified with this technology.

Cardiac Stress Testing

Cardiac stress testing can demonstrate the presence of functional ischemia. In such a test, stress on the heart may be induced by exercise such as walking on a treadmill or pedaling a bicycle while the patient is undergoing

TIP BOX 4-2

Cardiac Biomarkers

Troponin, a protein complex, is involved in the contractile process of skeletal and cardiac muscle. Cardiac troponins T and I are more specific to the heart. Each type of troponin demonstrates a characteristic rise and fall over time. That pattern allows for the diagnosis of an MI.

A single positive troponin test does not diagnose an MI, but it does help in risk stratifying patients according to whether they have an increased likelihood of ischemia or infarction. Troponins can be measured by using point-of-care (POC) tests in the EMS environment or using hospital lab equipment. Multiple types of troponin tests are available, and test results can be reported on different measurement scales. It is therefore important to know both which type of troponin is being measured and which scale the results are being reported on so that test results can be compared over time. Newer troponin tests called high-sensitivity cardiac troponin (Hs-cTn) have become available that allow for quicker evaluation of patients with chest pain. Given the large number of tests and testing strategies available, it is important to be familiar with the performance characteristics of the individual test being used.

Patients may have an elevated troponin level, without CAD, when their cardiovascular workload exceeds the metabolic support available. Disease processes such as sepsis, thyroid storm, and hypoxia can also result in decreased blood flow or oxygen delivery to the heart and cardiac ischemia, resulting in an elevated troponin level. Likewise, patients with renal failure often have elevated levels of troponin, which makes it difficult to determine if they have acute ischemia. Contrary to popular thought, troponin is not cleared by the kidneys and the elevation is not due to "backup" of troponin. In fact, renal patients with an elevated troponin level have increased long-term mortality and higher rates of adverse cardiac events and death at 30 days. Direct cardiac injury or inflammation, such as occurs with myocardial contusion, pericarditis, and myocarditis, also causes elevation of troponin levels.

POC troponin testing is possible in the prehospital environment, but research is needed to clarify how it would impact patient care or outcome. A thorough understanding and accurate interpretation of this laboratory marker are key in evaluating patients.

continuous cardiac monitoring in multiple leads. The ECG is then observed for signs of ischemia during exercise. Cardiac stress can also be induced by the administration of vasodilating medications such as adenosine.

Stress testing can be combined with echocardiography or nuclear imaging before and after the cardiac stress portion of the test. The imaging studies can then allow visualization of heart function that demonstrates compromised blood flow during exertion. Such compromise is usually caused by stenosis in the coronary arteries.

Refine the Differential Diagnosis

The history, physical exam, and 12-lead ECG are all key to early recognition of life-threatening conditions associated with chest pain. So far, you should have identified those life-threatening causes of chest pain that are initially suggested in the primary survey when the patient is complaining of pain with obvious shortness of breath and/or signs of shock.

For those patients whose conditions are more stable, or for those with conditions that cause fewer cardinal signs and symptoms, a more detailed history with the secondary exam will aid in making the diagnosis. When you are obtaining the patient's history, the following key findings may help narrow down the list of possible diagnoses:

- *Character of the pain.* Crushing or pressure-like pain versus tearing pain should lead you to think ACS versus thoracic aortic aneurysm. Patients with sharp pain may be suffering from a PE, pneumothorax, or a musculoskeletal cause. The complaint of burning or indigestion may lead you to think of gastrointestinal (GI) complaints in addition to ACS.
- *Activity with pain.* Pain with exertion that is relieved by rest is a classic symptom of ACS. When such pain occurs at rest, it suggests the presence of MI. A sudden onset of pain usually points to aortic dissection, PE, or pneumothorax. Pain after meals may indicate GI problems.
- *The 0-to-10 pain scale.* Obtain this information from the patient early during the assessment and management process. Onset and peak of pain should also be noted, along with ongoing assessment related to management.
- *Pain location.* Localized pain in a small area is usually somatic (the patient can point to it with one finger, and there is no radiation). Visceral pain, by comparison, is more difficult to localize (the patient circles the chest with one hand and talks about referral of pain). Localized chest wall pain is usually not cardiac in nature.
- *Radiation of pain.* Radiation into the back may guide you toward aortic dissection or GI causes. Pain located near the scapular area of the back and radiating into the neck suggests aortic dissection as well. Inferior and posterior MI may present as thoracic back pain. Any radiation of pain to the jaw, arms, or neck usually points toward cardiac ischemia.
- *Duration of pain.* Very short-lived (measured in seconds) pain is rarely due to cardiac ischemia. Pain that begins suddenly and is described as worst at the onset suggests aortic dissection. Pain that is constant and lasts for days is less commonly life threatening. Pain that is intermittent and fluctuates is more likely to have a serious cause.
- *Provocation/palliation.* Pain that worsens with exertion and improves with rest is usually coronary ischemia. Pain related to meals is associated with GI problems. Pain that worsens with a deep breath or cough is generally tied to pulmonary, pericardial, or musculoskeletal problems. These rules are generalizations, however—and when the history is suspicious for CAD, these factors are not always reassuring. For example, some cardiac pain can be reproduced with palpation of the chest wall. Likewise, antacid sometimes relieves cardiac chest pain while nitroglycerin sometimes relieves esophageal spasm from a GI cause.

Ongoing Management

Ongoing management of the patient's condition is accomplished en route to the hospital. Repeat the primary assessment. Vital signs should be obtained at a minimum of every 5 minutes for critical patients or every 15 minutes for patients in stable condition. The physical exam should be repeated, with the clinician noting any changes that have occurred or identifying any conditions that were missed in the initial exam. Assess the effectiveness of your interventions. For patients with ongoing symptoms concerning for ACS, obtain a repeat 12-lead ECG.

The choice of an appropriate method of transport for a patient with ACS should be based on the patient's needs. First you must decide whether the patient is critically ill, which modes of transportation the patient can tolerate, and which facility is best suited for the patient. A chest pain or heart attack center should be a consideration for patients with ACS. Altitude changes and the stress of flight can increase myocardial demand, so patients transported by air should be closely monitored and supported. Decreasing the transport time to the appropriate facility for patients with time-sensitive conditions such as STEMI may be a benefit of air transport in some situations. Patients with support devices may need additional space and teams for transport. Preparation of these resources should take place prior to transport to eliminate delays.

Life-Threatening Causes of Chest Pain

Life-threatening conditions associated with chest discomfort that require immediate treatment include tension pneumothorax, PE, esophageal rupture, acute pulmonary edema/HF, cardiac dysrhythmias, aortic dissection, cardiac tamponade, and ACS. Some of these conditions are observed in the primary survey as chest discomfort with respiratory distress, chest discomfort with altered vital signs, or a combination of those three chief complaints/cardinal signs and symptoms.

Tension Pneumothorax

Tension pneumothorax is a life-threatening cause of chest pain resulting from a progressive increase in size or worsening of a simple pneumothorax (an accumulation of air in the pleural space).

Pathophysiology

A tension pneumothorax is a life-threatening condition requiring emergent treatment to prevent death. The increased intrathoracic pressure arises due to an increasing volume of trapped air in the pleural space. The pressure of this pleural air can cause the affected lung to collapse and shift the heart toward the uncollapsed lung (mediastinal shift), compressing the unaffected lung and heart. As pressure increases in the thorax, venous blood return decreases to the heart. Without blood returning to the heart, systemic blood pressure drops.

Signs and Symptoms

In a patient with increased work of breathing, unilateral absence of or decreased breath sounds suggest a pneumothorax. If shock is also present, a tension pneumothorax must be immediately recognized and treated. Assessment of a patient with tension pneumothorax will reveal chest discomfort, severe respiratory distress, decreased or absent breath sounds on the affected side, and obstructive shock. JVD and tracheal shift can sometimes be seen as well, but are not always present or easily recognized.

Differential Diagnosis

The differential diagnosis for tension pneumothorax includes the following possibilities:

- Simple pneumothorax
- Acute coronary syndrome
- Acute respiratory distress syndrome
- Aortic dissection
- Heart failure and pulmonary edema
- Esophageal rupture and tears
- Myocardial infarction
- Pericarditis and cardiac tamponade
- Pulmonary embolism
- Rib fracture

Treatment

Treatment aims to relieve the pressure inside the chest by decompressing the affected side. The prehospital treatment of choice is needle decompression using a large-bore, over-the-needle catheter that is at least 3.25 inches (8.25 cm) in length. Needles that are specifically designed to relieve tension pneumothorax are preferred over a standard intravenous needle or catheter. Definitive treatment of a clinically significant pneumothorax entails placement of a chest tube. See Chapter 3, *Respiratory Disorders*, for more information on pneumothoraces and treatment.

Simple Pneumothorax

Pneumothorax refers to air in the pleural cavity. A small pneumothorax may cause mild symptoms and heal on its own. A larger pneumothorax generally requires treatment to remove the air and reestablish pulmonary negative pressure with inspiration.

Pathophysiology

A pneumothorax occurs when an air leak develops between the lung parenchyma and the pleural space. This condition can be seen after a traumatic injury or as the result of a bleb (a small air blister) that "pops," but other causes of barometric overpressure may also lead to the same effect. The pleural defect may function as a one-way valve, such that with each ensuing breath, more air becomes trapped in that space, causing the affected lung to collapse. A simple pneumothorax may occur spontaneously in patients with connective tissue diseases such as Marfan syndrome or in tall, slim males. In addition, it can occur as the result of barotrauma or other injuries to the chest. COPD; cystic fibrosis; cancers; smoking marijuana; and acute lung infections, such as pneumonia, or chronic lung infections, such as tuberculosis, may also cause a pneumothorax. The greatest threat associated with a pneumothorax is the development of a tension pneumothorax, which requires immediate intervention.

Signs and Symptoms

A person experiencing a spontaneous pneumothorax typically has a sudden onset of sharp chest pain and sudden shortness of breath. This diagnosis should be suspected in lanky young men as well as in patients with COPD who experience sudden decompensation. The physical exam classically reveals tympany to percussion on the affected side as well as decreased breath sounds. Clinical experience, however, suggests it can be difficult to hear chest percussion or the decrease in breath sounds in subtotal pneumothorax in the field.

Differential Diagnosis

Spontaneous pneumothorax and PE have similar clinical presentations; however, the context of each will often help differentiate these conditions. Bedside ultrasound is a sensitive and specific test for confirming pneumothorax, but its utility is dependent on operator skill. A chest radiograph is typically obtained to confirm a diagnosis of a simple pneumothorax but is not as sensitive as ultrasound. Computed tomography (CT) has been used in the past when simple chest radiograph was not sufficient.

Treatment

Treatment focuses on maintaining near-normal oxygen saturations by administering oxygen via nasal cannula or mask. Oxygen therapy does help the pneumothorax resorb in many cases. Assisting ventilations is usually not required and may even worsen the situation, increasing the likelihood of a tension pneumothorax. Some smaller simple pneumothoraces may seal on their own and require only conservative monitoring. Larger pneumothoraces may require needle aspiration or insertion of a chest tube to resolve the problem. Often monitoring is all that is required for the hemodynamically stable patient in the prehospital environment.

Table 4-3 Risk Factors for Pulmonary Embolism

Factors That Cause Venous Stasis	Hip or leg fracture Hip or knee replacement Major general surgery Trauma and spinal cord injury Long travel/plane flights
Factors That Cause Hypercoagulability	Chemotherapy Use of oral contraceptives Lupus Genetic hypercoagulopathy (e.g., factor V Leiden, protein C and protein S deficiency)
Factors That Result in Endothelial Injury	Trauma Prior venous thromboembolism Inflammatory vascular disease

Pulmonary Embolism

Clots (thrombi) that form and then break loose (emboli) from the deep vein system of the lower extremities or pelvis most commonly end up in the blood vessels of the lungs, where they are known as a **pulmonary embolism (PE)**. These venous thromboemboli can cause sudden, severe pleuritic chest pain; shortness of breath; and occasionally hemoptysis (the classic triad of PE). Large clots may occlude large pulmonary vessels, with the most dramatic being a saddle embolus that spans the pulmonary arteries as they leave the heart. These and other large proximal clots can cause rapid death.

Pathophysiology

PE occurs when a clot that has formed in those deeper veins (even weeks earlier) is dislodged and travels through the venous system (embolism), goes through the heart, and lodges in the pulmonary arteries. In the United States, 200,000 to 300,000 persons are hospitalized each year with PE. As many as one-third of these individuals will die. PE is often associated with the presence of risk factors (Table 4-3). When considering PE or deep vein thrombosis (DVT), remember Virchow's triad: hypercoagulability, venous stasis, and endothelial injury. These are the factors that increase risk of DVT formation.

Delayed or missed diagnosis of PE is more common in patients with complex clinical presentations and/or history, including coronary artery disease, COPD, asthma, or HF, relative to the patient's signs and symptoms and the more typical risk factor of prior immobilization or recent surgery.

Signs and Symptoms

The initial symptoms of DVT may be quite subtle and may be limited to pain or discomfort only, without outward signs. More commonly, however, swelling of an extremity is apparent when the clot is associated with the upper or lower limbs. Clots arising in the pelvis can be more difficult to detect.

The most frequently noted symptoms of PE include dyspnea, pleuritic chest pain, cough, palpitations, anxiety, and hemoptysis accompanied by tachycardia, tachypnea, and/or swelling of the legs. Patients with PE will normally have clear lungs on exam. They may experience sharp, localized pain that increases with a deep breath or cough (pleuritic) and leads to subsequent "splinting" of the patient's breathing.

To a large extent, the degree of the symptoms depends on the size and number of emboli in the lung, but another factor is the patient's prior cardiovascular reserve. Patients with preexisting lung or heart disease may not be able to compensate.

Approximately 90% of all patients with PE will have dyspnea, sometimes intermittently. This occurs because blood flow to certain areas of the lung is obstructed, preventing gas exchange in those areas despite adequate ventilation. This *ventilation–perfusion ($\dot{V}/\dot{Q}$) mismatch* (also called *dead space ventilation*) can lead to hypoxia. If the patient has hypoxia with no apparent physiologic explanation, you should consider PE. It is important to note that most pulmonary emboli are small and do not cause hypoxia. Do not dismiss the patient's subjective feeling of dyspnea even in the presence of otherwise normal vital signs. Also, bear in mind that patients with pulmonary emboli may be anxious and breathing fast; assuming the patient is having a panic attack is a grave error.

Elements of the patient history that suggest PE include an acute onset of shortness of breath, tachypnea, lightheadedness or syncope, chest pain, dry cough, and unexplained tachycardia. An acute onset of chest pain and hemoptysis in the same day suggest the possibility of a PE. There may be unilateral swelling of the leg and risk factors for DVT. Careful history taking and consideration of risk factors are especially important for patients with suspected PE because these are essential in expanding a differential to include a diagnosis of PE.

Approximately one-half of all patients with PE will have tachycardia. This can be driven by a response to hypoxia or to hypotension from poor left ventricular filling. CT, echocardiogram, or ECG may show signs of right heart strain due to increased pulmonary artery pressure. The classic $S_1Q_3T_3$ pattern on ECG is often mentioned but is an insensitive and nonspecific finding. An estimated 10% of patients with PE present with hypotension, which suggests a poor prognosis. Such a patient will be hemodynamically unstable if one of the main branches of the pulmonary artery is occluded with a saddle embolus, and cardiac arrest will usually present with pulseless electrical activity.

Differential Diagnosis

There are many differential diagnoses for PE, and these possibilities should be considered carefully with any patient suspected to have a PE. These patients also should have an alternative diagnosis confirmed, or PE should be excluded, before you conclude your evaluation. Additional problems to be considered include the following:

- Musculoskeletal pain
- Pleuritis
- Pericarditis
- Hyperventilation
- Spontaneous pneumothorax
- Pneumonia
- Thoracic aortic dissection
- Acute coronary syndrome

To help to confirm the diagnosis of PE, a 12-lead ECG should be completed as soon as feasible. In patients with chest pain or shortness of breath, this step is critical to evaluate for alternative diagnoses. The most common ECG finding in PE is sinus tachycardia. Other findings suggestive for PE, which are seen in a minority of cases, are related to pulmonary hypertension and right ventricular strain.

The prehospital approach to recognition and management of PE requires the clinician to understand the risk factors and the signs and symptoms of the condition sufficiently to strongly suspect the diagnosis, to provide stabilizing treatment, and to make the receiving facility immediately aware of a patient with a potential PE. Once at the hospital, the diagnosis is definitively made in most cases by CT angiogram of the chest. An alternative diagnostic test is a ventilation–perfusion scan (a nuclear imaging study). Other tests that may be done include a chest radiograph to exclude other causes as well as an ECG. Blood tests may be done to exclude a cardiac cause as well as a D-dimer test to assess for an active clotting process in the patient.

Treatment

Prehospital Setting

In the prehospital setting, the patient with acute chest pain, dyspnea, and/or alteration in vital signs should have oxygen, vascular access, continuous cardiac rhythm monitoring, and a 12-lead ECG. Beginning standard therapy for an ACS with aspirin is appropriate if the diagnosis is unclear. If the patient has been identified as having respiratory failure, airway control and ventilatory assistance are also required. Treatment for hypotension includes administration of crystalloid bolus and/or vasopressor infusion.

In-Hospital Setting

Once the patient enters the hospital, appropriate diagnostic tests should be performed. If the patient is in extremis, a bedside ultrasound showing a dilated right ventricle should be considered presumptive evidence of a severe PE in a patient with a suggestive history.

After diagnosing PE, hospital treatment usually involves initiation of anticoagulation therapy, but in extreme cases may involve administration of a fibrinolytic agent, emergent intravascular thrombus retrieval, or emergency surgery. The initial anticoagulant therapy given in the hospital is generally heparin or low-molecular-weight heparin. For a patient with a hemodynamically significant PE, thrombolytic therapy is an option. In some patients, this therapy can achieve faster results than anticoagulation therapy, but its benefits must be balanced with the increased risk for bleeding. Surgical embolectomy is performed by a cardiothoracic surgeon and requires placing the patient on cardiopulmonary bypass. In many centers, catheter thrombectomy can be performed by interventional radiology clinicians, providing an additional treatment option for patients with very large PEs. For patients with isolated DVTs or small uncomplicated PEs, therapy may be initiated in the emergency department and the patient discharged home with appropriate anticoagulant medications.

Esophageal Rupture

Spontaneous or effort-related rupture or perforation of the esophagus, also referred to as Boerhaave syndrome, most commonly results from forceful vomiting, but can occur from other conditions that lead to increased intra-esophageal pressure. These conditions include bearing down to defecate and weightlifting.

Pathophysiology

When the esophagus is torn, gastric contents enter the mediastinum, where an inflammatory and subsequent infectious process ensues. In addition to the spontaneous type just described, other common causes of esophageal perforation include iatrogenic injury from endoscopy or instrumentation, foreign bodies from poorly chewed food or sharp objects, caustic burns, blunt or penetrating trauma, and postoperative complications.

Signs and Symptoms

Chest pain with dyspnea may indicate esophageal rupture. Early clinical signs of esophageal rupture are vague. The patient may complain of pleuritic pain in the anterior part of the chest, with this pain becoming worse with swallowing when the head and neck are flexed. Dyspnea and fever often accompany the chest pain as the infectious process worsens.

As air and GI contents enter the mediastinum, subcutaneous air will gather around the patient's chest and neck. Palpable subcutaneous air may be felt (crunchy "Rice Krispies" feel). Pneumomediastinum and pneumopericardium may be apparent on the chest radiograph. Auscultation of heart sounds may pick up Hamman's sign, in which a crunching sound is heard during systole. As the inflammatory process begins because of mediastinal contamination, sepsis, fever, and shock will ensue. If the diagnosis is delayed for more than 24 hours, the patient's condition may deteriorate rapidly.

Differential Diagnosis

Esophageal rupture is a rare condition, but you should consider it in any patient initially seen with atypical chest or abdominal pain, especially after vomiting or in conjunction with the other related factors discussed earlier. The differential diagnosis may include, among other conditions, pericarditis, paracardial effusion with or without cardiac tamponade, thoracic aortic dissection, ACS, pneumonia, and PE.

Treatment

Management of this life-threatening condition begins with your ability to recognize its signs and symptoms and include esophageal rupture in your differential diagnosis, and the completion of a thorough history and physical exam. Patients will present with the previously described symptoms and have one of the common causes in their recent history. Prehospital care focuses on supportive care: supplemental oxygen administration, vascular access, application of monitors, obtaining a 12-lead ECG, and administration of intravenous (IV) fluids as needed to maintain a normal blood pressure. In-hospital management includes chest radiograph and CT, rapid initiation of antibiotics, volume replacement, and surgical consultation.

Acute Pulmonary Edema/Heart Failure

Pulmonary edema, an accumulation of fluid in the lungs, is categorized as either cardiogenic or noncardiogenic. *Noncardiogenic* pulmonary edema, as the name suggests, occurs despite adequate cardiac performance. Heart failure is a common cause of *cardiogenic* pulmonary edema. Pulmonary edema can also happen abruptly as a result of an acute coronary occlusion, severe hypertension, cardiac valve disfunction, dysrhythmia, or other sudden event, or gradually as a result of diet changes, medication noncompliance, or progression of underlying diseases causing worsening cardiac function. HF is a complication of nearly all forms of heart disease, both structural and functional; the ventricles are unable to fill or eject blood in amounts adequate to meet the body's needs.

Pathophysiology

Coronary artery disease is the most common underlying cause of HF. Poor ventricular pumping function leads to an overall decrease in cardiac output, and as more blood remains in the ventricle, the pressure in the ventricle builds. If the left ventricle fails, the pressure in the pulmonary veins then increases and blood backs up into the lungs, leading to pulmonary edema with poor gas exchange. This same pathophysiology can occur through several other mechanisms; as just one example, the somewhat paradoxical condition known as high-output failure occurs when the heart cannot keep up with the demand due to internal shunting of blood or very low blood counts. In a patient with chronic HF, compensatory mechanisms work to redistribute blood to critical organs and adapt the body to decreased cardiac output. If the right side of the heart is also involved, blood backs up into the venae cavae, causing congestion of the venous system, which may present as pedal edema, JVD, hepatic congestion, or sacral edema.

Signs and Symptoms

The signs and symptoms of pulmonary edema/HF include dyspnea, paroxysmal nocturnal dyspnea, fatigue, exercise intolerance, and peripheral fluid retention such as pedal or sacral edema. The clinician's ability to obtain a history may be limited depending on the severity of the patient's symptoms. It is important to inquire as to whether the patient's dyspnea is a first-time event or whether it is a recurrent problem. Does the patient have a history of HF, or this a new event? Is there chest pain suggestive of an MI? All practitioners are challenged by differentiating some cases of HF from exacerbations of COPD and other underlying pulmonary processes, therefore presence or absence of cough or sputum production should be sought when taking the history. Is there any evidence of pneumonia—for example, fever? Does the patient have a history of COPD, wheezing, or change in their normal cough/sputum? In patients with chronic HF, inquire about changes in medications, noncompliance with medications, and changes in diet.

When you arrive on scene, note whether the patient is sitting upright and leaning forward on one or both arms (tripod position), is working hard to breathe, or reports chest tightness or discomfort. Look for signs of poor perfusion (e.g., weak distal pulses, cool skin, delayed capillary refill, poor urinary output, and acidosis), as well as diaphoresis. Systemic and pulmonary congestion will also be present—tachypnea, labored breathing, bilateral crackles, pale or cyanotic skin, hypoxemia, and sometimes frothy, blood-tinged sputum.

In the primary survey, assess for clinical signs of shock even prior to obtaining vital signs and beginning monitoring. Note the patient's level of distress. Auscultate the heart for crackles and wheezing—but remember that wheezing can be found in patients with pulmonary edema as well as asthma, COPD, and some other conditions. A quick assessment of the patient's circulation can help you pinpoint the problem, especially if cardiogenic shock is also present.

Differential Diagnosis

The differential diagnosis may include HF due to high blood pressure, aortic or mitral valve disease, or cardiomyopathy. Pulmonary edema may be caused by an MI, lung infections, extensive burns, overdose, or liver or kidney disease.

Treatment

Prehospital Setting

In the prehospital setting, standard protocols for ACS should be followed if it appears to be the cause of the HF and pulmonary edema. Vital signs should be obtained. Acute HF has three major presentations: acute pulmonary edema, acute decompensated HF, and cardiogenic shock. In acute HF with pulmonary edema, onset is sudden, the blood pressure is typically significantly elevated (systolic values > 200 mm Hg are not unusual), and the patient has severe respiratory distress. The most severe form is sympathetic crashing acute pulmonary edema (SCAPE). Acute decompensated chronic HF typically develops over days, and is associated with volume overload (peripheral edema, possible mild to moderate pulmonary edema) and moderately elevated blood pressure. Patients with cardiogenic shock will usually have low blood pressure and may have associated pulmonary and peripheral edema.

SpO_2 should be assessed and oxygen used to treat hypoxemia; supplemental oxygen also should be used in normoxemic patients with air hunger. Cardiac rhythm monitoring should be instituted early in the patient's care, along with obtaining a 12-lead ECG.

Management of HF focuses on improving gas exchange and cardiac output. If the patient's blood pressure is adequate (systolic blood pressure > 100 mm Hg), help the patient get into a comfortable position. Many times, this can be done with the patient sitting with legs dependent (dangling). Supplemental oxygen should be provided if indicated.

The use of continuous positive airway pressure (CPAP) has had an immense impact on the treatment of pulmonary edema. In appropriately selected patients, the use of this technology significantly decreases the need for drugs and invasive ventilatory intervention. CPAP is a type of intervention broadly known as noninvasive positive-pressure ventilation (NIPPV), which also includes bilevel positive airway pressure (BiPAP). NIPPV can be therapeutic in the following two ways: (1) by decreasing venous return and preload, thereby reducing pulmonary edema; and (2) by decreasing alveolar edema, thereby improving gas exchange. The use of NIPPV is explained further in Chapter 3, *Respiratory Disorders*. One study on the use of CPAP in the treatment of HF concluded that prehospital use of CPAP in this context decreases the need for endotracheal intubation, improves vital signs during transport to the hospital, and reduces short-term mortality. If the patient has signs of respiratory failure along with altered mental status, intubation may be required.

Along with positive-pressure ventilation, nitroglycerin has emerged as the primary treatment for pulmonary edema if the patient's systolic blood pressure is > 100 mm Hg. This drug acts to decrease preload and afterload through peripheral vasodilation. In very hypertensive patients, high-dose nitroglycerin has been shown to be safe and effective, but caution must be exercised when employing these strategies simultaneously: Systemic blood pressure can drop quickly. Careful monitoring with frequent cycling of blood pressures is required.

Some cardiac patients may have an implanted pacemaker or automated internal cardioverter defibrillator (AICD), which you may find in the chest or abdominal wall. In patients with severe HF, left ventricular assist devices (LVADs) are increasingly being implanted to improve cardiac output or as a bridge to heart transplant. The management of these patients is complicated, and a review of the devices and management of patients with them is provided in **Tip Box 4-3**.

TIP BOX 4-3

Left Ventricular Assist Devices (LVADs)

LVADs are being implanted with increasing frequency and are increasingly encountered by EMS personnel. Many patients with worsening HF or awaiting heart transplant have an LVAD placed and are discharged home to pursue as normal a life as possible. In newer model LVADs, the pump is a frictionless electromagnetic engine that produces continuous blood flow, so a pulse may not be present. This can create confusion for patients and responders alike, as a patient with an LVAD who is unresponsive and without a pulse may be in cardiac arrest or may have hypoglycemia with adequate perfusion. These frictionless pumps decrease the risk of several complications, including thrombosis and hemolysis.

Management Steps

- The patient and family often are well versed in the operations of the pump and typically will have valuable information on troubleshooting, replacing batteries, and other functionality issues. Trust their guidance, as they are familiar with the operations of the pump and recognize that their loved one's life depends on its proper functioning. They should also be able to provide you with the contact information for the patient's LVAD coordinator, who can be an additional source of information.
- Vital signs may be difficult to ascertain in a patient with an LVAD. A pulse is normally not felt with the continuous-flow pump. In patients with nonpulsatile flow, blood pressure must be determined using a Doppler device, which is usually not available in the prehospital environment. A typical mean arterial pressure is 70 to 90 mm Hg in these patients. An SpO_2 probe may show a saturation and waveform, albeit often with artifact, and the results may be unreliable.
- Device malfunction typically results in the loss of a humming sound from the pump itself; an alarm or indicator may alert the patient as well. Specific guidance from the manufacturer or coordinator may be helpful. Possible catastrophic issues include massive pump thrombosis, cannula dislodgment, and tamponade. Early surgical coordination is required.
- Performing cardiac compressions is controversial. Early on in these devices' deployment, EMS clinicians were instructed to not perform compressions. If possible, consider discussion with the coordinator and implant team, although manufacturer recommendations typically say not to perform cardiopulmonary resuscitation.
- Right HF is treated essentially the same as in a non-LVAD patient (e.g., PE, ischemia, pulmonary hypertension).
- Hypoperfusion may be due to hypovolemia or pump thrombosis, which may require additional anticoagulation. Unless the patient has definitively been diagnosed with pulmonary edema, EMS clinicians should treat the patient with fluid boluses.
- Severe hypertension impedes pump outflow and should be treated with vasodilators.
- Severe bleeding may affect filling pressure of the heart, and patients should receive typical hemorrhage resuscitation therapies.
- Dysrhythmias are typically better tolerated by the patient with an LVAD. Supraventricular dysrhythmias are treated with an emphasis on rhythm control. Ventricular dysrhythmias are common, occurring in as many as 50% of patients with LVADs. Emergent cardioversion is typically not needed if the patient is stable (not the typical approach for a patient who may be pulseless and in ventricular fibrillation).

EMS should make sure to bring spare batteries and/or the LVAD plug adaptor (if available) in case of a dying or dead battery. Lack of power to the LVAD can be detrimental to the patient.

Patients with subacute HF who also experience volume overload may be given furosemide to initiate diuresis. However, use of furosemide in the field is controversial, as diagnosis of HF is difficult and the time to onset of action is relatively long for this agent. Therefore, furosemide is not routinely used to treat acute HF in the field or in the initial emergency department management of acute HF. Some EMS agencies also use ACE inhibitors as prehospital vasodilators for the treatment of acute HF.

Morphine has historically been used to treat acute HF, but is now recognized to have potentially severe side effects, including depression of the respiratory drive and hypotension. Its beneficial effects, such as mild venodilation and analgesia, can be achieved more effectively and safely with other medications and therapies.

If the patient's chest pain is complicated by low blood pressure, cardiogenic shock, and dyspnea, vasopressors may be needed to improve the blood pressure. Dobutamine or norepinephrine (in the field) and milrinone (in hospital settings) may be given to help increase blood pressure and inotropy/chronotropy. As of this writing, the current literature supports the safety of norepinephrine over DOPamine in the setting of cardiogenic shock.

In-Hospital Setting

In the hospital setting, patients require aggressive treatment while a history, physical exam, 12-lead ECG, chest radiograph, and laboratory assessment are completed. Arterial or venous blood sampling will help evaluate the patient's ability to oxygenate and ventilate. In addition to a routine laboratory analysis, an elevated level of brain natriuretic peptide (BNP) can be useful to help diagnose HF in unclear cases. BNP is released when there is greater than normal stretch in the ventricular muscle. A cardiac enzymes test should also be ordered to help evaluate for myocardial injury.

Echocardiograms or left- and right-sided hemodynamic monitoring can help evaluate the cause of HF along with treatment effectiveness. This type of monitoring can inform decision making as to whether pharmacologic intervention will likely be sufficient or whether some combination of pharmacologic and mechanical intervention might be necessary.

In patients with very severe HF that is refractory to other medical therapy, an intra-aortic balloon pump can be used to temporarily help reduce afterload and may improve overall perfusion. For long-term management, patients with ejection fractions of less than 30% and a life expectancy of greater than 6 months may receive implanted intracardiac devices, including LVADs and biventricular assist devices. Less-invasive biventricular pacemakers have been shown to improve quality of life, functional status, and exercise capacity, but do not affect mortality or morbidity.

Cardiac Dysrhythmias

Dysrhythmias can cause a wide spectrum of symptoms, ranging from palpitations to acute pulmonary edema and cardiogenic shock. The rapid identification and continuous monitoring of patients with cardiac dysrhythmias is extremely important.

Pathophysiology

Cardiac dysrhythmias can be broadly grouped into slow and fast dysrhythmias, and can result from a wide variety of causes, ranging from ACS and underlying cardiac structural abnormalities to medication side effects and electrolyte abnormalities. The resulting dysrhythmias can alter the volume of blood pumped per minute (**cardiac output**) by either reducing the heart rate or by reducing stroke volume. If the rate is too fast, there may not be enough time for blood to fill the ventricles, in which case the stroke volume decreases; if the rate is too slow, the volume delivered per minute may decrease to a critical level. Preexisting heart disease may cause early decompensation with relatively mild changes in rate. As cardiac output decreases, patients can develop pulmonary edema or syncope.

Signs and Symptoms

A patient who is experiencing a dysrhythmia may have the following signs and symptoms:

- Palpitations
- Chest discomfort
- Shortness of breath
- Syncope or near syncope
- Dizziness or lightheadedness
- Rapid or irregular heartbeat
- Increased awareness of heartbeats

Differential Diagnosis

A continuous cardiac recording in one or more leads is the preferred tool for diagnosing a cardiac dysrhythmia. A 12-lead ECG may offer additional insights.

Treatment

As the primary survey is being conducted, monitors should be applied by your team to obtain continuous vital signs and evaluate for dysrhythmias or acute myocardial injury. For treatment of bradycardia and tachycardia, follow the current guidelines and/or your protocols. The patient may also be experiencing ACS. A 12-lead ECG should be acquired early—as oxygen is applied and vascular access is obtained. If bradycardia is causing the patient to become clinically unstable (e.g., chest pain, dyspnea, acute pulmonary edema, shock), implement measures to increase the heart rate. Transcutaneous pacing should be considered as an initial intervention in the unstable patient with symptomatic bradycardia. American Heart Association (AHA) guidelines now include IV chronotropic medications as an alternative. Atropine can be of benefit in some cases but is unlikely to work in case of heart blocks below the atrioventricular node; even if it is successful, its effect on heart rate is not predictable. Challenging the heart by causing a too-high heart rate while the patient is experiencing ischemia may lead to myocardial injury.

For patients considered symptomatic from tachycardia (usually ≥ 150 beats/min) with a normal blood pressure (> 100 mm Hg systolic), treatment is based on the specific dysrhythmia present. Caution must be exercised in patients with atrial fibrillation or multifocal atrial tachycardia, as rhythm conversion may cause atrial clots to enter the systemic circulation; thus, rate control is preferred for these patients. For other supraventricular and most ventricular tachydysrhythmias, antidysrhythmic agents may be appropriate. If the patient with tachycardia has signs of alterations in mentation and evidence of cardiogenic shock, synchronized cardioversion may be necessary.

Aortic Dissection

The aorta arises from the outflow tract of the left ventricle; the right and left coronary arteries originate from the aortic root just above the aortic valve. The aorta, like all arteries, has three layers—the intima, media, and adventitia. The intima is the smooth, innermost lining, which is composed of endothelial cells; any significant disruption to this layer can lead to activation of clotting cascades. The media (middle layer) is made up of smooth muscle and some elastic tissue. The adventitia is the strong, fibrous outer layer, which is designed to withstand the forces exerted on this vessel. With normal aging, the adventitia loses its elasticity and the intimal layer weakens. If chronic hypertension is present, this deterioration may be intensified. Some patients have congenital changes in their aorta that also decrease wall strength and hasten the degeneration of the aortic wall. For example, Marfan and Ehlers-Danlos syndromes cause such changes.

Aortic dissection occurs when a tear in the vessel's intima allows blood under systolic pressure to dissect between the layers, tearing its way along the vessel and compromising the internal diameter. Such dissections can be isolated to the proximal aorta or distal aorta, or they may transverse both proximal and distal aortic regions. In contrast to aortic dissection, aortic aneurysm is the dilation of the entire wall of the aorta—like a garden hose with a weak side wall that creates a bulge in the hose. Aortic aneurysms are often found in the abdomen and are covered in more detail in Chapter 10, *Abdominal Disorders*.

Pathophysiology

Thoracic aortic dissection occurs when a failure of the intima allows blood under high pressure to enter the media, leading to a dissection of the area between the intima and the adventitia. The amount of dissection depends on where this tear is located, the degree of disease in the media layer, and the blood pressure. The injury may move up or down the aorta and extend back into the aortic root, affecting flow to the coronary arteries (usually right) and leading to an MI, and may rupture into the pericardial sac, or pleural cavity. More distally, the dissection can involve the carotid and/or subclavian arteries, leading to signs of a stroke, or it may occlude the spinal arteries or even extend to occlude the renal or iliac arteries, affecting blood flow to the lower extremities. Control of blood pressure and heart contractility are major factors in controlling the extension of the hematoma.

Signs and Symptoms

Chest pain is the most common complaint associated with aortic dissection, with patient descriptions including words such as "excruciating," "sharp," "tearing," or "ripping." The pain is often described as piercing through the chest into the back. If the patient indicates the pain is in the anterior part of the chest, the ascending aorta may be involved. Neck and jaw pain may be associated with injury to the aortic arch, and pain near the scapula may indicate dissection in the descending aorta.

The pain of aortic dissection is often associated with nausea, vomiting, a feeling of lightheadedness, anxiety, and diaphoresis. Syncopal episodes are not common but may be the only presentation in some patients. Other findings depend on which blood vessels are affected by the dissection. Compression or obstruction of a carotid artery will cause stroke-like findings, and if both carotids are involved, may lead to altered mental status. Involvement of one subclavian artery will cause pain and paresthesias in the associated upper extremity and asymmetric pulses and blood pressures.

Blood pressure may be interpreted in the following two ways:

1. Hypotension may indicate rupture of the dissection into the pericardium, with tamponade or hemorrhagic shock.
2. Hypertension is often an underlying cause and may be worsened by pain and anxiety.

Blood pressures should be checked in both the right and left arms, as a significant difference (> 20 mm Hg) in the setting of chest pain increases the concern for aortic dissection. Neurologic symptoms may indicate injury to the proximal aortic branches, which causes signs of stroke, or distal injury, which causes spinal cord signs and symptoms.

Differential Diagnosis

Suspicion of aortic dissection may be raised by the patient's history and physical exam, but diagnostic studies are needed to confirm the differential diagnosis. Other diagnoses include ACS, acute pericarditis, pneumothorax, PE, and Boerhaave syndrome.

Diagnostic Studies

The 12-lead ECG is not a specific diagnostic modality for aortic aneurysm, but should be obtained on all patients with chest pain. Suspicion of a thoracic aortic event occurring simultaneously with new ST-segment elevation should not delay referral of a patient to a facility with cardiac catheterization and cardiovascular surgery capabilities. The following diagnostic procedures contribute to the establishment of a diagnosis of aortic aneurysm:

1. *Chest radiography*. A chest radiograph is usually completed on all patients presenting with chest pain. Of the radiographs obtained, 12% are normal, even with aortic dissections. A widened mediastinum may be seen, along with other subtleties that may or may not point the clinician to this diagnosis.
2. *Echocardiography*. An echocardiogram can be obtained by two different techniques—transthoracic (where aortic regurgitation may be seen) or transesophageal (which allows a good view of the thoracic aorta).
3. *Computed tomography angiography (CTA)*. CTA is the primary diagnostic test chosen to find aortic dissection; the test uses iodinated IV contrast.
4. *Magnetic resonance imaging*. This modality is good at capturing the true image of an aortic dissection. However, because of the prolonged time required for obtaining images, it is not helpful when the patient's condition is unstable.
5. *Angiography*. An angiogram can also be used for diagnosing and evaluating this condition.

Treatment

In general, follow your protocol for chest pain, even when you suspect an aortic dissection. Oxygen, vascular access, and application of monitors are standard care. The use of antiplatelet therapy (e.g., aspirin) in patients with aortic dissection who require surgery is problematic, but not contraindicated. Transporting patients to a hospital with emergency cardiac capabilities is of high priority. Suspecting an aortic dissection and passing those signs and symptoms on to the in-hospital team may facilitate more rapid identification of this condition.

The most critical presentation of aortic dissection is the patient with hypotension due to aortic rupture and/or cardiac tamponade. Such a patient needs to be preferentially resuscitated with blood products while preparing for surgery. If tamponade is present, pericardiocentesis may afford the patient more time and lead to slight improvements in cardiac output until the definitive repair can be done in surgery.

Hospital-based stabilization of the patient's condition focuses on decreasing further shear stress on the aorta by decreasing the rate and force of cardiac contractions and systemic blood pressure. This typically has involved the use of IV vasodilators and beta blockers. These agents should be administered by medication infusion pumps and require continuous monitoring of blood pressure to allow fine adjustments of infusion rates. It is also important to aggressively treat the associated pain to lessen the stress forces, as it can drive a sympathomimetic response.

Definitive treatment of aortic dissection depends on the location of dissection. Those involving the root of the aorta are typically treated surgically, whereas those arising distal to the left subclavian artery are usually treated with medications or intravascular stents. It is important to note that thoracic aortic dissection at the root of the aorta can occlude coronary arteries, so that the ECG shows a STEMI. Empiric treatment of such conditions with anticoagulants, antiplatelet agents, or fibrinolytics can lead to disastrous consequences. Thus, a high index of suspicion is warranted if patients with STEMI have predominantly back pain or asymmetric blood pressures.

Cardiac Tamponade

The conditions previously described in this section involve a patient who presents with chest pain and increased work of breathing and/or chest pain and altered vital signs. One rare event that may present with chest pain, cough, or dyspnea is cardiac tamponade (also called *pericardial tamponade*).

Pathophysiology

Cardiac tamponade occurs when fluid accumulates inside the pericardial sac surrounding the heart. As this fluid accumulates and pressure builds, it causes compression of the thin-walled right ventricle, limiting its filling. Blood return to the right ventricle decreases, which decreases cardiac output, resulting in hypotension. Although you might think of cardiac tamponade as

Table 4-4 Common Medical Causes of Cardiac Tamponade	
Infectious	Bacterial Viral
Metabolic	Uremia
Inflammatory	Metastatic tumors Autoimmune disorders
Hemorrhagic	Aortic dissection Post-surgical Anticoagulation therapy

Data from Bodson L, Bouferrache K, Vieillard-Baron A. Cardiac tamponade. *Curr Opin Crit Care.* 2011;17(5):416–424.

a traumatic injury, many medical causes for this condition also exist (Table 4-4). The fluid that accumulates can come from cancer or infectious, inflammatory, and metabolic conditions. Rapid accumulation of even a small volume of fluid usually brings on signs and symptoms very quickly. Slower-accumulating fluid allows for adaptation, with a slower onset of signs and symptoms and a much larger amount of fluid within the space.

Signs and Symptoms

The classic signs and symptoms of cardiac tamponade are Beck's triad: hypotension, distended neck veins (high right-sided heart pressures), and muffled heart tones (fluid outside the heart). In a more subtle presentation (with slow accumulation), the patient may present with chest pain, cough, and dyspnea. Unfortunately, as is so often the case in medicine, many patients do not present with the classic signs, so a high degree of suspicion is required, particularly in cases of otherwise unexplained hypotension with preservation of visible neck veins on exam.

Other signs and symptoms that may indicate cardiac tamponade include the following:

- *Pulsus paradoxus, or paradoxical pulse.* Normally, the systolic blood pressure decreases slightly with each inhalation. When the heart is being squeezed in tamponade, this decrease is exaggerated. **Pulsus paradoxus** is found when the blood pressure decreases by more than 10 mm Hg during inhalation.
- *Kussmaul sign.* An increase in JVD during inspiration (Kussmaul sign) is also a paradox. Normally, during inspiration, JVD decreases.

Differential Diagnosis

The differential diagnosis for cardiac tamponade is a challenge and may include tension pneumothorax or acute HF with cardiogenic shock. The patient with cardiac tamponade presents with a complaint of chest pain and dyspnea, and possibly with a cough. A high index of suspicion must guide you toward this diagnosis while you are reviewing the patient's risk factors for development of a medical cardiac tamponade. To narrow down the list of possible diagnoses, the following tests need to be performed:

1. *Chest radiography.* A chest radiograph will show a large heart shadow if the fluid accumulation exceeds 200 to 250 mL, but in an acute effusion, the heart may look normal.
2. *ECG.* An ECG will show low amplitude (decreased voltage). Another diagnostic sign visible on the ECG is *electrical alternans*—a marker that is highly specific for a large, slowly developing pericardial effusion, but is rare in acute accumulation of pericardial fluid. The morphologic features and amplitude of the P waves, QRS complex, and ST-T waves in all leads will alternate in every other beat because of swinging heart phenomenon, during which the normal heart swings back and forth with each contraction but returns to the normal position before the next contraction. In patients with large pericardial effusions, the heart is too heavy to swing back to the normal position in time, and the continuous ECG "sees" the heart out of position for alternating contractions (**Figure 4-7**).
3. *Echocardiography.* The echocardiogram is the fastest means of making the diagnosis of pericardial fluid. It can easily be performed at bedside in the emergency department as well as by a growing number of EMS agencies using prehospital ultrasound. Evidence of right ventricular collapse is one of the hallmarks that pericardial fluid is causing the clinical syndrome of tamponade.

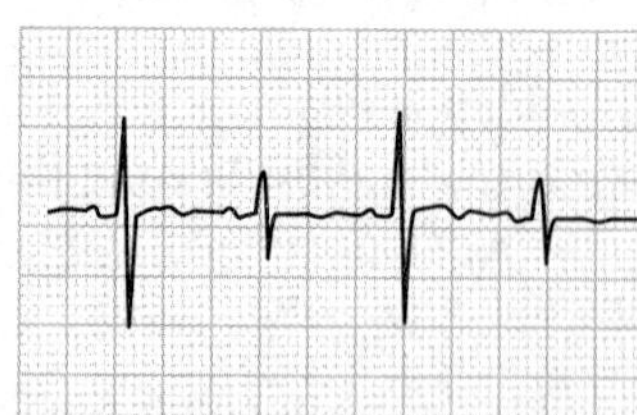

Figure 4-7 Electrical alternans may develop in patients with pericardial effusion and cardiac tamponade. Notice the beat-to-beat alternation in the P-QRS-T axis; this is caused by the periodic swinging motion of the heart in a large pericardial effusion. Relatively low QRS voltage and sinus tachycardia are also present.

Treatment

Applying oxygen, gaining vascular access, and applying monitors are standard care for patients with cardiac tamponade. Obtaining a 12-lead ECG is also necessary. Standard chest pain protocols in the prehospital setting are warranted, but signs of shock may prevent administration of nitrates.

If hypotension is present, fluid resuscitation with crystalloids for the obstructive shock state may initially help fill the right side of the heart and improve cardiac output. Fluid administration to the normotensive patient can negatively impact patient hemodynamics and should be avoided. These interventions serve as temporizing measures until the patient can undergo pericardiocentesis or surgical pericardiotomy.

Pericardiocentesis was previously taught with blind entry in the left subxiphoid area. In the era of readily available ultrasound, the preferred approach is now ultrasound-directed placement of a multifenestrated pigtail catheter. Depending on the cause and clinical factors, drainage may be accomplished surgically, by the creation of a pericardial window by a cardiac surgeon.

Figure 4-8 shows pericardiocentesis being used to remove blood from the pericardial sac (though not via an ultrasound-directed transthoracic approach). Enough fluid should be removed to improve the patient's condition. If tamponade recurs, the procedure may be repeated, and a catheter may be left in with a three-way stopcock. Surgical consultation is warranted if further drainage is required.

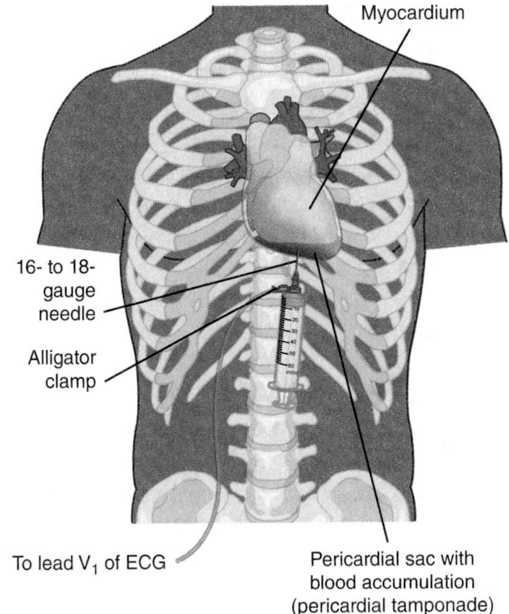

Figure 4-8 Pericardiocentesis to remove blood from the pericardial sac during tamponade.

Acute Coronary Syndrome

Acute coronary syndrome (ACS) is a group of conditions that involve decreased blood flow to the heart muscle. These conditions often share the common underlying pathology of atherosclerosis. *Atherosclerosis* comes from the Greek words *athero* (meaning "gruel" or "paste") and *sclerosis* (meaning "hardness"). In this case, the "gruel" or "paste" is made up of calcium, lipids, and fats and is called *plaque*. Plaque clings to the walls of coronary arteries, narrowing their lumens; this stenosis reduces the amount of blood (carrying nutrients and oxygen) reaching the heart muscle (**Figure 4-9**). The plaque may harden or remain soft.

Pathophysiology

When atherosclerosis occurs within the coronary arteries, it is referred to as *coronary artery disease (CAD)*. Patients with CAD are at increased risk for ACS. Certain risk factors place patients at a greater risk for developing ACS, and a larger number of these risk factors translates into a greater chance of developing ACS.

Risk factors that cannot be modified include age, sex, and heredity. The older a person is, the more likely their chance of experiencing CAD. Compared to women, men develop CAD at an earlier age and are more likely to die of ACS. However, heart disease remains the leading cause of death in women, particularly after menopause.

Modifiable risk factors include hypertension, smoking, high cholesterol, diabetes, obesity, stress, and lack of physical activity. Hypertension can usually be successfully managed with diet, exercise, and medications.

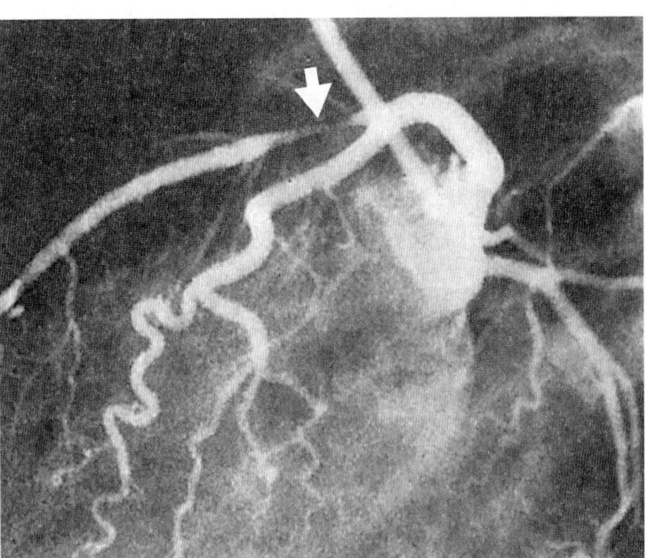

Figure 4-9 Coronary angiography shows stenosis (arrow) of the left anterior descending coronary artery.

Hypertension causes the heart to work harder than it should and, over time, causes it to enlarge and weaken. Smoking increases the risk of developing ACS. Smoking is the single most preventable risk factor leading to death in the United States. The risk of heart attack in smokers is more than twice that of nonsmokers. Quitting smoking reduces the risk of having ACS even after years of smoking. High cholesterol is another easily diagnosed problem that can be managed with diet, exercise, and medications. Diabetes greatly increases the risk of heart disease. Diabetes also affects the blood vessels themselves, accelerating atherosclerosis. Many people with diabetes also have high blood pressure, increasing their risk even more. Obesity, stress, and lack of exercise accelerate the atherosclerotic process, increasing the chances of having ACS.

Current AHA guidelines distinguish three categories of ACS: unstable angina, NSTEMI, and STEMI.

Acute Coronary Syndromes

Angina pectoris, which literally means "chest pain," is caused by an inadequate blood supply from a narrowed coronary artery filled with plaque. **Stable angina** usually occurs when a fixed plaque partially obstructs blood flow, and at times of increased metabolic demand, cardiac ischemia results in pain. This type of angina generally occurs with exercise or stress and resolves in 3 to 5 minutes, but sometimes up to 15 minutes, upon resting. In **unstable angina**, the patient's chest pain is different than normal (e.g., provoked by less exertion, lasts longer, more severe, or occurs at rest).

- *NSTE-ACS.* The AHA has formally associated the close relationship between unstable angina and NSTE-MI in terms of identifying at-risk patients and delineating their care. Patients presenting with NSTE-ACS exhibit ST-segment depression or prominent T-wave inversion. The presence of positive cardiac necrosis biomarkers distinguishes angina from MI. Unstable angina occurs at rest and is more severe than prior episodes of angina. Prolonged chest discomfort (lasting more than 15 minutes) that continues at rest and chest discomfort that awakens the patient at night (nocturnal) are features of unstable angina. The patient may describe the pain as increasing in duration and intensity over the last few days and is at risk for more serious complications such as plaque rupture. Patients with NSTEMI are diagnosed via cardiac biomarkers. They may also demonstrate ischemic changes on ECG. Blood flow through the coronary arteries can be diminished by various mechanisms, including thrombus, thromboembolism, vasospasm, arterial inflammation, and coronary artery dissection. Each of these conditions ultimately results in a greater demand for coronary oxygen than can be provided by the patient's obstructed coronary vasculature. Consistent with your local protocol and medical direction, patients with NSTE-ACS should be transported to a facility capable of monitoring patients for ischemia via serial 12-lead ECG and serial cardiac biomarker studies.
- *STEMI.* ST-elevation myocardial infarction is diagnosed based on symptoms characteristic of myocardial ischemia accompanied by regional ST elevation (STE) and release of cardiac biomarkers confirmed by laboratory tests. New or presumably new left bundle branch block in association with a patient presentation consistent with myocardial ischemia is no longer considered a STEMI equivalent (**Tip Box 4-4**). ST-segment depression in the precordial leads (V_1–V_4) may be indicative of a posterior wall MI, but direct assessment of posterior wall MI is possible utilizing leads V_7–V_9. Indeed, using V_7–V_9 can pick up approximately 20% to 30% of STEs otherwise not seen on routine 12-lead ECGs associated with lesions of circumflex coronary artery.

Myocardial Infarction

Myocardial infarction is most commonly caused by a clot or thrombus that forms in a narrowed coronary artery where the plaque has ruptured, causing platelets to aggregate and a clot to form. If the coronary artery becomes completely obstructed, the ischemic cells in the heart

TIP BOX 4-4

Modified Sgarbossa Criteria for Myocardial Infarction in Left Bundle Branch Block

Detecting a STEMI in a patient with ECG findings of a left bundle branch block (LBBB) can be difficult. A new LBBB is always considered pathologic and can be a sign of MI. Elena B. Sgarbossa first described ECG findings in 1996 that can help in the diagnosis of a STEMI in the setting of an LBBB. The *modified* Sgarbossa criteria are now used to assist in detecting a STEMI:

- Concordant ST elevation ≥ 1 mm in ≥ 1 lead
- Concordant ST depression ≥ 1 mm in ≥ 1 lead of V_1–V_3
- More than one lead anywhere with ≥ 1 mm STE and proportionately excessive discordant STE, as defined by ≥ 25% of the depth of the preceding S wave

The modified criteria are a little more complex (no scoring system), but also increase the sensitivity for identifying STE in LBBB. Additional research and validation are required for their widespread adoption.

muscle will begin to die. This event can cause permanent damage to the heart muscle and is often referred to by laypersons as a *heart attack*. As heart muscle dies, the muscle's cells lose their cellular membrane integrity. Biomarkers of this necrosis include the proteins known as troponins, some of which are specific to heart muscle and can be measured by simple blood tests, providing a rapid means of chemically confirming an MI. The detection of troponins in the serum often takes a few hours, so serial testing is commonly done. The type of troponin measured determines the intervals at which testing should be performed (see Tip Box 4-2).

Signs and Symptoms

Health care clinicians frequently receive calls for chest discomfort. Effective treatment for ACS is time sensitive, meaning it is important to recognize it quickly and provide essential treatment within the first hours of onset. Early intervention can reduce the likelihood of sudden cardiac death and/or myocardial damage. Quick recognition and diagnosis of ACS start with readily recognizing the signs and symptoms and obtaining a thorough history and physical exam.

The classic signs and symptoms of ACS may all be present, or only a few may be noted. Geriatric patients, patients with diabetes, and postmenopausal women older than 55 years may not experience any pain or discomfort, but instead present with a sudden onset of weakness. Women may also present with shortness of breath with or without chest discomfort. Likewise, nausea, vomiting, and back or jaw pain are more common in women. Failure to recognize weakness or dyspnea as ACS may lead to the development of serious and life-threatening consequences. These alternative presentations are termed *anginal equivalent symptoms*.

You can organize your approach to the patient with chest discomfort by using the SAMPLER history and the OPQRST mnemonic, as discussed in the AMLS Assessment Pathway. After completion of the OPQRST and SAMPLER, you will be prepared to narrow down the differential diagnosis and determine whether the patient is experiencing stable angina or an ACS, with special attention to the possibility of STEMI.

As an example, suppose a 57-year-old male patient states that he was shoveling heavy snow and suddenly developed chest discomfort. The pain is substernal and constant, and it radiates to the neck, jaw, and down the arms. He is having difficulty breathing because he feels pressure "like an elephant is sitting on his chest." When asked to rate his pain, he describes it as "greater than a 10." The pain has lasted for about an hour and has not been relieved by rest or nitroglycerin. Chances are that this patient is having an AMI.

Rapid acquisition of a 12-lead ECG is mandatory to determine whether a STEMI is present. Always consider obtaining serial ECGs, particularly in patients with compelling stories and symptoms but with no initial STEMI on ECG, as STEMI can be dynamic.

Differential Diagnosis

Importantly, the absence of a classic presentation should not falsely reassure the clinician. For example, the presence of tenderness to palpation of the chest, a pleuritic component, or presence of a cough does not rule out a cardiac etiology for the pain. Patients with these symptoms should be taken seriously and evaluated for possible ACS. Alternative diagnoses (**Tip Box 4-5**) such as GERD and musculoskeletal pain are diagnoses of exclusion and should be left to hospital staff to confirm.

TIP BOX 4-5

Takotsubo Cardiomyopathy: "Broken Heart Disease"

Takotsubo cardiomyopathy is an interesting clinical entity that is seen by EMS personnel but requires hospital evaluation to verify the diagnosis. It is often felt to be brought on by a stressful psychological or physical event. Patients demonstrate symptoms of ACS, which may include ST-segment elevation or new-onset HF and even elevated troponins. Nevertheless, no obstructive coronary lesion is identified on cardiac catheterization. This condition's name is Japanese for "octopus pot," which refers to how the heart looks on echocardiogram.

The Mayo Clinic criteria for Takotsubo cardiomyopathy include the following:

- Transient left ventricle dysfunction extending beyond a single coronary artery distribution or regional wall motion abnormality on cardiac ultrasound
- Absence of obstructive CAD on cardiac catheterization
- New ECG abnormalities or troponin elevation
- Absence of myocarditis or pheochromocytosis

In North America, 90% of patients diagnosed with Takotsubo cardiomyopathy are women (postmenopausal); in Japan, this condition is found predominantly in men. Some speculate that it is due to an excess of catecholamines, but this relationship has not been proven. Beta blockers are often prescribed, but ACE inhibitors have an improved mortality benefit. Although this diagnosis requires hospital evaluation, it may be responsible for some STEMI-alert false-positive results, as the patient may have ST elevation and elevated troponins but no coronary blockage.

Diagnostic Studies

Pulse oximetry should be used to monitor for hypoxemia ($SpO_2 < 94\%$). Hyperoxemia is thought to increase detrimental free-radical production in ischemic tissue and has been shown to worsen outcomes in patients with STEMI. Supplemental oxygen should be administered only to patients with demonstrated hypoxemia ($SpO_2 \leq 94\%$) or clinical dyspnea, and titrated to maintain 95% to 99% saturation.

A heart monitor with 12-lead ECG capabilities should be placed on all patients with suspected ACS prior to giving medications for suspected ischemia (e.g., nitroglycerin), when possible. A 12-lead ECG should be acquired immediately (within 10 minutes of patient contact) for all patients with symptoms consistent with ACS. In fact, early prehospital recording of a 12-lead ECG and subsequent alerting of the receiving facility is a Class I intervention in the 2020 AHA Guidelines. If STEMI is present, the patient should be transported following local guidelines. Ideally, these individuals will be transported to a Comprehensive Heart Attack Center (per Joint Commission certification) or a center capable of providing interventional care for STEMI.

For patients with STEMI, the AHA advocates PPCI within 90 minutes of first medical contact (FMC). The recommendations regarding fibrinolysis in the absence of a readily available PCI (< 120 minutes) have grown complex, and clinicians should follow their local guidelines. More details are available in the 2021 ACC/AHA/SCAI Guideline for Coronary Artery Revascularization. In general, in-hospital fibrinolysis is an acceptable alternative under some circumstances, but the estimated time of symptom onset and expected delay to PPCI drive decision making.

Medications may be administered en route to shorten on-scene times, as extended on-scene times do little more than increase the time to definitive therapy and reperfusion. Once the patient is stabilized, further scene time should be minimized. In some circumstances, field evacuation by helicopter transport of a patient to a PCI-capable center should be considered.

Treatment

Prehospital Setting

Prehospital clinicians should understand that early recognition of ACS, notification of the receiving facility, transport to a facility capable of coronary angioplasty, and recognition and defibrillation of ventricular dysrhythmias are key to patient survival. Record a 12-lead ECG as part of your initial set of vital signs and transmit it early if STEMI is present. The well-known mnemonic *MONA* (*morphine, oxygen, nitroglycerin,* and *aspirin*) is no longer appropriate because aspirin is the only component that may be helpful in decreasing morbidity and mortality in patients with ACS. Oxygen has been shown to worsen outcomes in such patients who are not hypoxemic; morphine has been shown to have no benefit in STEMI and to lead to worsened outcomes in NSTE-ACS; and administration of sublingual nitroglycerin has not been shown to have a survival benefit, though it may improve the patient's pain. Check with your medical director and review regional protocols for the medications preferred in your area. The following protocol is typical in describing the nuances in these treatments:

- Aspirin, 162 to 324 mg (2 to 4 baby aspirin), nonenteric coated, should be chewed (preferably) and swallowed at the earliest sign of ACS. Make sure the patient is not allergic to acetylsalicylic acid and has no recent GI bleeding. Aspirin administration prior to PCI is a Class I AHA recommendation. All patients complaining of chest pain should receive aspirin unless they are allergic to it. The AHA advocates that dispatchers give prearrival instructions to chew 162 to 325 mg of aspirin while awaiting the arrival of prehospital EMS clinicians. Aspirin suppositories (300 mg) are safe and can be considered for patients with severe nausea, vomiting, or disorders of the upper GI tract.
- Oxygen should be administered to patients with breathlessness, signs of HF, shock, or oxygen saturation < 94%. If the patient has signs of hypoxia, oxygen should be administered (goal: SpO_2 95% to 99%). If shortness of breath is severe or in the presence of acute pulmonary edema secondary to left-sided HF, oxygen should be administered with NIPPV (CPAP or BiPAP) or by using a bag-valve mask to provide positive pressure. In the absence of these conditions, the ILCOR/AHA 2015 review failed to identify any benefit of oxygen administration to normoxic patients with suspected or confirmed ACS.
- It is helpful to establish an IV of crystalloid prior to giving nitroglycerin, when possible. Rapid administration of a fluid bolus is indicated for patients with hypotension. If the patient has been administered nitroglycerin in the past without complications, then this agent can be given before obtaining vascular access.
- Nitroglycerin may be administered sublingually as a 0.4-mg tablet or metered-dose spray. It may be repeated every 3 to 5 minutes three times as long as the patient's systolic blood pressure remains > 90 mm Hg. AHA guidelines support 911 dispatchers advising patients who tolerate nitroglycerin to repeat nitroglycerin every 5 minutes while awaiting the arrival of EMS personnel. Nitroglycerin decreases the pain of ischemia by decreasing preload and cardiac oxygen

consumption, and it dilates coronary arteries, increasing cardiac collateral flow. Nitroglycerin should not be given to patients with hypotension, extreme bradycardias, or tachycardias. Do not administer nitroglycerin to patients who have taken a phosphodiesterase inhibitor for erectile dysfunction or other purposes (sildenafil within 24 hours; tadalafil or vardenafil within 48 hours). Watch for headache, decreased blood pressure, syncope, and tachycardia when nitroglycerin is given. The patient should sit or lie down during this agent's administration. Nitroglycerin may also be administered in small IV boluses and, with a medication pump, by infusion. Keep a close eye on the patient's blood pressure, as nitroglycerin infusion can lead to a dangerous drop in blood pressure.

- Relief of pain is important when caring for patients with ACS, as the associated emotional stress and sympathetic surge can worsen ischemia. Generally, this relief is achieved using opioids. FentaNYL is widely used in this setting due to its favorable cardiovascular profile. While morphine is still used by some agencies, it is more likely to cause a drop in blood pressure, especially in patients with volume depletion or with right ventricular infarction. All opioids have dose-related effects on respiratory drive, so monitor patients carefully, preferably incorporating waveform capnography as part of your clinical assessment.
- Prehospital administration of oral inhibitors of adenosine diphosphate (ADP)–associated platelet aggregation (e.g., ticagrelor and clopidogrel) has been recognized as potentially valuable for patients with STEMI as they are being transported to a receiving facility for PPCI. Studies have reported mixed results with prehospital administration of these medications. As they do have potent effects on clotting and may delay coronary revascularization when bypass is required (relatively infrequent), it is best to establish local protocols for field use that are compatible with the local cardiology and cardiovascular surgery practice.

Prehospital administration of fibrinolytics has been shown to be effective in the United States and Europe. This practice is relatively uncommon in the United States in ground ambulance agencies but is often used by air transport services. Provision of prehospital fibrinolytics should be considered when the FMC to mechanical intervention is anticipated to be greater than 120 minutes (**Tip Box 4-6**). The goal for "time to needle" in this case should be less than 30 minutes from FMC. Services offering out-of-hospital fibrinolytics require a strict adherence to protocols, 12-lead ECG acquisition and interpretation, experience in advanced cardiac life support, the ability to communicate with the receiving institution, and a medical director with experience in management of STEMI. A continuous quality improvement process to evaluate all calls where fibrinolytics are used is also required. Most EMS services have short enough transport times that they focus on making an early diagnosis with 12-lead ECG, completing a fibrinolytic checklist, administering first-line medications, and providing advance notification to the receiving facility to prepare

TIP BOX 4-6

ACCF/AHA Guideline for the Management of Patients with ST-Elevation Myocardial Infarction

1. In the absence of contraindications, fibrinolytic therapy should be administered to patients with STEMI at non-PCI-capable hospitals when the anticipated FMC-to-device time at a PCI-capable hospital exceeds 120 minutes because of unavoidable delays. (Class I, Level of Evidence: B)
2. When fibrinolytic therapy is indicated or chosen as the primary reperfusion strategy, it should be administered within 30 minutes of hospital arrival. (Class I, Level of Evidence: B)
3. In the absence of contraindications, fibrinolytic therapy should be given to patients with STEMI and onset of ischemic symptoms within the previous 12 hours when it is anticipated that primary PCI cannot be performed within 120 minutes of FMC. (Class I, Level of Evidence: A)
4. Fibrinolytic therapy should not be administered to patients with ST depression except when a true posterior (inferobasal) MI is suspected or when associated with ST elevation in lead aVR. (Class III, Level of Evidence: B)
5. In the absence of contraindications, fibrinolytic therapy should be administered to patients with STEMI and cardiogenic shock who are unsuitable candidates for either PCI or CABG. (Class I, Level of Evidence: B)

The proposed time windows are system goals. For any individual patient, every effort should be made to provide reperfusion therapy as rapidly as possible.

ACCF, American College of Cardiology Foundation; AHA, American Heart Association; CABG, coronary artery bypass graft; FMC, first medical contact; PCI, percutaneous coronary intervention; STEMI, ST-elevation myocardial infarction.

Source: American Heart Association, Inc.

for cardiac catheterization. However, in systems where prehospital fibrinolysis is a standard component of the care for patients with STEMI, and the alternative is hospital administration of fibrinolytic agents due to delayed or nonavailability of PCI, prehospital administration of fibrinolytics is reasonable when the transport time will exceed 30 minutes.

In-Hospital Setting

After initial field stabilization of patients diagnosed with STEMI, one or more of the following medications may be administered in the hospital setting:

- *Low-molecular-weight heparin.* Low-molecular-weight heparin, such as enoxaparin, is a convenient means of giving an anticoagulant, as it does not require a drip.
- *Unfractionated heparin.* When used as adjunctive therapy with fibrin-specific lytic agents in STEMI, current recommendations call for a bolus dose of 50 to 70 units/kg of unfractionated heparin, followed by infusion at a rate of 12 units/kg/h. While most ground services will not infuse heparin drips, some may give a bolus to patients with STEMI confirmed by history and 12-lead ECG. The local protocol, physician medical director involvement, and scope of practice within your state will determine if such treatment is appropriate for your service. Currently, most interfacility transfer services avoid infusion medications during transfer of care as changing over these lines and pumps can create excessive time delays.
- *Beta-receptor antagonist administration.* Beta blockers are part of standard care for patients following MI; however, their use in the acute management of patients with ACS requires careful consideration of the clinical situation. Agents used in the acute setting include metoprolol and esmolol. They decrease myocardial work by decreasing contractility and rate, and decrease cardiac electrical irritability when dysrhythmias are a problem. However, their effects on contractility and rate can significantly worsen the clinical situation if the patient-in-evolution develops complications such as cardiogenic shock or heart block. Contraindications to beta blockers include moderate to severe left ventricular failure and pulmonary edema, bradycardia, hypotension, signs of poor peripheral perfusion, second-degree or third-degree heart block, and asthma. Some jurisdictions may utilize metoprolol, atenolol, propranolol, esmolol, and labetalol in the field critical care setting. Paramedics should follow their local protocol.

  Vital signs should be taken between doses to ensure the patient's heart rate and blood pressure remain adequate. Sometimes, once discomfort is relieved, the catecholamine release stops. If IV beta blockers are in the patient's system, the patient then becomes hypotensive, and the condition may worsen. Be prepared to treat this reaction with an IV fluid bolus. The local protocol, physician medical director involvement, and scope of practice within your state will determine if such treatment is appropriate for your service.

Emergent Causes of Chest Pain

All complaints of chest discomfort and those patients presenting atypically with the associated signs and symptoms of an ACS should be assessed first for the presence of an ACS. After the initial evaluation, if ACS appears less likely, other differential diagnoses—both life threatening and non–life threatening—must be investigated (Table 4-5).

Table 4-5 Differential Diagnoses of Chest Discomfort

- Cardiovascular diseases
  - Acute coronary syndrome (acute ischemia related to coronary artery narrowing or occlusion from atherosclerosis, thrombus, embolus, dissection, or spasm)
  - Pulmonary embolism
  - Severe hypertension
  - Cardiac dysrhythmias
  - Structural abnormalities of the heart (congenital or acquired)
  - Viral myocarditis/pericarditis
  - Systemic vasculitis with coronary artery involvement
- Gastrointestinal diseases
  - Acute gastritis
  - Acute pancreatitis
  - Acid reflux, esophagitis
  - Peptic ulcer disease
  - Boerhaave syndrome
- Pulmonary diseases
  - Pneumonia
  - Pleurisy
  - Pneumothorax
- Toxic exposure (cyanide or carbon monoxide, for example)
- Anemia or red blood cell dysfunction (e.g., sickle cell)

Some emergent diagnoses include coronary spasm or Prinzmetal angina; stimulant-induced chest pain; infection (pericarditis, myocarditis); simple pneumothorax (see Chapter 3, *Respiratory Disorders*); and GI causes such as esophageal tear, cholecystitis, and pancreatitis (see Chapter 10, *Abdominal Disorders*).

Coronary Spasm or Prinzmetal Angina

A coronary spasm is a sudden narrowing of a coronary artery due to contraction of the muscular wall. Similar to an acute thrombosis, it deprives the heart muscle of blood and oxygen. A coronary spasm is also known as variant angina or Prinzmetal angina.

Pathophysiology

Prinzmetal angina results in chest pain at rest and is caused by coronary artery vasospasm. Although both men and women can experience Prinzmetal angina, it is more common in women in their 50s. People with Prinzmetal angina have an increased risk of experiencing ventricular dysrhythmias, MI, heart block, or sudden death.

Signs and Symptoms

Severe pain usually occurs while the person is resting at night or during the morning hours. The spasms may occur in cycles, with periods of no pain following an episode of pain.

Differential Diagnosis

Because this condition is difficult to differentiate from other forms of ACS, typical categorization, triage, and management should occur.

Treatment

Pain is often relieved with nitroglycerin. ECG may show transient ST depressions or elevations in a coronary artery distribution.

Stimulant Use

The dangerous consequences of using cocaine and crack cocaine are well documented. Recently, use of methamphetamine has increased, and multiple forms of cardiovascular disease can be found in regular users of this illicit substance.

Pathophysiology

Both cocaine and methamphetamine cause the release of catecholamines, and cardiac toxicity occurs because of the ensuing direct effects on the heart—namely, an increase in heart rate, blood pressure, and ventricular contractility (beta effect), resulting in increased myocardial oxygen demand. Additionally, coronary artery blood flow decreases, leading to a high risk for coronary vasospasm (alpha effect). In fact, coronary vasospasm is thought to be the primary cause of stimulant-induced MI. Dysrhythmia is also common after both cocaine and methamphetamine use. In 2018, methamphetamine use in the United States was found to be associated with a 25% increase in the risk of fatal dysrhythmia.

Signs and Symptoms

Patients who are using cocaine or methamphetamine may show signs of agitation, have dilated pupils, and exhibit behavioral changes such as paranoia and antisocial behavior. Methamphetamine use is more commonly associated with paranoia and audiovisual hallucinations than use of cocaine.

Differential Diagnosis

The differential diagnoses may include toxicity from other drugs (e.g., barbiturates, benzodiazepines, or alcohol), anxiety disorders (e.g., a panic attack), and depression.

Treatment

First-line treatment for stimulant-induced dysrhythmias and hypertensive episodes is usually benzodiazepine administration, which tempers the effects on the central nervous system and cardiovascular system. Benzodiazepines should be added to the standard ACS management protocols. Because of the risk associated with cocaine, use of fibrinolytics in patients using this drug is considered high risk. Beta blockers are contraindicated, as the resultant unopposed alpha effect can precipitate dangerous hypertensive states and/or coronary vasospasm.

Chronic cocaine/crack use accelerates atherosclerotic disease, so patients with pattern of usage may be at risk for ACS at younger ages than normal. A recently published registry study of more than 900 cocaine-positive patients showed them to be younger, male, and as a group exhibiting higher rates of STEMI and cardiogenic shock. Cocaine-positive patients with ACS were also less likely to have multivessel coronary artery disease.

Pericarditis

Pericarditis is an inflammation of the pericardium or pericardial sac. It can occur as an acute episode or a chronic condition.

Pathophysiology

Pericarditis is typically caused by a virus, but other etiologies include chronic renal failure, rheumatic heart disease, tuberculosis, leukemia, acquired immunodeficiency syndrome, and cancer, to name a few. Often the cause is unknown. The discomfort of pericarditis differs from ACS. It is often described as a dull ache that increases in intensity gradually over several days.

Signs and Symptoms

The classic pain of pericarditis is improved by leaning forward and worsened by lying back, presumably because the heart hangs in the chest and touches the posterior thorax when a person is supine. Pain may increase on inspiration. The lungs will be clear, with no JVD or pedal edema noted in the early stages. Additional symptoms may include fever, weakness, fatigue, malaise, and auscultation of a pericardial friction rub. If a pericardial effusion is developing as a result of the pericarditis, you might hear the friction rub or find pulsus paradoxus. A chest radiograph may show an enlarged cardiac silhouette due to pericardial effusion in patients with chronic pericarditis. The 12-lead ECG classically is said to have ST elevation in multiple leads and/or PR-segment depression, but a variety of findings could develop at different time points (**Figure 4-10**). Lab studies may show an elevated erythrocyte sedimentation rate (a test that indirectly measures inflammation in the body) and an elevated white blood cell count, which may indicate the presence of an infection.

Differential Diagnosis

The chest pain associated with pericarditis is differentiated from that of AMI based on its onset (usually gradual), pain type (sharp/somatic), and palliating/provoking features (leaning forward makes pain better), among other differentiators. Some patients may develop a form of pericarditis after MI or cardiac surgery known as post-MI pericarditis or Dressler syndrome.

Treatment

Management focuses on relieving discomfort with analgesics and nonsteroidal anti-inflammatory drugs (NSAIDs). Colchicine, a drug commonly used for gout, and steroids are also effective. The disposition of the patient depends on the severity of symptoms and any other related concerns or comorbidities.

Myocarditis

Myocarditis is defined as inflammation of the myocardial layer of the heart.

Pathophysiology

Often undiagnosed clinically, this inflammation is usually caused by a virus (e.g., Coxsackie B enterovirus,

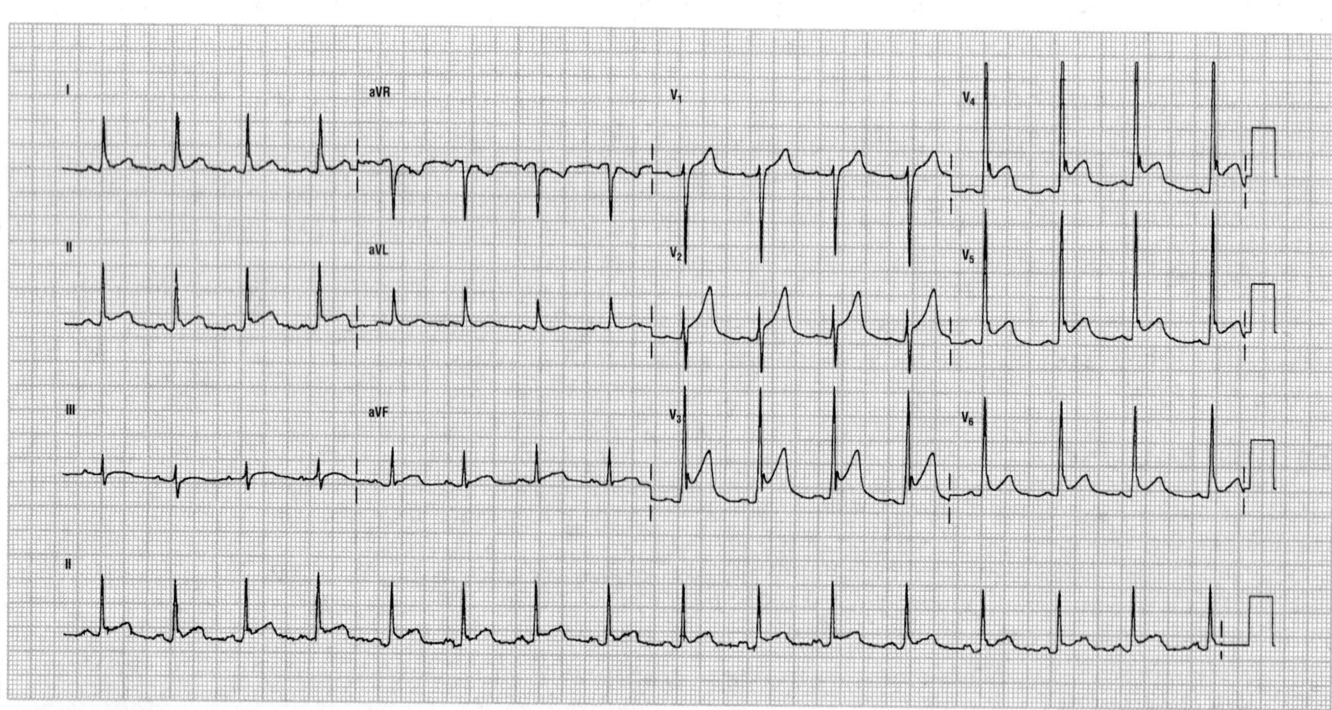

Figure 4-10 A 12-lead ECG showing pericarditis. ST elevation is present in leads I, II, aVF, and V_1–V_6. The QRS complexes are notched, indicating benign ST elevation.

Data from Garcia TB. *12-Lead ECG: The Art of Interpretation*. 2nd ed. Jones & Bartlett Learning; 2014.

adenovirus) in the summer months. The one-third rule applies to the prognosis for this disease: One-third of patients recover without consequences, one-third have chronic cardiac dysfunction, and one-third progress to have chronic HF and need a heart transplant or may die.

Signs and Symptoms

Patients with myocarditis may present with an influenza-like illness, including fever, fatigue, myalgia, vomiting, and diarrhea. Signs of myocarditis may also include tachycardia, and tachypnea, with 12% of patients complaining of chest pain. The ECG may show low voltage with a prolonged QT interval, atrioventricular block, or AMI patterns. Cardiac enzymes are usually elevated, along with the erythrocyte sedimentation rate.

Differential Diagnosis

Myocarditis can present like an AMI with HF, but the patient is usually young (< 35 years) and may not have risk factors for heart disease. No coronary obstruction is noted on cardiac catheterization. Other differential diagnoses may include cardiomyopathy, cardiac tamponade, and atherosclerosis.

Treatment

Management is supportive. In severe cases, patients may require a heart transplant.

Gastrointestinal Causes of Chest Pain

Because of the close proximity to the thorax and diaphragm, GI problems may also cause chest discomfort and pain. In addition, some GI conditions are associated with referred pain to the thorax. The following GI diseases that sometimes cause thoracic pain are covered in depth in Chapter 10, *Abdominal Disorders*: cholecystitis, pancreatitis, peptic ulcer disease, Boerhaave syndrome, and esophageal mucosal tear (Mallory-Weiss syndrome).

Structural Heart-Related Causes of Chest Pain

Other causes of chest discomfort may include structural changes in the heart such as valvular heart disease, aortic stenosis, mitral valve prolapse, and hypertrophic cardiomyopathy. All of these conditions may cause chest discomfort and pain similar to that in ACS. These structural heart and valvular disorders are generally nonemergent, but some can be associated with a life-threatening dysrhythmia.

Aortic Stenosis

As people age, the protein collagen that makes up the heart's valve leaflets becomes damaged, and calcium is deposited. Turbulence from blood flowing across the valve increases scarring, thickening, and stenosis (narrowing) of the valve. Why this aging process progresses to cause significant aortic stenosis in some patients but not in others is unknown. The progressive disease-causing aortic calcification and stenosis has nothing to do with healthy lifestyle choices, unlike the deposition of calcium in the coronary arteries that can cause heart attack.

Pathophysiology

One cause of valvular dysfunction is rheumatic heart disease, a condition resulting from untreated infection by group A streptococcal bacteria. Damage to valve leaflets from rheumatic fever causes stenosis (narrowing) or regurgitation (backward leakage). Under normal circumstances, the aortic valve closes to prevent blood in the aorta from flowing backward into the left ventricle. In aortic regurgitation, the diseased valve allows leakage of blood into the left ventricle as the ventricular muscles relax after pumping. Patients with rheumatic fever also have some degree of rheumatic damage to the mitral valve. Rheumatic heart disease has become uncommon in the United States, except in people who have emigrated from underdeveloped countries.

Signs and Symptoms

Chest pain may be the first symptom in patients with aortic stenosis. Chest pain in patients with aortic stenosis resembles the chest pain experienced by patients with angina. In both of these conditions, pain is described as substernal pressure brought on by exertion and relieved by rest. In patients with CAD, chest pain is due to inadequate blood supply to the heart muscles because of narrowed coronary arteries. In patients with aortic stenosis, chest pain occurs without any underlying narrowing of the coronary arteries. The thickened heart muscle must pump against high pressure to push blood through the narrowed aortic valve. This increases the heart muscle's demand for oxygen to a level exceeding the supply delivered in the blood, causing angina.

Syncope and hypotension may occur due to decreased cardiac output through the stenotic valve, particularly in the setting of vasodilation, such as during a vagal event or sepsis. Without effective treatment, the average life expectancy is less than 3 years after the onset of chest pain or syncope from aortic stenosis.

Shortness of breath from left HF—the most ominous sign—is caused by increased capillary permeability in the lungs due to the increased pressure required to fill the left ventricle. Initially, shortness of breath occurs only during activity, but as the disease progresses, it occurs at rest as well. Patients can find it difficult to lie flat without becoming short of breath. Strenuous activities should be avoided and may trigger syncope or angina, causing the patient to seek medical attention.

Differential Diagnosis

A thorough history and the presence of a murmur are key to identification of aortic stenosis.

Treatment

Acute care for the patient with aortic stenosis is similar to the therapy for the patient with angina, which is usually rest and oxygen. Use extreme caution with medications that decrease preload (e.g., nitroglycerin). Lack of sufficient preload in patients with syncope may lead to a significant drop in systolic blood pressure and worsening of their condition.

Because valve infection is a serious complication of aortic stenosis, patients are given antibiotics prior to any procedure in which bacteria may be introduced into the bloodstream. This recommendation previously included routine dental work and minor surgery. Today, however, there are very few indications for prophylactic antibiotics.

The definitive treatment is repair or replacement of the valve, which can be accomplished by either endovascular techniques or open-heart surgery depending on patient specifics. When symptoms of chest pain, syncope, or shortness of breath appear, the prognosis for patients with aortic stenosis without valve replacement surgery is poor.

Mitral Valve Prolapse

Mitral valve prolapse is the most common heart valve abnormality, affecting 5% to 10% of the world population. Evidence suggests that some types of mitral valve prolapse are associated with higher risk of arrhythmogenic sudden cardiac death.

A normal mitral valve consists of two thin leaflets located between the left atrium and the left ventricle of the heart. The leaflets, which are shaped like parachutes, are attached to the inner wall of the left ventricle by a series of strings called *chordae*. When the ventricles contract, the mitral valve leaflets close snugly and prevent the backflow of blood from the left ventricle into the left atrium. When the ventricles relax, the valves open to allow oxygenated blood from the lungs to fill the left ventricle.

Pathophysiology

In patients with mitral valve prolapse, the mitral valve leaflets and chordae degenerate, becoming thick and enlarged. When the ventricles contract, the leaflets prolapse (flop backward) into the left atrium, sometimes allowing leakage or regurgitation of blood through the valve opening.

Signs and Symptoms

Severe mitral regurgitation can lead to HF and abnormal heart rhythms. Most patients are unaware of the prolapsing of the mitral valve, but others may experience a number of symptoms such as palpitations, chest pain, anxiety, and fatigue. Some may report sharp chest pain that does not respond to nitroglycerin. Auscultation of heart sounds with a stethoscope might reveal a clicking sound that reflects the tightening of the abnormal valve leaflets against the pressure load of the left ventricle. If there is associated regurgitation of blood through the abnormal valve opening, a whooshing sound can be heard immediately following the clicking sound.

Differential Diagnosis

Generally, the only physical finding is a clicking sound during cardiac auscultation.

Treatment

Mitral regurgitation usually can be treated with medication, but some people need surgery to repair or replace the defective valve.

Cardiomyopathy

Cardiomyopathy generally refers to a group of conditions that weaken and enlarge the myocardium.

Pathophysiology

Most cardiomyopathies are classified into three groups—dilated, hypertrophic, and restrictive. Cardiomyopathy occurs when heart muscle myocytes are injured by various causes, and the heart remodels itself to accommodate these changes through hypertrophy or thickening of the muscle (**Figure 4-11**). Both genetic and immunologic causes of this debilitating disease process have been identified.

Signs and Symptoms

A common patient presentation includes chest pain, weakness, and dyspnea. Left-sided HF may be the first presentation, along with exertional chest pain. The ECG may be nonspecific, with ST-T wave changes and intraventricular conduction delay or left bundle branch block being noted. A chest radiograph will usually show a large heart, and the elevated BNP serum level reflects the degree of acute strain on the heart.

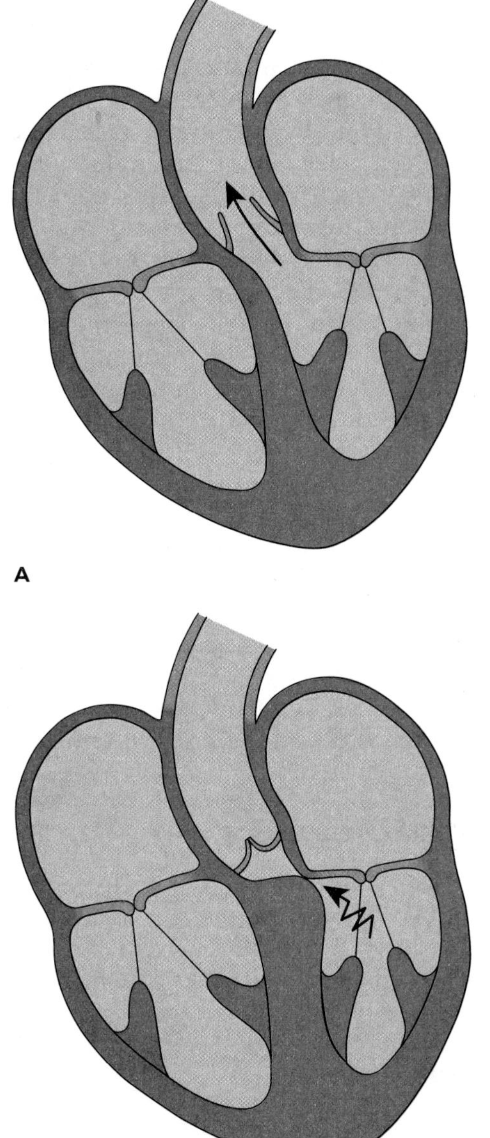

Figure 4-11 Comparison of normal cardiac function with the malfunction characteristic of hypertrophic cardiomyopathy. **A.** Normal heart—unobstructed flow of blood from the left ventricle into the aorta during ventricular systole. **B.** Hypertrophic cardiomyopathy—obstruction to the outflow of blood from the left ventricle by the hypertrophied septum, which impinges on the anterior leaflet of the mitral valve.

Differential Diagnosis

The differential diagnosis is one of exclusion.

Treatment

Management of cardiomyopathy is supportive and similar to that of HF. Acutely, care includes management of arrhythmias and hemodynamics, which may require preload reduction and vasodilation for hypertensive presentations with acute pulmonary edema or inotropic support and vasopressors for cardiogenic shock. Long-term management includes beta blockers, ACE inhibitors, and inotropic agents; implanted defibrillators are indicated for patients with severe systolic dysfunction. This disease is the leading indication for heart transplantation. As discussed earlier, ventricular assistive devices can be used as bridge therapy to transplantation or as sustained therapy.

Nonemergent Causes of Chest Pain

Some causes of chest discomfort and pain are neither emergencies nor life threats. Neurologic causes of chest discomfort include neuropathies, herpes zoster, and postherpetic neuralgia. Musculoskeletal causes of chest pain are likely the most common nonemergency etiologies for chest pain and include inflammation of the joints in the chest wall (costochondritis), such as the condition known as Tietze's syndrome. The many respiratory causes of chest discomfort include pneumonia, pleurisy, lung tumor, and pneumomediastinum, to name a few. Most conditions can be differentiated by the cause and description of the pain. Treatment is supportive, and finding the cause of the pain requires testing not routinely done in an ambulance. Diagnostic testing is often done as a follow-up to discharge from an emergency department after serious life threats have been ruled out.

Thoracic Outlet Syndrome

Thoracic outlet syndrome involves a compression of the brachial plexus (the nerves that pass into the arms from the neck) and/or the subclavian vein or artery by muscle groups in the chest, back, or neck. When compressed, these nerves produce chest discomfort that differs from ACS in that it is often associated with changes in position.

Pathophysiology

In thoracic outlet syndrome, the C8 and T1 nerve roots are usually affected, producing pain and tingling in the ulnar nerve distribution area (lower arm) or the C5, C6, and C7 nerve roots, with pain being referred to the neck, ear, upper part of the chest, upper part of the back, and outer arm. The people most likely to experience thoracic outlet syndrome are those with neck injuries from motor vehicle collisions and those who use computers in nonergonomic postures for extended periods of time. Young athletes (e.g., swimmers, volleyball players, and baseball pitchers) and musicians may also experience thoracic outlet syndrome, albeit significantly less frequently.

Signs and Symptoms

Signs and symptoms may include the following:

- Numbness and tingling in the hands, arms, or fingers
- Discoloration of the extremities due to poor circulation
- Pain in the neck, shoulder, or arms
- Weakness in the hands or arms

Differential Diagnosis

One physical test that may lead you toward this diagnosis is called the *elevated arm stress test* (*EAST*). Direct the patient to raise the arms to 90 degrees while seated, with elbows flexed 90 degrees. With shoulders back, ask the patient to open and close both fists slowly for about 3 minutes and describe the symptoms experienced. If the patient has thoracic outlet syndrome, this test will produce complaints of heaviness of the involved arm, gradual numbness of that hand, and progressive aching through the arm and top of shoulder. It is not unusual to see the patient drop the hand because of increasing pain. The involved arm and hand may have circulatory changes as well.

Treatment

Often, stretching, practicing proper posture, and treatments such as physiotherapy, massage therapy, and chiropractic care will resolve the pain of thoracic outlet syndrome. Cortisone and Botox (botulinum toxin A) injections will lessen the symptoms during a course of treatment. The recovery process, however, is long term, and a few days of poor posture can often lead to setbacks. Approximately 10% to 15% of patients undergo surgical decompression if 6 to 12 months of therapy fails to relieve the pain.

Herpes Zoster

Herpes zoster (shingles) is a painful rash due to reactivation of the varicella-zoster virus, which causes chickenpox at the time of initial infection. (See Chapter 7, *Infectious Diseases*, for further information on this condition.)

Pathophysiology

Herpes zoster results from the varicella-zoster virus, which is left dormant in the body following a case of the chickenpox, only to be later reactivated in a cranial nerve or spinal nerve dermatome. Herpes zoster can cause chest discomfort or pain before, during, or after the signature rash develops. Patients who are immunocompromised from human immunodeficiency virus or receiving chemotherapy are at a greater risk for herpes zoster outbreaks.

Signs and Symptoms

Unlike the pain of a heart attack, herpes zoster pain is described as severe burning pain, worsened by even light touch, that typically precedes a rash by several days. The pain can persist for several months after the rash disappears—a condition called postherpetic neuralgia. The pain and rash most commonly occur on the torso but can appear on the face, eyes, or other parts of the body; they always affect one or more adjacent dermatomes on one side of the body, appearing in a belt-like pattern and not crossing the midline. Initially, the rash consists of flat red spots, but it quickly forms small, fluid-filled blisters called vesicles. The patient may develop a fever and general malaise. The painful blisters eventually rupture, crust over within 7 to 10 days, and then fall off. Direct contact with or inhalation of droplets from the vesicles can spread the virus to a person who has never had chickenpox and is not vaccinated. Until the rash has developed crusts, a person is considered contagious. A person is not infectious before blisters appear or during postherpetic neuralgia (pain after the rash is gone). The pain may persist well after resolution of the rash and can be severe enough to require medications for relief.

Differential Diagnosis

Diagnosis is easy if the rash is present: Herpes zoster is the only rash that follows a dermatome and is limited to one side of the body. If no rash is present, as in the case of postherpetic neuralgia, blood tests may be needed for definitive diagnosis.

Treatment

Herpes zoster is usually treated with oral antivirals, which are most effective when started within 72 hours after the onset of the rash. The addition of an orally administered corticosteroid can provide modest benefits in reducing the pain of herpes zoster and the incidence of postherpetic neuralgia. Patients with postherpetic neuralgia may require narcotics for adequate pain control.

Musculoskeletal Causes of Chest Pain

As described in the assessment section, the thoracic cage is made up of musculoskeletal structures and can be a somatic cause for chest pain. Muscle strain, costochondritis, and nonspecific chest wall pain are usually well defined by the patient as sharp or aching. You must rule out all other causes for the patient's chest pain before deciding on these possibilities as a diagnosis. As with most inflammation, use of NSAIDs, heat or cold therapy, and rest are the most common tactics for management.

Other Pulmonary Causes of Chest Pain

The many respiratory causes of chest discomfort include pneumonitis, pleurisy, lung tumor, and pneumomediastinum, to name a few. Chapter 3, *Respiratory Disorders*, provides an in-depth review of these and other respiratory conditions responsible for chest discomfort.

Pneumonitis

Pneumonitis refers to any inflammation of lung tissue. It may be caused by a variety of conditions, including pneumonia, bronchitis, and aspiration. Productive cough and difficulty breathing are the most common symptoms of pneumonitis. Fever may occur with infection, and the cough may burn. Fatigue and malaise may also accompany pneumonitis.

Treatment of pneumonitis is generally supportive and focuses on finding the cause. Treatment may focus on avoiding the trigger, but may also include medications such as IV antibiotics. If the patient reports shortness of breath, administer oxygen to maintain SpO_2 at > 94%. An IV should be established, and a heart monitor applied. Place the patient in the position of greatest comfort. Obtain a complete blood count, chemistry panel, and chest radiograph to confirm or rule out pneumonia.

Pleurisy

Pleurisy—that is, painful respiration—should prompt the clinician to conduct a thorough assessment to find the cause of the pain. Pleuritic pain usually increases with respiration and is the result of pleuritis, inflammation of the parietal and visceral pleurae lining the chest wall and lungs; this pathologic process was described earlier in this chapter and is discussed in detail in Chapter 3, *Respiratory Disorders*. As the patient breathes, the inflamed pleurae rub against each other, causing a sharp pain that increases with inspiration. Fever and cough may be present if the inflammation is due to pneumonia or other infection. A possible exam finding is a pleural friction rub—the rough, scratchy sound heard with a stethoscope when the pleurae rub against each other. It often sounds like leather stretching when the patient inhales deeply.

A chest radiograph may show air or fluid in the pleural space. It also may show the cause of the pleurisy (e.g., pneumonia, a fractured rib, a lung tumor). If a significant amount of fluid is present, it may have to be removed with thoracentesis in the inpatient setting. The collected fluid will be tested to determine its origin; in some cases, fluid may accumulate from lung tissue disease or cancers.

Acetaminophen or NSAIDs may be used for pain relief. Treatment is generally supportive and focuses on finding the cause. As discussed earlier, life-threatening causes of heart-related chest pain will have been ruled out by this point.

Special Considerations

Older Adult Patients

Older patients may present with ACS, but the symptoms of this condition may not always be readily apparent. ACS in this population is commonly referred to as "silent MI" because symptoms can be completely absent or nonspecific, including fatigue or generalized weakness, dyspnea on exertion, and decreased appetite. Older persons may be taking medications (e.g., beta blockers) that decrease their ability to compensate for hemodynamic compromise. You must be prepared to address these issues. Many older patients have multiple medical conditions and are more sensitive to medications than younger individuals, making diagnosis and management challenging.

Bariatric Patients

Owing to the decreased mobility of obese persons, blood clots in their legs may contribute to pulmonary emboli. The complaint of chest pain may be altered because of nerve distribution in the tissues due to torso mass. The increase in myocardial workload puts obese patients at high risk for ACS. In addition, diabetes is more common in this population and may contribute to cardiovascular issues. Electrolyte imbalances may follow bariatric surgery and result in dysrhythmias that cause chest discomfort in postsurgery patients.

Obstetric Patients

PE should be high on your list of suspected diagnoses when assessing a pregnant patient; this condition may be due to the state of hypercoagulation and potential for developing blood clots associated with pregnancy. Pregnancy also places increased demands on the cardiovascular system and may exacerbate a previous diagnosed or undiagnosed condition. In addition, GERD is common during pregnancy and may contribute to chest discomfort. Consider transporting such patients to a facility that cares for high-risk obstetric patients. Postpartum cardiomyopathy can result in moderate to severe HF symptoms and is associated with high mortality.

Putting It All Together

Caring for a patient with chest pain begins with your initial observation. Your immediate goal is to determine whether the patient is sick or not sick. Your first impression should tell you whether you have time to continue the assessment or if you should intercede immediately. Evaluate the patient for life threats first, such as tension pneumothorax. Life-threatening conditions require immediate intervention. Evaluate the patient for other life-threatening conditions such as ACS, including obtaining a 12-lead ECG to look for STEMI, and acute aortic syndromes, including checking the patient's blood pressures and pulses in both upper extremities. Clues to many emergent conditions such as esophageal rupture and PE can be revealed during history taking, and using tools such as SAMPLER and OPQRST is helpful in obtaining this information. If the patient's condition is unstable or deteriorates, support the ABCs as you work through the AMLS patient assessment process.

At the receiving facility, chest radiographs, lab analyses, and CT scans are performed as indicated.

SCENARIO SOLUTION

- Differential diagnoses may include myocarditis, pneumonia, PE, ACS, cholecystitis, and pericarditis.
- To narrow your differential diagnosis, you will need to complete the patient's history of past and present illness. Obtain a more thorough history of her present illness. Perform a physical examination that includes vital signs assessment (considering blood pressure measurements in both arms) evaluation of heart and breath sounds, jugular vein assessment, ECG monitoring and 12-lead ECG, SpO_2, and blood glucose analysis.
- This patient has signs that may indicate ACS, infection, or HF. Administer oxygen if indicated. Establish vascular access. Monitor the cardiac rhythm, and obtain a 12-lead ECG. Further treatment will depend on the rest of your assessment findings. If you suspect ACS, treat the patient with aspirin and possibly nitroglycerin or fentaNYL. If the patient has signs of HF without shock, treat with CPAP and nitroglycerin. If the patient's examination points to GI or other causes, treat as appropriate. Transport the patient to the closest appropriate health care facility, emphasizing the appropriate destination for STEMI.

SUMMARY

- Your standard assessment practice for the patient with chest pain should include looking for life-threatening causes and managing them appropriately—even within the primary survey. In the patient with a patent airway, assessing for breath sounds and looking for shock are key considerations.
- Life-threatening causes of chest pain usually include diseases that produce both chest pain and increased work of breathing, or chest pain and alterations of vital signs (or a combination thereof).
- Standard protocols for chest pain include use of oxygen, vascular access, application of monitors, ECG, analgesia, chest radiography, and laboratory studies. Health care clinicians need to triage the patient to determine the need for additional resources (cardiac catheterization at a specialized heart center) and move the patient toward those specialties early in the process.
- Non–life-threatening causes of chest pain can arise from several body systems, including the cardiovascular, respiratory, gastrointestinal, immunologic, structural cardiac, neurologic, and musculoskeletal systems.

Key Terms

acute coronary syndrome (ACS) An umbrella term that refers to a group of conditions caused by myocardial ischemia (insufficient blood supply to the heart muscle that results from coronary artery disease), including unstable angina, ST-segment elevation myocardial infarction (STEMI), and non–ST-segment elevation myocardial infarction (NSTEMI).

acute myocardial infarction (AMI) Commonly known as a "heart attack"; occurs when the blood supply to part of the heart is interrupted, causing heart cells to die. This is most commonly due to blockage of a coronary artery following the rupture of plaque within the wall of an artery. The resulting ischemia and decreased supply of oxygen, if left untreated, can cause damage and/or death of heart muscle tissue.

cardiac output The volume of blood pumped by the heart over time. Cardiac output is often recorded in liters per minute. It can be calculated as the heart rate times the stroke volume (the volume of blood pumped in a single cardiac contraction).

cardiac tamponade Also known as "pericardial tamponade"; an emergent condition in which fluid accumulates in the pericardium (the sac that surrounds the heart) and restricts the amount of blood that can reenter the heart. If the amount of fluid increases slowly (such as in hypothyroidism), the pericardial sac can expand to contain a liter or more of fluid prior to tamponade occurring. If the fluid increases rapidly (as may occur after trauma or myocardial rupture), as little as 100 mL can cause tamponade.

ischemia Insufficient oxygen and nutrient delivery to an organ or tissue caused by decreased blood flow, severe anemia or hypoxia, or an increased metabolic demand, which leads to damage or dysfunction of the tissue.

non-ST-elevation myocardial infarction (NSTEMI) A type of myocardial infarction that is not associated with ST-segment elevation on electrocardiogram (ECG) recordings. It is diagnosed on the basis of laboratory tests for elevated cardiac enzymes.

pericarditis A condition in which the tissue surrounding the heart (pericardium) becomes inflamed. It can be caused by several factors, but is often related to a viral infection.

pleurae Thin membranes that surround and protect the lungs (visceral) and line the chest cavity (parietal).

pulmonary embolism (PE) The sudden blockage of a pulmonary artery by a blood clot, often originating from a deep vein in the legs or pelvis, that embolizes and travels to the lung. Symptoms include tachycardia, hypoxia, and hypotension.

pulsus paradoxus An exaggeration of the normal inspiratory decrease in systolic blood pressure, defined by an inspiratory fall of systolic blood pressure of > 10 mm Hg.

ST-elevation myocardial infarction (STEMI) A type of acute myocardial infarction associated with ST-elevation in a vascular distribution on 12-lead electrocardiogram (ECG) recordings. These attacks carry a substantial risk of death and disability and call for a quick response by a system geared toward reperfusion therapy.

stable angina Symptoms of chest pain, shortness of breath, or other equivalent symptoms that occur predictably with exertion, then resolve with rest, suggesting the presence of a fixed coronary lesion that prevents adequate perfusion with increased demand.

tension pneumothorax A life-threatening condition that results from progressive worsening of a simple pneumothorax (an accumulation of air under pressure in the pleural space). It can lead to progressive restriction of venous return, which leads to decreased preload, then systemic hypotension.

unstable angina Angina of increased frequency, severity, or occurring with less intensive exertion than the baseline. It suggests the narrowing of a static lesion, causing further limitations of coronary blood flow with increased demand.

Bibliography

Adam A, Dixon AK, Grainger RG, et al. *Grainger and Allison's Diagnostic Radiology.* 5th ed. Churchill Livingstone; 2008.

Aehlert B. *Paramedic Practice Today: Above and Beyond.* Jones & Bartlett Learning; 2011.

Aghababian R. *Essentials of Emergency Medicine.* 2nd ed. Jones & Bartlett Learning; 2011.

Akula R, Hasan SP, Alhassen M, et al. Right-sided EKG in pulmonary embolism. *J Natl Med Assoc.* 2003;95:714-717.

American Academy of Orthopaedic Surgeons: *Nancy Caroline's Emergency Care in the Streets.* 8th ed. Jones & Bartlett Learning; 2018.

American Heart Association. *2010 AHA Guidelines for CPR and ECC.* American Heart Association; 2010.

American Heart Association. *ACLS for Experienced Providers.* American Heart Association; 2013.

American Heart Association. Classes and stages of heart failure. Reviewed June 7, 2023. https://www.heart.org/en/health-topics/heart-failure/what-is-heart-failure/classes-of-heart-failure

American Heart Association. What is atherosclerosis? Reviewed November 6, 2020. https://www.heart.org/en/health-topics/cholesterol/about-cholesterol/atherosclerosis

Anderson JL, Adams CD, Antman EM, et al. 2012 ACCF/AHA focused update incorporated into the ACCF/AHA 2007 guidelines for the management of patients with unstable angina/non-ST-elevation myocardial infarction: a report of the American College of Cardiology Foundation/American Heart Association Task Force on Practice Guidelines. *Circulation.* 2013;127(23):e663-e828.

Black JM, Hokanson Hawks J. *Medical–Surgical Nursing.* 8th ed. Saunders; 2009.

Bledsoe BE, Anderson E, Hodnick R, et al. Low-fractional oxygen concentration continuous positive airway pressure is effective in the prehospital setting. *Prehosp Emerg Care.* 2012;16(2):217-221.

Bodson L, Bouferrache K, Vieillard-Baron A. Cardiac tamponade. *Curr Opin Crit Care.* 2011;17(5):416-424.

Braunwald E. *Heart Disease: A Textbook of Cardiovascular Medicine.* 4th ed. WB Saunders; 1992.

Damodaran S. Cocaine and beta blockers: the paradigm. *Eur J Intern Med.* 2010;21(2):84-86.

Dorland's Illustrated Medical Dictionary. Saunders; 2007.

Ferrari R, Guardigli G, Ceconi C. Secondary prevention of CAD with ACE inhibitors: a struggle between life and death of the endothelium. *Cardiovasc Drugs Ther.* 2010;24(4):331-339.

Field J. *Advanced Cardiac Life Support Provider Manual.* American Heart Association; 2006.

Field J, Hazinski M, Gilmore D. *Handbook of ECC for Healthcare Providers.* American Heart Association; 2008.

Frownfelter D, Dean E. *Cardiovascular and Pulmonary Physical Therapy.* 4th ed. Mosby; 2006.

Go AS, Mozaffarian D, Roger VL, et al. Heart disease and stroke statistics—2013 update: a report from the American Heart Association. *Circulation.* 2013;127(1):e6-e245.

Goldman L, Ausiello D. *Cecil Medicine.* 23th ed. Saunders; 2007.

Gulati M, Levy PD, Mukherjee D, et al. AHA/ACC/ASE/CHEST/SAEM/SCCT/SCMR guideline for the evaluation and diagnosis of chest pain: a report of the American College of Cardiology/American Heart Association Joint Committee on Clinical Practice Guidelines. *Circulation.* 2012;144(22):e368-e454.

Haji SA, Movahed A. Right ventricular infarction: diagnosis and treatment. *Clin Cardiol (Hoboken).* 2000;23(7):473-482.

Herlitz J, Bång A, Omerovic E, et al. Is pre-hospital treatment of chest pain optimal in acute coronary syndrome? The relief of both pain and anxiety is needed. *Int J Cardiol.* 2011;149(2):147-151.

Hiratzka LF, Bakris GL, Beckman JA, et al. 2010 ACCF/AHA/AATS/ACR/ASA/SCA/SCAI/SIR/STS/SVM guidelines for the diagnosis and management of patients with thoracic aortic disease: a report of the American College of Cardiology Foundation/American Heart Association Task Force on Practice Guidelines, American Association for Thoracic Surgery, American College of Radiology, American Stroke Association, Society of Cardiovascular Anesthesiologists, Society for Cardiovascular Angiography and Interventions, Society of Interventional Radiology, Society of Thoracic Surgeons, and Society for Vascular Medicine. *Circulation.* 2010;121(13):e266-e369.

Hoffman R, James SK. Routine oxygen supplementation in acute cardiovascular disease. The end of a paradigm? *Circulation.* 2018;137:320-322.

Ikematsu Y. Incidence and characteristics of dysphoria in patients with cardiac tamponade. *Heart Lung J Crit Care.* 2007;36(6):440-449.

Johnson D, ed. The pericardium. In: Standring S, et al., eds. *Gray's Anatomy.* Mosby; 2005.

Kevil C, Goeders N, Woolard M, et al. Methamphetamine use and cardiovascular disease. *Arterioscler Thromb Vasc Biol.* 2019;39(9):1739-1746.

Lange RA, Cigarroa RG, Yancy CW Jr, et al. Cocaine-induced coronary-artery vasoconstriction. *N Engl J Med.* 1989;321:1557-1562.

Lawton JS, Tamis-Holland JE, Bangalore S, et al. 2021 ACC/AHA/SCAI guideline for coronary artery revascularization: a report of the American College of Cardiology/American Heart Association Joint Committee on Clinical Practice Guidelines. *Circulation.* 2022;145:e18-e114.

Lazar DR, Lazar FL, Homorodean C, et al. High-sensitivity troponin: a review on characteristics, assessment, and clinical implications. *Dis Markers.* 2022;2022:9713326.

Manfrini O, Morrell C, Das R, et al. Management of acute coronary events study: effects of angiotensin-converting enzyme inhibitors and beta blockers on clinical outcomes in patients with and without coronary artery obstructions at angiography (from a register-based cohort study on acute coronary syndromes). *Am J Cardiol*. 2014;113(10):1628-1633.

Marx JA, Hockberger RS, Walls RM, et al. *Rosen's Emergency Medicine: Concepts and Clinical Practice*. 6th ed. Mosby; 2006.

National Association of Emergency Medical Technicians. *PHTLS: Prehospital Trauma Life Support*. 9th ed. Public Safety Group; 2019.

O'Connor RE, Ali Al AS, Brady WJ, et al. Part 9: acute coronary syndromes: 2015 American Heart Association guidelines update for cardiopulmonary resuscitation and emergency cardiovascular care. *Circulation*. 2015;132(18 suppl 2):S483-S500.

O'Gara PT, Kushner FG, Ascheim DD, et al. ACCF/AHA guideline: 2013 ACCF/AHA guideline for the management of ST-elevation myocardial infarction. *Circulation*. 2013;127:e362-e422.

Parikh R, Kadowitz PJ. A review of current therapies used in the treatment of congestive heart failure. *Expert Rev Cardiovasc Ther*. 2013;11(9):1171-1178.

Rezaie S. The death of MONA in ACS: part I—morphine. *REBEL EM*. November 5, 2017. https://rebelem.com/the-death-of-mona-in-acs-part-i-morphine

Rezaie S. The death of MONA in ACS: part II—oxygen. *REBEL EM*. November 5, 2017. https://rebelem.com/death-mona-acs-part-ii-oxygen

Rezaie S. The death of MONA in ACS: part III—nitroglycerin. *REBEL EM*. November 5, 2017. https://rebelem.com/death-mona-acs-part-iii-nitroglycerin

Rezaie S. The death of MONA in ACS: part IV—aspirin. *REBEL EM*. November 5, 2017. https://rebelem.com/death-mona-acs-part-iv-aspirin

Story L. *Pathophysiology: A Practical Approach*. 2nd ed. Jones & Bartlett Learning; 2015.

Torres-Macho J, Mancebo-Plaza AB, Crespo-Gimenez A, et al. Clinical features of patients inappropriately undiagnosed of pulmonary embolism, *Am J Emerg Med*. 2013;31(12):1646-1650.

Urden L, Stacy K, Lough M. *Critical Care Nursing: Diagnosis and Management*. 6th ed. Mosby; 2010.

U.S. Department of Transportation. *National Emergency Medical Services Education Standards: Paramedic Instructional Guidelines*. U.S. Department of Transportation; 2010.

U.S. Department of Transportation. *National EMS Education Standards: Paramedic*. U.S. Department of Transportation; 2010.

Webb SR. Takotsubo syndrome. American College of Cardiology. March 30, 2020. https://www.acc.org/latest-in-cardiology/ten-points-to-remember/2020/03/30/12/17/takotsubo-syndrome

Weitzenblum E. Chronic cor pulmonale. *Heart*. 2003;89(2):225-230.

Williams B, Boyle M, Robertson N, et al. When pressure is positive: a literature review of the prehospital use of continuous positive airway pressure. *Prehosp Disaster Med*. 2012;28:52-60.

Wilson SF, Thompson JM. *Mosby's Clinical Nursing Series: Respiratory Disorders*. Mosby; 1990.

CHAPTER 5

Shock

Chapter Editors
Stephen J. Rahm, NRP, FcEHS
Raymond L. Fowler, MD, FACEP, FAEMS
Melanie Lippmann, MD

This chapter takes a close look at perfusion, the physiologic function that fails in patients who are in shock. The chapter reviews the anatomy and physiology of tissue perfusion and describes the pathophysiology of hypoperfusion, or shock. The types and progression of shock are discussed and compared so you will be able to recognize shock from different causes at any stage. The AMLS Assessment Pathway offers tools for performing the assessment, building a differential diagnosis, and determining the emergency treatment of shock in general and of each particular type of shock.

LEARNING OBJECTIVES

At the conclusion of this chapter, you will be able to:

- Describe the anatomy and physiology of body systems as they relate to shock.
- Describe the pathophysiology of shock, including the progressive stages.
- Describe and compare the following types of shock: hypovolemic, distributive, cardiogenic, and obstructive.
- Identify the key features of each type of shock.
- Assess the patient for life-threatening findings during the primary and secondary surveys and ongoing management.
- List effective ways of obtaining information on a patient's allergies, current medications, incident and past medical history, and correlate them to each of the categories of shock.
- Describe laboratory and diagnostic tests used to verify diagnoses associated with shock.
- Apply appropriate treatment modalities for the management, monitoring, and continuing care of the patient in shock.
- Formulate a differential diagnosis, demonstrate sound clinical-reasoning skills, and apply advanced clinical decision making in caring for a patient in shock who has an emergent cardiovascular, respiratory, or hematologic condition.
- Describe how the AMLS Assessment Pathway can be used to address problems found during the assessment of the shock patient.

SCENARIO

Your patient is a 58-year-old man who presents with acute shortness of breath and lethargy. His radial pulses are absent, and his carotid pulse is weak. His skin is mottled and cool to the touch. His past medical history is significant for hypertension, coronary artery disease, and type 2 diabetes. His wife tells you that he had chest pain for the last several days but refused to go to the hospital. His blood pressure is 84/56 mm Hg; pulse rate, 130 beats/min; respirations, 26 breaths/min and labored; and oxygen saturation, 79%. Auscultation of his breath sounds reveals diffuse coarse crackles bilaterally.

- What is your initial impression?
- What immediate treatment is indicated for this patient?
- What do you suspect to be the primary cause of this patient's clinical presentation? Why?
- What specific treatment is indicated for this patient?

Shock is a progressive state of cellular hypoperfusion in which insufficient oxygen is available to meet tissue demands. Shock may be caused when oxygen intake, absorption, or delivery fails, or when the cells are unable to take up and use the delivered oxygen to generate sufficient energy to carry out cellular functions. It is key to understand that when shock occurs the body is in distress. The shock response is mounted by the body to attempt to maintain perfusion to vital organs during times of physiologic distress. This shock response can accompany a broad spectrum of clinical conditions that stress the body, ranging from acute myocardial infarctions, to major infections, to allergic reactions. Each year in the United States more than 1 million people arrive at emergency departments (EDs) in varying states of shock, making understanding of the pathophysiology, assessment, and management of this condition critical to the role of a health care clinician. Critical thinking and decision making are essential tools to use when encountering a patient in shock. This process involves performing rapid assessment, providing lifesaving treatment, and developing a differential diagnosis to determine the cause of the shock condition.

The initial signs of shock can be subtle and the progression of shock insidious. If not treated promptly, shock may injure the body's vital organs and ultimately lead to death. Rapid recognition of the signs and symptoms of shock is an essential skill for every health care clinician. It begins with an understanding of the anatomy and physiology of tissue perfusion.

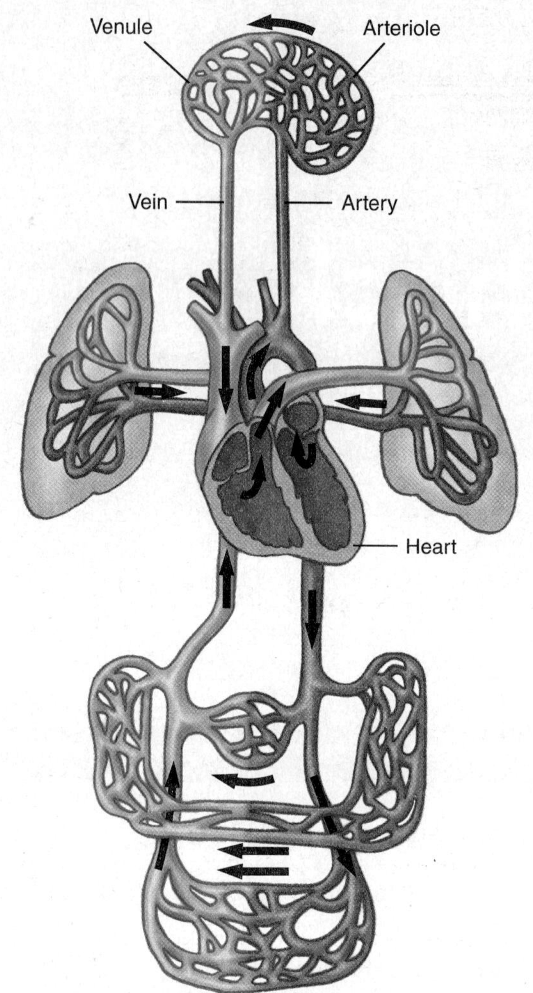

Figure 5-1 The cardiovascular system requires continuous operation of its three components: the heart (or pump), the blood vessels (or container), and the blood and body fluids (or fluid volume).

Anatomy and Physiology of Perfusion

The word **perfusion** derives from the Latin verb *perfundere*, meaning "to pour over." In the body, blood supplies oxygen to cells by way of the circulatory system. To keep the blood moving continuously through the body, the cardiovascular system requires three main components: a functioning pump (the heart); adequate fluid volume (the blood and body fluids); and an intact system of tubing (the blood vessels) capable of reflex adjustments, such as constriction and dilation, in response to changes in pump output and fluid volume (**Figure 5-1**). Intravascular volume is the amount of circulating blood in the vessels.

The Heart

The heart is a cone-shaped muscular organ situated in the mediastinum, posterior to the lower half of the sternum. It lies at an oblique angle, with two-thirds of its mass to the left of the body's midline and one-third to the right of the body's midline. The heart is composed of four chambers: the left and right atria are the upper chambers and are located at the base of the heart, and the left and right ventricles are the lower chambers and are located at the apex.

The atria are smaller than the more muscular ventricles. Venous blood enters the heart through the right atrium and then flows through the tricuspid valve into the right ventricle. From the right ventricle, the blood travels through the pulmonic valve into the pulmonary trunk, which branches into the left and right pulmonary arteries—the vessels that deliver deoxygenated blood to the lungs. Once the blood has been oxygenated in the lungs, it proceeds through the left and right pulmonary veins to the left atrium (the four pulmonary veins, two for each lung, are the only veins in the body that carry fully oxygenated blood). The mitral (bicuspid) valve allows blood to pass from the left atrium to the left ventricle, where the blood is then pumped to the aorta through the aortic valve to the remainder of the body.

A complete heartbeat is called a **cardiac cycle**. Systole (contraction) and diastole (relaxation) in all four chambers, both atria and ventricles, are the components of the cardiac cycle. The contraction of the heart occurs in stages. The ventricles relax (ventricular diastole), and the blood flows from the atria into the ventricles. Most ventricular filling occurs passively. Then the atria contract (atrial systole) to move additional blood into the ventricles. The contraction of the atria and its contribution to ventricular filling is called the atrial kick. As atrial contraction completes and the atrioventricular valves close and the atria relax (atrial diastole), the much stronger ventricles contract (ventricular systole) to pump blood to the lungs and body. The heart's structural and functional status, the volume of blood in the ventricle before systole, the autonomic nervous system, medications, and other factors affect its contractility, which determines the volume of blood it pumps with each contraction, also known as the **stroke volume**.

Cardiac Output

For blood to "pour" through the body, it must be pumped. In a healthy person, the heart is remarkably efficient at moving oxygenated blood through the body, ensuring adequate perfusion. **Cardiac output** is the volume of blood the heart can pump per minute and is dependent on several factors. First, the heart is a muscle and must have adequate strength, which is largely determined by the ability of the heart muscle to contract (**Figure 5-2**). Second, the heart must receive adequate blood to pump. As the volume of blood flowing to the heart increases, the precontraction pressure in the heart builds up. The precontraction pressure is known as **preload**. Lastly, the

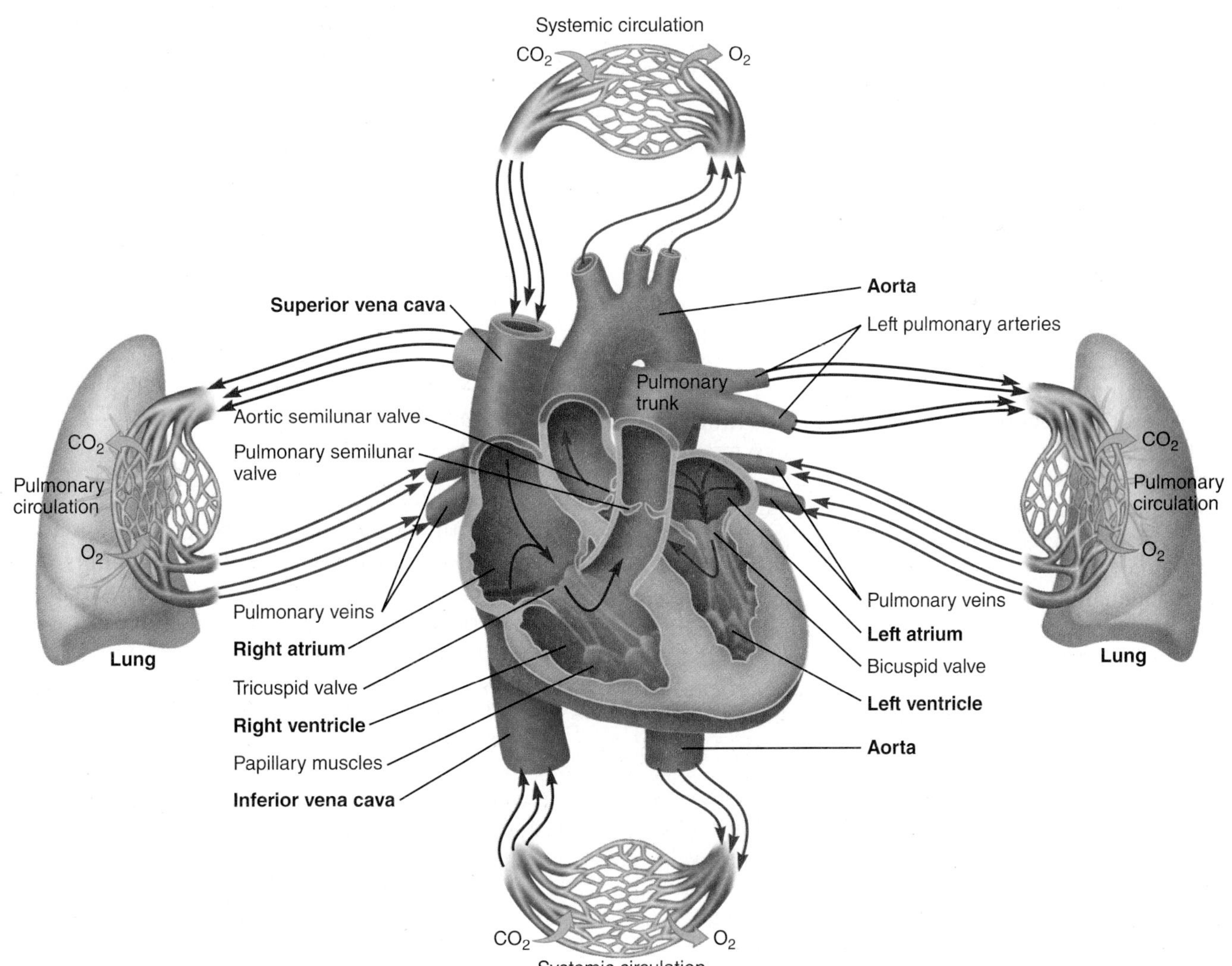

Figure 5-2 Circulation begins in the heart muscle.

resistance to flow in the peripheral circulation also affects cardiac output. The force or resistance against which the heart pumps is known as **afterload**.

Cardiac output is usually expressed as liters per minute (L/min). The cardiac output of a healthy adult varies from 3 to 8 L/min, with 5 L/min being the average. Cardiac output is determined by stroke volume—the volume of blood ejected with each contraction of the heart—and heart rate. The stroke volume of a healthy adult is typically about 70 mL, but the amount is variable because of individual physiologic differences. The equation is as follows:

Cardiac output = Stroke volume × Heart rate

The primary mechanical variable that affects stroke volume is explained by Starling's law, also known as the Frank-Starling mechanism. Starling's law describes the ability of cardiac muscle fibers to stretch and contract to regulate the strength of the heart's contraction. According to this law, the more the heart is stretched, the more forcefully it contracts, but only up to a point. Think of the heart as a rubber band: the farther you stretch it, the farther it will shoot when released. Once the heart muscle has stretched beyond its optimal elasticity (like an old rubber band), the contraction will become weaker and less effective.

Related to the stroke volume is the ejection fraction, or the percentage of blood that is ejected from the ventricle. A normal ejection fraction is 50% to 75%. For example, if the end-diastolic volume (preload) is 100 mL, and the ventricle ejects 70 mL (stroke volume), the ejection fraction would be 70%. Lower ejection fractions indicate decreased pumping force of the heart.

Neural and endocrine mechanisms also influence stroke volume through neurotransmitters. Sympathetic nerve fibers in the cardiac nerves release norepinephrine, and the adrenal medulla releases epinephrine. These two adrenergic agents boost the strength of cardiac contraction.

Inadequate cardiac output is one cause of hypoperfusion. To generate adequate cardiac output, the heart must be able to contract with sufficient force, and the heart rate must be within an effective range. Details of the primary factors determining stroke volume and cardiac output are as follows:

- *Preload*. The stretch of the myocardial tissue by the blood in the ventricles just before the start of a contraction. You can grasp the concept of preload by comparing it with the tension created when a bowstring is drawn back. If there is not enough tension on the string, the arrow will drop to the ground near the archer's feet. A strong pull, in contrast, will propel the arrow toward its target. In the heart, the pull or stretch on the muscle is from the volume of blood returning to the heart and accumulating in the ventricle prior to a contraction. Starling's law states the greater the stretch—up to a point—the stronger the cardiac contraction and the greater the stroke volume.
- *Afterload*. The force the ejected blood meets as it exits the ventricle. You can think about afterload as the pressure it takes to push through a swinging door. If someone or something is pushing against the other side of the door, it takes more pressure to open it. A major factor determining afterload is the transmural pressure, which is the difference between intrathoracic and intraventricular pressure. In the systemic circulation, afterload is also influenced by aortic systolic pressure and systemic vascular resistance. Increasing or decreasing the afterload alters the cardiac output. Another factor affecting afterload is the thickness or viscosity of the blood. When the blood is thicker, it can increase the afterload as well because it takes more force to move the thick blood through the vascular system.
- *Contractility*. The force of cardiac contraction for a given level of preload. Positive inotropic stimulation, such as what is provided by the administration of EPINEPHrine or DOPamine, increases the force and rate of contraction. This stronger contraction will, in turn, increase the stroke volume for a given level of preload. It is important to note that as cardiac contractility increases, the heart's demand for oxygen increases as well.
- *Synchrony*. To pump effectively, cardiac contractions must be synchronized to make the cycle function efficiently—the atria must contract to fill the ventricles, and the ventricles must contract to pump blood to the lungs and heart. Loss of atrioventricular synchrony, such as what occurs during atrial fibrillation or conduction disorders such as atrioventricular block, alters the effectiveness of the heart as a pump. Atrial fibrillation does not allow the atria to fully contract and pump blood to the ventricles, causing a decrease in ventricular preload (due to the loss of atrial kick) and potentially decreasing cardiac output. Conduction disorders such as atrioventricular blocks disturb coordination between the atrial and ventricular muscle fibers, reducing the efficiency of contraction, which may result in a decrease in cardiac output.

The Vascular System

The vascular system is a conduit for moving blood throughout the body. The arteries and arterioles, which make up the arterial vascular system, carry blood away from the heart; normally, this is oxygenated, nutrient-rich blood (except in the pulmonary arteries, which transport oxygen-poor blood to the lungs). The veins and venules, which make up the venous system, return blood to the heart; apart from the pulmonary veins, as discussed previously, the venous system contains deoxygenated blood and waste products to be eliminated from the body. The capillaries, which connect the arterial system to the venous system, are the smallest and thinnest-walled blood vessels. They are the site of the transfer of oxygen and other nutrients to the tissues and the removal of wastes from the tissues. The precapillary sphincters dilate to allow blood to flow into the capillaries when more oxygen is needed in the tissues.

In fact, all parts of the vascular system can contract (vasoconstrict) and dilate (vasodilate) in response to various stimuli. The arteries and arterioles constrict and dilate more vigorously than the veins and venules do because their vessel walls have more smooth muscle fibers and thus are stronger. The increased pressure of the blood in the arteries relative to the veins keeps the blood flowing quickly. Because the residual pressure is lower in the venous system, valves are necessary to prevent the backflow of blood into the periphery.

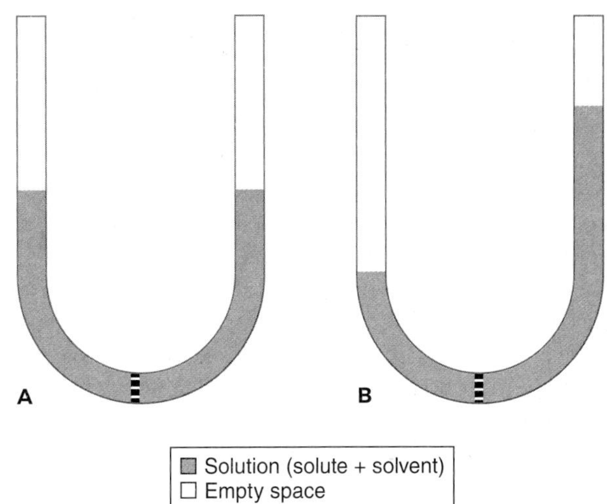

Figure 5-3 **A.** A U-tube, in which the two halves are separated by a semipermeable membrane, contains equal amounts of water and solid particles. **B.** If a solute that cannot diffuse through the semipermeable membrane is added to one side but not to the other, fluid will flow across the membrane to dilute the added particles. The pressure difference in the height of the fluid in the U-tube is known as osmotic pressure.

Blood

Blood has two important functions: transportation of oxygen and nutrients to the body's cells and removal of waste from the body. Hemoglobin, an iron-containing protein in red blood cells (RBCs), carries oxygen to the tissues. Carbon dioxide (CO_2), one of the primary waste products of metabolism, is principally dissolved in the plasma (though up to 25% is carried on hemoglobin) and must be eliminated quickly because a buildup of CO_2 contributes to a state of **acidosis**.

Other components of blood include the following:

- *White blood cells* (WBCs) help defend the body against infection by bacteria, fungi, and other pathogens.
- *Platelets* initiate the process of clotting.
- *Proteins* perform various functions involving blood clotting, immunity, wound healing, and transport.
- *Hormones* control organ system function, regulate growth and development, and perform other vital functions.
- *Nutrients* fuel cells so they can function properly (glucose, for example, is a nutrient carried by the blood to cells throughout the body).
- *Plasma* carries the formed components (i.e., RBCs, WBCs, platelets) in blood; this fluid is composed of about 92% water and 7% protein.

An equilibrium must be maintained between the interstitial (extracellular) fluid, which occupies the spaces between the cells, and the intracellular fluid, which remains inside the cells. Plasma proteins are critical in the regulation of fluid equilibrium. The plasma proteins albumin and globulin are large and cannot easily pass out of the vessels. Their presence within the vessels creates an osmotic pressure, drawing fluid back into the vasculature (**Figure 5-3**).

Blood Pressure

Blood pressure is the pressure the blood exerts against the walls of the arteries. Blood pressure is usually carefully controlled by the body so sufficient and consistent circulation in the various tissues and organs occurs; it is also considered a rough measure of perfusion. For perfusion to be effective, the heart must continue to force blood into the system, and the arterial vessels must maintain their vascular tone. This resistance to blood flow through the circulatory system is called systemic vascular resistance, and it is determined by the degree of vasoconstriction of distal arteries and arterioles. Vasoconstriction exerts compressive force on the blood, which maintains and increases pressure within the vascular space. When systemic vascular resistance increases, arterial blood pressure rises, promoting blood flow through capillary beds and effectively perfusing the tissues.

As vessels shrink in diameter, friction—and thus resistance—increases. Friction is created as blood, a viscous fluid, courses along the vessel walls and through the vessels. RBCs are responsible for much of the blood's viscosity, but protein molecules contribute as well. When the composition of blood changes, it becomes more or less viscous. For example, the percentage of the fluid component of blood, the plasma, may increase or decrease. If the plasma level drops, evidenced by an increased hematocrit (concentration of RBCs), the blood becomes more viscous because there is a greater ratio of RBCs to plasma. Conversely, if RBC levels drop, evidenced by a decreased hematocrit, the blood becomes less viscous because there is a greater ratio of plasma to RBCs. This gains significance when intravenous (IV) fluids (crystalloids such as saline) are administered in large amounts, decreasing blood viscosity and diluting clotting factors.

As the volume of blood ejected from the heart increases, so does the arterial blood pressure; therefore, arterial blood pressure is an indirect indicator of tissue perfusion. The amount of pressure exerted against the arterial wall, typically expressed as millimeters of mercury (mm Hg), determines the measured pressure. Blood pressure is expressed as the systolic pressure over the diastolic pressure. The systolic blood pressure represents the volume and pressure of blood ejected from the ventricle and the response of the arterial system to that ejection. The diastolic pressure represents the residual pressure in the arterial system after the ventricles relax.

Mean arterial pressure (MAP) is generally considered to be the patient's most important measure of blood pressure and takes into consideration both the systolic blood pressure and the diastolic blood pressure. MAP is ultimately the blood pressure required to sustain organ perfusion and is normally roughly 70 mm Hg. If the MAP falls significantly below 70 mm Hg for an extended amount of time, the result may be ischemia of the organs from lack of perfusion. Thus, the MAP generally needs to be greater than 60 mm Hg to ensure that the brain, heart, coronary arteries, and kidneys remain perfused. Patients may have higher or lower MAPs in response to various medical conditions. Patients with chronic hypertension may require a higher-than-average pressure to maintain adequate perfusion. Two formulae are used to calculate the MAP:

$$\textbf{MAP} = \textbf{Diastolic pressure} + \left(\frac{\textbf{Pulse pressure}}{\textbf{3}}\right)$$

$$\textbf{MAP} = \frac{[\textbf{Systolic pressure} + (\textbf{2} \times \textbf{Diastolic pressure})]}{\textbf{3}}$$

Pulse pressure is calculated by subtracting the diastolic pressure from the systolic pressure. The pulse pressure is normally about 40 mm Hg. Changes in cardiac output and/or vascular resistance are responsible for changes in pulse pressure. The body's response to hypovolemic shock is an example of the effect of each on pulse pressure. A decrease in cardiac output and an increase in peripheral vascular resistance produce a narrowing pulse pressure. As blood volume is lost, a decrease in blood returning to the heart causes a decrease in cardiac output. The body responds by activating the sympathetic nervous system, which stimulates secretion of epinephrine from the adrenal glands as well as norepinephrine from the nerve endings of the sympathetic nervous system, notably on the vascular contraction mechanism. This causes an increase in heart rate, an increase in heart contractility, and vasoconstriction. The result is an increase in diastolic blood pressure in the presence of a lower systolic blood pressure, causing a narrowing pulse pressure. The changes may be subtle and easily missed. For example, the blood pressure may change from 118/68 mm Hg to 108/82 mm Hg. This represents a decrease in pulse pressure of nearly 50% (50 to 26). When looking at the blood pressure alone, the decline in pulse pressure may not be noticed, but when the pulse pressure is calculated, a significant decrease is noted. A decline in pulse pressure greater than 50% indicates a 50% decrease in stroke volume. Pulse pressure is a helpful indicator of shock, especially when the measurement is taken repeatedly and an emerging pattern can be identified. Decreased pulse pressure produces a weaker pulse during the examination. Like any other sign or symptom, it should be a part of the whole assessment and be used to direct you to collect other findings to confirm the patient's status.

The Autonomic Nervous System

The body is perfused via the cardiovascular system. Control of the cardiovascular system is a function of the autonomic nervous system, which is composed of two competing subsystems. One of the subsystems, the sympathetic nervous system, helps maintain normal body functions and allows the body to respond to threats demanding an instant reaction—the so-called fight-or-flight response. During such events, the sympathetic nervous system plays a direct role in tissue perfusion by temporarily redirecting blood away from noncritical functions, such as digestion, and toward the heart and brain. The other subsystem of the autonomic nervous system is the parasympathetic nervous system, which is responsible for rest and regeneration. Table 5-1 summarizes the functions of the sympathetic and parasympathetic nervous systems.

Table 5-1 Functions of the Sympathetic and Parasympathetic Nervous Systems at Various Anatomic Structures

	Sympathetic System	Parasympathetic System
Cardiac muscle	Increased rate and strength	Decreased rate and strength
Blood vessels	Constriction (alpha receptors) Dilation (beta receptors)	Dilation
Bronchioles	Relaxation (beta receptors)	Constriction
Digestive tract	Decreased peristalsis	Increased peristalsis
Urinary bladder	Relaxation	Contraction
Skin	Sweat	No effect
Adrenal medulla	Increased adrenaline (hormone analog to the medication EPINEPHrine) secretion	No effect

Pathophysiology of Shock

Shock originates at the cellular level. The cellular changes that occur during shock have an impact on every system of the body, including the neurologic, gastrointestinal (GI), and endocrine systems. The symptoms of shock are consistent with the degree of metabolic impairment resulting from inadequate perfusion, but they are often similar regardless of etiology. In other words, the compensatory mechanisms of the body tend to respond in the same way to enhance organ and tissue perfusion no matter which type of shock is present. Shock can result from inadequate cardiac output, decreased peripheral vascular resistance, the inability of red blood cells to deliver oxygen to tissues, or any combination thereof. An important additional consequence of inadequate perfusion is a buildup of waste products such as CO_2 in the tissues. Accumulation of these dangerous waste products leads to cellular death and eventual death of the affected individual.

The mitochondria are some of the first cellular components to be affected by shock. Most of the oxygen in the body is consumed by mitochondria, which produce 95% of the aerobic energy used by every body system. When oxygen has been depleted in the mitochondria, the cells undergo anaerobic metabolism, resulting in an increased production of lactate, thereby creating an acidic environment. An elevated lactate level in the blood, therefore, is an indicator of shock.

Metabolic Acidosis

During normal cell metabolism of glucose, oxygen is consumed. This process is called *aerobic metabolism*. When insufficient oxygen is present, glucose is metabolized through an alternative pathway that does not require oxygen. This process is termed *anaerobic metabolism*. The anaerobic pathway is much less efficient, yielding less energy (in the form of adenosine triphosphate [ATP]) per molecule of glucose and generating many more waste products, primarily lactic acid.

When the body tissues are in shock due to insufficient oxygen perfusion, cells generate energy through anaerobic metabolism, resulting in the production of lactic acid and metabolic acidosis. If shock persists, the alternative pathway will eventually not be able to generate enough ATP due to the inefficiency of anaerobic metabolism. Deficiency of ATP impairs the function of the cellular membrane sodium-potassium pump, resulting in a buildup of sodium in the cell and a buildup of potassium in the serum. These changes in electrolyte levels can cause fluid shifts, resulting in edema forming within the cells and mitochondria, eventually damaging these components. Ischemic cells also create free radicals and inflammatory factors, increasing damage to the cells. These toxins are flushed back into the circulatory system when perfusion is restored, contributing to damage to other organs as well. If the damage is severe, no amount of reoxygenation and perfusion can repair the damage, and cellular death occurs.

As each stage advances, a greater response is activated. As the body's circulatory volume becomes compromised, the body responds by activating additional compensatory mechanisms.

Compensatory Mechanisms

When an event such as blood loss, septic shock, anaphylaxis, or tension pneumothorax results in decreased perfusion, the body must respond immediately to preserve the function of vital organs. Several compensatory mechanisms can be activated to help maintain adequate perfusion, including increasing cardiac output (increasing pulse rate and/or contractility), increasing vasoconstriction to shunt blood to the most vital organs, and increasing minute ventilation. Increased minute ventilation raises arterial oxygen content and facilitates CO_2 removal.

Compensatory mechanisms are effective only up to a point. Once a critical threshold has been reached, they are no longer able to compensate, and tissue hypoxia develops. At this point, the "shock state" begins to overtake the body. Ultimately, the oxygen levels available are insufficient to meet the oxygen demands throughout the body. This lack of oxygen and buildup of waste products and acidosis will result in multiple organ dysfunction and death.

Adrenal Response

The adrenal glands, located on top of the kidneys, release catecholamines (epinephrine and norepinephrine) in response to shock. These hormones stimulate alpha and beta receptors in the heart and blood vessels. Alpha-1 stimulation induces vasoconstriction, and beta-1 stimulation increases heart rate and cardiac contractility (Table 5-2). Receptor distribution usually leads to greater constriction in noncritical tissues such as fat, skin, and tissues of the digestive tract. Vasoconstriction also occurs within the kidneys.

Table 5-2 Catecholamine Receptor Actions

	Location	Action
Alpha 1	Arterioles in skin, viscera, mucous membranes Veins Bladder Sphincters	Constriction, increased systemic vascular resistance
Alpha 2	Digestive system	Decreased secretions and peristalsis
Beta 1	Heart Kidneys	Increased heart rate, force of contraction, and oxygen consumption Release of renin
Beta 2	Arterioles of the heart, lungs, and skeletal muscles Bronchioles	Dilation with increased organ perfusion Dilation

Pituitary Response

The posterior pituitary gland releases antidiuretic hormone (ADH) in response to shock. ADH, which is synthesized in the hypothalamus, is released during early shock when symptoms are less obvious. As it circulates to the distal renal tubules and the collecting ducts in the kidneys, ADH causes fluid to be reabsorbed. As a result, intravascular volume is maintained and urine output decreases. ADH is also called vasopressin (from the Latin *vaso-*, meaning "vessel," and *pressor*, meaning "to press"). ADH stimulates smooth muscle contraction in the digestive tract and blood vessels.

Renin-Angiotensin-Aldosterone System Activation

The kidneys are vital to maintaining blood pressure. When blood flow to the kidneys is reduced, the renin-angiotensin-aldosterone system (RAAS) is activated. Renin is an enzyme released from the juxtaglomerular cells in the kidneys. It converts angiotensinogen to angiotensin I (a vasodilator), which is, in turn, converted to angiotensin II (a vasoconstrictor) in the lungs by angiotensin-converting enzymes (ACEs). Angiotensin I and II also stimulate the production and secretion of aldosterone from the adrenal cortex, which causes the kidneys to reabsorb sodium, and thus water, from the renal tubules, thereby increasing vascular volume and increasing blood pressure. The release of aldosterone signals the kidneys to halt the release of renin and restore perfusion to the kidneys. Aldosterone secretion also creates the sensation of thirst, one of the early signs of shock.

Angiotensin II is a potent but short-lived vasoconstrictor that induces constriction of the arterioles farthest from the heart. This shunts blood from the less essential organs and leads to a greater return of blood to the heart, which increases preload and improves cardiac output. This selective perfusion also helps to maintain perfusion to vital organs.

The Progression of Shock

Shock occurs in three successive phases: compensated, decompensated, and irreversible (Table 5-3). The goal is to recognize the clinical signs and symptoms of shock in its earliest phase and begin immediate treatment before permanent damage occurs. To do so, all health care clinicians must be aware of the subtle signs exhibited while the body is compensating and treat the patient aggressively (Table 5-4). Begin by anticipating the potential for shock based on the scene size-up and evaluation of the mechanism of injury or nature of illness. As your assessment progresses, you must recognize the signs of poor perfusion that precede hypotension; you should not rely on any one sign or symptom to determine what phase of shock the patient is in. Always err on the side of caution when you are treating a potential shock patient by initiating rapid assessment, immediate intervention, and prompt transportation to preserve any chance of survival.

Altered mental status changes such as confusion and lethargy are late indicators because a key purpose of shock syndrome is to keep the brain well perfused. Sometimes "alert" patients may be agitated or anxious during the compensated phase, but this is not considered an altered mental status.

Compensated Shock

The earliest stage of shock, in which the body can still compensate for decreased perfusion, is called compensated shock. In compensated shock, the body responds to an insult causing anaerobic metabolism and a buildup of lactic acid by releasing chemical mediators. As discussed earlier, the chemical mediators, which are released by the autonomic nervous system, act to compensate for the decrease in perfusion. They stimulate the vascular system to contract, causing the arterial pressure to remain normal or slightly elevated. To address the need for oxygen and the developing acidosis, the brain increases the rate and depth of respirations

Table 5-3 Stages of Shock

Stage	Vital Signs	Signs and Symptoms	Pathophysiology
Compensated	Normal blood pressure Normal to slightly increased heart rate Tachypnea Delayed capillary refill Compensatory reserve index decreases	Cool hands and feet Pale mucous membranes Restlessness, anxiety Oliguria	Vasoconstriction maintains blood flow to essential organs, but tissue ischemia occurs in less essential areas.
Decompensated	Blood pressure decreasing Worsening tachycardia Worsening tachypnea Pulse pressure decreases	Mottled or pale, cool, clammy skin Pale or cyanotic mucous membranes Profound weakness Metabolic (lactic) acidosis Anxiety Absent or decreased peripheral pulses	Blood pressure decreases as vascular tone decreases. Dysfunction in all organs is imminent. Anaerobic metabolism ensues, causing lactic acidosis.
Irreversible	Profound hypotension	Lactate level may be > 8 mEq/L.	Metabolic acidosis causes postcapillary sphincters to open and release stagnant and coagulated blood. Excessive potassium and acidosis cause dysrhythmias. Cellular damage is irreversible. Free radicals released.

Table 5-4 Signs of Compensated vs. Decompensated Shock

Compensated Shock	Decompensated Shock
Agitation, anxiety, restlessness Sense of impending doom Weak, rapid (thready) pulse Clammy (cool, moist) skin Pallor with cyanotic lips Shortness of breath Nausea, vomiting Delayed capillary refill in infants and children Thirst Blood pressure is maintained	Altered mental status (response to verbal stimuli only or unresponsive)[a] Hypotension Labored or irregular breathing Thready or absent peripheral pulses Ashen, mottled, or cyanotic skin Dilated pupils Diminished urine output

[a]Mental status changes are late indicators.

to assist the body in bringing in more oxygen and removing more carbon dioxide. At this stage of shock, the body attempts to maintain the acid–base balance by creating respiratory alkalosis (through tachypnea, which blows off "respiratory acid" [CO_2]) to offset the metabolic acidosis. You may see this as a decrease in end-tidal CO_2 ($ETCO_2$) or partial pressure of CO_2 (pCO_2) readings and an elevated lactate level if these measurements are assessed. Some currently think that lactic acid production is a signal that the body's compensatory mechanisms are working, as you are still able to produce lactic acid.

During the compensated phase of shock, blood pressure is maintained. Blood loss in hemorrhagic shock can be estimated to be at 15% to 30% at this point. A narrowing of the pulse pressure (the difference between the diastolic and systolic pressures) also occurs, producing the narrow, threadlike (or "thready") pulse. The pulse pressure reflects the tone of the arterial system and is more indicative of changes in perfusion than the systolic or diastolic blood pressure alone. Patients in the compensated phase will also have a positive orthostatic test result. It is key to remember patients in compensated shock are *still in shock* and should be treated immediately. In fact, the more aggressively these patients are treated, the better the outcomes are. Preventing the transition to decompensated shock is paramount.

Decompensated Shock

The next stage of shock, when blood pressure is no longer maintained, is called decompensated shock. In hemorrhagic shock, decompensated shock occurs when blood volume drops by more than 30%. The compensatory mechanisms are no longer able to support the progressing catastrophic event, and signs and symptoms become more obvious. The cardiac output falls dramatically, leading to further reductions in blood pressure and cardiac function. The signs and symptoms become more obvious as blood is shunted to the brain and heart. The kidneys respond by autoregulating their blood flow. When the cardiac output drops, the arterioles (the afferent vessels) perfusing the capillaries of the kidneys dilate, and the arterioles leaving (efferent) the glomerular capillaries constrict. This helps maintain perfusion of the kidneys. Once the blood pressure drops, this process cannot be maintained, and perfusion of the kidneys is severely compromised. At this point, vasoconstriction can have a disastrous effect if allowed to continue. Cells in the nonperfused tissues become ischemic, leading to anaerobic metabolism and cell death. Timely and aggressive intervention at this stage may result in recovery.

Blood pressure may be the last measurable sign of change in shock. The body has several automatic mechanisms to compensate for the initial loss of perfusion and to help maintain blood pressure. Thus, by the time hypotension develops, shock is well established. This is particularly true in infants, children, and pregnant women, whose blood pressure may be maintained until they have lost more than 35% to 40% of their blood volume. For all hypotensive patients in whom you suspect shock, consider their situation an emergency; initiate lifesaving interventions, including IV fluids and/or vasopressors as indicated; and start transport, providing fluid resuscitation en route to the most appropriate hospital.

Irreversible (Terminal) Shock

The last phase of shock is irreversible shock, which is when the condition has progressed to a terminal stage. Arterial blood pressure is abnormally low (typically, in hemorrhagic shock there is a 40% or greater blood volume loss). A progressive deterioration of the cardiovascular system that cannot be reversed by compensatory mechanisms or medical interventions results in multisystem organ failure. Life-threatening reductions in cardiac output, blood pressure, and tissue perfusion are observed. Blood is shunted away from the liver, kidneys, and lungs to keep the heart and brain perfused. Cells begin to die. Even if the cause of shock is treated and reversed, vital organ damage often cannot be repaired, and the patient may eventually die. Providing aggressive treatment at this stage does not usually result in recovery; however, because the clinical differences between decompensated and irreversible shock may not be easily discerned, you should always provide aggressive treatment en route to the appropriate facility.

AMLS Assessment Pathway ▸▸▸▸

▾ Initial Observations

The AMLS Assessment Pathway for shock helps you quickly and efficiently recognize, evaluate, and manage a patient in shock. Early recognition of shock, immediate intervention, and prompt transport correlate directly with better patient outcomes. Your initial observations should focus on recognizing the presence of or potential for hypoperfusion. Because shock may be pronounced or insidious, you may recognize shock at multiple points during the assessment pathway. The key is maintaining a high level of suspicion for shock because it is a life threat that may progress rapidly.

Scene Safety Considerations

Scene safety is paramount when approaching any patient. When dealing with a patient who appears critical, it is easy to miss a safety issue, so take the time to ensure that the scene remains safe for you and all involved.

Patient Cardinal Presentation/ Chief Complaint

Cardinal presentations and chief complaints may vary in patients in shock. A patient with GI bleeding, for example, may complain of abdominal pain; a patient with a thoracic aortic dissection may complain of back pain; and a patient with a tension pneumothorax may complain of respiratory distress. All of these patients may be in shock, but each patient's cardinal presentation is different. Each patient's treatment evolves as new diagnostic information is discovered. For the patient whose condition is critical, your immediate focus should be on airway, breathing, and circulation until definitive care is reached.

For the patient suspected of shock, you must determine the following:

- Do I see any signs of a life threat as I approach my patient? Altered level of consciousness or respiratory distress?
- Does the patient's skin show signs of shock? Pale, ashen, diaphoretic, mottled, or hives?
- Do the surroundings suggest the possibility of shock? Vomitus? Blood?

Primary Survey

Particular attention to the primary survey will help you identify and treat life threats. Support oxygenation, ventilation, and circulation; keep the patient warm; and monitor the electrocardiogram (ECG), pulse oximetry, and capnography.

Level of Consciousness

Any patient who has an altered level of consciousness or seems anxious, combative, or confused should be evaluated for hypoxia and signs of shock. Assessing the patient using the AVPU (**A**lert, responsive to **V**erbal stimuli, responsive to **P**ain, **U**nresponsive) mnemonic can help you determine whether the patient has altered mentation. Consider oxygen administration, and carefully assess the patient for other signs of shock.

Airway and Breathing

If the patient is unable to maintain a patent airway, you should provide necessary airway management until definitive care is achieved, whether it is on scene or en route to the receiving facility.

Once you have secured the patient's airway, you should direct your attention to improving oxygenation. Remember, the patient's oxygen saturation may drop significantly before symptoms of hypoxia become apparent. An escalation in the rate and depth of respiration, often the earliest sign of shock, can be confused with anxiety. Increased work of breathing should lead you to rule out a life threat as well. The patient's breathing may provide you with clues to underlying conditions, such as acidosis. Prevention or prompt treatment of early acidosis can greatly improve patient outcomes. If the ventilatory rate is slow in the presence of shock, you should suspect shock has reached an advanced stage.

Circulation/Perfusion

Circulatory status can be rapidly assessed. Begin by looking for obvious bleeding as you approach the patient. Bloody vomitus or stool should raise suspicion of internal bleeding. Bright red blood in the stool indicates active bleeding from the lower GI tract. Dark red or black stool, called melena, is usually due to upper GI bleeding. Dark or black blood in the stool may indicate either old bleeding or the presence of digested blood. You may also smell the presence of GI bleeding before you see evidence. If the patient is unable to speak, ask bystanders what they have witnessed.

As you assess the patient's pulse, ask yourself the following questions:

- Are the radial, carotid, and femoral pulses strong, or are they weak and thready?
- Is the heart rate too fast or too slow?
- Is the pulse regular or irregular?

Because blood pressure is maintained in the early stages of shock, the quality of the pulse is a more useful tool when evaluating perfusion. Evaluating pulse quality will give you more information in less time. A weak, thready pulse is an indicator of hypoperfusion. A bounding, strong pulse suggests adequate perfusion but does *not* rule out compensated shock. As you assess the patient's pulse, note the color and temperature of the skin—cool, pale (or ashen) skin due to peripheral vasoconstriction is common in shock. Tachycardia indicates the sympathetic nervous system's compensatory response to shock. Patients with bradycardia may have a cardiac dysrhythmia contributing to shock. Bradycardia may also be present in neurogenic shock. Action should be taken to address the underlying cause of the abnormal heart rate.

If you must expose an area of the patient's body to assess properly for further illness or injury, take care to keep the patient warm. Shock causes diminished peripheral perfusion. Decreased energy production associated with the conversion to anaerobic metabolism makes it difficult for the patient to maintain normal body temperature. Consider placing blankets under and over the patient and administering warmed IV fluids to help maintain the patient's temperature. Hypothermia reduces the ability of the blood to clot, which can be catastrophic in patients with uncontrolled internal hemorrhage. Any IV fluid that is cooler than normal body temperature will further worsen hypothermia, putting additional demands on an already strained metabolism.

▼ First Impression

Your first impression is key to identifying a patient in shock. For example, the initial appearance of a prone patient who is pale and lethargic should warrant immediate movement to a supine position to rule out threats to the patient's life, including shock. Interventions focusing on life threats are a priority at this time.

▼ Detailed Assessment

History Taking

In a patient who appears critically ill, history taking can be done en route to the ED along with the secondary survey and any ongoing management. Time is of the essence in shock patients. On-scene care should focus on addressing airway, breathing, and circulation needs. Transport should then occur promptly, during which further history, exam, and management can be performed.

OPQRST and SAMPLER

Obtaining a thorough history, including an account of the present illness and relevant past medical history, is essential to determine the type of shock; interventions adding time to the scene must be justified by the benefits they will produce for the patient. The SAMPLER and OPQRST mnemonics can be used to obtain historical information. You may be selective initially. For example, in a patient with signs and symptoms of shock who is complaining of "trouble breathing," you may rapidly focus on allergies, recent medication, and foods ingested (allergies, medications, time last known well, and last meal from SAMPLER), and use OPQRST only if the patient complains of pain as you move to a physical exam and begin to initiate care. Historical data, in combination with physical exam findings, can help you modify your differential diagnosis and select appropriate interventions. Table 5-5 lists hypoperfusion considerations in the patient history, and Table 5-6 details medications affecting shock. Once all immediate life threats have been addressed, a complete history can be obtained.

Secondary Survey

Vital Signs

Vital signs (blood pressure, pulse rate, respiratory rate, and temperature) are essential to determining the patient's hemodynamic status and identifying the type of shock. Most types of shock are characterized by hypotension, tachycardia, tachypnea, and cool skin, but there are several exceptions. Because the blood vessels are dilated in distributive shock, the patient will have hypotension and tachycardia, but the skin may be warm and dry. In cardiogenic shock, the patient may be bradycardic or tachycardic, depending on the underlying cause. In neurogenic shock, the patient is often bradycardic and, because of vasodilation, the skin is often warm and dry. Vital signs will also help you determine the stages of shock and the patient's response to interventions, so monitoring trends in vital signs is important.

Physical Exam

Performing a physical exam on a patient with signs and symptoms of shock focuses on determining the cause and selecting the proper intervention. For example, as you approach a patient with an initial presentation of chest pain and signs of shock, you see distended neck veins. You know that jugular venous distension (JVD) may be observed with cardiac tamponade, tension pneumothorax, and cardiogenic shock due to right heart failure. Your next step may be to auscultate the lungs. You may note decreased breath sounds on one side. This points you to the possibility of a developing tension pneumothorax and obstructive shock.

Diagnostics

Diagnostic tools used to evaluate patients with signs of shock include pulse oximetry; electrocardiography, to

Table 5-5 Key Etiologies, History, Signs, and Symptoms for Hypoperfusion

Hypovolemic/Hemorrhagic Shock
■ Blood loss—internal or external (hemorrhagic) ■ Vomiting ■ Diarrhea ■ Excessive sweating ■ Excessive urination ■ Poor oral intake ■ Prolonged heat exposure
Obstructive Shock
Tension Pneumothorax ■ Breath sounds—decreased or absent on one side ■ Jugular venous distention (JVD) ■ Increasing respiratory distress ■ Cyanosis **Pulmonary Embolism** ■ Risk factors (e.g., immobilization, plane trip, genetic coagulopathy) ■ Sudden onset of chest pain and/or shortness of breath, pleuritic chest pain ■ Refractory hypoxemia (low oxygen saturation despite the administration of supplemental oxygen) ■ Cyanosis (in large pulmonary emboli) **Cardiac Tamponade** ■ Risk factors (e.g., recent cardiac surgery) ■ Muffled heart tones ■ JVD ■ Cyanosis ■ Narrowing pulse pressure
Distributive Shock
Neurogenic Shock ■ Spinal cord injury (traumatic and nontraumatic) ■ Flushed skin ■ Bradycardia (possible) **Anaphylactic Shock** ■ History of exposure to allergen ■ Angioedema ■ Wheezing and/or stridor ■ Hives **Septic Shock** ■ History of infection (e.g., pneumonia) ■ Receiving antibiotics ■ Fever ■ Wounds, Foley catheter, drains, IV, or venous access device ■ Depressed immune system
Cardiogenic Shock
■ History of heart failure ■ Acute myocardial infarction (AMI) ■ 12-lead ECG changes ■ Crackles (rales) in lungs ■ JVD ■ Peripheral edema
Various/Mixed Types
■ Toxic exposure ■ Drug overdose

include cardiac rhythm monitoring; laboratory testing; the compensatory reserve index; and the shock index. In the hospital, laboratory studies, ultrasonography, and radiographic studies are important in differentiating the cause of shock. Table 5-7 outlines laboratory studies typically used to evaluate patients in shock.

Pulse Oximetry

A pulse oximeter is one of the simplest assessment tools to use. It requires placing a sensor on the patient's skin, typically a finger, but despite its apparent straightforwardness, pulse oximetry presents many possibilities for error. If the pulse oximetry monitor does not display a waveform, you should question the accuracy of the reading. As shock progresses, peripheral vasoconstriction increases, which may make it difficult to obtain a pulse oximetry reading. Due to the time it takes for blood to circulate, a delay in a change of the reading may occur, so a patient may be more hypoxemic or less hypoxemic than the actual reading. Patient care should never be delayed or withheld based on a pulse oximetry reading when other signs and symptoms of poor tissue perfusion are present.

Capnography

When the cardiac output drops, less oxygen is delivered to the cells. Cellular CO_2 production requires oxygen, so if there is less oxygen at the cellular level, less CO_2 is made and returned to the lungs; as a result, capnography ($ETCO_2$) readings decrease. A drop in $ETCO_2$ reading also occurs when a ventilation-perfusion ($\dot{V}/\dot{Q}$) mismatch is present, such as with a large pulmonary embolism causing shock. Capnography has also been suggested as a tool in the identification of sepsis and is a predictor of mortality associated with shock. However, capnography is also quite nonspecific for assessing patients with shock. Patient baseline $ETCO_2$ can vary based on the presence of lung disease such as chronic obstructive pulmonary disease (COPD), and though, on average, the $ETCO_2$ may be lower with various types of shock, $ETCO_2$ readings among patients have significant overlap. In the ED, capnography is not generally used in assessing all patients who may have shock or respiratory disorders. Further research on capnography and its relationship to shock and metabolic acidosis may focus the use of capnography by identifying situations in which capnography can best change assessment, treatment, or patient outcomes.

Electrocardiogram

An ECG is helpful in assessing cardiac rhythm, as well as identifying ischemia, injury, and certain electrolyte abnormalities. Leads must be properly placed, and the findings interpreted or transmitted. The results are then used to guide transport of the patient to an appropriate health care facility. Because shock may be the result of acute

Table 5-6 Medication Considerations Related to Shock

Medication	Effect	Shock
Steroids	May mask signs of infection; decrease potential for early recognition.	Sepsis
Beta blockers	Blunt compensatory tachycardia, decreasing ability to compensate.	All types
Anticoagulants/antiplatelets	Increase potential for bleeding.	Hemorrhagic
Calcium channel blockers	Inhibit vasoconstriction and/or tachycardia, decreasing ability to compensate.	All types
Hypoglycemic agents	May impair blood glucose regulation.	All types
Herbal preparations	May exacerbate bleeding. May increase workload on the heart.	Hemorrhagic Cardiogenic specifically, but all types may be affected
Diuretics	Long-term diuretic therapy may cause hypokalemia and contribute to dehydration.	All types

Table 5-7 Laboratory Tests for Patients in Shock

Test	Normal Values	Abnormal Values	Indications for Test
Glucose	70–110 mg/dL (3.8–6.1 mmol/L)	Increase indicates hyperglycemia, HHNS, DKA, steroid use, or stress. Decrease indicates hypoglycemia.	If altered mental status is present
Hemoglobin (Hb)/hematocrit (Hct)	Hb, male: 14–18 g/dL (8.7–11.2 mmol/L) Hb, female: 12–16 g/dL (7.4–9.9 mmol/L) Hct, male: 42–52% (0.42–0.52) Hct, female: 37–47% (0.37–0.47)	Decrease indicates blood loss or loss of production. Increase indicates plasma loss, dehydration, underlying polycythemia vera.	All types of shock
Gastric/fecal occult blood	Negative	Positive result indicates presence of blood.	Suspected GI bleeding
Lactic acid	Venous: 5–20 mg/dL (0.6–2.2 mmol/L)	Increases due to tissue hypoperfusion, liver dysfunction, seizure, and certain medications (metformin) and toxins (cyanide).	All types of shock
Complete blood cell count	Total WBC 5,000–10,000/mm^3 (5–10 $\times$ 10^9/L)	Increased WBC suggests infection, inflammation, steroid use, or stress response. Decreased WBC indicates infection, immunocompromise, chemotherapy.	Septic shock

Test	Normal Values	Abnormal Values	Indications for Test
Acid–base balance	pH 7.35–7.45	Increased pH indicates alkalosis. Decreased pH indicates acidosis.	All types of shock
Bicarbonate (HCO_3)	21–28 mEq/L	Decreased bicarbonate levels indicate it is being lost in conditions such as diarrhea, or due to increased acid production such as shock, renal failure, DKA, or salicylate overdose. Increased bicarbonate levels indicate excessive intake of bicarbonate or antacids or loss of acid from conditions such as vomiting, gastric suctioning, potassium deficiency, or diuretic use.	All types of shock
Arterial blood gases	$PaCO_2$ 35–45 mm Hg PaO_2 80–100 mm Hg	Increased $PaCO_2$ levels indicate CO_2 retention, hypoventilation. Decreased $PaCO_2$ levels indicate decrease in CO_2 levels, hyperventilation; also occurs in response to metabolic acidosis (e.g., DKA). Decrease in PaO_2 levels indicates hypoxia.	All types of shock
Serum electrolytes	Na^+ 136–145 mEq/L (136–145 mmol/L) K^+ 3.5–5 mEq/L (3.5–5 mmol/L)	Increased Na^+ levels may be present with dehydration. Increased K^+ levels (hyperkalemia) are common in acute kidney injury, missed dialysis, and acidosis, such as DKA. Hyperkalemia may cause an abnormal ECG; peaked T waves, wide QRS complexes, bradycardia, or tachycardia may be present. Hypokalemia can occur with vomiting and excess diuresis.	All types of shock
Renal function	Serum urea nitrogen 10–20 mg/dL (3.6–7.1 mmol/L) Creatinine 0.5–1.2 mg/dL (44–97 mmol/L)	Increased levels of serum urea nitrogen indicate severe dehydration, shock, or sepsis. Increased serum creatinine levels ($>$ 4 mg/dL [0.2 mmol/L]) indicate impaired renal function.	All types of shock
Blood/urine cultures	Negative	Positive result indicates infection.	Septic shock
Compensatory reserve index	0.7–1.0	0.3–0.6 or trending downward indicates hypovolemia or blood loss. 0.1–0.3 nearing decompensated shock. 0 is decompensated shock.	Volume loss due to blood or fluids. Septic shock characteristics are unknown at this time.

DKA, diabetic ketoacidosis; HHNS, hyperglycemic hyperosmolar nonketotic syndrome; WBC, white blood cell.

Pagana KD, Pagana TJ. Mosby's *Diagnostic and Laboratory Test Reference*. 9th ed. Mosby; 2009.

myocardial infarction (AMI), a multilead, diagnostic ECG should be obtained in the secondary survey when the presentation suggests acute coronary syndrome—early enough to help determine the patient's destination for definitive care (e.g., cardiac catheterization lab for percutaneous coronary intervention). In a patient presenting with chest pain or discomfort and signs of shock, the 12-lead ECG should be one of the first interventions performed.

Laboratory Studies

Establish appropriate vascular access and draw blood for laboratory analysis according to local protocols if you can do so without delaying appropriate care. Point-of-care testing (POCT) is becoming more common in the prehospital setting; however, transporting a patient in shock to an appropriate facility is your priority. Because of an increase in metabolic demands during shock, hypoglycemia may result. If the patient's mental status is altered, a glucose test should be obtained. Elevated lactate levels may be indicative of shock. Suspect septic shock in patients with fever and elevated lactate levels.

In the hospital, interfacility, or critical care transport settings, urine output should be monitored and maintained at a minimum of 0.5 to 1 mL/kg/h in adults (1 to 2 mL/kg/h in children) who do not have kidney disease. Urine output is an important metric because it indicates renal perfusion status.

Compensatory Reserve Index

In 2017, the U.S. Food and Drug Administration (FDA) approved a new modality for determining how much compensatory capacity a patient has remaining in the setting of hypovolemic or hemorrhagic shock. A compensatory reserve index device is a noninvasive technology that uses pulse oximetry plethysmography to determine arterial waveform characteristics. The data undergo computer analysis and are displayed as a fuel gauge, showing capacity from 1 (normal volume status) to 0 (decompensated shock). This allows for advanced warning of changes in the body's compensatory capacity because compensatory reserve readings change before typical vital sign changes are detected. Additionally, this provides real-time monitoring and may provide feedback regarding interventions that have been administered (e.g., fluids, blood, or vasopressors).

Shock Index

The **shock index (SI)** is a mathematical quotient designed to improve detection of circulatory collapse in the setting of hypovolemia—either from water loss or blood loss. The SI is calculated from a simple equation relating heart rate and systolic blood pressure, as follows:

$$\textbf{SI} = \textbf{Heart rate} \div \textbf{Systolic blood pressure (mm Hg)}$$

A normal SI is 0.5 to 0.7. Higher values are more sensitive in the detection of occult shock than either vital sign in isolation. Any time the heart rate is greater than or equal to the systolic blood pressure, the SI will be 1 or greater.

SI is another tool in the resuscitation of medical and trauma patients. One study of 18,197 hospitalized patients found that a single SI ≥ 0.9 is a poor predictor of mortality, although persistent SI results ≥ 0.9 are associated with a higher risk of morbidity and mortality. The associations of in-hospital mortality were comparable for SI ≥ 0.9 or systolic blood pressure ≤ 100 mm Hg. Dynamic interactions between hemodynamic variables require further evaluation among critically ill patients.

Refine the Differential Diagnosis

You may have determined in your primary survey that the patient was in shock, but you may not have determined the underlying cause. The components of the secondary survey will facilitate your ability to determine the severity of the patient's condition and refine your differential diagnosis. It is important to move quickly through this assessment with *calculated purpose* to identify the cause of shock and initiate the necessary treatment. Some life-threatening conditions and signs of shock may not be obvious during the primary survey and may not be found until the secondary survey or as the patient progresses through the stages of shock. Regardless of when a life threat appears, it is essential to return to the ABCs of the primary survey, mitigate the life threat, and then progress through your secondary survey during transport to refine your differential diagnosis of the patient's condition and, if necessary, your treatment plan.

Ongoing Management

The rule of thumb of clinical care is to assess, intervene, and reassess. During your ongoing management, repeat the primary survey and vital signs, revisit the chief complaint, and monitor the patient's response to any treatment you have administered. Always consider the possibility of trauma. Proper positioning depends on initial complaints and symptoms. If a patient is unable to tolerate the supine position because of respiratory distress, intolerable pain, or other reason, then elevate the head and trunk to a tolerable position, recognizing that higher levels may decrease perfusion to the brain.

To ensure adequate perfusion, optimal oxygenation must be maintained. Some patients become hypoxic before the symptoms of shock are obvious. Patients with concern for shock should receive oxygen if they are hypoxic ($SpO_2 < 94\%$). If the patient is breathing adequately, deliver oxygen with a nasal cannula or nonrebreathing mask. Consider noninvasive positive-pressure ventilation (NIPPV) if indicated. If the patient is not breathing adequately, ventilate with a bag-valve mask and consider the need for advanced airway management such as intubation. Those with signs of hypoperfusion should receive high-flow oxygen unless there is a discrete tissue infarct occurring (e.g., ST-elevation MI [STEMI] or stroke), in which case oxygen should be titrated to an SpO_2 of 95% to 99%. Begin maintaining the patient's circulatory status by stopping any obvious bleeding. Although hemorrhagic shock is one of the most common types of shock, it is not the only cause of hypoperfusion. Many perfusion problems have complex causes that are difficult to reverse, so your treatment may be limited to resuscitation and symptomatic care until the underlying etiology can be addressed at the receiving facility. Patients in shock require immediate vascular access; however, if prehospital blood is not available and the patient has an uncontrollable ongoing medical hemorrhage, consider waiting to establish vascular access until en route to the hospital to reduce on-scene time.

Fluid Resuscitation

If the patient is in hypovolemic shock caused by loss of fluid other than blood (e.g., from severe vomiting or diarrhea), or from distributive shock, administer isotonic crystalloid fluids. An initial bolus of 20 mL/kg should be given if the patient shows no signs of fluid overload (e.g., crackles on lung auscultation). If the patient is at risk for fluid overload, a more modest bolus of 250 to 500 mL, followed by a reassessment, is appropriate. The purpose of fluid resuscitation should be to enhance perfusion to maintain MAP at > 65 mm Hg or a systolic pressure at > 90 mm Hg.

Note that crystalloid solutions do not carry oxygen, nor do they contain platelets, clotting factors, or many of the other essential blood components; as such, blood products (discussed in the next section) should be administered when possible, in cases of bleeding. Also, remember that isotonic crystalloid fluid works as a temporary volume expander, but if too much is administered the existing blood volume will become more dilute (hemodilution), and third-spacing such as pulmonary edema will occur. Frequent evaluation for signs of volume overload during administration is therefore essential. Colloids, dextran, and albumin are other volume expanders.

Administration of Blood Products

If bleeding is suspected, administration of blood products is indicated. Whole blood and blood products replace blood volume while offering the additional advantage of oxygen-carrying capacity (whole blood and packed RBCs) and hemostatic factors (platelets and fresh frozen plasma [FFP]), but the presence of antibodies in human blood presents some risk. It is preferred blood be typed and crossmatched, but if time does not allow, uncrossmatched type O-negative blood (or low-antibody O-positive whole blood) can be given. When massive transfusion is required, whole blood is preferred, but if packed RBCs are used, then concomitant administration of FFP and platelets has been shown to improve survival.

Low-titer Group O cold-stored whole blood is becoming the preferred initial therapy in hemorrhagic shock and has been implemented in some EMS systems in the United States. Table 5-8 describes available blood products and their clinical applications.

Table 5-8 Blood Products

Product	Clinical Application
Whole blood, low-titer O cold stored	Acute severe blood loss Note: Short shelf life
Packed red blood cells	Low hemoglobin level (usually < 7.0)
Platelets	Thrombocytopenia
Fresh frozen plasma (FFP)	Coagulation deficiencies in liver failure, warfarin overdose, disseminated intravascular coagulation, or massive transfusion
Freeze-dried plasma (not yet available in the United States; multiple products undergoing FDA submission)	Uses same as FFP Note: Stable shelf life at room temperature, requires reconstitution but easier administration process
Cryoprecipitate (cold FFP with fibrinogen, factor VIII, and von Willebrand factor)	Bleeding disorders, massive transfusion
Massive transfusion	Aggressively bleeding patients where > 10 units of blood are given over 24 hours Note: Coagulation factors and platelets added; patient at risk for hypothermia, hypocalcemia

Transfusion Reactions

Two complications can arise from blood product administration: infection and immune reactions. Improved methods of screening donors and blood products have decreased problems with the spread of infections. However, a small risk remains, especially for cytomegalovirus, a common virus that is rarely serious in the general population. Some pathogens can infect blood even during cold storage.

Hemolytic Reactions

When the recipient's antibodies recognize and react to transfused blood as an antigen, the donor RBCs are destroyed or hemolyzed. This hemolytic reaction can be quick and aggressive or slower, depending on the immune response.

Errors in the blood administration process can create fatal hemolytic reactions. When this occurs, most transfused cells are destroyed in an overwhelming immune response. When an immune response occurs, the coagulation cascade is also engaged, potentially creating bleeding disorders such as disseminated intravascular coagulation (DIC). With DIC and anaphylaxis, symptoms may include back pain, IV site pain, headache, chills and fever, hypotension, dyspnea, tachycardia, bronchospasm, pulmonary edema, bleeding, and renal failure.

At the first sign of a transfusion reaction, the blood products must be stopped and appropriate lab analysis completed. Immediate supportive treatment is initiated and the blood bank is notified. Every institution credentialing personnel to administer blood products has strict policies and procedures guiding the clinician in these cases.

Febrile Transfusion Reactions

During the transfusion or shortly thereafter, fever may develop (called a pyrogenic reaction); it is usually responsive to antipyretics. Monitoring the patient's temperature is a standard of care during blood administration. For patients who are prone to febrile reactions, diphenhydramine and acetaminophen administration may be considered as the transfusion is begun.

Allergic Transfusion Reaction

The onset of hives and/or rash is usually self-limiting during transfusion of blood products, but some cases will progress to bronchospasm and anaphylaxis. For limited, non–life-threatening reactions, administer antihistamines. For anaphylactic shock, administer EPINEPHrine.

Transfusion-Related Acute Lung Injury

Transfusion-related acute lung injury (TRALI) is a rare but complex immune response during or after transfusion, with subsequent development of noncardiogenic pulmonary edema or acute respiratory distress syndrome/acute lung injury (ARDS/ALI), which is described later in this chapter.

Transfusion-Associated Circulatory Overload

For those patients with limited cardiovascular reserve (elderly, infants), transfusion of blood products can increase circulating volume and create problems for the patient's cardiovascular system, a condition called transfusion-associated circulatory overload (TACO). Symptoms include dyspnea, hypoxia, and pulmonary edema.

Temperature Regulation

The body expends a great deal of energy to maintain a normal temperature. Vasoconstriction shunts blood away from peripheral tissues, and the body will expend valuable energy trying to stay warm. To help conserve metabolic reserves, keep the patient warm. The ambulance or resuscitation room should be kept warm, and the patient should be covered with a blanket when practical. This can be difficult during the physical exam, but it should be a high priority. Administration of warmed fluids will assist in maintaining body temperature and should be initiated when indicated and feasible.

Vasopressor Administration

Vasopressors, which are medications that cause arterial vasoconstriction and thereby increase blood pressure, are an efficient adjunct treatment in patients with distributive shock (septic, anaphylactic, and neurogenic) in addition to IV fluids. In cardiogenic shock, the heart is not functioning effectively, and inotropic agents can improve cardiac output by increasing cardiac contractility. It is essential to ensure that volume replacement has been initiated prior to vasopressor initiation. The following vasopressors and inotropes are commonly administered:

- Vasopressors
  - EPINEPHrine
  - Norepinephrine
  - DOPamine (at higher doses [> 10 mcg/kg/min])
  - Phenylephrine
- Inotropes
  - DOPamine
  - DOBUTamine (also causes vasodilation)
  - EPINEPHrine
  - Norepinephrine (preferred agent in most shock scenarios requiring vasopressors)

Pathophysiology, Assessment, and Management of Specific Types of Shock

Shock can be categorized into four types—hypovolemic, distributive, cardiogenic, and obstructive—depending on which portion of the cardiovascular system fails (Table 5-9).

Table 5-9 Types of Shock

Category	Initial Signs	Causes	Management
Hypovolemic Shock (Hemorrhagic/Nonhemorrhagic)			
	Cool, clammy skin Pale/ashen, cyanotic skin Decreased blood pressure (late sign) Altered level of consciousness Decreased capillary refill Tachypnea	Hemorrhage: trauma, GI bleeding, ruptured aortic aneurysm, pregnancy-related bleeding Severe dehydration: gastroenteritis, DKA	Stop the bleeding. Consider blood product transfusion if appropriate and available. Consider limited infusion of crystalloid IV fluids.
Distributive Shock			
Septic	Hyperthermia or hypothermia Decreased blood pressure (late sign) Tachycardia Altered level of consciousness	Infection	Give IV fluid bolus. Administer antibiotics. Consider vasopressors.
Anaphylactic	Pruritus, erythema, urticaria, angioedema Tachycardia Decreased blood pressure (late sign) Anxiety Respiratory distress, wheezing Vomiting, diarrhea	Antibody–antigen hypersensitivity response	Give EPINEPHrine (1 mg/mL), adult 0.3–0.5 mg intramuscular (IM), pediatric 0.01 mg/kg; may repeat. Give IV fluid bolus. Consider diphenhydrAMINE, 1–2 mg/kg IV (max, 50 mg). Consider corticosteroid treatment. Consider vasopressor infusion. Consider H2 receptor blocker administration.
Neurogenic	Warm, dry, flushed skin Decreased blood pressure (late sign) Alert Normal capillary refill time Normal or slow heart rate	Trauma	Give IV fluid bolus. Consider vasopressors.
Adrenal crisis	Shock symptoms	Due to adrenal failure of whatever cause	Patient must receive IV steroids.
Toxins	Based on specific agent		Provide based on specific agent.

(continues)

Table 5-9 Types of Shock (*continued*)

Category	Initial Signs	Causes	Management
Cardiogenic Shock			
	Cool, clammy skin Pale or cyanotic skin Tachypnea Tachycardia or other abnormal cardiac rhythm Decreased blood pressure (late sign) Altered level of consciousness Decreased capillary refill time	Pump failure: AMI, cardiomyopathy, myocarditis, papillary muscle dysfunction/ rupture, toxins, myocardial contusion, acute aortic insufficiency, ruptured ventricular septum Dysrhythmias	Administer oxygen as needed. Give IV fluid bolus. Correct heart rate/rhythm (medication or pacing/ cardioversion). Consider inotropes. Consider vasopressors. Consider intra-aortic balloon pump or LVAD.
Obstructive Shock			
	Decreased blood pressure (late sign) Difficulty breathing, tachycardia, tachypnea JVD, unilateral decreased or absent breath sounds, muffled heart tones Cyanosis may be present	Massive pulmonary embolus, tension pneumothorax, pericardial tamponade	Perform needle decompression for tension pneumothorax. Consider pericardiocentesis for pericardial tamponade. Transport to appropriate facility.

AMI, acute myocardial infarction; DKA, diabetic ketoacidosis; GI, gastrointestinal; JVD, jugular venous distension; LVAD, left ventricular assist device.

Failure can occur in any of the three major components of the cardiovascular system: the pump (the heart), the pipes (the blood vessels), or the fluid within them (the blood/ body fluids).

Hypovolemic Shock

It is easy to remember the cause of inadequate tissue perfusion in hypovolemic shock by taking a closer look at the term **hypovolemia** itself. The prefix *hypo-* means "below" or "low"; *vol* refers to volume; and the combining form *-emia* means "in or pertaining to the blood."

Inadequate circulating fluid leads to diminished cardiac output, which results in inadequate delivery of oxygen to the tissues and cells (**Figure 5-4**). The classic signs and symptoms of hypovolemic shock are tachycardia, hypotension, and increased respiratory rate, but signs will vary depending on how much fluid has been lost. Bleeding, vomiting, diarrhea, and many other conditions can lower the volume of circulating fluid. Hypovolemic shock has both hemorrhagic and nonhemorrhagic causes.

Hemorrhagic Shock

Hemorrhagic shock is a common cause of hypovolemic shock. Significant blood loss can occur without evidence of bleeding. Internal or external hemorrhage can accompany traumatic injuries or medical problems such as ruptured aortic aneurysm, ruptured spleen, ectopic pregnancy, GI bleeding, or other causes of significant blood loss. The bleeding may be obvious, as in a patient vomiting blood, or insidious, as in a patient with internal GI bleeding that has been occurring over time. In hemorrhagic shock, the oxygen-carrying capacity of the blood diminishes as red blood cells are depleted.

The severity of hemorrhagic shock depends on the percentage and rate of blood loss. Insidious blood loss gives the body time to compensate. In a healthy adult, a 10% to 15% blood loss is well tolerated. Children and older adults are more sensitive to even a small amount of blood loss, and compensatory mechanisms or medications may delay outward signs. Table 5-10 summarizes the classes of hemorrhagic shock.

Immediate treatment for hemorrhagic shock involves stopping all external bleeding. External bleeding can be more readily controlled in the prehospital setting than internal bleeding; however, in patients with suspected internal bleeding and signs of shock, administration of tranexamic acid (TXA) can be considered if the injury occurred within 3 hours. In the presence of external bleeding, direct pressure should be applied. If direct pressure to an extremity wound is not *immediately* effective, a tourniquet should be applied without delay. When possible, it is key to apply the tourniquet *before* signs and symptoms of shock are present to increase the rate of patient survival. If the wound is not amenable to a tourniquet, such as an injury high in the inguinal region or in the axilla, the wound should be packed with hemostatic-impregnated gauze and aggressive direct pressure methods used.

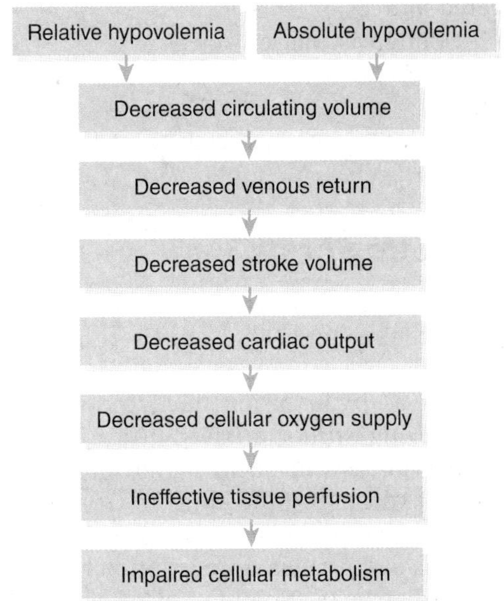

Figure 5-4 Pathophysiology of hypovolemic shock.

Reproduced from Urden LD. *Thelan's Critical Care Nursing: Diagnosis and Management*, 5th ed. Copyright Mosby 2006.

Nonhemorrhagic Hypovolemic Shock

Loss of fluids other than blood can also cause hypovolemic shock. For example, extreme fluid loss may follow vomiting and diarrhea in a patient with a severe GI infection (such as cholera) and massive diuresis in patients with diabetes mellitus or diabetes insipidus. Excessive plasma loss in patients with significant burn injuries and inadequate fluid replacement may result in shock. Shock in these patients is often delayed due to the time it takes for the fluids to shift.

Treatment

The treatment of hypovolemic shock depends on whether the cause is hemorrhagic or nonhemorrhagic. For

Table 5-10 Classes of Hemorrhagic Shock

	% Blood Loss	Stage of Shock	Mental Status	Blood Pressure	Pulse Rate	Respiratory Rate	Skin
Class I	< 15%	Compensated (early)	Slightly anxious	Normal	Normal	Normal	Normal
Class II	15% to 30%	Compensated (early)	Anxious and restless	Low normal	Mild tachycardia	Mild tachypnea	Pale, cool skin, > 2 sec capillary refill
Class III	30% to 45%	Decompensated (late)	Altered, lethargic	Hypotension	Marked tachycardia	Moderate tachypnea	Pale, mild cyanosis, cool, > 3 sec capillary refill
Class IV	> 45%	Irreversible	Extremely lethargic, unresponsive	Severe hypotension	Profound tachycardia to bradycardia	Severe tachypnea to agonal breathing	Pale, central and peripheral cyanosis, cold, > 5 sec capillary refill

nonhemorrhagic shock, administer isotonic crystalloid fluids via the IV or intraosseous (IO) route. Fluid should be administered in 500-mL increments in adults (20 mL/kg in children). It is important to reassess the patient after each bolus to determine how the patient is tolerating the fluids and whether the patient's condition is stabilizing. For hemorrhagic shock, blood products are preferred. As noted earlier, crystalloids do not carry oxygen, platelets, or other essential blood components. Furthermore, attempting to increase the blood pressure in a patient with a noncompressible hemorrhage (e.g., internal bleeding) can exacerbate their bleeding by diluting clotting factors and destroying clots that the body is attempting to make to achieve hemostasis. This reflects an increased emphasis on permissive hypotension in resuscitation.

Stabilization is indicated by a decrease in pulse rate and improvements in stroke index, peripheral pulse strength, mental status, and respiratory rate. For adults, fluid administration should be titrated to a systolic blood pressure > 90 mm Hg (> 80 mm Hg in noncompressible hemorrhage) in the absence of traumatic brain injury (TBI) and > 110 mm Hg in the context of evidence of significant TBI.

Distributive Shock

Distributive shock is also due to an inadequate volume of blood in the vascular space; however, the problem does not stem from blood or fluid *loss*, but rather from an *increase* in vascular capacity as blood vessels dilate and the capillaries leak fluid. This fluid leaks into extravascular and interstitial spaces, which is called the third space. Such vasodilation and capillary leakage can occur in sepsis, anaphylaxis, neurogenic shock, toxic shock syndrome, and toxin exposure. Too much vascular space translates into too little peripheral vascular resistance and a decrease in preload, which, in turn, reduces cardiac output and results in shock. Septic, anaphylactic, and neurogenic shock are discussed next. For shock related to toxins, please see Chapter 14, *Toxicology*.

Septic Shock

Septic shock is the result of a massive systemic inflammatory response to infection by bacteria, fungi, or viruses. Gram-negative bacteria appear to be the primary cause of sepsis, especially in hospitalized patients.

The following factors predispose a patient to sepsis:

- Inadequate immune response
  - Patients with diabetes mellitus, liver disease, or human immunodeficiency virus/acquired immunodeficiency syndrome (HIV/AIDS)
  - Neonates
  - Older adults
  - Pregnant women
  - Persons with alcoholism
- Primary infections
  - Pneumonia
  - Urinary tract infection
  - Cholecystitis
  - Peritonitis
  - Abscess
- Iatrogenic sources
  - Indwelling vascular catheter
  - Foley catheter
  - Surgery

Sepsis and septic shock are discussed in detail in Chapter 6, *Sepsis*.

Anaphylactic Shock

For patients with known hypersensitivities, anaphylaxis is a frightening possibility and is responsible for 400 to 800 deaths per year in the United States. Signs and symptoms such as hypotension, tachycardia, difficulty breathing, wheezing, stridor, anxiety, urticaria, vomiting, diarrhea, and pruritus can begin within minutes or up to 1 hour after exposure to the antigen. Gastrointestinal symptoms, such as vomiting, are often prominent. Atypical presentations of anaphylaxis (e.g., primary symptoms of vomiting or diarrhea) are often not recognized, especially in the prehospital setting. Symptoms may improve or even resolve after initial treatment but can return 1 to 12 hours later, at which time they may be either mild or more severe.

An antigen–antibody hypersensitivity response is the primary cause of anaphylactic shock. Not all hypersensitivity reactions evolve into shock. Most allergic reactions produce only mild symptoms such as pruritus and urticaria. Patients with allergic reactions may be managed with diphenhydramine and monitoring for additional symptoms. Not all people have repeated anaphylactic reactions to additional exposures, but of the 40% to 60% who do, the most common trigger is the sting of an insect belonging to the Hymenoptera order—wasps, bees, and ants. Almost any substance can provoke a reaction in a sensitive individual (Table 5-11), but some other common triggers of anaphylaxis are eggs, milk, shellfish, and peanuts.

Latex allergy is a trigger that has become increasingly common among patients and health care workers. Because of the risk associated with latex allergy, most medical equipment manufacturers have replaced latex with other substances in their products, and the use of latex examination gloves has become uncommon.

During anaphylaxis, biochemical mediators such as histamine, eosinophils, chemotactic factor of anaphylaxis, heparin, and leukotrienes are released. Vasodilation, increased capillary permeability (including pulmonary capillary permeability), bronchoconstriction, excessive mucus secretion, coronary vasoconstriction,

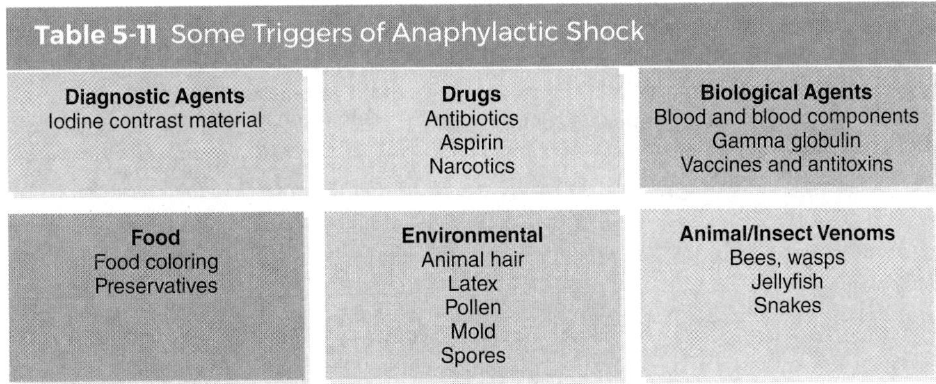

Table 5-11 Some Triggers of Anaphylactic Shock

Diagnostic Agents	**Drugs**	**Biological Agents**
Iodine contrast material	Antibiotics Aspirin Narcotics	Blood and blood components Gamma globulin Vaccines and antitoxins
Food	**Environmental**	**Animal/Insect Venoms**
Food coloring Preservatives	Animal hair Latex Pollen Mold Spores	Bees, wasps Jellyfish Snakes

inflammation, and cutaneous reactions ensue. The cutaneous reaction may be observed as flushed, warm skin resulting from vasodilation and urticaria. It is important to note that patients with anaphylactic shock do not always present with urticaria, and their skin may be cool, pale or ashen, and clammy. Do not rely on the absence of urticaria to rule out anaphylactic shock.

As with other causes of distributive shock, peripheral vasodilation in anaphylaxis causes a relative hypovolemia. This is due to vasodilation and leaking at the capillary level (third spacing). The sudden loss of volume and vascular resistance causes cardiac output to drop. Cardiovascular collapse and/or airway obstruction are typically the direct causes of death.

Because shock can quickly overwhelm such patients, prompt intervention is critical. As the ABCs—airway, breathing, circulation—are assessed and managed, it is important to ascertain the following:

- Does the patient have a history of previous allergic reactions? Does the patient use an EPINEPHrine autoinjector?
- Has the patient been exposed to an offending agent? If so, when?
- Is there a complaint of urticaria, rash, throat swelling, or shortness of breath? Laryngeal edema can have a rapid onset, so intervention must be swift.
- When did the symptoms begin? The more rapid the onset, the more likely it is the reaction will be severe.
- How long have the symptoms lasted? Symptoms typically resolve within 6 hours.

Treatment

The treatment of anaphylactic shock requires removing the allergen, when possible, and reversing the effects of the biochemicals that have been released (**Figure 5-5**). EPINEPHrine should be administered without delay and may be lifesaving. It may be necessary to support vital functions by providing oxygen, performing intubation or mechanical ventilation, and administering IV fluids (**Rapid Recall Box 5-1**). Corticosteroids can stabilize the capillary membranes and reduce angioedema and bronchospasm, but because their onset of action is somewhat delayed, their use is limited to preventing or ameliorating the late-phase component of anaphylaxis; they are not effective early during the initial attack. DiphenhydrAMINE is helpful for symptom relief in milder allergic reactions. It is often given with EPINEPHrine in severe reactions, but in true anaphylactic shock, EPINEPHrine and IV fluids are the mainstay of treating the shock. In patients receiving beta blockers, glucagon administration should be considered. Glucagon has ionotropic and chronotropic properties and can reverse bronchospasm. H2 receptor blockers (e.g., famotidine, cimetidine) may be used with diphenhydrAMINE to address GI and dermal manifestations of anaphylaxis (**Rapid Recall Box 5-2**). Patients with severe symptoms and/or sudden onset of anaphylaxis should be monitored for an extended period as a repeat onset of symptoms may occur and may require immediate intervention.

Anaphylaxis is one of the few disease entities where evidence-based guidelines are published for prehospital clinicians.

Neurogenic Shock

Neurogenic shock is a rare form of distributive shock. When signal transmission in the sympathetic nervous system is interrupted, the body cannot mount an appropriate fight-or-flight response. Spinal cord injury, usually at the sixth thoracic vertebra (T6) or higher, often leads to neurogenic shock. Vessels do not receive the sympathetic nervous system message to constrict and instead dilate due to the unopposed vagal stimulus. For this

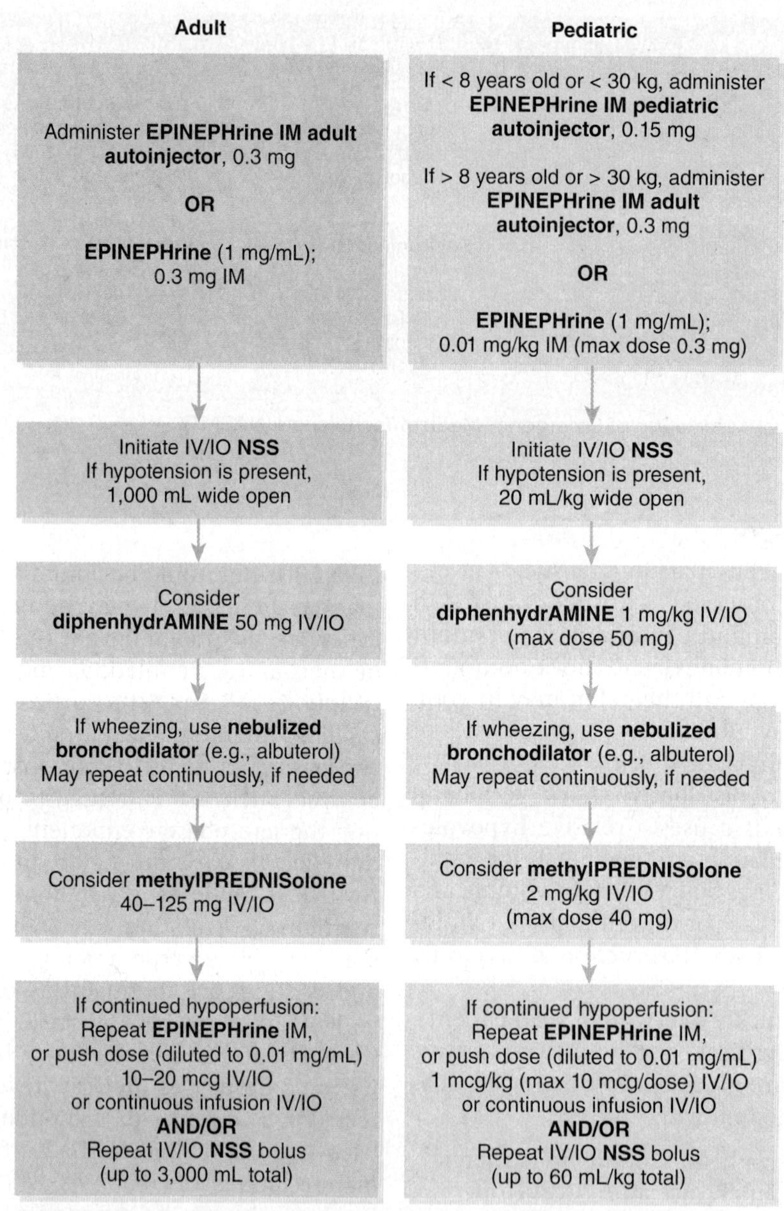

Adult
Administer **EPINEPHrine IM adult autoinjector**, 0.3 mg
OR
EPINEPHrine (1 mg/mL); 0.3 mg IM
Initiate IV/IO **NSS**
If hypotension is present, 1,000 mL wide open
Consider **diphenhydrAMINE** 50 mg IV/IO
If wheezing, use **nebulized bronchodilator** (e.g., albuterol)
May repeat continuously, if needed
Consider **methylPREDNISolone** 40–125 mg IV/IO
If continued hypoperfusion:
Repeat **EPINEPHrine** IM,
or push dose (diluted to 0.01 mg/mL)
10–20 mcg IV/IO
or continuous infusion IV/IO
AND/OR
Repeat IV/IO **NSS** bolus
(up to 3,000 mL total)
Pediatric
If < 8 years old or < 30 kg, administer **EPINEPHrine IM pediatric autoinjector**, 0.15 mg
If > 8 years old or > 30 kg, administer **EPINEPHrine IM adult autoinjector**, 0.3 mg
OR
EPINEPHrine (1 mg/mL); 0.01 mg/kg IM (max dose 0.3 mg)
Initiate IV/IO **NSS**
If hypotension is present, 20 mL/kg wide open
Consider **diphenhydrAMINE** 1 mg/kg IV/IO (max dose 50 mg)
If wheezing, use **nebulized bronchodilator** (e.g., albuterol)
May repeat continuously, if needed
Consider **methylPREDNISolone** 2 mg/kg IV/IO (max dose 40 mg)
If continued hypoperfusion:
Repeat **EPINEPHrine** IM,
or push dose (diluted to 0.01 mg/mL)
1 mcg/kg (max 10 mcg/dose) IV/IO
or continuous infusion IV/IO
AND/OR
Repeat IV/IO **NSS** bolus
(up to 60 mL/kg total)
Abbreviations: IM, intramuscular; IV, intravenous; IO, intraosseous; NSS, normal saline solution

Figure 5-5 Management of anaphylaxis.

reason, neurogenic shock is sometimes called vasogenic shock. The dilated vessels make the patient's skin warm and flushed. Blood pressure decreases, systemic vascular resistance decreases, and the circulatory system below the level of injury fails to return enough venous blood to the heart. Bradycardia is highly characteristic of neurogenic shock and is the result of a loss of sympathetic stimulation; however, it is not always present.

Treatment

Ensure that the airway is patent. Maintain oxygenation by providing supplemental oxygen and assist ventilation as indicated. Establish vascular access and initiate fluid resuscitation. If the patient does not respond to fluid resuscitation, consider vasopressor agents such as norepinephrine or DOPamine. Be sure to keep the patient warm and monitor for other neurologic dysfunction; associated head injury may be present. Transport the patient without delay.

Cardiogenic Shock

Cardiogenic shock occurs when the heart is unable to circulate sufficient blood to meet the body's metabolic

RAPID RECALL BOX 5-1

Push-Dose EPINEPHrine

Except in cases of cardiac arrest, EPINEPHrine should be diluted before administration. Mixing instructions are important as well. Here are four approaches that provide a diluted concentration of 0.01 mg/mL or 10 mcg/mL:

1. Start with EPINEPHrine 0.1 mg/mL in a prefilled 10-mL syringe, empty 9 mL of EPINEPHrine, refill it with 9 mL of normal saline, and label it "0.01 mg/mL Epi."
2. Start with EPINEPHrine 0.1 mg/mL in a prefilled 10-mL syringe, attach a three-way stopcock, attach a normal saline flush syringe with 9 mL, push 1 mL EPINEPHrine into the normal saline (NS) flush syringe, and label it "0.01 mg/mL Epi."
3. Start with a 50-mL bag of normal saline, add 0.5 mL of EPINEPHrine 1 mg/mL into that bag, then mix. Remove the needed dosing using a syringe.
4. Start with a 100-mL bag of normal saline, add 1 mL of EPINEPHrine 1 mg/mL into that bag, then mix. Remove the needed dosing using a syringe.

RAPID RECALL BOX 5-2

Pharmacology Review

EPINEPHrine

- Class: Catecholamine, sympathomimetic, adrenergic, inotropic, and bronchodilator
- Action: Binds with alpha and beta receptors, thereby increasing blood pressure, heart rate, and bronchodilation.
- Dosage:
  - Intramuscular (IM) dosing and autoinjector dosing
    - May repeat original IM dose
  - IV dosing, for life-threatening anaphylactic shock that does not respond to IM EPINEPHrine:
    - Use caution when giving IV EPINEPHrine to any patient with perfusing vital signs, especially those older than 50 years. Doses should be controlled, given slowly, and titrated only to adequate blood pressure. Higher doses may be needed in patients who are taking beta blocker medications. Generally, if the patient is not in cardiac arrest, IV EPINEPHrine should be diluted and given in titrated push doses or given by diluted continuous infusion. Avoid IV bolus of cardiac arrest concentration (0.1 mg/mL) EPINEPHrine.
  - Push-dose EPINEPHrine (diluted to 0.01 mg/mL) 10 to 20 mcg per dose titrated every 5 minutes to blood pressure as needed. Prepare by diluting 1 mL of 0.1 mg/mL solution in 9 mL normal saline (NS), which results in 10 mcg/mL.
    - For pediatrics, give 1 mcg/kg if < 10 kg and 10 mcg if > 10 kg.
- Adverse effects: Palpitations, tachydysrhythmias, hypertension, anxiety, nausea, vomiting

DiphenhydrAMINE

- Class: Antihistamine, anticholinergic, histamine 1 (H1) receptor antagonist
- Action: Binds and blocks H1 receptors. Provides symptomatic relief of urticaria and symptoms of histamine release but does not reverse anaphylaxis.
- Dosage: 1 to 2 mg/kg (maximum 50 mg) IM, IV, intraosseous (IO), oral every 4 to 8 hours.
- Adverse effects: Hypotension, palpitations

Glucagon

- Indication: May be ordered if patient is taking beta blocker and hypotension does not resolve with NSS bolus and EPINEPHrine.
- Dosage: 1 to 2 mg IV/IO in adults

needs. This can occur due to myocardial dysfunction (e.g., AMI, acute decompensated heart failure, Takotsubo cardiomyopathy), dysrhythmias (including atrioventricular heart block), a cardiac structural disorder such as chordae tendineae dysfunction or papillary muscle rupture, or the action of certain toxins. The most common cause is AMI, usually due to a massive infarction of the anterior wall of the heart. Risk factors for cardiogenic shock include advancing age, female sex, preexisting heart failure, previous myocardial infarction (MI), and diabetes.

In patients with cardiogenic shock, blood is no longer effectively pumped because of a diminished stroke volume or a heart rate that is too slow or too fast. When the left side of the heart fails, the blood overloads the pulmonary vasculature, causing pulmonary edema and impaired gas exchange.

Cardiogenic shock can present with diverse signs and symptoms and can be challenging to diagnose in the field. The patient is often tachypneic, and crackles caused by pulmonary edema can be heard on auscultation of the lungs. The patient is typically tachycardic with weak pulses, but may be bradycardic if the underlying cause is an atrioventricular heart block; other dysrhythmias may also be present. Hypotension occurs secondary to decreases in stroke volume and cardiac output. Poor peripheral perfusion results in cool, pale skin. JVD and cyanosis may be present. The patient may complain of chest pain and/or shortness of breath, and decreased cerebral perfusion may lead to an altered level of consciousness.

Cardiogenic shock requires early identification of the cause. Cardiac monitoring can identify dysrhythmias, and a multilead ECG can identify evidence of ischemia, injury, or infarct. At the receiving facility, a chest radiograph can be performed to detect pulmonary edema and pleural effusion. Cardiac markers such as troponin levels should be sent for laboratory analysis. In addition, a test for the presence of elevated levels of a hormone called brain natriuretic peptide (BNP) in the patient's serum may be performed, which may indicate heart failure. BNP is released in response to the stretch of the atria and ventricles. The vasodilation causes natriuresis (release of excessive sodium into the urine) and a reduction in blood volume. When BNP is elevated beyond the normal level as adjusted for age, it is typically a sign of acute decompensated heart failure.

Treatment

Initial treatment of a patient in cardiogenic shock must focus on stabilization of airway, breathing, and circulation. Managing the respiratory function and oxygenation is of paramount importance. Correct hypoxia as rapidly as possible. Rapid initiation of NIPPV for pulmonary edema may be lifesaving, but it is relatively contraindicated in shock. Establish vascular access.

If a STEMI is occurring, notify the appropriate receiving facility early so they can prepare to take the patient to the cardiac catheterization lab. Administer aspirin and heparin (if available) unless a contraindication exists. If an inferior wall MI is present, consider obtaining a right-sided ECG. ST elevation in lead V_4R indicates right ventricular infarction (RVI). Patients with RVI are preload dependent, and if hypotensive, should receive IV fluids. Nitroglycerin—a drug that reduces preload—can cause significant hypotension in this setting. In the absence of RVI, administer nitroglycerin if the patient's systolic blood pressure is adequate (> 100 mm Hg). Opiate analgesia (i.e., fentanyl) should also be provided if chest pain is not relieved with nitroglycerin, as long as the systolic blood pressure and level of consciousness are adequate. In a patient with cardiogenic shock because of a STEMI, timely transport to a cardiac center with percutaneous coronary intervention capabilities is essential and increases survival. In the hospital, an emergency ventricular assist device, such as an intra-aortic balloon or Impella pump, may be placed to improve cardiac output and perfusion.

If hypotension is present, consider initiating small isotonic fluid challenges, about 250 to 500 mL each, before progressing to a vasopressor infusion. Fluid must be administered cautiously, especially if high central venous pressure or pulmonary edema is present. If shock continues, initiate a vasopressor and titrate to a MAP of 65 to 70 mm Hg or systolic blood pressure > 90 mm Hg. If using dopamine, start at 5 mcg/kg/min and titrate to the lowest effective dose to minimize the increase in heart rate that dopamine may cause. If tachycardia is present with hypotension, consider using a norepinephrine or phenylephrine infusion. DOBUTamine and/or milrinone may be appropriate for inotropic support if the patient's systolic blood pressure is 80 to 100 mm Hg. However, these agents also cause vasodilation so the net effect on perfusion must be closely assessed and monitored. Some EMS agencies use push dose pressors by diluting EPINEPHrine to a concentration of 0.01 mg/mL and administering 1 to 2 mL (or 10 to 20 mcg) at a time and titrating to the target blood pressure (Rapid Recall Box 5-1).

Manage cardiogenic shock with signs of pulmonary congestion by placing the patient in semi-Fowler's position with the feet dependent unless this causes more severe hypotension. Oxygen should be administered to patients with dyspnea, signs of heart failure, shock, or an oxygen saturation < 94%. Use of continuous positive airway pressure (CPAP) or bilevel positive airway pressure (BiPAP) may assist in relieving pulmonary congestion at the alveolar level but is relatively contraindicated in hypotension. Follow local protocols and medical direction to guide this decision.

Obstructive Shock

Obstructive shock occurs when an obstruction to the forward flow of blood exists in the great vessels or heart. Significant causes are pericardial tamponade, massive pulmonary embolism, and tension pneumothorax. Common signs and symptoms of obstructive shock are shortness of breath, anxiety, tachypnea, and tachycardia. Breath sounds are usually unilaterally diminished if a tension pneumothorax is present. In later stages, the pulse pressure may narrow and the patient may become hypotensive. Cyanosis may be present, and the patient's level of consciousness may decrease. Pulsus paradoxus—a marked weakening or disappearance of a pulse during inspiration, which corresponds with a significant decrease in systolic blood pressure—may occur with cardiac tamponade or tension pneumothorax, and electrical alternans—beat-to-beat variations in the amplitude of the QRS complexes—may be observed in patients with pericardial tamponade.

Reversal of obstructive shock requires support of vital functions and treating the specific cause of blood flow obstruction. Initial management should focus on increasing vascular volume with fluid resuscitation and vasopressors as needed to maintain perfusion until a definitive diagnosis and treatment plan can be established.

Cardiac Tamponade

Cardiac tamponade is seen when fluid or blood accumulates in the pericardial sac surrounding the heart, diminishing the heart's ability to fill, thus reducing cardiac output (**Figure 5-6**). Trauma, ventricular rupture, infection, and metastatic cancer are possible causes of cardiac tamponade. The progression of cardiac tamponade depends on the speed of fluid accumulation (blood or effusion) in the pericardium. It may help to remember Beck's triad, the classic indicator of cardiac tamponade: JVD, shock, and muffled heart sounds. The classic Beck's triad is a late finding—present in only 10% to 40% of patients—and can be difficult to differentiate clinically, particularly in the out-of-hospital setting. With the use of point-of-care ultrasound, pericardial effusions are easily identified, and when available, this has supplanted the findings of Beck's triad.

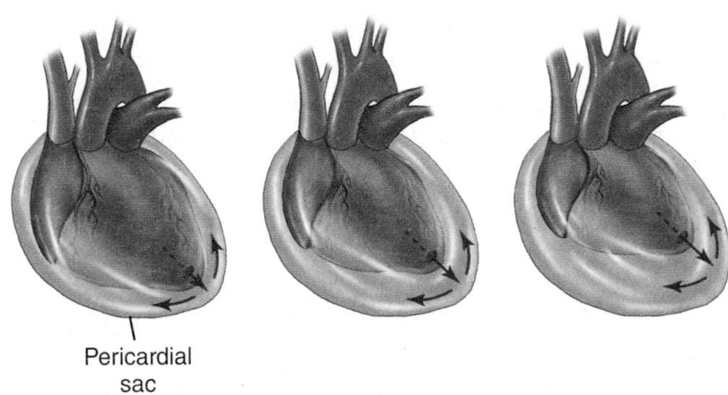

Figure 5-6 Cardiac tamponade. As blood courses from the cardiac defect into the pericardial space, it limits expansion of the ventricle. Therefore, the ventricle cannot fill adequately. As more blood accumulates in the pericardial space, less ventricular space is available to fill with blood, and cardiac output is reduced.

Treatment

Cardiac tamponade may be treated with fluid boluses, inotropic medications, and pericardiocentesis, the latter of which involves inserting a needle attached to a syringe into the chest far enough to penetrate the pericardium and then withdrawing fluid. Many recommend performing this procedure under ultrasound guidance. Another emergent method for draining the pericardial fluid is by surgically creating a pericardial window, usually performed in the operating theater. Definitive treatment depends on the cause and rate of fluid accumulation.

Pulmonary Embolism

Pulmonary embolism is a life-threatening condition that occurs when a thrombus (blood clot) travels through the vasculature and lodges in a pulmonary artery. If a large component of the pulmonary vasculature is occluded, reduced blood flow back to the heart decreases cardiac output, resulting in hypotension and shock.

Treatment

Treatment for shock related to pulmonary embolism focuses on oxygenation, ventilation, and supporting perfusion with fluid boluses. Pulmonary embolism causes right heart strain and makes the patient dependent on preload. The primary therapy is systemic anticoagulation with heparin or fractionated heparin medications such as enoxaparin. Fibrinolytics, endovascular clot retrieval (thrombectomy), or thoracic surgery may be considered for severe cases.

Tension Pneumothorax

The most immediately treatable cause of obstructive shock is tension pneumothorax. A tension pneumothorax develops when air becomes trapped outside the lung between the visceral and parietal pleurae and applies pressure to the contents of the chest cavity. This pressure causes the mediastinum to shift to the unaffected side and interferes with ventilation and perfusion. The increased intrathoracic pressure causes compression of the vena cava, diminishing venous return to the heart, which leads to inadequate cardiac output. Although trauma is a common cause of pneumothorax, the condition can develop spontaneously or as a result of positive-pressure ventilation. Patients with COPD have weakened areas of the lungs called blebs, which may rupture and are thus vulnerable to the effects of excessive pressure. Pneumothorax can also be caused by overzealous ventilation in an otherwise healthy patient. Patients being ventilated with positive pressure are at increased risk for a pneumothorax, which, if left untreated, can progress to a tension pneumothorax.

Treatment

The *only* intervention that can prevent death from a tension pneumothorax is decompression of the injured side of the chest. Thoracostomy must be performed on patients with this life-threatening emergency. In the prehospital setting, this has traditionally been done with needle decompression. Finger thoracostomy is another option for EMS clinicians with proper training. In the hospital, tube thoracostomy is the most common intervention.

Complications of Shock

Shock is a serious disorder with a high mortality. The complications from shock include:

- Acute renal failure
- ARDS/ALI
- Coagulopathies (including DIC)
- Hepatic dysfunction
- Multiple organ dysfunction syndrome

Population-Specific Considerations

Older Adult Patients

Older adults are living longer and staying more active into their later years. Paradoxically, living longer makes a person more likely to become severely ill or injured.

The use of medications to control chronic disease states can complicate both the body's ability to heal itself and your ability to recognize disorders such as shock. Platelet-inhibiting drugs can cause bleeding, even when therapeutic levels are present; for example, GI bleeding may develop. Excessive bleeding may result if too much medication is taken or if trauma occurs. Because platelet-inhibiting drugs affect hemostasis—the body's ability to stop bleeding—it is important to identify these or any other drugs that may prolong bleeding time and understand their potential to contribute to shock. Recognizing the need to control bleeding and possibly reverse the effects of certain drugs with antagonists or blood products is part of early intervention. Ask older patients whether they take any drugs inhibiting platelet activity, including acetylsalicylic acid (aspirin) and clopidogrel. Many older adults are also on anticoagulation therapy with drugs such as warfarin, dabigatran, rivaroxaban, and apixaban. Early notification of the receiving facility of the use of these medications is important if bleeding is suspected, to allow the facility time to prepare interventions. Patients may also be taking supplements that increase bleeding, including vitamin E, ginkgo biloba, ginseng, dong quai, feverfew, garlic, ginger, and omega-3 fatty acids, so be sure to specifically inquire about their use as well, as some patients may not consider supplements to be drugs and may not mention them if asked about their medications.

Some antihypertensive and vasoactive drugs limit the ability of the heart to increase its rate in response to shock. Beta blockers and calcium channel blockers are two examples of medications that may keep the patient's pulse rate low despite normal compensation mechanisms creating tachycardia.

Other factors can complicate the early diagnosis of shock in an older adult patient. As a person ages, pulmonary and cardiac reserves diminish. The alveoli stiffen, and tidal volume is reduced. Resting cardiac output declines, as does the basal metabolic rate. Shock-related compensatory mechanisms are more sluggish and less effective, and this may cause the patient to decompensate rapidly. The amount of adipose tissue decreases, muscle mass begins to atrophy, and it becomes more difficult to maintain body heat.

Obstetric Patients

When caring for a pregnant patient, it is important to realize the survival of both the fetus and the pregnant patient depends on maintaining adequate perfusion in the pregnant patient. Pregnancy normally lasts about 40 weeks, during which the woman's body undergoes significant physiologic changes. The maternal heart rate accelerates by 10 to 15 beats/min to compensate for the additional perfusion demands of the fetus. Blood volume expands by almost 50%, and cardiac output increases by 30%.

As the fetus grows, it places additional pressure on the internal organs, diaphragm, and inferior vena cava. Because of the increased cardiac output and intravascular volume, signs of hypoperfusion in pregnant patients may be delayed. Vascular changes attributable to pregnancy can mask early signs of shock.

When managing a pregnant patient who is 20 weeks or greater into a pregnancy (the uterine fundus is palpable at the umbilicus by the 20th week), place the patient in the left-lateral recumbent position to avoid hypotension caused by pressure by the enlarged uterus on the inferior vena cava. Maintain adequate oxygenation, and initiate IV fluid therapy.

Pediatric Patients

Children have a great capacity for compensation when in shock due to their ability to increase cardiac output by robustly increasing their heart rate; as a result, hypotension in pediatric patients may be a late finding. Fluid replacement with boluses of isotonic fluids such as normal saline or lactated Ringer's solution is necessary until the patient is at the hospital for definitive care and blood transfusions. Other diseases also predispose children to shock.

Putting It All Together

Early, accurate identification of the patient's stage and type of shock is essential in managing this condition. Sound clinical reasoning skills, a thorough assessment, and careful but expedient interpretation of diagnostic findings are necessary to provide effective treatment for the patient in shock.

SCENARIO SOLUTION

- Your patient is in decompensated shock, as evidenced by his significant hypotension, lethargy, mottled skin, and absent radial pulses. He is also in respiratory failure, as evidenced by his labored breathing and severe hypoxemia.
- Your patient is in a periarrest situation and requires immediate and aggressive intervention. Begin your focus on supporting oxygenation and ventilation. Given the coarse crackles in his lungs, continuous positive airway pressure would ordinarily be indicated; however, his lethargy and hypotension contraindicate this therapy. Start by placing him in a position that better facilitates breathing. Providing the patient with 100% oxygen via a nonrebreather mask would not be unreasonable, but he will likely need ventilation assistance with a bag-valve mask, and the use of advanced airway management must be considered. Use extreme caution, however, because positive-pressure ventilation can have a negative effect on cardiac output. You must next address his perfusion failure; establish vascular access and consider a brief, conservative trial of crystalloid solution. Again, you must exercise great caution to avoid fluid overload (remember the coarse crackles in his lungs?).
- Given his recent history of chest pain and his past medical history of hypertension and coronary artery disease, you should suspect that he is in cardiogenic shock (pump failure). He likely experienced an AMI; however, because he did not seek timely care, a significant amount of cardiac muscle has been damaged. When the left heart fails, forward blood flow is impaired, which would explain his signs of poor systemic perfusion. If blood cannot move forward, then it will move backward into the lungs, causing pulmonary edema and eventually ventilation and oxygenation compromise. You should obtain a multilead ECG as soon as feasible to assess for evidence of ischemia, acute injury, or infarct (new or old). Given his prearrest condition, you should also consider applying the defibrillation pads.
- In addition to the interventions previously discussed, medication therapy will be needed to increase and maintain cardiac output and, therefore, systemic perfusion. DOPamine, starting at 5 to 10 mcg/kg/min, or norepinephrine, starting at 0.05 mcg/kg/min, should be initiated without delay. If you do not have an infusion pump available, then administer push-dose EPINEPHrine (0.01 mg/mL) 10 to 20 mcg every 2 to 5 minutes as needed. This is a very complex patient who has several imminently life-threatening problems that must be simultaneously managed. Minimize your scene time as much as possible and transport without delay for definitive care. Depending on what the multilead ECG reveals (e.g., evidence of acute injury), he may be taken straight to the cardiac catheterization lab. Furthermore, he may be a candidate for an intra-aortic balloon pump or ventricular assist device.

SUMMARY

- Understanding inadequate tissue perfusion requires a thorough knowledge of the anatomy, physiology, and pathophysiology of shock.
- Shock is a progressive state of cellular hypoperfusion in which too little oxygen and too little energy are available to meet tissue demands in multiple organ systems.
- The three stages of shock are compensated, decompensated, and irreversible.
- The three main determinants of cellular perfusion are cardiac output, intravascular volume, and vascular capacitance.
- Cardiac output is determined by stroke volume and heart rate.
- The four primary determinants of stroke volume are preload, afterload, contractility, and synchrony.
- Mean arterial blood pressure is an indirect indicator of tissue perfusion. Higher mean arterial pressures may be required for adequate perfusion in patients with a history of hypertension.
- Narrowing pulse pressures are indicators of decreased cardiac output and a helpful indicator of shock.
- Blood transports oxygen to and wastes from the body's cells. Hemoglobin, an iron-containing protein in RBCs, is the primary carrier of oxygen.
- Underlying chronic medical illnesses, age, and immunosuppression adversely affect compensatory mechanisms of shock.
- Compensatory mechanisms include increasing minute ventilation, increasing cardiac output, and vasoconstriction.
- The types of shock are hypovolemic, obstructive, distributive, and cardiogenic.
- When the body no longer has ample oxygen and cells begin producing lactic acid as a by-product of anaerobic metabolism, metabolic acidosis occurs.
- During the compensated phase of shock, perfusion of the brain, heart, lungs, and liver is enhanced, while less essential organs become ischemic.
- Anxiety, combativeness, and confusion may be early signs of shock.
- Most types of shock are characterized by tachycardia, tachypnea, cool skin, and hypotension. In distributive shock, however, the skin may be warm. Bradycardia can accompany cardiogenic or neurogenic shock.
- Assessment tools used to evaluate patients suspected of being in shock include pulse oximetry, electrocardiography, serum glucose testing, capnography, shock index, and lactate levels. In the hospital, laboratory studies, CT, ultrasonography, and radiographic studies are used.
- Complications of shock include acute renal failure, ARDS, coagulopathies, hepatic dysfunction, and multiorgan system failure.
- Initial treatment of shock consists of supportive measures, supplemental oxygen, fluid resuscitation, temperature regulation, and administration of vasopressors. Specific interventions are based on the underlying cause.

Key Terms

Acidosis An abnormal increase in the hydrogen ion concentration in the blood resulting from an accumulation of an acid or the loss of a base; indicated by a blood pH below the normal range.

afterload In the intact heart, the pressure against which the ventricle ejects blood. It is impacted by the transmural pressure, peripheral vascular resistance, and the physical characteristics and volume of blood in the arterial system.

cardiac cycle A complete cardiac movement or heartbeat. The period from the beginning of one heartbeat to the beginning of the next; from diastole through systole.

cardiac output The effective volume of blood expelled by either ventricle of the heart per unit of time (usually volume per minute). It is equal to the stroke volume multiplied by the heart rate.

hypovolemia Abnormally decreased volume of circulating blood in the body, due to loss of either blood or plasma.

perfusion The delivery of oxygenated blood to body tissues.

preload The volume of blood in the ventricle at the end of diastole. It reflects venous return and the stress or stretch on the ventricular wall. Also called end-diastolic volume.

pulse pressure The difference between the systolic and diastolic blood pressures.

shock A condition of profound hemodynamic and metabolic disturbance characterized by failure of the circulatory system to maintain adequate perfusion to vital organs. It may result from inadequate blood volume, cardiac function, or vasomotor tone or from obstruction to blood flow.

shock index (SI) A measure of hemodynamic status particularly useful in patients with compensated shock. It is calculated by dividing the heart rate by the systolic blood pressure, with a normal range of 0.5 to 0.7. Increasing values, particularly > 0.9, indicate worsening hemodynamic status.

stroke volume The amount of blood ejected by the ventricle during each heartbeat.

Bibliography

Aehlert B. *Paramedic Practice Today: Above and Beyond*. Mosby/JEMS; 2009.

American Academy of Orthopaedic Surgeons. *Nancy Caroline's Emergency Care in the Streets*, 8th ed. Jones & Bartlett Learning; 2018.

American College of Surgeons. *ATLS Student Course Manual*, 10th ed. American College of Surgeons; 2018.

Cairns CB. Rude unhinging of the machinery of life: metabolic approaches to hemorrhagic shock. *Curr Opin Crit Care*. 2001;7(6):437–443.

Centers for Disease Control and Prevention. Guide to infection prevention for outpatient settings: minimum expectations for safe care. Last reviewed September 9, 2014. https://www.cdc.gov/HAI/settings/outpatient/outpatient-care-guidelines.html

Copstead-Kirkhorn LE, Banasik JL. *Pathophysiology*. Saunders; 2010.

Darovic GO. *Handbook of Hemodynamic Monitoring*, 2nd ed. Saunders; 2004.

Gaugler MH. A unifying system: does the vascular endothelium have a role to play in multi-organ failure following radiation exposure? *Br J Radiol*. 2005;78:100–105.

Hamilton GC. *Emergency Medicine: An Approach to Clinical Problem-Solving*, 2nd ed. Saunders; 2003.

Hirschl M, Wollmann C, Mayr H. 30 day survival of patients with STEMI and cardiogenic shock. *Crit Care Med*. 2013;41(12), 2013. doi:10.1097/01.ccm.0000439211.53447.b9

Hudak CM, Gallo BM, Morton PG. *Critical Care Nursing: A Holistic Approach*, 7th ed. Lippincott; 1998.

Hunter CH. End-tidal carbon dioxide may be used in place of lactate to screen for severe sepsis. *JEMS*. 2014;3:134.

Hunter CL, Silvestri S, Dean M, et al. End-tidal carbon dioxide levels are associated with mortality in emergency department patients with suspected sepsis. October 1, 2011. http://med.ucf.edu/media/2011/10/i2-poster-dean-matthew.pdf

Hunter CL, Silvestri S, Ralls G, et al. The sixth vital sign: prehospital end-tidal carbon dioxide predicts in-hospital mortality and metabolic disturbances. *Am J Emerg Med*. 2014;32(2):160–165.

Japp A, Robertson C, Wright R, et al. *Macleod's Clinical Diagnosis*, 2nd ed. Elsevier; 2018.

Kolecki P. Hypovolemic shock treatment and management. Updated October 13, 2016. http://emedicine.medscape.com/article/760145

Kragh JF Jr, Walters TJ, Baer DG, et al. Survival with emergency tourniquet use to stop bleeding in major limb trauma. *Ann Surg*. 2009;249:1–7.

Maheshwari K, Nathanson BH, Munson SH, et al. Abnormal shock index exposure and clinical outcomes among critically ill patients: a retrospective cohort analysis. *J Crit Care*. 2020;57:5–12, 2020. doi:10.1016/j.jcrc.2020.01.024

Marx JA, Hockberger RS, Walls RM. *Rosen's Emergency Medicine: Concepts and Clinical Practice*, 6th ed. Mosby; 2006.

McCance KL, Huether SE. *Pathophysiology: The Biologic Basis for Disease in Adults and Children*, 5th ed. Mosby; 2006.

Miller RD, Eriksson L, Fleisher L, et al. *Miller's Anesthesia*, 7th ed. Churchill Livingstone; 2009.

Moultan SL, Mulligan J, Grudic GZ, et al. Running on empty? The compensatory reserve index. *J Trauma Acute Care Surg*. 2013;75(6): 1053–1059.

Mustafa S, Kaliner A. Anaphylaxis medication. Updated May 16, 2018. http://emedicine.medscape.com/article/135065-medication

National Association of Emergency Medical Technicians. *PHTLS: Prehospital Trauma Life Support*, 10th ed. Public Safety Group; 2023.

Pagana KP. *Mosby's Diagnostic and Laboratory Test Reference*, 9th ed. Mosby; 2008.

Panchal AR, Bartos JA, Cabañas JG, et al. Part 3: Adult Basic and Advanced Life Support: 2020 American Heart Association Guidelines Update for Cardiopulmonary Resuscitation and Emergency Cardiovascular Care. *Circulation*. 2020;142(16 Suppl2):S366–S468. doi.org/10.1161/CIR.0000000000000916

Patton KT, Thibodeau GA. *Anatomy and Physiology*, 7th ed. Mosby; 2010.

Seif D, Perera P, Mailhot T, et al. Review article: Bedside ultrasound in resuscitation and the rapid ultrasound in shock protocol. *Crit Care Res Pract.* 2012;2012:503254. doi:10.1155/2012/503254

Society of Critical Care Medicine. Surviving sepsis: bundles. http://www.survivingsepsis.org/Bundles/Pages/default.aspx

Solomon EP. *Introduction to Human Anatomy and Physiology*, 3rd ed. Saunders; 2009.

Stanton BA, Koeppen BM. *Berne and Levy Physiology*, 6th ed. Mosby; 2008.

Swan KG Jr, Wright DS, Barbagiovanni SS, et al. Tourniquets revisited. *J Trauma.* 2009;66:672–679.

Tintinalli JE, Kellen GD, Stapczynski S, et al. *Tintinalli's Emergency Medicine: A Comprehensive Study Guide*, 6th ed. McGraw-Hill; 2003.

Urden LD, Stacy KM, Lough ME. *Thelan's Critical Care Nursing: Diagnosis and Management*, 5th ed. Mosby; 2006.

Wallgren UM, Castrén M, Svensson AEV, et al. Identification of adult septic patients in the prehospital setting: a comparison of two screening tools and clinical judgment. *Eur J Emerg Med Off J Eur Soc Emerg Med.* 2013;28(6):573–579.

CHAPTER 6

Sepsis

Chapter Editors
Karin H. Molander, MD, FACEP
Rommie L. Duckworth, MPA, LP, EFO

In this chapter, the pathophysiology of sepsis is discussed, along with common pathogens triggering sepsis, populations particularly vulnerable to sepsis, sepsis alert criteria, advanced treatment options, and methods to effectively coordinate sepsis care with in-hospital colleagues. Clinicians will be asked to apply their knowledge to patient assessment, determine whether sepsis is present, differentiate between sepsis and septic shock, and apply clinical reasoning to select the best treatment plan for the patient.

LEARNING OBJECTIVES

At the conclusion of this chapter, you will be able to:

- Explain the anatomy, physiology, and pathophysiology of both sepsis and septic shock.
- Describe how to obtain a thorough history from a patient with suspected sepsis.
- Carry out a comprehensive assessment of a patient with suspected sepsis or septic shock using the AMLS Assessment Pathway.
- Form an initial impression and generate differential diagnoses on the basis of a patient's history, signs, and symptoms.
- Select appropriate diagnostic tests, and apply the results to aid in diagnosis.
- Follow accepted evidence-based practice guidelines for the overall management of sepsis and septic shock.
- Provide an ongoing assessment of the patient, revising your clinical impression and treatment strategy on the basis of the patient's response to interventions.
- Describe differences in the identification, assessment, and treatment of sepsis and septic shock in special patient populations.

SCENARIO

You are called to a private residence for an 81-year-old female who has fallen. As you greet the patient, you find her sitting upright on the floor in her bedroom in obvious distress. The caregiver advises you she came into the room and the patient needed to use the restroom urgently, attempted to walk without assistance, and lost her footing and fell. The caregiver explains the patient has been more lethargic as of late and has not been making sense. The patient is not cooperative during the exam and complains of "not feeling right"; she is unable to give any specific information or a timeline of the events. As you obtain a history from the caregiver, you learn the patient has a history of atrial fibrillation, heart failure, hypertension, and hyperlipidemia and has been prescribed appropriate medications for each of these conditions. Initial vital signs include blood

(continues)

SCENARIO (CONTINUED)

pressure of 74/44 mm Hg; pulse rate of 149 beats/min, regular, but weak; and respirations of 24 breaths/min. Diagnostic tests reveal an $ETCO_2$ of 23 mm Hg (3.1 kPa), blood glucose of 234 mg/dL (13 mmol/L); temperature of 38.3°C (100.9°F), and lactate of 55 mg/dL (6.4 mmol/L).

- What differential diagnoses are you considering?
- What additional information will you need to narrow your list of possible diagnoses?
- What are your initial treatment priorities as you continue your patient care?

Sepsis: A Complex Syndrome

Sepsis, a potentially life-threatening reaction, is due to an overwhelming host response to infection. Sepsis involves the activation of both pro- and anti-inflammatory responses along with major dysfunctions in cardiovascular, neuronal, autonomic, hormonal, metabolic, and coagulation responses, leading to end-organ damage. Depending on geographic location, age, comorbidities, time of year, and predominance of local pathogens, the primary cause of sepsis can differ. Sepsis can be triggered by bacterial, viral, parasitic, or fungal infections, leading to an improper and overwhelming response. The sepsis response works in much the same way as an anaphylactic reaction: an improper physiologic response to stimuli. A patient does not need to be stung a minimum of 50 times, nor do they need to eat an entire jar of peanut butter before they have an anaphylactic reaction. Similarly, the physiologic reaction that is sepsis can be triggered by a small infection, and thus easily remain unrecognized until the signs and symptoms of septic shock are both obvious and severe. However, sepsis is arguably a more complex and insidious response than anaphylaxis because sepsis typically involves more body systems and is more challenging to recognize early on, when treatment is more likely to be successful.

Prior to 2019, the most common cause of sepsis in the United States was bacterial infection, and thus the Surviving Sepsis Campaign's focus on rapid antibiotics was pertinent. However, not all sepsis is caused by bacterial infections. During the COVID-19 pandemic, the virus SARS-CoV-2 became a common cause of sepsis (and antibiotics would prove futile), leading to the death of many patients. In sub-Saharan Africa, common contributors to sepsis are the parasites *Plasmodium falciparum, P. vivax, P. ovale, P. malariae,* and *P. knowlesi,* all of which cause malaria. Patients who are on chronic immunosuppressive agents, such as organ transplant recipients, are susceptible to fungal causes of sepsis.

Sepsis is one of the leading causes of death, especially in hospitals. In the United States, one out of three hospital deaths is attributed to sepsis. Early recognition of sepsis—even though its presentation may be subtle—is crucial for patients to have positive responses to interventions. This is particularly challenging because the clinical presentation of sepsis can change based on the pathogen, age, site of infection, acute illness, long-standing comorbidities, medications, and interventions.

The Immune System: Innate Immune Response and Adaptive Immune Response

The **immune system** is the body's method of combating infection and preventing sepsis and septic shock. The immune system consists of multiple defenses, including the **innate immune response** and the **adaptive immune response**. The innate immune response is the body's first line of defense against infection. It comprises intrinsic barriers to infection (stomach acid, respiratory system mucus, sweat and sebum from skin); **complement** proteins; and innate immune cells such as natural killer cells, **monocytes**, mast cells, and polymorphonuclear leukocytes (PMNs; also called **granulocytes**). The adaptive immune response takes longer to develop and involves interactions among the pathogen, two classes of lymphocytes (**T cells** and **B cells**), and the creation of **antibodies** (by B cells) against the pathogen.

When a microbe penetrates the typically sterile environment of the human body, a cascade of events occurs, which may differ slightly depending on the pathogen (bacterium, virus, parasite, or fungus), whether the body has previously encountered this invasive pathogen, the general health and age of the patient, and the portal of entry.

The innate immune response is the initial defense system we have at birth. This response is immediate. It has no memory. The receptors on our cells can recognize general patterns of pathogens and initiate this first response. The later, more specific stage of the immune response is the adaptive immune response. Adaptive immunity is acquired and can take days to develop T cells and B cells specific to the invading pathogen. The adaptive immune response can build memory from prior exposures, and thus generate a strong and rapid response on re-exposure to the offending agent. Vaccines are an attempt to help the body develop an adaptive immune response. The vaccine will trigger the innate response and then the adaptive response so that when the offending pathogen is encountered again, the host is better prepared to more rapidly fight it and contain the infection.

The following information is somewhat in-depth and provides details at the cellular level of the immune response. Although much of this material may not have been covered in initial education programs, it provides a means of understanding the body's complex immune response and how it responds to pathogens. The information provided hopefully offers an opportunity to see how the complex physiology and pathophysiology of the human body relate to disease and the body's disease response. The information will also help you better understand new advances in early diagnostics and therapeutics currently being developed and tested.

The Innate Immune Response

Natural Barriers to Infection

The human body has many natural barriers to infection (**Figure 6-1**). All humans have a rich biome of microbes (primarily bacteria and viruses) coexisting within us, assisting, for example, with the digestion of food. We have multiple methods of preventing pathogenic (disease-causing) microbes such as bacteria, parasites, fungi, or viruses from penetrating our body's internal environment. Barriers to infection include the multiple layers of epithelial cells making up the skin surface, subcutaneous glands secreting fluid to maintain an acidic environment on the skin surface, and mucous membranes producing mucus to trap microbes. The production of saliva, mucus, tears, and urine helps to lubricate and continuously flush environments prone to attack, such as the mouth, nose, eyes, and bladder.

Cilia (minuscule hairlike fibers) that line the respiratory tract are continuously moving foreign agents out. The natural sneeze and cough reflex also protects the body's airways. Saliva and mucus contain enzymes, such as lysozyme, that can kill bacteria. Surfactant on the surface of lung cells covers invading microbes and increases the activity of phagocytic cells in the area.

In addition, native populations of flora may exist in portions of the body and prevent colonization by invading species. For example, *Lactobacillus* are common bacteria in the vagina and prefer the low pH of this environment. Its presence can prevent other bacteria from invading and populating the vagina. *Escherichia coli* commonly exist in the gut to assist with digestion, but would be seen as a foreign invader when present in the bladder.

Innate Immune Cells

A key component of the innate immune system is the activation of innate immune cells by the circulating complement proteins. Complement proteins play a role in both the innate immune response and the adaptive immune response. They do not require previous exposure to a pathogen to initiate the activation of defense mechanisms. Complement proteins can activate the following types of innate immune cells:

- Natural killer cells play a key role in the destruction of transformed (by infection or mutation, such as cancer) host cells and are important in the destruction of those transformed or infected cells.

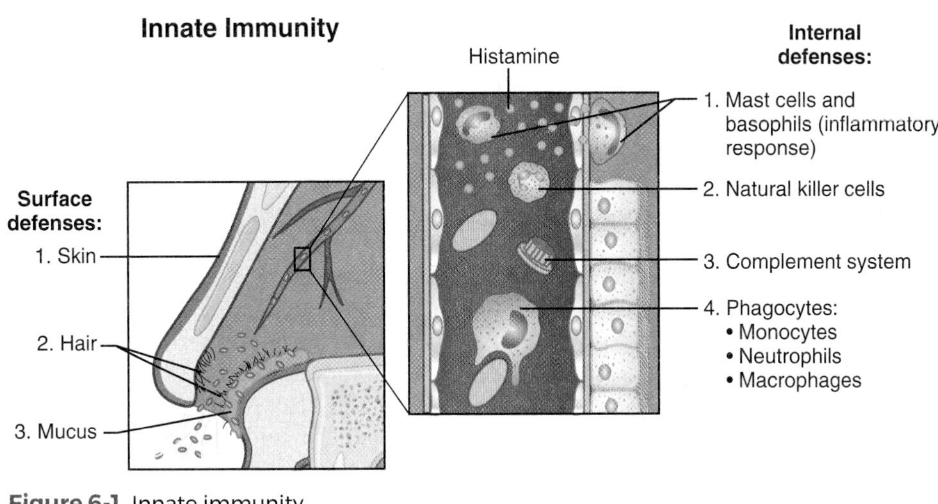

Figure 6-1 Innate immunity.

A type of lymphocyte (white blood cell), natural killer cells assist in attacking cells deemed foreign by our bodies.
- Mast cells are present in large numbers on the mucosal surfaces. They release a large quantity of histamine upon activation, causing vasodilation and inflammation. This increases the permeability of the tissues, which then allows for additional **phagocytes** to penetrate the infected area. Mast cells also play a large role in allergic reactions.
- Monocytes are cells that are capable of differentiating into **macrophages** or **dendritic cells**. They can engulf an invading microbe and secrete a number of cytokines and **chemokines** upon activation, such as tumor necrosis factor-alpha (TNF-alpha) and interleukin-6 (IL-6), accelerating the host response to the foreign invader. Dendritic cells can further differentiate depending on their location in tissue or blood and cause the further release of **cytokines**, such as IL-12 or interferon alpha.
- Polymorphonuclear granulocytes can differentiate into **eosinophils**, **basophils**, or **neutrophils**.
  - Eosinophils play a role in parasitic infections and allergic reactions. They release histamine and other immune-modulating chemicals.
  - Basophils play a role in parasitic infections and allergic reactions. They release histamine and heparin.
  - Neutrophils comprise approximately 50% of all circulating leukocytes and are typically the first to encounter a foreign microbe from a bacterial, fungal, or viral infection. They can surround the offending agent, ingest it (phagocytosis), and release enzymes to destroy the organism.

The Acquired Immune Response

The acquired immune response, also known as the adaptive immune response, takes days to months to develop. Two types of granulocytes called **lymphocytes** play key roles in this response: cell-mediated T cells and humoral-mediated B cells. The T cells mature in the thymus, whereas B cells mature in the bone marrow. The cytotoxic T cells directly kill the infected cells by causing **apoptosis** (cell death), which causes the release of certain cytokines and chemokines that help moderate the reaction to the infection. However, if a cell dies from infection caused by cell **necrosis**, rather than apoptosis, a different cascade of chemokines and cytokines is released, accelerating the immune response.

The helper T cells activate other immune cells (T and B cells) and will assist them in maturing more rapidly or becoming more effective. Mature B cells, also called plasma cells, secrete antibodies that directly attach to the invading microbe or diseased host cell, assisting in their rapid identification and destruction by the cytotoxic T cells. Plasma cells may actually change to secrete antibodies, indicating early infection (immunoglobin M [IgM]) or late infection (IgG), or can differentiate to secrete IgA, which concentrates in the mucus, saliva, and tears as an effective first line of attack should reinfection occur. Plasma cells can also secrete IgE, which binds to mast cells and basophils and plays a role in parasitic infections and allergic reactions.

T cells that mature in the thymus are able to travel to the site of the infection and further assist in eradicating the invading pathogen. These activated killer T cells locate the body's cells that are infected with the microbe and target these cells to die. Helper T cells can further activate macrophages to target pathogens, or they can help B cells produce antibodies to the offending pathogen (**Figure 6-2**).

The Role of Cytokines in the Innate and Adaptive Immune Responses and the Coagulation Cascade

Cytokines are chemicals released by certain cell lines that further activate or slow the body's initial immune response. Cytokines are released as part of the innate immune response and can also initiate the adaptive immune response. They can also create a counterbalance by assisting the body in deactivating or slowing its immune response.

For example, in the innate immune response, IL-8 strongly attracts phagocytic cells (such as neutrophils) to the site of the infection. IL-12 will activate natural killer cells. Interferon alpha and beta also activate natural killer cells and increase the cell's ability to resist attack from foreign pathogens.

Some of these cytokines (such as TNF-alpha, IL-1, and IL-6) can also lead to activation and dysfunction of the **coagulation cascade**, leading to both clotting and bleeding. This disorder is known as disseminated intravascular coagulation (DIC).

In some cases, the cascade of events causes increased capillary permeability; vasodilation, leading to low blood pressure; and activation of the coagulation cascade by release of certain cytokines, such as IL-6, to a hyperinflammatory state, causing blood clots and further cell death from poor perfusion. Further cell death causes the release of additional cytokines, which can indiscriminately injure both the pathogen and host cells, and the cycle continues, leading to sepsis, organ dysfunction, and septic shock. Tissue hypoxia can also independently activate inflammation and release of cytokines through the production of nitric oxide and induction of the coagulation cascade through the activation of certain cytokines. Lab tests are currently being developed that look for the protein components or genetic material (messenger RNA) being

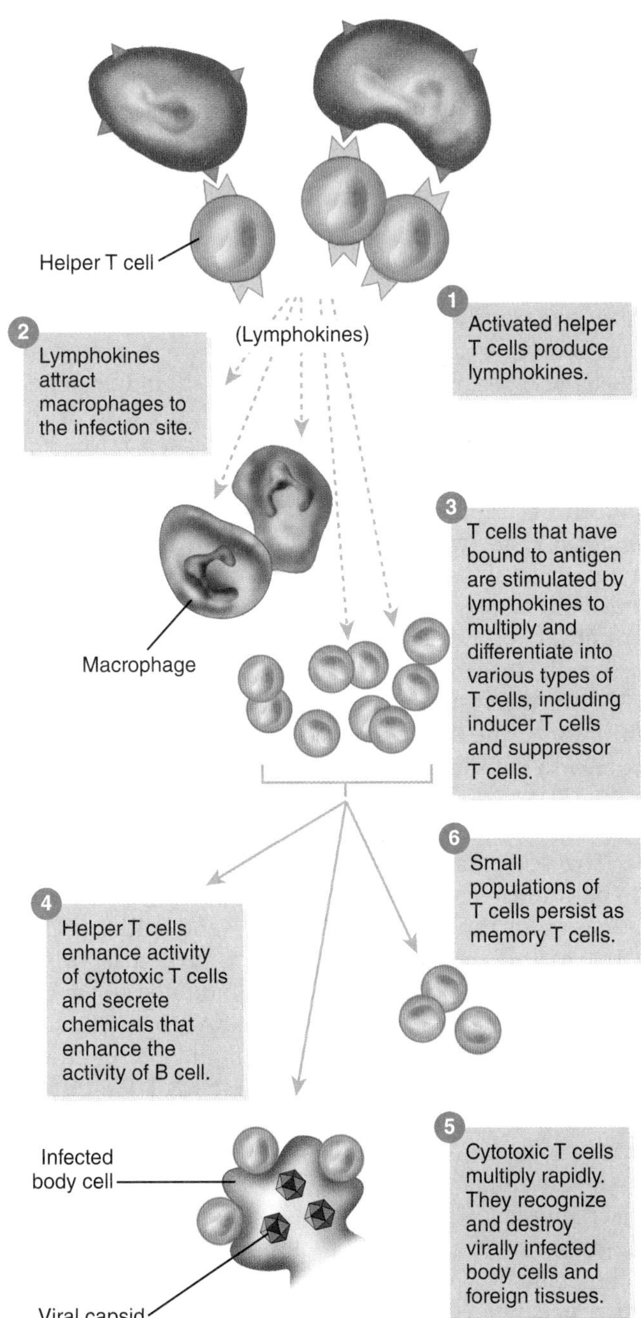
Helper T cell
(Lymphokines)
1 Activated helper T cells produce lymphokines.
2 Lymphokines attract macrophages to the infection site.
3 T cells that have bound to antigen are stimulated by lymphokines to multiply and differentiate into various types of T cells, including inducer T cells and suppressor T cells.
Macrophage
6 Small populations of T cells persist as memory T cells.
4 Helper T cells enhance activity of cytotoxic T cells and secrete chemicals that enhance the activity of B cell.
Infected body cell
5 Cytotoxic T cells multiply rapidly. They recognize and destroy virally infected body cells and foreign tissues.
Viral capsid

Figure 6-2 The cell-mediated immune response.

produced by the body to try and recognize (long before blood cultures show results 48 hours later) whether the patient has a dysregulated inflammatory response due to a viral, bacterial, parasitic, fungal, or autoimmune cause.

Inflammatory cytokines trigger peripheral vasodilation and damage endothelial barriers, especially in capillaries, resulting in "leaky blood vessels." As hypotension and vascular permeability continue, systemic vascular resistance decreases, and the body compensates by increasing cardiac output by increasing the heart rate. At this point, the patient is progressing to septic shock. Unlike hypovolemic shock from blood and fluid loss where the vascular smooth muscle response can help compensate, in septic shock there is a loss of smooth muscle reactivity. Furthermore, when cytokines and microthrombi cause endothelial injury leading to increased capillary leakage, significant shifts in fluid can occur, including third-spacing and tissue edema. This combination of low perfusion and increased pressure on vessels leads to organ hypoperfusion, damage, and death.

Role of Complement Proteins in the Innate and Adaptive Immune Response

The liver produces complement proteins that circulate within the bloodstream. Approximately 30 of these complement proteins are inactive. Some complement proteins are activated by the presence of foreign proteins from microbes. These complement proteins bind to the microbes or antigens, coating them so that phagocytes (natural killer cells, monocytes, and PMNs) can recognize them as foreign. This is called **opsonization**. Other complement proteins may be activated when they encounter products from destroyed cells, such as mitochondria or cytoplasm. This initiates a cascade of events that leads to increased complement activation and increased chemical signaling for phagocytes to gather.

As part of the adaptive immune response, the **complement cascade** leads to complement attachment to the invading microbe's cell wall, disrupting the phospholipid bilayer and causing the foreign cell's death. The increased chemical signaling allows phagocytic neutrophils, monocytes, and killer cells to enter the area of infection. They then attack and envelope the invading microbes.

The immune system has two complement pathways. The alternate pathway plays a vital role during the innate immune response. The classic pathway is part of the adaptive response and involves the interaction of multiple complement proteins to perforate an invading pathogen's cell wall or an infected host's cell wall and lead to its destruction.

The History of Sepsis

Sepsis is when an infection, large or small, triggers an inappropriate systemic inflammatory response, resulting in poor perfusion through a variety of physiologic mechanisms. The concept of sepsis has been attributed to Hippocrates, who described it in his writings. It is derived from the Greek term *sipsi*, which means "to make rotten." Blood putrefaction was also linked to fever in the early BCE period. However, it was not until the 1800s that links were made between poor hand hygiene and fever by the obstetrician Ignaz Semmelweis. At around the same time, Louis Pasteur was developing the germ theory. Pasteur was the first to use a microscope to visualize the single-celled organisms that had been associated with putrefaction. He called these organisms *bacteria*. Pasteur also discovered that high heat could kill the bacteria, leading to the concept of sterilization. Although the link between fever and putrefaction was well known, it was not until the development of modern-day antibiotics, such as penicillin in 1928 and sulfa in 1935, that survivability from bacterial sepsis was seen in any significant fashion.

Sepsis remained a loosely defined term until 1989, when Dr. Roger Bone, an intensive care physician at Rush Medical College, stated, "Sepsis is defined as an invasion of microorganisms and/or their toxins into the bloodstream along with the organism's reaction against this invasion." Dr. Bone noted that the body sometimes responds to infection with an increased heart rate, elevated or lowered body temperature, elevated respiratory rate or increased oxygen demand, and elevated or lowered white blood cell count, all of which put the patient at an increased risk of death. He termed this the systemic inflammatory response syndrome (SIRS). SIRS can also be triggered by pancreatitis, burns, or trauma, but when SIRS is triggered by infection, it is called sepsis.

In 1992, the first major consensus conference on the definition of **sepsis** was held, incorporating SIRS criteria. Sepsis was defined as when two or more of the SIRS criteria are seen in the setting of infection.

SIRS criteria are as follows:

- Temperature > 38°C (100.4°F) or < 36°C (96.8°F)
- Heart rate > 90 beats/min
- Respiratory rate > 20 breaths/min (or arterial carbon dioxide [CO_2] < 32 mm Hg or need for mechanical ventilation)
- White blood cell count > 12 cells/cmm (cubic millimeter) or < 4 cells/cmm or > 10% immature bands

Screening and Prognostic Tools in Sepsis

The International Sepsis Definitions Conference has met multiple times since 1992, incorporating and expanding the view of sepsis based on additional research. We have known for decades that certain populations are at higher risk of death from infection. In 1988, Sorensen and colleagues showed adoptive children had a 5.81-fold increased risk of dying from infection if their biological parents died from sepsis. Since then, we have discovered genetic links with the body's ability to recognize invading microbes, produce certain cell lines, or manufacture cytokines—increasing the risk of death from sepsis.

The 2001 conference developed the concept of PIRO to delineate the risk factors:

- **P**: predisposition (preexisting comorbid conditions)
- **I**: insult/infection (noting that some organisms are more lethal than others)
- **R**: response to the infectious challenge (including SIRS)
- **O**: organ dysfunction and coagulation system failure

During the Third International Consensus Definitions for Sepsis and Septic Shock (Sepsis-3), Singer and colleagues recommended that "[s]epsis should be defined as life-threatening organ dysfunction caused by a dysregulated host response to infection." They refuted the previously held belief that there was progression on a continuum from sepsis to severe sepsis to septic shock, and the term *severe sepsis* was eliminated. The poor sensitivity and specificity of SIRS in the septic patient were shown, and so the Sepsis-3 indicators instead focused on *prognostic* indicators: They showed that if a patient had changes in certain organ systems, such as hepatic, renal, cardiovascular, and respiratory function, they had an *increased risk of death*. The Sepsis-Related Organ Failure Assessment score, also known as the Sequential Organ Failure Assessment (SOFA) score, is commonly incorporated into the intensive care unit care of the septic patient.

This score has been further modified for use outside of the intensive care unit, such as the fast-paced environments of the prehospital setting and initial presentation to the emergency department (when laboratory studies may not be available). The modified qSOFA (or quickSOFA) includes respiratory rate > 22 breaths/min, systolic blood pressure < 90 mm Hg, and altered mental status, and again serves as a quick method of determining patients with a high likelihood of decompensation and death.

Research has shown that whereas SIRS was superior at screening for sepsis, *qSOFA was superior at predicting mortality*. However, neither tool provides great sensitivity and specificity when it comes to identifying patients with sepsis or septic shock. Additional screening tools have been tested and compared to qSOFA and SIRS, such as the Modified Early Warning Score (MEWS) and the National Early Warning Score version 2 (NEWS2). The key component to remember with these screening and scoring systems is that they *incorporate vital signs and mental status*. NEWS2 is a mandatory screening tool used in the United Kingdom that checks seven parameters: temperature, respiratory rate, pulse, oxygen level, systolic blood pressure, mental status, and hypercapnia (hypercarbia). MEWS includes temperature, pulse, blood pressure, respiratory rate, mental status, and urine output, providing a scoring system of 0–3 for each measure to help determine who is at high risk for decompensation and death. Table 6-1 presents a comparison of these scores.

Table 6-1 Comparison of Critical Illness Scores

	SIRS	qSOFA	MEWS	NEWS2
Pulse	X		X	X
Respiratory rate	X	X	X	X
Temperature	X		X	X
Systolic blood pressure		X	X	X
Mental status		X	X	X
Oxygen saturation				X (+ hypercapnia)
Use of supplemental oxygen				X
Urine output			X	
Leukocyte count	X>			

SIRS, systemic inflammatory response syndrome; qSOFA, Quick Sequential Organ Failure Assessment; MEWS, Modified Early Warning Score; NEWS2, National Early Warning Score version 2.

Data from Churpek MM, Snyder A, Han K, et al. Quick sepsis-related organ failure assessment, systemic inflammatory response syndrome, and early warning scores for detecting clinical deterioration in infected patients outside the intensive care unit. *Am J Respir Crit Care Med.* 2017;195(7):906–911. doi:10.1164/rccm.201604-0854OC.

The AMLS Assessment Pathway ▶▶▶▶

▼ Initial Observations

The AMLS Assessment Pathway for sepsis will help you recognize, evaluate, differentiate, and care for a patient with sepsis or septic shock. An organized and systematic assessment is crucial to identify sepsis early, when signs and symptoms may be very subtle but more opportunity exists for intervention. By the time shock becomes clearly recognizable, organ dysfunction may have already occurred or the effectiveness of interventions may be severely limited.

Scene Safety Considerations

Sepsis itself does not generally present any inherent scene safety issues, but a strict focus on the patient can lead you to miss critical environmental clues and cues indicating safety issues, as well as information important to your assessment. Some agents, such as anthrax, tuberculosis, Ebola, meningococcus, COVID-19, and Middle East respiratory syndrome (MERS), can be highly infectious, so maintaining respiratory and droplet precautions is always advised. If the patient is having a significant productive cough, but not showing signs of respiratory distress, placing a mask on the patient may prevent spread of infection to first responders. Universal precautions should always be followed.

Following verification of scene safety, investigate whether the patient has an advance directive. Portable medical orders or POLST are helpful in clarifying the patient's goals for care. (POLST once stood for Physician Orders for Life-Sustaining Treatment, but National POLST no longer uses this definition.) Some states use different names for POLST forms or may allow nonphysicians to complete a POLST form. If possible, promptly locate the person named on a durable power of attorney for health care. This person can help guide whether care should focus on maximal resuscitation efforts or patient comfort.

Patient Cardinal Presentation/ Chief Complaint

Sepsis can often masquerade as other illnesses, so a detailed history and physical exam are vital. For example, a patient who presents with altered mental status may initially appear to be experiencing a stroke, but a urinary tract infection may, in fact, be causing the confusion. Some common cardinal presentations and chief complaints related to sepsis include the following (**Figure 6-3**):

- Pneumonia
- Urinary tract infection

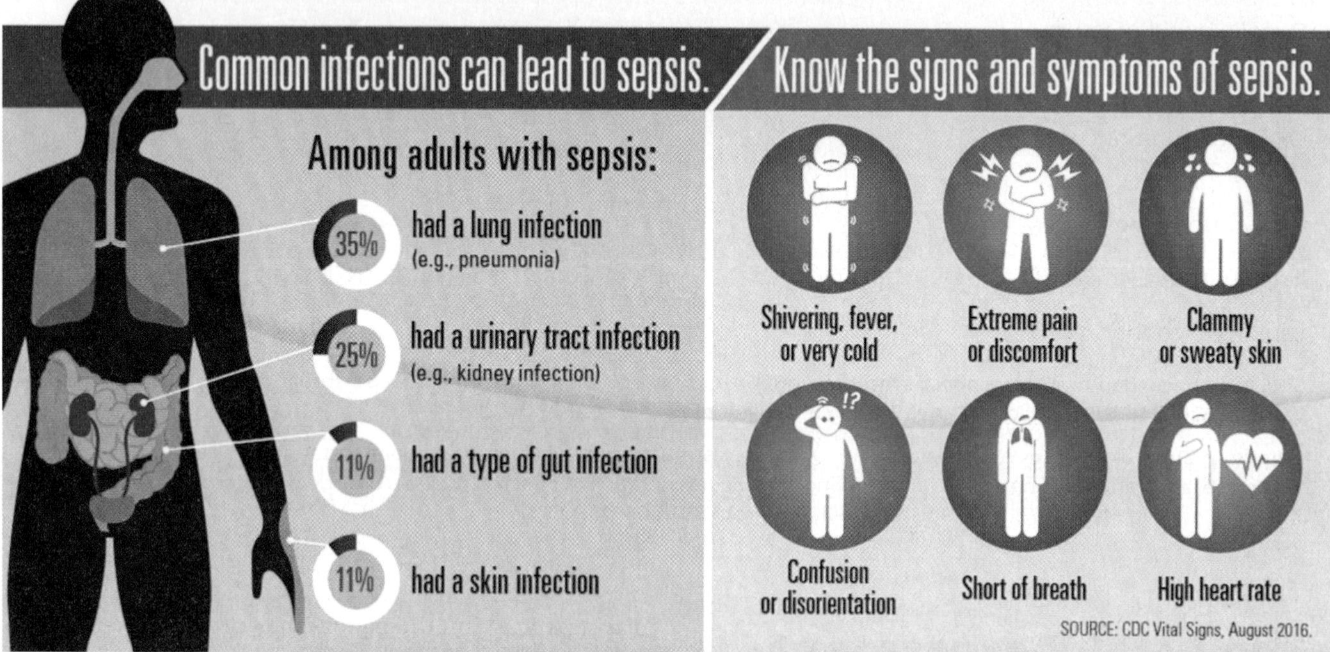

Figure 6-3 Some common causes and presentations of sepsis.

Reproduced from National Center for Emerging and Zoonotic Infectious Diseases. Healthcare providers are key to preventing infections and illnesses that can lead to sepsis. Centers for Disease Control and Prevention. August 23, 2016. https://stacks.cdc.gov/view/cdc/59352

- Cellulitis (skin infections)
- Intra-abdominal infections: appendicitis, diverticulitis, cholecystitis, intussusception, pelvic inflammatory disease, bowel obstruction.
- Meningitis
- Recent failure of outpatient treatment for an infection

Primary Survey

As with every patient you encounter, start with the primary survey to identify any immediate life threats. Is the patient maintaining the airway? How is the breathing and circulation? Are there any signs of disability, such as change in level of consciousness? Expose the patient to see if there are signs of skin infection, recent surgery, or indwelling devices. Look at the patient's environment. Is the patient covered in emesis or cold to touch? Has the patient been on the ground for an extended period following a fall? Has there been exposure to excessive heat or cold? How may the environment have played a role in the patient's presentation?

Level of Consciousness

Many patients with sepsis and septic shock present with an altered level of consciousness. Use of a standardized assessment tool may help clinicians better quantify changes in level of consciousness over time, an important indicator of deterioration or improvement. Asking family members, friends, or care providers about the patient's *baseline mental status* and *how it has changed* is very important—for example, if a patient is normally able to complete activities of daily living such as eating and dressing, but was unable to do so today. Family members may recognize subtle changes in confusion that may be important indicators of sepsis, such as a patient who normally manages their medications is confused about how to take them. AVPU (**A**lert, responsive to **V**erbal stimuli, responsive to **P**ain, **U**nresponsive) is a mnemonic used frequently in the EMS setting to track changes in mental status and is part of MEWS and NEWS2.

Airway and Breathing

Respiratory rate and work of breathing are often the first signs of the increased metabolic demands as the body begins to fight an infection, regardless of whether the infection involves the respiratory system. In addition to possible respiratory infections, such as pneumonia, that may trigger sepsis, the excessive response from inflammatory mediators may cause acute respiratory distress syndrome (ARDS). If the patient is experiencing metabolic acidosis from infection, then they may have a compensatory increase in breathing rate to try and return the body to equilibrium, as discussed in detail in Chapter 3, *Respiratory Disorders*, and Chapter 11, *Endocrine and Metabolic Disorders*. The infectious agent may also exacerbate underlying disease processes such as heart failure (HF) or chronic obstructive pulmonary disease (COPD). Efficient treatment of the underlying disease as well as timely identification and treatment of sepsis can potentially stop the exacerbation of HF or COPD or the development of ARDS. As with any airway and respiratory issue, this begins with identifying a compromised airway or deficient breathing. When a patient reports dyspnea or has an observable increased work of breathing, you must pause and ask yourself, "Is this patient in respiratory distress, or is the patient exhibiting signs of respiratory failure? Could there be another cause?" If the patient improves with simple resuscitation maneuvers, then respiratory distress is the answer. If, however, the patient does not improve with basic interventions (such as supplemental oxygen or a breathing treatment), or if any patient with respiratory distress has signs of fatigue or altered mental status, then respiratory failure may be imminent. Immediate resuscitation measures should be implemented to support the patient's airway and ventilation. The following lists some of the indicators of impending respiratory failure:

- Respiratory rate > 24 or < 6 breaths/min
- Oxygen saturation < 94%
- End-tidal carbon dioxide ($ETCO_2$) < 25 mm Hg (3.3 kPa)
- Changes in skin color, including cyanosis of the lips
- Tracheal tugging
- Nasal flaring
- Intercostal retractions or subcostal retractions
- Adventitious lung sounds
- Inability to clear oral secretions
- Changes in body position to sniffing or tripod positions

First, ensure that the patient is protecting their airway. If there is concern the patient cannot maintain a patent airway, immediate actions may include inserting a nasopharyngeal or oropharyngeal airway; placing a more advanced airway adjunct, such as an extraglottic tube; or performing endotracheal intubation. Once the airway is secured, focus on improving oxygenation to at least 94%. Actions may include providing supplemental oxygen, continuous positive airway pressure, or ventilation via bag-valve mask. Please refer to Chapter 3, *Respiratory Disorders*, for additional information.

Circulation/Perfusion

Sepsis may decrease perfusion through distributive, hypovolemic, and obstructive shock in a variety of combinations. Signs of poor perfusion include the following:

- Weak or thready pulses
- Pulse rate > 120 or < 60 beats/min
- Irregular pulse rate
- Systolic blood pressure < 90 mm Hg
- Mean arterial pressure (MAP) < 65 mm Hg
- Shock Index ≥ 1
- Capillary refill > 2 seconds
- $ETCO_2$ < 25 mm Hg (3.3 kPa)
- Changes in skin color

Due to the multiple mechanisms through which sepsis produces shock, the patient must be monitored carefully for early signs of decompensation. Evidence of compromised perfusion should prompt immediate life-saving intervention. Intravenous (IV) or intraosseous (IO) access should be obtained, and rapid, but measured, fluid resuscitation should be initiated. If the patient is initially unresponsive to fluids, vasopressors such as norepinephrine or push-dose sequential boluses of dilute epinephrine should be considered while fluids are continued. Reevaluate how the patient is tolerating these interventions. Is the patient feeling better? Have the patient's vital signs improved? Does the patient appear more awake, alert, and better able to follow commands? A sepsis alert should be declared as soon as you determine the patient meets criteria, to provide as much advance notice to the receiving hospital as possible.

▾ First Impression

In the early phases, sepsis is as subtle and difficult to diagnose as it is easy to treat. As it progresses to the point where it is so severe that diagnosis is obvious, sepsis becomes far more difficult to treat. Your knowledge of anatomy, physiology, pathophysiology, and screening tools for sepsis is the first step in being able to recognize when sepsis is the cause of the patient's illness, even when it is not obvious. If you suspect sepsis, you should consider the patient to be sick and high priority even if there are not yet overt signs of shock.

Although not its original intention, PIRO can provide a good framework to focus patient assessment.

- *Predisposition*: Assess for any predispositions the patient has toward infection, such as indwelling catheters, immunosuppressant medications, or lack of vaccinations, or predispositions to shock, such as any diseases or disorders that compromise the patient's cardiac or respiratory capacity.
- *Infection*: Assess for any known or suspected infections, including obviously infected wounds, current or recent courses of antibiotics, or signs and symptoms such as cough and congestion or nausea and vomiting.
- *Response*: Assess vital signs to look for subtle indications of compromised perfusion, including not only mentation, respirations, pulse oximetry, pulse rate, and blood pressure, but also MAP, lactate, and urine output.
- *Organ dysfunction*: Assess key indicators of organ failure, especially those that will trigger a sepsis alert or code sepsis at a receiving facility. In addition to altered mental status and compromised cardiorespiratory vital signs, symptoms of organ failure include jaundice, low urine output, fluid retention, bleeding disorders, and sudden gastrointestinal pain or problems.

The initial presentation of a patient with sepsis or septic shock often focuses on an infection. In some cases, the presentation may focus on signs and symptoms of shock. A patient with sepsis may initially present simply with unexplained altered mental status or other ambiguous signs and symptoms. With the primary survey and associated interventions complete, a patient with a presentation of infection, shock, or nonspecific complaints should be evaluated to rule out sepsis and/or septic shock as a differential diagnosis. Sepsis is more common than stroke or heart attack in the prehospital setting; therefore, the EMS clinician should have a high index of suspicion in assessing the undifferentiated patient.

▼ Detailed Assessment

History Taking

History taking for patients where sepsis or septic shock is a potential diagnosis should focus on the presence or risk of infection and the presence or risk of shock. When managing high-priority patients or patients who are at risk of rapid deterioration, it is of the utmost importance to gather key information from the patient history in the most effective manner possible.

OPQRST and SAMPLER

Begin with clarification of the history of present illness, moving on to the past medical history. Use the OPQRST and SAMPLER formats to efficiently obtain and quantify information that will be key to your differential diagnosis. If the patient has a history of similar complaints, ask how today's symptoms compare with those experienced previously—are they the same or different from the last time? If they are different, how so? Similarly, with a potential differential diagnosis of sepsis or septic shock, it is important to develop a timeline of events. When did events occur? When did signs or symptoms change and how? Remember: Even though the timeline of events may have taken a while to get to this point, the patient may now be approaching rapid deterioration. This systematic approach will provide you with information crucial to differentiating the patient's priority problem, and it will help direct the rest of your detailed assessment as well as the priority treatments you provide. Table 6-2 outlines some key findings from the patient history that may contribute to a differential diagnosis of sepsis. Here again it can be helpful to consider the key elements of sepsis as PIRO: Predisposition, Infection, Response to the infection, and Organ dysfunction.

Secondary Survey

Vital Signs

Baseline vital signs for patients with suspected sepsis include pulse, respiration, blood pressure, MAP, oxygen saturation, temperature, $ETCO_2$ measurements, mental status (AVPU), urine output, and blood glucose and blood lactate levels. Start with simple diagnostics such as basic vital signs, systolic blood pressure, AVPU, and respiratory rate. Measurement and trending of other vital signs such as MAP, $ETCO_2$, and blood lactate, if available, can help improve the accuracy of your differential diagnosis as well as your ability to prioritize and focus patient care.

Whereas the primary survey focused on rapidly identifying and addressing life threats, the secondary survey will require more in-depth measurement and analysis to provide a clear picture of the patient's condition and priority needs, as well as the patient's response, or lack of response, to interventions. Remember that the early presentation of sepsis can be very nonspecific, so ensure that you maintain a high level of suspicion. Frequent reassessment, especially of critical patients, will provide key information on the trends of patient vital signs as deteriorating, stabilizing, or improving. This will help you with rapid clinical decision making and rapid priority interventions. It will also help you determine when interventions need to be scaled back or discontinued in order to provide maximum benefit with minimum unwanted effects.

Table 6-2 History Taking for Sepsis

Common Chief Complaints (Commonly presenting with infection or organ dysfunction)
■ Flulike symptoms ■ Fever or hypothermia ■ Nausea/vomiting/diarrhea ■ Pus/discharge/skin discoloration ■ Dysuria or cloudy, foul-smelling urine ■ Cough or shortness of breath
Common Sites of Infection
■ Respiratory tract (approximately 35% of sepsis cases) ■ Intra-abdominal ■ Urinary tract ■ Soft tissues/wounds
Age Factors (Predispositions)
■ Younger than 1 year ■ Older than 65 years
Risk Factors (Predispositions)
■ Immunocompromised (patients receiving immunotherapy, chemotherapy, antirejection medications, anti-inflammatory medications or steroids; human immunodeficiency virus [HIV] infection) ■ Diabetes ■ Chronic liver disease ■ Chronic renal disease ■ Cancer ■ Chronic lung disease ■ Cerebrovascular accident (e.g., impaired swallowing, hemiparesis with risk for decubitus ulcers) ■ Open wounds or indwelling tubes or catheters ■ Recent hospitalization, surgery, or medical procedure ■ Intravenous drug abuse
Past Medical History
■ Current or recent infection ■ Acquired immunodeficiency syndrome (AIDS) ■ Use of immunosuppressive agents (e.g., in rheumatoid arthritis, psoriasis, chemotherapy) ■ Cancer ■ Diabetes ■ Sickle cell disease or splenectomy* ■ Cystic fibrosis ■ Liver or splenic or renal dysfunction ■ Poor cardiac function ■ Poor respiratory function ■ Recent trauma or surgery ■ Pregnancy or recent delivery ■ Breaches of the skin, including burns, trauma, or IV drug abuse ■ Presence of indwelling catheters ■ Lack of current immunizations

*A nonfunctioning spleen increases a person's risk for infection, especially from encapsulated bacteria such as *Streptococcus* and *Meningococcus* (Waterhouse-Friderichsen syndrome).

Physical Exam

Through the course of your primary survey, you will have already performed an assessment of the patient's physical state. It is important to remember this is not the same as the physical exam that is part of the detailed assessment. The detailed physical exam can reveal a variety of key clinical findings indicating the presence and severity of both infection and shock.

Neurologic Exam

Assessing level of consciousness and cognitive function is crucial in patients with suspected sepsis or septic shock. Mental status is a good rough indicator of adequate perfusion and oxygenation of the central nervous system. In patients with sepsis, it is thought that metabolic encephalopathy may further contribute to findings of mild to severe confusion often accompanied by anxiety and agitation. These are common neurologic findings in septic patients, especially the elderly.

A detailed neurologic evaluation can be especially helpful in narrowing a differential diagnosis. Was the onset of the neurologic deficit sudden? Is the neurologic deficit focused on a particular part of the body? This may lead to stroke rising to the top of the differential diagnosis, but do not completely discount the possibility of sepsis.

Evaluation of mental status is an important part of patient examination. Assess the patient's orientation to person, place, and time. Assess clarity of speech, verbal coherence, and response time. Frequent reassessment is important to determine deterioration, stabilization, or improvement of the patient's condition. Any changes to a patient's mental status are significant to the patient picture.

Head and Neck Exam

Signs of infection of the head and neck include severe headache; stiff neck; earache; sore throat; sinus pain, especially with discharge; and swelling of the lymph nodes of the neck, known as submandibular, anterior cervical, or posterior cervical lymphadenopathy. With narrowing of the airway in the neck, you may hear stridor (commonly seen in pediatric croup infections).

Chest Exam

Chest infections may present with mild to severe symptoms such as nonproductive or productive cough, pleuritic chest pain, dyspnea, bronchial breath sounds, localized crackles, or decreased breath sounds as evidence of pulmonary consolidation (where an area of lung tissue becomes filled with liquid, as usually evident on chest x-rays).

Cardiac infections, including pericarditis, endocarditis, and myocarditis, may present with muffled heart sounds, rub, or murmur. These infections are more commonly seen in patients with indwelling catheters or a history of IV drug use. Patients with an inflamed cardiac lining (pericarditis) may complain of pain relieved with sitting upright and leaning forward. In the case of infected lining and valves of the heart (endocarditis), an infected heart valve may be throwing septic emboli throughout the body. This can manifest as splinter hemorrhages to the fingernails, stroke, pulmonary emboli, ischemic bowel, or a skin rash. They may also have a murmur on exam because the heart valve works less efficiently. If the heart muscle itself is infected (myocarditis), the patient may present with signs of cardiogenic shock (crackles on lung exam, low blood pressure, increased jugular venous distension).

Abdominal Exam

Infections of the abdomen may present with findings of abdominal pain: tenderness on palpation, especially point tenderness; guarding; distention; vomiting; constipation; diarrhea; and referred pain to the shoulder, chest, or back.

Pelvic and Genitourinary Exam

Signs and symptoms of infections of the genitourinary tract may include pelvic or flank pain; vaginal, penile, urethral, or anal discharge; dark or discolored urine; pain on urination, especially accompanied by frequency and urgency; or referred pain to the abdomen.

Examination of the Soft Tissues and Extremities

Infections of the skin, soft tissues, and bones commonly present with focal pain, edema, redness/discoloration, blotchiness, purpura, ulceration, formation of bullae, and discharge of purulent material or other fluids.

Diagnostics

Because sepsis can present with very subtle signs and symptoms initially, as it progresses to septic shock it is important to frequently reassess the patient and make use of additional diagnostic tools in patient assessment and reassessment. Although no specific set of diagnostic criteria has been definitively shown to identify sepsis in the prehospital environment, significant evidence exists to show that educated and sepsis-aware clinicians can improve their differential diagnoses and clinical decision making through proper use of diagnostic equipment.

It is always important to start with a *complete set* of vital signs. One should be concerned about sepsis in an adult patient if the heart rate is noted to be > 90 beats/min or < 60 beats/min; breathing rate is noted to be > 20 breaths/min or < 6 breaths/min; temperature is > 38°C (100.4°F) or < 36°C (96.8°F); systolic blood pressure is < 90 mm Hg, or 40 mm Hg lower than the patient's baseline; or MAP is < 65 mm Hg. Detecting sepsis is much more challenging in a pediatric patient because vital signs change with age. Consider consulting the Pediatric Surviving Sepsis Guidelines or use available apps to determine abnormal vital signs in the pediatric population and risk of sepsis.

Thermometry

When envisioning sepsis or septic shock, the picture almost always includes a patient with an obvious fever. This is one of the most important myths of sepsis to break and highlights the importance of correct use and interpretation of diagnostic equipment and the information it can provide.

Although it is true that many patients with sepsis present with a fever, the lack of fever most definitely *does not* rule out sepsis. In fact, several studies have shown quite the opposite, finding that patients with sepsis who are *hypothermic* (< 35°C [< 95°F]) have a *higher mortality* than patients who have a mild to moderate fever (37.0–39.5°C [98.6–103.1°F]). In fact, patients with the highest fevers (> 39.5°C [103.1°F]) were found to have the lowest mortality of all groups. Whether this is because a high fever may provide or indicate a particularly effective physiologic response to sepsis, or patients with especially high fevers are more easily identified as potentially septic, or possibly for other reasons, is unknown. What is clear is that obtaining initial and ongoing patient temperature can be an important adjunct to direct patient care and can predict patient outcome.

A variety of thermometer types are currently used in the prehospital environment, including sensors to detect oral, rectal, tympanic, and temporal artery temperatures. These have varying degrees of accuracy, and EMS agencies and their medical directors should evaluate the most appropriate type of thermometer for their use. Regardless of the sensor you use, ensure that you can obtain a reading of clinical usefulness. Follow manufacturer's instructions on the care, maintenance, and operation of your particular device, paying special attention to the following:

- The device must be stored in the vehicle in such a way that minimizes the amount of impact, vibration, and temperature extremes that may cause the device to produce unreliable readings.
- Some devices require regular calibration to ensure they produce clinically reliable readings.
- Some devices cannot be used under field conditions of environmental heat or cold.
- Place and maintain the probe in the exact position the sensor needs to read the temperature. For example, for an oral probe this would be in the sublingual pocket, as opposed to simply under the tongue.

Pulse Oximeter

One of the most common and useful noninvasive diagnostic devices applicable for the evaluation of patients with suspected sepsis or septic shock is the pulse oximeter. Although the operation and function of the pulse oximeter is no different for patients with suspected sepsis than it is for anyone else under your care, it is especially important to ensure that the readings you receive are not subject to error. In order to provide a viable reading, you must ensure that the plethysmograph (pulse oximeter waveform) is showing an adequate waveform. Keep in mind that the pulse oximeter reading can be inaccurate if the probe is poorly connected or if the patient has dark skin pigmentation; has poor perfusion, especially to the site where the probe is attached; is significantly hypotensive, hypovolemic, or hypothermic; is moving or in bright light; is on vasoactive drugs; or has sickle cell anemia, dysrhythmia, or an SpO_2 (oxygen saturation) of < 70%.

Blood Pressure

Although blood pressure is an important vital sign, the diagnostic value of trending repeated blood pressure measurements can make a noninvasive blood pressure (NIBP) cuff a useful diagnostic adjunct for patients with suspected sepsis. In addition, NIBP monitors often automatically calculate a patient's MAP, which is the average arterial blood pressure in a single cardiac cycle. This pressure is calculated as systolic blood pressure added to two times the diastolic pressure (because the diastolic portion of the cycle is twice as long as the systolic portion), divided by three (to get the average of two parts diastolic and one part systolic of the cardiac cycle):

$$\mathbf{MAP} = \frac{\left[\mathbf{Systolic} + (\mathbf{2} \times \mathbf{Diastolic})\right]}{\mathbf{3}}$$

MAP can give a clinician a more complete picture of a patient's circulatory status than that of a simple blood pressure. In addition, because MAP uses only a single number, it can make it easier to observe positive or negative trending of the patient's circulatory status. A normal range for MAP is between 70 and 110 mm Hg. The target MAP for patients experiencing sepsis is > 65 mm Hg. This target can be used to guide fluid resuscitation.

Waveform Capnography

$ETCO_2$ monitoring is not only a method of assessing a patient's ventilatory status, but it can also provide useful information about the patient's metabolism and circulatory status. The human body functions ideally with a pH of 7.35–7.45. The kidneys and lungs act in concert to prevent an acidotic or alkalotic state. In sepsis, patients have an overactive metabolic state, leading to lactate buildup in areas of poor perfusion and metabolic acidosis. The body's method of compensating for this metabolic acidosis is to increase ventilation to blow off CO_2.

$ETCO_2$ has been closely correlated with the presence of lactate, showing an inverse relationship: An $ETCO_2$ < 25 mm Hg (3.3 kPa) closely correlates with a serum lactate > 4 mmol/L (36 mg/dL). $ETCO_2$ provides a rapid, noninvasive diagnostic tool for the identification and evaluation of patients with undifferentiated shock, as well as patients with identified sepsis or septic shock. Although capnography may indicate a low $ETCO_2$ level that is consistent with metabolic acidosis, EMS clinicians should understand that there is significant overlap in levels based upon respiratory and metabolic factors in any given patient, and these nonspecific findings are not reliable to make diagnoses of sepsis or metabolic acidosis.

Point-of-Care Ultrasound

Prehospital point-of-care ultrasound (POCUS) is the natural extension of diagnostic technology from the emergency department, where its use has expanded rapidly in recent years. Prehospital POCUS can be a critical diagnostic tool to help differentiate patients with hypotension or shock of unknown origin using the Rapid Ultrasound for Shock and Hypotension (RUSH) protocol, which uses a phased array probe and linear probe to rapidly examine potential sources of shock and hypotension, including the heart, inferior vena cava, Morrison's abdominal view (right upper quadrant), aorta, and pneumothorax. Specific to sepsis and septic shock, the RUSH exam is looking for identifiers of distributive shock such as a heart in a hyperdynamic state (walls move > 90% or touch at the end of systole), indicating possible early sepsis, or a heart in a state of poor contractility, indicating possible late sepsis. Prehospital POCUS can also help clinicians identify other sources of shock coexisting with sepsis. Accurate use of POCUS requires significant training and experience before a clinician is capable of identifying various diagnoses on these exams. EMS agencies that utilize POCUS need to be committed to significant training and quality improvement reviews to ensure competence.

Laboratory Studies

Blood Cultures

Although blood cultures obtained in the prehospital environment will not provide any immediate diagnostic information to EMS clinicians, they may be important in altering antimicrobial treatments during a patient's hospitalization. To date, although studies have shown an association of early antibiotics with improved patient outcomes, they have not yet identified the optimal approach in balancing early antibiotics with the value of obtaining accurate blood cultures for use in altering care later. Logistical concerns include how to store supplies and train personnel. Additional challenges include multiple hospitals or hospital systems using different types of blood culture collection systems. Regional solutions may be possible, but given the complexities of multiple hospital systems having to agree on one system, this is a significant barrier in most prehospital environments. Most hospital systems are concerned about meeting and reporting core measures, of which obtaining blood cultures before antibiotics is one. Unfortunately, these core measures rarely take into consideration the prehospital phase of care, and thus a mismatch of priorities is identified.

Lactate

Lactic acid, or lactate, is a compound formed as a result of anaerobic metabolism. Lactate is thought to arise as a function of anaerobic metabolism resulting from shock and, more important, be produced by the body as cellular fuel in response to stimulation of the beta-2 adrenergic receptors. This stimulation upregulates glycolysis, generating more pyruvate than can be used by the cell's mitochondria, resulting in a rise in lactate.

One form of lactate, L-lactate, is sensitive but not specific to the presence of sepsis. This means that measure of lactate is not a test that can determine sepsis the way a glucometer can determine hypoglycemia. However, lactate can serve as an important indicator of the presence and level of tissue hypoperfusion and physiologic stress. As with the use of other diagnostics, measurements of blood lactate must be put together with other parts of the patient assessment to facilitate pattern recognition and allow effective clinical decision making. For example, lactic acid levels may be elevated in cases of hypoperfusion (from myocardial infarction, blood loss, or sepsis), poor mitochondrial function, liver dysfunction, and metformin metabolism. Multiple studies have shown that the higher the lactate level initially measured, and the slower the lactate clearance, the greater the mortality, prompting its use as a nonspecific measure of hypoperfusion and risk of death.

Septic shock can be identified in patients with organ failure caused by a dysregulated response to infection that requires vasopressors to maintain a MAP > 65 mm Hg and who have a serum lactate > 2 mmol/L (18 mg/dL). Lactate is useful not only for initial identification and assessment of sepsis and septic shock, but it can also be used as a guide for ongoing resuscitation.

One must keep in mind that any state of hypoperfusion can lead to an elevated lactate level. So, although sepsis must be strongly considered, other sources of hypoperfusion must also be explored. For example, patients with end-stage liver disease or those with diabetes on chronic metformin may present with elevated lactic acid from a nonseptic cause.

Beyond blood cultures, additional bloodwork for laboratory analysis may be appropriate. Likewise, some patients may have recent laboratory studies presented as part of their medical history. Although these may not be of priority for treatment in the prehospital environment, they may be of significant value for clinical decisions further down this patient's continuum of care. In addition to point-of-care testing of lactate, point-of-care glucose monitoring may also be of value for patients with sepsis.

Refine the Differential Diagnosis

Septic shock is not simply the occurrence of acute circulatory failure in the presence of infection. Septic shock is a subset of sepsis in which intense circulatory, cellular, and metabolic abnormalities occur, producing a higher risk of mortality than with sepsis alone. Septic shock is a severe illness demanding more intense assessment and coordinated treatment.

Septic shock is clinically defined by the need for vasopressor administration to maintain a MAP $\geq$ 65 mm Hg and the presence of a serum lactate level $>$ 2 mmol/L (18 mg/dL) despite fluid resuscitation. This combination is associated with hospital mortality rates greater than 40%. If the patient has a change in vital signs and mental status associated with infection, suspect sepsis and voice your concerns to emergency department staff.

Ongoing Management

In addition to the challenge of identifying sepsis early, when the presentation is subtle but the opportunities for intervention are greater, there is the challenge for management where treatment must be aggressive but guided by frequent reassessment to avoid over-resuscitation. The differing presentations of sepsis and septic shock will require varied approaches to resuscitation. Not all treatments outlined in this section will be appropriate for all patients and, again, even treatments requiring aggressive intervention must be applied carefully to avoid causing more harm than good.

Ongoing management can follow the same basic systematic approach of evaluating and addressing primarily issues of airway, breathing, and circulation/perfusion, as needed. Secondary issues, including glucose and electrolyte disturbances, temperature regulation, and administration of antibiotics, may also be considered. Finally, but perhaps most importantly, is the effective coordination of ongoing management with colleagues in the emergency department, not only through use of some form of a sepsis alert, but also through an effective patient hand-off process so that hospital care can maintain the patient care progress and momentum prehospital care has achieved.

Airway Management

With some exceptions noted here, basic and advanced airway management for patients with sepsis should be approached in the same way as for all other patients. Evaluate the patient's current and near-future ability to manage their airway and provide interventions as appropriate to ensure patency. Traditional interventions such as suctioning and the insertion of oropharyngeal and nasopharyngeal airways, supraglottic/extraglottic airways, or endotracheal intubation may be appropriate.

When considering rapid sequence, delayed sequence, or medication-facilitated intubation, use caution with any medications that may precipitate hypotension. Ketamine is an induction agent that maintains cardiovascular stability and has a neutral effect on the immune system. Etomidate may block the body's normal stress response.

Respiratory Management

The multiorgan dysfunction occurring during sepsis may produce inadequate oxygenation and ventilation through a variety of pathways. Supportive oxygen is appropriate if the patient is hypoxemic ($SpO_2 < 94\%$). If ventilatory assistance is needed, it may be provided through use of a manual bag-valve device or automatic transport ventilator. Ventilatory assistance may be particularly effective to increase ventilation and oxygenation and reduce the patient's workload and oxygen demand.

Positive-pressure ventilation may increase intrathoracic pressure, which will decrease cardiac preload and potentially worsen hypotension and shock. This highlights the challenges of providing interventions for these patients. Patients with sepsis, and especially septic shock, may be far more fragile than they initially present. Interventions intended to improve one aspect of the patient's condition may have unintended consequences on other aspects of the patient's condition. This is why reassessment and consideration of the full patient picture are crucial after initiating any intervention.

Fluid Resuscitation

Rapid vascular access, either IV or IO, is important for fluid resuscitation and medication administration in patients with sepsis. For patients who are hypotensive or with a lactate $\geq$ 2 mmol/L (18 mg/dL), recommended resuscitation is rapid infusion of 30 mL/kg of crystalloid fluids until any of the following occur:

- MAP $>$ 65 mm Hg
- Systolic blood pressure $>$ 90 mm Hg
- Crackles on lung auscultation
- Shortness of breath and hypoxia
- Lactate $<$ 2 mmol/L (18 mg/dL)

Although rapid fluid administration has been shown to improve patient outcome, frequent reassessment is crucial as the risks of fluid overload include pulmonary edema, lung injury, HF, abdominal compartment syndrome, and cerebral edema.

Vasopressor Administration

Vasopressor medications are indicated for patients who remain hypotensive after initial fluid resuscitation. Pressor medications, in order of preference, include norepinephrine or combinations of norepinephrine, EPINEPHrine, and/or vasopressin administered to a target MAP of > 65 mm Hg. Norepinephrine is the pressor of choice for patients in septic shock. You may consider early addition of norepinephrine as your IV fluid bolus is infusing. DOPamine most likely should be avoided as a pressor agent because it has been shown to result in a higher incidence of cardiac dysrhythmias and greater mortality than the use of norepinephrine. Some EMS agencies use "push-dose EPINEPHrine," which is the administration of small boluses of dilute EPINEPHrine that are titrated to the patient's MAP or systolic blood pressure.

Glucose and Electrolyte Disturbances

Far below the priority level of management of airway, breathing, and circulatory disturbances, patients may be evaluated by point-of-care testing for abnormal electrolyte or glucose levels. Correction of hypoglycemia through the administration of 10% dextrose may be appropriate.

Antipyretics

Although it may be tempting to administer an antipyretic medication to control fever for patient comfort, current research suggests that administration of an antipyretic medication to patients with sepsis or septic shock does not significantly change outcomes.

Antibiotic Administration

Research has shown early administration of antibiotics contributes to improved outcomes for patients with sepsis. Standard treatment includes initiating broad-spectrum antibiotics covering all likely pathogens within 1 hour of recognition. As such, in some areas, paramedics have been educated to effectively identify critically ill septic patients; perform diagnostics, including lactate testing; draw blood cultures; and administer broad-spectrum antibiotics in the field. Although drawing blood cultures in the field prior to administration of broad-spectrum antibiotics may be considered best practice, it is important to note that it is clinically appropriate to proceed with administration of antibiotics without blood cultures if the drawing of blood cultures would result in a substantial delay. As a delay per hour in antibiotic administration has been shown to have a 4% mortality increase, it is reasonable to consider empiric antibiotic administration in the prehospital environment. A previous randomized controlled trial in the prehospital environment with the administration of cefTRIAXone did not demonstrate a benefit; however, research is ongoing, and several prehospital care programs across the globe currently administer antibiotics to help expedite control of the infection for patients suffering from sepsis and septic shock. Additional study will continue to help clarify this issue.

Calling a Sepsis Alert

Worldwide, a variety of criteria exist to trigger prehospital sepsis alerts to notify the receiving hospital of a possible patient with sepsis and to mobilize their bundles of care. The differences among the criteria used in these systems usually reflect an attempt to use the current equipment and capacities of the EMS clinicians to improve the sensitivity and specificity of detecting patients with sepsis. In this way, patients receive the most appropriate prehospital care, and prehospital healthcare clinicians coordinate effectively with clinician colleagues in the receiving emergency department.

Effective use of a sepsis alert protocol may decrease time to treatment in the emergency department and may improve patient mortality. Although a seamless transfer of care is essential in all hand offs between EMS and the receiving facility, this transfer of care report is particularly critical in patients with serious time-sensitive illnesses such as sepsis.

Special Populations

A common factor among older, pregnant, and younger patients putting them at risk for sepsis is a less-effective immune system, making it more likely for them to get an infection and more likely for these infections to be severe. Furthermore, although it is for different reasons among these special populations, they are all likely to have comorbid factors contributing to the rapid progression of shock should sepsis develop.

Older Adult Patients

Although people aged 65 years and older make up approximately 12% of the U.S. population, they make up 65% of sepsis cases in hospitals. This may be due to a variety of factors. As people age, their immune systems become less effective, resulting in more frequent and more severe infections. This can be compounded by other risk factors common among older adults, such as skin tears and sores, which can provide greater opportunity for infectious agents to enter the body than in younger adults with healthy integumentary systems. Furthermore, frequent and prolonged hospitalizations (due to other causes such as myocardial infarction or stroke) and recovery periods can contribute to the increased likelihood and severity of infections and development of sepsis.

The most common causes of infection among older adults include pneumonia and urinary tract infections. Although the chief complaint of an older patient or their caregiver may focus on discomfort caused by the infection itself, clinicians must be sure to follow the systematic AMLS Assessment Pathway to develop a complete clinical picture so that subtle changes in vital signs, mental status, diagnostic test results, and so forth do not get missed or misattributed as simply signs of old age. A high index of suspicion must be maintained to sort out the often-ambiguous clinical picture, which can delay the identification and initiation of treatment for sepsis in the elderly patient. These patients may not have the cardiovascular reserves to compensate for long periods of time if their condition progresses to septic shock.

Sepsis risk factors specific to older adult patients include the following:

- Older than 80 years
- Obesity
- Poor functional status
- Placement of indwelling devices such as catheters
- History of cancer
- History of diabetes
- Endocrine deficiency
- Residence in a skilled nursing facility
- Recent hospitalization
- Any condition, therapy, or treatment impairing the immune system

Although the treatment for older adult patients with sepsis identified in the prehospital environment is much the same as it is with younger adult patients, the key to improving outcomes for these patients lies in identifying sepsis early and coordinating effective treatment rapidly, because the worsening of sepsis to septic shock may be masked by a variety of other preexisting conditions, and these older adult patients are less likely to have the functional reserve capacity to survive prolonged periods of shock.

Obstetric Patients

According to the World Health Organization, approximately 20% of all-cause global deaths are due to sepsis, disproportionately affecting neonates, pregnant or recently pregnant women, and people living in low-resource settings.

Sepsis accounts for 13.9% of maternal mortality in the United States. Pregnant patients have weakened immune systems to prevent rejection of the fetus. In addition, these patients have baseline increased respiratory rate and lower blood pressure due to increased blood volume, making use of standard sepsis identification criteria less useful. Although obstetric-specific sepsis criteria have been developed outside of the United States, to date none have proven superior to use of standard sepsis scores. The Maternal Early Warning Trigger tool has been shown to reduce mortality among pregnant patients with sepsis, cardiopulmonary dysfunction, preeclampsia/hypertension, and hemorrhage; however, measurement of the criteria is not well suited for use in the prehospital environment.

Pediatric Patients

Worldwide, 7.5 million children die from sepsis annually, making it the leading cause of morbidity and mortality in children. The low frequency of pediatric patient encounters in the United States, combined with the increased fragility of patients with sepsis, can present some of the biggest challenges any clinician may face. The initial presentation of sepsis in pediatric patients is often nonspecific, especially in children younger than 3 years. Compounding this problem, changes in vital signs as sepsis progresses may be subtle and can go undetected unless trends are being very closely monitored. Patient care references such as pediatric vital sign charts, tapes, wheels, and software applications can be helpful in rapidly identifying deviations from acceptable vital sign and diagnostic test ranges. If subtle changes are not put together early to form a clinical picture of sepsis and organ dysfunction, it may progress as the patient moves rapidly to potentially irreversible cardiovascular collapse.

Common infection sources for sepsis in pediatric patients include *E. coli* infection and respiratory syncytial virus infection.

Pediatric-specific risks include the following:

- Younger than 90 days
- Immunotherapy
- Chemotherapy
- Regular use of steroids
- Known B- or T-cell deficiency
- AIDS
- Any condition, therapy, or treatment impairing the immune system

Risks factors specific to neonatal pediatric patients include the following:

- Maternal rupture of membranes (water breaks) > 24 hours before birth
- Limited/no prenatal care
- Premature birth
- Very low birth weight
- Maternal TORCH infections untreated at the time of birth
  - Toxoplasmosis
  - Other (SARS-CoV-2, syphilis, varicella-zoster, parvovirus, mumps, HIV, Zika)
  - Rubella
  - Cytomegalovirus
  - Herpes simplex

Sepsis developing from congenital infections (generally acquired before or during the delivery process) within the first 72 hours of birth is considered early-onset neonatal sepsis. Sepsis presenting more than 72 hours after birth and up to 28 days of life usually develops from a nosocomial (hospital-acquired) or community-acquired infection and is considered late-onset neonatal sepsis.

Not every infection a child gets will lead to sepsis, but when sepsis occurs, the mixture of inflammatory, immune, and coagulation responses can trigger a complex and deadly combination of distributive, hypovolemic, and obstructive shock pathways. Sepsis in pediatric patients often goes unrecognized until the patient is at an extremely challenging, if not irreversible, stage of shock. Early recognition relies on a good systematic assessment and sound clinical judgment rather than any one single identifying clinical marker or blood test.

Fluid resuscitation for pediatric patients should include 20 mL/kg of crystalloid solution over 5 to 10 minutes. Total fluid administration may approach 200 mL/kg, but the risks of fluid overload, especially in children, demand reassessment between each fluid bolus.

Just as in adults, if fluid administration is inadequate to maintain effective circulatory pressures, pressor medications should be administered. For hyperdynamic (warm) shock, the recommended pressor is norepinephrine at 0.1–2 mcg/kg/min IV/IO, titrating to effect. For the later hypodynamic (cold) shock phase, EPINEPHrine at 0.1–1 mcg/kg/min IV/IO may be used, titrating to effect.

Although hyperglycemia is a more common finding in pediatric patients with sepsis, EMS clinicians should check for low blood sugar (neonates < 2.5 mmol/L [45 mg/dL], infants and children < 3.3 mmol/L [60 mg/dL]) and correct as necessary with 0.5–1 g/kg (or 5–10 mL/kg) of 10% dextrose IV/IO.

Putting It All Together

Sepsis is an insidious pathology, often presenting subtly, masking itself behind the same comorbidities that can worsen and accelerate the progress of septic shock. Efficient use of the AMLS Assessment Pathway can help the prehospital clinician with early and accurate identification of sepsis so that effective prehospital care can begin and be coordinated with colleagues in the emergency department.

SCENARIO SOLUTION

As you recall, our patient from the chapter introduction, an 81-year-old female, was found down and confused and had complained of an urgent need to use the restroom prior to the fall.

- Differential diagnoses may include sepsis of many possible origins, gastrointestinal hemorrhage, coagulopathy, and stroke.
- To narrow your differential diagnosis, you will need to complete a detailed history of the patient's condition, including all events leading up to her current condition. Perform a detailed physical exam. Between the detailed history and detailed physical exam, you should be able to identify if the patient has any indications of an infection. This patient was urgently needing to go to the restroom. Evaluating this further could lead to critical information about the possibility of urosepsis or gastrointestinal-based sepsis. The detailed physical exam could yield indications of a wound- or skin-based sepsis, but can also help identify indications of pneumonia. Detailed history taking could yield information that this patient's fall was witnessed, the patient did not strike her head, and the patient is not taking any blood thinners. A proper stroke assessment is paramount in this patient.
- The patient has clear evidence of SIRS. Furthermore, the patient is hemodynamically unstable and requires immediate stabilization. Immediate vascular access and fluid resuscitation are warranted. Consideration of early empiric antimicrobial therapy is important, where possible. In this situation, if the patient's hemodynamic status does not respond quickly to aggressive fluid resuscitation, early administration of vasopressors (such as norepinephrine) is paramount. Careful monitoring of mental status and airway protection is important, because intubation may quickly become warranted given the patient's condition. Most important, this patient is critically ill, and frequent reassessment should be performed. Treatment plans should be updated accordingly.

SUMMARY

- Sepsis is life-threatening organ dysfunction due to a dysregulated host response to infection.
- Sepsis must be recognized early, when the presentation may be subtle but the clinician has more chance of a positive patient response to interventions.
- A variety of screening and prognostic tools have been developed for sepsis, including SOFA, qSOFA, MEWS, and NEWS2.
- Many patients with sepsis and septic shock present with an altered level of consciousness.
- Sepsis can often masquerade as other illnesses, so a detailed history and physical are vital.
- Sepsis may decrease perfusion through distributive, hypovolemic, and obstructive shock in a variety of combinations.
- In the early phases, sepsis is as difficult to diagnose as it is easy to treat.
- Assessing level of consciousness and cognitive function is crucial in patients with suspected sepsis or septic shock.
- Signs and symptoms of infection include severe headache; stiff neck; earache; sore throat; sinus pain, especially with discharge; swelling of the lymph nodes of the neck, such as submandibular, anterior cervical, or posterior cervical lymphadenopathy; cough; shortness of breath; fever; rhonchi; pain with urination or urinary frequency; or signs of skin infections or abscesses.
- Because sepsis can present with very subtle signs and symptoms initially, as it progresses to septic shock it is important to frequently reassess the patient and make use of additional diagnostic tools in the assessment and reassessment of the patient.
- Septic shock is a subset of sepsis in which intense circulatory, cellular, and metabolic abnormalities occur, producing a higher risk of mortality than with sepsis alone.
- Norepinephrine is the pressor of choice for patients in septic shock.
- The hospital-based standard of care is to initiate broad-spectrum antibiotics covering the most likely pathogens within 1 hour of recognition of septic shock.
- Effective use of a sepsis alert protocol may decrease time to treatment in the emergency department and may improve patient mortality.
- A common factor among older, pregnant, and younger patients putting them at risk for sepsis is a less-effective immune system, making it more likely for them to get an infection and more likely for these infections to be severe.

Key Terms

adaptive immune response The body's secondary response to infection. It has memory. It uses T cells (helper and killer) and B cells and their antibodies and the classic pathway of the complement cascade to accelerate or potentiate (slow) the response to infection.

antibodies Proteins produced by plasma cells/B cells in response to a specific antigen. Also known as immunoglobulins, they are the key component of the adaptive immune response.

apoptosis Programmed cell death. Cytokines signal an infected or damaged host cell to die, preventing further escalation of infection to additional host cells.

B cells Lymphocytes that mature in the bone marrow and play an important role in the adaptive immune response. Also known as plasma cells, they produce antibodies (IgA, IgE, IgG, and IgM) that play a role in the body's immune response.

basophils Cells containing secretory granules that release histamine and heparin. They play a key role in the innate immune response.

chemokines A subclass of cytokines (signaling proteins) released by cells that cause the attraction of other cells to the area (i.e., chemotaxis).

coagulation cascade Causes clot formation and regulation after exposure to tissue damage. It can be triggered by the extrinsic or intrinsic pathway and by platelet or cell damage.

complement Inactive proteins produced by the liver that play a key role in the innate and adaptive immune responses.

complement cascade Complement can be triggered to be activated indirectly by exposure to a pathogen in the innate immune response, causing opsonization of the invading microbe, sending additional signals in the area to cause inflammation and phagocytosis. It can also be triggered directly by exposure to specific antibodies to the invading pathogen. This leads to formation of the membrane attack complex under the classic complement cascade in the adaptive immunity response.

cytokines Signaling proteins released by cells that initiate further response by the surrounding cells.

dendritic cells Act as a messenger between the innate immune response and the adaptive immune response. They present pieces of the invading microbe, known as antigens, along their cell surface.

eosinophils Cells containing secretory granules that release histamine and cytokines. They play a key role in parasitic infections and allergic reactions.

granulocytes A type of a white blood cell with secretory granules in its cytoplasm, that is, a neutrophil, basophil, or eosinophil.

immune system Protects the body from invading pathogens; includes the spleen, thymus, bone marrow, lymphatic system, T cells, and B cells.

innate immune response The body's initial response to a foreign microbe. It has no memory and is nonspecific. The type of response incorporates the alternative complement pathway, natural killer cells, granulocytes, monocytes, and mast cells.

lymphocytes White blood cells that are part of the immune system; they are differentiated as B cells and T cells.

macrophages Monocytes capable of engulfing an invading pathogen or infected host cell.

monocytes White blood cells that can differentiate into macrophages or dendritic cells. They play a key role in the innate immune response.

necrosis Unregulated cell death caused by factors external to the cell, such as bacterial toxins or injury.

neutrophils Cells containing secretory granules and comprising greater than 50% granulocytes. They play a key role in the innate immune response by enveloping invading pathogens and releasing enzymes and cytokines to destroy the invading microbe and alert the host immune response.

opsonization The act of marking a foreign microbe or antigen for phagocytosis or a dead cell for recycling. Surfactant in the lung can cover invading microbes and mark them for phagocytosis as part of the innate immune response. Complement proteins can also cover or mark an invading microbe or antigen as part of the innate immune response. Antibodies can identify and mark an invading microbe as part of the adaptive immune response.

phagocytes Cells that can engulf a foreign cell or an infected host cell. Include macrophages and neutrophils.

sepsis The body's response to potentially life-threatening infection.

T cells Lymphocytes that mature in the thymus and play an important role in escalating the adaptive immune response. There are two types: helper and cytotoxic/killer.

Bibliography

Alam N, Oskam E, Stassen PM, et al. Prehospital antibiotics in the ambulance for sepsis: a multicenter, open label, randomised trial. *Lancet Respir Med.* 2018;6(1):40–50. doi:10.1016/S2213-2600(17)30469-1

Arefian H, Heublein S, Scherag A, et al. Hospital-related cost of sepsis: a systematic review. *J Infect.* 2017;74(2):107–117. doi:10.1016/j.jinf.2016.11.006

Báez A, Giraldez E, Peña J. Precision and reliability of the Glasgow Coma Scale Score among a cohort of Latin American prehospital emergency care providers. *Prehosp Disaster Med.* 2007;22:230–232. doi:10.1017/S1049023X00004726

Band RA, Gaieski DF, Hylton JH, et al. Arriving by emergency medical services improves time to treatment endpoints for patients with severe sepsis or septic shock. *Acad Emerg Med.* 2011;18:934–940. doi:10.1111/j.1553-2712.2011.01145.x

Beglinger B, Rohacek M, Ackermann S, et al. Physician's first clinical impression of emergency department patients with nonspecific complaints is associated with morbidity and mortality. *Medicine.* 2015;94(7):e374.

Beloncle F, Radermacher P, Guerin C, et al. Mean arterial pressure target in patients with septic shock. *Minerva Anestesiol.* 2016;82(7):777–784.

Bisarya R, Song X, Salle J, et al. Antibiotic timing and progression to septic shock among patients in the ED with suspected infection. *Chest.* 2022;161(1):112–120. doi:10.1016/j.chest.2021.06.029

Bone RC, Balk RA, Cerra FB, et al. Definitions for sepsis and organ failure and guidelines for the use of innovative therapies in sepsis. The ACCP/SCCM Consensus Conference Committee. American College of Chest Physicians/Society of Critical Care Medicine. *Chest.* 1992;101(6):1644–1655. doi:10.1378/chest.101.6.1644

Bone RC, Fisher CJ Jr, Clemmer TP, et al. Sepsis syndrome: a valid clinical entity. Methylprednisolone Severe Sepsis Study Group. *Crit Care Med.* 1989;17(5):389–393.

Caputo ND, Fraser RM, Paliga A, et al. Nasal cannula end-tidal CO_2 correlates with serum lactate levels and odds of operative intervention in penetrating trauma patients: a prospective cohort study. *J Trauma Acute Care Surg*. 2012;73(5):1202–1207. doi:10.1097/TA.0b013e318270198c

Chakraborty RK, Burns B. Systemic inflammatory response syndrome. In *StatPearls*. NCBI Bookshelf version. StatPearls Publishing, 2022. http://www.ncbi.nlm.nih.gov/books/NBK547669/

Churpek MM, Snyder A, Han X, et al. Quick sepsis-related organ failure assessment, systemic inflammatory response syndrome, and early warning scores for detecting clinical deterioration in infected patients outside the intensive care unit. *Am J Resp Crit Care Med*. 2017;195(7):906–911. doi:10.1164/rccm.201604-0854OC

Cully M, Treut M, Thompson AD, et al. Exhaled end-tidal carbon dioxide as a predictor of lactate and pediatric sepsis. *Am J Emerg Med*. 2020;38(12):2620–2624. doi:10.1016/j.ajem.2020.07.075

Dantes RB, Epstein L. Combatting sepsis: a public health perspective. *Clin Infect Dis*. 2018;67(8):1300–1302. doi:10.1093/cid/ciy342

Denver Metro EMS Medical Directors. Protocols. Published January 15, 2023. https://www.dmemsmd.org/protocols

Drewry AM, Ablordeppey EA, Murray ET, et al. Antipyretic therapy in critically ill septic patients: a systematic review and meta-analysis. *Crit Care Med*. 2017;45(5):806–813. doi:10.1097/CCM.0000000000002285

Duckworth RL. Recognizing pediatric sepsis with CHART mnemonic. *JEMS*. September 1, 2016. https://www.jems.com/patient-care/recognizing-pediatric-sepsis-with-chart-mnemonic/

Duckworth RL. Five ways to perfect the patient handoff: it's a perilous transition for the patient; here's how to help it go smoother. *EMS World*. 2016;45(11):38–44, 64.

Dwyer J. In Rory Staunton's fight for his life, signs that went unheeded. *New York Times*. July 11, 2012. https://www.nytimes.com/2012/07/12/nyregion/in-rory-stauntons-fight-for-his-life-signs-that-went-unheeded.html

Eperjesiova B, Bogaard J, Rubin G, et al. Mortality outcome of patients in septic and hypovolemic shock associated with prolonged norepinephrine, phenylephrine, epinephrine, vasopressin and/or dopamine use. In *D51. Critical Care: The Fountainhead—Fluids, Monitoring and Management of Shock*, 2019. American Thoracic Society International Conference Abstracts. doi:10.1164/ajrccm-conference.2019.199.1_MeetingAbstracts.A6698

Femling J, Weiss S, Hauswald E, et al. EMS patients and walk-in patients presenting with severe sepsis: differences in management and outcome. *Southern Med J*. 2014;107(12):751–756. doi:10/f6vrjw

Fingar K, Washington R. *Trends in hospital readmissions for four high-volume conditions, 2009–2013*. Statistical Brief #196. Healthcare Cost and Utilization Project (HCUP). November 2015. Agency for Healthcare Research and Quality, Rockville, MD. https://www.hcup-us.ahrq.gov/reports/statbriefs/sb196-Readmissions-Trends-High-Volume-Conditions.jsp

Gao Y, Zhu J, Yin C, et al. Effects of target temperature management on the outcome of septic patients with fever. *Biomed Res Int*. 2017;2017:3906032. doi:10.1155/2017/3906032

Guerra WF, Mayfield TR, Meyers MS, et al. Early detection and treatment of patients with severe sepsis by prehospital personnel. *J Emerg Med*. 2013;44:1116–1125. doi:10.1016/j.jemermed.2012.11.003

Halimi K, Freeman-Garrick J, Agcaoili C, et al. Prehospital identification of sepsis patients and alerting of receiving hospitals: impact on early goal-directed therapy. *Crit Care*. 2011;15:P26. doi:10.1186/cc10395

Herlitz J, Bång A, Wireklint-Sundström B, et al. Suspicion and treatment of severe sepsis. An overview of the prehospital chain of care. *Scand J Trauma Resusc Emerg Med*. 2012;20:42. doi:10.1186/1757-7241-20-42

Hunter CL, Silvestri S, Dean M, et al. End-tidal carbon dioxide is associated with mortality and lactate in patients with suspected sepsis. *Am J Emerg Med*. 2013;31:64–71. doi:10.1016/j.ajem.2012.05.034

Hunter CL, Silvestri S, Ralls G, et al. Comparing quick sequential organ failure assessment scores to end-tidal carbon dioxide as mortality predictors in prehospital patients with suspected sepsis. *Western J Emerg Med*. 2018;19(3):446–451. doi:10.5811/westjem.2018.1.35607

Hunter CL, Silvestri S, Ralls G, et al. A prehospital screening tool utilizing end-tidal carbon dioxide predicts sepsis and severe sepsis. *Am J Emerg Med*. 2016;34(5):813–819. doi:10.1016/j.ajem.2016.01.017

Itenov TS, Johansen ME, Bestle M, et al. Induced hypothermia in patients with septic shock and respiratory failure (CASS): a randomised, controlled, open-label trial. *Lancet Respir Med*. 2018;6(3):183–192. doi:10.1016/S2213-2600(18)30004-3

Janagama SR, Newberry JA, Kohn MA, et al. Is AVPU comparable to GCS in critical prehospital decisions?—A cross-sectional study. *Am J Emerg Med*. 2022;59:106–110. doi:10.1016/j.ajem.2022.06.042

Jordan A. 16 most common EMS emergencies for EMTs & paramedics. *Unitek EMT*. Published November 5, 2020. Available at: https://www.unitekemt.com/blog/most-common-ems-emergencies-for-emts-and-paramedics/

Kaplan L. Systemic inflammatory response syndrome. *Medscape*. Updated November 12, 2020. https://emedicine.medscape.com/article/168943-overview

Kumar A, Safdar N, Kethireddy S, et al. A survival benefit of combination antibiotic therapy for serious infections associated with sepsis and septic shock is contingent only on the risk of death: a meta-analytic/meta-regression study. *Crit Care Med*. 2010;38(8):1651–1664. doi:10.1097/CCM.0b013e3181e96b91

Levy B, Buzon J, Kimmoun A. Inotropes and vasopressors use in cardiogenic shock: when, which and how much? *Curr Opin Crit Care*. 2019;25(4):384–390. doi:10.1097/MCC.0000000000000632

Levy MM, Fink MP, Marshall JC, et al. 2001 SCCM/ESICM/ACCP/ATS/SIS International Sepsis Definitions Conference. *Crit Care Med*. 2003;31(4):1250–1256. doi:10.1097/01.CCM.0000050454.01978.3B

Lewis AJ, Griepentrog JE, Zhang X, et al. Prompt administration of antibiotics and fluids in the treatment of sepsis: a murine trial. *Crit Care Med*. 2018;46(5):426–434. doi:10.1097/CCM.0000000000003004

Martín-Rodríguez F, Sanz-García A, del Pozo Vegas C, et al. Time for a prehospital-modified sequential organ failure assessment score: an ambulance-based cohort study. *Am J Emerg Med*. 2021;49:331–337. doi:10.1016/j.ajem.2021.06.042

McGillicuddy DC, Tang A, Cataldo L, et al. Evaluation of end-tidal carbon dioxide role in predicting elevated SOFA scores and lactic acidosis. *Intern Emerg Med.* 2009;4(1). doi:10.1007/s11739-008-0153-z

Mellhammar L, Linder A, Tverring J, et al. NEWS2 is superior to qSOFA in detecting sepsis with organ dysfunction in the emergency department. *J Clin Med.* 2019;8(8). doi:10.3390/jcm8081128

Middleton DJ, Smith TO, Bedford R, et al. Shock index predicts outcome in patients with suspected sepsis or community-acquired pneumonia: a systematic review. *J Clin Med.* 2019;8(8). doi:10.3390/jcm8081144

Muldoon KM, Fowler KB, Pesch MH, et al. SARS-CoV-2: is it the newest spark in the TORCH? *J Clin Virol.* 2022;127:104372. doi:10.1016/j.jcv.2020.104372

National Highway Traffic Safety Administration. V2 911 call complaint vs. EMS provider findings dashboard. *NEMSIS.* 2023. https://nemsis.org/911-call-complaint/

Nuttall A, Paton K, Kemp A. To what extent are GCS and AVPU equivalent to each other when assessing the level of consciousness of children with head injury? A cross-sectional study of UK hospital admissions. *BMJ Open.* 2018;8:e023216. doi:10.1136/bmjopen-2018-023216

Polito CC, Bloom I, Dunn C, et al. Implementation of an EMS protocol to improve prehospital sepsis recognition. *Am J Emerg Med.* 2022;57:34–38. https://doi.org/10.1016/j.ajem.2022.04.035

Radius Global Market Research. *Sepsis annual study: Sepsis awareness.* 2017. http://sepsis.us2.list-manage2.com/track/click?u=909d224c892e0a0d4a712fdc9&id=6dc6cbed3d&e=61fb2a1d7e

Ramzy M. Early sepsis screening in the emergency department. *REBEL EM Emergency Medicine Blog.* Published December 10, 2018. https://rebelem.com/early-sepsis-screening-in-the-emergency-department/

Reinhart K, Daniels R, Kissoon N, et al. Recognizing sepsis as a global health priority—A WHO resolution. *New Engl J Med.* 2017;377(5):414–417. doi:10.1056/NEJMp1707170

Reith FC, Synnot A, van den Brande R, et al. Factors influencing the reliability of the Glasgow Coma Scale: a systematic review. *Neurosurgery.* 2017;80(6):829–839. doi:10.1093/neuros/nyw178

Romaine ST, Sefton G, Lim E, et al. Performance of seven different paediatric early warning scores to predict critical care admission in febrile children presenting to the emergency department: a retrospective cohort study. *BMJ Open.* 2021;11(5):e044091. doi:10.1136/bmjopen-2020-044091

Rumbus Z, Garami A. Fever, hypothermia, and mortality in sepsis: comment on: Rumbus Z, Matics R, Hegyi P, Zsiboras C, Szabo I, Illes A, Petervari E, Balasko M, Marta K, Miko A, Parniczky A, Tenk J, Rostas I, Solymar M, Garami A. Fever is associated with reduced, hypothermia with increased mortality in septic patients: a meta-analysis of clinical trials. *PLoS One.* 2017;12(1):e0170152. doi:10.1371/journal.pone.0170152. *Temperature.* 2019;6(2):101. doi:10.1080/23328940.2018.1516100

Rusmawatiningtya D, Rahmawati A, Makrufardiet F, et al. Factors associated with mortality of pediatric sepsis patients at the pediatric intensive care unit in a low-resource setting. *BMC Pediatr.* 2021;21:471. doi:10.1186/s12887-021-02945-0

Sepsis Alliance. Fifty-five percent of Americans have heard of sepsis—nation's third leading killer—Sepsis Alliance survey reveals. Sepsis Alliance. Published August 23, 2016. https://www.sepsis.org/sepsis-alliance-news/fifty-five-percent-americans-heard-sepsis-nations-third-leading-killer-sepsis-alliance-survey-reveals/

Seymour CW, Band RA, Cooke CR, et al. Out-of-hospital characteristics and care of patients with severe sepsis: a cohort study. *J Crit Care.* 2010;25:553–562. doi:10.1016/j.jcrc.2010.02.010

Seymour CW, Rea TD, Kahn JM, et al. Severe sepsis in prehospital emergency care. *Am J Resp Crit Care Med.* 2012;186(12):1264–1271. doi:10.1164/rccm.201204-0713OC

Shi C, Goodall M, Dumville J, et al. The accuracy of pulse oximetry in measuring oxygen saturation by levels of skin pigmentation: a systematic review and meta-analysis. *BMC Med.* 2022;20(1):267. doi:10.1186/s12916-022-02452-8

Simpson SQ. Prehospital antibiotics for sepsis. *Chest.* 2018;153(3):588–589. doi:10/gf85qd

Singer M, Deutschman CS, Seymour CW, et al. The Third International Consensus Definitions for Sepsis and Septic Shock (Sepsis-3). *JAMA.* 2016;315(8):801–810. doi:10.1001/jama.2016.0287

Society of Critical Care Medicine. *Surviving Sepsis Campaign COVID-19 Guidelines.* Updated January 29, 2021. https://sccm.org/COVID19RapidResources/Resources/Surviving-Sepsis-Campaign-COVID-19-Guidelines

Society of Critical Care Medicine. *Surviving Sepsis Campaign Guidelines 2021.* October 4, 2021. https://sccm.org/Clinical-Resources/Guidelines/Guidelines/Surviving-Sepsis-Guidelines-2021

Spigner M, O'Connell A. Prehospital sepsis alerts: a STEMI or stroke equivalent? *EM Resident.* June 5, 2017. http://www.emra.org/emresident/article/preshospital-sepsis-alerts-a-stemi-or-stroke-equivalent/

Studnek JR, Artho MR, Garner Jr CL, et al. The impact of emergency medical services on the ED care of severe sepsis. *Am J Emerg Med.* 2012;30:51–56. doi:10.1016/j.ajem.2010.09.015

Tahotná A, Brucknerová J, Brucknerová I. Zika virus infection from a newborn point of view. TORCH or TORZiCH? *Interdiscip Toxicol.* 2018;11(4):241–246. doi:10.2478/intox-2018-0023

Tisdale JE, Patel R, Webb CR, et al. Electrophysiologic and proarrhythmic effects of intravenous inotropic agents. *Prog Cardiovasc Dis.* 1995;38(2):167–180. doi:10.1016/s0033-0620(05)80005-2

Topeli A, Baspinar B, Ortac Ersoy E. In search of the ideal risk score in sepsis. *Am J Resp Crit Care Med.* 2020;202(1):152–153. doi:10.1164/rccm.202002-0315LE

Tufan Z, Kayaaslan B, Mer M. COVID-19 and sepsis. *Turk J Med Sci.* 2021;51(7):3301–3311. doi:10.3906/sag-2108-239

Villar J, Ariff S, Gunier RB, et al. Maternal and neonatal morbidity and mortality among pregnant women with and without COVID-19 infection: the INTERCOVID Multinational Cohort Study. *JAMA Pediatr.* 2021;175(8):817–826. doi:10.1001/jamapediatrics.2021.105

Walchock JG, Pirrallo RG, Furmanek D, et al. Paramedic-initiated CMS sepsis core measure bundle prior to hospital arrival: a stepwise approach. *Prehospital Emerg Care.* 2016;21(3):291–300. doi:10.1080/10903127.2016.1254694

Wang HE, Weaver MD, Shapiro NI, et al. Opportunities for emergency medical services care of sepsis. *Resuscitation*. 2010;81:193–197. doi:10.1016/j.resuscitation.2009.11.008

Weiss SJ, Guerrero A, Root-Bowman C, et al. Sepsis alerts in EMS and the results of pre-hospital $ETCO_2$. *Am J Emerg Med*. 2019;37(8):1505–1509. doi:10.1016/j.ajem.2018.11.009

Wiryana M, Sinardja IK, GedeBudiarta I, et al. Correlation of end tidal CO_2 ($ETCO_2$) level with hyperlactatemia in patient with hemodynamic disturbance. *J Anesth Clin Res*. 2017;8(7). doi:10.4172/2155-6148.1000741

World Health Organization. *Global report on the epidemiology and burden of sepsis*. September 9, 2020. https://www.who.int/publications/i/item/9789240010789

Yealy DM, Mohr NM, Shapiro NI, et al. Early care of adults with suspected sepsis in the emergency department and out-of-hospital environment: a consensus-based task force report. *Ann Emerg Med*. 2021;78(1):1–19. doi:10.1016/j.annemergmed.2021.02.006

CHAPTER 7

Infectious Diseases

Chapter Editors
Matthew R. Neth, MD
Jonathan Jui, MD, MPH

Health care clinicians come into daily contact with patients who may have a wide range of illnesses and infections, some of which may be contagious. Patients may or may not know they have a communicable disease, may have an altered level of consciousness that prevents recognition of such a disease, or may choose not to reveal such information to you. This chapter will give you more knowledge in recognizing and understanding the nature and communicability of infectious diseases. Safe practice and standard precautions are reviewed, as are the signs, symptoms, and treatment of a number of infectious diseases.

LEARNING OBJECTIVES

At the conclusion of this chapter, you will be able to:

- Define specific terminology associated with infectious diseases.
- Explain how health care clinicians and the general public are protected from communicable and infectious diseases through regulations developed by various federal, state, and local governmental agencies.
- Outline primary, secondary, and ongoing assessment strategies for the patient with an infectious disease using the AMLS Assessment Pathway.
- Identify the links in the chain of infection, and describe how bacteria, viruses, fungi, and parasites cause disease.
- Explain how an exposure to a pathogen may evolve into an infection, and describe how each body system responds to this process.
- Identify and discuss the epidemiology; pathophysiology; methods of transmission; clinical manifestations; and treatment and prevention protocols and strategies for common infectious diseases, bloodborne diseases, enteric (intestinal) diseases, parasites, zoonotic (animal-borne) diseases, vector-borne diseases, infection with multidrug-resistant organisms, communicable diseases of childhood, and emerging diseases.
- Explain the rationale for the various types of personal protective equipment, and describe proper disinfection of patient care equipment.
- Describe the health care clinician's responsibilities in preventing communicable and infectious diseases and maintaining patients' confidentiality.
- Formulate provisional diagnoses on the basis of assessment findings for a variety of infectious diseases.
- Identify your local protocol for reporting and documenting a communicable disease.

SCENARIO

You and your partner are called to the local bus station, where you find a 56-year-old female complaining of chest tightness, shortness of breath, and generalized weakness. She is outside, sitting on the sidewalk and leaning against the building. She tells you that she has been staying in the women's shelter a few blocks away for about 2 months. The patient says that she has been feeling progressively worse over the last 2 weeks and left the shelter tonight to "catch my breath and get some fresh air." She is speaking in full sentences with frequent coughing. During your interview, she begins coughing forcefully; she is now visibly short of breath, with rapid, shallow respirations at 40 breaths/min, and begins complaining of dizziness and significant increase in chest pain.

Assessment is as follows:

- Blood pressure: 104/64 mm Hg
- Pulse rate: 106 beats/min
- Respirations: Shallow, 40 breaths/min
- SpO_2 on room air: 94%
- SAMPLER
  - Chest pain, shortness of breath, productive cough, worsening weakness for 2 weeks.
  - Allergies: angiotensin-converting enzyme (ACE) inhibitors, penicillin, ragweed.
  - Medications: abacavir/dolutegravir/lamivudine, metoprolol, duloxetine, methadone.
  - Past medical history: human immunodeficiency virus (HIV), hypertension, history of intravenous (IV) drug use, compliant on methadone regimen for 3 months, depression, chronic back pain.
  - Patient had a small dinner at the shelter 2 hours ago.
  - Patient has been feeling worse over 2 weeks; symptoms were exacerbated with mild exertion. She felt as if she would not be able to walk back to the shelter. Worsening of chest tightness triggered her calling 911.
  - Risk factors: lack of stable housing/homelessness, HIV status, history of IV drug use.
- Given this information, what differential diagnoses are you considering?
- What additional historical and physical exam information will you need to narrow your differential diagnosis?
- What are your initial treatment priorities as you continue your patient care?
- How can you decrease your risk of acquiring infection if you are exposed to blood, body fluids, and respiratory droplets during your care of this patient?

The incidence of infectious and communicable diseases is on the rise because of both globalization and the re-emergence of diseases once thought to have been eradicated. Health care clinicians must maintain awareness of the risks of disease transmission when assessing patients and their environment. When responding to a call, emergency medical services (EMS) clinicians typically arrive to an uncontrolled environment. They must recognize that transmission of a communicable disease is more likely in situations where people live in close proximity to each other, such as dormitories, military barracks, shelters, and prisons. Clinicians may not be aware the patient has an infectious disease, so it is crucial to perform a risk assessment anytime clinicians care for patients. Prearrival dispatch information may provide clues to the presence of a potentially infectious condition and prompt consideration of appropriate precautionary measures.

Their caution, however, must be tempered by clinicians' obligation to give the best possible care to all who request it. Having a fundamental knowledge of disease processes, understanding the transmission cycle of infectious organisms, and observing universal, standard, and transmission-based precautions will allow clinicians to provide care without incurring undue risks.

Infectious and Communicable Diseases

Infectious diseases are illnesses caused by pathogenic organisms such as bacteria, viruses, fungi, parasites, and, rarely, protein chains called prions. Most infectious diseases, such as the common cold and gastrointestinal (GI) viruses, are not life threatening in otherwise healthy patients. **Communicable diseases** are a subset of infectious diseases consisting of illnesses transmitted directly from person to person; they pose a potential threat to the health care clinician. Not all infectious diseases are directly communicable from person to person.

Modes of Transmission

Infectious diseases are spread by several specific mechanisms, which can generally be divided into direct and indirect methods.

Direct Transmission

- *Contact transmission.* Direct contact with an infected person may be brief, such as touching a patient. Most cases of the common cold are thought to be transmitted through casual direct contact. Other infections, such as syphilis and gonorrhea, are transmitted principally by direct sexual contact. Direct contact also includes puncture by a contaminated needle or other sharp instrument and transfusion of contaminated blood products from one patient to another. Indirect contact occurs by touching or handling an object that carries the infectious agent or by coming in contact with a person who is contaminated with pathogens from a person or their excretions. When indirect transmission occurs, the organism survives for at least a brief period outside the human host. A **fomite** is an inanimate object that allows for the transmission of an infectious disease. For example, methicillin-resistant *Staphylococcus aureus* (MRSA)—a type of bacteria—can be transferred onto gym equipment and subsequently transmitted by direct contact to another person. Factors influencing contact transmission include community prevalence, stability of the infectious disease, the amount of pathogen expelled, environmental factors, time on the fomite prior to contact, and needed mucous membrane exposure.
- *Droplet transmission.* Droplet transmission of a communicable disease occurs when the droplets (particles > 5 nm in diameter) emitted by an infected person reach another person. Droplet particles spread during close person-to-person contact within a relatively close distance (approximately a 3- to 6-foot [0.9- to 1.8-m] radius). These heavy particles do not become aerosolized, so they cannot hang suspended in the air for any appreciable length of time or distance. Exposure to a disease that is communicable by droplet transmission is defined as direct contact with a patient's oronasal secretions. Such contact may occur, for example, during coughing, sneezing, talking, unprotected mouth-to-mouth ventilation, suctioning, or spraying of secretions with no facial protection during nebulization of medications or intubation.
- *Oral transmission.* Oral transmission of pathogenic organisms can occur by ingesting contaminated food or water, by any oral exposure (e.g., licking or chewing), or by ingesting something from contaminated objects or surfaces. Examples of organisms that are transmitted by this method include norovirus, *Giardia*, *Campylobacter*, *Escherichia coli*, *Salmonella*, or *Shigella* gastroenteritis.

Indirect Transmission

- *Airborne transmission.* A common mode of transmission of communicable pulmonary diseases is inhalation of airborne pathogens (particles ≤ 1 nm in diameter). A vapor containing infectious particles can remain suspended in the air for long periods and can drift to new locations far from its source. Patients with compromised immune systems and people who live and work in densely populated areas are at increased risk of acquiring these types of diseases. Health care clinicians must maintain a vigilant awareness of the potential risk of these types of diseases and ensure they use appropriate personal protective equipment (PPE) and ventilation systems (i.e., negative-pressure rooms).
- *Vector or zoonotic transmission.* A vector is an organism that harbors pathogens that are harmless to the host organism but cause disease to a human host. For example, a mosquito infected with West Nile virus that bites a susceptible person may transmit the pathogen to that person.

Infectious Agents

Bacteria

Bacteria are single-celled microorganisms that live in water, inside the human body, in organic matter, and on inorganic surfaces or objects (fomites). Antibiotics are effective against most bacterial infections, though the problem of antibiotic resistance continues to grow. Aerobic bacteria, such as those causing tuberculosis and plague, can survive only in the presence of oxygen. In contrast, anaerobic bacteria, such as *Clostridium* strains, which cause botulism and tetanus, can survive and carry out their cellular functions without oxygen.

Most bacteria are fastidious, requiring specific conditions to grow, reproduce, and flourish. Certain bacteria, for example, require a narrow temperature range or must be supplied with particular nutrients to survive.

Viruses

Viruses, one of the smallest infectious agents, must grow and multiply inside the living cells of a host. Viruses can cause minor illnesses, such as the common cold, or life-threatening diseases, including acquired immunodeficiency syndrome (AIDS), Ebola virus disease, coronavirus disease 2019 (COVID-19), and smallpox.

Supportive care is required to treat most viral illnesses. Viruses are not susceptible to antibacterial or antifungal medications, although some viruses are susceptible to antiviral drugs. Antiviral drugs are available for the treatment of herpes, HIV, COVID-19, influenza, hepatitis B and C, respiratory syncytial virus (RSV; in selected cases), smallpox, mpox (formerly known as monkeypox), and cytomegalovirus (CMV). Vaccines against certain viruses have been and are being developed to prevent lethal viral infections or to moderate the severity of symptoms and reduce the length of illness (e.g., measles, mumps, rubella, influenza, COVID-19, herpes zoster).

Fungi

Fungi are plantlike microorganisms, most of which are not pathogenic. Examples of fungi include yeast, mold, mildew, and mushrooms. Those of particular importance to humans and the illnesses they cause include the following pathogens:

- Dermatophytes (skin infections such as tinea corporis, also called *ringworm*)
- *Aspergillus* species (pulmonary aspergillosis and infections of the external ear, sinuses, and subcutaneous tissues)
- *Blastomyces dermatitidis* (blastomycosis, which causes abscesses of skin and subcutaneous tissue)
- *Histoplasma capsulatum* (histoplasmosis)
- *Coccidioides immitis* or *Coccidioides posadasii* (coccidioidomycosis)
- *Candida* species (vaginal candidiasis and oral candidiasis, also called *thrush*)
- *Pneumocystis jirovecii* (*P. jirovecii* pneumonia [PJP])
- *Cryptococcus neoformans* and *Cryptococcus gattii* (cryptococcosis, which may infect the brain, lungs, and spinal cord)
- Mucormycetes (a group of molds that cause mucormycosis).

Antifungal agents have been developed to treat most of these infections.

Parasites

Parasites live within or on the host and feed on the host or the host's nutrient supply. Parasitic infections are frequently seen in areas where sanitation is poor, generally in developing countries, but are also still found in developed countries. They are found in locations where the parasite can coexist with humans. Although they are most frequently seen in tropical environments, they can be found in more temperate environments as well. Unlike viruses, parasites are living organisms. Like viruses, however, they must have a living host to survive and reproduce. Examples of parasitic infections include malaria, GI parasites (hookworms, tapeworms, *Giardia*), and skin parasites (lice and mites).

Antiparasitic medications are available for some parasites. For example, effective treatments are available for malaria and certain GI and skin parasites. These medications include antiprotozoal (e.g., malaria), anthelmintic (e.g., tapeworms), and ectoparasitic (e.g., lice, scabies) agents.

Treatment focuses on agents that will relieve symptoms and eradicate developing eggs and live parasites. Antihistamines may be used to relieve urticaria. Insecticides, acetylcholinesterase inhibitors, ovicides, and pediculicides can be effective at decreasing parasite infections.

Stages of the Infectious Process

Disease progression varies greatly depending on the pathogen dose (the number of organisms present), the **virulence** of the organism, and the susceptibility of the host. Several conditions must be met for infection to occur.

A key concept in infection control is that exposure to a pathogen will not necessarily cause infection or symptoms—it simply means the pathogen entered the host. Whether infection occurs depends on the factors previously described. Postexposure prophylaxis can also decrease the likelihood of an infection or the severity of illness if it does occur.

Communicable diseases go through stages (i.e., periods) that are identified based on the components of the infectious process: the incubation period, prodromal period, illness period, decline period, and convalescence period (Table 7-1).

Incubation Period

The incubation period is the interval between the exposure to the pathogen and the onset of symptoms. Its length varies from one organism to another, ranging from hours to years. During the incubation period, the pathogen reproduces in the host, which mobilizes the body's immune system to fight the infection.

Prodromal Period

During the prodromal period, the individual is between the incubation and illness periods. The virus continues

Table 7-1 Stages of the Infectious Process

Stage	Begins	Symptoms
Incubation period	With invasion, when disease process begins	No symptoms
Prodromal period	After invasion	Before symptoms of infection occur; patient may be infectious during this phase
Illness period	After prodromal	When symptoms appear; patient is usually infectious during this phase
Decline period	Immune system mounts a successful defense	Symptoms will gradually improve
Convalescence period	Symptoms resolve	Patient is usually not infectious during this phase

to replicate, and the individual may be infectious at this point. The body's immune response is triggered, leading to nonspecific signs of infection—fever, fatigue, headache, and malaise. At this point, the individual does not yet exhibit the full symptoms that are characteristic of the illness.

Illness Period

The clinical disease follows the prodromal period. Its duration depends on the particular pathogen. This stage may not be associated with any symptoms, or it may produce obvious symptoms such as skin lesions, GI illness, cough, or respiratory failure. The body may be able to destroy the pathogen and eliminate the disease, although some pathogens cannot be removed despite the immune system's best efforts. They may lie dormant, causing a latent infection. Pathogens such as HIV and human herpesviruses (HSVs) remain in the body indefinitely once an infection has occurred.

Decline Period

In this stage, the immune system mounts a successful defense against the infectious agent. Generally, the number of infectious particles declines and symptoms usually improve. Depending on the pathogen, a patient may still be infectious during this period. Some patients may also develop secondary infections during the decline period.

Convalescence Period

During this phase, symptoms improve and the patient enters a period of recovery. In most cases, the patient is not infectious during this stage. This period may last for an extended time, depending on the severity of the infection.

Public Health and Safety Regulations

The public health and safety system is responsible for ensuring the general health of the population by means of education, disease reduction and surveillance, sanitation, and pollution control. Public health comprises a number of basic services, including those focusing on vital statistics; diseases and conditions (e.g., communicable and chronic diseases); environmental health; public health laboratory services; healthy people and families (e.g., maternal and child health); and public education, preparedness, prevention, and wellness. An important segment of public health is **epidemiology**, the branch of medicine concerned with studying the causes, distribution, and control of disease in a population. Applied epidemiology also helps public health officials prevent or identify and control trends in the spread of infectious diseases.

The *2050 EMS Agenda for the Future* notes that EMS systems are an integral component of the public health system and are necessary to optimize patient-centered outcomes. In particular, EMS systems assist with data collection and monitoring of disease. Some EMS systems within the United States have incorporated mobile-integrated health care and community paramedicine programs designed to optimize long-term, patient-centered outcomes through assessing and improving social needs, providing needs-based care and preventive services, and preventing unnecessary hospital readmissions. EMS clinicians also contribute to the reduction of disease spread through their involvement in community vaccination programs. This aspect of EMS care delivery is especially important when a large number of vaccinations need to be administered, as was the case in the COVID-19 pandemic.

Agencies

At the local level, EMS agencies, EMS clinicians, health departments, health care facilities, and hospital and public health laboratories are the first line of defense in disease surveillance, pandemic planning, and outbreak identification. Local agencies also support efforts to reduce the incidence and prevent the spread of infectious diseases by collecting and sharing data related to illness and injury; organizing those data according to geographic region, race, age, sex, sexual practices and ethnicity; and implementing priority initiatives such as community education.

Many countries have their own national health agencies that monitor the incidence of infectious diseases and provide standards of care. Regional and local agencies may be involved as well. In the United States, the Centers for Disease Control and Prevention (CDC) provides these guidelines along with other agencies, such as the Department of Health and Human Services (DHHS) and the Department of Labor's Occupational Safety and Health Administration (OSHA).

At the international level, the United Nations' World Health Organization (WHO) coordinates worldwide disease prevention efforts for members of the United Nations by providing leadership on global health issues and technical and logistical support for health research. WHO also establishes evidence-based standards related to health trends.

U.S.-Specific Requirements

In the United States, public health and safety initiatives at the national level are executed primarily by DHHS. The following agencies operate under its auspices:

- The CDC in Atlanta, Georgia, is the chief national agency responsible for tracking and preventing morbidity and mortality associated with infectious disease. It is the most visible epidemiologic agency in the international medical community. The CDC monitors national infectious disease data and distributes this information to all health care clinicians and to the community through publications such as *Morbidity and Mortality Weekly Report* (*MMWR*) and *Emerging Infectious Diseases*, as well as via its website (www.cdc.gov).
- The DHHS's Administration for Strategic Preparedness and Response (ASPR) leads the nation's medical and public health preparedness for, response to, and recovery from disasters and public health emergencies, such as the COVID-19 pandemic.
- The Office of the Surgeon General oversees the U.S. Public Health Service and spearheads risk-reduction activities, such as promoting childhood immunization, and addressing disparities in rates of infectious disease and access to treatment among various racial, ethnic, and socioeconomic patient population groups.
- The Food and Drug Administration (FDA) is responsible for ensuring the safety, efficacy, and security of human and veterinary drugs, biologic products, and medical devices, including those associated with transmission of infectious disease, such as indwelling catheters.
- The National Institute for Occupational Safety and Health (NIOSH) was established in 1970 as a research and education agency with the mission of advancing knowledge in the field of occupational safety and health to create safe and healthy workplaces.

In addition, the Department of Homeland Security's Federal Emergency Management Agency (FEMA) works with the CDC, the Office of the Surgeon General, ASPR, and other agencies to coordinate emergency preparedness for hurricanes, earthquakes, and other natural disasters that foster outbreaks of a variety of diseases. For example, infectious diseases are associated with floodwater, sewer line breaks, and crowded living conditions in shelters.

Standards, Guidelines, and Statutes

OSHA is an office within the Department of Labor. Under the Occupational Safety and Health (OSH) Act of 1970, OSHA was charged with the responsibility of creating enforceable safety rules. OSHA oversees compliance, enforcement, inspection, tracking, and reporting related to infection control practice in the workplace. This agency establishes guidelines for preventing transmission of airborne and **bloodborne pathogens (BBP)** and develops postexposure protocols for use in occupational settings. OSHA standard 1910.120 specifies the PPE that must be available in given occupational settings and dictates how employees must be educated on its use to protect themselves from the hazards they are likely to encounter during the normal course of their work.

The OSHA regulation that is most important to health care workers is 29 CFR 1910.1030, which is intended to reduce the number of **exposure incidents**. Such an incident is defined as the transmission of bloodborne pathogens through **parenteral** contact between blood or other potentially infectious materials and the eyes, mouth, or other mucous membranes or nonintact skin during the performance of an employee's duties.

The Ryan White CARE Act, passed by the U.S. Congress in 1990 and reappropriated in September 2009, constitutes Part G of the law. The Ryan White CARE Act authorization officially expired in 2013; however, the legislation continues in effect as long as Congress appropriates funds for it. It contains a provision requiring each emergency response agency to have a designated infection control officer who is notified in the event of an exposure. The designated infection control officer acts as a liaison between the exposed employee and the medical facility to ensure proper notification, testing, and reporting of results.

Immunization Schedule

A recommended immunization schedule can be obtained from the CDC, which publishes both childhood and adolescent (birth to 18 years) and adult schedules (19 years or older). **Figure 7-1** shows the adapted 2023 immunization schedule for adults.

OSHA Bloodborne Pathogens Standard

The OSHA standards for bloodborne pathogens (29 CFR 1910.1030) and PPE (29 CFR 1910 Subpart I) require employers to protect workers from occupational exposure to infectious agents. This standard applies whenever workers have occupational exposure to human blood or other potentially infectious materials (OPIM).

Since 1991, when OSHA first issued its BBP standard to protect health care personnel from blood exposure, the focus of regulatory and legislative activity has been on implementing such control measures, including removing sharps hazards by developing and using engineering controls. The BBP standard and the CDC's recommended standard precautions both include PPE such as gloves, gowns, masks, and eye protection.

Since 1991, each fire/rescue department has been required to formulate a comprehensive plan to address these issues. Exposure control plans are summarized in **Table 7-2**.

Infection Control

Infection control always centers on early recognition through proficient assessment. Health care clinicians are obligated to protect themselves and others from infectious hazards while they provide patient care. When patients with communicable diseases are being treated, clinicians should always consider the impact of the disease process not only on the infected patient, but also on the clinicians themselves and the community. The risk of transmission can be limited by taking a few simple precautions:

- Receive vaccinations (the process of using vaccines to trigger an immune response to protect against infections) and/or immunizations (the process of making a person resistant to an infectious disease, usually through vaccination).
- Practice appropriate hand hygiene and respiratory hygiene/cough etiquette.
- Gain a broad comprehension of typical disease progression and recommended supportive management of the common conditions for which patients seek care.
- Use PPE consistent with the signs and symptoms and transmission mechanism of an infectious disease.
- Pursue immediate postexposure medical reporting and follow-up.

Standard Precautions

Employers and workers should be familiar with the following approaches to infection control and know which precautions are engineered to protect exposure to blood and body fluids:

- Universal precautions: Recommended in the 1980s, this approach treats all blood and body fluids as if they are known to be infectious.
- **Standard precautions**: Introduced in the CDC's 1996 *Guidelines for Isolation Precautions in Hospitals*, this infection control approach added to the universal precautions. Standard precautions include hand hygiene, use of certain types or levels of PPE based on anticipated exposure, safe injection practices, and safe management of a contaminated patient environment and contaminated equipment.
- Transmission-based precautions: Additional controls to interrupt transmission for contact-, droplet-, and airborne-transmissible diseases. These precautions are applied based on what is known or suspected about the infectious agent and the patient.

In addition to using PPE, safe work practices can help to protect mucous membranes and nonintact skin from exposure. They include keeping gloved and ungloved hands that may be **contaminated** from touching your mouth, nose, eyes, or face, and positioning patients so as to direct any sprays and spatters of droplets from them away from your face. Carefully selecting and gathering PPE before direct patient contact occurs will help you avoid the need to make PPE adjustments, reduce the likelihood of face or mucous membrane contamination during use, and reduce the possibility of contaminating gloves before you have contact with the patient. In areas where the need for resuscitation is unpredictable, mouthpieces, pocket resuscitation masks with one-way valves, and other ventilation devices provide an alternative to mouth-to-mouth ventilation, preventing exposure of your nose and mouth to the patient's oral and respiratory secretions during the procedure.

Table 1 Recommended Adult Immunization Schedule by Age Group, United States, 2024

Vaccine	19–26 years	27–49 years	50–64 years	≥65 years
COVID-19	1 or more doses of updated (2023-2024 Formula) vaccine (See Notes)			
Influenza inactivated (IIV4) or **Influenza recombinant** (RIV4)	1 dose annually			
or	or			
Influenza live, attenuated (LAIV4)	1 dose annually			
Respiratory Syncytial Virus (RSV)	Seasonal administration during pregnancy. See Notes.			≥60 years
Tetanus, diphtheria, pertussis (Tdap or Td)	1 dose Tdap each pregnancy; 1 dose Td/Tdap for wound management (see notes) 1 dose Tdap, then Td or Tdap booster every 10 years			
Measles, mumps, rubella (MMR)	1 or 2 doses depending on indication (if born in 1957 or later)			For healthcare personnel, see notes
Varicella (VAR)	2 doses (if born in 1980 or later)		2 doses	
Zoster recombinant (RZV)	2 doses for immunocompromising conditions (see notes)		2 doses	
Human papillomavirus (HPV)	2 or 3 doses depending on age at initial vaccination or condition	27 through 45 years		
Pneumococcal (PCV15, PCV20, PPSV23)				See Notes See Notes
Hepatitis A (HepA)	2, 3, or 4 doses depending on vaccine			
Hepatitis B (HepB)	2, 3, or 4 doses depending on vaccine or condition			
Meningococcal A, C, W, Y (MenACWY)	1 or 2 doses depending on indication, see notes for booster recommendations			
Meningococcal B (MenB)	19 through 23 years 2 or 3 doses depending on vaccine and indication, see notes for booster recommendations			
***Haemophilus influenzae* type b** (Hib)	1 or 3 doses depending on indication			
Mpox				

- Recommended vaccination for adults who meet age requirement, lack documentation of vaccination, or lack evidence of immunity
- Recommended vaccination for adults with an additional risk factor or another indication
- Recommended vaccination based on shared clinical decision-making
- No recommendation/Not applicable

Figure 7-1 Adult immunization schedule.

Reproduced from Centers for Disease Control and Prevention. Recommended adult immunization schedule for ages 19 years or older. 2023. https://www.cdc.gov/vaccines/schedules/downloads/adult/adult-combined-schedule.pdf

Table 2 Recommended Adult Immunization Schedule by Medical Condition or Other Indication, United States, 2024

Always use this table in conjunction with Table 1 and the Notes that follow. Medical conditions or indications are often not mutually exclusive. If multiple medical conditions or indications are present, refer to guidance in all relevant columns. See Notes for medical conditions or indications not listed.

VACCINE	Pregnancy	Immunocompromised (excluding HIV infection)	HIV infection CD4 percentage and count		Men who have sex with men	Asplenia, complement deficiency	Heart or lung disease	Kidney failure, End-stage renal disease or on dialysis	Chronic liver disease; alcoholism[a]	Diabetes	Healthcare Personnel[b]
			<15% or <200mm	≥15% and ≥200mm							
COVID-19		See Notes									
IIV4 or RIV4	1 dose annually										
LAIV4					1 dose annually if age 19 - 49 years		1 dose annually if age 19 - 49 years				
RSV	Seasonal administration. See Notes	See Notes				See Notes					
Tdap or Td	Tdap: 1 dose each pregnancy	1 dose Tdap, then Td or Tdap booster every 10 years									
MMR	*										
VAR	*			See Notes							
RZV		See Notes									
HPV	*	3 dose series if indicated									
Pneumococcal											
HepA											
Hep B	See Notes									Age ≥ 60 years	
MenACWY											
MenB											
Hib		HSCT: 3 doses[c]				Asplenia: 1 dose					
Mpox	See Notes				See Notes						See Notes

Legend:
- Recommended for all adults who lack documentation of vaccination, **OR** lack evidence of immunity
- Not recommended for all adults, but recommended for some adults based on either age **OR** increased risk for or severe outcomes from disease
- Recommended based on shared clinical decision-making
- Recommended for all adults, and additional doses may be necessary based on medical condition or other indications. See Notes.
- Precaution: Might be indicated if benefit of protection outweighs risk of adverse reaction
- Contraindicated or not recommended *Vaccinate after pregnancy, if indicated
- No Guidance/ Not Applicable

a. Precaution for LAIV4 does not apply to alcoholism.

b. See notes for influenza; hepatitis B; measles, mumps, and rubella; and varicella vaccinations.

c. Hematopoietic stem cell transplant.

Figure 7-1 *(Continued)*

Table 7-2 Elements of an Agency Exposure Control Plan

- Policy for health maintenance and surveillance.
- Program administration. Appointment of a designated infection control officer to serve as a liaison between the agency and health care facilities. Procedure for identifying and evaluating exposures and a strategy for postexposure counseling, medical care, and documentation (as required by the Ryan White Emergency Response Notification Act, Part G).
- Identification of work functions when a risk of exposure to pathogens exists.
- Policy for use of PPE and availability of PPE to health care workers.
- Effective plan for decontaminating personnel and for disinfecting and storing equipment.
- Education regarding disease transmission, cleaning and disinfection procedures, use of PPE, and the purpose of immunization.
- Steps for complying with medical waste regulations.
- Strategy for compliance monitoring.
- Recordkeeping policies and procedures.

PPE, personal protective equipment.

Needlesticks

The federal Needlestick Safety and Prevention Act, signed into law in November 2000, authorized OSHA to revise its BBP standard to require more explicitly the use of safety-engineered sharps devices.

After a needlestick exposure, the risk of infection depends on the pathogen involved, the person's immune status, the type of needlestick injury (e.g., needle used in a blood vessel, depth of needle puncture, visible blood on the needle), the type of needle (e.g., size of needle, hollow versus blunt), the amount of circulating virus in the source patient, and the availability and use of appropriate postexposure prophylaxis. Needlesticks and cuts should be immediately washed with soap and water. Mucosal or cutaneous exposures should be flushed with water, and ocular exposures should be irrigated with clean water, saline, or sterile irrigation solutions. The exposure should subsequently be reported to the agency supervisor or infection control officer per the local protocol.

Common pathogens that may be encountered during a needlestick injury include HIV, hepatitis B virus (HBV), and hepatitis C virus (HCV). The decision to begin postexposure prophylaxis (PEP) is based on the factors noted previously. Initiation of PEP is time sensitive. The optimal timing is within a few hours of exposure, with the outer limit of benefit being 72 hours. Additional information regarding PEP can be found in agency policy and at the National Clinician Consultation Center (https://nccc.ucsf.edu).

Preventing Sharps Injuries

The prevention of sharps injuries has always been an essential element of standard precautions. Needles and other sharp devices must be handled in a way that will prevent injury to the user and to others who may encounter the device during or after the procedure.

The passage of the Needlestick Safety and Prevention Act of 2000 prompted the development of many engineering controls, including self-capping IV catheter needles, needleless IV tubing, resheathing scalpels, and safety syringes for medication administration. OSHA requires that sharps and other disposal containers be easily accessible at their sites of use.

Special Considerations

Patients with methicillin-resistant *Staphylococcus aureus* (MRSA) and vancomycin-resistant *Enterococcus* (VRE) may be protected by the Americans with Disabilities Act (ADA), so it is important to exercise sensitivity with the use of unnecessary PPE, which may be considered by some as discriminatory. The ADA also requires employers to maintain a safe environment for their workers.

Agency personnel should be updated annually on new information about diseases, technology, equipment modifications, agency exposure rates, and number of infectious disease transmissions and tuberculosis (TB) contacts during the previous year. This information serves to place risk in a proper perspective. Risk of disease transmission is always present, but this risk is low when proper protective measures are followed by health care clinicians. OSHA has framed such risk-reduction and education requirements as a right-to-know issue.

Responsibilities of Health Care Clinicians

Employers are required to establish specific policies and procedures to protect personnel during the course of their duties. However, employees and volunteers play a role in protecting themselves as well. Employee self-protection responsibilities include the following:

- Giving full consideration to participation in vaccination/immunization programs
- Attending required education and training programs
- Using PPE properly
- Promptly reporting exposures
- Complying with all aspects of the agency's exposure control plan

Hand Washing

The best means of preventing transmission of infectious agents remains the most basic one—effective hand washing. No barrier is 100% effective; therefore, hands should be washed before and after caring for each patient and after removing gloves. Alcohol-based antimicrobial products may be used when no gross contamination is visible or when conventional soap and water are not available.

Personal Protective Equipment

Protective barriers offer a second line of defense to block entry of pathogens. These barriers include gloves, gowns, masks, protective eyewear, sharps containers, and engineering controls that limit needlesticks. Gloves reduce contamination of hands but do not prevent penetrating injuries by needles or other sharp objects. Gowns prevent saturation of clothing and contact of skin with body fluids during procedures and patient care, although they can still be compromised by sharp objects. Masks, face shields, and other protective eyewear reduce the likelihood of contamination of mucous membranes of the mouth, nose, and eyes.

PPE selection should be task specific (Table 7-3). Local protocols, policies, and procedures should be followed.

PPE and Procedures for Airborne Risks and Aerosol-Causing Procedures

Specific attention to respiratory PPE is required when EMS clinicians treat a patient suspected of having a disease that is spread by droplets or aerosol. Furthermore, various respiratory procedures have been shown to generate aerosolized pathogens. These procedures include endotracheal intubation, manual ventilation, airway suctioning, cardiopulmonary resuscitation (CPR), and possibly administration of nebulized medications.

Table 7-3 Recommendations for Application of Standard Precautions for the Care of All Patients in All Healthcare Settings

Component	Recommendations
Hand hygiene	After touching blood, body fluids, secretions, excretions, contaminated items; immediately after removing gloves; between patient contacts.
	Personal protective equipment (PPE)
Gloves	For touching blood, body fluids, secretions, excretions, contaminated items; for touching mucous membranes and nonintact skin
Gown	During procedures and patient-care activities when contact of clothing/exposed skin with blood/body fluids, secretions, and excretions is anticipated.
Mask, eye protection (goggles), face shield	During procedures and patient-care activities likely to generate splashes or sprays of blood, body fluids, secretions, especially suctioning, endotracheal intubation. During aerosol-generating procedures on patients with suspected or proven infections transmitted by respiratory aerosols wear a fit-tested N95 or higher respirator in addition to gloves, gown and face/eye protection.
Soiled patient-care equipment	Handle in a manner that prevents transfer of microorganisms to others and to the environment; wear gloves if visibly contaminated; perform hand hygiene.
Environmental control	Develop procedures for routine care, cleaning, and disinfection of environmental surfaces, especially frequently touched surfaces in patient-care areas.
Textiles and laundry	Handle in a manner that prevents transfer of microorganisms to others and to the environment
Needles and other sharps	Do not recap, bend, break, or hand-manipulate used needles; if recapping is required, use a one-handed scoop technique only; use safety features when available; place used sharps in puncture-resistant container

(continues)

Table 7-3 Recommendations for Application of Standard Precautions for the Care of All Patients in All Healthcare Settings (*continued*)

Component	Recommendations
Patient resuscitation	Use mouthpiece, resuscitation bag, other ventilation devices to prevent contact with mouth and oral secretions
Patient placement	Prioritize for single-patient room if patient is at increased risk of transmission, is likely to contaminate the environment, does not maintain appropriate hygiene, or is at increased risk of acquiring infection or developing adverse outcome following infection.
Respiratory hygiene/cough etiquette (source containment of infectious respiratory secretions in symptomatic patients, beginning at initial point of encounter e.g., triage and reception areas in emergency departments and physician offices)	Instruct symptomatic persons to cover mouth/nose when sneezing/coughing; use tissues and dispose in no-touch receptacle; observe hand hygiene after soiling of hands with respiratory secretions; wear surgical mask if tolerated or maintain spatial separation, >3 feet if possible.

Reproduced from Siegel JD, Rhinehart E, Jackson M, Chiarello L, and the Healthcare Infection Control Practices Advisory Committee, 2007. Guideline for Isolation Precautions: Preventing Transmission of Infectious Agents in Healthcare Settings. Centers for Disease Control and Prevention. July 2023. https://www.cdc.gov/infectioncontrol/guidelines/isolation/index.html

When caring for patients with infections that may be spread in this manner and when performing aerosol-generating procedures on these patients, EMS clinicians should wear an N95 respirator (or better), gown, gloves, and eye protection. This level of PPE provides adequate protection against infection, and medically indicated procedures should not be avoided if the clinician is properly protected.

In addition to personal PPE, EMS clinicians should consider performing aerosol-generating procedures before placing the patient in the confined space of an ambulance compartment. During transport, the ventilation system in the patient compartment of the ambulance should have the fan turned on in the "high" setting. The ambulance exhaust fan in some ambulances can replace contaminated air with fresh air as efficiently as a negative-pressure system in a hospital room.

Cleaning and Decontamination Procedures for Equipment and Vehicles

All potentially contaminated durable (reusable) medical equipment and vehicle surfaces should be immediately decontaminated according to the manufacturer's and CDC's decontamination guidelines and in keeping with local requirements. **Decontamination** of equipment should be performed only in marked, designated areas. Each area should have an appropriate ventilation system and adequate drainage. Clinicians should always wear gloves, a cover gown if their uniform might become contaminated, and protective eyewear or a full-face mask if blood or other potentially infectious materials might be splashed when decontaminating equipment.

Begin decontamination by removing gross dirt and debris with soap and a copious amount of water, then disinfect as appropriate. Aerosol-generating decontamination devices can apply disinfectant to difficult-to-reach surfaces of vehicles or equipment. It is important to follow the manufacturer's recommendations for each piece of equipment.

Postexposure Procedures

In the event you experience an exposure to a communicable or infectious disease while on duty, report the occurrence without delay to your supervisor or infection control officer per protocol and follow your organization's procedures for testing and possible prophylactic or empiric treatment. Patient care should continue as appropriate. Hand washing and proper disposal of contaminated items should continue.

Emergency Medical Dispatch

EMS dispatch plays an important role not only in recognizing a potential infectious disease, but also in notifying EMS personnel about potential hazards so they can prepare themselves by donning appropriate PPE. Dispatch screening tools can be used to help recognize patients who are at high risk for COVID-19 or other community-based infections.

Epidemics and Pandemics

An **endemic** disease is one that is present in the community at a constant baseline level over time. Examples of endemic diseases include the viruses responsible for the common cold, herpes simplex, and varicella zoster virus (VZV).

An **epidemic** is a disease outbreak in which many more than the baseline number of people in a community or region become infected with the same disease. Epidemics may occur in a setting where the disease has been brought into a new community by an outside source, such as an infected traveler, or because a pathogen (in this case, a bacterium or virus) has mutated in a way that either has enabled it to evade the immune system or has made it more virulent. Some epidemics occur when an entirely new disease emerges in humans, as occurred with HIV and severe acute respiratory syndrome (SARS). Others begin when a new version of an old disease reemerges, as was the case with influenza A strains H1N1 and H5N1.

A **pandemic**, such as the devastating 1918 influenza pandemic or the COVID-19 event, is an epidemic that spreads over several countries or continents. As might be expected, a pandemic may result in a high death toll. Like an epidemic, a pandemic may arise from an old disease, such as smallpox or the bubonic plague, or from the development of a new disease or a new form of an old disease.

If the source of the pandemic is a virulent new pathogen or a new form of a pernicious old pathogen, very few people, if any, will have intrinsic immunity that makes them resistant to the disease. Consequently, the rates of illness and death may be catastrophic unless effective prevention strategies are developed and implemented rapidly. Although immunization is often an effective prevention strategy, developing a vaccine and ensuring its safety and efficacy in humans is usually a protracted process. A pathogen may also evolve over time, making vaccination less effective. The purpose of a vaccination is to induce a protective immune response to prevent severe consequences of disease in a healthy individual receiving the vaccine. Evolving technology has begun to compress the amount of time necessary to develop, manufacture, and distribute new vaccines, as was seen with the COVID-19 vaccines.

AMLS Assessment Pathway ▶▶▶▶

▼ Initial Observations

The AMLS assessment process for a patient suspected of having an infectious disease relies on a thorough, comprehensive, and efficient approach to diagnosing and managing associated medical emergencies.

Scene Safety Considerations

In assessing any patient, clinicians must maintain a keen awareness of the risk for transmission of an infectious disease, not only from patient to clinician but also from clinician to patient. Appropriate precautions must be followed to minimize the risk of disease transmission through selection of proper PPE and other infection-control strategies.

Patient Cardinal Presentation/Chief Complaint

As you begin to assess the patient, the scene, and the situation, note the character and severity of the patient's signs and symptoms as clues to the possible presence of an infectious process. Typical chief complaints include fever, malaise, fatigue, nausea or vomiting, cough, rash, chest pain, difficulty breathing, diarrhea, or urinary symptoms. It is essential to be able to recognize the cardinal presentation/chief complaint of a wide variety of infectious diseases and to know how they are most effectively treated or prevented. This can be accomplished by exploring signs and symptoms, diagnostic studies, and assessment and management strategies for the infectious diseases likely to be encountered in the prehospital setting.

Primary Survey

At the start of the primary survey, perform a risk assessment for possible exposure and take the appropriate standard precautions. Next, assess for and treat any immediate life threats, including ensuring the patient has a patent airway, efficient respiratory effort, and adequate perfusion. For example, respiratory infections may cause severe hypoxia or respiratory failure. Rapid recognition during the primary survey and immediate intervention with continuous positive airway pressure (CPAP) and supplemental oxygen may be lifesaving. Likewise, patients with severe infectious diseases may present with life-threatening hypoperfusion, and rapid IV fluid infusion may prevent morbidity.

First Impression

Identify how sick the patient appears to be. Focus on addressing any life-threatening conditions (e.g., impending need for airway protection, respiratory failure, hypoperfusion). Generate differential diagnoses based on the cardinal presentation/chief complaint, with a focus on both life-threatening presentations and the most common presentations.

Detailed Assessment

History Taking

The differential diagnosis and subsequent working diagnosis should be refined based on the following:

- Incident and past medical history taken using the OPQRST and SAMPLER mnemonics
- History of travel
- A focused physical examination
- Interpretation of diagnostic findings

OPQRST and SAMPLER

The OPQRST mnemonic will help you elaborate on the patient's chief complaint. Be sure to obtain a SAMPLER history, paying particular attention to medications the patient is currently taking, the events leading up to the current presentation, recent infections or known exposures, and recent travel history. Risk factors such as a compromised immune system, age, comorbidities, current medications, or indwelling devices should also be taken into consideration during this component of the history collection.

Secondary Survey

The secondary survey of a patient suspected of having an infectious disease should be approached much like that of any other medical patient. Vital signs should be obtained to determine the patient's overall stability. Perform an examination to evaluate the function of specific body organ systems, as detailed in Chapter 1, *Advanced Medical Life Support Assessment for the Medical Patient.*

Diagnostics

Clinical reasoning and the patient's response to treatment should guide you in determining which laboratory or radiographic diagnostic tools might help confirm or rule out potential infectious disease processes, enabling you to arrive at a definitive diagnosis.

Refine the Differential Diagnosis

As you perform your reassessment, you will continually work to rule in or rule out certain conditions from your differential diagnosis. Keep an open mind as you gather all your patient information and modify your differential diagnosis based on new findings. Avoid implicit bias and premature anchoring when making diagnostic impressions.

Ongoing Management

Continue to monitor the patient's condition. Obtain another complete set of vital signs as needed and compare them with the expected outcomes from your therapies. Document all of your findings with each reassessment so that your medical record is accurate and complete for handoff at the emergency department. It is important to report suspicion of infection or sepsis to the receiving facility so as to not delay administration of antibiotics or other essential treatments for infectious diseases.

The Chain of Infection

Infection involves a chain of events through which the communicable disease spreads (**Figure 7-2**). Microorganisms residing in the human body without causing disease are part of the body's normal flora and constitute one layer of the host's defenses. Normal flora help keep the host free of disease by creating environmental conditions inhospitable to pathogens—that is, disease-causing microorganisms that rely on a host to supply their needs.

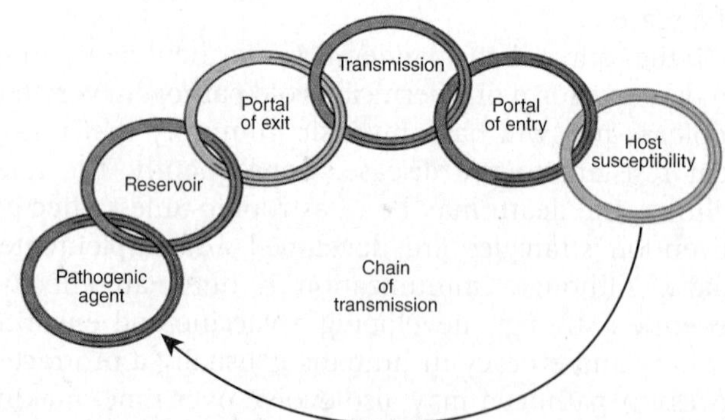

Figure 7-2 Chain of transmission for infection. The chain must be intact for an infection to be transmitted to another host. Transmission can be controlled by breaking any link in the chain.

Reservoir/Host

Pathogens may live and reproduce on and within humans, animal hosts, other organic substances, or inanimate objects. Once infected, the human host may show clinical signs of illness, or the individual may become an asymptomatic carrier who has no signs or symptoms of infection, but is capable of transmitting the pathogen to another person. The life cycle of the pathogen depends on several factors: demographics of the host (e.g., age), genetic factors, temperature, and the efficacy of any therapeutic measures initiated once the infection has been recognized.

Portal of Exit

A portal of exit is necessary if a pathogenic agent is to leave one host to invade another. The organism may exit the body by a single portal or several points, such as the oral cavity, respiratory tract, open skin lesion, GI tract, or genitourinary tract.

Transmission

Direct or indirect transmission may occur from the portal of exit to the portal of entry. Modes of direct and indirect transmission, with examples of each, are listed in Table 7-4.

Table 7-4 Modes of Transmission of Infectious Diseases

Mode	Examples of How Contact Might Occur	Selected Infectious Diseases Transmitted by This Mode
	Direct Transmission	
Touching an infected person	Shaking hands	Influenza, chickenpox (VZV), common cold viruses (coronaviruses and rhinoviruses), scabies
Oral transmission	Kissing	Mumps, pertussis, infectious mononucleosis, herpes simplex virus
Droplet transmission	New host inhales droplets (usually larger > 5 microns) produced by coughing or sneezing	Rubeola, mumps, pertussis, respiratory syncytial virus, SARS, COVID-19 (SARS-CoV-2), influenza, bacterial meningitis (*Neisseria meningitidis*), *Mycoplasma*, parvovirus, rhinovirus, streptococcal pharyngitis
Airborne	New host inhales small particles (< 1 micron) produced by coughing, sneezing, and talking	Measles, COVID-19 (SARS-CoV-2), aspergillosis, TB, hantavirus, mpox (monkeypox), VZV
Fecal contamination	Contact with feces	Enteroviral meningitis, hepatitis A virus, CMV, norovirus
Sexual contact	Contact with genitalia without condom use	HIV, human herpesviruses, chlamydia, gonorrhea, syphilis, HPV
	Indirect Transmission	
Food	Consumption of raw shellfish	Hepatitis A virus, *Vibrio cholerae* or other *Vibrio* species (e.g., *V. parahaemolyticus*)
Biologic matter	Needle sharing, needlestick injuries, tattooing, and body piercing	HIV, hepatitis B virus, hepatitis C virus, MRSA
	Touching an infected surface such as a bed rail	Rubeola, respiratory syncytial virus, MRSA, VRE

(*continues*)

Table 7-4 Modes of Transmission of Infectious Diseases *(continued)*

Mode	Examples of How Contact Might Occur	Selected Infectious Diseases Transmitted by This Mode
	Contact with fomites such as towels and linens	Scabies, MRSA, VRE
	Health care clinician who has had contact with an infected patient touches another patient without washing their hands	*Clostridioides* (formerly called *Clostridium*) *difficile*
Soil/ground surfaces	Puncture wound Contact of nonintact skin with field turf	*Clostridium tetani* (tetanus disease), MRSA
Air	Cleaning a basement or barn that contains infected rodent feces	Hantavirus

CMV, cytomegalovirus; HIV, human immunodeficiency virus; HPV, human papillomavirus; MRSA, methicillin-resistant *Staphylococcus aureus*; SARS, severe acute respiratory syndrome (caused by a coronavirus); TB, tuberculosis; VRE, vancomycin-resistant *Enterococcus*; VZV, varicella zoster virus.

Portal of Entry

The portal of entry is the site at which the pathogenic agent enters a new host. The organism may be ingested, inhaled, or injected through the skin, or it may cross a mucous membrane, the placenta, or nonintact skin. The amount of time it takes for the infectious process to begin in a new host after the pathogen enters varies with the organism and the host's susceptibility. In fact, exposure to an infectious agent often does not produce illness in a healthy person, because the immune system is able to destroy the pathogen before it can multiply to cause an infection. The duration of exposure and the quantity of pathogens required to produce infection in the host differ for each pathogen.

Host Susceptibility

In healthy individuals, the immune system usually subdues the pathogen and protects the host from infection. However, certain factors can impair the immune system's ability to prevent infection following exposure to a pathogen, making some people more susceptible to illness than others. These factors are summarized in Table 7-5.

Table 7-5 Factors That Increase Host Susceptibility to Infection

- *Age.* The very young and the very old are at greater risk of contracting an infectious disease.
- *Use of drugs.* Taking immunosuppressive medications, steroids, or other drugs may affect immune response.
- *Chronic disease.* Chronic diseases, such as diabetes and kidney disease, can impair immune functions, resulting in functional immunodeficiency.
- *Genetics.* Primary immunodeficiency disorders, sickle cell disease, and cystic fibrosis are inherited diseases that reduce the ability to defend against infection.
- *Malnutrition/obesity.* Poor nutrition weakens the immune system. Obesity is often associated with multiple chronic disease processes and places patients at risk for infection due to a compromised immune system.
- *Trauma.* Trauma usually involves disruption of the normal protective skin barriers.
- *Smoking.* Tobacco smoking has been shown to impair the lungs' protective mucociliary clearance mechanism.

Natural Defenses of the Body

The body is equipped with natural defenses that counteract pathogen invasion. An immune response is activated once an unrecognized **antigen** (e.g., a structural component of a pathogen, a toxin, a blood product transfused into the body) enters the body. First, the pathogen is recognized by a variety of immune cells such as macrophages and dendritic cells. These immune cells then release intracellular signaling molecules, ultimately

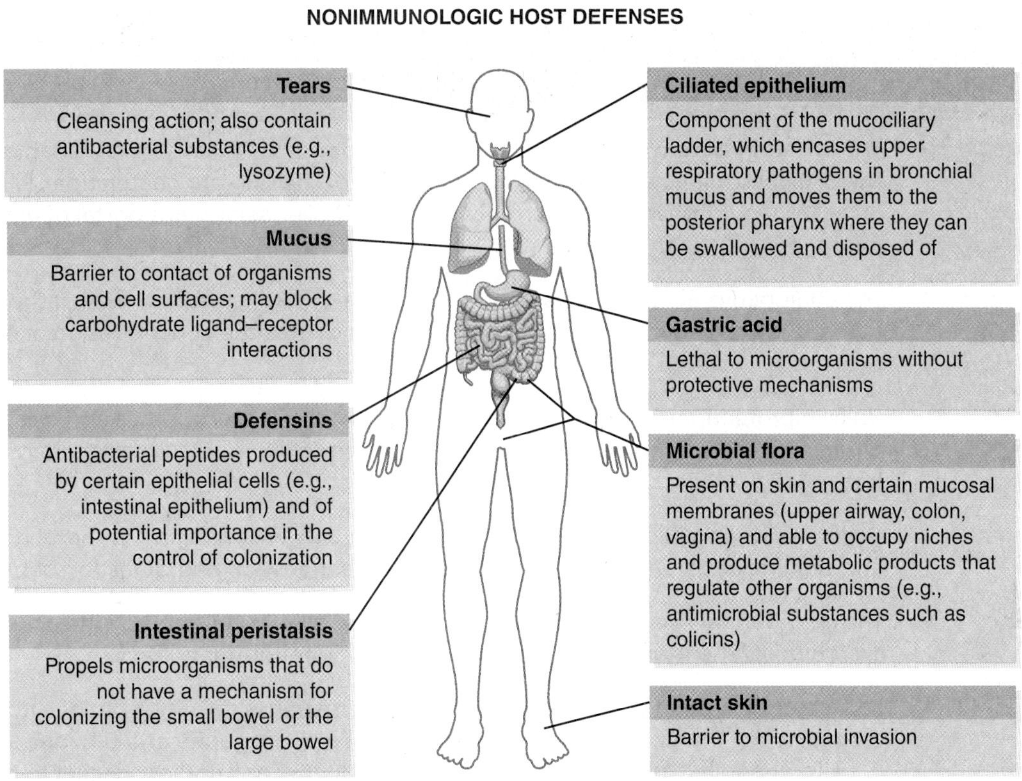

NONIMMUNOLOGIC HOST DEFENSES

Tears
Cleansing action; also contain antibacterial substances (e.g., lysozyme)

Mucus
Barrier to contact of organisms and cell surfaces; may block carbohydrate ligand–receptor interactions

Defensins
Antibacterial peptides produced by certain epithelial cells (e.g., intestinal epithelium) and of potential importance in the control of colonization

Intestinal peristalsis
Propels microorganisms that do not have a mechanism for colonizing the small bowel or the large bowel

Ciliated epithelium
Component of the mucociliary ladder, which encases upper respiratory pathogens in bronchial mucus and moves them to the posterior pharynx where they can be swallowed and disposed of

Gastric acid
Lethal to microorganisms without protective mechanisms

Microbial flora
Present on skin and certain mucosal membranes (upper airway, colon, vagina) and able to occupy niches and produce metabolic products that regulate other organisms (e.g., antimicrobial substances such as colicins)

Intact skin
Barrier to microbial invasion

Figure 7-3 The body has a number of defense mechanisms to prevent infection.

culminating in the expression of a variety of proinflammatory molecules, which together orchestrate the early host response to infection.

This nonspecific inflammatory response results in neutrophil migration and release of inflammatory mediators in an effort to contain and inactivate the pathogen. A more specific response progresses as T lymphocytes develop receptors for a specific antigen on the pathogen. This allows the T cells to attach to and ingest the pathogen. B lymphocytes are activated and begin to produce **antibodies** (free-floating proteins) with an affinity for the specific antigen. These circulating antibodies then bind to the antigen on the pathogen, either rendering the pathogen ineffective or allowing other body defenses to inactivate or destroy it. Some cloned B cells become memory cells, which generate specific antibodies quickly in the event of a reexposure to the pathogen. This reaction supports immunity to certain diseases by targeting specific antigens and disabling them when they make a reappearance.

The human body has many other nonspecific protective mechanisms, such as the skin, mucus, and cilia that trap organisms (**Figure 7-3**). Acidic secretions, such as those found in the intestinal tract, inhibit organism growth. Several body systems also have mechanisms affecting immunity (Table 7-6).

Physiologic Response to Infections by Body System

Respiratory System

Respiratory infections are a common cause of illness in the United States. Notably, acute respiratory infections are the leading cause of death in children younger than 5 years throughout the world. A variety of organisms can infect the respiratory system, with viral infections being more common than bacterial infections. Respiratory infections can occur in the upper or lower respiratory tract.

Upper respiratory illnesses include infections of the nose, sinuses, throat, tonsils, larynx, epiglottis, and trachea. Signs and symptoms of upper respiratory infection include fever, nasal congestion/drainage, sore throat, painful swallowing/speaking, and nonproductive cough. Upper respiratory infections are typically caused by viruses.

Lower respiratory infections include bronchitis and pneumonia. Bronchitis occurs when the large airways of the lung become inflamed, causing cough (often lasting for more than 5 days) and occasional sputum production, but typically without fever. Viruses are the most common cause of bronchitis. Pneumonia involves an infection and

Table 7-6 The Role of Body Systems in Immunity

System	Role
Integumentary system	The immune system's first line of defense is intact skin. Organisms are unable to pass through intact skin, and the normal secretions of the skin are bactericidal, killing off many would-be invaders. Nonintact skin, however, serves as a portal of entry for pathogens.
Ocular system	The conjunctiva are protective in two ways. First, blinking sweeps away pathogens before they can enter the eye. Second, tear film dilutes the concentration of organisms present.
Respiratory system	Built-in protections in the lungs include moist mucous membranes and cilia that trap organisms entering during inhalation. The cough reflex expels the pathogens from the body.
Gastrointestinal tract	Gastric acids and juices, along with helpful microorganisms living in the GI tract, serve as another line of defense. Phagocytes assist in the ingestion and digestion of bacteria.
Genitourinary system	The genitourinary system is protected by a thick layer of cells and by the acidic secretions of the mucous membranes lining the genitourinary tract.
Immunologic system	Leukocytes initiate a nonspecific inflammatory response involving phagocytosis (cell eating), while T lymphocytes (T cells) initiate cellular immunity and B lymphocytes (B cells) generate the humoral response by producing antibodies specific to the invading organism.

GI, gastrointestinal.

inflammation of the actual lung tissue. Signs and symptoms of pneumonia include fever, chills, pleuritic chest pain, and productive cough. Bacteria are common causes of pneumonia, and treatment often involves antibiotics. For patients with compromised immune function, respiratory infections may exacerbate underlying pulmonary conditions and progress to a more severe infection. Management focuses on supporting oxygenation, ventilation, and hydration while preventing spread of the pathogen.

Cardiovascular System

Fever increases the body's metabolic needs, so that a larger supply of oxygen and nutrients is required to carry out physiologic functions. Fever is also associated with an increased heart rate. Hypotension may develop in a severe infection (e.g., septic shock) owing to the intravascular volume depletion and vasodilation associated with this illness.

Clinicians should identify and treat hypotension promptly and aggressively by administering IV or intraosseous (IO) isotonic fluids and vasoactive medications (e.g., norepinephrine, epinephrine), depending on the etiology of hypotension. In cases of suspected severe dehydration, IV/IO isotonic fluids are indicated. If volume overload is a concern (e.g., pulmonary edema with hypoxia, missed hemodialysis), administration of large amounts of isotonic fluids should be avoided. Sepsis and septic shock are discussed in more detail in Chapter 6, *Sepsis*.

Neurologic System

Neurologic infections can be caused by viruses, bacteria, or fungi, and their severity ranges from virtually innocuous to life threatening. Central nervous system (CNS) infections can involve the brain (encephalitis), the coverings that surround the brain and spinal cord (meninges), or the spinal cord itself. Symptoms of CNS viral infections can be mild and self-limiting, as seen with viral meningitis that involves inflammation limited to the cerebrospinal fluid (CSF), or they can cause permanent neurologic injury, as in meningitis, which affects the meninges, or encephalopathies with direct brain tissue invasion. Viral, bacterial, and fungal infections affecting the spinal cord may cause transverse myelitis, which can cause pain, muscle weakness or paralysis, sensory loss, and bladder or bowel dysfunction. Early diagnosis and management of these severe CNS infections is essential if the patient is to have a favorable outcome.

Genitourinary System

Infection of the genitourinary system (e.g., urinary tract infection) causes inflammation and symptoms of the specific anatomy involved. Bladder infection leads to painful urination (dysuria), increased urinary frequency, bloody urine, and urinary malodor. Back/flank pain and fever can develop with ascending infection in the kidneys. Simple bladder infections (e.g., uncomplicated cystitis) are especially common in female patients, given their anatomy. Risk factors for complicated urinary infections include indwelling catheters, urinary obstruction, and immunosuppression.

Integumentary System

The skin serves as a barrier to pathogens, ultraviolet radiation, and loss of body fluids. It also helps regulate body temperature and maintain an internal homeostatic environment. Wounds (e.g., burns, pressure sores, diabetic ulcers) can predispose a person to skin infection by breaking the continuity of the skin structures and creating a portal for infection. Superficial soft-tissue infections (e.g., cellulitis) can be recognized by redness, tenderness, warmth, drainage, and induration. Infections involving structures deeper below the skin (e.g., fascia, muscle, bone) are often life threatening (e.g., necrotizing fasciitis, bacterial myositis) and require prompt diagnosis and treatment. Individuals without stable housing, those in congregate living facilities, and socially disadvantaged patients are especially susceptible to ectoparasites such as scabies, bedbugs, and lice, which can be diagnosed on the basis of a visual inspection and the patient's history (e.g., nocturnal pruritus).

Common Infectious Diseases—Respiratory

COVID-19

COVID-19 coronavirus disease is caused by the SARS-CoV-2 virus, a novel virus that was first discovered in late 2019. SARS-CoV-2 is an RNA virus, which is known to undergo multiple mutations. Since the start of the COVID-19 pandemic, multiple mutations of SARS-CoV-2 (labeled as "variants") have emerged, complicating the development of effective vaccines and monoclonal antibodies for treatment.

Pathophysiology/Transmission

Transmission is primarily by respiratory droplets.

Signs and Symptoms

Symptoms include cough, shortness of breath, sore throat, nasal discharge, diarrhea, and anosmia (loss of smell), along with indications of systemic illness such as fever, headache, myalgia, fatigue, nausea, and vomiting. Mild COVID-19 appears like any other "viral illness" and usually has minimal physical findings. Severe COVID-19 exam findings may include confusion or coma, fever, hypotension, tachycardia, tachypnea, hypoxia, signs of heart failure, and inspiratory crackles (rales) on pulmonary exam. Some patients may have a variable rash as well.

Differential Diagnosis

The differential diagnosis for COVID-19 includes other viral upper respiratory illnesses, influenza, and bacterial pneumonia. Also consider time-sensitive emergencies such as acute decompensated heart failure, chronic obstructive pulmonary disease (COPD)/asthma exacerbation, acute myocardial infarction, acute myocarditis, acute pulmonary embolism, sepsis, and viral or bacterial gastroenteritis.

Diagnosis

Rapid COVID-19 Antigen Tests

Rapid antigen tests are available for both at-home use by patients and medical clinician use. Antigen tests detect structural features of the virus's exterior (antigens), indicating current viral infection. They do not detect the RNA of the SARS-CoV-2 virus. Antigen tests are less sensitive than a nucleic acid amplification test (NAAT) based on **polymerase chain reaction (PCR)**. A single, negative antigen test result should not be used to rule out infection. Results of these tests are often available within 10 to 20 minutes.

PCR (NAAT Nucleic Acid Amplification Test)

Nucleic acid amplification tests for SARS-CoV-2 specifically identify the genetic RNA of the virus. NAATs are effective because of their ability to detect very small concentrations of a virus that other tests might miss. One such test, called an rt-PCR test, uses a nasal swab to detect the presence of COVID-19. NAATs often take 12 to 24 hours to process, but rapid NAAT tests are also available.

Treatment

Patients with very mild cases of COVID-19 require only supportive treatment. COVID-19 treatment during the pandemic led to the development of treat-in-place strategies by many EMS agencies, including ambulance services and community paramedicine/mobile integrated health care services. Protocols allowed EMS clinicians to screen for low-risk patients and provide instructions for home care without transport to an emergency department. Options available to individuals at higher risk include the following:

- Outpatient antiviral agents: Two oral antiviral medications for COVID-19 are currently available—nirmatrelvir ritonavir (Paxlovid) and molnupiravir. Both have been approved in the United States for use in adults. Children ages 12 years or older are eligible for Paxlovid treatment. Both of these antivirals must be started within 5 days of symptom onset.
- Remdesivir: The antiviral remdesivir is available only via IV and must be started within 7 days of symptom onset. A total of three single IV doses must be administered over 3 consecutive days. This medication has been approved for use in all adults and children.
- Monoclonal antibody therapy: Prior to the emergence of the COVID-19 variants, monoclonal antibody therapy (IV infusion of specific antibodies targeted for the antigens) was very effective in decreasing morbidity and mortality among individuals affected with COVID-19. Monoclonal antibody therapy (IV infusion of specific antibodies targeted for the antigens) was initially very effective in decreasing morbidity and mortality among individuals affected by COVID-19. However, COVID-19 variants became resistant to the initial monoclonal agents. Currently, two monoclonal therapies are approved for treating COVID-19 in the United States. Tocilizumab is a humanized interleukin-6 receptor-inhibiting monoclonal antibody that is administered intravenously. Baricitinib is a janus kinase (JAK) inhibitor used to treat rheumatoid arthritis; it is administered orally.
- In-hospital medications: Depending on the severity of illness and the patient's oxygen requirements, respiratory support may be necessary (e.g., high-flow nasal cannula, ventilator, extracorporeal membrane oxygenation [ECMO]). The specific treatment varies depending on the patient presentation and degree of illness. Options include dexaMETHasone, remdesivir, and monoclonal antibody therapy.

Prevention

As with most infectious diseases, the mainstays of prevention efforts are hand hygiene and respiratory hygiene/cough etiquette. In case of exposure to a patient with known or suspected COVID-19 infection, surgical, N95, or higher-level masks and gloves should be worn, with clinicians taking care not to touch their face. N95 or greater respirators and eye protection should be worn during close or extended exposure to respiratory secretions or aerosol-generating procedures. Having the patient don a mask is also preferred. Some organizations recommend the use of gowns as well to minimize fomite spread.

The COVID-19 vaccine is intended to both prevent disease spread and reduce the severity of illness if it occurs. After vaccinations were introduced, hospitalizations and mortality from this disease declined. EMS clinicians should consider obtaining vaccinations against COVID-19 and other infectious diseases to reduce their chance of serious infection and to protect their families and close contacts from these infections.

Influenza

Influenza (flu) is an acute respiratory illness, caused by influenza A or B viruses, that occurs in outbreaks and epidemics worldwide, mainly during the winter season. On average, approximately 35,000 Americans have died annually from influenza over the past 10 years, according to CDC statistics. The disease burden from influenza has been less than average since the emergence of SARS-CoV-2 in late 2019, likely due to the masking and social distancing initiatives that were implemented to prevent the spread of COVID-19. The CDC estimates 5,000 flu deaths occurred in 2021–2022 in the United States.

Pathophysiology/Transmission

Transmission is primarily by respiratory droplets, mostly within 6 feet (1.8 m), but also by contact with surfaces contaminated with respiratory droplets. The incubation period is 1 to 4 days. Once the virus has entered the body, it attaches to the epithelial host cells of the respiratory tract, causing inflammation of the trachea and bronchi. The individual is usually contagious 1 day prior to the onset of symptoms, with the duration of contagiousness approximately 5 to 7 days after symptom onset.

Signs and Symptoms

Symptoms include cough, sore throat, and nasal discharge, along with indications of systemic illness such as fever, headache, myalgia, and fatigue. Exam findings may include fever, tachycardia, tachypnea, and red throat; the lungs are usually clear to auscultation but in more severe cases, crackles may be present. Although acutely debilitating, influenza is a self-limited infection in the general population (uncomplicated influenza). However, it is associated with increased morbidity and mortality in certain high-risk populations (complicated influenza). Table 7-7 summarizes the groups considered to be at high risk for complications of influenza. The major complication of influenza is bacterial pneumonia, which usually presents as an exacerbation of fever and respiratory symptoms several days after initial improvement in the symptoms of acute influenza.

Differential Diagnosis

The differential diagnosis for influenza includes other viral upper respiratory illnesses and bacterial pneumonia.

Table 7-7 People at High Risk for Developing Complications of Influenza

Children < 5 years of age, but especially < 2 years
Adults ≥ 65 years of age
Women who are pregnant or up to 2 weeks postpartum
Residents of nursing homes and long-term care facilities
Some racial/ethnic populations (e.g., non-Hispanic Black persons, Hispanic or Latino persons, and American Indians and Alaska Natives)
People with certain medical conditions, including: ■ Asthma ■ Chronic lung disease (e.g., chronic obstructive pulmonary disease, cystic fibrosis) ■ Heart disease (e.g., congenital heart disease, heart failure, coronary artery disease) ■ Blood disorders (e.g., sickle cell disease) ■ Endocrine disorders (e.g., diabetes mellitus) ■ Liver disorders ■ Kidney diseases ■ Metabolic disorders (e.g., mitochondrial disorders) ■ Weakened immune system due to disease (e.g., HIV, AIDS, cancer) or medication (e.g., chronic glucocorticoids) ■ Extreme obesity (BMI ≥ 40) ■ Stroke

AIDS, acquired immunodeficiency syndrome; BMI, body mass index; HIV, human immunodeficiency virus.

Modified from Centers for Disease Control and Prevention. People at higher risk of flu complications. n.d. https://www.cdc.gov/flu/highrisk/index.htm

Also consider time-sensitive emergencies such as acute decompensated heart failure, COPD/asthma exacerbation, acute myocardial infarction, acute pulmonary embolism, and sepsis.

Diagnosis

Most clinical sites use the rapid influenza antigen test (RIDT) to diagnose this disease; the test takes 15 minutes to perform. RIDTs work by detecting the parts of the virus (antigens) that stimulate an immune response and have a pooled sensitivity of approximately 53%. Rapid molecular assays detect genetic material of the flu virus, produce results in 15–20 minutes, and are more accurate than RIDTs. Hospitals and public health laboratories occasionally perform more accurate tests including reverse transcription PCR (RT-PCR), viral culture, and immunofluorescence assays.

During known influenza outbreaks, most patients can be diagnosed clinically as having influenza (see the signs and symptoms section).

Treatment

All children or adults with severe disease (hospitalized) or who are at increased risk for complications (Table 7-7) should receive antiviral agents (e.g., oseltamivir, peramivir, zanamivir, baloxavir), ideally as soon as possible and within 48 hours of symptom onset. According to a CDC report, treatment with oseltamivir reduces the duration of symptoms by approximately 1 day.

Prevention

The influenza vaccine is one of the best public health measures for prevention. Two types of vaccines are widely available: inactivated influenza vaccines and live attenuated influenza vaccines. Recombinant influenza (flu) vaccines are produced using recombinant technology, which does not require an egg-grown vaccine virus.

Oseltamivir, zanamivir, and baloxavir have been approved as prophylaxis for adults. They may be used in pediatric patients depending on the specific antiviral agent.

In case of exposure to a coughing patient during an influenza outbreak, surgical masks and gloves should be worn, with clinicians taking additional care not to touch their face. Asking the patient to don a mask as well is preferred.

Pneumonia

Pneumonia is an inflammation and infection of the lung tissue caused by pathogens including bacteria, viruses, and fungi. Pneumonia is a leading cause of morbidity and mortality worldwide, and is responsible for approximately 4.5 million outpatient and emergency department visits and 47,000 deaths each year. Risk factors for this disease include older age, smoking, alcohol overuse, and chronic medical conditions (e.g., asthma, COPD, diabetes, heart failure, and immunosuppression).

Pneumonia can be further classified based on its presumed etiology and likely causative agent.

- Community-acquired pneumonia (CAP) occurs when a person develops pneumonia in the community, outside of the hospital setting. Common causative pathogens include *Streptococcus pneumoniae, Haemophilus influenzae, Staphylococcus aureus, Mycoplasma pneumoniae, Legionella species, Chlamydia pneumoniae, Moraxella catarrhalis,* and viruses including influenza A and B, SARS-CoV-2, and respiratory syncytial virus.

- Hospital-acquired pneumonia (HAP) occurs when pneumonia develops during or following a stay in a hospital (usually 48 hours after admission).
- Ventilator-associated pneumonia (VAP) occurs when pneumonia develops during or after a person was on a mechanical ventilator.

Common causative pathogens for both hospital- and ventilator-acquired pneumonia include MRSA, *Pseudomonas aeruginosa*, and non-pseudomonal gram-negative bacteria.

Signs and Symptoms

Common symptoms of pneumonia include fever, cough, sputum production, shortness of breath, and pleuritic chest pain. Patients may be febrile, hypotensive, tachypneic, hypoxic, and confused. Crackles may be auscultated during the pulmonary assessment. Be cognizant of the patient's work of breathing and oxygenation to determine the severity of illness.

Cough, dyspnea, purulent sputum, and pleuritic chest pain are the symptoms most commonly associated with CAP. Clinicians may also see tachypnea, increased work of breathing, and pulmonary crackles and rhonchi on lung exam. Chills, malaise, and loss of appetite may be present as well. Because CAP is a leading cause of sepsis, the initial presentation may include hypotension and altered mentation. Some of these signs may be less developed and thus more subtle in elderly patients. The clinical presentation of CAP varies widely, so it should be considered in the differential diagnosis of almost all respiratory illnesses.

Diagnosis

Both CAP and HAP are most frequently diagnosed by chest x-ray. For some patients with multiple comorbidities or lung scarring, computed tomography (CT) scan may be required to make the diagnosis. Recently, bedside ultrasound has proved useful in the early diagnosis of CAP.

HAP requires a much more intensive diagnostic workup. Cultures of blood, sputum, pleural fluid, and urine are frequently obtained. For immunocompromised patients, a complete viral panel may be helpful as well.

Treatment

Most patients with CAP are treated empirically with bacterial antimicrobials. Treatment usually consists of a combination of a beta lactam (cefTRIAXone, ampicillin–sulbactam, or a third- or fourth-generation cephalosporin) plus a macrolide or doxycycline. Rapid tests for viral organisms (influenza, COVID-19, and RSV) may assist clinicians in deciding whether to add antiviral agents to the treatment regimen. For more seriously ill ambulatory patients, blood cultures and sputum cultures may be helpful.

For patients with HAP, empiric coverage with a third- or fourth-generation beta lactam plus macrolide or doxycycline is usually initiated pending culture results.

Once cultures or immunologic testing is available, targeted antibiotic therapy can then be initiated.

Respiratory Syncytial Virus

Respiratory syncytial virus (RSV) is the leading cause of bronchiolitis (inflammation of the small airways) and pneumonia in the United States in children younger than 1 year. It can also occur in adults. Outbreaks generally occur in the late fall and peak in the winter. Most healthy adults recover from RSV infection in 1 to 2 weeks, and often experience mild or no symptoms. However, young infants (especially those ages 6 months and younger) are at risk for severe infection and may develop apnea (respiratory pause for more than 10 seconds). Adults ages 65 years and older or with chronic medical conditions are also at risk of severe infection.

Pathophysiology/Transmission

Transmission of RSV occurs by direct contact with contaminated surfaces and respiratory droplets. The portal of entry is usually the eyes, nose, or mouth. RSV is a large-particle virus that travels only about 3 feet (0.9 m). Recent evidence suggests that in certain situations, RSV may also be transmitted by aerosol. This virus is stable on fomites, with reports indicating that RSV can be cultured more than 5 hours after it has transferred to an impervious surface (e.g., bed rail). The virus has an incubation period of 2 to 8 days.

Signs and Symptoms

Symptoms of RSV include runny nose, nasal congestion, sneezing, wheezing, cough, irritability, possible fever, and decreased appetite. Hypoxemia and apnea are common in infants (typically younger than 6 months) with RSV and constitute the primary reason for hospitalization. Patients suspected of having RSV should be assessed for a history of exposure to the virus with an evaluation of ventilation and breath sounds (fine crackles or wheezing). Concerning signs include wheezing, tachypnea, cyanosis, retractions, and apnea.

Differential Diagnosis

The differential diagnosis includes other viral upper respiratory illnesses, influenza-like illness, bacterial pneumonia, asthma/COPD exacerbations, and upper airway obstruction.

Testing is usually done during the RSV season to help diagnose the illness in patients who have moderate to severe symptoms and lower respiratory tract involvement. Testing is ordered primarily on young children between ages 6 months and 2 years, elderly patients, and patients with compromised immune systems, such as those with preexisting lung disease and recipients of organ transplants. Rapid molecular testing is now available for RSV, and recent studies have demonstrated it has a very high sensitivity rate (100%).

Treatment

The mainstay of treatment is supportive care with rehydration, nasal suctioning, and respiratory support (supplemental oxygen, nebulized hypertonic saline). Some high-risk patients (e.g., premature infants, patients with congenital heart disease or lung disease) are eligible to receive palivizumab (a monoclonal antibody), which has been shown to prevent severe infection. Ribavirin (orally or aerosolized) has been used in adults and children with good results. The use of bronchodilators such as albuterol in the treatment of RSV remains controversial.

Prevention

Prevention requires following standard precautions, including frequent hand washing and cleaning contaminated surfaces. In May 2023, an RSV vaccine (Arexvy) was approved by the FDA, and there are recommendations that it should be offered to all individuals over 60 years of age. It can also be given to pregnant females after 32 weeks of gestation to protect the infant up to 6 months of age.

Tuberculosis

Tuberculosis (TB) is caused by *Mycobacterium tuberculosis*, an aerobic bacterium that typically attacks the lungs, although it can affect other organ systems as well (e.g., spine, brain, kidneys). After exposure to the TB bacterium, a person may or may not develop active infection. Exposure to *M. tuberculosis* that does not make a person ill is termed *latent TB*. People with latent TB are asymptomatic and cannot spread the TB bacterium to others, but may develop TB disease if they do not receive treatment for their latent TB. The majority of persons develop latent TB. *TB disease* refers to active TB illness, which occurs once the bacterium becomes activated and the immune system cannot impede its replication. People with TB disease are symptomatic and feel unwell. Individuals with compromised immune systems are at highest risk for developing active TB disease.

In 2021, 7,882 cases of active TB infections were reported in the United States. U.S. infection rates have been declining since the 1950s. The incidence of TB infections is more common in congregate living facilities and developing countries.

Pathophysiology/Transmission

M. tuberculosis is spread through the air rather than by direct contact, and airborne precautions are essential when caring for anyone with suspected active TB. Transmission occurs when a person with active TB disease speaks, sneezes, or coughs, emitting respiratory particles in the air that are inhaled by another person. Transmission typically requires prolonged exposure to an infected individual. Patients are no longer considered to have communicable disease when they have three appropriately collected negative sputum smears that are collected in 8- to 24-hour intervals and/or until 14 days after the initiation of appropriate treatment with clinical improvement.

Signs and Symptoms

Signs and symptoms of TB disease include a persistent cough, sputum production, night sweats, fever, weight loss, hemoptysis, and chest pain.

Differential Diagnosis

The differential diagnosis for TB includes upper respiratory infection, bronchitis, COVID-19, influenza, and pneumonia. Other time-sensitive emergencies (e.g., acute decompensated heart failure, COPD/asthma exacerbation, acute myocardial infarction, and acute pulmonary embolism) should also be considered. If the infection involves the CNS, meningitis, encephalitis, spinal infection, and stroke can occur and should be considered.

Diagnosis

The Mantoux tuberculin skin test and interferon-gamma release assays (e.g., QuantiFeron TB or T-SPOT.TB) are screening tests commonly performed to determine exposure to TB. If the initial testing is positive or there is high suspicion of TB disease, a chest x-ray can be obtained to support the diagnosis of active disease. Sputum testing with cultures and NAAT are also used to diagnose active TB disease.

TB testing for health care clinicians depends on risk assessment in the workplace. Testing is conducted on newly hired employees and for health care clinicians known to have been exposed to TB. In prehospital care settings, annual testing is often mandated.

Treatment

Even though EMS clinicians will not be able to make a new diagnosis of TB in the field, when TB is suspected, standard care for respiratory infection should be provided. When indicated, this care includes supplemental oxygen, CPAP, and manual ventilation. Appropriate use of respiratory PPE is essential and is described in the prevention section.

Definitive treatment of both latent TB and active TB disease comprises a prolonged course of antibiotics, usually ranging from 4 to 9 months depending on the drug regimen and active infection. The 4-month TB treatment regimen consists of high-dose daily rifapentine with moxifloxacin, isoniazid (INH), and pyrazinamide (PZA). The most common treatment for active TB is INH in combination with rifampin, PZA, and ethambutol, for 6 to 9 months.

Drug-resistant TB has increasingly become a problem. It typically involves a more complicated course and a different antibiotic regimen chosen based on expert consultation.

Prevention

Place a surgical mask on the patient if there is concern for TB infection. During transport, an N95 respirator or higher should be worn and vehicle exhaust fans in the patient compartment may be employed to optimize air flow. If preventive measures are not taken, the clinician may be exposed to the TB bacterium. A clinician who suspects they have been exposed to TB should report this incident to the agency infection control officer (or designated personnel) for follow-up. At the conclusion of patient care, contaminated surfaces (e.g., stretchers) and reusable medical equipment (e.g., blood pressure cuffs) should be decontaminated using an approved method.

The bacille Calmette-Guérin (BCG) vaccine is commonly used outside of the United States, in countries with higher incidence of TB disease, as a means to prevent severe forms of TB. In the United States, this vaccine is only considered for high-risk individuals. Recent evidence suggests that the BCG vaccine provides significant protection against TB disease, but only for children younger than 5 years. The vaccine does not provide any protection for adolescents or adults.

Meningitis

Meningitis is an inflammation of the membranes covering the brain and spinal cord. It is typically caused by viruses or bacteria, but may also be caused by fungi, parasites, amoebae, or noninfectious etiologies. Viral and bacterial meningitis occur worldwide. The bacterial organisms most often associated with meningitis are *Neisseria meningitidis*, *Haemophilus influenzae* type b (Hib), and *Streptococcus pneumoniae*. More than 90% of meningitis cases have a viral etiology, with the highest incidence of viral meningitis occurring in the first year of life. Bacterial meningitis from Hib and *S. pneumoniae* can be prevented by vaccination. The incidence of bacterial meningitis has greatly diminished since immunization programs have been initiated. The most common bacterial organisms are discussed in detail here.

Neisseria meningitidis *(Meningococcal Meningitis)*

N. meningitidis is a gram-negative organism that is part of the normal flora of the nasopharynx in many people. In certain circumstances, such as in the setting of weakened host resistance, the bacteria can enter the bloodstream and gain access to the CNS, including the meninges, causing meningococcal meningitis. Meningococcal meningitis is a seasonal disease that tends to occur in the early spring and fall; it is observed worldwide, especially in sub-Saharan Africa. Globally, meningococcal meningitis is fatal in 50% of cases if untreated. Each year in the United States, 2,500 to 3,500 cases of *N. meningitidis* infection are diagnosed, 10% to 14% of which are fatal. Persons at increased risk of contracting meningococcal meningitis include infants and young children, refugees living in crowded or unsanitary conditions, military recruits, college students living in dormitories, high school students, and the household contacts of individuals who have the illness.

Pathophysiology/Transmission

Transmission of meningococcal meningitis occurs by direct contact with droplets from the oronasal secretions of an infected person. This pathogen is not passed by airborne transmission. The virulent components of *N. meningitidis* bind with the host's cellular receptors, triggering an inflammatory response. The blood–brain barrier, which normally protects the brain from pathogens, is compromised in meningococcal meningitis, allowing microorganisms to reach the brain and meninges.

Signs and Symptoms

The classic symptoms of meningococcal meningitis are a petechial rash that rapidly develops into purpura, accompanied by high fever, headache, symptoms of upper respiratory infection, nausea and vomiting, and photophobia (light sensitivity) (**Figure 7-4**). Neurologic symptoms of meningococcal meningitis, which can occur within 48 hours of the onset of the illness, include mental status changes, seizures, and coma. Specific exam findings for meningitis include neck muscle rigidity with flexion (nuchal rigidity), pain with knee extension when the hip is flexed at 90° (Kernig sign), and involuntary lifting of the legs with passive neck flexion (Brudzinski sign). While the Kernig and Brudzinski signs are considered the classic signs of meningitis, the absence of either finding is not sensitive enough to exclude the diagnosis of meningitis. When two of the four symptoms are present (headache, altered mental status, neck stiffness, and fever), the vast majority of patients are ultimately diagnosed with meningitis.

Ask the patient or their family about vaccination status. Check for evidence of an earlier infection, such as aches, rash, and flu-like symptoms.

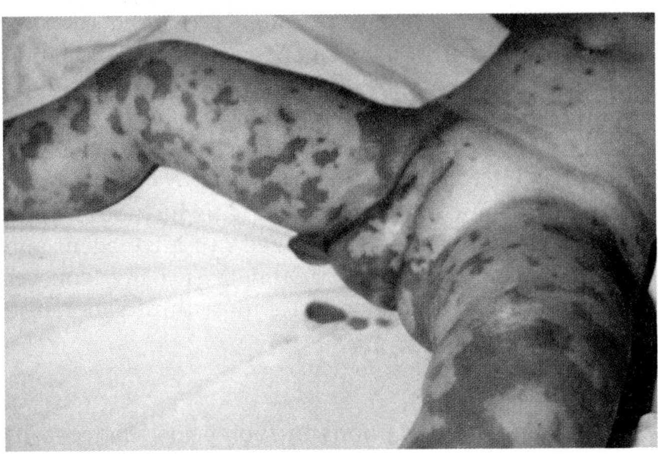

Figure 7-4 Purpura in a child with meningococcal sepsis.
Courtesy of Ronald Dieckmann, MD.

Differential Diagnosis

The differential diagnosis includes other forms of meningitis or brain infection, sepsis, flu-like illness, subarachnoid hemorrhage, and some stroke presentations.

The diagnosis of *meningococcal meningitis* is confirmed through CSF sampling. CSF should be analyzed based on Gram stain of the fluid, cell count, and chemistries (glucose and protein). Additional CSF studies include PCR and latex agglutination tests to confirm *N. meningitidis* infection.

Treatment

Treatment should be initiated quickly; it includes antibiotics targeted toward the presumed causative agent and sometimes steroids (dexaMETHasone). Depending on the patient's age, preemptive empiric antibiotics may include a third-generation cephalosporin such as cefTRIAXone or cefotaxime.

Prevention

Vaccination is recommended for people in high-risk groups: children aged 2 to 18 years, college students living in dormitories, and military recruits. Two types of meningococcal vaccines are available in the United States:

- Meningococcal conjugate or MenACWY vaccines
- Serogroup B meningococcal or MenB vaccines

All 11- to 12-year-olds should get a MenACWY vaccine, with a booster dose at 16 years of age. Teens and young adults (16 to 23 years old) also may get a MenB vaccine. In addition, the CDC recommends meningococcal vaccination for other children and adults who are at increased risk for meningococcal disease.

Postexposure treatment should be considered for close contacts of cases. It consists of either one dose of intramuscular cefTRIAXone, one dose of oral ciprofloxacin, or oral rifampin for 2 days. Prophylaxis should be started within 24 hours of the exposure (confirmed cases).

Haemophilus influenzae *Type b Meningitis*

Haemophilus influenzae type b (Hib) can cause serious illness in humans. In infants and young children, Hib causes bacteremia, pneumonia, acute bacterial meningitis, epiglottitis, and joint infections. The incubation period for Hib meningitis is unknown, but may be approximately 2 to 4 days. Before 1985, when a vaccine became available, 1 in 200 children was believed to have had Hib meningitis by 2 months of age. Given the high rates of childhood vaccination in the United States, *H. influenzae* meningitis has been rarely seen since 1985.

Pathophysiology/Transmission

Hib is transmitted through respiratory secretions.

Signs and Symptoms

The signs and symptoms of Hib meningitis are similar to those of other types of meningitis:

- Fever
- Severe headache
- Irritability and crying (common in babies and young children)
- Bulging fontanelles
- Stiff neck (not as common in babies and young children)
- Photophobia (not as common in infants and young children)
- Tiredness, drowsiness, or difficulty waking up
- Vomiting
- Refusing food and drink
- Convulsions or seizures
- Loss of consciousness

As many as 50% of patients with meningitis may have long-term neurologic involvement. Hib epiglottitis, a dangerous infection that may accompany meningitis, causes noisy, labored breathing and should be monitored closely (see Chapter 3, *Respiratory Disorders*).

Differential Diagnosis

Other forms of meningitis or brain infection, flu-like illness, and subarachnoid hemorrhage are all part of the differential diagnosis. The diagnosis is confirmed through CSF sampling.

Treatment

Treatment includes antibiotics (most commonly a third-generation cephalosporin) targeted toward the presumed causative agent. Steroids (most commonly dexaMETHasone) have been shown to reduce the cerebral edema associated with inflammation of the meninges and to reduce complications such as hearing loss and other neurologic sequelae. For steroids to be beneficial, they must be administered prior to or along with parenteral antibiotics.

Prevention

Children are immunized against Hib using a series of vaccines, beginning at 2 months of age. Doses are given at 2, 4, and 6 months, followed by another dose at 12 to 15 months, depending on the vaccine used. When treating a child suspected of having bacterial meningitis, use good hand washing practices. Postexposure treatment with rifampin should be considered for all members of a household if the family includes children younger than 4 years of age without full vaccination or individuals who are immunocompromised and younger than 18 years of age.

Streptococcus pneumoniae (*Pneumococcal Meningitis*)

Streptococcus pneumoniae (often called pneumococcus) is a bacterium that can be cultured from the nasopharynx of most healthy people. The presence of pneumococcus in the nasopharynx is referred to as *carriage*. Most people have been carriers of *S. pneumoniae* at some point in their lives. Carriage is more common in young children and generally causes no illness.

Worldwide, *S. pneumoniae* is the most common cause of bacterial meningitis, CAP, bacteremia, and otitis media. More than 90 serotypes of *S. pneumoniae* have been identified. Certain populations in the United States, including Alaska Natives, have high rates of pneumococcal disease.

Pathophysiology/Transmission

S. pneumoniae is an exclusively human pathogen that is spread from person to person by respiratory droplet transmission. Carriers of *S. pneumoniae,* while generally healthy themselves, often infect others. *S. pneumoniae* sometimes causes disease by spreading from the nasopharynx of a colonized person to other parts of the body, such as the middle ear (otitis media), nasal sinuses (sinusitis), and lungs. Meningitis is the result when the bacteria colonize the brain and spinal cord. The bacteria may also reach the bloodstream, causing bacteremia.

Signs and Symptoms

Symptoms include fever, headache, neck pain/stiffness, and photophobia (light sensitivity). Neurologic symptoms include mental status changes, seizures, and coma. Specific exam findings for meningitis include nuchal rigidity, Kernig sign, and Brudzinski sign.

Ask the patient or their family about vaccination status. Check for evidence of an earlier infection, such as aches, rash, and flu-like symptoms.

Differential Diagnosis

The differential diagnosis list includes other forms of meningitis or brain infection, flu-like illness, and subarachnoid hemorrhage.

Diagnosis is confirmed through CSF sampling (see the previous discussion). Gram stain, latex agglutination test (LAT), culture, and PCR are available to assist in the diagnosis of *S. pneumoniae* in CSF.

Treatment

Treatment of pneumococcal meningitis includes antibiotics targeted toward the presumed causative agent and dexaMETHasone. Empiric treatment usually consists of vancomycin in combination with a third-generation cephalosporin.

Prevention

Observe standard precautions, including good hand washing practices. Pneumococcal vaccination has been shown to decrease the incidence of pneumococcal meningitis.

Viral Meningitis

Compared to bacterial meningitis, viral meningitis is more common and typically has a less severe course of illness. Neonates, geriatric patients, and immunocompromised patients are more likely to develop severe illness. The most common cause of viral meningitis is non-polio enteroviruses. Other causes include adenovirus, mumps virus, human herpesviruses, measles virus, influenza, arboviruses (e.g., West Nile virus, dengue, Zika, chikungunya), and lymphocytic choriomeningitis virus.

Pathophysiology/Transmission

Viral infections are spread through contact with infected feces or respiratory/mucosal secretions, airborne droplets (e.g., measles), and reactivation (e.g., herpes [HSV1 and HSV2]). Viruses spread most rapidly among young children and persons in group living situations.

Signs and Symptoms

Symptoms include fever, headache, neck pain/stiffness, photophobia (light sensitivity), and nausea and vomiting. Neurologic symptoms include mental status changes, seizures, and coma. Specific exam findings for meningitis include nuchal rigidity, Kernig sign, and Brudzinski sign. Some strains of viral meningitis cause a rash, which may cover either most of the body or just the arms and legs. This rash is red and mostly flat, but may be raised in some areas. It is not the same as the rash seen in meningococcal meningitis (see the section on meningococcal meningitis), which is initially characterized by small, bright-red pinpoint spots covering most of the body.

Ask the patient or their family about vaccination status. Check for evidence of an earlier infection, such as aches, rash, and flu-like symptoms.

Differential Diagnosis

The differential diagnosis includes other forms of meningitis or brain infection, flu-like illness, and subarachnoid hemorrhage. The diagnosis is confirmed through CSF sampling, and by viral swabs and PCR testing for some viruses.

Treatment

There is no specific treatment for most cases of viral meningitis, and patients typically recover within 7 to 10 days. Antiviral treatment is indicated in cases of suspected herpesvirus (IV acyclovir) and influenza infections (oseltamivir or baloxavir).

Prevention

Prevention through vaccination is the ideal way to prevent meningitis. Vaccinations are available for measles, mumps, varicella, and influenza.

Use proper PPE when treating a patient suspected of having viral meningitis and follow standard precautions, including practicing scrupulous hand hygiene. It is also important to avoid contact from mosquitoes, other insects, and rodents to decrease the chances of zoonotic disease transmission.

Bloodborne Diseases

Human Immunodeficiency Virus and Acquired Immunodeficiency Syndrome

Although human immunodeficiency virus (HIV), the virus that causes acquired immunodeficiency syndrome (AIDS), was first identified in 1983, it has been found in a human specimen dating from 1959. Thus, it has a longer history than was initially suspected in the 1980s. A double-stranded RNA **retrovirus**, HIV attacks the immune system by infecting and destroying CD4 lymphocytes, which reduces the body's ability to fight off infection.

In 2019, there were approximately 37,000 new diagnoses of HIV and 15,815 HIV-related deaths in the United States. An estimated 13% of people infected with HIV are unaware of their disease status.

Pathophysiology/Transmission

A healthy person has 500 to 1,500 CD4 (helper T cells) cells/mm^3. These specialized lymphocytes are an important component of the body's cellular immune system. The CD4 count is reduced during the first 6 weeks after HIV infection because of the uncontrolled replication of the virus, called the *initial phase* (i.e., primary HIV infection). This initial phase is characterized by flu-like symptoms, which can be confused with mild viral illness. This phase is followed by mobilization of a cellular and humoral response to the presence of HIV. If the infection is left untreated, the number of CD4 cells slowly declines over several years. Seroconversion (i.e., detection of antibodies in the blood) usually occurs within the first 3 months following the primary HIV infection. Positive results on other diagnostic tests, such as HIV RNA, can be detected 7 to 14 days post infection.

AIDS is the end-stage disease process caused by HIV. A patient with AIDS is extremely vulnerable to numerous opportunistic infections that would not affect a person with an intact immune system. The incubation period of AIDS spans the time between the initial HIV infection and the development of advanced disease, which is determined by the CD4 cell count and the presence of opportunistic infections.

HIV cannot survive outside the human host. Persons are able to transmit the virus once they have become infected with HIV. Transmission occurs primarily during sexual contact and via inoculation of infected blood directly into the bloodstream of an uninfected person, as occurs when IV drug users share needles.

Signs and Symptoms

Primary HIV infection (i.e., acute retroviral syndrome) is usually clinically asymptomatic, but can present with fever, headache, rash, mouth ulcers, and swollen lymph nodes. This initial phase is often misdiagnosed as a nonspecific viral illness. After the primary infection subsides, the infection is usually asymptomatic for years until significant CD4 depletion occurs. Individuals may experience more frequent herpes simplex outbreaks or an outbreak of herpes zoster during this latent phase. Despite the individual being clinically asymptomatic in this phase, there is widespread HIV replication and risk of transmission to others. Opportunistic infections that develop over time (e.g., PJP, CMV, lymphoma, *Cryptococcus*, *Cryptosporidium*, toxoplasmosis, CMV retinitis, and *Mycobacterium avium* complex) are characteristic of AIDS.

Differential Diagnosis

Primary HIV infection can be confused with mononucleosis and influenza-like illness. The differential diagnosis also includes nonspecific viral illness, anemia, cancer, and other immunosuppressive disorders.

Diagnosis is made when blood testing detects the presence of HIV. A CD4 count and HIV viral load are also obtained to guide treatment. AIDS is diagnosed in a person who is HIV positive and who has a CD4 count less than 200 cells/mm^3 or develops an opportunistic infection.

Treatment

Treatment of HIV with antiretrovirals has dramatically changed the nature of the HIV epidemic and the manifestations of the illness. With appropriate prolonged treatment, the infected patient's viral load may be significantly reduced, minimizing that person's ability to infect others.

Prevention

To protect yourself from HIV infection, use gloves when you are in contact with a patient's nonintact skin, mucous membranes, blood, or OPIM. Use needle-safe devices and wear eye, nose, and mouth protection when you intubate a patient or suction the airway. Routine use of a mask is not necessary. Good hand washing, however, is an important part of risk reduction.

The use of postexposure rapid HIV testing is encouraged (in the United States, it is enforced by OSHA). If the source patient tests negative for HIV, no testing of the exposed clinician is needed or recommended. If the source patient tests positive, the clinician may be offered antiretroviral drugs as a preventive measure. However, because these agents have substantial side effects, such treatment is given only to patients who meet certain risk criteria. The exposed clinician should be counseled regarding the risks and benefits of the treatment. Any EMS clinician exposed to body fluids must follow their agency policy for exposures. The EMS agency infection control officer can provide information regarding the proper procedure.

Preexposure prophylaxis (PreP) with a single emtricitabine/tenofovir pill daily has been available since 2014. It can dramatically reduce the risks of HIV transmission through the sexual contact and IV routes.

Hepatitis B Virus Infection

Hepatitis B virus (HBV) is a small DNA virus that infects the liver. Such an infection could result in acute and chronic liver injury (cirrhosis) and is associated with liver cancer. HBV is a global problem, with an estimated 240 million people being infected with chronic HBV.

Pathophysiology/Transmission

Transmission of HBV occurs primarily through exposure to infected blood products, sexual contact, or perinatal exposure. Activities linked to higher risk for HBV infection include passage through the birth canal of an infected mother, IV drug use, multiple sexual contacts, and hemodialysis. Needles, including those used for tattooing and acupuncture, and occasionally other objects, such as shared razors, have been implicated in the transmission of HBV.

Limited data suggest the HBV can survive outside the body in the medium of dried blood for as long as 7 days. The incubation period varies widely, from 30 to 200 days. The communicable period starts weeks before the first symptoms appear and may persist for years in chronic carriers. An estimated 2% to 10% of all people infected with HBV will become chronic carriers.

Signs and Symptoms

Signs and symptoms of HBV infection occur in two phases. During the first phase, a large amount of virus is present in circulating blood. The patient has flu-like symptoms, including fever, nausea, diarrhea, and abdominal pain. During the second phase, the patient's skin and eyes become jaundiced (**Figure 7-5**), the stools become whitish, and the urine becomes almost brown. The viral load drops, and antibodies appear in the blood. Approximately 10% of all people with HBV infection will become chronically infected, and the disease may progress to liver failure or liver cancer. The risk for chronic infection varies with the age of the patient when infected; it is greatest among young children.

For patients in both stages of infection, assessment is primarily visual, but also depends on taking a thorough history. Ask the patient when symptoms began and the character and location of any pain.

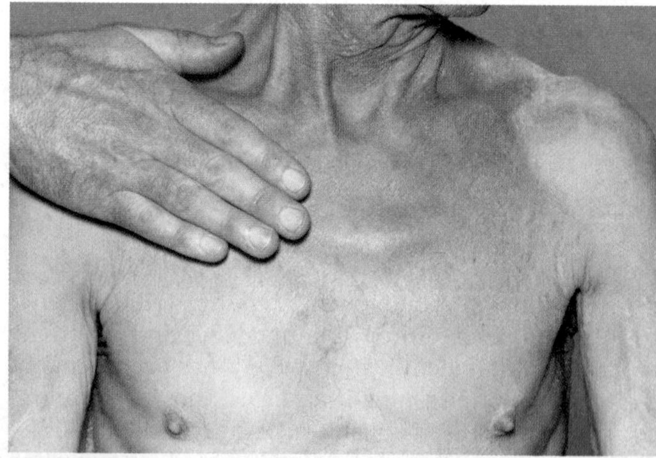

A

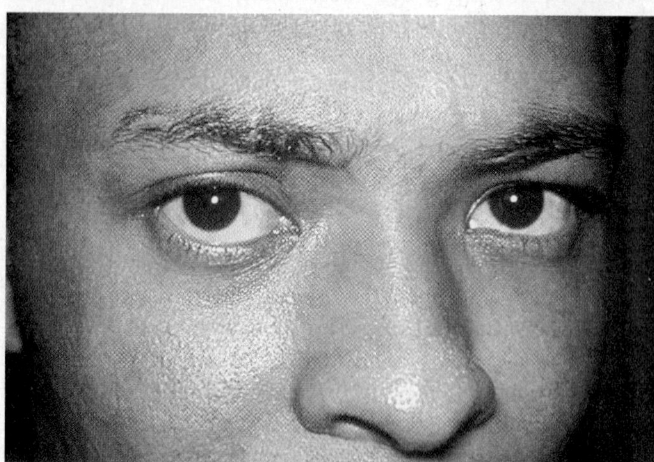

B

Figure 7-5 Signs of HBV infection. **A.** Jaundice. **B.** Scleral icterus.

Differential Diagnosis

Any other cause of hepatitis or liver failure should be considered in the differential diagnosis for HBV infection, including other hepatitis viruses, toxins (e.g., acetaminophen), alcohol, and autoimmune and other liver diseases.

Diagnosis is made through serologic testing for HBV antigens and antibodies. Additional blood tests and imaging are performed to assess the extent of liver injury.

Treatment

Treatment of HBV infection can take the form of immunomodulation (e.g., interferon), with the aim of boosting the immune response to rid the body of the virus. Antiviral drugs (e.g., entecavir, tenofovir, lamivudine, adefovir, telbivudine), which inhibit the virus from replicating, are also used. Treatment is most effective for individuals with active liver disease, with the goal of reducing the risk of liver disease and the virus's transmissibility.

Prevention

HBV vaccination is the primary method of protection for all people in the United States, where immunization is universal. Since 1991, all newborns have been vaccinated within 12 hours of birth. As of 2000, all middle school, high school, and college students were required to have been vaccinated before enrolling in school. Most health care personnel have been vaccinated since 1982. Recommendations for preventing and controlling hepatitis B can be obtained from WHO. Thanks to these measures, the risk for and incidence of HBV have declined precipitously in the United States. Full vaccination generally confers lifetime protection from the illness, so no booster or routine titer testing is required or recommended. Clinicians can also protect themselves from HBV infection by following standard precautions when they must be in contact with blood.

For unvaccinated or incompletely vaccinated health care clinicians, the source patient should be tested for hepatitis B surface antigen (HBsAg) as soon as possible after an exposure. If the source patient is HBsAg positive or has an unknown HBsAg status, the health care clinician should receive one dose of hepatitis B immune globulin (HBIG) and one dose of HepB vaccine administered as soon as possible after the exposure. The HepB vaccine may be administered simultaneously with HBIG at a separate anatomic injection site (e.g., separate limb). The health care clinician should then complete the HepB vaccine series according to the vaccination schedule.

Hepatitis C Virus Infection

Hepatitis C virus (HCV) is the most common chronic bloodborne infection and the leading cause of liver transplantation in the United States. This single-stranded RNA virus was first identified in 1988, and testing became available in 1992. HCV infection affects an estimated 1.5% of the U.S. population and 3% of the world population. Its incidence has declined by 80% in the United States since 1990.

Pathophysiology/Transmission

HCV transmission occurs through injection of contaminated blood, chiefly among IV drug users who share needles. Occasionally, the virus is spread in other ways:

- Tattooing or body piercing
- Needlestick injury
- Organ transplantation
- Transfusion of blood or blood products
- Sexual contact
- Passage through the birth canal

Transmission though mucous membranes or nonintact skin exposure is rare. The virus cannot survive in the environment long enough to pose a risk of transmission by any means except bloodborne contact. The incubation period for HCV infection is 6 or 7 weeks, but appears to be shorter when exposure occurs through transfusion of blood products.

Signs and Symptoms

Early signs and symptoms of HCV infection are the same as those for HBV infection, including fatigue, abdominal pain, and hepatomegaly (an enlarged liver). In general, primary HCV produces mild effects. Only 20% of patients with HCV infection experience symptoms associated with the second phase of hepatitis: jaundice, whitish stools, and dark urine. Chronic infection develops in approximately 20% of these patients, and 30% become carriers of the illness.

Differential Diagnosis

Any other causes of hepatitis or liver failure should be considered in the differential diagnosis for HCV infection, including other hepatitis viruses, toxins (e.g., acetaminophen), alcohol, and autoimmune and other liver diseases.

Diagnosis is made through serologic testing for HCV antigens and antibodies. Additional blood tests and imaging are performed to assess the extent of liver injury.

Treatment

Many antiviral options are available to cure HCV infection (e.g., elbasvir/grazoprevir, glecaprevir/pibrentasvir, sofosbuvir/ledipasvir, sofosbuvir/velpatasvir), based on the HCV genotype involved. Treatment duration is typically 8 to 12 weeks, but may be longer (up to 24 weeks) depending on the extent of liver damage.

Prevention

Clinicians can reduce their risk of contracting HCV by following standard precautions, including good hand washing practices, when in contact with a patient's blood or other potentially infectious materials. Promptly report any exposure so the source patient can be tested. If the source patient tests positive for HCV, the following steps should be taken:

- Perform baseline source-patient testing for anti-HCV (antibody), with subsequent testing for hepatitis C RNA if the test for antibody is positive. Another option is to test the source patient for hepatitis C RNA initially.
- Perform a baseline test for the person exposed to an HCV-positive source, which includes anti-HCV and alanine aminotransferase (ALT) activity baseline testing. Follow-up initial testing is performed in 3 to 6 weeks (if the source patient is positive for hepatitis C), and final testing at 4 to 6 months. Testing for HCV RNA may be performed at 4 to 6 weeks if earlier diagnosis of HCV infection is desired.
- To confirm the diagnosis, perform supplemental anti-HCV testing (usually molecular HCV RNA testing) of all anti-HCV results reported as positive by enzyme immunoassay.

Currently, no medication can be given for postexposure prophylaxis, and no HCV vaccine has been developed. If an individual tests positive for HCV at 4 weeks after exposure, referral for treatment is needed.

Enteric (Intestinal) Diseases

Hepatitis A Virus Infection

Hepatitis A virus (HAV), also known as infectious hepatitis, is the most common type of hepatitis in the United States. HAV is a single-stranded RNA virus found in the feces of infected people. This virus replicates in the liver, but usually does not directly result in permanent damage to the liver. Infection with HAV is often described as a benign disease, because acquiring it provides lifelong immunity to the virus.

Infection rates in the United States have declined considerably since a vaccine for HAV became available in 1995. In 2018, 12,474 cases were reported in the United States. HAV is present throughout the world, although the incidence of this infection is not well tracked. Acute HAV outbreaks have been associated with unsheltered homeless populations. Younger patients either have mild symptoms or are asymptomatic; in contrast, older children and adults commonly experience symptomatic disease. Hepatitis A resolves completely in more than 99% of cases. However, mortality has been described in older patients (age > 50 years).

Pathophysiology/Transmission

Transmission of HAV occurs by the fecal–oral route. The virus colonizes the GI tract and is detectable in the blood 4 weeks before symptoms of infection become apparent. The incubation period is 2 to 4 weeks. The communicable period starts toward the end of the incubation period and continues for a few days after the patient becomes jaundiced.

Signs and Symptoms

Patients with HAV may initially experience malaise, fatigue, anorexia, nausea, vomiting, diarrhea, fever, or abdominal discomfort. Signs and symptoms during the second phase of the illness are the same as those for any type of hepatitis: jaundice, icterus, dark urine, and whitish stools.

Differential Diagnosis

Other causes of hepatitis or liver failure should be considered in the differential diagnosis for HAV infection, including other hepatitis viruses, toxins (e.g., acetaminophen), and liver diseases. Other diagnoses to consider are viruses that cause gastroenteritis (e.g., norovirus).

To help refine the diagnosis, ask the patient about any recent travel outside the United States, possible intake of contaminated water or food (e.g., raw shellfish), and similarly sick contacts. Laboratory tests can detect the presence of anti-HAV and immunoglobulin M (IgM) antibodies within 3 weeks of exposure.

Treatment

Treatment is supportive and centers on providing good nutrition and administering IV fluids.

Prevention

Preexposure prophylaxis with intravenous immunoglobulin (IVIG) is approved for individuals who have not been immunized against HAV and are traveling to areas in which hepatitis A is endemic. The dose depends on the duration of travel and the timing of administration prior to travel. All susceptible people (i.e., those who are unvaccinated or have never been infected) traveling or working in countries that have high or intermediate HAV disease risk should be vaccinated or receive immunoglobulin before departure.

Hepatitis A vaccine, if administered within 2 weeks of exposure, is the preferred prophylaxis. It has been shown to be as effective as IVIG.

Clinicians should follow standard precautions, including good hand washing practices, when in direct contact with a patient's stool.

Norovirus

Norovirus causes GI inflammation leading to hemorrhage and erosion of the mucosal layers of the GI tract, affecting absorption of water and nutrients. What is typically called *acute gastroenteritis*, or "stomach flu," is a viral infection of the stomach and intestines leading to abdominal cramping, vomiting, and diarrhea. Noroviruses are the most common cause of acute gastroenteritis, with some strains causing symptoms for 1 to 3 days. The most important treatment is maintaining good hydration.

Norovirus infection is an international problem, as this pathogen is extremely contagious. The infectious dose of norovirus is extremely low, with as little as 18 viral particles being capable of causing infection. Outbreaks are common in semiconfined communities such as schools, cruise ships, nursing homes, hospitals, hotels, and restaurants.

Pathophysiology/Transmission

Norovirus, or Norwalk-like virus, also known as "winter vomiting disease," is caused by nonenveloped, single-stranded RNA viruses from the genus *Norovirus*. It is primarily spread by the fecal–oral route. However, severe vomiting from patients infected with norovirus can create aerosols, which can be inhaled or contaminate mucosal surfaces and cause disease.

When norovirus enters the body, it begins to multiply in the small intestines. The incubation period is 12 to 48 hours, and the virus can be transmitted from infected persons, via contaminated food or water, or by touching contaminated surfaces. The virus can be shed for weeks after infection. Norovirus has been documented to cause asymptomatic infections, with the highest prevalence occurring in younger individuals (especially $<$ 5 years of age).

Signs and Symptoms

Patients will present with GI complaints including abdominal pain, vomiting, projectile vomiting, diarrhea, and fever. Symptoms usually last 1 to 2 days, and then most patients recover fully. However, norovirus can be devastating for young children, older adults, and immunocompromised patients.

Differential Diagnosis

Other conditions that may present with similar symptoms include acute gastritis; bacterial gastroenteritis, including *Campylobacter*, *Escherichia coli*, *Salmonella*, *Shigella*, and *Vibrio* infections; rotavirus; *Cryptosporidium*; Crohn disease; food allergies; diverticulitis; irritable bowel syndrome; *C. difficile*; and inflammatory bowel disease. A diagnosis is made based on the patient's signs and symptoms, obtained by taking a thorough patient history.

Treatment

Care is supportive and focuses on oral or IV rehydration. Antimotility agents are not recommended in children younger than 3 years. In older children and adults, antimotility and antiemetic agents may be useful in supporting rehydration. Antibiotics are not useful in treating gastroenteritis caused by norovirus. Vaccines for norovirus are not available. Individuals can contract norovirus multiple times in their lifetime.

Prevention

Following standard enteric precautions—including good hand washing practices and face and eye protection when indicated—can reduce the risk of contracting norovirus. Ensure the water supply is safe and appropriate facilities are available for disposal of feces. Rooms, vehicles, and equipment must be cleaned thoroughly per local protocols. According to the CDC, a high concentration of domestic bleach (5 to 25 tablespoons bleach per gallon of water) may be used for disinfection. Soiled articles of clothing should be washed at the maximum available cycle length and machine-dried at high heat. When outbreaks occur in semi-closed environments such as cruise ships, patients should be isolated to prevent spread of the disease.

Escherichia coli Infection

Although most strains of *E. coli* are harmless, some strains cause serious foodborne illnesses. *E. coli* has been recognized as a major cause of colonization and infection in cattle, which can contaminate food. The first serious outbreak caused by the O157:H7 subtype occurred in a fast-food restaurant in Washington State in 1993. Epidemiologists estimate that this specific bacterium is the cause of more than 75,000 cases of illness each year, resulting in more than 3,000 hospital stays and 60 deaths. Illness occurs mostly in young children and in older adults. Although the disease is a problem worldwide, it is not well tracked in developing countries, so data on its incidence are limited.

Pathophysiology/Transmission

E. coli is a gram-negative bacterium belonging to the Enterobacteriaceae family. More than 30 serotypes of *E. coli* have been identified. Of these, *E. coli* O157:H7 has been the most notable in recent years for being found in improperly cooked meat, municipal water supplies, milk, raw vegetables, unpasteurized apple cider, lettuce, and products contaminated by cattle waste. Transmission is via the fecal–oral route after consumption of undercooked foods or contaminated liquids. The organism has an incubation period of 1 to 9 days. The Shiga toxin–producing strain of *E. coli* (i.e., O157:H7) is one of the most potent toxins known to humans.

Signs and Symptoms

Infection with *E. coli* O157:H7 begins with abdominal pain and tenderness, myalgia, and headache. Vomiting may also occur, followed by diarrhea ranging from watery diarrhea to hemorrhagic colitis, which causes visible blood in the stool. This stage may last 3 to 7 days and occurs mostly in people aged 65 years or older. A grave complication of this illness is hemolytic uremic syndrome, a life-threatening condition that affects approximately 10% of patients infected with *E. coli* O157:H7. Hemolytic uremic syndrome is now recognized as the most common cause of acute kidney failure in infants and young children. Adolescents and adults are also susceptible, and older adults often succumb to the disease.

Differential Diagnosis

The differential diagnosis includes gastroenteritis caused by other bacterial or viral pathogens, parasites, chemical toxins, allergies, or immune disorders.

To refine the diagnosis, ask patients whether they might have eaten any uncooked or undercooked meat. Question the patient about the appearance of their stool. Watery, yellow-green, or bloody stool, or stool that contains pus, is a clue to this illness: 90% of bloody stools will culture positive for *E. coli* bacteria. Check for signs of dehydration or shock. Diagnosis is made on the basis of a special stool culture and/or the presence of *Shigella* (Shiga) toxin.

Treatment

Supportive treatment (e.g., hydration, pain/nausea control) is the mainstay of treatment. Antibiotics have not been effective against the O157:H7 strain of *E. coli* and are typically not recommended. Likewise, antimotility agents such as loperamide or dicyclomine, which slow peristalsis, are not recommended and should be avoided.

Transfusion may be indicated if the patient becomes severely anemic. Dialysis may be indicated if acute renal failure develops.

Prevention

The best prevention is education on hand washing, appropriate preparation of raw and cooked foods, proper storage of all foods, and drinking treated water. Standard precautions, including the use of gowns to protect clothing, are recommended. As always, follow thorough hand washing practices. Rooms, vehicles, and care equipment must be cleaned thoroughly per local protocols.

Shigellosis

Shigellosis is a highly infectious, acute bacterial enteritis affecting the large and small intestines. Only a small number of bacteria—possibly as few as 10 to 100 organisms—is needed to cause infection. This disease is believed to be responsible for more than 600,000 deaths each year worldwide. Most infections and deaths occur in children younger than 10 years, the elderly, and immunocompromised individuals.

Pathophysiology/Transmission

Shigella is a genus of gram-negative, non–spore-forming, rod-shaped bacteria closely related to *E. coli* and *Salmonella*. *Shigella* species are transmitted by the fecal–oral route. Failing to wash hands or not doing so properly after defecation is an easy way to spread this infection. The incubation period may be as brief as 12 hours but can extend to 96 hours. A person can harbor this disease for as long as 4 weeks.

Signs and Symptoms

The *Shigella* bacteria multiply in the small intestine and enter into the colon. These pathogens cause cell injury and death both by direct cell invasion and by production of enterotoxins. *Shigella* strains can produce three different enterotoxins, which have enterotoxic, cytotoxic, and neurotoxic effects. Patients infected with *Shigella* have watery diarrhea, fever, vomiting, and cramps, and rehydration may be necessary. Convulsions are a complication sometimes seen in young children. Other symptoms may include nausea, vomiting, high fever, abdominal cramping, and lethargy. In mild infection, the only sign may be watery diarrhea, whereas other patients may have bloody diarrhea. Other signs include hypotension, tachycardia, and abdominal tenderness. Illness lasts about 4 to 7 days.

Differential Diagnosis

The differential diagnosis includes gastroenteritis caused by other bacterial and viral pathogens, parasites, chemical toxins, allergies, or immune disorders. Diagnosis is made based on the patient's history, signs and symptoms, stool sample culture, and assays for enterotoxin and cytotoxins.

Treatment

Most illness is self-limited, although antibiotics are often administered to patients with a positive stool culture. In adults, fluoroquinolone is recommended for patients with no risk factors for resistance, whereas a third-generation cephalosporin is recommended for high-risk patients. In pediatric patients, the first-line drug is azithromycin if antibiotic susceptibility is unknown.

Supportive treatment (e.g., hydration, pain/nausea control) is also an essential component of treatment.

Prevention

Following standard precautions, including good hand washing practices, can reduce the risk of contracting shigellosis. Ensure that the water supply is safe and that appropriate facilities are available for disposal of feces. Chlorination of the water supply also reduces risk.

Clostridioides (formerly Clostridium) difficile (Pseudomembranous Colitis)

Rates of *C. difficile* (*C. diff*) infection in the United States have tripled since 2000, and mortality from this disease has increased. Toxic strains are now widespread in both North America and Europe. This illness is usually a direct result of antibiotic therapy, which suppresses the normal flora in the GI tract and allows *C. diff* to predominate. Although it is classified as a hospital-acquired infection (HAI), this disease is also associated with outpatient antibiotic therapy. Community-acquired *C. diff* has been reported as well. High-risk environments include acute-care and long-term facilities. Increased incidence rates in pediatric patients who are immunocompromised and peripartum women who have had cesarean sections have been reported. Nevertheless, the highest incidence rates continue to be seen in the elderly population.

Pathophysiology/Transmission

C. diff is a gram-positive spore-forming anaerobic bacillus that produces two large toxins, A and B. The spores are noninfectious until ingested, but remain dormant in the colon until the normal bowel flora are disrupted. At that point, the spores germinate into the pathogenic bacteria, which then release the two toxins.

C. diff is often found in the environment and can survive for long periods as spores. Spore production causes heavy contamination of environmental surfaces. Transmission usually occurs via the fecal–oral route and most often after contact with contaminated surfaces or hands. As a result, health care clinicians' unwashed hands are a major means of *C. diff* transmission.

Signs and Symptoms

Patients with this illness have watery, nonbloody diarrhea that has a characteristic foul odor. Fever, abdominal pain and cramping, anorexia, and nausea and vomiting may also be present. If these signs and symptoms are present, ask the patient about any recent hospital stays or antibiotic therapy. Rarely, potentially life-threatening complications such as toxic megacolon may develop (**Figure 7-6**).

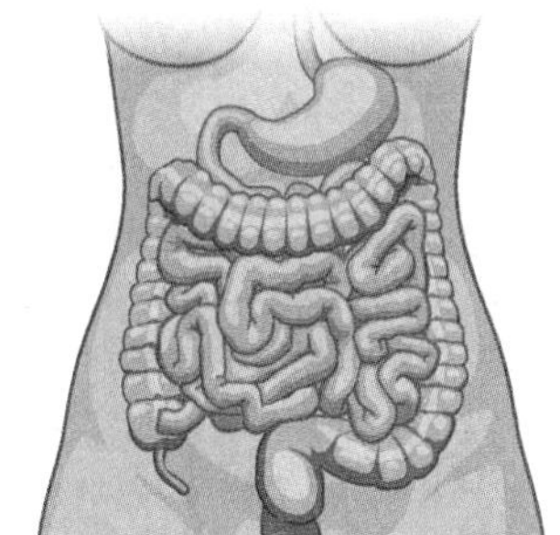

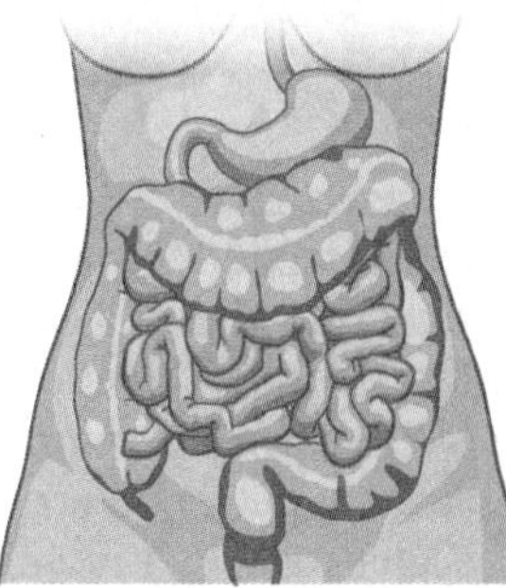

Figure 7-6 The image on the right shows a dilated colon associated with toxic megacolon.

Differential Diagnosis

The differential diagnosis includes gastroenteritis caused by other bacteria, viral pathogens, parasites, chemical toxins, allergies, and immune disorders. Acute abdominal emergencies (e.g., acute appendicitis, diverticulitis, intra-abdominal abscess, ischemic bowel) should also be considered.

To refine the diagnosis, check the odor of the stool and assess the patient for the presence of fever. The diagnosis of *C. diff* infection may be suspected based on a thorough history, a focused physical exam, and an increased index of suspicion (e.g., knowing the patient has taken antibiotics in the previous 3 months). An increased white blood cell count is associated with most severe infection. A positive stool assay for *C. diff* toxin A and B or the toxigenic *C. diff* bacillus is most commonly used to confirm the diagnosis.

Treatment

Stopping any unnecessary antibiotics is the first step of treatment. Antibiotic selection then depends on recurrence of infection and illness severity. Preferred antibiotics include fidaxomicin or oral vancomycin, given the bacterium's resistance to metroNIDAZOLE. Fecal microbiota transplant to restore the bowel ecology has also emerged as an effective treatment for some patients.

Prevention

Follow standard contact precautions, including good hand washing practices with soap and vigorous rubbing. Alcohol-based gels do not eradicate the spores and should not be relied upon when treating a patient with diarrhea. A chlorine-based solution must be used to clean equipment, because *C. diff* is a spore-forming organism. Avoiding the use of unnecessary antibiotics is essential.

Ectoparasites

Scabies

Scabies is caused by the parasitic mite *Sarcoptes scabiei*. A scabies "infection" is actually an infestation with the organism itself; the scabies mite is not a vector for transmission of other infectious agents. The scabies mites can survive outside the human body and remain infectious for 24 to 36 hours at normal room temperature.

Scabies is a worldwide problem and can have devastating effects if not treated, particularly in developing countries. Scabies infestation can affect families and children, sexual partners, patients who have chronic illnesses or are hospitalized, and people who live in group homes or in close proximity to others.

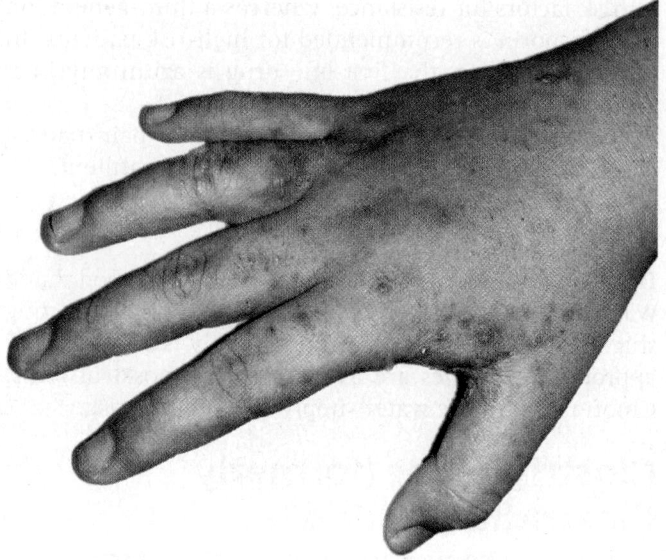

Figure 7-7 Rash produced by scabies.

Pathophysiology/Transmission

Transmission of scabies occurs by direct skin-to-skin contact. It can also occur when an uninfected person has contact with fomites such as undergarments, towels, and linens. The transmission of a single pregnant mite, or several larvae, can infect another human host. Typically, this requires close skin-to-skin contact of at least 5 to 10 minutes' duration.

The incubation period for people with no previous exposure is 2 to 6 weeks. The disease is communicable until the mites and their eggs have been destroyed by treatment. If treated early, few complications are likely. If the disease persists, skin infections leading to ulcers, soft-tissue infections, sepsis, and cardiovascular and renal complications may occur.

Signs and Symptoms

Signs and symptoms of scabies infestation include nocturnal itching and the presence of a rash (**Figure 7-7**) in any of the following areas:

- Hands and interdigit web spaces
- Flexor aspects of the wrists
- Axillary folds
- Ankles or toes
- Genital area
- Buttocks
- Abdomen

Differential Diagnosis

Other diagnostic considerations include insect bites, impetigo, cellulitis, atopic dermatitis, drug rash, and herpes.

In the vast majority of cases presenting to the emergency department, the diagnosis is "suspected scabies," a category based on the presence of typical lesions in a typical distribution and one history feature, or atypical lesions or atypical distribution and two history features. Confirmation of the scabies diagnosis is made by microscopic examination of the mite. Specimens are taken by using a needle or scalpel to remove mites that have burrowed into the skin.

Treatment

Permethrin is a topical treatment for scabies. Reapplication of this medication may be required to treat the infestation effectively in children. Lindane lotion may be prescribed as a second-line treatment, although toxicity has been reported with overuse of this agent.

For severe cases, ivermectin tablets have been used successfully. With this therapy, repeated treatment is required in 7 to 14 days after the first treatment.

It is also critical to decontaminate all clothing and bedding and treat close contacts at the same time as treatment is instituted to prevent reinfection.

Prevention

Prevention requires wearing gloves and following good hand washing practices. Cleaning of linens requires only routine washing in hot water (10 minutes at 122°F [50°C]). Routine cleaning of rooms or vehicles after patient contact is sufficient.

If clinicians are concerned that they may have been exposed, they should follow the established notification guidelines. If a clinician has been exposed, treatment will be indicated, and work restrictions limiting patient care may be necessary. Treatment of the entire household may be indicated, depending on the clinician's living conditions and the extent of infestation. This is also true for institutional incidents.

Pediculosis (Lice)

Pediculus humanus capitis (head louse), *Pediculus humanus corporis* (body louse, clothes louse), and *Pthirus pubis* (pubic lice) are parasites that, like scabies, cause infestations rather than true infections. Each type of lice is different and typically infests different parts of the body. Lice can be easily transmitted among people who live in group homes, have poor hygiene, or have multiple sexual partners.

Head and pubic lice live on the skin; body lice live and lay their eggs in the stitching of clothing or bedding, moving to the skin only to feed. Unlike the other types of lice, body lice can transmit bacterial diseases—specifically, trench fever, relapsing fever, and epidemic typhus—to humans. Head lice, however, are not a primary health hazard.

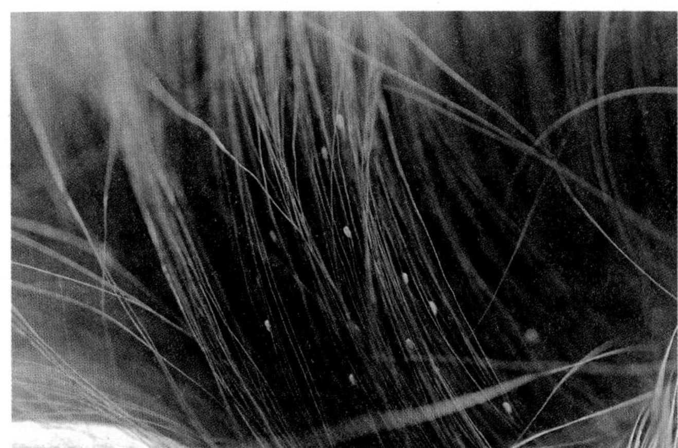

Figure 7-8 Lice nits (eggs) are visualized on the hair shafts in this photo.

Pathophysiology/Transmission

Transmission of lice occurs through physical contact or contact with clothing or shared bedding. Transmission of head lice is thought to occur by head-to-head contact, sharing of headgear, or other direct contact with fomites. Pubic lice are transmitted through sexual contact or through bedding or clothing. Body lice spread primarily by direct contact in populations with poor hygiene.

Trench fever and epidemic typhus are transmitted through infected feces of the louse, not via a bite. Relapsing fever, caused by *Borrelia recurrentis*, is transmitted when a person crushes an infected louse; the bacteria then invade the bite site or the skin of the fingers or hand that crushed the louse.

The incubation period is about 8 to 10 days after the eggs hatch. The lice are communicable until all mites and their eggs or their empty egg cases (nits), including those in infested clothing, are destroyed by treatment. Humans are the only reservoir for lice.

Signs and Symptoms

Signs and symptoms of lice include mild to severe itching and visible nits clinging to hair. Head lice infest the head and neck. Body lice are found on the body, but usually lay their eggs on clothing. Pubic lice are found on pubic, perianal, or perineal areas, and may infest the eyelashes, eyebrows, axillae, scalp, and other hair-covered body areas.

Differential Diagnosis

Other diagnostic considerations for lice include insect bites, bed bugs, ticks, fleas, and scabies.

Diagnosis of head and pubic lice is usually made by a visual observation of nits (white eggs) attached to hair shafts (**Figure 7-8**). The presence of nits indicates a past infestation, not necessarily a current infection. Diagnosis of active lice infestation requires the detection of a living louse. Infection with body lice is typically diagnosed by finding eggs and lice in the seams of clothing rather than on the skin, so careful inspection of clothing is critical.

Treatment

Manual removal of the nits and lice and application of pediculicides is the recommended treatment. Among the various topical agents, pyrethroids (e.g., permethrin 1% is a synthetic pyrethroid) are one of the most frequently used treatments for lice. Permethrin is available over the counter in the United States. Lindane is another topical treatment that kills lice, but is absorbed into the bloodstream and carries a risk of neurotoxicity. Although sometimes used in adults, this medication is not recommended for children, the elderly, or small adults.

Prevention

Prevention requires wearing gloves and practicing good hand washing techniques. Routine cleaning of the room and vehicle after contact is sufficient. Washing infested clothing and bedding with hot water at 126°F (52°C) for 30 minutes is necessary to destroy all stages of lice. If an actual exposure occurred, treatment with permethrin cream may be ordered, and restrictions from patient care may be indicated.

Zoonotic (Animal-Borne) Diseases

Rabies

The rabies virus is a bullet-shaped, single-stranded RNA virus that reaches the CNS by way of the peripheral nerves. Infection with this virus causes a progressive encephalomyelitis that is almost always fatal. In the United States, rabies is common in wild and domesticated mammals (e.g., bats, raccoons, skunks, foxes, dogs, cats). Rodents (e.g., rats, mice, squirrels, hamsters) are rarely infected by rabies and have not been known to transmit the virus to humans. Animal immunization programs have reduced the incidence of rabies and the number of deaths attributable to the disease to one or two per year.

Hawaii is the only state whose animal population is free of rabies. Rabies is found on all continents except Antarctica, with the majority of deaths from this cause occurring in Africa and Asia, where canine rabies is endemic (generally resulting from dog bites or scratches). Bats account for most cases in the Americas. Worldwide, most rabies deaths occur in countries with inadequate public health resources, limited access to preventive treatment, few diagnostic facilities, and virtually nonexistent rabies surveillance programs.

Pathophysiology/Transmission

Rabies is an acute viral infection of the CNS, primarily affecting animals, that is transmitted to humans through the virus-laden saliva of an infected animal. Incubation can range from days to years.

Once the virus enters the body, it travels through the peripheral nervous system targeting the central nerves, which then leads to encephalomyelitis. Transmission from person to person has never been documented. All animals found outside their natural habitat or behaving abnormally or aggressively should be presumed to be infected with rabies.

Signs and Symptoms

Two types of rabies may occur—encephalopathic and paralytic. In the encephalopathic form, patients show signs of hyperactivity, excited behavior, anxiety, confusion, hydrophobia, and sometimes aerophobia.

One-fourth to one-third of cases present as paralytic rabies. This form of the disease presents more gradually and is more prolonged. Muscles become gradually paralyzed, moving outward from the site of the bite or scratch. Coma develops, and death occurs. Paralytic rabies is often misdiagnosed, leading to underreporting of the disease. Early symptoms are nonspecific, consisting of fever, headache, and general malaise. As the disease progresses, depending on the form, patients will present with neurologic symptoms, including insomnia, anxiety, confusion, slight or partial paralysis, excitation, hallucinations, agitation, hypersalivation, and difficulty swallowing. Contrary to popular belief, rabies does not make the infected person afraid of water. Patients will be averse to drinking water, however, because doing so induces agonizing throat spasms. This condition is called *hydrophobia,* a term formerly synonymous with rabies itself. Death may occur within days of the onset of symptoms.

Differential Diagnosis

Early in the prodrome phase, patients present with nonspecific symptoms similar to those associated with flu-like illnesses, including GI symptoms, myalgias, and fevers. In later stages, when neurologic symptoms are present, the differential diagnosis consists of tetanus, delirium tremens, drug toxicity, stroke, CNS infection, or seizure. For patients presenting with the paralytic form, the differential diagnosis consists of botulism, tickborne diseases, Guillain-Barré syndrome, and diphtheria.

Humans are very susceptible to rabies infection after exposure to virus-laden saliva in a bite or scratch from an infected animal. The diagnosis of rabies is facilitated by a high clinical suspicion usually based on history of clinical exposure along with presenting symptoms.

Rabies can be diagnosed through multiple routes, including CSF, blood, saliva, tears, and tissue biopsies (neck, immunofluorescent stain).

Treatment

Clean the wound area thoroughly; irrigate it copiously and scrub for at least 15 minutes with soap and water, detergent, iodine, or a solution known to kill rabies. For high-risk exposures (see the local health guidelines), rabies immune globulin and rabies vaccines are the foundation of rabies prevention.

For individuals who have not previously received the rabies vaccine series, rabies vaccination in the United States consists of intramuscular injections starting on the day of injury or within 10 days, with follow-up injections on days 3, 7, and 14, for immunocompetent patients. One additional dose is recommended for immunocompromised patients on day 28. Human rabies immunoglobulin (HRIG) is also given with the first dose of vaccine, with the whole or majority of the dose to be infiltrated around the wound (if feasible). The remainder should be administered in the same extremity. HRIG should never be administered in the same extremity as the rabies vaccine. The HRIG dosage is 20 IU/kg of body weight administered on day 0. For individuals who have received prior rabies preexposure vaccination, HRIG is not indicated; instead, they should receive booster doses of the rabies vaccine on days 0 and 3.

Prevention

The incubation period for the rabies virus ranges from 9 to 30 days. In 1% of cases, the incubation period may last more than 1 year, with one possible case of 25 years' incubation having been reported. Vaccination of domestic animals is essential. When treating a patient with suspected rabies exposure, observe standard precautions, including wearing gloves and using good hand hygiene. Preexposure rabies vaccination is available through public health programs, although the criteria for administering this vaccine to at-risk individuals have changed because of its reduced availability. Routine vaccination of health care clinicians in the United States as a preventive measure is not recommended.

Hantavirus

The *Hantavirus* genus of rodent-borne viruses is distributed worldwide and causes a group of related hantavirus diseases. These diseases include hantavirus pulmonary syndrome (HPS), which is seen in the Americas, and hemorrhagic fever with renal syndrome (HFRS), which is seen primarily in Europe and East Asia. Both clinical presentations are associated with fever with acute thrombocytopenia and changes in vascular permeability, and both may produce renal and/or pulmonary symptoms.

Hantavirus occurs in Asia, western Russia, Europe, the United States, and South and Central America. Worldwide, approximately 150,000 to 200,000 cases are reported annually. The disease was first described in Korea in the early 1950s. There are two seasonal peaks for almost all outbreaks of hantavirus disease: A small outbreak appears in the spring, and a more substantial spike occurs in fall. Epidemiologists suspect that these upturns correspond with farming cycles and with seasonal increases in the infection rate of the rodents that carry the disease. The virus is spread by the deer mouse, the white-footed mouse, and the cotton rat, as well as by city rats.

Pathophysiology/Transmission

Transmission of hantavirus occurs by inhalation of aerosolized rodent waste. The virus is shed into the urine, feces, and saliva of chronically infected rodents. The incubation period usually lasts about 12 to 16 days, but may be as short as 5 days or as long as 42 days. Although human-to-human transmission of hantavirus has been reported in Argentina and Chile, this disease is rarely transmitted from person to person, so there is no period of communicability.

Signs and Symptoms

HFRS is divided into five phases: febrile, hypotensive, oliguric, polyuric, and convalescent. HFRS signs and symptoms begin with the sudden onset of fever, which lasts 3 to 8 days. The fever is accompanied by headache, abdominal pain, loss of appetite, and vomiting. Facial flushing is characteristic, and a petechial rash usually appears (generally limited to the axillae). Sudden and extreme albuminuria on about day 4 is a cardinal sign of severe HFRS. The patient may also have ecchymosis and scleral injection (bloodshot eyes). Additional symptoms include hypotension, shock, respiratory distress or failure, and renal impairment or failure. The characteristic damage to the renal medulla is unique to hantaviruses. HFRS has a mortality rate as high as 15%.

HPS, also known as hantavirus cardiopulmonary syndrome (HCPS), is a febrile illness. HCPS develops in three phases:

1. *Prodrome.* After the incubation period, patients may present with flu-like symptoms including fever, myalgia, headache, cough, chills, muscle aches, abdominal pain, diarrhea, and malaise.
2. *Cardiopulmonary phase.* In this phase, which occurs 4 to 10 days after the initial onset, symptoms may include shortness of breath and tachypnea. Capillary leak leads to decreased cardiac output and a state of shock. This phase is also marked by pulmonary edema, arrhythmias, and coagulopathy.
3. *Convalescent phase.* Resolution of symptoms occurs following the oliguria and diuretic phases of the disease.

Ask the patient about exposure to mice or other rodent droppings if you observe symptoms consistent with hantavirus. HPS (or HCPS) has a mortality rate as high as 50%.

Differential Diagnosis

The differential diagnosis for HFRS includes other causes of hemorrhagic fever, including yellow fever, Ebola, septicemia, dengue, leptospirosis, and severe fever with thrombocytopenia syndrome. The differential diagnosis for HCPS includes severe generalized pneumonia, interstitial pneumonia, eosinophilic pneumonia, septic shock, cardiogenic shock, severe dengue infection, tularemia, and yellow fever.

Diagnosis is confirmed by IgM antibody response or a rising immunoglobulin G (IgG) titer, or by PCR testing for the virus. Viral RNA is detected only in the early days of infection; a negative test cannot rule out the disease. Chest radiographs may reveal a diffuse interstitial infiltrate.

Treatment

No specific treatment is available other than supportive measures, including oxygen administration, respiratory status monitoring, fluid and electrolyte balance maintenance, and blood pressure support.

Prevention

Follow standard safety precautions; hantavirus is not transmitted from person to person. Routine cleaning of the vehicle is sufficient. Public health officials will assess the need for cleaning out areas of rodent infestation.

Tetanus (Lockjaw)

Tetanus is caused by the gram-positive anaerobic bacterium *Clostridium tetani*. According to the CDC, from 2000 to 2019, a total of 597 cases of tetanus were reported in the United States. More than half of these cases occurred in people 20 to 59 years of age, with 30% of all cases occurring in patients who were aged 60 or older. However, tetanus occurs worldwide and affects all age groups, with the highest prevalence on a global basis being found in neonates and young people. It is one of the diseases targeted by WHO's Expanded Program on Immunization.

Tetanus is more common in agricultural areas and in underdeveloped areas. Cases are usually isolated to rural areas where contact with animal waste is common and immunization is inadequate. The tetanus bacillus is found in the intestines of horses and other animals and in contaminated soil. Some cases of tetanus have been linked to IV drug use.

Pathophysiology/Transmission

Transmission of tetanus occurs when tetanus spores enter the body by way of a puncture wound contaminated with animal feces, street dust, or soil; by the injection of contaminated street drugs; or in neonates delivered in settings without adequate sterile procedures. Occasionally, cases have occurred postoperatively or after minor injuries that were left untreated. The incubation period is thought to be about 14 days from the exposure, but a period of as little as 3 days has been reported. A short incubation period is associated with a higher level of contamination. Tetanus is not transmitted from person to person, so there is no period of communicability. A decrease in the incidence of tetanus has occurred worldwide with the institution of immunization programs.

Signs and Symptoms

Signs and symptoms—which result from the neurotoxin that is released as the bacteria begin to grow—start at the site of the wound, followed by painful muscle contractions in the neck and trunk muscles. The most common initial sign is a spasm of the jaw preventing the person from opening the mouth; this effect is why tetanus is referred to as *lockjaw*. Another form of tetanus is localized tetanus, in which muscle spasms occur in a confined area close to the site of the injury.

Differential Diagnosis

Other diagnostic considerations include rabies, drug toxicity, electrolyte disturbances, stroke, CNS infection, and seizure.

The diagnosis of tetanus is made on the basis of signs and symptoms. No laboratory testing for tetanus has been developed.

Treatment

Tetanus immunoglobulin should be injected directly into the wound to bind the circulating toxin. The wound must be cleaned and surgically debrided. An antibiotic (e.g., metroNIDAZOLE,, clindamycin) may be prescribed to prevent associated infection.

Supportive treatment is critical to survival; it consists of agents to control muscle spasm and aggressive wound care. Clinicians must not forget to initiate active immunization during the convalescence period.

Prevention

Anyone presenting with a tetanus-prone wound should have their tetanus vaccination status reviewed and receive tetanus immunoglobulin and vaccination if appropriate. Prevention of tetanus requires vaccination during childhood and booster doses every 10 years. If a patient has not undergone primary vaccination as a child, immune globulin may be indicated as well. Wear gloves when handling any patient who has a draining wound. No special cleaning of the room or vehicle is necessary after caring for a patient with tetanus.

Vector-Borne Diseases

Lyme Disease

Lyme disease, which is caused by the spirochete *Borrelia burgdorferi*, is the most common tickborne disease in the United States. The number of reported cases has increased since 1982, when a national reporting system was established. Lyme disease is found worldwide, with most cases occurring in forested areas of Asia, Europe, and the northeastern/upper midwestern United States. The disease occurs most often in children younger than 10 years and in middle-aged adults.

Pathophysiology/Transmission

Lyme disease is transmitted by tick (*Ixodes scapularis*) bite. The peak season for cases is between June and August, with the incidence of the disease receding in early fall. The incubation period ranges from 3 to 32 days. The disease has no period of communicability, because it is not transmitted from person to person.

Signs and Symptoms

Lyme disease primarily affects the skin, heart, joints, and nervous system. Some patients are asymptomatic. The disease is usually divided into three stages:

1. *Early localized*. In the early localized stage, a round, slightly irregular, red skin lesion called *erythema migrans* appears 3 to 32 days after

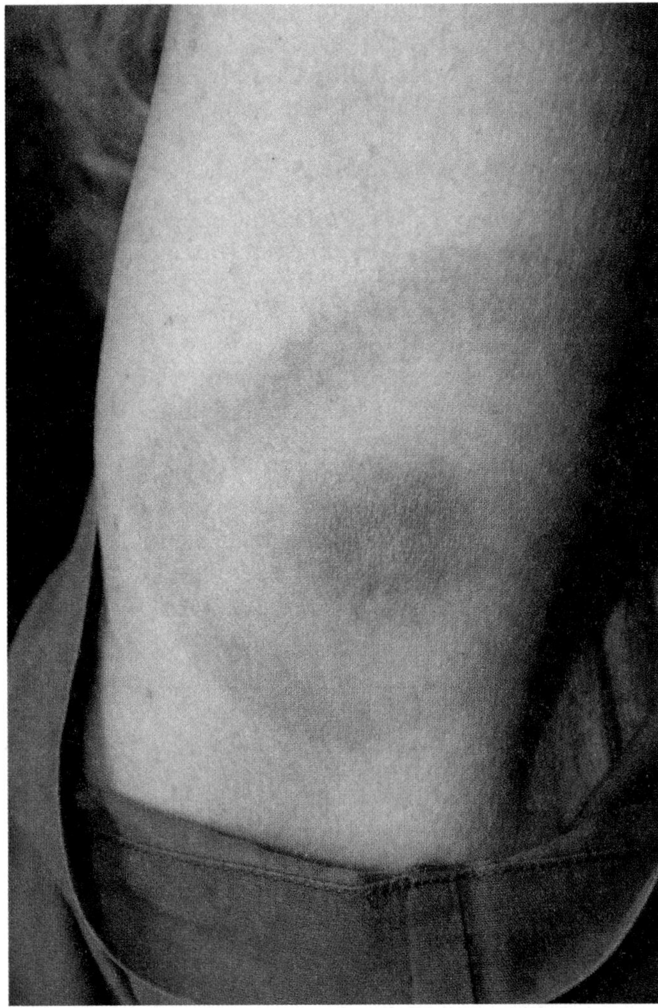

A

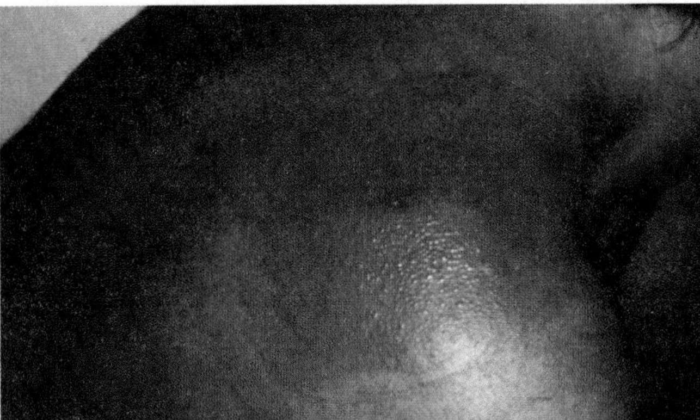

B

Figure 7-9 The bull's-eye rash of Lyme disease is most commonly seen in the area of the groin, thigh, or axilla.

A. Courtesy of CDC/James Gathany; **B.** Courtesy of the Centers for Disease Control and Prevention.

the tick bite. This lesion is often described as a bull's-eye rash, because it consists of a central necrotic spot surrounded by an area of clearing, around which a dark-red ring appears, with lighter erythema around the periphery (**Figure 7-9**). The rash is more than 5 cm in diameter. It usually appears on the skin of the groin, thigh, or axilla and is easy to miss. The skin is warm to the touch and may be blistered or covered with a scab.

2. *Early disseminated*. The second, early disseminated stage may develop within days. This stage is characterized by secondary lesions and flu-like symptoms such as fever, chills, headache, malaise, and muscle pain. The patient may also have a nonproductive cough, sore throat, enlarged spleen, or enlarged lymph nodes. Neurologic involvement occurs in 15% to 20% of untreated patients within 8 weeks and can lead to many vague neurosensory complaints. Cardiac involvement, usually in the form of heart block, appears in approximately 10% of untreated patients.
3. *Late manifestations*. In the final phase of the illness, which may begin days or years after the second phase, arthritis occurs in approximately 60% of untreated patients. Intermittent joint pain lasting days or months occurs in about half of patients. Chronic neurologic symptoms are uncommon.

Differential Diagnosis

Diagnostic considerations include nonspecific viral illness, rheumatic fever, and vasculitis. Other tickborne illnesses (e.g., babesiosis, ehrlichiosis, Rocky Mountain spotted fever) should also be considered.

In later stages of the disease, the differential diagnosis is greatly increased, as it is directly related to the presenting symptoms (cardiac, neurologic, arthritis, dermatologic).

Diagnosis

The diagnosis of Lyme disease is usually based on a simple history and physical examination. In obvious cases, in which the diagnosis can be based on the history, signs, and symptoms, treatment should be given without checking antibodies, as the Lyme antibody can take weeks to develop and a negative result could confuse the clinician and delay treatment.

Treatment

There is minimal risk of transmission when the tick remains attached to the skin for less than 24 hours, although the definitive timing is unknown. The mainstay of treatment is oral doxycycline for 10 to 21 days, depending on the patient's age. Amoxicillin or a third-generation cephalosporin (cefTRIAXone or cefuroxime) is preferred in children younger than age 8 and in pregnant patients. As many as 20% of patients, predominantly those with a late diagnosis and those who received antibiotic treatment, may have persistent or recurrent symptoms (referred to as posttreatment Lyme disease syndrome) that respond to oral antibiotic treatment as well. Patients who experience neurologic or cardiac forms of the disease may require IV treatment with drugs such as cefTRIAXone or penicillin.

Prevention

Wear long sleeves and trousers when you must work in tick-infested areas. Repellents such as diethyltoluamide (DEET) can deter these insects, but such chemicals can be toxic and must be used judiciously, especially around young children. In a randomized, controlled trial involving persons 12 years of age or older, a single prophylactic 200-mg dose of doxycycline administered within 72 hours after removal of a deer tick was 87% effective in preventing Lyme disease.

Rocky Mountain Spotted Fever

Rocky Mountain spotted fever (RMSF) is a tickborne illness caused by *Rickettsia rickettsii*, a small bacterium that grows inside the vascular endothelial cells lining the small and medium blood vessels of its hosts. The disease was first recognized in 1896, in the Snake River Valley of Idaho. It was originally given the foreboding name *black measles*. RMSF has been a reportable disease in the United States since the 1920s. Despite its name, this disease can be found throughout most of the country, including the District of Columbia and states in the south Atlantic (Delaware, Maryland, Virginia, West Virginia, North Carolina, South Carolina, Georgia, and Florida), Pacific (Washington, Oregon, and California), and west south-central (Arkansas, Louisiana, Oklahoma, and Texas) regions. Worldwide, infection with *R. rickettsii* has been documented in Argentina, Brazil, Colombia, Costa Rica, Mexico, and Panama.

About two-thirds of RMSF cases occur in children younger than 15 years, with a peak at ages 5 to 9. People who are often around dogs or who live close to wooded areas or patches of tall grass are also at increased risk of infection. American Indians have the highest incidence of RMSF. Only about 60% of people diagnosed with RMSF recall having had a tick bite.

Pathophysiology/Transmission

More than 20 species are currently classified in the genus *Rickettsia*, but not all are known to cause disease in humans. The rickettsia grow in the cytoplasm or in the nuclei of host cells. The organisms multiply, damaging or destroying those cells and causing blood to leak through tiny holes in vessel walls into adjacent tissues. This mechanism is responsible for the characteristic rash associated with RMSF. The incubation period is 3 to 14 days after the tick bite. The illness is not transmissible from person to person.

Signs and Symptoms

Initial symptoms of RMSF may include fever, nausea, vomiting, severe headache, muscle pain, and lack of appetite. A rash appears 2 to 5 days after the onset of fever, often appearing initially as a smattering of small, flat, pink, nonpruritic spots (macules) on the wrists, forearms, and ankles. Some patients may present with confusion, nuchal rigidity, or cardiovascular instability.

RMSF can be a life-threatening illness because *R. rickettsia* infects the cells lining blood vessels throughout the body. Severe manifestations of this disease may involve the respiratory or renal system, the CNS, or the GI tract. Patients with illness severe enough to require hospital care may have the following long-term effects:

- Partial paralysis of the lower extremities
- Gangrene requiring amputation of fingers, toes, arms, or legs
- Hearing loss
- Loss of bowel or bladder control
- Movement or language disorders

Differential Diagnosis

Diagnostic considerations include nonspecific viral illness, rheumatic fever, and vasculitis. Depending on the patient's travel and exposure history, other tickborne (e.g., babesiosis, ehrlichiosis, Lyme disease), viral (e.g., enteroviruses, Epstein-Barr virus, dengue, influenza), bacterial (e.g., leptospirosis, disseminated gonococcal infection), and parasitic (e.g., malaria) diseases should be considered. A detailed travel history and presence of a rash are important in making the diagnosis of RMSF.

Most cases of RMSF are diagnosed based on IgM and IgG serologic responses (via indirect immunofluorescent antibody) to *R. rickettsii*, in conjunction with a high degree of clinical suspicion. IgG antibodies are more specific and reliable, because other bacterial infections can also cause elevations in rickettsial IgM antibody titers. Other diagnostic options include molecular tests, such as PCR, in some centers, and skin biopsy.

Treatment

It is critical that treatment not be delayed while awaiting confirmatory laboratory testing in a patient with a suspected rickettsial infection due to the high mortality rates, up to 20% to 30%, in untreated patients.

Doxycycline (100 mg every 12 hours for adults or 4 mg/kg of body weight per day in two divided doses for children $<$ 45 kg [100 lb]) is the drug of choice for patients with RMSF. Therapy is continued for at least 3 days after fever subsides and until there is unequivocal evidence of clinical improvement, generally for a minimum total course of 5 to 10 days. Severe or complicated disease may require a longer course of treatment.

Prevention

Good hand washing is essential for health care clinicians. Risk of contracting RMSF can be limited by reducing exposure to ticks. When individuals are exposed to ticks, careful inspection and removal of crawling or attached ticks is a simple but important way of preventing disease.

When the presence of ticks is recognized, they should be removed. Ticks are easily removed with tweezers or forceps by identifying and grabbing the tick's mouth, very close to the person's or animal's skin. The entire tick should be gently removed. To prevent further contamination, the body of the tick should not be squeezed (**Figure 7-10**). The area should be cleaned and an antiseptic applied.

West Nile Virus

West Nile virus is a *Flavivirus* (a genus of viruses) that is commonly found in Africa, Europe, the Middle East, North America, and West Asia. The disease derives its name from the place of its origin, along the Nile River. West Nile virus was first discovered in Uganda in the 1930s. Its first appearance in the Western Hemisphere came in 1999, when it was identified in New York City, marking the beginning of the largest outbreak of mosquito-borne illness in U.S. history. Other outbreaks of West Nile virus have been reported in Russia, Israel, and Romania. In most cases, the disease is mild and uneventful. In fact, approximately 80% of all people infected with this virus are not aware that they have acquired the disease.

Pathophysiology/Transmission

Transmission of West Nile virus occurs when a person is bitten by a mosquito carrying the virus. Only about 1% of mosquitoes are vectors for this pathogen. The primary mosquitos in North America are the *Culex* species and *Aedes albopictus* (Asian tiger) mosquito. The disease is not transmitted from person to person, but it has been transmitted by donor blood, through organ transplantation, and by needlestick injury among laboratory workers handling the virus. The incubation period is 2 to 14 days after the bite, during which time the virus multiplies in the dermal cells and lymph nodes before entering the bloodstream. Symptoms typically last 3 to 6 days.

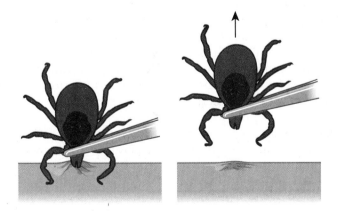

Figure 7-10 Proper tick removal.

Courtesy of CDC.

Signs and Symptoms

Approximately 80% of all people infected with West Nile virus are asymptomatic. The remaining 20% develop mild signs and symptoms such as fever, headache, body rash, and swollen lymph glands. About 1 in 150 will go on to have severe signs and symptoms, such as encephalitis and meningitis, resulting in inflammation and loss of neurons that can lead to neurologic complications and death.

Differential Diagnosis

Other diagnostic considerations include meningitis, other viral encephalitis, subarachnoid hemorrhage, endocarditis, Lyme disease, and toxic/metabolic encephalopathy.

Diagnosis

Keen observation of signs and symptoms is the key to making a preliminary diagnosis. Ask the patient about recent mosquito bites if cases have been reported in the area. Ask about risks for exposure, such as work and travel history. Observe the patient for severe signs and symptoms that suggest meningitis or encephalitis, such as loss of consciousness, confusion, stiff neck, and muscle weakness.

Laboratory diagnosis is accomplished by identification of West Nile virus–specific IgM antibodies through serum or CSF testing. Immunoassays for West Nile virus–specific IgM are available commercially and through state public health laboratories.

Treatment

Supportive treatment for the disease is offered. No prescribed treatment is available for West Nile virus.

Prevention

As West Nile virus is transmitted almost exclusively by mosquitos, avoiding mosquito bites is the primary prevention method. The public can assist in controlling the spread of this infection by draining standing pools of water, using insect repellent, wearing long sleeves after dusk, and reporting dead birds to local authorities, as birds are carriers of West Nile virus. These precautions will reduce the virus's reproduction capabilities and, in turn, individuals' risk of exposure.

Use needle-safe device systems to avoid a contaminated sharps injury. No particular medical follow-up treatment is recommended if a needle exposure occurs. In addition, no special cleaning of the vehicle or equipment is needed or recommended after transporting a patient suspected of having West Nile virus.

Infection with Multidrug-Resistant Organisms

Methicillin-Resistant *Staphylococcus aureus*

Methicillin-resistant *Staphylococcus aureus* (MRSA) is a bacterium that is resistant to several antibiotics. Infection with this pathogen can affect several body systems (e.g., skin, lungs, and bloodstream). An estimated 5% of hospitalized patients in the United States have nasal colonization with MRSA.

MRSA is often classified based on antibiotic resistance and infection patterns. Community-associated MRSA (CA-MRSA) is most commonly seen in skin and soft-tissue infections. Health care–associated MRSA (HA-MRSA) is most commonly seen in postoperative infections, urinary catheter–associated infection, and ventilator-associated infections. HA-MRSA typically has more antibiotic resistance than does CA-MRSA.

Pathophysiology

MRSA is spread by direct contact from contaminated hands or objects via an active infected wound or colonization.

Signs and Symptoms

MRSA commonly causes a skin infection that can present with pain, redness, warmth, and swelling. An abscess may also develop. Symptoms of a more systemic infection (e.g., sepsis, bacteremia, pneumonia, endocarditis, osteomyelitis, joint infection) include fever, chills, sweats, malaise, nausea and vomiting, shortness of breath, chest pain, and joint and bone pain.

Differential Diagnosis

Other diagnostic considerations include other causes of soft-tissue infection, sepsis, bacteremia, pneumonia, endocarditis, osteomyelitis, nonspecific viral illness, and vasculitis.

Diagnosis

Diagnosis of MRSA is confirmed by culture. A rapid test for MRSA produces results in 2 hours, whereas a culture may take as long as 48 to 72 hours. DNA PCR for MRSA is available and may be useful in settings where cultures are inconclusive.

Treatment

Antibiotics used to treat MRSA infections include trimethoprim–sulfamethoxazole, clindamycin, doxycycline, vancomycin, daptomycin, and linezolid. Treatment is based on local sensitivities and culture results. Telavancin, ceftaroline, and quinupristin–dalfopristin have been used successfully in some patients.

Prevention

Measures such as wearing gloves and practicing good hand hygiene should be employed to prevent infectious spread. No prophylactic medical treatment is recommended after exposure to MRSA. MRSA is a slow-growing bacterium that is easily destroyed by routine approved cleaning solutions. Clean the room, vehicle, and patient care equipment after each use. Shower after physical activity, and clean exercise equipment before use. Cover open skin areas with a dressing.

Vancomycin-Resistant *Enterococcus*

Enterococcus is a group of common bacteria that constitute part of the normal flora of the GI tract, urinary tract, and genitourinary tract. This genus includes more than 400 species, many of which are resistant to antibiotics. A cagey organism, it flourishes equally well under conditions of scarce or abundant oxygen. When this organism becomes resistant to vancomycin (the primary drug used to treat *Enterococcus* infection), the result is vancomycin-resistant *Enterococcus* (VRE). VRE infection is primarily an HAI.

Pathophysiology/Transmission

The pathogenic organisms are found in the GI tract and may present in patients with urinary tract or bloodstream infections. Patients identified with VRE infection outside the hospital setting often reside in nursing homes or spend time at hemodialysis centers. VRE can live on surfaces for long periods of time, so thorough cleaning of devices used in health care settings is important.

Transmission occurs by direct contact with contaminated surfaces or equipment. The bacteria may also spread by direct contact of an open cut or sore with a draining wound.

Signs and Symptoms

VRE infections have a varied presentation. They can take the form of a urinary tract infection, an intra-abdominal infection, bacteremia, or infective endocarditis. Signs and symptoms include fever or chills; abdominal pain; wound infection with redness, tenderness, or purulence; and signs of a urinary infection (e.g., an unusual urine color or odor and pain on urination).

Differential Diagnosis

Other causes of sepsis or endocarditis, as well as abdominal, soft-tissue, surgical-related, and urinary infections, should be considered. To refine the diagnosis, ask the patient about recent medical history, particularly any hospital stay for surgery and any prolonged antibiotic treatment. The diagnosis is confined by culturing a wound, urine, blood, or stool.

Treatment

Antibiotics used to treat VRE infections include daptomycin, linezolid, beta lactams (e.g., ceftaroline), and gentamycin or other aminoglycosides. Tigecycline has been used successfully for VRE disease as well for intra-abdominal infections. Treatment is based on local sensitivities and culture results.

Prevention

Clinicians should follow standard precautions, including wearing gloves and using good hand washing techniques when they come in contact with wound drainage. A gown is needed only if wound drainage may contaminate the clinician's uniform. Clean all areas with which the patient had contact; no special cleaning solution is needed. Direct contact between an open wound and VRE-infected body fluids should be reported according to the organization's infection control policy. An exposure report will need to be completed, but no postexposure medical treatment is indicated.

Communicable Diseases of Childhood

Immunizations have dramatically reduced the incidence of communicable diseases in both children and adults. It is important to understand the clinical presentations of these diseases to implement appropriate PPE and interventions.

The measles, mumps, and rubella (MMR) and measles, mumps, rubella, and varicella (MMRV) vaccines use live, weakened viral strains to confer immunity to these childhood diseases. First approved as a combined vaccine in 1971, MMR contains the safest and most effective forms of each vaccine. Considerations for administration of the appropriate vaccine depend on the patient's specific health history and underlying health factors. Vaccination is recommended for all health care clinicians who do not have proof of immunity. Vaccination is not recommended for pregnant women, however, and women of childbearing age who are offered the MMR vaccine must be counseled not to become pregnant for 3 months after being vaccinated.

Rubeola (Measles)

Rubeola is an illness caused by the measles virus, which can be found in an infected person's blood, urine, and pharyngeal secretions.

Pathophysiology/Transmission

The rubeola virus resides in the mucus of the nose and throat of the infected person. When the person sneezes or coughs, droplets spray into the air. The virus spreads by direct contact as well as airborne spread.

The virus remains active and contagious on infected surfaces for as long as 2 hours. Measles is one of the most contagious respiratory viruses: A single person can infect as many as 90% of the individuals in close proximity to them. The virus is usually passed directly or indirectly through contact with infected respiratory secretions. The resulting illness lasts for about 9 days. In severe cases, seizures may occur, or the illness may prove fatal. Serious complications are more common among children younger than 5 years and in adults older than 20 years. Patients are contagious from about 4 days before to 4 days after the onset of the measles rash. Despite immunizations, measles outbreaks continue to occur, and are usually linked to unvaccinated children.

Signs and Symptoms

One of the first signs of measles is often a high fever that develops 7 to 14 days after exposure to the virus. Koplik spots (whitish-gray spots visible on the buccal mucosa) develop 2 to 3 days after symptoms begin. The pathognomonic rash (small raised bumps starting on the face and spreading downward to the trunk and extremities) develops 3 to 5 days after symptoms onset. Other signs and symptoms include diarrhea, conjunctivitis, cough, and coryza (nasal congestion and discharge). Complications such as otitis media, pneumonia, myocarditis, and encephalitis are reported in approximately 20% of measles cases.

Differential Diagnosis

Other diagnostic considerations include nonspecific viral illness, rubella, scarlet fever, smallpox, varicella, roseola infantum, hand–foot–mouth disease, parvovirus B19, drug rash, dermatitis, infectious mononucleosis, and vasculitis.

Serologic testing for the measles virus and antigens is helpful for diagnosis and treatment. IgM is the antibody first produced in an immune response. If an IgM blood test is positive, viral cultures are performed.

Treatment

Treatment for measles is supportive, with the emphasis on maintaining hydration and considering antibiotics for associated ear and eye infections or pneumonia, should they occur. In developing countries, children should receive two doses of vitamin A supplements 24 hours apart. Vitamin A administration has been shown to decrease mortality from measles by 50%.

Prevention

If you are caring for a patient with rubeola and you have not been vaccinated or are not immune to rubeola, place a surgical mask on the patient. If you are unsure whether you are immune, a serologic blood test should be performed. If the results indicate nonimmunity, consider being vaccinated.

Rubella

Rubella, or German measles, is caused by a virus found in respiratory secretions. This illness lasts for about 3 days. Rubella contracted during pregnancy may cause miscarriage, premature birth, or a low-birth-weight infant. If this infection is passed from the mother to fetus during the first trimester of pregnancy, anomalies in fetal development can occur, including intellectual disability, deafness, and an increased risk of congenital heart disease and sepsis during the first 6 months of life. Collectively, these developmental anomalies are known as congenital rubella syndrome.

Pathophysiology/Transmission

Transmission occurs by direct contact with the nasopharyngeal secretions of the infected person—by droplet spread or by touching the patient or articles freshly contaminated with the patient's secretions. An infected individual is contagious from 8 days before to 8 days after the onset of the rubella rash.

Signs and Symptoms

Small raised bumps starting on the face and spreading downward to the trunk and extremities are usually the first sign of rubella and last for approximately 3 days. Other symptoms include low-grade fever, headache, cough, coryza, malaise, and swollen lymph nodes. Onset of symptoms is usually 2 to 3 weeks after exposure. Rubella produces minimal or no symptoms in more than 50% of people infected with this virus.

Differential Diagnosis

Other diagnostic considerations include nonspecific viral illness, rubeola, scarlet fever, smallpox, varicella, roseola infantum, hand–foot–mouth disease, drug rash, dermatitis, infectious mononucleosis, and vasculitis.

Serologic tests are performed to identify antibodies. The most common diagnostic test for recent infection focuses on detection of rubella-specific IgM antibodies with an enzyme immunoassay. PCR identification is done to confirm the virus.

Treatment

Treatment is supportive. It includes analgesic/antipyretic medication and maintaining hydration.

Prevention

Practice standard precautions. Clinicians can reduce their risk of contracting rubella by taking respiratory precautions such as placing a surgical mask on the patient, but vaccination is the key to risk reduction for health care personnel. As with measles, the only certain protection against rubella is immunity. Immunity acquired after recovering from natural infection or through vaccination is lifelong; however, reinfection has been reported with wild-type virus and in persons who received only one dose of the rubella vaccine.

Mumps

Mumps is an acute, communicable, systemic illness caused by the mumps virus. It occurs most commonly in winter and spring. Anyone who has not been vaccinated is at risk for developing this disease.

Pathophysiology/Transmission

The mumps virus is transmitted by droplet spread or direct contact with the saliva of an infected person. The virus has an incubation period of 12 to 26 days and a communicable period ranging from 7 to 9 days after the onset of symptoms.

Signs and Symptoms

Mumps is characterized by swelling and tenderness of the parotid salivary glands, affecting one or both sides of the neck, and a fever. The patient may have a history of exposure to another person with mumps. Mumps orchitis (inflammation of testes) is rarely seen when infection occurs before puberty. Of affected testicles, 30% to 50% show a degree of testicular atrophy. Rare complications include meningitis, hydrocephalus, hearing loss, Guillain-Barré syndrome, pancreatitis, and myocarditis.

Differential Diagnosis

Other diagnostic considerations include viral parotitis, salivary stones, autoimmune disorders, soft-tissue infection, and nonspecific viral illness.

An assessment for parotid swelling should be performed to help determine whether the patient may have mumps. Serologic tests are not necessarily done for mumps (or measles). For selected patients, RT-PCR and viral culture are used to confirm the infection. IgM serology can also aid in diagnosing mumps infection.

Treatment

Treatment is supportive. It includes analgesic/antipyretic medication and maintaining hydration.

Prevention

Clinicians should take respiratory droplet precautions (place a surgical mask on the patient) when transporting a patient suspected of having mumps. Vaccination is the key to risk reduction among health care personnel.

Pertussis (Whooping Cough)

The gram-negative bacterium *Bordetella pertussis* causes pertussis, also called whooping cough. The primary risk group for this disease is children and adolescents, although adults with waning immunity are also at increased risk of infection. Complications of pertussis include pneumonia, seizures, and (rarely) encephalitis.

Pathophysiology/Transmission

Pertussis has an insidious onset and is characterized by an irritating cough. The organism that causes pertussis can survive outside the respiratory tract for only a short period of time. When it does gain entry to the respiratory tract, it attaches to cilia, immobilizing them. The bacteria produce toxins, causing systemic illness. The incubation period is 7 to 10 days, and transmission occurs by direct contact with oral or nasal secretions.

Signs and Symptoms

Signs and symptoms during the first stage of whooping cough, known as the catarrhal phase, include fever, malaise, sneezing, anorexia, and conjunctival injection. This stage lasts several days.

The second stage, the paroxysmal coughing phase, is the key to identifying the disease. The patient may have 50 or more episodes of spasmodic coughing per day. When each convulsive cough subsides, a whooping sound emerges. In very young patients, the coughing may be followed by episodes of apnea. Assess for vomiting, low oxygen saturation, convulsions, and coma.

During the third stage, the convalescent phase, the coughing begins to subside, becoming less frequent and intense. The illness may last for several weeks.

Differential Diagnosis

Other diagnostic considerations include foreign body airway obstruction, structural airway obstruction, tracheitis, croup, epiglottitis, retropharyngeal abscess, and peritonsillar abscess.

The diagnosis of pertussis is often clinically based on the patient history and examination, combined with the pathognomonic cough. Assessing for known close infected contacts should be considered. Laboratory testing for rising antibody titers can assist in making the diagnosis, but results may be negative initially, early in the course of illness, and become useful only later (generally 2 to 8 weeks following onset of cough).

Nasopharyngeal culture and PCR may allow for laboratory confirmation of pertussis. Cultures are typically not positive for 3 to 7 days; they are used primarily within the first 2 weeks following cough onset. PCR (when available) is a rapid test that has excellent sensitivity; it is useful for confirming the diagnosis of pertussis 3 to 4 weeks after cough onset.

Treatment

Treatment is primarily supportive. Close monitoring of respiratory status is indicated, and ventilation support should be initiated as needed. In the early phase of the disease (catarrhal phase), antibiotics (azithromycin) are often prescribed, which may not impact the severity of illness, but can decrease infectivity and symptom severity. In the later phases of pertussis, antibiotics may not alter the course of illness or prevent transmission.

Prevention

A pertussis vaccine became available in 1940, and childhood vaccination remains the primary means of prevention and control. Take droplet precautions when caring for a patient suspected of having whooping cough. Place a surgical mask or an oxygen mask on the patient, and follow standard precautions.

Vaccination does not provide lifetime immunity to pertussis as previously believed, so all adults should receive a one-time booster dose of the Tdap (tetanus, diphtheria, acellular pertussis) vaccine. Report any exposure as soon as possible to ensure prompt administration of postexposure antibiotics.

Varicella-Zoster Virus Infection (Chickenpox)

Chickenpox is a highly contagious disease caused by the varicella-zoster virus, a member of the human herpesvirus family. Chickenpox occurs worldwide, affecting people of all races, all ages, and both sexes, but is more common in children younger than 10 years. An estimated 60 million cases occur worldwide each year. Chickenpox is often mild in children and more severe in adults. Infection with the varicella-zoster virus may result in chickenpox or, later in life, shingles.

Once a person has had chickenpox, they are unlikely to contract the illness again because natural infection is thought to provide lifelong immunity in most people. Persons with a compromised immune system who are exposed to the virus are susceptible to infection regardless of their medical history, and actions to either prevent or modify the course of the disease should be taken in such cases.

In some people, the varicella-zoster virus is retained in the spinal dorsal nerve root ganglia after having chickenpox and reappears later in life as herpes zoster (shingles) infection (**Figure 7-11**). Reactivation of the virus may occur during a period of physical or emotional stress and causes a rash following dermatomal patterns. The herpes zoster lesions drain live virus and are extraordinarily painful.

Pathophysiology/Transmission

Transmission of the varicella-zoster virus may occur in one of two ways: inhalation of airborne respiratory droplets or contact with drainage from vesicles. The portal of entry is usually the conjunctival or upper respiratory mucosa.

The disease presents in stages. Viral replication takes place in regional lymph nodes 2 to 4 days after exposure, after which a primary viremia occurs (4 to 6 days after inoculation). The virus then replicates in the liver and spleen, and possibly in other organs. Secondary viremia occurs 14 to 16 days after the initial exposure and is characterized by the spread of viral particles to the skin, which causes the typical vesicular rash. The rash initially appears on the covered areas of the body and spreads to the face and scalp, and sometimes the mucous membranes of the mouth or genitals. The shallow vesicles progress to become deeper pustules. As they heal, the lesions dry up and crust over, leaving scabs. The usual incubation period for the varicella-zoster virus is 10 to 21 days. The patient is contagious from 1 to 2 days before the rash appears until all the lesions are dry and crusted.

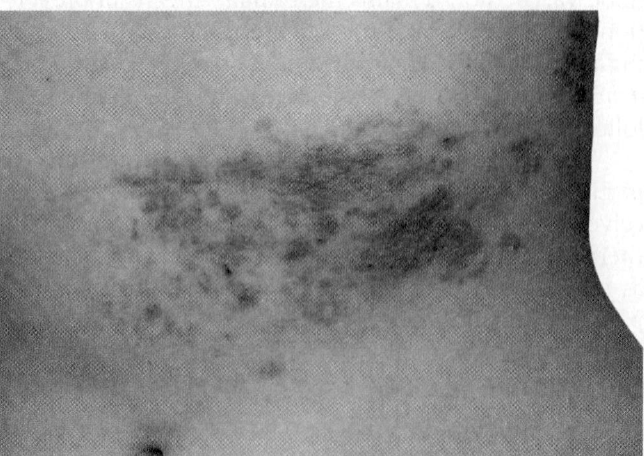

Figure 7-11 Herpes zoster (shingles).

Signs and Symptoms

Prodromal symptoms of chickenpox include fever, malaise, anorexia, and headache. The rash typically begins as pruritic, red, flat lesions that spread to the extremities. After about one day, vesicles develop on this red base, often described as a "dew drop on a rose."

Differential Diagnosis

Patients should be assessed for signs of superinfection, including impetigo, cellulitis, necrotizing fasciitis, and arthritis.

Diagnosis

Laboratory testing is generally not performed for patients with suspected chickenpox. Instead, diagnosis is made on the basis of the clinical presentation. For patients requiring confirmatory testing, diagnosis by PCR is the best option, though direct fluorescent antibody test is a good alternative. Serology (IgM and IgG) is also available to assist in the diagnosis but is less reliable.

Treatment

Treatment for patients with chickenpox is symptomatic. Oral antihistamines or lotion can be prescribed to relieve itching. Fever should be treated with antipyretic medications. In children, aspirin should not be given as a fever-reducing medication, because its use is associated with a risk of Reye syndrome. Fingernails may be trimmed to prevent skin excoriation from scratching. Antiviral medications and corticosteroids may be prescribed to shorten the duration of symptoms. Patients should be monitored for skin infections and pneumonia.

In patients with a severe disease (varicella pneumonia, immunocompromised patients, reactivation infection [shingles], or disseminated herpes zoster), antiviral agents (acyclovir or valacyclovir) are prescribed to reduce illness severity and the risk of developing postherpetic pain.

Prevention

Vaccination is the primary means of protecting both patients and health care clinicians from varicella-zoster virus infection. Droplet precautions should include placing a surgical mask on the patient, if possible. If the patient is unable to tolerate or wear a mask, the clinician should don one. Gloves should be worn when in direct contact with draining lesions. Routine cleaning of the vehicle, rooms, or equipment is adequate, and no airing of the vehicle is needed.

If an exposure occurs, follow-up is recommended because postexposure medical treatment may be indicated. Clinicians who are vaccinated after a potential exposure may be restricted from work from days 10 to 28 post exposure to prevent possible transmission to others. Studies have found transmission to household members who have not had the disease is highly likely (90% infection incidence).

For immunocompromised patients, varicella zoster immune globulin (VZIG) is recommended by the CDC as postexposure prophylaxis.

Bioterrorism Syndromes

Anthrax

Anthrax is caused by *Bacillus anthracis*, a gram-positive, rod-shaped bacteria. Naturally found in the soil and more commonly affecting animals, anthrax has been used as a biologic terrorism weapon directed against human populations. There are four types of anthrax exposure: cutaneous, inhalation, gastrointestinal, and injection. The focus here is on the three major syndromes—*cutaneous, inhalation, and gastrointestinal tract anthrax.*

Cutaneous anthrax, the most common and least deadly form of the disease, occurs when spores of *B. anthracis* are introduced subcutaneously, usually as the result of a cut or a scrape when handling infected animals or animal products (e.g., wool, hides). Its incubation period usually has a range of 1 to 7 days.

More than 90% of cutaneous anthrax lesions occur in exposed areas of the skin, primarily the upper extremities and face. Initially, the disease appears as a small, painless, often pruritic papule that enlarges over 24 to 48 hours and develops a central blister, followed by erosion, leaving a painless necrotic ulcer with a black, depressed eschar. An eschar with extensive surrounding edema is the hallmark of cutaneous anthrax.

In addition to the papule, patients may experience lymphadenopathy, which, if near the upper airway, may cause respiratory compromise. Occasionally, systemic symptoms, including fever, malaise, and headache, can accompany the cutaneous lesion. (*Injection anthrax* behaves similarly to cutaneous anthrax.) Most cases of cutaneous anthrax are cured with antibiotic therapy, although mortality can be as high as 20% without treatment.

Inhalation anthrax results from the inhalation of particles containing *B. anthracis* spores. People who work in tanneries, slaughterhouses, or wool mills with contaminated animal products such as wool, hair, or hides may breathe in the spores. Infection has also resulted from inhalation of weaponized and intentionally released spore preparations. Symptom onset has a wide range—from several hours to 2 months. During the anthrax bioterrorism event in the United States in 2001, the time between known exposure and symptom onset ranged from 4 to 6 days.

The course of the disease has two phases. Prodromal symptoms of inhalation anthrax may be vague and nonspecific, which can complicate assessment and diagnosis. Early symptoms, such as myalgia, fever, and malaise, may mimic those associated with influenza. However, a variety of symptoms less suggestive of influenza may also be present, such as nausea, hemoptysis, dyspnea, odynophagia, confusion, dysphagia, and chest pain. Prodromal symptoms last, on average, 4 to 5 days and are followed by a hyperacute phase marked by the development of progressive respiratory symptoms, including severe dyspnea, high fever, cyanosis, hypoxemia, and shock. A widened mediastinum due to hemorrhagic mediastinitis may be seen on chest x-ray, contributing to the clinical suspicion. CT scan may reveal hilar adenopathy, pleural effusions, and mediastinal hemorrhage. Accompanying meningitis has been reported in a high percentage of cases of inhalation anthrax. This type of anthrax is usually fatal without treatment, but approximately 55% of patients are cured with aggressive antibiotic therapy.

Gastrointestinal tract anthrax presents as one of two clinical forms: oropharyngeal or gastrointestinal. *B. anthracis* has been reported to infect all regions of the alimentary tract, from the mouth to the ascending colon. Patients with oropharyngeal anthrax complain of difficulty swallowing and develop lymphadenopathy with multiple superficial lesions that are ulcerative with surrounding edema. Patients with GI anthrax develop fever, abdominal pain, nausea, vomiting, diarrhea (sometimes bloody), and, on occasion, ascites. In some cases, lesions become hemorrhagic, resulting in the patient's death. This disease results from consumption of undercooked meat from animals infected with anthrax and tends to occur in family clusters or point-source outbreaks. GI anthrax is highly fatal without treatment, although approximately 60% of affected patients will survive with aggressive antibiotic therapy.

Differential Diagnosis

- Cutaneous anthrax: The differential diagnosis includes staphylococcal skin sepsis, cat-scratch disease, and zoonotic viral infections.
- Inhalation anthrax: The differential diagnosis includes acute bacterial or viral pneumonia, TB, plague, and tularemia.

- GI anthrax: The differential diagnosis includes bacterial diarrhea (*Shigella, E. coli, Salmonella, Campylobacter, Yersinia*) and parasitic infections.

Diagnosis

The diagnosis of anthrax is made by PCR, Gram stain, and cultures of the respective clinical specimens (blood, pleural fluid, stool, CSF, skin site, ascites). Laboratory staff must be warned of the potential presence of anthrax in the received specimen so they can take appropriate precautions. Additionally, identification of antibodies or toxin with the enzyme-linked immunosorbent assay (ELISA) technique can assist in the diagnosis.

Treatment

All forms of anthrax should be treated with antibiotics. Options include doxycycline, ciprofloxacin, or another quinolone. If the anthrax isolate is susceptible, penicillin and clindamycin are alternative medications. For patients with meningitis, the carbapenem class of antimicrobial drugs is highly resistant to beta lactamase enzymes, which degrade the antibiotic, and provides good CNS penetration.

Protein synthesis inhibitors (e.g., linezolid or clindamycin) should be added to decrease toxin production. Antitoxin (monoclonal and polyclonal) agents should be considered in addition to antibiotics for individuals with suspected systemic anthrax. Anthrax immune globulin is available and should be considered in collaboration with the CDC.

Prevention

A vaccine is available to prevent anthrax, although it is usually recommended only for high-risk groups (e.g., military, lab workers).

Postexposure prophylaxis should be started as soon as possible and continued for minimal of 60 days for short-term prophylaxis. The anthrax vaccine is used for long-term protection.

Smallpox

The variola virus is the causative agent of smallpox, a highly infectious disease characterized by fever, rash, and a high mortality rate. The two strains of variola (major and minor) differ greatly in their mortality rates (30% versus 1%, respectively).

In 1980, the 33rd World Health Assembly announced the global eradication of smallpox as a result of worldwide vaccination efforts; this feat is considered one of the greatest achievements of modern medicine. There have been no reported cases of naturally occurring smallpox since its eradication.

Pathophysiology/Transmission

Smallpox is transmitted through direct contact as well as airborne transmission. Transmission can occur from the onset of lesions until the crusting stage. Airborne transmissions have been well documented in hospital and laboratory settings. The virus may be able to survive in the right conditions for months and even many years.

Clinical Features

Two clinical forms of smallpox disease are distinguished: variola major and variola minor. Variola minor is the less common of the two. There are four types of variola major smallpox: ordinary, modified, flat, and hemorrhagic. In the past, more than 70% of smallpox cases worldwide were of the ordinary type, which was further subdivided into three categories according to the type of rash:

- Confluent rash present on face and forearms
- Semiconfluent rash present on the face with discrete rash elsewhere
- Discrete rash on all involved areas with normal skin between pustules

The clinical outcome for ordinary type smallpox was closely linked to the type of accompanying rash. As an example, in unvaccinated patients, mortality was 62% for infection with confluent rash, 37% for semiconfluent rash, and 9% for discrete rash. Death from smallpox occurs secondary to coagulopathy, hypotension, and multiorgan failure.

Differential Diagnosis

Other diagnostic considerations include herpes simplex, herpes varicella, mpox (monkeypox), eczema herpeticum, disseminated gonococcal disease, soft-tissue infection, drug rash, and nonspecific viral illness.

Diagnosis can be made based on clinical examination. The rash of smallpox is defined by blister lesions that are all in the same phase of blistering (**Figure 7-12**). Definitive diagnosis should be made based on detection of the virus by culture or PCR, or identification of viral antibodies from lesion or blood testing.

Treatment

The currently recommended smallpox vaccines are based on attenuated vaccinia viruses that are much less virulent and carry lesser side effects. The attenuated viruses may be either replicating or nonreplicating.

Vaccines can be administered 3 to 4 days after an exposure (before rash develops) and may lessen the severity of illness. Supportive care and wound care are the primary treatments for active illness. Two antiviral medications (tecovirimat and brincidofovir) are approved by the FDA to treat smallpox. Of the two, most experts

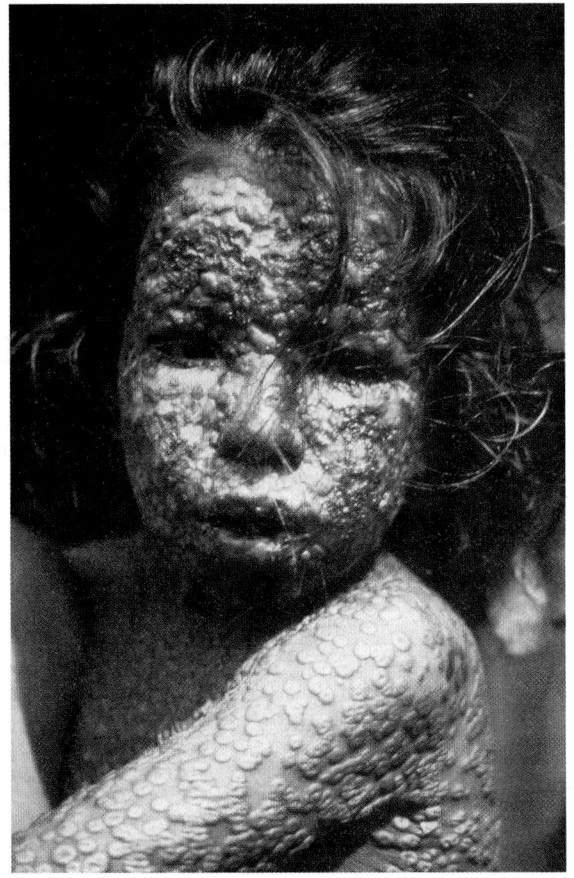

A

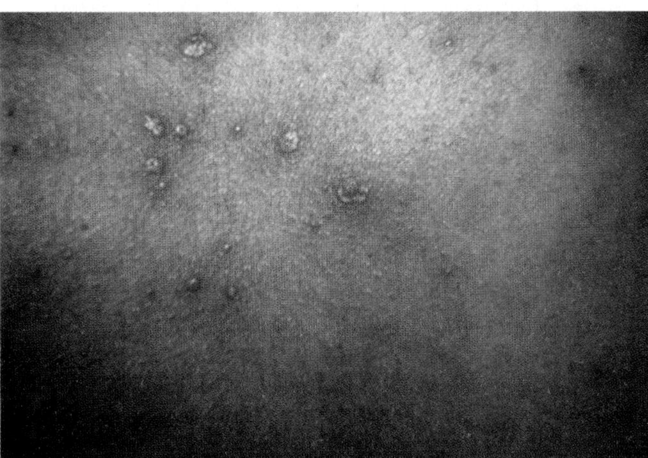

B

Figure 7-12 **A.** The vesicles (blisters) in smallpox are all in the same phase of blistering. **B.** The blisters of chickenpox are in various stages of formation of papule, vesicle, and crusting.

Courtesy of CDC.

recommend use of tecovirimat due to its efficacy and lack of side effects.

Prevention

Prior to the worldwide eradication of the disease, vaccinations were routinely administered before exposure to smallpox. If there is concern for smallpox, hospital, local, and state public health agencies and the CDC should be contacted immediately. In such a case, contact and airborne precautions should be implemented immediately, including use of an N95 or higher respirator.

Monkeypox Virus

The monkeypox virus causes the disease known as mpox (formerly called monkeypox). Mpox was first discovered in 1958 in a colony of monkeys shipped from Singapore to Copenhagen, although the first reported human case occurred in 1970 in the Democratic Republic of Congo. Mpox has predominately been observed in central and western Africa, but was reported globally (including in the United States) in 2022. Two forms of the monkeypox virus exist, Clade I (Central African) and Clade II (West African). Clade I has a fatality rate of about 10% and Clade II is less than 1% fatal.

Pathophysiology/Transmission

Mpox is a zoonosis—that is, a disease spread from animals to humans. The animal reservoir for the disease is thought to be rodents, with the infection spreading through primate contact with rodents. Monkeypox virus is predominately transmitted through direct contact with an mpox lesion or mucosa and respiratory secretions, or indirectly through contact with fomites. Activities that increase the risk of transmission between humans include sexual intercourse, prolonged face-to-face contact, hugging, and kissing. An infected person is communicable from the time of symptom onset until the mpox skin lesions have fully healed and new skin has formed.

Signs and Symptoms

Mpox presents similarly to smallpox, with a pox skin eruption that develops a few days after fever eruption. Skin lesions can be seen over the entire body (including the genitalia), but predominately appear on the face, hands, and feet. Oral mucosa lesions are also seen. Associated symptoms include headache, muscle aches, and swollen lymph nodes. Symptoms are self-limiting, lasting about 2 to 4 weeks. In the 2022 outbreak in Europe and North America, atypical presentations of mpox were observed, including lesions at different stages of evolution (i.e., vesicles, pustules, and crust) and presentations with skin lesions primarily in the genital region, often without febrile prodromes.

Differential Diagnosis

Other diagnostic considerations include herpes simplex and varicella, smallpox, disseminated gonococcal disease, syphilis, scabies, generalized vaccinia, eczema herpeticum, soft-tissue infection, drug rash, and nonspecific viral illness.

The diagnosis of mpox can be made based on clinical examination. Definitive diagnosis should be based on detection of the virus by culture or PCR, or identification of viral antibodies from lesion or blood testing.

Treatment

Supportive care and wound care are the primary treatments for active illness. Currently, there is no approved treatment, although medications approved for smallpox (e.g., tecovirimat, vaccinia immune globulin) can be considered for use in severe cases.

Prevention

If there is concern for mpox, contact precautions and quality hand hygiene should be followed.

Ebola Virus Disease

Ebola virus disease is caused by the Ebola virus, an RNA-based filovirus. Ebola was first discovered in 1976 in Africa near the Ebola River (Democratic Republic of the Congo). The majority of cases and outbreaks have been reported in Africa. Recent modern outbreaks include the 2014–2016 West African outbreak, which accounted for an estimated 11,325 deaths. Localized transmission occurred in the United States, with four suspected/confirmed cases and one death. In 2022, another outbreak was reported in the Democratic Republic of the Congo and Uganda. The bat is thought to be the reservoir for the virus.

Pathophysiology/Transmission

The Ebola virus is spread through direct contact with broken skin or mucous membranes. The virus can be transmitted via the following pathways:

- Blood and body fluids (e.g., urine, feces, vomit, salvia, sweat, semen, amniotic fluid, breast milk) of an infected or diseased person
- Contaminated objects (e.g., clothing, medical equipment)
- Infected bats or nonhuman primates

Signs and Symptoms

Symptoms occur, on average, 8 to 10 days after viral contact, but may appear as soon as 2 days after transmission. These symptoms are the same as those associated with viral hemorrhagic fevers. The primary symptoms include fever, body aches, headache, fatigue, decreased appetite, abdominal pain, nausea/vomiting/diarrhea, and unexplained bleeding or bruising.

Differential Diagnosis

Other diagnostic considerations include malaria, dengue, typhoid fever, yellow fever, bacterial gastroenteritis, disseminated intravascular coagulation, and viral hemorrhagic fevers.

Diagnosis may be suspected based on the patient history and examination, especially if there is a known close exposure. Blood samples are needed to confirm the diagnosis—most commonly via PCR or ELISA, or immunofluorescence, and serologic antibody assays.

Treatment

Two medications, both monoclonal antibodies, are approved to treat Ebola virus disease; both have demonstrated the ability to improve survival in recent outbreaks. However, neither of these agents has been evaluated against the Clade 1 (Central African) variant. Supportive care, including optimizing fluid status, repletion of electrolytes, and treating concomitant infections, is also essential.

Prevention

Physical agents that can eradicate Ebola virus include bleach, strong disinfectants that destroy nonenveloped viruses, heat, sunlight, ultraviolet (UV) light, electron beam, and gamma rays. The virus is resistant to intense heat and requires high doses of UV light or gamma radiation to inactivate it.

It is recommended that people with confirmed or suspected Ebola virus infection be transported to designated Ebola assessment and treatment centers using specially outfitted transport vehicles. The personnel responsible for their transport should have specialized training in the following areas: communications, transport patient care, infection control, PPE selection and donning/doffing, and decontamination. Required PPE commonly includes a powered air-purifying respirator (PAPR) hood and coveralls. High-quality hand and respiratory hygiene practices must also be followed.

Two vaccines against the Ebola virus are available: Ervebo and Ad26.Zebov-gp. They have been found to be safe and efficacious, although the extent of protection afforded by the vaccines is not currently known. Both the Ervebo and Ad26.Zebov-gp vaccines are specific to the Zaire ebolavirus (Clade 2); their protection against Clade 1 viruses is not proven.

Special Populations

Older Adult Patients

As people age, their physiologic reserves decline. The following changes are associated with normal aging:

- Challenges with temperature regulation
- Osteoporosis with increased risk of fractures
- Reduced cardiac and pulmonary reserves
- Reduced kidney renal function

- Decreased visual acuity and hearing
- Decreased muscle mass and strength
- Skin thinning, which renders it more prone to ulcers and skin tears

Geriatric patients are more vulnerable to infection than younger patients, and they tend to suffer greater morbidity and a higher rate of mortality from infectious disease given the diminished functioning of their immune systems as they age. They are also more likely to use multiple medications (polypharmacy), and some may experience altered baseline mental status. Aging lowers the primary antibody response and cellular immunity and increases susceptibility to infection and autoimmune disorders. The following factors increase the risk of infection among older adults:

- The frequent existence of comorbid conditions, such as diabetes and neurologic diseases
- The living conditions inherent to group living situations such as nursing care facilities
- The higher rate of hospitalization among this population, which significantly increases the risk of contracting a **hospital-acquired infection/health care–associated infection (HAI)** (formerly called **nosocomial infection**)
- An increased incidence of malnutrition, which directly impairs the immune response

Assessment of older adults with infections may be challenging because of the difficulty of obtaining a thorough, accurate history and the absence of fever in nearly one-half of older adults with bacterial infections. An older patient may not exhibit the typical signs and symptoms of infection because of difficulties regulating body temperature and a depressed immune system due to medications that may impact the physiologic response. Pneumonia, urinary tract infections, and sepsis occur more often in older adult patients.

Bariatric Patients

Obesity has now become a global problem. During an infection, the complications of obesity, such as hypertension, stroke, heart disease, and diabetes, can impact the immune system and exacerbate serious illness.

Patients Who Are Technology Dependent

Increasingly, many patients with complicated acute and chronic medical conditions who are often dependent on technologically advanced monitoring and care are cared for at home in structured "Hospital-at-Home" or "acute care at home programs." The trend of caring for such patients in the home setting is gaining momentum because of burdensome hospital costs, insurance limitations placed on length of hospital stays, a desire to treat patients in their home environment, and the goal of reducing the risk of HAIs. Some patients with infectious diseases (e.g., cellulitis or community-acquired pneumonia) who previously were treated in the hospital are now treated at home through these programs. The medical needs of patients served by such programs, most of whom have neuromuscular and respiratory disorders, include mechanical ventilation, tracheostomy care, administration of IV medications, maintenance of feeding tubes, administration of oxygen, and wound care. Decubitus ulcers are more prevalent in patients who are immobile and have compromised immune systems; this complication increases the patient's risk of acquiring an infection. Vascular access devices, urinary catheters, and a compromised immune system from treatments such as chemotherapy increase susceptibility to viral and bacterial infections as well.

Putting It All Together

Understanding the epidemiology and pathophysiology of a variety of infectious disease processes is essential to ensure early identification of the cause of an illness. In addition, becoming aware of an abrupt increase in the number of patients with similar common presentations will help you and your public health colleagues pinpoint geographic trends that might need to be reported to the appropriate local, state, and federal authorities.

Identification of the patient's cardinal presentation or chief complaint, a thorough history, a focused physical exam, and evaluation of diagnostic findings as you work through the AMLS Assessment Pathway will help you recognize that the patient has a communicable or infectious disease. Early recognition can help prevent the spread of the disease by enabling you to choose the appropriate PPE early in patient contact. The health care team's assessment and early interventions are critical strategies in preventing the transmission of infectious diseases. However, the health care environment is often unpredictable, and disease identification may not occur until after you have rendered care. Fortunately, researchers continue to make progress in identifying communicable and infectious diseases and developing new vaccines, medications, and treatment protocols.

SCENARIO SOLUTION

- Differential diagnoses may include pulmonary embolism, myocardial infarction, congenital heart failure, pulmonary edema, pleural effusion, pneumonia, inhalation injury, tuberculosis, influenza, and COVID-19.
- To narrow your differential diagnosis, you will need to obtain the patient's history of past and present illness. Assess her temperature. Asking about recent exposure to other individuals who are ill is key. You may also want to inquire about other people with similar symptoms in the shelter. Ask about the patient's vaccine history (influenza, COVID-19, pneumococcal). Inquiring about symptoms of insomnia, difficulty sleeping, or orthopnea may be helpful as well. Assess if there is increased sputum production or hemoptysis. Does she have a history or treatment or diagnosis of tuberculosis?
- This patient would benefit from supplemental oxygen administered by nasal cannula. If this intervention is ineffective, consider alternatives including a nonrebreather (NRB) mask and noninvasive positive-pressure ventilation. Initiate a 12-lead electrocardiogram, and transport the patient to the appropriate facility.
- Use standard precautions with all patients. Place a surgical mask on the patient and yourself. Use rapid air exchange in the transport unit (exhaust fan). A fit-tested N95 mask or higher should be considered if there is concern for airborne transmission. Report your exposure immediately to the health care clinician at the receiving facility. Notify your designated infection control officer. Complete the necessary reports and follow-up. Good hand washing and cleaning any contaminated equipment are essential.

SUMMARY

- Exposure to an infectious agent does not necessarily mean that a person has acquired the disease and can pass it on to others.
- PPE is a secondary barrier that complements the protection the body already offers.
- PPE should be selected with an understanding of the mode of transmission for the diseases you expect to encounter.
- Vaccination is essential for risk reduction in the health care setting.
- Health care clinicians can decrease their risk of exposure to infectious diseases by using standard precautions and implementing thorough hand washing techniques.
- Local and federal governmental agencies establish standards and guidelines geared toward reducing the risk of infection for health care clinicians and the communities in which they serve.
- Prevention of transmission of infectious diseases can result from an understanding of the pathophysiology, clinical manifestations, and treatment strategies for communicable and infectious diseases.

Key Terms

antibodies Immunoglobulins produced by lymphocytes in response to bacteria, viruses, or other antigenic substances.

antigen A substance, usually a protein, that the body recognizes as foreign and that can evoke an immune response.

bloodborne pathogens (BBP) Pathogenic microorganisms that are transmitted via human blood and cause disease in humans; examples include hepatitis B virus and human immunodeficiency virus.

communicable diseases Any disease transmitted from one person or animal to another either directly, by contact with excreta or other discharges from the body; or indirectly, by means of substances or inanimate objects such as contaminated drinking glasses, toys, or water, or by vectors such as flies, mosquitoes, ticks, or other insects.

contaminated A condition of being soiled, stained, touched, or otherwise exposed to harmful agents, making an object potentially unsafe for use as intended or without barrier techniques; for example, entry of infectious or toxic materials into a previously clean or sterile environment.

decontamination The process of removing foreign material such as blood, body fluids, or radioactivity; it does not eliminate microorganisms, but is a necessary step preceding disinfection or sterilization.

endemic A disease that is present in the community at a given baseline level over time, such as herpes or chickenpox.

epidemic A disease that affects a significantly large number of people at the same time and spreads rapidly through a demographic segment of the human population.

epidemiology The study of the determinants of disease events in populations.

exposure incidents Being in the presence of or subjected to a force or influence (e.g., viral exposure, heat exposure).

fomite An inanimate object that can become contaminated with an infectious pathogen and spread disease.

hospital-acquired infection/health care–associated infection (HAI) An infection acquired from exposure to an infectious agent at a health care facility, defined as at least 72 hours after hospitalization.

infectious diseases Diseases caused by another living organism or virus, which may or may not be transmissible to another person.

nosocomial infection *See* hospital-acquired infection/health care–associated infection (HAI).

pandemic A disease occurring throughout the population of a large part of the world.

parenteral Pertaining to treatment other than through the digestive system.

polymerase chain reaction (PCR) A laboratory method used to replicate DNA that is leveraged to test for the presence of genetic material from organisms, including viruses.

retrovirus Any of a family of ribonucleic acid (RNA) viruses containing reverse transcriptase, an enzyme, in the virion; examples include human immunodeficiency virus (HIV1, HIV2) and human T-cell lymphotropic virus.

standard precautions Guidelines recommended by the Centers for Disease Control and Prevention for reducing the risk of transmission of bloodborne and other pathogens in hospitals. Standard precautions apply to (1) blood; (2) all body fluids, secretions, and excretions except sweat, regardless of whether or not they contain blood; (3) nonintact skin; and (4) mucous membranes.

virulence The power of a microorganism to produce disease.

Bibliography

Aehlert B. *Paramedic Practice Today: Above and Beyond*. Mosby; 2009.

Albright A, Gross K, Hunter M, O'Connor L. A dispatch screening tool to identify patients at high risk for COVID-19 in the prehospital setting. *West J Emerg Med*. 2021;22(6): 1253-1256.

Alter MJ, Kuhnert WL, Finelli L, et al. Guidelines for laboratory testing and result reporting of antibody to hepatitis C virus. *MMWR Recomm Rep*. 2003;52(RR-3):1-13.

American Academy of Orthopaedic Surgeons. *Nancy Caroline's Emergency Care in the Streets*. 7th ed. Jones & Bartlett Learning; 2013.

American Academy of Pediatrics Committee on Infectious Diseases and Committee on Fetus and Newborn. Revised indications for the use of palivizumab and respiratory syncytial virus immune globulin intravenous for the prevention of respiratory syncytial virus infection. *Pediatrics*. 2003;112(6 pt 1): 1442-1446.

Association for Professionals in Infection Control and Epidemiology, Inc. *APIC Text of Infection Control and Epidemiology*. APIC; 2009.

Baeten JM, Donnell D, Ndase P, et al. Antiretroviral prophylaxis for HIV prevention in heterosexual men and women. *N Engl J Med*. 2012;367(5):399-410.

Blain A, Tiwari TSP. Chapter 16: Tetanus. In: *Manual for the Surveillance of Vaccine-Preventable Diseases*. Reviewed February 6, 2020. Accessed October 9, 2023. https://www.cdc.gov/vaccines/pubs/surv-manual/chpt16-tetanus.html

Bragg BN, Wills C. Pediculosis. *StatPearls*. Updated March 14, 2023. Accessed October 9, 2023. https://www.ncbi.nlm.nih.gov/books/NBK470343

Camejo Leonor M, Mendez MD. Rubella. *StatPearls*. Updated August 8, 2023. Accessed October 9, 2023. https://www.ncbi.nlm.nih.gov/books/NBK559040

Centers for Disease Control and Prevention. Guideline for isolation precautions: preventing transmission of infectious agents in healthcare settings. Published 2007. Accessed October 9, 2023. http://www.cdc.gov/hicpac/2007IP/2007isolationPrecautions.html

Centers for Disease Control and Prevention. CDC research confirms benefits of flu antiviral drugs, even beyond 2 days after symptoms start. Reviewed November 22, 2013.

Accessed October 9, 2023. https://www.cdc.gov/flu/spotlights/2013-2014/flu-antiviral-benefits.htm

Centers for Disease Control and Prevention. Chickenpox (varicella), clinical overview. Updated August 22, 2013. Accessed October 9, 2023. https://www.cdc.gov/chickenpox

Centers for Disease Control and Prevention. Controlling tuberculosis in the United States. Published 2005. Accessed October 9, 2023. https://www.cdc.gov/mmwr/preview/mmwrhtml/rr5412a1.htm.

Centers for Disease Control and Prevention. Disease burden of flu. Last reviewed October 4, 2022. Accessed October 9, 2023. https://www.cdc.gov/flu/about/burden/index.html

Centers for Disease Control and Prevention. Ebola disease. Reviewed March 23, 2023. Accessed October 9, 2023. https://www.cdc.gov/vhf/ebola/index.html

Centers for Disease Control and Prevention. 2009 H1N1 flu. Accessed October 9, 2023. https://www.cdc.gov/h1n1flu

Centers for Disease Control and Prevention. Hand hygiene in healthcare settings. Last reviewed April 28, 2023. Accessed October 9, 2023. https://www.cdc.gov/Handhygiene

Centers for Disease Control and Prevention. Hantavirus. Last reviewed September 16, 2022. Accessed October 9, 2023. https://wwwnc.cdc.gov/travel/diseases/hantavirus

Centers for Disease Control and Prevention. Hantavirus pulmonary syndrome (HPS). Reviewed February 6, 2013. Accessed October 9, 2023. https://www.cdc.gov/hantavirus/hps/index.html

Centers for Disease Control and Prevention. Hepatitis A questions and answers for health professionals. Reviewed July 28, 2020. Accessed October 9, 2023. https://www.cdc.gov/hepatitis/hav/havfaq.htm

Centers for Disease Control and Prevention. Hepatitis B. Last reviewed March 9, 2023. Accessed October 9, 2023. https://www.cdc.gov/hepatitis/hbv

Centers for Disease Control and Prevention. Hepatitis C questions and answers for health professionals. Reviewed August 7, 2020. Accessed October 9, 2023.https://www.cdc.gov/hepatitis/HCV/HCVfaq.htm

Centers for Disease Control and Prevention. HPV and men: fact sheet. Reviewed April 18, 2022. Accessed October 9, 2023. https://www.cdc.gov/std/hpv/stdfact-hpv-and-men.htm

Centers for Disease Control and Prevention. Human papillomavirus (HPV) vaccination: what everyone should know. Updated November 16, 2021. Accessed October 9, 2023. https://www.cdc.gov/vaccines/vpd/hpv/public

Centers for Disease Control and Prevention. Immunization schedules. Last reviewed February 10, 2023. Accessed October 9, 2023. https://www.cdc.gov/vaccines/schedules

Centers for Disease Control and Prevention. Influenza ACIP vaccine recommendations. Last reviewed August 23, 2023. Accessed October 9, 2023. https://www.cdc.gov/vaccines/hcp/acip-recs/vacc-specific/flu.html

Centers for Disease Control and Prevention. Lyme borreliosis (Lyme disease), Last reviewed May 1, 2023. Accessed October 9, 2023. https://wwwnc.cdc.gov/travel/yellowbook/2024/infections-diseases/lyme-disease

Centers for Disease Control and Prevention. Lyme disease. Updated January 19, 2022. Accessed October 9, 2023. https://www.cdc.gov/lyme

Centers for Disease Control and Prevention. Mumps. Last reviewed March 8, 2021. Accessed October 9, 2023. https://www.cdc.gov/mumps/travelers.html

Centers for Disease Control and Prevention. The national plan to eliminate syphilis from the United States. Published May 2006. Accessed October 9, 2023. https://www.cdc.gov/stopsyphilis/SEEPlan2006.pdf

Centers for Disease Control and Prevention. Parasites: Lice. Updated September 11, 2019. Accessed October 9, 2023. https://www.cdc.gov/parasites/lice

Centers for Disease Control and Prevention. Pertussis surveillance and reporting. Reviewed August 4, 2022. Accessed October 9, 2023. https://www.cdc.gov/pertussis/surv-reporting.html

Centers for Disease Control and Prevention. Pneumonia can be prevented—vaccines can help. Reviewed September 30, 2022. Accessed October 9, 2023. https://www.cdc.gov/pneumonia/prevention.html

Centers for Disease Control and Prevention. Pre-exposure prophylaxis (PrEP). Reviewed July 5, 2022. Accessed October 9, 2023. https://www.cdc.gov/hiv/risk/prep/index.html

Centers for Disease Control and Prevention. Rabies. Reviewed December 8, 2022. Accessed October 9, 2023. https://www.cdc.gov/rabies

Centers for Disease Control and Prevention. Rocky Mountain spotted fever (RMSF). Reviewed May 7, 2019. Accessed October 9, 2023. https://www.cdc.gov/rmsf

Centers for Disease Control and Prevention. Syphilis & MSM (men who have sex with men): CDC fact sheet. Reviewed April 11, 2023. Accessed October 9, 2023. https://www.cdc.gov/std/syphilis/stdfact-msm-syphilis.htm

Centers for Disease Control and Prevention. Treatment for TB disease. Reviewed March 22, 2023. Accessed October 9, 2023. https://www.cdc.gov/tb/topic/treatment/tbdisease.htm

Centers for Disease Control and Prevention. Trends in tuberculosis—United States, 2008, *MMWR*. 2009;58(10):249-253.

Centers for Disease Control and Prevention. Tuberculosis: Data and statistics. Updated March 23, 2023. Accessed October 9, 2023. https://www.cdc.gov/tb/statistics/default.htm

Centers for Disease Control and Prevention. Updated U.S. public health service guidelines for the management of occupational exposures to HBC, HCV, and HIV, recommendations for postexposure prophylaxis.Published 2013. Accessed October 9, 2023. https://npin.cdc.gov/publication/updated-us-public-health-service-guidelines-management-occupational-exposures-hiv-and

Centers for Disease Control and Prevention. Viral hemorrhagic fevers. Last reviewed September 2, 2021. Accessed October 9, 2023. https://www.cdc.gov/vhf

Centers for Disease Control and Prevention. West Nile virus. Reviewed June 13, 2023. Accessed October 9, 2023. https://www.cdc.gov/ncidod/dvbid/westnile/index.htm

Centers for Disease Control and Prevention. West Nile virus: diagnostic testing. Reviewed April 25, 2023. Accessed October 9, 2023. https://www.cdc.gov/westnile/healthcareproviders/healthCareProviders-Diagnostic.html

Centers for Disease Control and Prevention, Division of Bacterial and Mycotic Diseases. *Streptococcus pneumoniae* disease prevention and control of meningococcal disease:

Recommendations of the Advisory Committee on Immunization Practices (ACIP). *MMWR Recomm Rep*. 2000;49(RR-9): 1-35.

Chippendale J, Lloyd A, Payne T, et al. The feasibility of paramedics delivering antibiotic treatment pre-hospital to "red flag" sepsis patients: a service evaluation. *Br Paramed J*. 2018;2(4):19-24.

Cohen J, Powderly WG. *Infectious Diseases*. 2nd ed. Mosby; 2004.

Cross JR, West KH. Clarifying HIPAA and disclosure of disease information. *JEMS*. Published August 31, 2007. Accessed October 9, 2023. https://www.jems.com/operations/clarifying-hipaa-and-disclosur

Dailey A, Gant Z, Lyons SJ. *HIV Surveillance Report, 2019*. Vol. 32. Published May 2021. Accessed October 9, 2023. https://www.cdc.gov/hiv/pdf/library/reports/surveillance/cdc-hiv-surveillance-report-2018-updated-vol-32.pdf

Evans L, Rhodes A, Alhazzani W, et al. Surviving Sepsis campaign: international guidelines for management of sepsis and septic shock 2021. *Intens Care Med*. 2021;47(11):1181-1247.

Giersing BK, Karron RA, Vekemans J, et al. Meeting report: WHO consultation on respiratory syncytial virus (RSV) vaccine development, Geneva, 25–26 April 2016. *Vaccine*. 2019;37(50):7355-7362. doi:10.1016/j.vaccine.2017.02.068

Henderson DA. The looming threat of bioterrorism. *Science*. 1999;283(5406):1279.

Hunter CL, Silvestri S, Stone A, et al. Prehospital sepsis alert notification decreases time to initiation of CMS sepsis core measures. *Am J Emerg Med*. 2019;37(1):114-117.

Immunize.org. Hepatitis B and healthcare personnel. Published August 16, 2023. Accessed October 9, 2023. https://www.immunize.org/catg.d/p2109.pdf

Inglesby TV, O'Toole T, Henderson DA, et al. Working Group on Civilian Biodefense: anthrax as a biological weapon, 2002: updated recommendations for management. *JAMA*. 2002;287(17):2236.

Institute of Medicine. Respiratory protection for healthcare workers in the workplace against novel H1N1 influenza A: a letter report. Published 2009. Accessed October 9, 2023. https://www.ncbi.nlm.nih.gov/books/NBK219940

Jefferson T, Jones MA, Doshi P, et al. Neuraminidase inhibitors for preventing and treating influenza in adults and children. *Cochrane Database Syst Rev*. 2014;4:CD008965.

Jefferson T, Rivetti A, Di Pietrantonj C, Demicheli V. Vaccines for preventing influenza in healthy children. *Cochrane Database Syst Rev*. 2018;2:CD004879.

Juneau C, Mendias EP, Wagal N, et al. Community-acquired *Clostridium difficile* infection: awareness and clinical implications. *J Nurse Pract*. 2013;9(1):1-6.

Khattak ZE, Anjum F. *Haemophilus influenzae* infection. *StatPearls*. Updated April 27, 2023. Accessed October 9, 2023. https://www.ncbi.nlm.nih.gov/books/NBK562176

Koury R, Warrington SJ. Rabies. *StatPearls*. Updated October 31, 2022. Accessed October 9, 2023. https://www.ncbi.nlm.nih.gov/books/NBK448076

Kretsinger K, Broder KR, Cortese MM, et al. Preventing tetanus, diphtheria, and pertussis among adults: use of tetanus toxoid, reduced diphtheria toxoid, and acellular pertussis vaccine; recommendations of the Advisory Committee on Immunization Practices (ACIP) and recommendation of ACIP. *MMWR Recomm Rep*. 2006;55(RR-17):1-37.

Kulkarni H, Smith CM, Lee DDH, et al. Evidence of respiratory syncytial virus spread by aerosol: time to revisit infection control strategies? *Am J Respir Crit Care Med*. 2016;194(4): 308-316.

Kushel M. Hepatitis A outbreak in California: addressing the root cause. *N Engl J Med*. 2018;378;3.

Lessa FC, Gould CV, McDonald LC. Current status of *Clostridium difficile* infection epidemiology. *Clin Infect Dis*. 2012;55 (suppl 2): S65-S70. Accessed October 9, 2023. https://cid.oxfordjournals.org/content/55/suppl_2/S65.full

Mandziuk J, Kuchar EP. Streptococcal meningitis. *StatPearls*. Updated April 10, 2023. Accessed October 9, 2023. https://www.ncbi.nlm.nih.gov/books/NBK554448

Martinez L, Cords O, Liu Q, et al. Infant BCG vaccination and risk and pulmonary and extrapulmonary tuberculosis throughout the life course: a systematic review and individual participant data meta-analysis. *Lancet Glob Health*. 2022;10(9):e1307-e1316.

Masarani M, Wazait H, Dinneen M. Mumps orchitis. *J R Soc Med*. 2006;99(11):5730-5575.

Mast EE, Weinbaum CM, Fiore AE, et al. A comprehensive immunization strategy to eliminate transmission of hepatitis B virus infection in the United States: recommendations of the Advisory Committee on Immunization Practices (ACIP) part II: immunization of adults. *MMWR*. 2007;56(42):1114.

McCance KL, Huether SE. *Pathophysiology: The Biologic Basis for Disease in Adults and Children*. 5th ed. Elsevier; 2006.

McCann-Pineo M, Li T, Barbara P, et al. Utility of emergency medical dispatch (EMD) telephone screening in identifying COVID-19 positive patients. *Prehosp Emerg Care*. 2021;1-10. doi:10.1080/10903127.2021.1939817

Medical News Today. Where did HIV come from? Updated February 16, 2023. Accessed October 9, 2023. https://www.medicalnewstoday.com/articles/etiology-hiv

Memoli MJ, Athota R, Reed S, et al. The natural history of influenza infection in the severely immunocompromised vs nonimmunocompromised hosts. *Clin Infect Dis*. 2014; 58(2):214.

Meningitis Research Foundation. *Haemophilus influenzae* type b (Hib) meningitis. Accessed October 9, 2023. https://www.meningitis.org/meningitis/causes/haemophilus-influenzae-type-b-(hib)-meningitis

Mizra S, Hall AJ. Norovirus. *CDC Yellow Book 2024*. Reviewed May 1, 2023. Accessed October 9, 2023. https://wwwnc.cdc.gov/travel/yellowbook/2024/infections-diseases/norovirus

Monto AS, Gravenstein S, Elliott M, et al. Clinical signs and symptoms predicting influenza infection. *J Arch Intern Med*. 2000;160(21):3243

Nadelman RB, Nowakowski J, Fish D, et al. Prophylaxis with single-dose doxycycline for the prevention of Lyme disease after an *Ixodes scapularis* tick bite. *N Engl J Med*. 2001;345: 79-84.

National Highway Traffic Safety Administration, Office of EMS. Planning for the future: EMS agenda 2050. Updated December 8, 2022. Accessed October 9, 2023. https://www.ems.gov/issues/planning-for-the-future-ems-agenda-2050

Needlestick Prevention Act, public law 106–430, U.S. Congress, March 2000.

Nguyen N, Ashong D. *Neisseria meningitidis*. *StatPearls*. Updated September 26, 2022. Accessed October 9, 2023. https://www.ncbi.nlm.nih.gov/books/NBK549849

Occupational Safety and Health Administration. 29 CFR 1910.1020: access to employee exposure and medical records. Accessed October 9, 2023. https://www.osha.gov/laws-regs/regulations/standardnumber/1910/1910.1020

Occupational Safety and Health Administration. 29 CFR 1910.1030: bloodborne pathogens standard. Accessed October 9, 2023. https://www.osha.gov/laws-regs/regulations/standardnumber/1910/1910.1030

Occupational Safety and Health Administration. *CPL 2-2.69: Enforcement Procedures for the Occupational Exposure to Bloodborne Pathogens*. Occupational Safety and Health Administration; November 27, 2001.

Occupational Safety and Health Administration. OSHA's bloodborne pathogens standard: OSHA fact sheet. Published January 2011. Accessed October 9, 2023. https://www.osha.gov/sites/default/files/publications/bbfact01.pdf

Peltan ID, Mitchell KH, Rudd KE, et al. Prehospital care and emergency department door-to-antibiotic time in sepsis. *Ann Am Thorac Soc*. 2018;15(12):1443-1450.

Polito CC, Bloom I, Dunn C, et al. Implementation of an EMS protocol to improve prehospital sepsis recognition. *Am J Emerg Med*. 2022;57:34-38.

Powers J, Badri T. *Pediculosis corporis*. *StatPearls*. Updated June 12, 2023. Accessed October 9, 2023. https://www.ncbi.nlm.nih.gov/books/NBK482148

Romero MG, Anjum F. Hemorrhagic fever renal syndrome. *StatPearls*. Updated July 19, 2022. Accessed October 9, 2023. https://www.ncbi.nlm.nih.gov/books/NBK560660

Roome AJ, Hadler JL, Thomas AL, et al. Hepatitis C virus infection among firefighters, emergency medical technicians, and paramedics—selected locations, United States, 1991–2000. *MMWR*. 2000;49(29):660-665.

Ryan White CARE Act, S. 1793, part G, §2695, notification of possible exposure to infectious diseases, September 30, 2009—reauthorization.

Sanders MJ. *Mosby's Paramedic Textbook*. 3rd ed. rev. Mosby; 2007.

Schille S, Vellozzi C, Reingold A, et al. Prevention of hepatitis B virus infection in the United States: recommendations of the Advisory Committee on Immunization Practices. *MMWR Recomm Rep*. 2018;67(1):1-31.

Shankar SK, Mahadevan A, Dias Sapico S, et al. Rabies viral encephalitis with proable [sic] 25-year incubation period! *Ann Indian Acad Neurol*. 2012;15(3):221-223. Accessed October 9, 2023. http://www.ncbi.nlm.nih.gov/pmc/articles/PMC3424805

Siddiqui AH, Koirala J. Methicillin-resistant *Staphylococcus aureus*. *StatPearls*. Updated April 2, 2023. Accessed October 9, 2023. https://www.ncbi.nlm.nih.gov/books/NBK482221

Siegel JD, Rhinehart E, Jackson M, et al. 2007 guideline for isolation precautions: preventing transmission of infectious agents in healthcare settings. https://www.cdc.gov/infection control/pdf/guidelines/isolation-guidelines-H.pdf

Snowden J, Simonsen KA. Rocky mountain spotted fever (*Rickettsia rickettsii*). *StatPearls*. Updated July 17, 2023. Accessed October 9, 2023. https://www.ncbi.nlm.nih.gov/books/NBK430881

Staub LJ, Mazzali, Biscaro RR, Kaszubowski E, Maurici R. Lung ultrasound for the emergency diagnosis of pneumonia, acute heart failure, and exacerbations of chronic obstructive pulmonary disease/asthma in adults: a systematic review and meta-analysis. *J Emerg Med*. 2019;56(1):53-69.

Tiwari T, Murphy TV, Moran J, et al. Recommended antimicrobial agents for treatment and postexposure prophylaxis of pertussis. *MMWR Recomm Rep*. 2005;54(RR-14):1-16.

U.S. Department of Transportation, National Highway Traffic Safety Administration. *EMT-Paramedic National Standard Curriculum*. U.S. Department of Transportation; 1998.

U.S. Department of Transportation, National Highway Traffic Safety Administration. *National EMS Education Standards, Draft 3.0*. U.S. Department of Transportation; 2008, The Department.

U.S. Food and Drug Administration. FDA approves expanded use of Gardasil 9 to include individuals 27 through 45 years old. Published October 5, 2018. Accessed October 9, 2023. https://www.fda.gov/NewsEvents/Newsroom/PressAnnouncements/UCM622715.htm?utm_campaign=10052018

Walchok JG, Pirrallo RG, Furmanek D, et al. Paramedic-initiated CMS sepsis core measure bundle prior to hospital arrival: a stepwise approach. *Prehosp Emerg Care*. 2017;21(3):291-300.

West KH. *Infectious Disease Handbook for Emergency Care Personnel*. 3rd ed. ACGIH; 2001.

Wooten J, Benedyk K, Patel M, et al. EMS incorporation in mass-vaccination: a feasibility study. *Am J Emerg Med*. 2021;49:424-425.

Workowski KA, Berman SM. Sexually transmitted diseases treatment guidelines, 2006. Published 2006. Accessed October 9, 2023. https://www.cdc.gov/mmwr/preview/mmwrhtml/rr5511a1.htm

World Health Organization. Global burden of dog-transmitted human rabies. Accessed October 9, 2023. https://www.who.int/teams/control-of-neglected-tropical-diseases/rabies/epidemiology-and-burden

World Health Organization. *Global Incidence and Prevalence of Selected Curable Sexually Transmitted Infections, 2008*. World Health Organization; 2012.

World Health Organization. Global tuberculosis report 2022. Published 2022. Accessed October 9, 2023. https://www.who.int/publications/i/item/9789240061729

World Health Organization. Hepatitis C. Reviewed July 18, 2023. Accessed October 9, 2023. https://www.who.int/news-room/fact-sheets/detail/hepatitis-c

World Health Organization. Immunization coverage. Reviewed July 18, 2023. Accessed October 9, 2023. https://www.who.int/en/news-room/fact-sheets/detail/immunization-coverage

World Health Organization. Measles: fact sheet No. 286. Reviewed August 9, 2023. Accessed October 9, 2023. https://www.who.int/en/news-room/fact-sheets/detail/measles

World Health Organization. Obesity. Reviewed June 9, 2021. Accessed October 9, 2023. https://www.who.int/news-room/facts-in-pictures/detail/6-facts-on-obesity

World Health Organization. Pneumonia. Accessed October 9, 2023. https://www.who.int/teams/immunization-vaccines-and-biologicals/diseases/pneumonia

World Health Organization. Rabies. Updated September 20, 2023. Accessed October 9, 2023. https://www.who.int/en/news-room/fact-sheets/detail/rabies

World Health Organization. Scabies. Updated May 31, 2023. Accessed October 9, 2023. https://www.who.int/news-room/fact-sheets/detail/scabies

World Health Organization. Tetanus. Updated August 24, 2023. Accessed October 9, 2023. https://www.who.int/news-room/fact-sheets/detail/tetanus

World Health Organization. Tuberculosis. Reviewed April 21, 2023. Accessed October 9, 2023. https://www.who.int/en/news-room/fact-sheets/detail/tuberculosis

World Health Organization. West Nile virus. Reviewed October 3, 2017. Accessed October 9, 2023. https://www.who.int/news-room/fact-sheets/detail/west-nile-virus

CHAPTER 8

Neurologic Disorders

Chapter Editors
Cecilio Padrón, MD
Christian Martin-Gill, MD, MPH
Benjamin Smith, MD

Assessing and treating patients with neurologic disorders (acute or chronic) can be some of the most challenging cases you will encounter. This is particularly true of the patient with an altered mental status. Altered mental status is a common symptom of many neurologic disorders. The many causes of altered mental status and the frequent inability of patients to communicate effectively can present unique difficulties. This chapter will assist you by providing tools to complete a basic neurologic exam and formulate a differential diagnosis using the AMLS Assessment Pathway.

LEARNING OBJECTIVES

At the conclusion of this chapter, you will be able to:

- Recognize the signs and symptoms of altered mental status and abnormal neurologic function.
- Gather pertinent historical data related to neurologic complaints.
- Perform a basic neurologic exam.
- Recognize and treat immediate life threats.
- Recognize life-threatening, emergent, and nonemergent patient presentations and be able to anticipate when a stable patient has the potential to become unstable.
- Provide physical and emotional supportive care on the scene and en route.
- Apply the neurologic exam findings to help formulate a diagnosis using the AMLS Assessment Pathway.
- Consider the appropriate differential diagnosis.
- Explain the importance of performing a blood glucose test on patients with an altered mental status to rule out the possibility of hypoglycemia.
- Consider special transport and destination alternatives based on clinical findings and diagnosis.

SCENARIO

As you arrive on scene to a private residence, a woman approaches you outside and states that her mother "isn't acting right." The daughter came to check on her when she did not come to church this morning. She goes on to tell you that her mother is normally "sharp as a tack" and is able to care for herself. Upon entering the home, you find a disheveled 72-year-old female wearing a nightgown and heels stumbling around the home. She does not seem to notice you have entered. Her daughter gives you a short list of medications and says she is "pretty healthy for her age" and that she has never seen her act this way. When you attempt to get the woman's attention, she looks at you with eyebrows crinkled in annoyance. You recognize that this patient encounter will be challenging.

- What specific assessments should you perform on this patient?
- What conditions are in your differential diagnosis?

This chapter builds on your current knowledge foundation for patients with altered mental status to develop the clinical judgment necessary to form a differential diagnosis, treat immediate life threats, monitor a patient's status, and intervene with appropriate treatment. Any decrease in a person's alertness, difficulty with cognition, or behavior that departs from what is normal for that person constitutes **altered mental status**. Behavior that is normal for one person might not be typical of another, so altered mental status manifests differently from one individual to the next. The signs of altered mental status range from mild confusion to significant cognitive deficit.

Altered mental status is a common sign of morbidity in the prehospital setting, and early recognition and treatment of its underlying cause can be lifesaving. The condition is often associated with comorbid conditions such as trauma and infection. Identification of the underlying condition(s) is necessary to determine the appropriate course of treatment.

Patients with neurologic issues are vulnerable and at risk for decompensation. Many of the reflexes that protect an awake person can temporarily become inactive when the nervous system is depressed by any cause: The eyelids may not blink away dust and irritants, or the larynx may not cause gagging and coughing in reaction to secretions draining down into the airway, which can place the patient at risk for injury.

Providing appropriate emergency care and formulating a differential diagnosis for any patient depends on having a fundamental understanding of anatomy and pathophysiology and performing a methodical, detail-oriented assessment. To carry out an adequate neurologic assessment of the patient with altered mental status, you cannot rely on vital signs alone. Close observation of the patient's symptoms and behavior, a skillful physical examination, and additional diagnostic tests, such as blood glucose, can help give you a clearer picture of the cause of a patient's distress.

Anatomy and Physiology

The brain represents only 2% of body weight, yet it defines who we are. Billions of neurons allow us to interact with the world around us, regulate our thoughts and behavior, determine our intelligence and temperament, make it possible for us to perceive pleasure and pain, mold our personalities, and store a lifetime of memories. The brain is not fully developed until after 20 years of life, and new evidence suggests an adult brain can create new neurons in a process called *neurogenesis*. Thanks to advances made in neurologic research—including revolutionary functional and structural imaging modalities—we now know more about the brain than at any other time in human history.

Protective Anatomic Structures

The central nervous system (CNS), which consists of the brain and spinal cord, accounts for 98% of all neural tissues of the body. The brain itself is composed of nervous tissue (called white matter or gray matter, depending on its location and function) and occupies about 80% of the cranial vault, or skull. The average adult brain weighs about 1.5 kg (approximately 3 lb) and is cushioned inside the skull by **cerebrospinal fluid (CSF)**. CSF is a transparent, clear fluid that acts as a shock absorber and energy source for the brain. It is made up primarily of water but also contains proteins, salts, and glucose. The flow of CSF within the skull is shown in **Figure 8-1**.

Additional protection for the brain and spinal cord is provided by the three membrane layers called *meninges* (**Figure 8-2**). Each layer of the meninges is called a *meninx*, from a Greek word meaning "membrane." The innermost meninx, which attaches directly to the brain's surface, is a delicate membrane called the *pia mater* (meaning "tender mother" or "soft mother"). The pia mater is highly vascular, containing the blood vessels supplying the surfaces of the brain and spinal cord. The middle layer of the meninges is a tangle of collagen and elastin fibers that takes its name from its appearance. The meshlike vascular network of this meninx resembles a cobweb, so it is known as the *arachnoid* (meaning "spiderlike") *membrane*. CSF circulates in the space between the arachnoid and the pia mater

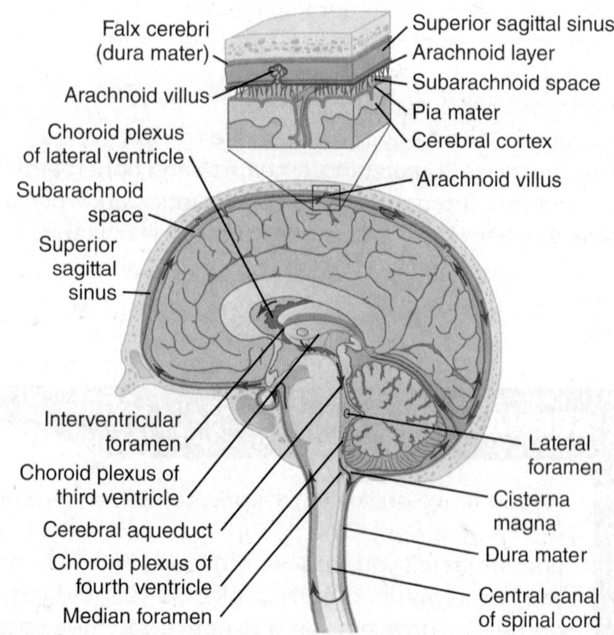

Figure 8-1 Flow of cerebrospinal fluid. Red arrows indicate cerebrospinal fluid and blue arrows show blood in the dural venous sinuses.

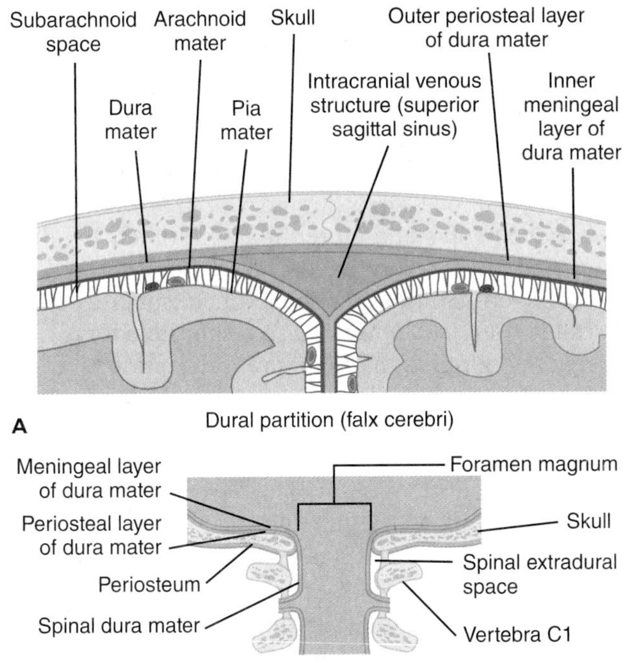

Figure 8-2 The dura mater, arachnoid mater, and pia mater are the three layers of the meninges. **A.** Superior coronal view. **B.** Continuity with the spinal meninges.

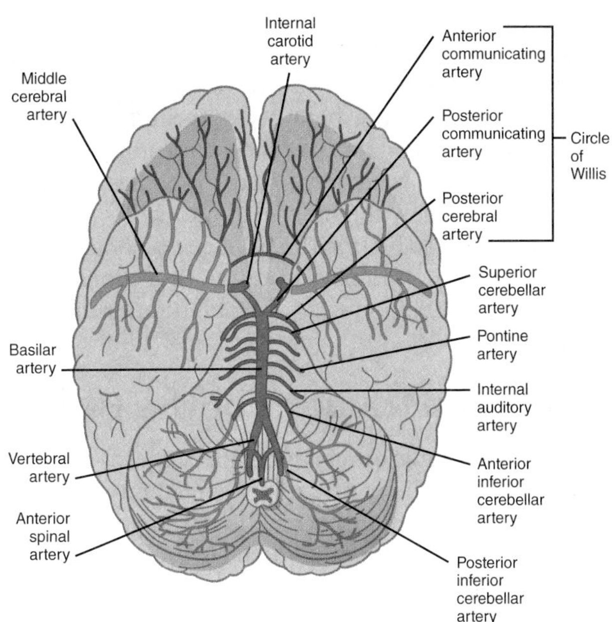

Figure 8-3 Cerebral circulation and the circle of Willis at the base of the brain.

(the subarachnoid space), protecting the brain against mechanical injury and providing an immunologic shield. The outermost meninx, which lines the cranial vault, contains arteries that supply the bones of the skull. It is called, appropriately, the *dura mater*—"tough mother." Composed of two fibrous layers, the dura mater is the most impregnable layer of the meninges. The epidural space is between the dura mater and the skull, and the subdural space is between the dura and the subarachnoid membrane.

Blood Supply

Maintaining the critical functions of the brain requires that adequate perfusion is maintained. The brain requires a constant supply of oxygen and glucose to function properly and does not have any storage capability.

Four major arteries supply blood to the brain: two internal carotid arteries anteriorly and two vertebral arteries posteriorly. The vertebral arteries merge to become the basilar artery just inside the base of the skull, which provides branches to the brainstem and cerebellum. The basilar artery divides and joins branches of the internal carotid arteries to form the circle of Willis on the undersurface of the brain, as shown in **Figure 8-3**.

Cerebral blood flow (CBF) is dependent on adequate **cerebral perfusion pressure (CPP)**, defined as systemic **mean arterial pressure (MAP)** minus **intracranial pressure (ICP)**, but normally is maintained and regulated independently of systemic blood pressure both globally and regionally based on metabolic demands by constriction or dilation of cerebral vessels. This regulation of CBF can be maintained with systemic MAPs between 60 and 160 mm Hg. However, this autoregulatory function is often compromised in the setting of traumatic brain injury or other acute intracranial events. When this occurs, CBF becomes more dependent on the direct relationship between systemic blood pressure and ICP. This explains the phenomenon of **Cushing triad** during head trauma or intracranial hemorrhages in which systolic blood pressure begins to increase as ICP increases to maintain the same CPP.

CBF is also affected by the serum level of carbon dioxide (CO_2). Hypocapnia (hypocarbia) (such as with hyperventilation) causes cerebral vasoconstriction but also decreased ICP due to a decrease in total intracranial blood. The net effect on cerebral perfusion is thus variable, but in general, hypocapnia leads to decreased CBF and should be avoided. Alternatively, hypercapnia causes vasodilation, leading to increased CBF and increase in total intracranial blood, and potentially increased ICP. The net effect is difficult to predict and must be determined based on clinical exam findings. In hospital, ICP can be measured directly, but CBF is more difficult to quantitate. Thus, close monitoring of end-tidal carbon dioxide ($ETCO_2$) during any positive-pressure ventilation by EMS clinicians is important to avoid an unwanted impact on cerebral perfusion. Understanding cerebral vasoactivity, which is the constriction or dilation of blood vessels, is important in managing patients with altered mental status, suspected traumatic brain injury, or stroke.

The capillaries that nourish the brain have a special lining with tight junctions between cells forming a protective barrier, known as the **blood–brain barrier**, between blood and the brain's extracellular fluid. This barrier prevents certain particles (including bacteria, some proteins and toxins, but also antibodies and many antibiotics) from flowing into the brain while still allowing and actively facilitating the passage of oxygen, water, and glucose. Head trauma and certain infections and illnesses disrupt the blood–brain barrier, often causing secondary brain injury.

Functional Regions of the Brain

The brain is a complex organ with many components and functional areas. The brain can be divided into four main regions: the cerebrum, the cerebellum, the diencephalon, and the brainstem. **Figure 8-4** depicts the cerebrum and the other major structures of the brain.

Cerebrum

The cerebrum is composed of the cortex (divided into lobes) and subcortex. The cortex, also called the *neural cortex* or *gray matter*, is the outermost layer of the cerebrum and is the highest-functioning part of the brain, comprising more than two-thirds of its mass. Because of its many convolutions, grooves, and ridges, the surface area of the cerebral cortex is actually 30 times larger than the space it occupies. Each ridge, or gyrus, and groove, or fissure, is associated with a specific cognitive function.

The structure and function of the brain hemispheres and lobes are as follows:

- *Right and left hemispheres*. The cerebrum is divided into left and right hemispheres. Structurally and functionally, they control opposite sides of the body. The hemispheres are interconnected by constantly communicating nerve fibers (in the corpus callosum) that transmit as many as 4 billion impulses per second.
- The brain's structure is not identical from one individual to the next. In more than 90% of right-handed people and more than 70% of left-handed people, the interpretive speech center is located in the left hemisphere. The left hemisphere, often called the *logical brain*, is also responsible for reading, writing, mathematical calculation, and sequential and analytic tasks. The right hemisphere, known as the *creative brain*, interprets sensory information and processes spatial awareness. Interestingly, many musicians, dancers, and artists are left-handed, and the right hemisphere of the cerebral cortex in such people appears to be more active than the left.
- *Lobes*. The cerebrum is further subdivided into lobes, each of which is named for the cranial bone that lies above it. For example, the frontal lobe lies beneath the frontal bone. The other lobes are the parietal, temporal, and occipital. Each lobe and its corresponding region of the cerebral cortex have a specific function. The frontal lobe controls motor function, determines personality, and elaborates thought and speech; the parietal lobe interprets bodily sensations; the temporal lobe stores long-term memory and interprets sound; and the occipital lobe is responsible for sight.

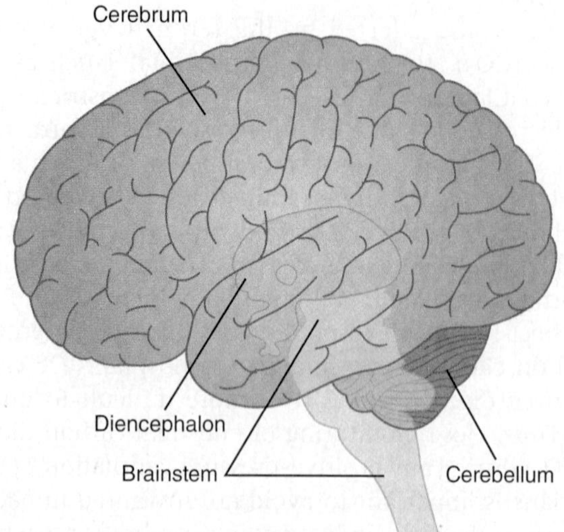

Figure 8-4 The four primary areas of the brain are the brainstem, diencephalon, cerebrum, and cerebellum.

Cerebellum

The second largest part of the brain, the cerebellum, lies above the brainstem and posterior to the cerebrum (see Figure 8-4). The cerebellum coordinates movements, balance, and posture.

Diencephalon

Near the center of the brain is the diencephalon (see Figure 8-4). The diencephalon includes the thalamus and the hypothalamus. The thalamus, composed of gray matter, connects sensory input between the spinal cord and the cerebral cortex and houses much of the reticular activating system, which is responsible for arousal (sleep–wake transitions). The tiny hypothalamus, not much bigger than a cherry pit, is responsible for maintaining homeostasis in the body. It links the sympathetic and parasympathetic nervous systems by way of the pituitary gland. The hormones of the hypothalamus stimulate or inhibit the release of hormones from the pituitary gland to regulate circadian rhythm (the body's innate sleep cycle), thirst and hunger, and other functions.

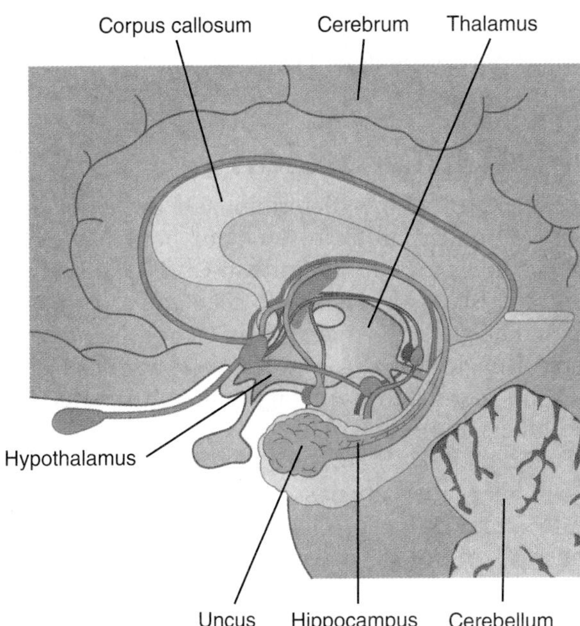

Figure 8-5 The limbic system.

Surrounding the thalamus are the structures of the primitive brain, known collectively as the *limbic system* (**Figure 8-5**). The limbic system is composed of two structures: the amygdala and the hippocampus. The system is connected to the prefrontal cortex of the frontal lobe.

The limbic system is referred to as the *primitive brain* because it controls basic survival instincts and many of the behavioral responses that constitute key features of our personalities, such as whether we have a positive or negative outlook. The system is responsible for intense feelings—fear, frustration, anxiety, tension, anger, rage, sexual desire, appetite, the desire or ability to bond, and the storage of our emotional memories. The limbic system allows us to interpret events as they are happening and helps us predict the consequences of actions or events.

Brainstem

Connecting the spinal cord to the brain is the brainstem, which includes the medulla, midbrain, and pons (see Figure 8-4). The medulla controls basic physiologic functions such as breathing and heart rate. The midbrain is involved in regulation of vision, hearing, and body movement. The pons (meaning "bridge") connects the cerebellum to the medulla and is involved in posture and movement, as well as sleep.

Ventricles

The ventricles (meaning "little bellies") are cavity-like spaces filled with circulating CSF, which is constantly produced by the capillary network within the ventricles.

AMLS Assessment Pathway ▸▸▸▸

▾ Initial Observations

Scene Safety Considerations

In situations where patients are acting aggressive, confused, or violent, make sure the scene is safe, and if necessary, that the scene has been secured by law enforcement personnel before you approach. As you approach, observe the patient from a distance and note any physical movements and verbal comments. If the patient is becoming agitated or aggressive, take this behavior into account as part of your scene safety evaluation and immediately call for appropriate backup or assistance.

Patient Cardinal Presentation/ Chief Complaint

A brief overview of some of the most common cardinal presentations or chief complaints in patients with neurologic dysfunction follows. Many disease processes have similar presentations, or one finding may mask another. For example, hypoglycemia may lead to delirium, hypoglycemia may cause a seizure, and a seizure may mask a stroke. In addition, although a patient's neurologic symptoms may seem pressing, sometimes they indicate other serious medical conditions that should be considered in the differential diagnosis. Syncope (fainting), for example, may be due to a pulmonary embolism or a dysrhythmia.

Primary Survey

The primary survey includes an evaluation of the patient's airway, breathing, and circulation, as well as interventions for immediate life threats. Blood glucose levels should be checked in *every patient* with any change in mental status or behavior, even if another cause seems obvious.

Level of Consciousness

A rapid assessment of consciousness can be achieved using the AVPU mnemonic as described in Chapter 1 and also by evaluating whether a person can follow commands (verbal component of GCS). If the patient has a decreased level of consciousness, the airway may also be compromised. In most cases, a patient who is able to speak has a patent airway, but any neurologic condition that impairs mental status may quickly progress to the patient being unable to maintain a functional airway.

Airway and Breathing

Evaluation of the patient's respiratory rate, depth, and pattern may also indicate the underlying cause of altered mental status. Acidosis, stroke, metabolic disease, and other pathologic conditions cause changes in breathing patterns. Hypoventilation may indicate CNS depression, which might be attributable to drug overdose, stroke, or intracranial swelling. If possible, obtain a baseline oxygen saturation (SpO_2) measurement (with the patient breathing ambient air) before you provide oxygen or ventilatory support, but in cases of severe respiratory distress, do not delay treatment just to obtain a baseline reading. Provide oxygen and ventilatory support to maintain an oxygen saturation of at least 95%. Monitor the patient's response to oxygenation and ventilation. Adequacy of ventilation (minute ventilation) is best assessed by measuring the partial pressure of carbon dioxide ($PaCO_2$) in blood. In the field and in other emergency settings, you can approximate $PaCO_2$ by measuring the $ETCO_2$ in patients with an advanced airway in place. In intubated patients in particular, there is a strong tendency for clinicians to hyperventilate the patient, which directly correlates with increased brain injury from decreased cerebral perfusion due to cerebral vasoconstriction.

Circulation/Perfusion

In this component of the primary survey, you first want to ensure the patient has a palpable pulse. As blood pressure drops, pulses are usually lost first in the distal extremities (radial and pedal); then more proximally (brachial); and, last, the central pulses of the carotid and femoral. One can assess the strength of the pulse and also check for other signs of adequate perfusion, including capillary refill, skin color, and temperature. Mental status is usually a good indicator of adequate perfusion, but as outlined in this chapter, there are many other causes of altered mental status besides inadequate perfusion.

Assessment of pulse rate and rhythm can also help you pinpoint the cause of an altered mental status. Primary dysrhythmias such as atrial fibrillation with rapid ventricular response, tachydysrhythmias, and bradydysrhythmias can directly cause hypoperfusion. Tachycardia (rapid pulse rate) could be a sign of infection, temperature elevation, postictal (postseizure) state, drug withdrawal or toxicity, or hypovolemia (low blood volume). Bradycardia may suggest cerebral herniation, hypothermia, or drug toxicity. An irregular pulse should lead you to consider cardiac dysrhythmia, which may be triggered by acute coronary syndrome, electrolyte disturbance, acidosis, hypoxia, or ingestion of a toxic substance.

Blood pressure is relied on heavily in determining the cause of an altered mental status, and this should be obtained as part of your examination, but it is important to not use this parameter alone to confirm adequate perfusion. You must rely on all the manifestations of perfusion as previously described.

▼ First Impression

When you are trying to determine whether your patient has a neurologic problem, look for both obvious and subtle changes that can indicate disease. Take in the surroundings. Being alert will help keep you safe and could suggest a diagnosis. Is there any evidence the patient is a victim of neglect or abuse? Send your partner to investigate (ask permission of a family member if necessary) the cabinets and refrigerator to see whether there seems to be enough food. If not, or if the food on hand appears to be spoiled, the patient's condition could be attributable to malnutrition or electrolyte abnormalities. Look for insulin or oral hypoglycemic medications. Are there empty or nearly empty pill bottles lying scattered about? Are the prescription labels out of date? If so, an accidental or intentional overdose might be responsible for the patient's altered mental status. Who is the patient's caregiver if the patient does not live independently or is a minor? Be alert to objects in the patient's environment (e.g., oxygen canisters or drug paraphernalia). This situational awareness and these observations can significantly improve your ability to identify your patient's medical condition and contributing issues. After you have stabilized the patient and treated any life threats, form a general impression of the patient's status and develop a list of possible differential diagnoses.

Life-Threatening Presentations

Hypoventilation (CO_2 Narcosis)

A patient requires ventilatory assistance if respiratory effort is compromised, which may be due to a stroke, accidental or intentional medication overdose, trauma, or a medical event. When ventilation is impaired, $PaCO_2$ climbs to dangerous levels, causing confusion, drowsiness, tremors, and seizures. This condition is known as *CO_2 narcosis*, and it will lead to death if ventilatory assistance is not provided. It is often overlooked during the initial evaluation. Although elevated $ETCO_2$ values can be measured with capnography, ventilatory assistance with a bag-valve mask (BVM) should not be delayed while attempting to measure $ETCO_2$ in a patient who is clinically hypoventilating.

Hypoxia

Severe hypoxia may lead to confusion and a decrease in mental status, so the measurement of SpO_2 is an essential component of the assessment of every patient with altered mental status. Supplemental oxygen will be required if the SpO_2 is $< 94\%$, and assisted ventilation must be provided if the patient is hypoventilating, which may be the cause of the hypoxia.

Clinicians should be aware of several situations in which SpO_2 is not accurate. Perhaps the most common of these is related to carbon monoxide poisoning, in which case pulse oximetry readings show hemoglobin bound to carbon monoxide as being oxygenated. When carbon monoxide is suspected, the patient should receive high-flow oxygen by the device that will give the highest concentration. Methemoglobinemia, which is caused by certain drugs such as benzocaine, also leads to a slightly higher than actual reading, with a characteristic reading of 85% despite supplemental oxygen therapy in severe cases. Finally, cyanide may block oxygen utilization at the cellular level despite fully oxygen-saturated blood.

Hypoperfusion with Cerebral Ischemia

Many acute medical conditions, major trauma, and certain kinds of medications can cause hypoperfusion that leads to global cerebral hypoperfusion and altered mental status. The cause of the shock should be quickly discerned, and targeted treatment implemented when possible. Chapter 5, *Shock*, offers an in-depth discussion of what to do in cases of shock.

Intracranial Hypertension

Elevated ICP can compromise perfusion to the brain as it decreases the CPP, especially with acute elevations. ICP elevation may be due to mass effect, such as from acute hemorrhage, edema, or malfunction of a ventriculoperitoneal shunt. If the pressure becomes too high, the brain may herniate into the lower skull or through the foramen magnum. This condition is often characterized by a unilateral dilated pupil and unconsciousness and has a high mortality.

Treating intracranial hypertension with hyperventilation must be managed more cautiously and judiciously than was recommended in the past. Hyperventilation decreases the amount of CO_2 dissolved in the blood, which induces cerebral vasoconstriction, decreasing the blood volume in the brain, and thus reducing ICP. However, vasoconstriction also decreases blood flow. The net effect on perfusion is difficult if not impossible to predict, so the patient's neurologic status must be monitored closely. In deciding whether it is appropriate to perform hyperventilation, follow local protocol in life-threatening clinical scenarios.

Hypoglycemia

A patient with hypoglycemia often presents with confusion and abnormal behavior but may also seem depressed or sluggish. The patient may have focal weakness, seizure, or be completely unresponsive. Skin findings include pallor and diaphoresis. In patients with dark skin tones, pallor may be difficult to detect; assess the patient's mucous membranes, nail beds, and palmar surface for indications of pallor. If the patient is awake enough to swallow without risk of aspiration, oral glucose in some form may be given. When the patient has a decreased level of consciousness, dextrose should be administered intravenously (IV) according to local protocol. Many EMS agencies use lower concentrations of dextrose (e.g., 10%) instead of the more viscous 50% concentration. The lower concentrations are equally effective in reversing hypoglycemia just as quickly, but they do not have the issues of tissue necrosis if the IV infiltrates or of giving too high a concentration to pediatric patients. When IV access is not available, glucagon by intramuscular (IM) injection should be considered.

Detailed Assessment

Before you perform the secondary survey and the detailed physical exam, you should try to get an idea of how distressed the patient is, considering your general assessment findings as well as vital signs, the results of the serum glucose test, and pulse oximetry readings. Decide whether the patient must be immediately transported to the hospital or if you can take more time for evaluation on scene. Remain alert for traumatic injuries and for any information that could prove diagnostically useful, such as unusual sights, sounds, and odors. Note the patient's positioning and any clues in visual appearance that may suggest causes of distress.

History Taking

Patients with altered mental status may not be able to give a clear history or understand the EMS clinician. It is helpful to have other family members around, if possible, to collect additional information at the scene. If the patient can give some history, it should be obtained as soon as possible before further deterioration in the patient's mental status. If you are working with a partner, the history and physical exam can often be conducted simultaneously.

When you treat a patient with altered mental status, gather information from witnesses or bystanders that might help describe the patient's baseline mental status and how it has changed recently. Ask about the degree of change, and inquire when the patient was last seen or known to be acting normal. Collect any other potential clues to the cause of the mental status change, such as information about the patient's medication regimen, blood pressure, and any recent trauma that might have been sustained. Ask about and observe for signs of abnormal body movements, smells, speech, or automatisms. Witnesses may also be able to provide history that can point toward the underlying cause of the patient's altered mental status.

OPQRST and SAMPLER

The OPQRST and SAMPLER mnemonics should be used to obtain the patient's complete history using a systematic approach. Talk to the patient directly when the neurologic status allows. Ask the patient about what is wrong and allow the patient to describe concerns in an open-ended fashion. Patients, family, and bystanders may give you valuable historical clues that will help generate your differential diagnosis. While all aspects of the SAMPLER history may provide helpful information, the L ("Last known well" time) is of critical importance for patients suspected of experiencing stroke who may be candidates for fibrinolytic therapy or thrombectomy. Likewise, the time of last oral intake can be important in evaluating patients who may have hypoglycemia.

Secondary Survey

The secondary survey is meant to be a more comprehensive physical exam than performed in the primary survey. The findings will help to generate a more complete set of differential diagnoses.

During the physical examination, identify any injuries or other abnormalities in the patient's physical condition, and complete as much of a neurologic exam as possible. During your initial contact with the patient, you will have completed your evaluation of the patient's level of consciousness, ability to speak, and general orientation. The easiest and most widely used means of evaluation is the AVPU mnemonic, which classifies the patient's level of consciousness as alert, responsive to verbal stimuli, responsive to pain, or unresponsive. Other neurologic functions should be tested, including the presence or absence of cranial nerve functions (pupil reaction, extraocular eye movements, facial droop, etc.), motor function in the upper and lower extremities, and sensation and strength in those extremities. Document incontinence if present and, if the patient can walk, whether the gait is normal.

Diagnostics

The diagnostic tools in an ambulance or helicopter are limited, but the tools you do have, along with careful observation, often allow you to detect critical and treatable conditions. The Glasgow Coma Scale is a tool used to evaluate level of consciousness and mental status (Table 8-1). Scores are obtained on the basis of three responses: eye opening, motor response, and verbal response. This tool is often used to assess for brain injury in patients with head trauma. It is only validated as a means of standardized communication of the conscious state in trauma patients, but it has also reached widespread use in medical patients.

As noted earlier, take and record vital signs, including temperature when possible, blood glucose level, and SpO_2 measurements when applicable, and administer appropriate treatment. Perform cardiac monitoring and, if indicated, a 12-lead electrocardiogram (ECG). Some blood analyses may be carried out using a portable device. In addition, some services may be equipped with portable ultrasound.

Table 8-1 Glasgow Coma Scale

Eye Opening	Score	Best Verbal Response	Score	Best Motor Response	Score
Spontaneous	4	Oriented and converses	5	Follows commands	6
To verbal command	3	Disoriented conversation	4	Localizes pain	5
To pain	2	Speaking but nonsensical	3	Withdraws to pain	4
No response	1	Moans or makes unintelligible sounds	2	Decorticate flexion	3
		No response	1	Decerebrate extension	2
				No response	1

Scores:
15: Normal GCS
13–14: Mild dysfunction
9–12: Moderate to severe dysfunction
8 or less: Severe dysfunction (The lowest possible score is 3.)

Refine the Differential Diagnosis

The components of the primary and secondary surveys will help you refine your differential diagnosis and determine the severity of the patient's condition. Manage any life threats as they appear during the assessment process. Remember that most diseases or conditions, including neurologic disorders, are caused by more than one factor. The specific conditions described later will provide an approach for helping you determine the differential diagnosis and recognize key findings.

The mnemonic SNOT (**Rapid Recall Box 8-1**) may assist you in refining a differential diagnosis in patients with altered mental status, on the basis of history, physical exam, and laboratory findings. A mnemonic used in the hospital setting, where more diagnostic testing is available, is AEIOU-TIPS (**Rapid Recall Box 8-2**).

RAPID RECALL BOX 8-1

Initial Assessment of Altered Mental Status: SNOT

Remember this mnemonic when performing initial assessment in the prehospital setting:

S Sugar, stroke, seizure
N Narcosis (CO_2, opiates)
O Oxygen
T Trauma, toxins, temperature

Be aware that this list is not a comprehensive survey of all possible causes of altered mental status.

RAPID RECALL BOX 8-2

Causes of Decreased Level of Consciousness Altered Mental Status: AEIOU-TIPS

A Alcohol, anaphylaxis, acute myocardial infarction
E Epilepsy, endocrine abnormality, electrolyte imbalance
I Insulin (glucose)
O Opiates
U Uremia
T Trauma
I Intracranial (tumor, hemorrhage, or hypertension), infection
P Poisoning
S Seizure, stroke, syncope

Altered Mental Status

Patients with altered mental status may show signs of confusion or exhibit changes in their typical behavior. In a patient with altered mental status, it is often difficult to sort out cause and effect. A patient who has a seizure will likely be altered after the seizure, but an underlying illness leading to a seizure such as hypoglycemia or alcohol withdrawal can also cause an altered mental status. Such behavioral alterations should be confirmed by a family member or someone else who knows the patient well. They may also be able to provide history that can point toward the underlying cause of the patient's altered mental status. A patient who has a significantly depressed mental status or is comatose and cannot give a history requires immediate resuscitation. A mental decline of this sort can be ominous and attributable to hemorrhagic stroke, overdose, and other grave conditions.

Delirium

Delirium is an acute alteration in mental status characterized by waxing and waning impairment of awareness, orientation, and cognition and sometimes is associated with hallucinations or delusions. It is most often associated with an acute illness in older adults. These alterations can cause decrements in alertness, orientation, emotional or behavioral response, perception, language expression, judgment, and activity. The EMS clinician must understand that patients with delirium are not capable of reasoning, and it is fruitless to expect the patient to understand or for the clinician to become angry with a delirious patient who is not cooperating. Common causes of delirium include infection, intoxication, trauma, the postictal state after a seizure, endocrine disorders, organ failure, stroke, shock, and tumors. Medications are also a common cause of delirium.

In a patient with delirium, short-term memory becomes clouded, and the person becomes disoriented to time or place. Level of awareness may fluctuate over brief periods, and speech may be incoherent, tense, or rambling. The patient usually has no discernible focal neurologic deficit. Nevertheless, infection, intoxication with alcohol or other drugs, dehydration, cardiac dysrhythmia, thyroid problems, and prescription medication issues (such as overdosing and underdosing) may cause alterations in vital signs and physical exam findings.

The patient who demonstrates any level of delirium must be fully assessed. Appearance, vital signs, hydration, and evidence of trauma or infection should all be taken into account. When you encounter an individual in an acute delirious state, remember that the patient is confused and is likely to have poor judgment. Your safety and that of the patient are the highest priorities. Patients with delirium and agitated or combative behavior should be treated with dignity. Physical restraint and pharmacologic management with sedation may be necessary to permit the required medical assessment and treatment of the patient in a safe manner.

Provide supplemental oxygen if oxygen saturation is < 94% or the patient appears to be in respiratory distress. If you suspect spinal cord trauma, take precautions to provide spinal motion restriction. Test the patient's serum glucose level. The patient will be evaluated in the emergency department (ED) with additional laboratory and radiologic studies.

Delirium is categorized as hypoactive, hyperactive, or mixed. Hypoactive delirium is the most common form of delirium, comprising more than three-fourths of cases, and is often missed because the presentation can be subtle. In contrast, patients with hyperactive delirium are more apparent and may exhibit agitation or combative or violent behaviors, especially in the setting of specific toxidromes. The Richmond Agitation Sedation Scale (RASS) is helpful in objectively measuring the degree of agitation that a patient has at baseline and serially following changes after treatment (Table 8-2). Oftentimes, law enforcement involvement is required when responding to these patients for the safety of both the clinicians and the patient. The term *excited delirium* is not broadly recognized as a diagnosis within various fields of medicine, so it should not be used. Instead, it is best to describe the patient as having delirium with agitated behavior or hyperactive delirium.

When law enforcement is required to restrain combative patients to allow proper assessment and care, the roles of law enforcement and EMS must be understood by both groups. When an individual has delirium and requires medical assessment and treatment, law enforcement's role is to provide safety for the patient and rescuers to facilitate patient assessment, treatment, and transport. The EMS clinicians must work cooperatively with other public safety entities, but EMS clinicians must ensure that restraint procedures allow for rapid patient assessment and appropriate treatment.

Efforts should be made to control the environment and verbally de-escalate patients to cooperate. The patient may be extremely distraught, hyperthermic, hyperstimulated, and uncontrollable. Attempts to physically restrain a patient with delirium and agitated behavior, although necessary, may worsen the patient's combativeness. Physical restraint can also result in the sudden cessation of struggling; this could be because the patient voluntarily stops, but it could also be that the restraint position compromises adequate respiration and the patient's condition rapidly deteriorates. Inadequate respiratory efforts and metabolic acidosis from the struggling can lead to respiratory arrest, cardiac arrest, and death. Cardiac dysrhythmias have been noted in patients who

Table 8-2 Richmond Agitation Sedation Scale

RASS Score	Term	Description
+4	Combative	Overtly combative, violent; immediate danger to staff
+3	Very agitated	Pulls on or removes tube(s) or catheter(s), or has aggressive behavior toward staff
+2	Agitated	Frequent nonpurposeful movement, fights ventilator
+1	Restless	Anxious or apprehensive but movements not aggressive
0	Alert and calm	Alert and calm, spontaneously pays attention to caregiver
−1	Drowsy	Not fully alert but has sustained awakening(> 10 seconds) with eye contact to voice
−2	Light sedation	Briefly (< 10 seconds) awakens with eye contact to voice
−3	Moderate sedation	Any movement (but no eye contact) to voice
−4	Deep sedation	No response to voice, but any movement to physical stimulation
−5	Unarousable	No response to voice or physical stimulation

Modified from Sessler CN, Gosnell MS, Grap MJ, et al. The Richmond Agitation-Sedation Scale: validity and reliability in adult intensive care unit patients. *Am J Respir Crit Care Med*. 2002;166(10):1338-1344. doi:10.1164/rccm.2107138 are restrained and bradyasystole is often the rhythm if cardiac arrest occurs. These patients may be hyperthermic and often have elevated circulating levels of adrenaline and a metabolic acidosis. All patients who exhibit signs of delirium with agitated behavior must be medically evaluated and should not be restrained in a prone position any longer than necessary to safely maintain control. Patients who are restrained by law enforcement in the prone position should be placed in a supine or sitting position as soon as feasible to maintain respiratory effort and effective tidal volume, which buffers the underlying acidosis. Avoid excessively tight straps around the thorax. Pharmacologic sedation using medications such as a benzodiazepine, a neuroleptic, or ketamine is often appropriate. Monitor the patient's cardiac rhythm, oxygen saturation, and $ETCO_2$ continuously, and frequently check vital signs and circulation in restrained extremities. If active struggling stops abruptly, or if the patient's mental status declines acutely, evaluate for respiratory and/or cardiac arrest. Aggressive airway management and cardiac support may prevent cardiac arrest. The safe management of a patient with delirium with agitated behavior requires coordination and communication between law enforcement and EMS personnel. This is a vulnerable period for patients and unrecognized hypoventilation or sudden cardiac arrest can occur rapidly.

Dementia

In contrast to delirium, dementia is a chronic and insidious process. All reversible causes should be ruled out before assuming that any neurologic or psychiatric symptom is due to underlying dementia. Patients with dementia exhibit a slow decline in memory and cognitive function over the course of months to years. *Dementia* is a broad term that defines a set of disorders that lead to gradual neurologic decline. The most common disorders in the United States are Alzheimer dementia, vascular dementia, frontotemporal dementia, and Lewy body dementia. Classically, dementia is grouped into three general categories: mild/early, moderate/middle, and severe/late-stage dementia. The various disorders affect different parts of the brain, and therefore, have different presentations during the earlier stages. However, as disease progresses and more brain tissue is affected, the symptoms begin to have significant overlap at the moderate to severe/late stage.

Alzheimer dementia is the most common form and is caused by the deposition of amyloid plaques and the development of neurofibrillary tangles in the cerebral cortex, typically affecting the parietal and temporal lobes. Early-stage patients are still able to function independently but will exhibit signs of short-term memory loss. Patients will typically have difficulty recalling the location of objects, recalling people's names, and remembering things they recently read. As the disease progresses, patients begin to present more classically with middle-stage symptoms, including forgetfulness of personal information, sleep pattern changes, tendencies to wander and get lost, and repetitive speech and behaviors. Middle- or moderate-stage dementia is the longest form and can last several years. Patients can typically perform most of their activities of daily living (ADLs) with assistance and will often live with relatives or in assisted living facilities. Late-stage Alzheimer disease is characterized by patients who are no longer able to respond to their environment and require continuous care. They have difficulty communicating thoughts such as pain and gradually lose their basic physical abilities, becoming much more susceptible to infections such as urinary tract infections (UTIs) and pneumonia.

The formal diagnosis of dementia is usually made after several rounds of outpatient testing. Quality care is demonstrated by documenting a baseline of a patient's abilities with caregivers at the scene, including orientation status, physical abilities such as walking independently versus with assistance, and capabilities of performing ADLs. Several tools, such as the Short Blessed Test and the Mini Mental State Exam have been validated for screening for dementia. The priority in evaluation of patients with dementia is in keeping a wide differential and evaluating for acute on chronic delirium, trauma, sepsis, acute coronary syndrome (ACS), stroke, and other acute conditions.

Syncope/Light-Headedness

Syncope, a transient loss of consciousness associated with loss of postural tone and rapid return to baseline, has many possible causes. A transient episode of near-syncope, or feeling like one is about to pass out but without loss of consciousness, has the same differential diagnosis as syncope because the pathophysiology is similar. It includes conditions such as cardiac dysrhythmia, hypovolemia/orthostasis (e.g., gastrointestinal bleeding, dehydration, ruptured ectopic pregnancy, ruptured aortic aneurysm), CNS event (e.g., subarachnoid hemorrhage), pulmonary embolism, aortic valve stenosis, hypertrophic cardiomyopathy, and vasovagal reflex (often due to situational or emotional triggers). Hospital-based evaluation may only determine the etiology of syncope in 50% of patients. Emphasis is on excluding life-threatening causes such as dysrhythmia, ischemia, hemorrhage, trauma, etc. Patients who have a syncopal episode can also have myoclonic jerking that may look like seizure activity, so it is important to obtain history regarding any prodromal symptoms, the duration of shaking, and the rapidity of the return to baseline to help differentiate between a seizure and a syncopal episode.

Dizziness/Vertigo

When patients complain of dizziness, it is essential to differentiate whether the patient is referring to a feeling of light-headedness (or near-syncope) versus vertigo. Vertigo is a patient's sensation of spinning or moving—the patient can feel like they are moving or they can feel like the environment/room is moving. Light-headedness or near-syncope is typically more concerning for a nonneurologic cause of the patient's symptoms such as a cardiac etiology, dehydration, or infection.

Patients who report alterations in **proprioception** (awareness of the spatial orientation of one's own body) and balance are usually able to give a history of such experiences. You may not be able to assess intermittent alterations such as those secondary to transient ischemic attack (TIA). Many patients, however, including those with cerebellar/posterior strokes, positional vertigo, overdose, vertebral artery dissection, and electrolyte abnormalities, may still be symptomatic as you complete your assessment.

Vertigo is a symptom. It originates in the CNS or in the vestibular organs of the peripheral nervous system. Central vertigo may be caused by hemorrhagic or ischemic insult (stroke), concussion, tumors, infection, migraine headache, multiple sclerosis, toxic ingestion or inhalation, or lesion of the eighth cranial nerve nucleus in the brainstem. Wernicke-Korsakoff syndrome is a cause of vertigo in patients with chronic alcohol abuse. Peripheral vertigo is due to a disruption in the vestibular system or eighth cranial nerve.

A patient with vertigo has a feeling of imbalance or difficulty maintaining an upright posture and may complain of feeling drunk or that the room is spinning. The patient frequently has nausea or vomiting. Vertigo may have an abrupt onset, and the patient may also complain of tinnitus, a buzzing or ringing in the ears. It is important to question the patient about a history of stroke, atrial fibrillation, and hypertension because this history can suggest stroke-related vertigo. A patient may have a decreased level of consciousness, or the eyes may be moving quickly back and forth, a condition known as *nystagmus*. Nystagmus may be horizontal, vertical, or rotatory and may or may not diminish spontaneously. Nystagmus can result from a lesion in the cerebellum, brainstem, or vestibular organs.

Patients who have vertigo lasting longer than 24 hours, accompanied by a loss of balance and difficulty maintaining their posture, standing, and walking, are often found to have a cerebellar stroke. Transient symptoms not triggered by motion may indicate a TIA. The patient who has other cranial nerve deficits needs to be evaluated for brainstem or cerebellar issues.

Vertigo may also be due to dysfunction of the vestibular system, usually the inner ear. This is commonly referred to as *peripheral vertigo*. Symptoms may be more acute, abrupt, severe, and of shorter duration than central vertigo and are often worsened or triggered by movement or change in position of the head. Brief, recurrent episodes of vertigo associated with a change in position that resolves with cessation of movement suggest benign positional vertigo. Patients may prefer to face one side or the other during transport and may not want to turn toward you to answer questions because it exacerbates symptoms.

Ataxia/Gait Disturbance

Ataxia refers to a loss of muscular control and coordination causing truncal instability, gait unsteadiness, abnormal eye movements, or difficulty with precision of movements of the extremities, such as distance-finding or rapid alternating movements. This may be due to dysfunction of the cerebellum, spinal cord, peripheral nerves, or inner ear. The patient or a family member may report that the patient is unable to walk normally, and any of the following may be noted:

- Has trouble coordinating movements
- Double vision or irregular eye movements
- Feels weak or unstable (off balance or about to fall) when walking or standing

Associated symptoms such as incontinence or altered mentation (as occurs with normal-pressure hydrocephalus) or nausea, vomiting, and visual changes (as may occur with a posterior-circulation stroke) may also be present. Causes of ataxia include intoxication, peripheral neuropathy, stroke, Parkinson disease, medication side effect, spinal or brain injury/abscess/tumor, multiple sclerosis, and Guillain-Barré syndrome.

Focal Neurologic Deficit

Focal neurologic deficit refers to any localized loss of neurologic function, such as weakness or numbness/sensory deficit in part or all of an extremity or one side of the face. Unless the patient has an associated neurologic insult that hinders speech, a condition known as **expressive aphasia**, the patient will probably be able to describe the onset of the deficit. Stroke is a particularly time-sensitive etiology of focal neurologic deficits. The history may reveal a preceding illness (e.g., Guillain-Barré syndrome) or chronic neurologic disorder (e.g., neuromuscular degenerative disease such as amyotrophic lateral sclerosis [ALS], also known as Lou Gehrig's disease; multiple sclerosis; or myasthenia gravis). Bowel and bladder dysfunction such as incontinence and urinary retention typically accompany the lower extremity weakness of cauda equina syndrome, which is a compression of the nerve roots from the lowest portion of the spinal cord. Note any change in the patient's ability to understand or follow instructions. Such deficit may indicate a stroke, intoxication, electrolyte abnormality, or hepatic encephalopathy.

Ongoing Management

Managing patients with suspected neurologic dysfunction should be approached in a systematic manner. During your ongoing management, revisit the primary assessment, the vital signs, the cardinal presentation/chief complaint, and any treatment you have administered, including oxygen administration. As always, you should monitor airway, breathing, and circulation. Maintain the patient's oxygenation (in stroke patients, supplemental oxygen should be given if needed to maintain an SpO_2 goal of 95% to 99%). Capnography is helpful in monitoring respiration in patients with an advanced airway in place, patients receiving positive-pressure ventilation, or patients who have been sedated with medication. Check for hypoglycemia, which can mimic many neurologic disorders, and even if IV fluids are not needed, consider placing an IV with a saline lock if the patient has a risk of decompensation. If you have any suspicion the patient may have suffered traumatic injury, protect the cervical spine with spinal motion restriction.

A calm, supportive, professional demeanor is of the utmost importance because the patient is usually frightened. A physiologic function the patient may have taken for granted is not working properly or no longer working. In addition, the patient may be confused and lash out physically or verbally. Use a composed, reassuring manner at all times.

Your team must decide which hospital can best treat the patient. You may select a **stroke center**, a trauma center, or another center offering advanced specialized care. If the patient's condition is life threatening, transport the patient to the closest appropriate facility, where the medical staff can stabilize and transfer the patient for more definitive care if needed. If the decision is made not to transport the patient to the nearest hospital, the destination should be chosen on the basis of local protocols, each hospital's respective capabilities, and the patient's medical needs. A patient's informed choice should be respected and considered. Online medical direction can be a resource for additional guidance if needed.

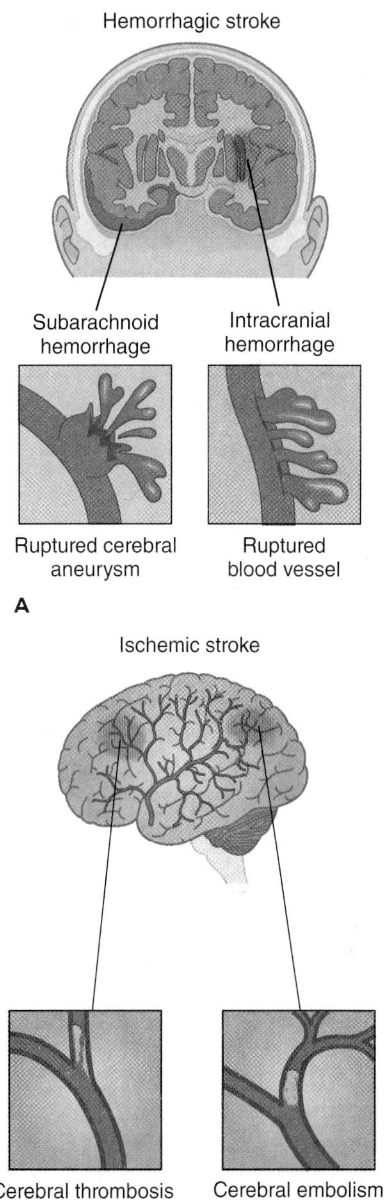

Figure 8-6 Causes of stroke. **A.** Hemorrhagic stroke is the result of bleeding, either an intracerebral hemorrhage or a subarachnoid hemorrhage, usually a result of a ruptured cerebral aneurysm. **B.** Ischemic stroke is the result of a blocked blood vessel caused by a cerebral thrombosis or cerebral embolism.

Specific Diagnoses

Stroke

A **stroke**, sometimes called a *brain attack*, is a brain injury occurring when blood flow to the brain is obstructed or interrupted, causing brain cells to die. According to the National Stroke Association, the term *cerebrovascular accident* (CVA) is no longer used by the medical community because stroke is considered to be a preventable event, not an accident.

Strokes are classified as either ischemic or hemorrhagic (**Figure 8-6**). An **ischemic stroke** occurs when a thrombus or embolus obstructs a vessel, diminishing blood flow to the brain. A **thrombus** is a blood clot forming in an artery at the site of the occlusion, whereas an **embolus** is a clot that forms elsewhere in the circulatory system, breaks off, and obstructs blood flow when it becomes lodged in a smaller artery. Rarely, an embolus may be composed of fat from a broken bone, amniotic fluid related to labor, or an air bubble introduced during IV therapy, surgery, trauma, or severe decompression sickness. Ischemic stroke is much more common than **hemorrhagic stroke**, which occurs when a diseased or damaged vessel ruptures.

Key features of a stroke include a sudden onset of neurologic impairment associated with a specific vascular distribution in the brain. If the impairment resolves spontaneously within 24 hours, then it is termed a **transient ischemic attack (TIA)**; however, the patient is at high risk for stroke in the near future.

Stroke Scales

Stroke identification scales are widely used in the assessment of potential stroke patients to recognize the likelihood that a patient with neurologic symptoms is or is not having a stroke. Examples of these scales include the following:

- The Cincinnati Prehospital Stroke Scale (CPSS), which identifies the presence of facial droop, arm drift on one side of the body, or slurred speech (Table 8-3). The CPSS has been further operationalized by adding time last known well and using the FAST mnemonic for ease of remembering the criteria:
    - **F**acial droop
    - **A**rm drift
    - **S**lurred speech
    - **T**ime last known well
- The Los Angeles Prehospital Stroke Screen (LAPSS), which evaluates smile or grimace, hand grip, and arm weakness on each side of the body, while factoring in historical information about age, presence of a seizure disorder, duration of symptoms, glucose measurement, and ambulation at baseline (Table 8-4).
- The Miami Emergency Neurologic Deficit (MEND) prehospital checklist, which contains the CPSS and additional components to detect both anterior and posterior circulation strokes (Table 8-5).

Stroke severity scales have been developed to identify the likelihood that a large vessel occlusion (LVO) is causing the suspected stroke. These scales assist in determining which patients may benefit from advanced procedures, including endovascular therapy aimed to directly remove the clot. Stroke severity scales typically use a numerical scoring system, where higher scores signify a

Table 8-3 Cincinnati Prehospital Stroke Scale (CPSS)

Assessment	Normal	Abnormal
	Facial droop	
Ask the patient to smile and show the teeth.	Both sides of the face move equally.	One side of the face does not move as well as the other side.
	Arm drift	
Ask the patient to close the eyes and hold the arms out with palms up for 10 seconds.	Both arms move the same or neither arm moves. (If neither arm moves, then this may indicate the patient did not understand the instructions. Perform the test again.)	One arm does not move, or one arm drifts down compared with the other.
	Speech	
Ask patient to say, "The sky is blue in Cincinnati."	The patient uses correct words with no slurring.	Patient slurs words, uses inappropriate words, or is unable to speak.

Interpretation: If any one item is abnormal, then the probability of a stroke is 72%.

Table 8-4 Los Angeles Prehospital Stroke Screen (LAPSS)

Criteria	Yes	Unknown	No
1. Age > 45 years	☐	☐	☐
2. History of seizures or epilepsy absent	☐	☐	☐
3. Symptoms < 24 hours	☐	☐	☐
4. At baseline, patient does not use a wheelchair or is not bedridden.	☐	☐	☐
5. Blood glucose level between 60 and 400 mg/dL	☐	☐	☐
6. Obvious asymmetry (right versus left) in any of the following three exam categories (must be unilateral):	☐	☐	☐
	Equal	**Right Weak**	**Left Weak**
Facial smile/grimace	☐	☐ Droop	☐ Droop
Grip	☐	☐ Weak grip ☐ No grip	☐ Weak grip ☐ No grip
Arm strength	☐	☐ Drifts down ☐ Falls rapidly	☐ Drifts down ☐ Falls rapidly

Interpretation: If patient has unilateral motor deficit on exam and criteria 1–6 are marked yes, then the probability of a stroke is 97%.

Table 8-5 Miami Emergency Neurologic Deficit (MEND) Examination

Mental status		
▪ Level of consciousness (AVPU)	☐	
▪ Speech (repeat “You can’t teach an old dog new tricks”) Abnormal = wrong words, slurred speech, no speech	☐	
▪ Questions (age, month)	☐	
▪ Commands (open and close eyes)	☐	
Cranial nerves		
▪ Facial droop (show teeth and smile) Abnormal = one side does not move as well as other	☐ R	☐ L
▪ Visual fields (sees fingers in all four quadrants)	☐ R	☐ L
▪ Horizontal gaze (side to side)	☐ R	☐ L

(continues)

Table 8-5 Miami Emergency Neurologic Deficit (MEND) Examination (*continued*)

Limbs		
▪ Motor: arm drift (close eyes and hold out both arms) Abnormal = one side does not move as well as other	☐ R	☐ L
▪ Motor: leg drift (open eyes and lift each leg separately)	☐ R	☐ L
▪ Sensory: arm and leg (close eyes and touch, pinch)	☐ R	☐ L
▪ Coordination: arm (finger to nose)	☐ R	☐ L
▪ Coordination: arm (finger to nose) Coordination: leg (heel to shin)	☐ R	☐ L

Table 8-6 Cincinnati Prehospital Stroke Severity Scale (CPSSS)

Assessment	Points
Gaze palsy	2
Arm weakness	1
Abnormal levels of consciousness	1

Interpretation: When number of points is ≥ 3, then the likelihood of an LVO is 72%.

Table 8-7 Los Angeles Motor Scale (LAMS)

Assessment	Points
Facial strength	1
Arm strength	2
Grip strength	2

Interpretation: When number of points is ≥ 4, then the likelihood of an LVO is 85%.

higher stroke severity and higher likelihood of LVO. Examples of stroke severity scales for use in the prehospital setting include the following:

- The Cincinnati Prehospital Stroke Severity Scale (CPSSS), which builds on the CPSS and incorporates a numerical scale to identify stroke severity and likelihood of LVO (Table 8-6). Meeting one of the CPSS criteria for stroke increases the suspicion for stroke, but having two of the three criteria is more sensitive for an LVO.
- The Los Angeles Motor Scale (LAMS), which was derived from the motor components of the LAPSS (Table 8-7).
- The Rapid Arterial Occlusion Evaluation Scale (RACE), a six-part score that was developed from components of the National Institutes of Health Stroke Scale (Table 8-8).

Table 8-8 Rapid Arterial Occlusion Evaluation (RACE) Scale

Assessment	Points
Facial palsy	2
Arm motor function	2
Leg motor function	2
Gaze palsy	1
Aphasia/agnosia	2

Interpretation: When number of points is ≥ 5, then the likelihood of an LVO is 42%.

In hospital settings, the National Institutes of Health Stroke Scale is commonly used for detailed evaluation of the neurologic and neuromotor deficits in stroke patients (Table 8-9). It also allows hospital providers to follow the patient's course by identifying improvement or worsening of the patient's condition as measured by the numerical scale.

Administer stroke scale items in the order listed. Record performance in each category after each subscale exam. Do not go back and change scores. Follow directions provided for each exam technique. Scores should

Table 8-9 National Institutes of Health Stroke Scale

Instructions	Scale Definition
1a. Level of Consciousness: The investigator must choose a response if a full evaluation is prevented by such obstacles as an endotracheal tube, language barrier, or orotracheal trauma/bandages.	**0** = **Alert;** keenly responsive **1** = **Not alert but arousable** by minor stimulation **2** = **Not alert;** requires repeated stimulation to attend **3** = **Responds** only with reflex motor or autonomic effects or totally unresponsive, flaccid, and areflexic
1b. Level of Consciousness Questions: The patient is asked the month and his/her age. The answer must be correct—there is no partial credit for being close.	**0** = **Answers** both questions correctly **1** = **Answers** one question correctly **2** = **Answers** neither question correctly
1c. Level of Consciousness Commands: The patient is asked to open and close the eyes and then to grip and release the nonparetic hand. Substitute another one-step command if the hands cannot be used.	**0** = **Performs** both tasks correctly **1** = **Performs** one task correctly **2** = **Performs** neither task correctly
2. Best Gaze: Only horizontal eye movements will be tested. Voluntary or reflexive (oculocephalic) eye movements will be scored, but caloric testing is not done.	**0** = **Normal** **1** = **Partial gaze palsy;** gaze abnormal in one or both eyes **2** = **Forced deviation,** or total gaze paresis not overcome by the oculocephalic maneuver
3. Visual: Visual fields (upper and lower quadrants) are tested by confrontation, using finger counting or visual threat, as appropriate.	**0** = **No visual loss** **1** = **Partial hemianopia** **2** = **Complete hemianopia** **3** = **Bilateral hemianopia (blind)**
4. Facial Palsy: Ask—or use pantomime to encourage—the patient to show teeth or raise eyebrows and close eyes.	**0** = **Normal** symmetrical movements **1** = **Minor paralysis** (asymmetry on smiling) **2** = **Partial paralysis** (total or near-total paralysis of lower face) **3** = **Complete paralysis** of one or both sides
5. Motor Arm: The limb is placed in the appropriate position: extend the arms (palms down) 90 degrees (if sitting) or 45 degrees (if supine). Drift is scored if the arm falls before 10 seconds. **5a.** Left arm **5b.** Right arm	**0** = **No drift;** limb holds position for 10 seconds **1** = **Drift;** limb holds position but drifts down before full 10 seconds **2** = **Some effort against gravity;** limb cannot get to or maintain position, drifts down to bed, some effort against gravity **3** = **No effort against gravity;** limb falls **4** = **No movement** **UN** = **Amputation** or joint fusion
6. Motor Leg: The limb is placed in the appropriate position: hold the leg at 30 degrees (always tested supine). Drift is scored if the leg falls before 5 seconds. **6a.** Left leg **6b.** Right leg	**0** = **No drift;** leg holds position for full 5 seconds **1** = **Drift;** leg falls by the end of the 5-second period but does not hit bed **2** = **Some effort against gravity;** leg falls to bed by 5 seconds, has some effort against gravity **3** = **No effort against gravity;** leg falls to bed immediately **4** = **No movement** **UN** = **Amputation** or joint fusion

(continues)

Table 8-9 National Institutes of Health Stroke Scale (*continued*)

Instructions	Scale Definition
7. Limb Ataxia: The finger-nose-finger and heel-shin tests are performed on both sides with eyes open.	0 = **Absent** 1 = **Present in one limb** 2 = **Present in two limbs** UN = **Amputation** or joint fusion
8. Sensory: Sensation or grimace to pinprick when tested, or withdrawal from noxious stimulus in the obtunded or aphasic patient.	0 = **Normal;** no sensory loss 1 = **Mild to moderate sensory loss;** feels pinprick is less sharp or is dull on the affected side; or there is a loss of superficial pain with pinprick, but aware of being touched 2 = **Severe to total sensory loss;** patient is not aware of being touched in the face, arm, and leg.
9. Best Language: Patient is asked to describe what is happening in an attached picture, to name the items on an attached naming sheet, and to read from an attached list of sentences. Comprehension is judged from responses here, as well as to all of the commands in the preceding general neurologic exam.	0 = **No aphasia;** normal 1 = **Mild to moderate aphasia;** some obvious loss of fluency or facility of comprehension, without significant limitation on ideas 2 = **Severe aphasia;** all communication is through fragmentary expression; great need for inference, questioning, and guessing by the listener 3 = **Mute, global aphasia;** no usable speech or auditory comprehension
10. Dysarthria: An adequate sample of speech must be obtained by asking patient to read or repeat words from a list.	0 = **Normal** 1 = **Mild to moderate dysarthria;** patient slurs some words; can be understood with some difficulty. 2 = **Severe dysarthria;** patient's speech is so slurred as to be unintelligible; or is mute/anarthric. UN = **Intubated** or other physical barrier
11. Extinction and Inattention (Formerly Neglect): Sufficient information to identify neglect may be obtained during prior testing. If the patient has a severe visual loss preventing visual double simultaneous stimulation, and the cutaneous stimuli are normal, the score is normal.	0 = **No abnormality** 1 = **Visual, tactile, auditory, spatial, or personal inattention** or extinction to bilateral simultaneous stimulation in one of the sensory modalities 2 = **Profound hemi-inattention or extinction to more than one modality;** does not recognize own hand or orients to only one side of space

Modified from NIH stroke scale. National Institute of Neurological Disorders and Stroke, National Institutes of Health website. https://www.ninds.nih.gov/health-information/public-education/know-stroke/health-professionals/nih-stroke-scale. 2004.

reflect what the patient does, not what the clinician thinks the patient can do. The clinician should record answers while administering the exam and work quickly. Except where indicated, the patient should not be coached (i.e., repeated requests to patient to make a special effort).

Many of the stroke scales perform well at identifying middle cerebral artery distribution strokes but may be limited in identifying posterior circulation strokes. Compared to strokes of the anterior circulation (e.g., middle cerebral artery), strokes impacting other cerebral artery distributions may have a variety of clinical symptoms that can be difficult to distinguish. Posterior circulation strokes may have isolated vision changes, dizziness, or vertigo. The BE-FAST (Balance, Eyes, Face, Arm, Speech, Time) exam combines the elements of the FAST scale with an assessment of balance and vision change to identify posterior circulation strokes. However, cerebellar testing by assessing balance may be difficult to perform in the EMS environment. Testing for ataxia (poor muscle control that causes clumsy movements) by having the patient rub one leg on the other while they are supine may also help distinguish a posterior stroke.

Ischemic Stroke

Pathophysiology

During an ischemic stroke, blood flow to a portion of the brain is disrupted, and ischemia of the brain occurs (see Figure 8-6B). Ischemia is insufficient blood flow to an organ or tissue—in this case the brain—causing inadequate perfusion (oxygen delivery to the tissue). When lack of perfusion to a portion of the brain causes infarction (cell death or necrosis), there is often an area of potentially reversible ischemia surrounding the infarct (the penumbra) (**Figure 8-7**). An important goal of stroke treatment is to restore perfusion to this region in order to preserve associated neurologic function. Rapid recognition of stroke symptoms, which is one of the goals of this course, can help facilitate rapid treatment.

Strokes in the middle cerebral artery territory typically produce **hemiparesis** (unilateral weakness) and/or numbness on the side of the body opposite to the brain lesion (**Figure 8-8**). Patients often show a gaze preference toward the side of the lesion. If the ischemic lesion is in the dominant hemisphere, the patient may have receptive or expressive aphasia, which is an inability to comprehend or express language. A stroke in the nondominant hemisphere may cause neglect of or inattention to one side of the body. Usually, weakness is more pronounced in the arm and lower face than in the lower extremity. A stroke in the distribution of the anterior cerebral artery can cause altered mental status and impaired judgment, opposite-side weakness (greater in the leg than in the arm), and urinary incontinence.

Posterior cerebral artery occlusion impairs thought processes, clouds memory, and causes visual field deficits. Finally, vertebrobasilar artery occlusions may cause vertigo; syncope; ataxia; and cranial nerve dysfunction, including nystagmus, double vision, and difficulty swallowing. For this reason, stroke should always be on the differential diagnosis for the patient with vertigo.

Patients with atherosclerosis may have turbulent blood flow, which increases the risk of blood clot formation and platelet adherence within the arteries. In addition, patients who have blood disorders such as sickle cell anemia, protein C deficiency, and polycythemia (a hereditary disorder characterized by an abundance of circulating red blood cells) also have properties of the blood that increase the risk of stroke.

Signs and Symptoms

Any patient who presents with an acute neurologic deficit should be evaluated for a stroke, whether the deficit

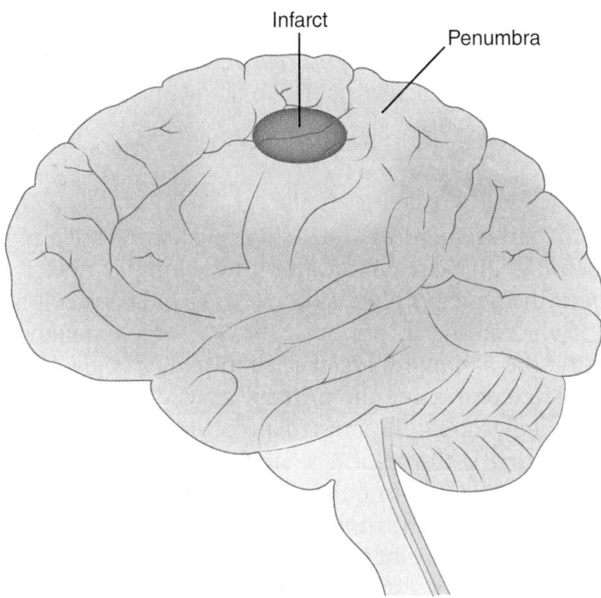

Figure 8-7 Following a thrombotic or embolic stroke, an area of ischemia–the penumbra–surrounds the infarction. The ischemia is potentially reversible with rapid diagnosis and treatment.

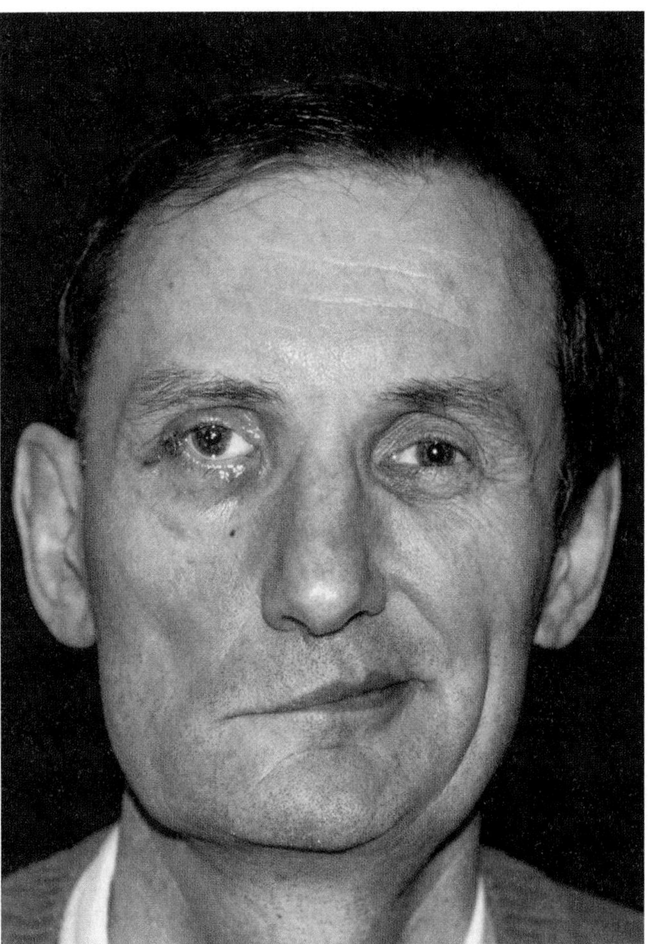

Figure 8-8 Facial droop.

is focal, such as a loss of strength or sensation in a particular body region, or diffuse, such as altered mental status. Stroke may present with very mild and nonspecific symptoms or life-threatening or deadly symptoms.

A patient having a major stroke often experiences an abrupt onset of significant weakness, numbness, or tingling on one side of the face, in one arm or leg, or on the entire one side of the body. A sudden decrease in or loss of consciousness may also occur. A patient may lose vision in one or both eyes and have nausea or vomiting, a headache, or trouble speaking. This difficulty speaking may take the form of **dysarthria** (an inability to control the muscles used in speech causing garbling or slurring) or expressive or receptive aphasia (an inability to express or understand language).

Other patients with stroke may have more subtle presentations and can experience an array of symptoms. A stroke can also occur while sleeping, and the patient may only notice symptoms upon waking. Sometimes the symptoms are incapacitating, and the patient cannot use a telephone or summon other help because of an altered mental status, aphasia, or **hemiplegia** (paralysis on one side of the body). Alternatively, something as mild as vague numbness, dizziness, blurred vision, vertigo, or a clumsy hand may be a symptom of a stroke. EMS personnel should recognize patients with these subtle presentations of stroke. Key findings include the following:

- Unilateral weakness
- Speech disturbance
- Vertigo or loss of balance
- Altered mental status

A very important point is to differentiate between the time the patient was last seen acting normally (or "last known well") and the time the symptoms are discovered. If a patient is sitting with a family member and suddenly cannot speak or has acute weakness on one side of the body (or other stroke symptoms), the time of discovery of symptoms and the time last seen normal are the same. If the patient went to bed the night before and was acting normally but woke up in the morning with stroke symptoms, the time the patient was last seen acting normally was the night before. The same applies if a patient seemed normal when a family member left the house to go out but was showing symptoms of a stroke when the family member returned a few hours later. The time the patient was last seen normal is prior to the family member's leaving the house, not the time of arrival home. The time that the patient was last known well is a critical part of the SAMPLER history for time-sensitive innovations in patients with conditions such as stroke and ST-elevation myocardial infarction. In stroke, the time last known well is important in evaluating whether the patient is a candidate for medications that cause fibrinolysis or for interventional thrombectomy. Further, if a patient has suffered a stroke in the past, it is important to know the patient's baseline level of function and mental status. At the hospital, the patient will probably undergo a computed tomography (CT) scan and/or magnetic resonance imaging (MRI), and the physician will decide whether to administer a fibrinolytic agent.

Differential Diagnosis

It is difficult to distinguish one kind of stroke from another in the field, but certain other causes of altered mental status can be quickly ruled out. A hypoglycemic episode, for example, can mimic a stroke. For this reason, blood glucose level should be checked in any patient who exhibits altered mental status or weakness. The symptoms of traumatic brain injury may also be like those of a stroke. Migraine headaches or migraine equivalents; electrolyte abnormalities; CSF infections, such as encephalitis and meningitis; demyelinating diseases of the nervous system, such as multiple sclerosis or Guillain-Barré syndrome; and psychiatric disorders may also have strokelike symptoms but making these diagnoses will require further testing at the hospital.

Other diagnoses to consider include acute intoxication with alcohol or other drugs, Bell palsy, abscess or other infection, delirium, amnesia, carotid or vertebral artery dissection, intracranial bleeding attributed to trauma, and postictal state following a seizure.

A TIA mimics a stroke, but the symptoms resolve within 24 hours, with a majority resolving in 1 hour. According to the National Stroke Association, about 10% of these patients will suffer a stroke in 90 days and about one-half of those do so within 2 days. A TIA is a red flag that should not be ignored. However, a TIA precedes only one of every eight strokes. For most people, a stroke occurs without warning.

Treatment

Initial management should include evaluating the airway, breathing, and circulation and intervening as necessary. Check the patient's blood glucose level and correct if necessary, according to protocol. Provide supplemental oxygen if the patient's oxygen saturation dips below 94%.

After completing the primary survey and evaluating for hypoglycemia, the immediate priority in the prehospital setting is to perform a rapid but thorough evaluation for stroke and to quickly transport the patient with suspected stroke to the most appropriate stroke center. Stroke scales have been developed to help identify the likely presence of a stroke, as well as whether a suspected stroke patient is likely to have an LVO. Strokes due to an LVO involve occlusions in the proximal, larger vessels (internal carotid and proximal middle cerebral artery). These strokes may require treatment at interventional stroke centers.

Hemorrhagic Stroke

The two types of hemorrhagic stroke (see Figure 8-6A) are intracerebral hemorrhage and subarachnoid hemorrhage. In a hemorrhagic stroke, small arteries spontaneously rupture and bleed directly into the tissues of the brain itself or the subarachnoid space. This is differentiated from bleeding into the subdural or epidural spaces, which is often caused by trauma (**Figure 8-9**).

Intracerebral Hemorrhage

Intracerebral hemorrhage accounts for 10% to 15% of all strokes and carries a higher likelihood of mortality than ischemic stroke. Mortality during the first month after this kind of stroke ranges from 40% to 80%. About half of all deaths, however, occur within 48 hours of presentation. Only 20% of patients with intracranial hemorrhage regain full functional independence.

Certain conditions place people at higher risk of intracerebral hemorrhage: anticoagulation; hypertension; atherosclerosis; and use of stimulant drugs, such as cocaine, synthetic cathinones (bath salts), or methamphetamine.

Pathophysiology

The stage is set for intracerebral hemorrhage when small intracerebral arteries—that is, arteries within the brain rather than on its surface—are damaged by disease processes such as hypertension and atherosclerosis. In patients who have had a previous stroke, the vascular tissue may be weaker and more friable and bleed more readily. Smoking may also weaken blood vessels. In fact, smokers with a systolic blood pressure > 150 mm Hg are nine times more likely to suffer a hemorrhagic stroke than nonsmokers.

Bleeding most often occurs in the thalamus, putamen, cerebellum, or brainstem. Brain tissue beyond the immediate area of the bleeding may be damaged by pressure produced by the mass effect of the hemorrhage itself. This mass effect increases ICP, which may cause symptoms such as nausea, vomiting, altered mental status, coma, respiratory depression, and/or death.

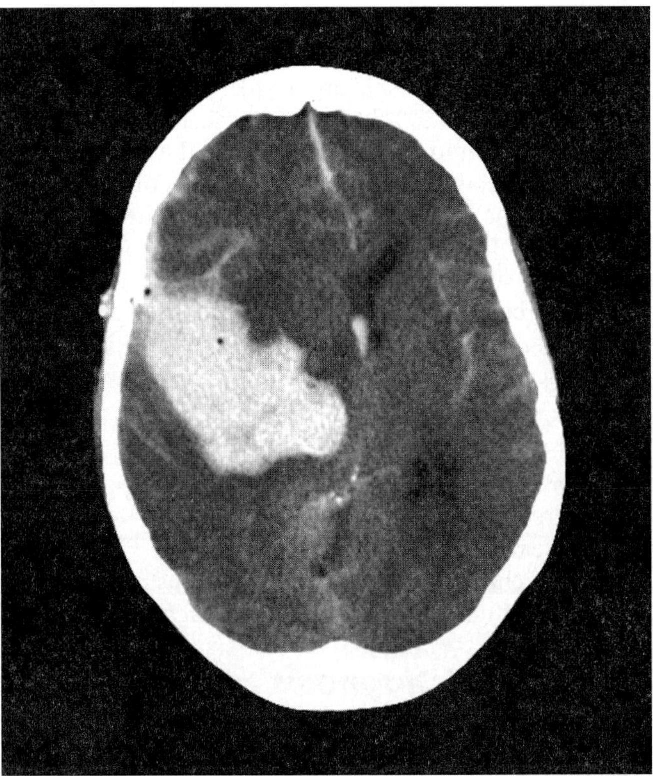

Figure 8-9 Magnetic resonance imaging (MRI) of an intracerebral hemorrhage.

Signs and Symptoms

A patient with intracerebral hemorrhage is likely to have an altered mental status. Frequent complaints include headache, nausea, and vomiting. The patient may have a seizure, with or without marked hypertension. However, in the prehospital setting it is very difficult to distinguish between intracranial bleeding and an ischemic stroke. That determination will have to be made on arrival at the emergency department by obtaining a CT scan of the brain. Key findings include the following:

- Alteration in vital signs (hypertension, pulse, and respiration changes)
- Altered level of consciousness
- Headache
- Focal neurologic deficit (weakness, gaze preference)
- Difficulty with gait, fine motor control
- Nausea, vomiting
- Dizziness or vertigo
- Abnormal eye movements

Differential Diagnosis

The differential diagnosis of intracerebral hemorrhage includes ischemic stroke, subarachnoid hemorrhage, migraine headache, hypertensive emergency, tumor, and metabolic abnormalities. Vomiting may be gastrointestinal in origin, but it may also suggest increased ICP, as occurs with an intracerebral hemorrhage.

Treatment

The most important thing to do when hemorrhagic stroke is suspected is to transport the patient as quickly as possible to a hospital with emergent neurosurgical capabilities. Recognize the signs and symptoms of stroke and be able to take control of any difficulties that arise with airway, breathing, or circulation. Patients who do not have a patent airway or who have signs of respiratory dysfunction, including apnea, require intervention. You should use a stroke scale and ask specific questions about anticoagulation and bleeding problems, but treating life-threatening problems takes precedence over gathering information.

Many patients who have intracerebral bleeding also have hypertension. In general, blood pressure will not be treated in the field unless confirmatory imaging has been obtained. However, you should minimize stimuli that could further increase the patient's intracranial pressure. Monitor the patient, elevate the head of the gurney to 30 degrees, establish IV access, and check the blood glucose level because hypoglycemia may mimic stroke symptoms and has been associated with poor outcomes in stroke patients. Treatment of nausea and vomiting, either via local protocol or online medical oversight, can help prevent further increases in intracranial pressure.

Patients with intracranial bleeding may have ECG changes or seizures. The receiving hospital will perform an immediate CT scan on the patient. Other possible imaging includes CT angiography, CT perfusion, and MRI (including MR angiography and venography). Patients who are on anticoagulants or are hypocoagulable from other causes may be treated by a number of different modalities. Vitamin K, prothrombin complex concentrate, fresh-frozen plasma, recombinant factor VIIa, or other reversal agents may be administered in an attempt to limit bleeding. Blood pressure may be tightly controlled for the same reason. Emergent neurosurgical consultation may be necessary.

Patients believed to have had a hemorrhagic stroke should be brought to a stroke center with neurosurgical capabilities.

Subarachnoid Hemorrhage

Subarachnoid hemorrhage (SAH) occurs when arteries on the brain's surface bleed into the subarachnoid space, the area between the pia mater and the arachnoid mater. This kind of bleeding can be triggered by trauma such as a car accident, but more often occurs when a cerebral aneurysm or arteriovenous malformation ruptures (see Figure 8-6A).

Pathophysiology

A cerebral aneurysm is a pouch that develops in the weakened wall of a diseased or damaged vessel. An arteriovenous malformation is a genetic developmental defect of the vascular system in which certain arteries connect directly to veins rather than to a capillary bed, creating a tangle of vessels that can rupture. However, any part of the brain that has a tumor, a thrombosis, or an abnormal blood vessel malformation may bleed. Uncontrolled hypertension and congenital aneurysms can be predisposing factors. Patients who have certain systemic diseases, such as Ehlers-Danlos syndrome, Marfan syndrome, aortic anomalies, or polycystic kidney disease, may also be at increased risk of SAH. Patients with vessel-wall deficits due to age, hypertension, smoking, or atherosclerosis are also at risk.

SAH may enter the ventricular system of the brain and cause obstruction of CSF, leading to increased ICP. The resultant decrease in CBF may cause neurologic dysfunction, including a decrease in responsiveness.

Signs and Symptoms

SAH should be suspected in any patient who describes a sudden, severe headache, often described as a thunderclap. Patients should be specifically asked how long it took from the start of pain until pain became maximally intense. Shorter times (seconds to minutes) are more suggestive of SAH. Loss of consciousness may have occurred. About half of patients who present with subarachnoid bleeding have elevated blood pressure. Middle cerebral artery bleeding may cause seizures, motor deficits, nausea and vomiting, neck stiffness, back pain, photophobia, and visual changes. Given that the bleeding is usually within the subarachnoid space rather than the brain parenchyma, focal neurologic signs are less common than in intracerebral hemorrhage. Cranial nerve findings can be present, most frequently oculomotor nerve palsy, causing the affected eye to be displaced downward and outward. Diplopia is a common complaint if nerve palsy is present, and patients should be asked about double vision. Onset of pain during exertion or sexual activity should also increase the index of suspicion of SAH.

About 30% to 50% of patients have a sentinel hemorrhage, a small amount of bleeding into the subarachnoid space. The headache that accompanies sentinel hemorrhage often has the same characteristics as that of a larger SAH, particularly a sudden onset and pain perceived as worse than usual, but may improve fairly quickly and there may be no evident neurologic deficits or symptoms. It is critical to recognize this event as an anticipatory sign of a subsequent, often catastrophic larger hemorrhage.

Key findings include the following:

- Sudden onset of severe headache
- Weakness (focal) or neglect
- Altered mental status
- Nausea/vomiting
- Vision changes, diplopia, or nystagmus
- Neck stiffness with associated headache

Differential Diagnosis

The differential diagnosis for SAH includes any pathologic occurrence that could lead to headache, nausea and vomiting, loss of consciousness, and altered mental status, including stroke, migraine headache, tumor, infection, medication use, overdose, and trauma.

Treatment

During prehospital treatment, support of the patient's airway, breathing, and circulation is of utmost importance. If at all possible, do not sedate the patient en route. Obtain IV access, elevate the head of the bed up to 30 degrees, and prepare to secure the airway if the patient exhibits an acute change in mental status or consciousness. Blood pressure control is usually not recommended in the field, but any stimuli that might increase the patient's ICP should be minimized, so be sure to institute aggressive control of nausea and vomiting if present.

At the hospital, a CT scan will be performed, and perhaps an MRI or cerebral angiogram will be done to locate the source of the bleeding. A patient with no obvious bleeding on initial imaging studies may receive a lumbar puncture to look for blood in the CSF or for changes consistent with blood being degraded in the CSF (xanthochromia), which is usually seen 12 hours after the onset of bleeding. If SAH is found in the hospital, antihypertensives will typically be administered to prevent worsening bleeding. If the hemorrhage is from an aneurysm, the patient will require neurosurgery to repair the aneurysm.

Appropriate triage and transport of the patient to a hospital that has CT scanning and neurosurgical support capabilities are critical.

The use of both a stroke identification and a stroke severity scale, along with establishing a last known well time, are critical to both identify patients with stroke and to identify those stroke patients who may benefit from specialized interventions. Patients with stroke who can be treated within 3 to 4.5 hours of the last time they were last known well may benefit from treatment with fibrinolytic agents, which have been associated with improved neurologic functioning and a lower mortality rate. Fibrinolytic agents also carry a risk of causing intracranial hemorrhage, and patients with contraindications to fibrinolytic treatment generally require more specialized interventions and facilities capable of thrombectomy. Some EMS agencies are using a fibrinolytic checklist to identify patients who likely would not be eligible for this therapy and then transport those patients directly to an interventional stroke center (Table 8-10).

Table 8-10 Fibrinolytic Therapy Checklist for Ischemic Stroke

All of the "**YES**" boxes and all of the "**NO**" boxes must be checked before a patient is transported to a "Designated Stroke Center."

INCLUSION CRITERIA
(All of the "**YES**" boxes must be checked)

YES

- ☐ 18 years of age or older
- ☐ Signs and symptoms of stroke with neurologic deficit (abnormal Cincinnati Stroke Scale)
- ☐ Patient can be delivered to a stroke center within 4.5 hours of sign/symptom onset

EXCLUSION CRITERIA
(All of the "**NO**" boxes must be checked)

NO

- ☐ Active internal bleeding (e.g., GI or urinary bleeding within the last 21 days)
- ☐ Known bleeding disorder
- ☐ Within 3 months of intracranial surgery, serious head trauma, or previous stroke
- ☐ Within 14 days of major surgery or serious trauma
- ☐ History of intracranial hemorrhage
- ☐ Witnessed seizure at stroke onset
- ☐ History of cancer of the brain

Additionally, new treatment modalities have been developed for LVO strokes. Patients who present with LVO typically have ischemia to a larger area of the brain, with significantly more neurologic disability on examination. Interventional techniques involving removal of the clot directly from the artery by aspiration or use of a removable stent have been demonstrated to improve the functional outcome of stroke patients with LVO when performed up to 24 hours after onset of symptoms. These specialized techniques are being done at certain medical centers (most commonly at comprehensive stroke centers or thrombectomy-capable stroke centers) and are not available at most primary stroke centers. The stroke severity scores outlined previously can help to identify patients with LVO and facilitate appropriate destination decisions.

Currently, no consensus exists on which stroke identification or severity scale is best or most reliable for EMS use. Each of the scales outlined has been implemented in multiple EMS systems. It is important for EMS personnel to refer to the stroke scales implemented through their local, regional, or state protocols and ensure that they are used to best evaluate and triage patients within their regional stroke system. Furthermore, because eligibility for each of these interventions is determined from the time the patient was last seen without symptoms, the time when the patient was last seen well is a critical aspect of the history that should be obtained and communicated to the receiving stroke center.

EMS clinicians should be aware of the stroke designation of hospitals within their EMS system and transport patients to the appropriate center based on the patient's clinical findings and timing of symptoms and using established protocols or local medical direction. The Joint Commission, in collaboration with The American Heart

Association/American Stroke Association, has identified and provided accreditations for various levels of stroke centers:

- Acute Stroke Ready Hospital, capable of the early evaluation and management of stroke patients, including initial administration of fibrinolytics. Neurology consultation at Acute Stroke Ready Hospitals is often available through a telehealth video connection.
- Primary Stroke Center, capable of the early evaluation and management of stroke patients, including administration of fibrinolytics and continued care and admission for noncomplicated stroke patients.
- Thrombectomy-Capable Stroke Center, in addition to the capabilities of a Primary Stroke Center, capable of performing endovascular interventions for LVO.
- Comprehensive Stroke Center, capable of all current treatments for ischemic strokes, including fibrinolytics and endovascular interventions, as well as the comprehensive management of hemorrhagic strokes.

Stroke center certifications and the optimal triage of patients to these centers based on clinical findings, timing, and distance are continuously evolving and areas of active research. Patients who are believed to be having a stroke should be transported to a stroke center. For patients with symptoms of less than 3 hours, it is usually best to go to the closest primary stroke center. Patients who have acute symptoms of longer duration or who are not eligible for peripheral fibrinolytic therapy, particularly those who screen positive for LVO, may benefit from transport to a comprehensive stroke center or hospital where additional intravascular interventions can be performed. *Local triage and destination protocols should be used to guide patient destination for suspected stroke patients.* Those who have a severe headache or known intracerebral lesion (e.g., tumor, arteriovenous malformation, or aneurysm) may be transported to a hospital with neurosurgical capabilities, such as a Comprehensive Stroke Center, in the event the stroke is found to be hemorrhagic and the patient requires emergency surgery. Considering the continuing evaluation of stroke destination algorithms, it is essential for EMS medical directors, EMS agency directors, and EMS personnel to continually participate in the development of regional stroke systems.

During transport, patients should be kept in a comfortable position, either a low-Fowler's or supine position with head elevation of 30 degrees if an ischemic stroke is suspected. Regulate the patient's blood pressure to maintain a MAP of at least 65 mm Hg, which will facilitate adequate CBF. In general, blood pressure should not be purposefully lowered for patients with suspected stroke, but in the situation where the patient's blood pressure exceeds the limit for fibrinolysis administration (> 185/110 mm Hg), the prehospital administration of a medication such as labetalol may be helpful. Treatment of severe hypertension with stroke symptoms should be guided by EMS protocols or direct consultation with a physician. Seizure-control medications may be administered as directed by medical control or per local protocol. Targeted temperature management or purposefully reducing a patient's temperature to reduce brain cell injury from ischemia has been used in patients who are post–cardiac arrest, and this treatment is being studied for patients with stroke.

An evolving prehospital approach in a few locations comprises deployment of a mobile stroke response unit with CT imaging, fibrinolytic administration capability, and telecommunication with a stroke specialist. The incremental morbidity and mortality benefit and cost-effectiveness for this approach is currently being studied.

Seizures

A **seizure** is a transient occurrence of abnormal excessive or synchronous neuronal activity in the cerebral cortex of the brain that can cause loss of or alteration in consciousness, convulsions or tremors, incontinence, behavior changes, subjective changes in perception (taste, smell, fears), and other symptoms.

Seizures are a common nonspecific manifestation of neurologic injury and disease and may occur as a primary condition or secondary to an underlying abnormality. Seizures can be caused by fever, infection, drug ingestion/withdrawal, acute neurologic insult (e.g., stroke, trauma), structural changes (e.g., brain tumor, degenerative diseases), pregnancy complications, metabolic disturbances, electrolyte imbalances, and congenital conditions. Seizures (reflex seizures) can also be caused by light flickers, certain visual patterns, or even brushing the teeth. Nearly 70% of all seizures have no known cause (idiopathic).

Common triggers for those with a history of seizures are failure to take medication correctly, changing from a brand name to generic medication, sleep deprivation/fatigue, stress/illness, and even dehydration. Females of childbearing age may have seizures associated with menstrual periods (catamenial epilepsy).

Epilepsy is a condition in which a persistent abnormality in the brain leads to recurrent seizures; this may be a congenital or acquired structural, metabolic, or genetic abnormality. Seizures due to transient abnormalities such as hyponatremia are not considered epilepsy.

Seizures can be classified as generalized or focal. A generalized seizure quickly involves both cerebral hemispheres and is associated with loss of consciousness. A focal seizure involves only or primarily one cerebral hemisphere, so wakefulness is usually maintained, but there may be changes in mentation, responsiveness, or behavior. Within generalized seizures are absence, atonic,

tonic, clonic, and tonic-clonic types. The classification of focal seizures is discussed later.

Pathophysiology

Seizures are thought to occur when there is an imbalance between the excitatory and inhibitory forces within the brain, and the scales tip in favor of the excitatory forces. Researchers believe seizures are caused by either a decrease of gamma-aminobutyric acid (GABA), an inhibitory neurotransmitter in the cerebral cortex of the brain, or by an increase of glutamate, an excitatory neurotransmitter. Benzodiazepines, which are commonly used to stop active seizure activity, increase GABA release, and thus inhibit neuronal activity.

Seizures have three distinct phases: preictal, ictal, and postictal. Depending on the type of seizure, not all phases are observed. Some patients may even experience a symptom several hours or days before a seizure, warning them that a seizure will occur. The preictal phase is the period immediately prior to observable seizure activity and may include an aura or warning of the impending seizure. The aura is a very small focal seizure lasting only a few seconds or minutes. Although antiseizure medications may obscure or alter the aura, patients may say they felt weak, hot, or cold or had abnormal epigastric sensations just prior to the seizure. Others describe their auras to be a sudden sense of fear, with difficulty speaking or understanding speech, a headache, hearing sounds and smelling unpleasant odors that are not there, a tongue-tingling sensation, or visual hallucinations. The ictal phase is the actual seizure activity, when the transient occurrence of abnormal excessive, usually synchronous neuronal activity in the cerebral cortex takes place and can be recorded on an electroencephalogram (EEG). The various observable clinical manifestations are related to the location of the abnormal electrical activity. The postictal phase immediately follows the ictal phase as seizure activity subsides and is considered the recovery period after the seizure. Some patients recover immediately, whereas others may take minutes to hours to feel and act like their usual selves, depending on the type of seizure, how long it lasted, and the location of the activity within the brain. Patients can be aware of the seizure or wake up afterward not knowing what happened. Generalized seizures involve complete loss of consciousness, whereas focal seizures typically do not. During a generalized seizure, the patient cannot talk, reach out, or perform purposeful activity. Following a generalized tonic-clonic seizure, the postictal phase is more severe and may manifest as amnesia, confusion, fatigue, or coma.

Most seizures, including generalized tonic-clonic seizures, terminate prior to 2 minutes, with a small percentage prolonged up to 5 minutes or more. A single, short-duration seizure is usually not a life-threatening event. However, a prolonged seizure, called *status epilepticus* (discussed later in this chapter), is a life-threatening medical and neurologic emergency that requires prompt diagnosis and immediate treatment.

Signs and Symptoms

Most often, a family member or bystander will call EMS to report a person exhibiting convulsive activity, acting confused or disoriented, or wandering aimlessly. People may activate EMS if they believe they are about to have a seizure. For many years, seizures were classified as generalized or partial, but in 2010 the International League Against Epilepsy (ILAE) Commission published a revised classification, which was updated again in 2017 (Table 8-11), that retains the term *generalized seizure* but changed *partial* to *focal*, added unknown onset, and replaced subtypes of focal with subcategories of motor or nonmotor, with retained or impaired awareness for focal seizures.

Generalized seizures, according to the 2017 ILAE classifications, originate at some point within, and rapidly engage, bilaterally distributed networks. Generalized seizures initially start with a loss of consciousness, which may be brief or extended, but continues through to the postictal phase.

There are multiple subtypes of generalized seizures. The tonic-clonic form tends to start out tonic (flexion or extension of the head, trunk, or extremities), then become clonic (rhythmic motor jerking of the extremities or neck), and then resolve with the patient becoming postictal. Other forms of generalized seizure include tonic only, clonic only, myoclonic jerking, atonic, and absence.

During a generalized seizure, the patient may experience airway obstruction or may not breathe adequately. Clinicians should be prepared to maintain the airway, administer oxygen, and assist ventilation.

Focal seizures originate within one hemisphere, and may remain localized or become more widely distributed. Focal seizures are the most common type of seizure experienced by people with epilepsy and usually last only 1 to 3 minutes. The two subsets of focal seizures are as follows:

- *Focal seizure with retained consciousness and awareness.* This seizure usually starts and stays within a very small, defined area of one hemisphere, leading to abnormalities that can be identified as coming from that area of the brain. For example, a seizure starting and staying within the right motor area of the cerebral cortex may cause rhythmic movement in the left arm, leg, or face. The patient will be awake and aware of the seizure activity. If the patient is unconscious or has altered mental status, consider and investigate other causes for the decreased consciousness state.
- *Focal seizure with impaired consciousness or awareness or responsiveness.* This seizure (old terminology was

Table 8-11 Classification of Seizures

Generalized Onset
Motor ▪ Tonic-clonic (in any combination) ▪ Atonic ▪ Epileptic spasms ▪ Myoclonic-atonic ▪ Myoclonic-tonic-clonic ▪ Clonic ▪ Tonic ▪ Myoclonic
Nonmotor (absence) ▪ Typical ▪ Atypical ▪ Myoclonic ▪ Eyelid myoclonia
Focal Onset
Motor Onset ▪ Automatisms ▪ Atonic ▪ Clonic ▪ Epileptic spasms ▪ Hyperkinetic ▪ Myoclonic ▪ Tonic
Nonmotor Onset ▪ Autonomic ▪ Behavior arrest ▪ Cognitive ▪ Emotional ▪ Sensory
Unknown Onset
Motor ▪ Tonic-clonic ▪ Epileptic spasms
Nonmotor ▪ Behavior arrest

Modified from Fisher RS, Cross JH, French JA, et al. Operational classification of seizure types by the International League Against Epilepsy: position paper of the ILAE Commission for Classification and Terminology. *Epilepsia*. 2017;58(4): 522–530.

complex partial seizure) also takes place in only one hemisphere, but usually involves a larger area or the entire hemisphere. This leads to some alteration in normal responsiveness and may include odd behavioral activities.

Focal seizures, especially with altered consciousness, may be an indication of a space-occupying lesion in the brain. As these patients may still be awake and able to control movements of the unaffected parts of the body, they may be confused for patients who are intoxicated or under the influence of illicit substances.

Although consciousness is maintained during a focal seizure, a focal seizure may evolve into unconsciousness and generalized seizure. Key findings of a focal seizure include the following:

- Focal or generalized rhythmic, uncontrolled movements
- Staring spell or drop attack, eyelid flutter
- Alteration in mental status or behavior, such as:
  - Grunting sounds, repeating of words or phrases, laughter, screams, crying
  - Taking clothes off, walking into traffic, wandering about without purpose
- Automatisms
- Postictal state described by family, friends, or caregivers

Status Epilepticus

Status epilepticus (SE) is defined as continuous convulsions lasting for 5 or more minutes or recurrent episodes of convulsions in a 5-minute interval without return to preconvulsive neurologic baseline. SE is further classified into convulsive and nonconvulsive types, based on the presence of tonic and/or clonic movement of the patient's extremities. SE is a life-threatening medical and neurologic emergency that requires prompt diagnosis and immediate treatment. During SE, cerebral glucose and oxygen supplies can be depleted. Systemic hypoxia, hypercapnia, acidosis, blood pressure changes, hyperthermia, neurogenic pulmonary edema, and rhabdomyolysis can occur. After 30 minutes of SE, pathologic changes in the brain take place, and after 60 minutes neurons start to die, independent of maintenance of systemic homeostasis.

Nonconvulsive SE (NCSE) is defined as a mental status change from baseline of at least 30 to 60 minutes' duration associated with continuous or near-continuous ictal discharges on an EEG. This type of seizure occurs frequently after acute traumatic brain injury, certain toxic ingestions and toxidromes, and some variants of epilepsy. It has been reported in 8% to 20% of critically ill patients. Delayed diagnosis and treatment of NCSE may lead to increased mortality.

NCSE may present as continuous observable motor activity (in nonparalyzed, including pharmacologically induced paralysis, patients) or only observed on an EEG. For this reason, if there is no improvement in level of consciousness or awareness after 5 to 10 minutes postictal, the EMS clinician should consider the possibility of the patient being in NCSE and treat per protocol and/or contact medical control.

Psychogenic Nonepileptic Seizure

A psychogenic nonepileptic seizure (PNES), also known as *nonepileptic behavioral spell* (NEBS) and previously termed *pseudoseizure*, may look like generalized seizure activity with abnormal motor movements and altered mentation, but it is not caused by abnormal neuronal activity. A PNES is considered primarily due to stress-related or emotional causes, but is not an intentional act. Without EEG monitoring, a PNES is nearly impossible to diagnose and, as such, it is the most common condition misdiagnosed as epilepsy. It is also possible to have an EEG-diagnosed seizure disorder and still exhibit a PNES at other times. Withholding treatment and antiseizure medication believing your patient to be "faking a seizure," however, could be dangerous and is not recommended. Treat a presumed seizure per protocol and/or contact online medical oversight.

A PNES should not affect the medulla or a patient's respirations because it is not caused by a generalized seizure or abnormal electrical discharges. The patient will usually continue to breathe. The use of capnography to monitor the patient's respirations and CO_2 status is an excellent assessment tool to potentially help differentiate seizure-like activity.

Differential Diagnosis

The differential diagnosis for seizure includes stroke, dysrhythmia, eclampsia, hypoglycemia, hyperthermia, migraine, amnesia, hemorrhage, tumor, metabolic abnormalities, sleep disorders, movement disorders, PNES, and psychiatric or substance-use conditions. Additionally, cardiac arrest, vasovagal symptoms, and administration of etomidate often present with myoclonic jerking, which is often confused for seizure activity. When a patient in cardiac arrest is not correctly identified by an EMS dispatch point, seizure is frequently a mistaken dispatch category, because during the initial phases of a cardiac arrest, the lack of blood flow to the brain often causes some myoclonic jerking movements. EMS dispatchers and medical directors of dispatch centers should be aware of this and provide training specific to recognizing cardiac arrest and providing prearrival instructions to initiate cardiopulmonary resuscitation when appropriate.

Treatment

Oxygenation, ventilation, and protection from harm are the most important interventions in the prehospital setting. Protect the patient from injury by placing padding or removing hazards. Administer oxygen via blow-by for infants and/or cannula for all others. Oxygen masks strapped down to the patient should be used cautiously due to the possibility of vomiting and aspiration. Suction equipment should be at hand. Consider the placement of a nasal airway. Provide ventilatory assistance if the patient's respiratory rate or ventilatory effort is inadequate or if the patient becomes hypoxic despite oxygen therapy. Obtain IV access if the seizure is prolonged or after the seizure if transporting so recurrent seizures can be treated. Blood glucose levels should be checked in all patients, and dextrose administered as needed. If the patient is hyperthermic and thought to have heatstroke, begin active cooling. Placing patients on their side or in the recovery position helps to protect the airway from aspiration while they are seizing and during the postictal period. As with any patient with an uncontrolled airway, never give oral antiseizure medication to an actively seizing patient.

Patients actively seizing for more than 5 continuous minutes or recurrent seizure without returning to baseline should be considered to be in SE and treated aggressively with a benzodiazepine to stop the seizure. Patients in SE may require repeat doses of benzodiazepines per local protocols or in consultation with direct medical oversight. If an attempt to start an IV has not been successful or is delayed, consider other routes for initial medication administration, including IM, intranasal (IN), intraosseous (IO), and rectal. This should be based on the specific benzodiazepine used. Clinicians should know the characteristics of the specific drugs they have available, such as that midazolam is preferred over diazepam for IM administration. The RAMPART (Rapid Anticonvulsant Medication Prior to Arrival Trial) trial found IM midazolam and IV lorazepam were equally safe and effective in adults. Intranasal administration of specific benzodiazepines, such as midazolam, has also been shown to be a safe and effective means of managing acute repetitive seizures in children and adults. Another route often used by parents and childcare providers for infants and young children is rectal administration of diazepam gel. As all benzodiazepines can cause respiratory depression, EMS clinicians should ask about any medications or treatments given to the patient prior to their arrival and be prepared to manage the airway of all seizure patients.

If adequate and repeated doses of benzodiazepine are not effective at stopping the seizure activity, then second-line agents such as levetiracetam, phenytoin, and PHENobarbital should be administered. Although very high levels of lidocaine can cause seizures, at typical cardiac doses lidocaine has antiseizure properties. Except for lidocaine, these medications are typically not carried by ground EMS but may be available in air medical and critical care transport units. Ketamine can effectively control status epilepticus, especially if it is resistant to PHENobarbital. The last resort is general anesthetic agents, including propofol.

During the postictal state, supportive care is the best treatment. Postictal patients will often be confused, upset, and perhaps aggressive or violent. Be reassuring and try to explain what happened. If the patient is in public, consider the patient's need for privacy and the possibility of incontinence and opened or torn clothes. Not all adult patients with an out-of-hospital seizure need to be transported to the hospital for evaluation. If the postictal patient is regaining their level of consciousness, some EMS systems allow crews to stay on-scene for a short period of time to monitor the patient's return to baseline behavior. If the patient is of legal age, returns to an awake stage, is fully oriented and mentating normally, and is judged to understand and accepts the risks of not going to the hospital for evaluation, the patient has the right to refuse transport. Ideally, the patient is under current medical care for seizure disorder and is taking medications and has a plan of action for when "breakthrough" seizures occur. EMS crews should encourage the patient to contact their personal physician to inform them of this seizure episode. Patients should be counseled against operating heavy machinery or a motor vehicle until reevaluated by their physician. It is possible, due to a number of factors (e.g., illness, exercise, diet, etc.), that the antiepileptic drug the patient has been prescribed is no longer at a therapeutic level and needs to be adjusted. EMS clinicians should follow local protocols and contact medical direction as needed to determine which patients should be transported to an emergency department for stabilization or reevaluation of their seizure disorder. Some states may require reporting to the Department of Motor vehicles or similar agency.

Patients who suffered a seizure for the first time should always be transported to a hospital for evaluation. Similarly, if the seizure is due to trauma; if possible aspiration occurred or the seizure took place in water; if the patient is older, diabetic, or pregnant; if the seizure lasted longer than 5 minutes or multiple seizures occurred in series; or if during the postictal phase there is no obvious improvement in the level of consciousness within a short time (approximately 5 to 10 minutes), the patient should be transported. If the seizure is thought to have been precipitated by trauma, the patient should be transported to a trauma center. Patients who are pregnant with a gravid abdomen and seizures should be considered to be in eclampsia, and magnesium administration should be initiated.

Febrile seizures are convulsions brought on by a fever in children between the ages of 6 months and 5 years and are particularly common in toddlers. The vast majority of febrile seizures are harmless. Most last for only a few seconds to a few minutes, with the majority lasting less than 2 minutes. There is no evidence that short febrile seizures cause brain damage, although certain children who have febrile seizures face an increased risk of developing epilepsy. As the child does not breathe during the seizure, the child's color can turn dark or cyanotic. This observation, along with the seizure activity, can be very scary for parents and observers who have never witnessed a seizure before.

Responding EMS clinicians should be aware that a seizure thought to be due primarily to hyperthermia (e.g., illness, infection) might be caused by another disorder (e.g., hypoglycemia, trauma, drug exposure), so considering and assessing for other pathologies causing seizures are important. Maintain airway, give oxygen, and monitor that the child is continuing to improve.

If the seizure has continued longer than 5 minutes, consider the patient to be in febrile status epilepticus (FSE) and aggressively treat per protocol. Give benzodiazepines by IM, IN, IO, or rectally if unable to start or there is a delay in starting an IV. Maintain airway control and respiratory status. Monitor oxygen saturation and waveform capnography. Early aggressive treatment results in shorter total seizure duration. Contact online medical direction if FSE continues after initial treatment.

In general, all pediatric patients who have had a seizure should be transported by advanced life support personnel to an ED for evaluation. For further information about febrile seizures, please refer to the NAEMT Emergency Pediatric Care (EPC) course materials.

Meningitis

Meningitis is an inflammation of the meninges, the membranes surrounding the brain and spinal cord. By extension, the CSF will also show signs of infection and inflammation. Meningitis has many different infectious and noninfectious causes, but life-threatening acute meningitis is frequently due to a bacterial infection. Meningitis can be caused by viral infections, though these are often self-limited and less likely to be life threatening than bacterial meningitis.

Pathophysiology

Bacterial meningitis usually occurs when bacteria migrate from the bloodstream to the CSF. If there is not an obvious source of infection, invasion of the CSF is usually presumed to have been caused by the bacteria that colonize the nasopharynx. In some cases, bacteria may spread from contiguous structures (e.g., sinuses, nasopharynx) that are infected or have been disrupted by trauma or surgical instrumentation. Once again, these historical factors can be important clues to the differential diagnosis.

Once in the CSF, the lack of antibodies and white blood cells allows bacteria to proliferate. The presence of bacterial components in the CSF makes the blood–brain barrier more permeable and allows toxins to enter. As the bacteria multiply, inflammatory cells respond, changing the cell count, pH, lactate, protein, and glucose composition of the CSF. ICP may rise as inflammation develops, causing occlusion of CSF outflow.

At a certain point, pressure in and around the brain reverses the flow of CSF. This development is associated with further deterioration of mental status. Ongoing damage to the brain triggers vasospasm, thrombosis, and septic shock, and the patient usually dies from diffuse ischemic injury.

Meningitis in neonates and infants is usually caused by group B streptococcus or *Escherichia coli*. In children beyond the first year, *Streptococcus pneumoniae* and *Neisseria meningitidis* become increasingly common; these bacteria are the most common in adult meningitis as well. *Haemophilus influenzae* type B, once the most prevalent cause in children, is rarely seen since the advent of immunization for this organism, but there are some cases caused by different *Haemophilus* subtypes in children and adults. Other causative bacteria in adults include *Listeria monocytogenes* (particularly in older persons), *Staphylococcus aureus*, various other streptococci, and gram-negative species. A different spectrum of bacteria is seen in meningitis after neurosurgical procedures; these include various staphylococci, streptococci, and gram-negative rods, including *Pseudomonas* and *Aeromonas*.

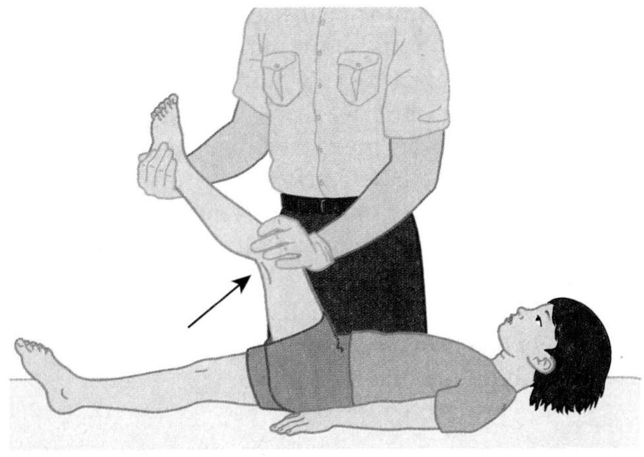

A

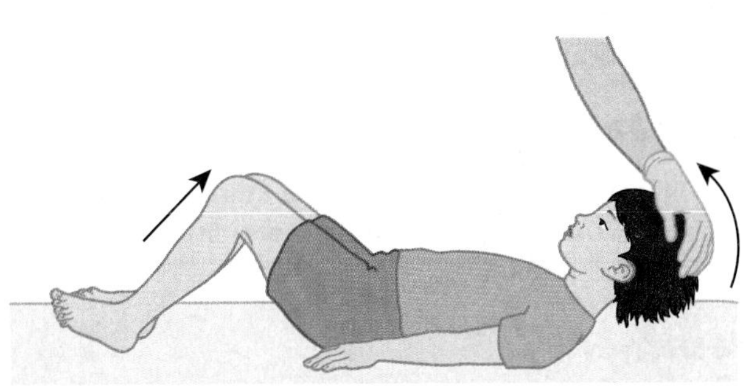

B

Figure 8-10 **A.** Kernig's sign. Meningeal irritation results in the inability to straighten the leg with the hips flexed. **B.** Brudzinski's sign. Meningeal irritation results in an involuntary flexion of the knees when the head is flexed toward the chest.

Signs and Symptoms

Patients with acute bacterial meningitis may decompensate quickly and require emergency care and antibiotics. The classic symptoms of meningitis include headache, nuchal rigidity (resistance to flexing/extending the neck), fever and chills, and photophobia. The infection can also cause seizures, altered mental status, confusion, coma, and death. The condition is sometimes precipitated by an upper respiratory illness.

Nearly one-fourth of patients with bacterial meningitis present acutely within 24 hours of onset of symptoms. Most patients with viral meningitis have symptoms that develop slowly over the course of days or a week. Patients who have a fever and headache should be examined for nuchal rigidity or discomfort with flexion of the neck, Kernig's sign (positive when the leg is flexed at the hip and knee, and subsequent extension of the knee is painful, leading to resistance and flexion of the torso), and Brudzinski's sign (involuntary flexing of the legs in response to flexing of the neck). These findings are positive in less than half of patients diagnosed with meningitis in the hospital, and are less useful if they are negative, thus the clinician must maintain a high level of suspicion in any patient presenting with headache, fever, and neck pain (**Figure 8-10**).

Altered mental status is often seen in patients with meningitis and can range from irritability or confusion to coma. Because of the effect of the infection on the CNS, the patient may become agitated or violent. Remember that any patient with psychiatric symptoms may have an underlying medical problem, and the psychiatric diagnosis should be one of exclusion, once organic causes have been evaluated. In infants, the patient may present with a bulging fontanelle, decreased tone, and paradoxical irritability (calm when left alone, crying when held). Meningitis should be considered in older adults and in young children, especially those with diabetes, renal insufficiency, or cystic fibrosis. Patients with immune system suppression, those who live in crowded conditions (e.g., military recruits, inmates at correctional facilities, and college dorm residents), splenectomy patients, patients with alcoholism or other cirrhotic liver disease, patients receiving chemotherapy, patients who use IV drugs, and patients who have been exposed to others with meningitis are all at high risk of contracting this illness.

If you suspect the patient has meningitis, you should protect yourself using droplet precautions, including a mask, gown, and gloves, to prevent airborne or droplet transmission of respiratory particles. Potential exposures of crew members should be reported immediately to a supervisor or the agency's infection control officer. Prophylactic antibiotics are needed if there is a high likelihood a clinician has been exposed to bacterial meningitis due to meningococcus (*N. meningitidis*); prophylaxis for meningitis due to other organisms is not indicated. Additionally, close contacts and persons living with the patient will typically be informed by the local health department of the indication for prophylactic antibiotics if the patient is ultimately diagnosed with meningococcal meningitis.

Key findings include the following:

- Fever
- Altered mental status, especially confusion or diminished level of consciousness
- Meningismus (a triad of nuchal rigidity, photophobia, and headache)

Differential Diagnosis

The differential diagnosis for meningitis includes brain abscess or tumor, encephalitis, intracranial or spinal bleeding, and stroke.

Treatment

Be sure the patient's airway, breathing, and circulation have been stabilized, and begin IV fluids to treat the patient for shock or hypotension. Because patients with meningitis are at high risk for seizures, take seizure precautions, and administer treatment according to protocol. If the patient does have altered mental status, consider airway protection. If the patient is alert and may have an early stage of meningitis, monitor closely, administer oxygen, establish IV access, and transport rapidly to the ED. A patient with meningitis may decompensate en route, so be prepared to control airway and breathing and treat seizures if they occur.

Patients with suspected meningitis can be treated in most EDs. If the patient is younger than 14 years of age, consider transport to a pediatric hospital if within reasonable distance. While at the ED, the patient will be stabilized, and a head CT scan may be performed to rule out stroke, bleeding, and abscess. Testing will usually include a lumbar puncture for evaluation of CSF. If bacterial meningitis is suspected, the patient will receive IV antibiotics. The patient may also receive corticosteroids.

Encephalitis

Encephalitis is a general inflammation of the brain causing focal or diffuse brain dysfunction. This disorder has signs and symptoms similar to those of meningitis, including lethargy and headache. The key distinguishing feature is that encephalitis usually causes some alteration of brain function—disorientation, behavior change, motor or sensory deficits—whereas meningitis does not. However, keep in mind patients may have both conditions at once.

Pathophysiology

Encephalitis is most often a viral infection that damages brain parenchyma. A virus can enter the body through many different vectors. Some viruses are transmitted by humans, some are mosquito or tick borne, and some are transmitted by animal bites. A common culprit is herpes simplex virus type 1, known more commonly for causing cold sores. Patients with compromised immune systems are more likely to contract certain viruses, such as cytomegalovirus and varicella zoster. This latter virus, also known as *herpes zoster*, lies dormant in sensory nerve ganglia after initial infection (chickenpox) and is reactivated under circumstances that are still obscure, causing shingles. Rabies must be considered if there was potential exposure such as an animal bite or contact with a bat. Geography plays a role as well, with persons in North America at risk for St. Louis encephalitis and those in Asia for Japanese encephalitis.

Usually, the virus replicates outside the CNS and enters through the bloodstream or a neural pathway. Once the virus has crossed over into the brain and entered the neural cells, the cells begin to malfunction. Hemorrhage, inflammation, and perivascular congestion all occur more frequently in the gray matter.

The body can also create antibodies to the brain tissue that cause the immune system to attack the brain, resulting in encephalitis. This autoimmune encephalitis can happen due to tumors, after viral infections, or without clear causes. Encephalitis is difficult to distinguish clinically from acute viral infection at the time of initial presentation as symptoms are nearly identical.

Signs and Symptoms

The course of encephalitis varies widely among patients. The acuity and severity of the presentation usually correlates with the prognosis. Generally, the patient reports a history of having a virus consistent with the common cold or flu as an early symptom. It might include fever, headache, nausea and vomiting, myalgia, or lethargy. The patient may also have behavioral or personality changes, decreased alertness or altered mental status, a stiff neck, photophobia, lethargy, generalized or focal seizures, confusion or amnesia, or flaccid paralysis. In the case of encephalitis associated with one of the viruses that causes chickenpox, measles, mumps, cold sores, or Epstein-Barr, the patient may have a rash, lymphadenopathy, or glandular enlargement. Because of the effect of the infection on the CNS, the patient may be agitated or violent. Remember that any patient with psychiatric symptoms may have an underlying medical problem. Infant patients may have skin, eye, or mouth lesions; a rash; decreased alertness; increased irritability; seizures; poor feeding; and shocklike symptoms. HIV infection may predispose patients to encephalopathy secondary to toxoplasmosis infection. Key findings include the following:

- Fever
- Altered mental status, such as confusion or diminished level of consciousness
- Headache

Differential Diagnosis

The differential diagnosis for encephalitis includes bacterial, viral, fungal, and protozoal infections; reactive autoimmune disease; and noninfectious illnesses and conditions that can cause encephalopathy, such as renal failure, liver failure, chronic autoimmune diseases, seizures, cerebral hemorrhage/edema, electrolyte abnormalities, intoxication, stroke, and trauma.

Treatment

The mortality rate for encephalitis is up to 75%, and those fortunate enough to survive often have long-term motor or mental disabilities. In the case of rabies encephalitis, the mortality is thought to be nearly 100%.

Patients with encephalitis may decompensate quickly, so be ready to take control of the airway and provide resuscitative support of blood pressure. Patients who have a seizure or are in status epilepticus should be treated according to local protocol. Antiviral medications will usually be given in the ED early in the course of treatment. Signs of hydrocephalus and increased ICP will usually be treated conservatively at first, and then with more aggressive methods, including diuresis, mannitol or hypertonic saline, corticosteroids, and placement of an external ventricular drain.

If you suspect a patient has encephalitis, protect yourself by wearing a mask, gown, and gloves to prevent airborne transmission of particles. As with any patient who may have an infectious disease, the prehospital clinician should practice strict blood and body fluid isolation precautions and should wear a mask at all times. For additional safety, a mask should also be placed on the patient.

In the hospital, the patient will undergo a series of blood tests, radiologic and other imaging studies, and CSF studies, including viral serologies. A brain biopsy may be performed.

Bell Palsy

Bell palsy is a unilateral facial paralysis that has an abrupt onset and uncertain cause. It is one of the most common cranial neuropathies, but it may frighten the patient by mimicking a stroke. Bell palsy accounts for about half of cases of peripheral facial nerve palsy, with the other half associated with specific causes.

Pathophysiology

Bell palsy refers to unilateral facial weakness due to dysfunction of the peripheral portion of the seventh cranial nerve, as opposed to the nucleus of the nerve, which lies in the brainstem. Inflammation and swelling of the sheath of the nerve are typically present where it passes through the temporal bone. By definition, when the etiology is unknown, the condition is termed *Bell palsy*, and there is increasing evidence of specific causes, most notably infection, particularly due to herpes simplex, a variety of other viruses, and Lyme disease (neuroborreliosis).

Signs and Symptoms

A patient with Bell palsy typically calls EMS or comes to the ED after having facial weakness that leads the person to believe they are having a stroke. Some patients have pain in the mastoid region or external ear, decreased tearing of the eye on the affected side, and an altered sense of taste.

On exam, weakness or paralysis of the entire face including the forehead on the affected side may be present, and the eye may not close completely on that side (**Figure 8-11**). If you watch carefully, you may see that the eye on the affected side rolls upward and inward.

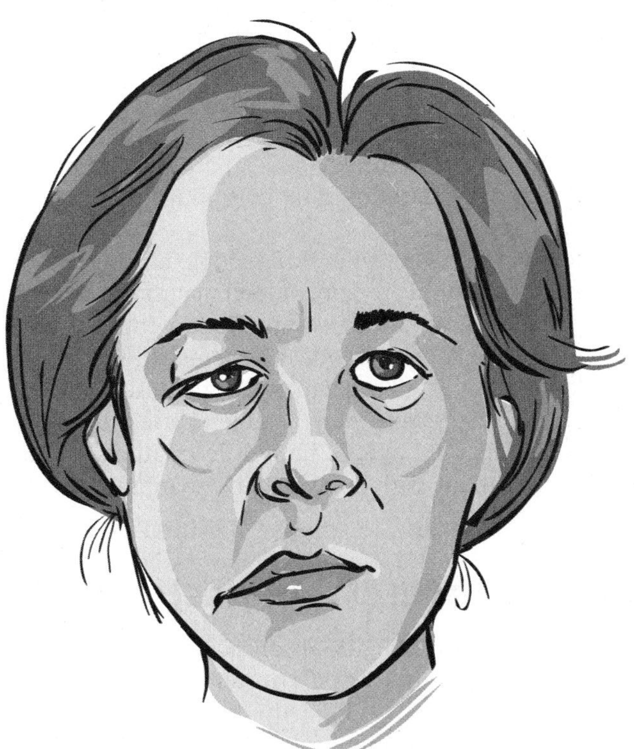

Figure 8-11 A patient with Bell palsy may present with weakness or paralysis on one side of the face, often with difficulty closing the eye on the affected side, leading the patient to believe that the condition is a stroke.

Facial signs of a stroke differ in that with a stroke only the lower half of the face will be weak and the forehead and upper eyelid retain normal motor function. In some patients, this can be difficult to differentiate, and in these cases, the patient should be treated as having had a stroke until proven otherwise. Key findings include the following:

- Unilateral weakness of entire side of face
- No arm or leg weakness
- Difficulty closing eyes

Differential Diagnosis

Facial nerve palsy has a variety of potential causes other than Bell palsy. These include Lyme disease, shingles, acute HIV infection, tumor, and otitis media. It is important to rule out a CNS cause such as stroke. A person who has had a stroke will usually have some wrinkling of the forehead.

Treatment

The management of Bell palsy in the prehospital setting is primarily providing patient transport, supporting vital signs, and offering emotional support to the patient. Because of the impaired eyelid closure on the affected side, you should protect the affected eye with an eye shield or gauze taped lightly over the eye to keep it closed. Periodically placing a small amount of normal saline in the eye or on the gauze to keep it moist is also an acceptable option. In the ED, after ruling out other causes previously mentioned, corticosteroids and antiviral agents may be prescribed, with neurologic follow-up for further testing and observation.

Bell palsy is not life threatening and is usually self-limiting. For this reason, emergency transport is not necessarily indicated, but differentiation from a stroke may be difficult and, in most systems, these patients should be transported urgently to the nearest stroke center. Some EMS systems may be able to use a telehealth video examination or alternative destinations to help identify and treat patients who have symptoms consistent with Bell palsy.

Herpes Zoster (Shingles)

Herpes zoster—or shingles—is an acute neuritis caused by reactivation of the varicella-zoster virus (also known as human herpes virus-3) in the dorsal root ganglion. The disorder causes significant dermatomal neuropathic pain prior to or concomitant with a characteristic rash. Routine childhood vaccination began in 1995, and currently, a booster vaccine is recommended for adults older than 50 years of age, thus decreasing the incidence of the disease every year.

Pathophysiology

Varicella zoster virus causes primary infection in unvaccinated patients via transmission through direct contact with vesicular fluid. Disseminated shingles leads to greater risk of airborne and droplet transmission. The virus then spreads, causing the primary infection known as chickenpox. After the primary infection resolves, the virus remains latent in the dorsal root ganglion. As immunity from primary infection wanes, the virus may reactivate, causing shingles along a single or multiple dermatomes with associated pain and loss of function. It is possible to develop shingles after having been vaccinated for chickenpox as a child but there is significantly less risk for these patients.

Signs and Symptoms

As shingles can affect any dermatome in the body, and the pain and nerve dysfunction typically precede the characteristic rash, patients will call EMS with a variety of symptoms that may all be presentations of herpes zoster. Patients typically have a prodrome of headache and malaise. Then they develop pain, described as burning or itching, and paresthesia in a unilateral dermatomal fashion. The chest and abdomen are commonly affected areas, and as such, may possibly be the cause of chest and abdominal pain. The face is another commonly affected area and has specific associated conditions that may require subspecialty care.

Patients will eventually develop a characteristic vesicular rash in a dermatomal fashion (**Figure 8-12**). The rash does not cross the midline. Zoster that affects the forehead and eyelid may cause zoster opthalmicus, leading to corneal damage. Zoster oticus can cause Ramsay-Hunt syndrome and lead to facial nerve palsy, resembling a stroke, and hearing damage. Zoster that affects three or more dermatomes, especially in an immunocompromised patient, should raise suspicion for disseminated varicella, which is a life-threatening systemic viral infection.

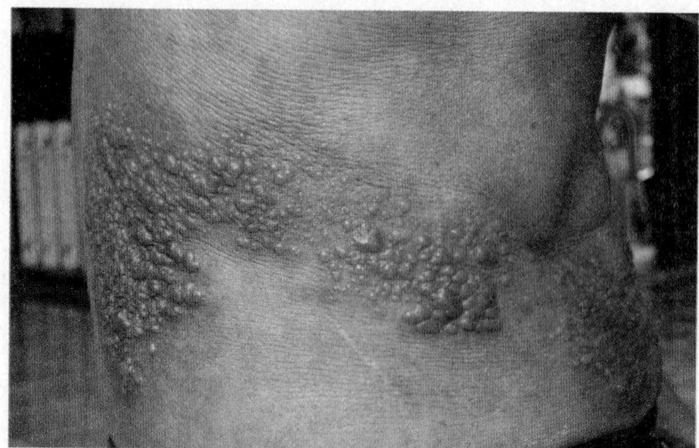

Figure 8-12 Shingles rash.

Differential Diagnosis

Shingles is a very specific rash and therefore is usually diagnosed clinically. Other causes of painful/itchy vesicular rash include poison ivy/oak contact dermatitis, chickenpox, monkeypox, and herpes gladiatorum. Shingles should also be in the differential for headache, chest pain, abdominal pain, back pain, or any extremity pain in a dermatomal fashion.

Treatment

Most patients who exhibit symptoms limited to dermatomal pain and rash do not have a life-threatening condition, and the role of the EMS clinician is to evaluate for other life-threatening disorders, transport to an appropriate location, and provide symptomatic care such as pain control. The rare presentation of disseminated varicella can cause end-organ damage, including pneumonitis, leading to respiratory failure, encephalitis, and hepatitis requiring resuscitative measures and airway/respiratory support.

Spinal Epidural Abscess

Spinal epidural abscess is a condition where purulent infectious material is present in the space between the spinal column and the dural layer of the spinal cord. This can cause compression of the spinal cord and spinal nerve roots, causing paralysis, weakness, pain, and loss of function. Abscesses usually present with fever, but an absence of fever does not rule out this diagnosis. This diagnosis is often not considered, even though it is a potential cause of severe permanent disability. The astute medical clinician will incorporate the features of this diagnosis into the history and physical examination and can potentially prevent lifelong disability if the abscess is identified in time to allow for appropriate antibiotic and surgical intervention.

Pathophysiology

The spinal cord lies in the bony spinal canal and, like the brain, is covered by a protective layer (the dura mater) that sequesters the nerve tissue from surrounding tissues. Spinal epidural abscess develops when infection occurs between the dura and the spinal canal. This can occur from local spread related to cellulitis of the back, discitis, or vertebral osteomyelitis or from hematogenous spread of bacteria from remote or systemic infections or illicit IV substance use. As purulent material accumulates in the epidural space, compression of the spinal cord, nerve roots, or the blood vessels may occur.

Risk factors for the development of spinal epidural abscess include any form of immunocompromise, including alcohol use disorder, diabetes mellitus, HIV/AIDS, cancer, chemotherapy, chronic corticosteroid use, and any pharmacologic forms of immunosuppression. This can include known immunosuppressive agents for the transplant patient or immunomodulating agents used for conditions such as rheumatoid arthritis and Crohn disease. Additionally, patients with a history of recent spinal trauma, surgery, or instrumentation (including injections, epidural anesthesia, or lumbar puncture); IV substance use; indwelling catheter; dental infection or procedures; septicemia/bacteremia; overlying cellulitis; or vertebral osteomyelitis are also at risk.

Signs and Symptoms

Patients typically present with back pain, which can occur at any spinal level. Given that abscesses can form in multiple locations and are not necessarily contiguous, patients can have pain in multiple locations of the spinal column. Patients usually also present with infectious-type symptoms, including generalized malaise, fever, chills/rigors, and headache. Those with more progressive disease and spinal compression may show signs/symptoms of neurologic impairment, with weakness, numbness, paresthesias, and rapidly progressive paraparesis or paraplegia. Bowel and bladder incontinence may or may not be present, depending on the level of the compressive lesion. Key findings include the following:

- Back pain, present at any or multiple sites in the spine
- Neurologic deficit (weakness, numbness, tingling, paraparesis)
- Recent instrumentation of the spine (epidural anesthesia, injections, or surgery)
- Immunocompromise or IV substance use

Differential Diagnosis

The differential diagnosis for spinal epidural abscess includes tumor, hematoma, Guillain-Barré syndrome, myelitis, spinal infarct, spinal cord syndrome, meningitis, trauma, and other compressive lesions.

Treatment

Prehospital treatment of spinal epidural abscess is predominantly supportive. Patients who meet sepsis criteria should be treated according to local sepsis protocol. Pain control will be important, with an emphasis of establishing a realistic pain goal with the patient. This will be especially important in the chronic opioid user, who may not respond to standard doses of opioid analgesia. The definitive diagnostic test is MRI, and the definitive treatment is usually surgical in addition to antibiotics. Patients should be transported to a facility with neurosurgical and MRI capability.

Migraine Headaches

Migraine headaches are mild to severe recurrent headaches sometimes accompanied by neurologic symptoms such as cognitive or visual disturbances, dizziness, nausea, and vomiting. The headache may be either unilateral or bilateral. Migraines often begin in childhood and become more frequent during adolescence or early adulthood. About 80% of patients experience their first migraine before age 30 years, and the headaches tend to become less frequent after age 50 years. Common migraine triggers include the following:

- Stress
- Illness
- Physical activity
- Changes in sleep pattern
- High altitude and other barometric pressure changes
- Skipping meals
- Use of certain medications (such as oral contraceptives)
- Ingestion of caffeine, alcohol, and certain foods
- Exposure to bright lights, loud noises, or unpleasant odors

Pathophysiology

The pathophysiology of migraine headaches is not completely understood. Research suggests that **neurotransmitters** in the brain, such as serotonin and dopamine, stimulate an inflammatory cascade that causes vasodilation, which is responsible for the pain. Some of the symptoms associated with migraine headaches, such as nausea and vomiting, are also associated with dopamine receptor activation. Many dopamine antagonists have been clinically shown to be effective in treating migraines.

Signs and Symptoms

An aura consisting of dizziness, tinnitus, and a perception of flashing lights or zigzagging lines in the visual field may signal or accompany the migraine. The headache is often described as throbbing and unilateral and accompanied by photophobia and/or phonophobia, although a wide variety of neurologic symptoms have been associated with or attributed to migraine syndrome. Subtypes of migraine may include ocular (scotomata or transient blindness), hemiplegic (some of which lead to permanent weakness with brain infarction), and brainstem (associated with vertigo, dysarthria, tinnitus, diplopia, or ataxia). Migraines usually last 4 to 72 hours, and the patient often prefers to be in a quiet, dark room and may initially attempt to treat the headache with over-the-counter medication. Key findings include the following:

- Headache
- Photophobia
- Nausea/vomiting
- Increased sensitivity to sound or smell
- History of migraines

Differential Diagnosis

The differential diagnosis for migraine headaches includes other primary headache (such as cluster or tension), infections (such as meningitis and sinusitis), temporal arteritis, and ischemic or hemorrhagic stroke or bleeding. In addition, increased ICP from a brain tumor, idiopathic intracranial hypertension, a leaking aneurysm, or opiate withdrawal may also cause headaches that resemble migraines. Given the broad differential diagnosis for migraine headache, care should be taken to not presume headaches with associated neurologic symptoms are "only" migraines without further evaluation and testing. In other words, an "atypical" or "subtype" migraine headache as described previously should only be diagnosed after other concerning diagnoses, such as acute stroke, are ruled out.

Treatment

Although patients may appear to be uncomfortable, their conditions are usually stable. Opioid analgesia is not indicated. Treatment with antiemetics may help break the cycle and intensity of the migraine as well as treat accompanying nausea. Medications that are frequently used in the ED to treat migraine headaches are also available to some EMS clinicians. These include IV prochlorperazine, droPERidol, or ketorolac. IV fluids may be helpful if the patient has been vomiting.

Patients with a history of migraine headaches may mistake a stroke or other emergent condition for an especially bad migraine or complex migraine. Be alert for sudden changes in neurologic status should one of these other conditions be present.

Because the differential diagnosis includes stroke and intracranial hemorrhage, transport the patient to a facility that can care for these medical conditions. Patients may prefer to be transported without lights or siren or with their eyes closed or covered because they may be highly sensitive to light and sound. Supportive care is usually all that is necessary during transport.

Carotid Artery Dissection

The internal carotid arteries supply the brain with oxygenated blood. Carotid artery dissection begins with a tear in the innermost layer of the artery. Circulating blood enters the tear, quickly dissecting (separating) the innermost and middle layers. This mechanical process compresses the lumen (the hollow interior space) of the artery so blood flow is partially or completely obstructed, potentially triggering an ischemic stroke.

Carotid artery dissection is an unusual cause of ischemic stroke (see Figure 8-6B). This kind of stroke can occur in any age group but tends to appear most often in people younger than age 50 years. Carotid artery dissection represents about one-fourth of all strokes that occur in teens and young adults, often striking while they are engaged in physical activity. Men and women are roughly equally affected.

Pathophysiology

The initial tear in the inner layer of the artery wall may be attributable to traumatic injury, connective tissue disease, hypertension, atherosclerosis, or some other pathologic process. The false lumen created by the dissection may be on the inside of the middle layer leading to stenosis and obstruction of the true lumen or on the outside of the middle layer leading to aneurysm and possible rupture.

The dissection of the internal carotid artery can occur inside or outside the skull. Extracranial dissection occurs most frequently because the skull tends to absorb the force of any traumatic impact. Sophisticated imaging studies are often required to make this diagnosis, because the signs and symptoms of the condition are ambiguous.

Signs and Symptoms

Patients with carotid artery dissection may complain of unilateral headache, neck, or facial pain, and they may report a recent traumatic injury. You may note a Horner syndrome on the affected side, characterized by ptosis (drooping) of the eyelid, miosis (a constricted pupil), and facial anhidrosis (a lack of perspiration). The syndrome is usually the result of unilateral sympathetic nerve compression due to tumor, trauma, or vascular disorders.

The patient may present after physical activity or after an event that is normally innocuous, such as coughing or sneezing; neck extension, such as when painting a ceiling; or chiropractic adjustment. Pain, usually in the head, back, or face, is often the initial symptom of a spontaneous, nontraumatic dissection. The headache is described as constant, severe, and unilateral. Patients may present with pulsatile tinnitus (a sensation of hearing or feeling the pulsation of each heartbeat in the ear). Physical findings may include hemiparesis, cervical spine trauma, cervical bruit, or cranial nerve palsy. Key findings include the following:

- Unilateral pain in head or neck
- Vision changes
- Pupil constriction, especially unilaterally

Differential Diagnosis

The differential diagnosis for a carotid artery dissection includes neck trauma, other causes of stroke (either hemorrhagic or ischemic), subarachnoid hemorrhage, TIA, electrolyte abnormality, headache, cervical spine fracture, near-hanging injury, and direct neck trauma from a "clothesline-type" injury.

Treatment

If trauma preceded the dissection, restrict movement of the patient's spine. Provide supportive care, and monitor airway, breathing, and circulation. The patient should be transported to a hospital with neurologic and vascular capabilities and able to perform interventional radiologic procedures.

Tumors

A brain tumor, or intracranial neoplasm, is the inappropriate proliferation of cells forming a mass that invades and compresses the surrounding healthy parenchymal tissue. Tumors are classified as either primary or metastatic and benign or malignant. *Primary* means the tumor originates in the brain. A metastatic tumor arises when cells migrate from a tumor elsewhere in the body, such as cutaneous melanoma or lung cancer, travel through the bloodstream, and begin to grow in the brain. Primary malignant lesions account for about half of all intracranial tumors and tend to be aggressive, invasive, and life threatening. Primary benign tumors tend to grow more slowly and are less aggressive, but they can still be life threatening if they arise in vital areas such as the brainstem.

Tumors are often classified by cell type, such as meningioma or glioma, but prehospital treatment is the same regardless of cell type.

Pathophysiology

Brain tumors may damage neural pathways by mass effect or infiltration of normal brain tissue. Tumors that arise near the third and fourth ventricles may obstruct the flow of CSF, causing hydrocephalus. Blood vessels that form to support the tumors may disrupt the blood–brain barrier and cause edema or may rupture, leading to hemorrhage.

Signs and Symptoms

The signs and symptoms of a brain tumor are nonspecific. The patient may have headaches, altered mental status, nausea, vomiting, weakness, alterations in gait, or even subtle behavioral changes. Focal seizure, visual changes, speech deficit, and sensory abnormalities are also possible. The patient may not notice symptoms, even as the tumor grows rather large, but often seeks treatment when an acute change in symptoms occurs. Such a change is often precipitated by an obstruction of CSF flow or hemorrhage.

Key findings may differ depending on where the tumor is located (Table 8-12). Other signs and symptoms include the following:

- Focal weakness
- Visual changes
- Dizziness/vertigo
- Nausea/vomiting

Differential Diagnosis

The differential diagnosis for brain tumor includes infection, stroke, and intracranial bleeding.

Treatment

Provide supportive care on the basis of the patient's symptoms. Edema, hydrocephalus, intracranial hemorrhage, pituitary infarction, infarction of the parenchyma (usually caused by compression of blood vessels), and seizures can cause the patient to deteriorate abruptly. Be prepared to intervene in the event the patient's level of consciousness suddenly diminishes or a seizure occurs.

Patients with a suspected brain tumor should be brought to a hospital that has oncology and neurosurgical backup. If the patient has rapid decompensation and the treating team is concerned for edema/swelling, hypertonic saline or mannitol may be given to reduce ICP until the patient can receive neurosurgical intervention. Steroids may also be given to reduce swelling.

Table 8-12 Key Findings of Brain Tumors by Location

Location of Tumor	Key Findings
Frontal lobe	Behavioral disinhibition Memory loss Decreased alertness Diminished sense of smell
Temporal lobe	Emotional changes Behavioral disturbances
Pituitary	Visual changes Impotence Changes in the menstrual cycle
Occipital lobe	Visual field deficits
Brainstem or cerebellum	Cranial nerve palsies Reduced coordination Nystagmus Sensory deficits on either side of the body

Idiopathic Intracranial Hypertension

Idiopathic intracranial hypertension used to be known as *pseudotumor cerebri* or *false tumor* because its symptoms mimic those of a brain tumor. The condition is characterized by the poor resorption of CSF from the subarachnoid space. Idiopathic intracranial hypertension predominantly affects obese women in their childbearing years. Papilledema, or the swelling of the optic nerve, is the most worrisome problem and is due to chronically elevated ICP. Papilledema leads to progressive optic nerve atrophy and blindness.

Pathophysiology

The cause of idiopathic intracranial hypertension, as its name suggests, remains elusive. Some studies have found a decreased outflow of CSF into the dural venous sinus. Others suggest that increased blood flow impedes the brain's ability to drain CSF.

Signs and Symptoms

Elevated ICP may lead the patient to seek medical attention for headaches that are nonspecific and tend to vary in type, location, and frequency but are often worse when lying flat. Pulsatile tinnitus (ringing or sensation of vibration in the ears with each heartbeat) and horizontal diplopia (double vision) are other symptoms. Uncommonly, the patient may have pain that radiates into the arms. Affected individuals may have orthostatic hypotension after bending over and standing up again, causing episodes of syncope. Papilledema may lead to blurriness, intermittent dimming, or blacking out of vision in one or both eyes. The patient may have progressive loss of peripheral vision, usually starting in the nasal lower quadrant and then moving to the central visual field, followed by loss of color vision. Key findings include the following:

- Headache
- Vision disturbance and papilledema
- Younger, obese female patients

Differential Diagnosis

The differential diagnosis for idiopathic intracranial hypertension includes aseptic meningitis, Lyme disease, vascular tumors such as meningioma, arteriovenous malformation, stroke, hydrocephalus, intracranial abscess, intracranial bleeding, migraine headache, and lupus.

Treatment

Little can be done for the patient in the prehospital arena. Prehospital care is typically supportive only.

At the hospital, visual acuity testing, ophthalmologic examination, lumbar puncture, and imaging studies may be required. Blood and CSF must be examined to rule out differential diagnoses. The patient may be placed on medication and may require drainage of CSF by lumbar puncture or surgical care, including placement or adjustment of an intracranial shunt.

Brain Abscess

A brain abscess is an infection that begins when an organism from a site outside the CNS penetrates the blood–brain barrier to enter the brain. Initially, inflammation occurs, turning into a collection of pus around which a well-vascularized capsule usually forms.

Pathophysiology

Certain bacteria (*Streptococcus, Pseudomonas, Bacteroides*) typically enter from the sinuses, mouth, middle ear, or mastoid (area located behind the ear) through veins draining directly into the brain from these sites. Other bacteria (*Staphylococcus, Streptococcus, Klebsiella, Escherichia, Pseudomonas*) enter via the arteries from distant sites. Direct spread from penetrating trauma or surgical procedures may also be a source of bacterial infection (*Staphylococcus, Clostridium, Pseudomonas*) in the brain. Include surgical history and history of trauma, history of indwelling catheters, and recent ear infection in the history of present illness. About one-fourth of abscesses have no clear source. Patients who have compromised immune systems, use IV drugs, have prosthetic valves, or are chronic steroid users, as well as patients with near drowning or submersion injury and patients who have had extensive dental procedures are at risk for brain abscesses caused by the spread of bacteria.

Signs and Symptoms

A patient who has a brain abscess most often complains of a headache. A focal neurologic deficit consistent with the site of infection may be present. The triad of headache, fever, and focal neurologic deficit is seldom seen. Seizures, altered mental status, nausea or vomiting, and stiff neck may also indicate a brain abscess. A sudden worsening of the headache may indicate rupture of the abscess into the CSF. Patients who are immunocompromised, either due to medication or underlying illness such as HIV/AIDS, are at particular risk of having a brain abscess. Immunosuppression is becoming more common, especially with the development of multiple immunomodulating agents for disorders such as Crohn disease, ulcerative colitis, and rheumatoid arthritis, among other conditions. Index of suspicion must be increased in this patient population. Key findings include the following:

- Fever
- Altered mental status, such as confusion or diminished level of consciousness
- Neck stiffness/meningismus
- Headache
- Nausea/vomiting
- Focal deficit consistent with the location of the abscess

Differential Diagnosis

Beyond the wide range of bacterial infections that must be considered, the differential diagnosis for a brain abscess includes headache, hypertension, intracranial bleeding, viral and bacterial meningitis, fungal infection, and tumor.

Treatment

Brain abscesses are life threatening. With early recognition and intervention, however, morbidity and mortality have declined. Provide supportive care for the patient. Monitor the patient's airway, breathing, and circulation; administer oxygen; and give IV fluids. If the patient has a seizure or decompensates, be prepared to provide the appropriate interventions. Although these patients are at risk of dying as a result of the mass effect of the abscess, its interference with brain function, and sepsis, this rarely happens acutely. Nevertheless, the abscess may rupture or cause bleeding in the brain, and the patient's condition may quickly deteriorate.

At the hospital, laboratory and radiologic studies and possibly a lumbar puncture or brain biopsy will be performed, and antibiotics will be administered.

Normal-Pressure Hydrocephalus

Normal-pressure hydrocephalus (NPH) is characterized by an excessive volume of CSF in the ventricles but normal CSF pressure when determined by lumbar puncture. The classic triad of symptoms includes urinary incontinence, abnormal gait, and cognitive disturbance, which are often reversible. The average age of onset is over 60 years and the overlap of symptoms with chronic dementia make it a commonly missed diagnosis.

Pathophysiology

A patient with NPH has an increased volume of CSF in the ventricles. The excess CSF is believed to put pressure on the nerve fibers exiting the cerebral cortex, leading to clinical findings. The exact cause of NPH is not known but is thought to be an imbalance between the rate of CSF production and CSF resorption.

Signs and Symptoms

The patient with NPH typically presents with the triad of gait disturbance, urinary incontinence, and cognitive impairment. The patient tends to have a shuffling, widened gait and usually has difficulty taking the first step, much like a patient with Parkinson disease. Urinary incontinence is experienced, and, in the early stages, the patient may have urinary urgency and frequency. Cognitive impairment typically consists of apathy, psychomotor slowing, decreased attention span, and inability to concentrate. Key findings include the following:

- Altered gait
- Urinary incontinence
- Altered mental status

Differential Diagnosis

The differential diagnosis for NPH includes Alzheimer disease and other causes of dementia, stroke, Parkinson disease, electrolyte abnormalities, toxicity, and idiopathic increased ICP.

Treatment

On the scene and during transport, provide physical and emotional support to the patient. Once the diagnosis has been made by means of radiologic and laboratory studies in the ED setting, the patient may have CSF removed and a shunt placed to allow continuous CSF shunting to decrease volume and pressure.

Careful monitoring and documentation of vital signs, historical data, and physical exam findings will be useful to the ED team at the receiving facility. Emergency interventions are usually not necessary but remain alert in case the patient has a seizure.

Transport the patient to a hospital that offers neurosurgical support.

Cerebral Venous Thrombosis

Cerebral venous thrombosis (CVT) is a blood clot that forms in the veins and dural sinuses of the brain. The condition, once thought to be rare because it was diagnosed only at autopsy, has been shown with advanced imaging techniques to be more common than previously believed. It affects women more often than men, and it tends to occur in early adulthood or middle age.

Pathophysiology

CVT typically occurs in persons with an underlying risk factor, such as a hypercoagulable state (an abnormally increased tendency to form blood clots, which can occur during pregnancy, malignancy, and with the use of oral contraceptives), facial or sinus infection, or head trauma. The clotted blood can be in a localized area or involve large areas of the venous system. CVT can lead to cerebral edema and/or increased ICP and thereby result in global or focal neurologic dysfunction.

Signs and Symptoms

The most common chief complaint, occurring in 90% of patients with CVT, is headache, which may be localized initially and then more diffuse as the condition progresses. Local effects on the brain can lead to strokelike symptoms, particularly ophthalmoplegia (dysfunction of eye movement), whereas increased ICP will lead to more generalized effects and visual disturbances. Cranial nerve palsies can be seen with cavernous sinus thrombosis. Nausea and vomiting are frequently present, and seizures may occur. Other symptoms may include hemiparesis, aphasia, ataxia (altered gait), dizziness, tinnitus (ringing in the ears), diplopia (double vision), and facial weakness. Key findings include the following:

- Headache
- Nausea/vomiting
- Visual changes
- Tinnitus

Differential Diagnosis

The differential diagnosis for CVT includes acute stroke, head injury, idiopathic intracranial hypertension, optic neuritis, nerve palsy, seizure, infection, and lupus.

Treatment

Provide supportive care en route to the hospital. As with a stroke, airway patency and adequate ventilation should be ensured. To prevent aspiration if the patient has an altered mental status or cranial nerve palsy, do not provide the patient with anything to eat or drink. Fluids may be given intravenously, and supplemental oxygen may be provided for hypoxia. Treat seizures according to protocol.

At the hospital, the patient will usually undergo CT or MRI imaging, and infectious processes will be ruled out. Laboratory studies, including a lumbar puncture, may be done, and the patient may be placed on blood thinners to prevent further clotting. Because patients with blood clots in the venous sinuses are often given thrombolytic agents using a surgically placed microcatheter, interventional radiology or neurosurgery backup at the hospital is recommended.

Hypertensive Encephalopathy and Malignant Hypertension

Hypertensive emergencies involve dysfunction of the brain, kidney, or heart in the setting of severe hypertension. *Hypertensive encephalopathy* describes the neurologic symptoms associated with extremely elevated blood pressure; malignant hypertension further includes retinal hemorrhage and papilledema. These symptoms are usually reversible when blood pressure is lowered.

Most patients with hypertensive encephalopathy already have a history of hypertension. For those who do not, history taking may require specifically focused questions to identify the cause of the high blood pressure, including the use of drugs.

Pathophysiology

In healthy patients, cerebral autoregulation preserves steady-state cerebral blood flow through a range of MAP, roughly from 50 to 150 mm Hg. In chronically hypertensive patients, the range of effective autoregulation is shifted to a higher range to allow protection at higher blood pressures. When blood pressure elevates dramatically, cerebral autoregulation is overcome, leading to increased pressure in the intracranial vessels, vascular damage, and compromise of the blood–brain barrier. These events lead to capillary fluid leak and resultant cerebral edema. In the eye, increased ICP can cause retinal hemorrhages and lead to papilledema.

Signs and Symptoms

The patient may have a headache, confusion, visual disturbances, seizure, nausea, or vomiting. Be alert for other end-organ damage, such as aortic dissection, acute heart failure, ACS, palpitations, papilledema, or hematuria (blood in the urine).

Key findings include the following:

- Hypertension
- Headache
- Nausea/vomiting
- Visual changes
- Altered mental status or focal neurologic deficits

Differential Diagnosis

A patient who has symptoms consistent with hypertensive encephalopathy may also have renal disease, pheochromocytoma, or preeclampsia or eclampsia (in pregnant patients). The patient may have ingested a specific food or medication that caused a blood pressure spike or may be in withdrawal from antihypertensive agents or alcohol. However, hypertension can be an effect of another pathologic process or even simply due to pain, rather than a cause of symptoms. Bleeding in the brain, trauma, and stroke should also be considered as part of the differential diagnosis.

Treatment

Give supplemental oxygen if indicated and start an IV. Specific intervention to lower blood pressure is generally warranted only if the systolic blood pressure $>$ 220 mm Hg or the diastolic blood pressure is $>$ 120 mm Hg. For most ground EMS, the only medication available is nitroglycerin, although some clinicians are now carrying angiotensin-converting enzyme (ACE) inhibitors such as captopril, for sublingual administration, and enalapril, which is given by the IV route. Treatment on critical care ambulances and in the hospital may include IV vasodilators and beta blockers. Remember to be cautious if antihypertensive medications are initiated, because lowering blood pressure rapidly can cause serious complications such as ischemic stroke or myocardial infarction. Blood pressure should not be lowered by more than 25% acutely, with a diastolic blood pressure of 100 mm Hg a reasonable goal within 6 hours.

Because patients who are acutely hypertensive may have a sudden intracranial hemorrhage and lose consciousness or become unable to protect their own airway, be prepared to take appropriate steps if the airway is lost.

Wernicke Encephalopathy and Korsakoff Syndrome

Wernicke encephalopathy and Korsakoff syndrome are thought to be different stages of the same pathologic process, with the former progressing to the latter. Acute deficiency of thiamine, or vitamin B_1, can cause the disorder known as **Wernicke encephalopathy**, which is characterized by a triad of symptoms: acute confusion, ataxia, and **ophthalmoplegia** (abnormal function of the eye muscles). However, only one-third of affected patients demonstrate all three features of the triad.

Korsakoff syndrome is the term for the late stages of the disease, especially memory loss. The syndrome is often seen in alcoholics, but it can occur in any patient who has malnutrition, such as those on long-term hemodialysis and patients with AIDS. The average age at diagnosis of the syndrome is about 50 years, but the syndrome can occur in younger patients who have metabolic disorders, receive parenteral nutrition, or have a diet deficient in thiamine or other vitamins.

Pathophysiology

Thiamine plays a key role in the metabolism of carbohydrates. If too little thiamine is available, these cellular systems fail, leading to inadequate usable energy and subsequent cell death. The systems most critically affected are those that have high metabolic needs, such as the brain. Energy production decreases and neuronal damage occurs, causing cellular edema and further nervous system injury.

Signs and Symptoms

A diagnosis of Wernicke encephalopathy should be considered for any patient who has evidence of alcohol overuse or malnutrition and acute symptoms of confusion, ocular dysfunction, and memory disturbance. The ocular problems most commonly seen are nystagmus, bilateral lateral rectus palsies, and dysconjugate gaze. Blindness is not usually seen.

The encephalopathy may manifest as global confusion, apathy, agitation, or inattentiveness. Significant mental status changes, such as coma or unresponsiveness, are rarely seen. About 80% of patients have some peripheral neuropathy. Hypotension, nausea, and temperature instability may also be caused by thiamine deficiency. Infants may have constipation, agitation, vomiting, diarrhea, anorexia, eye disorders, or altered mental status, including seizures and loss of consciousness. Key findings include the following:

- Confusion or behavioral changes
- Eye movement abnormalities, particularly nystagmus

Differential Diagnosis

The differential diagnosis for Wernicke encephalopathy includes alcohol or illicit drug intoxication, delirium, dementia, stroke, psychosis, closed head injury, encephalopathy secondary to liver failure, and postictal state.

Treatment

At the hospital, the patient will undergo an array of possible laboratory and radiologic tests, such as blood tests, electrolyte measurement, lumbar puncture, arterial blood gas readings, and a CT scan and MRI to evaluate differential diagnoses.

In the prehospital setting, focus on stabilizing the airway, ensuring oxygenation, and maintaining blood pressure and volume control. If the condition is suspected, empirical thiamine replacement should be initiated. Thiamine can be given orally, but to ensure absorption, it is often administered IV or IM. The initial dose of thiamine is typically 100 mg, but over time as much as 500 mg may be needed to reverse the encephalopathy.

Some clinicians have expressed concern about giving patients dextrose before administering thiamine if they are in a thiamine-deficient state. The concern is that dextrose will exacerbate the encephalopathy. However, this effect is seen only in patients receiving long-term dextrose administration without concurrent thiamine administration. It is safe to give dextrose alone in the prehospital setting for hypoglycemic events, even if thiamine is not immediately available.

Thiamine and glucose should be given to patients who have an altered mental status if there is a chance that Wernicke encephalopathy is being considered as a diagnosis. Previously, this therapy was given empirically in the prehospital setting. Currently, it is rarely administered by EMS. No special transport decisions must be made. The patient may be brought to any hospital, but children should be brought to a pediatric specialty center if one is available.

Temporal Arteritis

Temporal arteritis, also known as *giant cell arteritis*, is an inflammation of the temporal arteries that causes throbbing or burning pain in the area of the temples, often accompanied by jaw pain when chewing, visual disturbances, and other symptoms. Other arteries may be inflamed as well. The condition tends to affect adults age 50 years and older, especially women in their 70s.

Pathophysiology

The exact pathophysiology of temporal arteritis is unknown. Some researchers speculate it has an infectious cause, but this has never been proven. Another hypothesis implicates an autoimmune response that stimulates T-cell proliferation in the arterial walls.

Signs and Symptoms

The patient usually reports a headache and scalp tenderness in the area of the temporal artery. The headache has a subacute onset and, although often in the temporal area, it may be in any region or generalized. In addition, about half the patients have jaw claudication (pain that worsens when chewing). Fever is also common. A frequent and very concerning complication is visual disturbance in the ipsilateral eye, including transient (amaurosis fugax) or permanent vision loss. Sometimes the patient reports hearing loss or vertigo. Other signs and symptoms include diaphoresis, anorexia (loss of appetite) with accompanying weight loss, muscle aches, fatigue, weakness, mouth sores, and bleeding gums. Key findings include the following:

- Headache (usually unilateral and temporal)
- Temporal scalp tenderness and/or erythema
- Visual changes (usually in one eye)
- Older adult

Differential Diagnosis

The differential diagnosis for temporal arteritis includes other inflammatory rheumatic diseases, malignancies, migraine headache, tumor, and infection.

Treatment

Provide supportive care. At the receiving facility, the patient may undergo a battery of tests, including blood tests, radiologic studies, and temporal artery biopsy. Patients who are believed to have temporal arteritis are usually prescribed a high dose of corticosteroids to reduce vascular inflammation.

Cauda Equina Syndrome

Cauda equina syndrome is a disorder in which the nerve roots exiting from the end of the spinal cord in the lower lumbar and sacral region of the spine become compressed, causing lower extremity pain, weakness, or paralysis; bladder and bowel incontinence or retention; and loss of sexual function. This syndrome is an emergent condition, and surgical intervention is necessary to prevent permanent loss of function.

Pathophysiology

Anatomically, the cauda equina resembles a horse's tail. It is formed by the nerve roots in the spinal canal distal to the spinal cord, which ends at the L1–L2 level. Cauda equina syndrome is due to compression of the nerve roots, which may be caused by trauma, disk herniation, tumors and other spinal cord lesions, and spinal stenosis (narrowing of the spinal canal). The nerve roots in the lumbar part of the spinal cord are susceptible to injury because they lack a well-developed covering, or epineurium, which may protect against stretch and compression injury.

Signs and Symptoms

The patient affected by cauda equina syndrome may have low back pain, radicular pain in the buttocks or lower extremities unilaterally or bilaterally, saddle sensory disturbances in the perineum, and bowel or bladder dysfunction. Variable lower extremity motor and sensory changes caused by compression of the nerve roots may also be present, and lower extremity reflexes may be diminished or absent. Back pain is the most common complaint. If the patient does not voluntarily relate a history of urinary or bowel incontinence or retention, or of weakness, numbness, and tingling in lower extremities, be sure to ask. An accurate medical history is key to making the diagnosis, and discretion and confidentiality may be required to elicit important historical factors. Key findings include the following:

- Low back pain, often with radiation down the legs
- Bowel or bladder incontinence or retention
- Recent manipulation of the spine (such as during a lumbar puncture or surgery)
- Trauma

Differential Diagnosis

The differential diagnosis includes back pain attributable to trauma and other causes, tumor, epidural abscess, transverse myelitis, Guillain-Barré syndrome, spinal cord compression, metabolic abnormalities, and other nerve disorders.

Treatment

Prehospital care is mainly supportive, including pain control if needed. A patient suspected of having cauda equina syndrome may require spinal motion restriction for transport if there is an underlying traumatic cause that could be worsened with movement.

Although prehospital intervention is not usually necessary, and cauda equina syndrome is not fatal, the neurologic impairment may be permanent, causing significant disability if not treated with emergency surgery. Therefore, with any possible suspicion of cauda equina syndrome or undifferentiated low back pain, transport to the ED should be recommended. MRI is the definitive diagnostic test.

Parkinson Disease

Parkinson disease is a chronically progressive neurologic movement disorder caused by a decrease of functional dopamine in the brain. The disorder is rather common, affecting nearly 1 million people in the United States. Symptoms progress from a resting tremor to late-stage dementia.

Pathophysiology

Parkinson disease is characterized by the progressive loss of neurons in the substantia nigra, the part of the brain that produces dopamine. Dopamine serves as a neurotransmitter in signaling intended motor activity. The dead neurons contain clumps of abnormal protein called *Lewy bodies*, the significance of which is still poorly understood.

Signs and Symptoms

As symptoms of Parkinson disease develop slowly, patients can often go years before being formally diagnosed. A vague premotor phase may include constipation, restless legs, decreased smell, and difficulty with sleep, but these are nonspecific. Initial motor symptoms are usually subtle such as mild tremors, mild weakness such as difficulty getting up from a chair, and lack of normal facial expression. As symptoms progress, diagnosis is made based on the four hallmark neurologic symptoms characterized by the mnemonic TRAP:

- Resting **tremor** (flapping motion of distal extremities at rest)
- Cogwheel **rigidity** (rigidity of muscles with both flexion and extension)
- **Akinesia** or bradykinesia (inability to perform or slowly performing certain movements such as rapid alternating movements)
- **Postural** impairment or disequilibrium (leads to shuffling gait)

This middle stage is highly responsive to medications, and patients who are compliant can often live near-normal lives. After medical and surgical therapies have been maxed out, patients enter late-stage Parkinson disease, which is characterized by severe motor disability unresponsive to medications, incontinence, orthostatic hypotension, and Parkinson dementia.

Differential Diagnosis

Parkinsonism is a set of symptoms characteristic of Parkinson disease but attributable to another disorder, the most common being drugs or medications. Other conditions causing parkinsonism include AIDS, neurosyphilis, and brain tumors.

Treatment

Patients' symptoms are typically well controlled on medications for some time; however, as the disease progresses, various complications emerge, including dyskinesias, depression, hallucinations, and dementia. Respiratory failure is the most common cause of death. Prehospital care requires transport of the patient and support of the patient's airway, breathing, circulation, and vital signs. Administer oxygen, airway and ventilatory support, and fluid resuscitation per local protocol.

Because patients are on medications that increase dopamine levels in the brain, they are at risk for developing dopaminergic toxicity. Dopaminergic toxicity resembles the positive symptoms of schizophrenia, such as hallucinations, nightmares, sleep disturbances, paranoia, and acute psychosis, in addition to cardiac dysrhythmias, dystonia, and orthostatic hypotension. Patients may require sedation, but note that antipsychotics with antidopaminergic properties, particularly butyrophenones, such as haloperidol and droPERidol, and phenothiazines, such as prochlorperazine, should be avoided because they can worsen dystonia.

Abrupt withdrawal of a patient's dopaminergic medications can lead to parkinsonism-hyperpyrexia syndrome, which is similar in presentation to neuroleptic malignant syndrome. Patients will require cooling measures for hyperthermia, respiratory and circulatory support for dysautonomia, and possibly sedation for altered mental status.

Multiple Sclerosis

Multiple sclerosis (MS) is one of the most common causes of nontraumatic neurologic disease in younger patients. It affects females more often than males in a 3:1 ratio and is characterized by intermittent periods of acute neurologic dysfunction lasting weeks to months with gradual return to at or near baseline function. Some forms of multiple sclerosis are chronically progressive. The exact cause of MS is not well understood; however, advances in immunomodulators and suppression therapy, such as steroids, have improved morbidity significantly, and patients only have a mild reduction in life expectancy of 5 to 10 years.

Pathophysiology

MS is caused by an autoimmune phenomenon by which T cells attack the myelin sheath and oligodendrocytes, which are the cells of the CNS responsible for producing and maintaining the myelin sheath around cells and axons. Myelin acts as insulation for the axons, decreasing resistance and increasing the velocity of nerve signal transmission. The inflammatory/immune response leads to scar formation around the axons, thereby causing neurologic dysfunction.

Signs and Symptoms

Consistent with other upper motor neuron disorders, patients will present with weakness, sensory deficits, and hyperreflexia/spasticity. MS can affect any part of the CNS system and therefore can present differently from patient to patient. Optic neuritis, a painful eye condition with vision loss, is the initial presentation in almost one-third of patients. Other characteristic findings of MS are worsening of symptoms with increased body temperature, such as running, and Lhermitte sign, an electric shock sensation running down the spine and extremities with flexion of the neck.

Patients may have organ dysfunction such as respiratory distress from respiratory muscle dysfunction, cardiovascular collapse, incontinence from bladder or urethral dysfunction, and constipation or diarrhea from gastrointestinal dysfunction. Patients can also have hearing loss, vertigo, truncal ataxia, and many other CNS symptoms. Cognitive decline and seizures occur in a subset of patients with MS. Most patients who have been formally diagnosed with MS are very knowledgeable about their disorder and can describe an MS flare when it is occurring.

Differential Diagnosis

The differential diagnosis for MS includes intracranial hemorrhage, cervical artery dissection, Guillain-Barré syndrome, spinal cord tumor, anterior or central cord syndrome, and stroke.

Treatment

Prehospital care requires transport of the patient and support of the patient's airway, breathing, circulation, and vital signs as well as evaluating for other emergent neurologic disorders, such as a stroke. Administer oxygen and fluids for general weakness according to protocol.

At the hospital, the patient with MS will typically have a baseline evaluation in the ED with stabilization, including airway management, management of hypotension/shock, and evaluation for underlying sepsis (e.g., from urinary tract infection in patients with bladder dysfunction). IV steroid therapy may be initiated in the ED. However, most evaluation and management is guided by neurologists. Patients frequently have an MRI performed to look for new lesions around nerve cells and lumbar punctures to look for specific proteins associated with MS when the diagnosis is uncertain. Patients with vison complaints will also be evaluated by ophthalmology.

Amyotrophic Lateral Sclerosis (ALS)

Amyotrophic lateral sclerosis (ALS), also known in the United States as Lou Gehrig's disease, is characterized by degeneration of the upper and lower motor neurons causing voluntary muscles to weaken or atrophy. Onset peaks around age 60 years for the sporadic form (~90%) and around age 50 years for the familial form. It is more common in men and in Caucasian and non-Hispanic people. Patients usually die 3 to 5 years after diagnosis, although recent multidisciplinary approaches show some benefit. Death is attributable to respiratory muscle weakness, aspiration pneumonia, and malnutrition. Medical complications of immobility add to the morbidity and mortality of patients with this disorder.

Pathophysiology

ALS has no specific known cause. Scientists have recently identified a mutation in a gene that controls protein synthesis and synaptic function of motor neurons in some patients. However, this explanation accounts for only a small percentage of cases. Glutamate toxicity, mitochondrial dysfunction, and autoimmunity may all play a role in ALS, but researchers are still trying to find out precisely how.

Signs and Symptoms

Upper motor neuron findings in patients with ALS include spasticity and hyperreflexia. Lower motor findings include weakness, ataxia, and fasciculations. A bulbar form of the disease affects swallowing and speech.

The patient may seek acute medical care for limb weakness, difficulty speaking and swallowing, visual disturbances, and limb spasticity. Motor problems typically present from the periphery inward, starting with wrist drop, loss of finger dexterity, foot drop, and tongue fasciculations. The patient's lack of control over emotions may be present and may cause the patient to overreact to sad or humorous events or comments. Ocular, sensory, and autonomic dysfunction occur late in the disease, usually in patients who require ventilatory support. Weakness is often asymmetric and begins in the arms or legs. Difficulty chewing and swallowing occur late in the illness. Key findings include the following:

- Ascending and peripheral weakness moving upward and inward
- Mixed upper and lower motor neuron findings

Differential Diagnosis

The differential of ALS includes other types of neuromuscular disease, Guillain-Barré syndrome, multiple sclerosis, myasthenia gravis, spinal cord tumor, and stroke.

Treatment

Prehospital care requires support of the patient's airway, breathing, circulation, and vital signs. Administer oxygen and fluids for general weakness according to protocol.

At the hospital, the patient will undergo a battery of tests, including neurology consults and nerve conduction studies. Care is mainly symptomatic, and emotional support should be available to the patient and family. The patient's living will or do-not-resuscitate (DNR) orders should be followed. Complications such as pneumonia or other infections, deep vein thrombosis, or respiratory problems are common. These problems should be managed according to protocol.

Patients with ALS may decompensate from extreme weakness in the respiratory muscles, and corrective action must be taken. Airway management should proceed based on the patient's advance directives.

Guillain-Barré Syndrome

Guillain-Barré syndrome refers to a group of acute immune-mediated polyneuropathies, demyelinating disorders that cause weakness, numbness, or paralysis throughout the body. In the United States, the incidence of Guillain-Barré is 1 to 3 per 100,000 people. Although the syndrome can occur at any age, it is usually found in young adults and older adults. The condition affects men and women equally.

Pathophysiology

Guillain-Barré syndrome is believed to represent an autoimmune response to a recent infection or to many different types of medical problems. Researchers believe the body forms antibodies against the peripheral nerves, in particular the axons, which become demyelinated, leading to motor weakness and in some cases sensory loss. Recovery is typically associated with a brief remyelination period. It has been shown that many patients with Guillain-Barré syndrome are seropositive for *Campylobacter jejuni*.

Signs and Symptoms

The patient with Guillain-Barré often is seen initially with lower extremity muscle weakness, mainly in the thighs. The weakness usually appears a few weeks after a respiratory or gastrointestinal illness. Over the course of hours to days, the weakness may progress to involve the arms and chest muscles, facial muscles, and respiratory muscles. Approximately 12 days from onset, most patients will be at their worst and then will gradually begin to improve during the next few months.

Many patients with Guillain-Barré syndrome require mechanical ventilation during their illness to compensate for respiratory muscle weakness. In many cases, patients cannot stand or walk even though they feel strong. Loss of deep tendon reflexes is typical due to lower motor neuron involvement. In addition, the patient may initially have paresthesias in the feet, and then the hands. Pain may be present with the most minimal movements and is most impressive in the shoulder, back, buttocks, and thighs. The patient may experience a loss of ability to sense vibration; loss of proprioception and touch; and impressive autonomic dysfunction, including wide variation in vital signs, heart rate, and blood pressure. The patient may also have urinary retention, constipation, facial flushing, hypersalivation, anhidrosis, and tonic pupils. Key findings include the following:

- Progressive, symmetric weakness of legs, arms, face, and trunk
- Areflexia (absence of reflexes)
- Preceding illness

Differential Diagnosis

The differential diagnosis of Guillain-Barré is the same as that of a spinal cord infection or injury. Electrolyte abnormalities, including deficiencies of magnesium, potassium, and calcium, can cause muscle weakness. Infections such as meningitis, encephalitis, and botulism, as well as tickborne infections, also mimic this disease. In the early stages of the disease, Guillain-Barré may also be mistaken for MS; myasthenia gravis; toxic ingestion of alcohol, heavy metals, or organophosphates; diabetes; and HIV neuropathy.

Treatment

In the prehospital setting, management of airway, breathing, and circulation; administration of oxygen; and assisted ventilation (if needed) are of primary importance. If the patient has autonomic dysfunction, hypertension is best treated with short-acting agents; symptomatic bradycardia is best treated with atropine, and hypotension usually responds to IV fluids. Temporary cardiac pacing may be required if the patient has a second- or third-degree heart block. Because this is a rapidly progressing disease, it is important to recognize the likelihood that a patient will decompensate. Provide airway control and maintenance as necessary.

Myasthenia Gravis

Myasthenia gravis is a neuromuscular disorder that causes weakness due to impaired signal transmission from the motor neurons to the muscles at what is called the *neuromuscular junction*. Symptoms can be mild and limited to weakness of the muscles around the eyes, resulting in drooping eyelids or double vision, or severe enough to result in weakness of respiratory muscles.

Pathophysiology

When electrical impulses reach the end of motor neurons, the signal is passed to muscle cells at the neuromuscular junction. The nerve impulse causes release of acetylcholine from the presynaptic nerve cell that binds to acetylcholine receptors on the postsynaptic muscle cell, causing the muscle to contract. In myasthenia gravis, the immune system develops antibodies to the postsynaptic acetylcholine receptors. When these antibodies bind the receptors, the acetylcholine from the motor nerve is unable to bind the receptors on the muscle fibers, resulting in the inability to trigger muscle contraction.

Signs and Symptoms

Typically, the first symptom of myasthenia gravis is drooping eyelids, or ptosis. Further weakness of the extraocular muscles can result in diplopia, or double vision, which typically is more noticeable when looking sideways. The next symptoms are often related to weakness of facial and neck muscles, including difficulty swallowing and speaking. Weakness may spread to upper and lower extremities and to muscles of respiration. One characteristic finding with myasthenia gravis is progressive muscular fatigue, where the weakness worsens with repetitive muscle contraction and later in the day.

Patients' clinical course typically begins with fluctuating symptoms. Initially, mild symptoms may be ignored, and the diagnosis delayed because the symptoms improved. The diagnosis is often not recognized until symptoms become more severe. When patients experience severe weakness or respiratory impairment, this is called *myasthenic crisis*. This can be the result of acute infection, medication tapering, or other metabolic derangements. Many medications can precipitate a myasthenic crisis. Be sure to ask about any new medications the patient may be taking.

Differential Diagnosis

The differential diagnosis of myasthenia gravis includes other causes of weakness. Electrolyte abnormalities; Guillain-Barré syndrome; MS; toxic ingestion of alcohol, heavy metals, or organophosphates; diabetes; and HIV neuropathy can all cause similar symptoms.

Treatment

In the prehospital setting, management of airway, breathing, and circulation is of utmost importance. The most life-threatening complication of myasthenia gravis is respiratory failure, so care should be taken to monitor the patient's respirations, including pulse oximetry and capnography. Given the patient's weakness, the patient may have difficulty managing secretions and may be at risk for aspiration, so be prepared to assist with suctioning or potentially manage the airway. If there are signs of hypoventilation, assist ventilations as necessary. Because infections or other metabolic disturbances can cause myasthenic crisis, be prepared to provide fluid resuscitation for tachycardia or hypotension.

Care should be taken when administering any medication that can decrease respiratory drive, such as opioids or benzodiazepines. Similarly, if rapid sequence intubation is to be performed, the neuromuscular blocking agent will have a prolonged effect and a smaller dose can be used. The clinician should be cognizant of ensuring adequate postintubation sedation because the paralytic agent will have a prolonged effect.

If the patient does not have a diagnosis of myasthenia gravis, the evaluation in the ED will likely be extensive, including bloodwork, imaging, and likely lumbar puncture. Treatment for myasthenic crisis typically includes steroids, IV immune globulin to bind antibodies, and plasmapheresis to remove antibodies. Patients will often be placed on chronic immune suppression and will sometimes receive a thymectomy.

Peripheral Neuropathy (Diabetic)

Peripheral neuropathy, often shortened to *neuropathy*, is any disorder of the peripheral nervous system. Many of the previously described disorders, including Guillain-Barré, are considered peripheral neuropathies. However, diabetes is the most common cause of neuropathy in the United States and is a frequent cause of chronic pain and neurologic disability.

Pathophysiology

The pathophysiology behind diabetic neuropathy is multifactorial but it is primarily caused by an inflammatory response to chronically high circulating levels of glucose leading to oxidative stress. Patients will typically develop the disease over the distal-most, longest nerve fibers of the lower extremities. As the disease becomes chronic, it progresses to the larger, more proximal nerves.

Signs and Symptoms

Several syndromes are associated with peripheral nervous system disease in diabetics. Diabetic peripheral neuropathy is the most common form, appearing in chronic diabetics, with classic glove-and-stocking distribution primarily affecting the feet and lasting longer than 6 months. Symptoms consist of pins and needles sensation, burning, and decreased pain and temperature sensation. When patients experience pain for longer than 6 months, it is termed *chronic diabetic neuropathy*. Hyperglycemia neuropathy is often seen in recently diagnosed diabetics with high circulating glucose levels. This neuropathy improves with gradual correction. Alternatively, patients can experience a painful disorder from the rapid reduction in glucose levels called *insulin neuritis*. Patients can have muscle wasting and chronic wounds associated with neuropathy. Profound sensory deficits can cause patients to have unrecognized wounds on their feet that may lead to infections, such as cellulitis, osteomyelitis, and septic shock.

Differential Diagnosis

In patients with chronic diabetic neuropathy, care must be given to evaluate for other coexisting acute neuropathies, especially with profound sensory deficits or any motor deficits, including Guillain-Barré syndrome, as well as tickborne infections that may cause tick paralysis. Multiple sclerosis, myasthenia gravis; toxic ingestion of alcohol, heavy metals, or organophosphates; and HIV neuropathy are also possible differentials.

Treatment

The most common neuropathy-related complaint in the prehospital setting is an acute exacerbation, typically severe pain. The role of the EMS clinician is to evaluate for acute neurologic dysfunction that may indicate an acute disorder such as acute cord compression, Guillain-Barré, or anterior/central cord syndrome from trauma. Remove the patient's shoes and socks to evaluate feet for wounds, infections, and retained foreign bodies and evaluate for signs of infection and sepsis.

In regard to pain management in the prehospital setting, nonsteroidal anti-inflammatory drugs are of little effect in the treatment of neuropathic pain. Severe pain should be guided by local pain protocols. Analgesics with some evidence of effect include opioids, ketamine, pregabalin, gabapentin, and capsaicin.

Subdural Hematoma

A subdural hematoma is a collection of blood between the dura mater and arachnoid membrane (**Figure 8-13**). The hematoma may be acute, subacute, or chronic. The acute period is measured from the time of the injury to the third day. The subacute period lasts from day 3 to about 2 weeks after the injury, and the chronic phase begins 2 to 3 weeks after the injury. Subdural hemorrhage

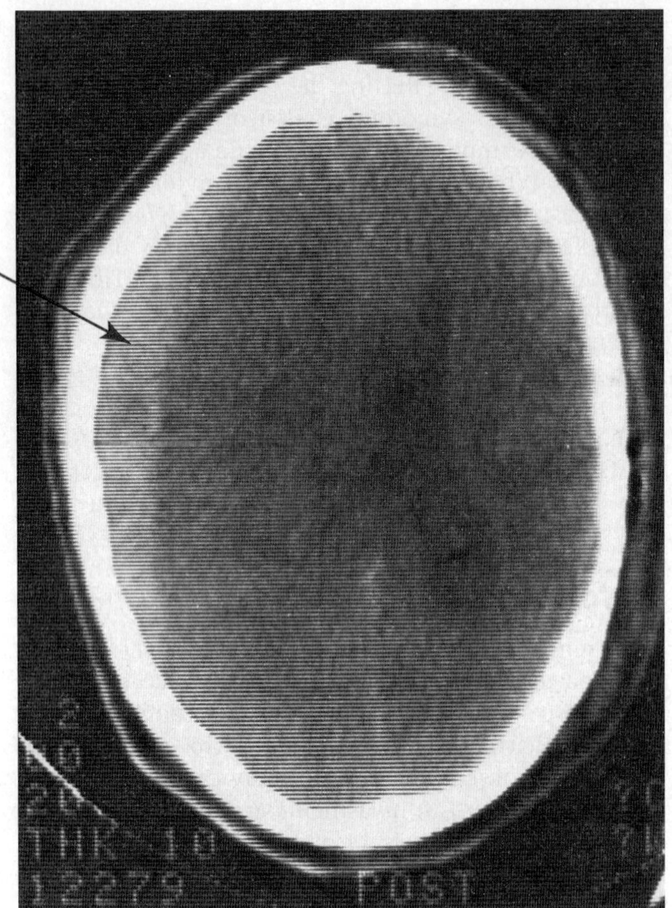

Figure 8-13 Computed tomography (CT) scan of a subdural hematoma.

Courtesy of Peter T. Pons, MD, FACEP.

has a mortality rate of about 20% and usually occurs in patients older than age 60 years.

Pathophysiology

Subdural hemorrhage is usually caused by a tearing of the bridging veins that communicate between the cerebral cortex and the venous sinuses. This is usually precipitated by direct trauma or acute deceleration. The blood then clots in the subdural space. In the subacute phase of a subdural bleed, the clotted blood may liquefy and thin out. In the chronic phase, the blood has disintegrated, and serous fluid remains in the subdural space until it is resorbed.

The phenomenon of coup–contrecoup injury can lead to subdural hematoma. The coup, or blow, causes trauma to the brain directly under the area of the skull that absorbs the direct force of impact. After the impact, the brain recoils within the closed container of the skull and is injured on its opposite side (contrecoup) when it rebounds against the cranium. This may cause bleeding or neurologic damage on both sides of the brain and generate separate but distinct findings on physical exam and imaging studies of the brain.

Older persons may have a smaller brain volume as a result of the aging process and be at greater risk for tearing of the bridging veins between the skull and brain during any type of traumatic or deceleration injury, leading to subdural bleeding. Additionally, because of cerebral atrophy, patients who chronically consume large quantities of alcoholic beverages are at similar risk. Because there is increased empty intracranial space, the hemorrhage may also be less symptomatic, and focal signs/symptoms or coma may not appear for hours to days post injury. These patients should be transported to evaluate for occult hematoma.

Signs and Symptoms

After blunt head trauma, the patient may present with a subdural hematoma, often accompanied by loss of consciousness or amnesia for the event. The patient may either be asymptomatic or have personality changes, signs of increased ICP (headache, visual changes, nausea, or vomiting), hemiparesis, or hemiplegia. Patients with bleeding abnormalities, such as hemophilia, and patients taking anticoagulant medications may develop a subdural hematoma after only minor trauma, as can alcoholics and older adults. In some patients, there is no history of trauma. Key findings include the following:

- Headache
- Loss of consciousness or alteration in level of consciousness
- Focal or general weakness
- History or signs of trauma

Differential Diagnosis

The differential diagnosis for subdural hematoma includes other types of intracranial hemorrhage, intracranial mass, infections such as meningitis, and ischemic stroke.

Treatment

If the patient has any alteration in mental status, check the patient's blood glucose level and correct it if necessary. Ensure that the patient's airway and breathing are intact. Place a cervical collar and maintain spinal motion restriction as indicated by mechanism of injury and clinical findings. Because of the potential for a worsening mental status, watch carefully for any signs of increasing confusion, respiratory depression, or airway compromise.

The patient should be transported to a trauma center or, if that is not possible, taken to a hospital where neurosurgical backup is available.

Epidural Hematoma

An epidural hematoma is an accumulation of blood between the inner table of the skull and the dura mater, the

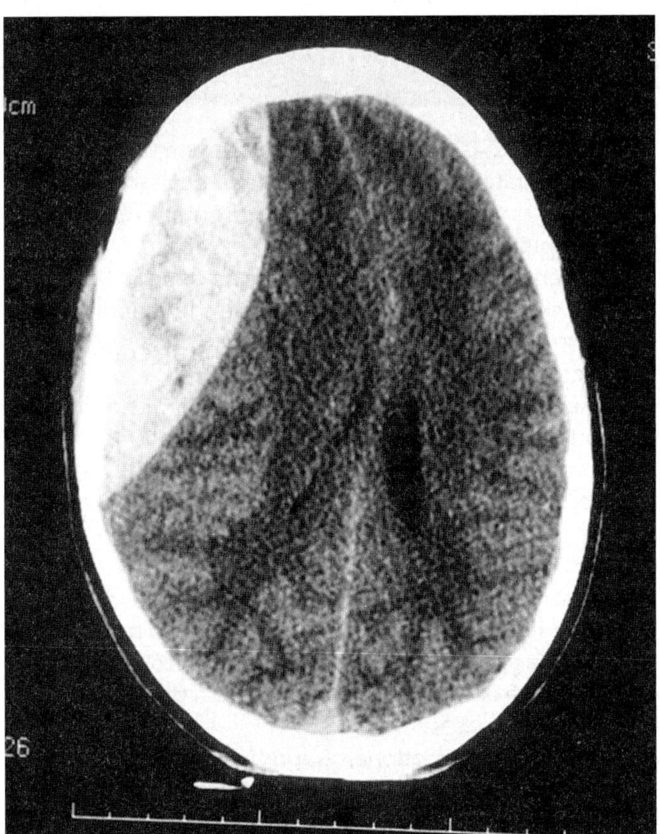

Figure 8-14 CT scan of an epidural hematoma.
Courtesy of Peter T. Pons, MD, FACEP.

outermost of the meninges (**Figure 8-14**). This condition is usually caused by trauma to the arteries in the epidural space, and thus leads to high-pressure mass effect. Frequently, there is an associated skull fracture, usually in the area of the middle meningeal artery on the temporal aspect of the skull. Prompt surgical decompression is necessary for patients with significant neurologic dysfunction. The likelihood of recovery is directly related to the patient's preoperative neurologic condition. Typically, trauma is the only etiology of an epidural hematoma; it is included in this AMLS text as a matter of completeness regarding bleeding types of the brain. Intracranial hemorrhages from trauma and the identification and management of traumatic brain injuries are covered in detail in the Prehospital Trauma Life Support (PHTLS) course.

Putting It All Together

The patient with alterations in mental status or acute neurologic changes is often challenging for healthcare clinicians. When a person's mental function is altered, it is difficult to obtain an accurate history and perform a reliable examination, so you must be especially observant and astute in looking for diagnostic clues and interpreting the information obtained. After assessing the patient's airway, breathing, and circulation for life threats, it is critically important to check every patient for those fundamental conditions that can be rapidly identified and managed. The SNOT mnemonic (Rapid Recall Box 8-2) was developed specifically for prehospital clinicians for this purpose. Once screening for these threats has been completed, more detailed evaluation guided by the patient's chief complaint and using the SAMPLER/OPQRST mnemonic for history should be performed. The secondary survey should be conducted, and a differential diagnosis developed. This stepwise process allows prioritization of diagnostic testing and treatment interventions and, in the prehospital setting, determination of the most appropriate transport destination. Repeated reassessment, vigilance for life threats, and reconsideration of differential diagnoses until care is transferred at the receiving facility is particularly important in patients with acute neurologic conditions and accompanying altered mental status.

SCENARIO SOLUTION

- After you ensure that the patient has a patent airway, is breathing adequately, and has adequate perfusion, you should obtain her vital signs. Your full-body assessment should include examination of pupils, vision (including peripheral vision), and extraocular movements. Ask if she has photophobia. Note any nodular swellings or tenderness over the temporal arteries on the sides of the head. Evaluate the symmetry of her face. Auscultate her carotid arteries for bruits. Determine if she has any nuchal rigidity. Assess extremities for pulse, sensory function, and motor strength. Obtain additional history to determine whether she has sustained trauma. Evaluate her medications to obtain clues regarding her past medical history. Assess the patient with a stroke scale. Consider other diagnostic tests based on your findings. The blood glucose level should be checked in *every patient* with any change in mental status or behavior, even if another cause seems obvious.
- Differential diagnoses for this patient include ischemic stroke, hemorrhagic stroke, temporal arteritis, meningitis, and migraine headache.

SUMMARY

- Neurologic disorders can involve life threats due to loss of airway reflexes and effects on ventilation and circulation.
- The central nervous system has two structures, the brain and the spinal cord, which account for 98% of all neural tissues of the body.
- Each portion of the brain is responsible for specific functions. The occipital lobe receives and stores images. The temporal lobe makes language and speech possible. The frontal lobe controls voluntary motion. The parietal lobe allows for the perception of the sensations of touch and pain. The diencephalon filters out unneeded information from the cerebral cortex. The midbrain helps to regulate the level of consciousness. The brainstem regulates the blood pressure, pulse rate, and respiratory rate and pattern. The hypothalamus and pituitary control the release of multiple hormones from the endocrine system. The cerebellum allows coordination of complex motor activity.
- The AMLS Assessment Pathway can be used to evaluate the likelihood of specific diagnoses based on a patient's cardinal presentation/chief complaint.
- It is critical to determine when the patient was last seen acting normally because the amount of time elapsed since the onset of symptoms will dictate the treatments available.
- The neurologic exam findings will help refine the differential diagnosis.
- A variety of disease processes can cause neurologic dysfunction, including cancer, degenerative conditions, developmental anomalies, infectious diseases, and vascular conditions.
- Most neurologic diseases are thought to be multifactorial—that is, a number of factors combine to induce vulnerability to a particular disease process.
- Physical and emotional supportive care are vital on the scene and en route to the treatment facility.

Key Terms

altered mental status Any decrease in normal level of wakefulness, change in mentation, or behavior that is not normal for a particular patient.

ataxia Loss of coordination of muscle control, which can lead to gait disturbance or extremity clumsiness. May be due to many causes, including peripheral nerve, spinal cord, or brain dysfunction, often of the cerebellum, which controls coordination.

blood-brain barrier A filtering mechanism of the capillaries that carry blood to the brain and spinal cord tissue, blocking the passage of certain substances.

cerebral perfusion pressure (CPP) Represents the pressure gradient driving cerebral blood flow (CBF) and therefore oxygen and metabolite delivery; it is the difference between the mean arterial pressure (MAP) and the intracranial pressure (ICP). CPP = MAP – ICP.

cerebrospinal fluid (CSF) A transparent, slightly yellowish fluid in the subarachnoid space around the brain and spinal cord.

Cushing triad Hypertension; bradycardia; and rapid, deep, or irregular respirations.

dysarthria Garbled speech (but of one's intended words) due to cranial nerve motor dysfunction (distinguish from expressive and receptive aphasia).

embolus A particle that travels in the circulatory system and obstructs blood flow when it becomes lodged in a smaller artery. A blood clot is the most common type of embolus, but fat (after long bone fracture), atherosclerotic, and air (diving) emboli can also occur.

expressive aphasia Inability to speak intended words due to dysfunction of the cerebral speech center (Broca's area) in the left frontal lobe (distinguish from dysarthria).

hemiparesis Unilateral mild to moderate weakness, usually occurring on the opposite side of the body from the stroke (distinguish from hemiplegia).

hemiplegia Paralysis or severe weakness on one side of the body (distinguish from hemiparesis).

hemorrhagic stroke Damage to the brain from bleeding in the brain tissue (intracerebral), most commonly related to hypertension, or into the subarachnoid space, often due to rupture of an aneurysm or arteriovenous malformation.

intracranial pressure (ICP) A measure of the hydrostatic pressure of the intracranial CSF fluid. Swelling (cerebral edema), increased volume of CSF (hydrocephalus), tumor, and intracranial hemorrhage can increase the ICP. If ICP is increased significantly, perfusion to the brain can be impaired and brain structures can herniate, causing severe neurologic impairment and death.

ischemic stroke A stroke that occurs when a thrombus or embolus obstructs a blood vessel, diminishing blood flow to and causing injury to the affected area of the brain.

Korsakoff syndrome Chronic and irreversible condition involving cognitive dysfunction, especially memory loss, due to prolonged thiamine deficiency.

mean arterial pressure (MAP) The average pressure in a patient's arteries during one cardiac cycle, an indicator of perfusion to vital organs; to calculate MAP: SBP + (2 x DBP) / 3

neurotransmitters Chemical substances that are released at the end of a nerve fiber by the arrival of a nerve impulse (action potential) and, by diffusing across the synapse or junction, cause the transfer of the impulse to another nerve fiber, a muscle fiber, or some other structure.

ophthalmoplegia Abnormal function of the eye muscles.

proprioception Sensory function that provides the awareness of the location of one's own body parts relative to the rest of the body.

seizure An episode of abnormal neuronal activity in the cerebral cortex that can cause loss of or alteration in consciousness, convulsions or tremors, incontinence, behavior changes, subjective changes in perception (taste, smell, fears), and other symptoms.

stroke A brain injury that occurs when blood flow to a part of the brain is obstructed or interrupted or when nontraumatic bleeding in the brain damages brain cells from increased pressure. (See ischemic stroke and hemorrhagic stroke.)

stroke center Hospital or receiving facility that is designated as an appropriate facility with appropriate resources to receive, assess, and treat patients with suspected stroke. Regional authorities that designate stroke centers often use outside accrediting organizations to ensure that the center meets standards for preparedness and care.

thrombus A blood clot that forms in a blood vessel and causes obstruction where it forms.

transient ischemic attack (TIA) Sometimes referred to as a "mini stroke," TIA is a condition of low or interrupted blood flow to a part of the brain, causing transient ischemia and strokelike symptoms that resolve within 24 hours. A TIA is considered a warning sign of an impending stroke.

Wernicke encephalopathy A disorder caused by deficiency of thiamine (vitamin B_1) and characterized by a triad of symptoms: acute confusion, ataxia, and ophthalmoplegia.

Bibliography

American Academy of Orthopaedic Surgeons. *Nancy Caroline's Emergency Care in the Streets*, 8th ed. Jones & Bartlett Learning; 2018.

American Brain Tumor Association. About brain tumors. A primer for patients and caregivers. Modified January 2015. https://www.abta.org/wp-content/uploads/2018/03/about-brain-tumors-a-primer-1.pdf

Arzimanoglu A, Blast T, Jaume C, et al., eds. Prolonged epileptic seizures: identification and rescue treatment strategies. *Epilept Disord*. 2014;16(suppl 1):1.

Baslet G. Treatment of psychogenic nonepileptic seizures: updated review and findings from a mindfulness-based intervention case. *Neuroscience*. 2014;46(1):54–64.

Borris DJ, Bertram EH, Kapur J. Ketamine controls prolonged status epilepticus. *Epilepsy Res*. 2000;42(2–3):117–122.

Brandt J, Puente A. Update on psychogenic nonepileptic seizures. *Psychiatr Times*. 2015;32(2).

Buck ML. Intranasal administration of benzodiazepines for the treatment of acute repetitive seizures in children. *Pediatr Pharm*. 2013;19(10).

Devinsky O, Cilio MR, Cross H, et al. Cannabidiol: pharmacology and potential therapeutic role in epilepsy and other neuropsychiatric disorders. *Epilepsia*. 2014;55(6):791–802.

Dobson R, Giovannoni G. Multiple sclerosis—a review. *Eur J Neurol*. 2019;26(1):27–40.

England MJ, Liverman CT, Schultz AM, et al., eds. *Epilepsy Across the Spectrum: Promoting Health and Understanding*. National Academies Press; 2012.

Gammicchia C, Johnson C. Autism information for paramedics and emergency room staff. Safe & Sound Autism Society. https://www.admboard.org/Data/Sites/25/Assets/pdfs/cit/7-Autism-Spectrum/7-3-Autism-Paramedics-and-Emergency-Room-Staff-signed.pdf

Hackam DG, Kapral MK, Wang JT, et al. Most stroke patients do not get a warning: a population-based cohort study. *Neurology.* 2009;73:1074.

Han JH, Zimmerman EE, Cutler N, et al. Delirium in older emergency department patients: recognition, risk factors, and psychomotor subtypes. *Acad Emerg Med.* 2009;16(3):193–200.

Hills F. The psychological and social impact of epilepsy. *Neurol Asia.* 2007;12(suppl 1):10–12.

Kapur J. Prehospital treatment of status epilepticus with benzodiazepines is effective and safe. *Epilepsy Curr.* 2002;2(4):121–124.

Klein P, Tyrlikova I, Mathews GC. Dietary treatment in adults with refractory epilepsy: a review. *Neurology.* 2014;83(21):1978–1985.

Laccheo I, Sonmezturk H, Bhatt AB, et al. Non-convulsive status epilepticus and non-convulsive seizures in neurological ICU patients. *Neurocrit Care.* 2015;22(2):202–211.

Lee J, Huh L, Korn P, et al. Guidelines for the management of convulsive status epilepticus in infants and children. *BCMJ.* 2011;53(6):279–285.

National Stroke Association. *National Stroke Association's Complete Guide to Stroke.* National Stroke Association; 2003.

National Stroke Association. Transient ischemic attack. National Strock Association. https://www.stroke.org/en/about-stroke/types-of-stroke/tia-transient-ischemic-attack

Oh ES, Fong TG, Hshieh TT, Inouye SK. Delirium in older persons: advances in diagnosis and treatment. *JAMA.* 2017;318(12):1161–1174.

Pearce JMS. Meningitis, meninges, meninx. *Eur Neurol.* 2008;60:165. doi:10.1159/000145337

Ruoff G, Urban G. Standards of care for headache diagnosis and treatment. National Headache Foundation. Published 2007. https://headaches.org/2007/11/19/standards-of-care-for-headache-diagnosis-and-treatment/

Ryvlin P, Nashef L, Lhatoo SD, et al. Incidence and mechanisms of cardiorespiratory arrests in epilepsy monitoring units (MORTEMUS): a retrospective study. *Lancet Neurol.* 2013;12(10):966–977.

Scheffer IE, Berkovic S, Capovilla G, et al. ILAE classification of the epilepsies: position paper of the ILAE Commission for Classification and Terminology. *Epilepsia.* 2017;58(4):512.

Seinfeld S, Shinnar S, Sun S, et al. Emergency management of febrile status epilepticus: results of the FEBSTAT study. *Epilepsia.* 2014;55(3):388–395.

Shrestha GS, Joshi P, Chhetri S, et al. Intravenous ketamine for treatment of super-refractory convulsive status epilepticus with septic shock: a report of two cases. *Indian J Crit Care Med.* 2015;19(5):283–285.

Silbergleit R, Durkalski V, Lowenstein D, et al. Intramuscular versus intravenous therapy for prehospital status epilepticus. *N Engl J Med.* 2012;366(7):591–600.

Silbergleit R, Lowenstein D, Durkalski V, et al. RAMPART (Rapid Anticonvulsant Medication Prior to Arrival Trial): a double-blind randomized clinical trial of the efficacy of intramuscular midazolam versus intravenous lorazepam in the prehospital treatment of status epilepticus by paramedics. *Epilepsia.* 2011;52(suppl 8):45–47.

Simon RP, Aminoff MJ, Greenberg DA. *Clinical Neurology*, 10th ed. McGraw-Hill; 2018. (See chapters "Coma," "Headache & Facial Pain," "Motor Disorders," and "Stroke.")

Theodore W, Spencer S, Wiebe S, et al. Epilepsy in North America: a report prepared under the auspices of the Global Campaign against Epilepsy, the International Bureau for Epilepsy, the International League Against Epilepsy, and the World Health Organization. *Epilepsia.* 2006;47(10):1–23.

Thurman DJ, Hesdorffer DC, French JA. Sudden unexpected death in epilepsy: assessing the public health burden. *Epilepsia.* 2014;55:1–7.

Vespa PM, McArthur DL, Xu Y, et al. Nonconvulsive seizures after traumatic brain injury are associated with hippocampal atrophy. *Neurology.* 2010;75(9):792.

Warden CR, Zibulewsky J, Mace S, et al. Evaluation and management of febrile seizures in the out-of-hospital and emergency department settings. *Ann Emerg Med.* 2003;41(2):215–222.

Zeiler FA, Zeiler KJ, Kazina CJ, Teitelbaum J, Gillman LM, West M. Lidocaine for status epilepticus in adults. *Seizure.* 2015;31:41–48. doi:10.1016/j.seizure.2015.07.003

CHAPTER 9

Mental Health Disorders

Chapter Editors
Lauren Young Work, MSW, LCSW
Priyanka Amin, MD
Scott T. Youngquist, MD, MSc

This chapter is intended to explore mental health crises in the community and how patients who are living with a mental health disorder or experiencing psychological distress may present to emergency medical services (EMS) clinicians during such episodes. Mental health conditions are, at their core, medical issues requiring the same approach to assessment and treatment as any other chronic disease or medical condition.

Although many factors may contribute to, or trigger, the onset of a mental health crisis or disorder, pathology of the brain is the underlying reason patients experience the symptoms observed during mental health emergency and crisis calls. Just like individuals with diabetes or high blood pressure, patients who live with mental health disorders require appropriate medical care and mental health resources and support to ensure they remain safe, functional, and healthy. Preventing episodes or crises that may cause patients to feel vulnerable or become a safety risk to themselves or others is an important part of empowering those living with mental health disorders (or associated symptomology) to achieve the highest wellness level possible. The manner in which EMS clinicians approach patients with mental health disorders (whether or not the disorder is causing the specific encounter at that time) can significantly affect these patients' condition and ability to engage in their own care.

EMS clinicians can play a vital role in providing nonjudgmental medical and community paramedicine interventions for patients with mental health disorders and conditions by understanding both the medical and psychosocial factors that contribute to mental health crises and emergencies. This requires that EMS clinicians be familiar with assessment and intervention techniques on the scene of both frontline emergent calls and community paramedic visits.

Along with training and protocols, EMS clinicians may need to employ in-the-moment, sometimes outside-the-box, critical thinking and decision making during mental health crisis episodes to ensure the safety and care of the patient, the patient's caregivers, the community, and EMS personnel. As with other clinical conditions, EMS personnel must be sensitive to religious and cultural components of their mental health patients' lives. It is also critical for them to be well versed in the mental health resources that are available in their community, for both their patients and themselves.

LEARNING OBJECTIVES

At the conclusion of this chapter, you will be able to:

- Define mental health, including common disorders and their symptoms.
- Discuss the impact of stigma on the patient experience during a mental health crisis or EMS call.
- Understand how neurobiology plays a role in mental health.
- Recognize the signs of substance use and alcohol use disorders.
- Provide nonjudgmental and ethical care and interventions on scene and while transporting patients experiencing a mental health crisis or emergency.
- Consider mental health crises among special populations, including pediatric, adolescent, and older adult patients.
- Apply interventions to ensure the safety of the patient, bystanders, and prehospital clinicians on scene and while transporting the patient.
- Consider safety on scene and while transporting for patients who are experiencing suicidal thoughts, self-harming, experiencing psychosis, and/or becoming violent.
- Demonstrate awareness of treatment options and resources for patients and families who are living with a mental health disorder.

SCENARIO

You are dispatched on a call for an individual with altered mental status. As you arrive on scene, you see a 22-year-old male who appears agitated and is pacing in his driveway. As you approach, the patient asks who you are and why you are at his home. After you identify yourself as an EMS clinician who wants to see if you can help, the patient warns you may be in danger because "they are looking" for him. You recognize the patient is experiencing paranoia and may be a safety risk to himself or others.

- What should you rule out before you assume this patient is experiencing a mental health emergency?
- What issues should you consider on scene and while transporting the patient to ensure the safety of the patient and those caring for him?

Prevalence of Mental Health Disorders in the United States

Mental health conditions are very common. In fact, it is likely that you or someone you know is living with a mental health disorder:

- 1 in 5 U.S adults experiences mental illness each year.
- 1 in 6 U.S. youth aged 6 to 17 experiences a mental health disorder each year.
- 1 in 20 U.S. adults experiences serious mental illness each year.
- 1 in 15 U.S. adults experiences both a substance use disorder and mental illness.
- 155 million people live in a designated Mental Health Professional Shortage Area.
- 37.9% of the 20.3 million adults living with a substance use disorder also have a co-occurring mental illness.
- 46.2% of U.S. adults who are diagnosed with a mental illness over their lifetime received mental health services in the past year.

Factors Contributing to Mental Illness

Mental health disorders cause impairment in functioning by altering emotion regulation, cognition, and behaviors. Several factors can contribute to mental health disorders. In general, both genetic and environmental factors play a role in the development of mental illness.

Neurologic factors play a significant role in mental health, as several neurologic pathways, structures, and neurotransmitters are involved in the pathogenesis of mental health disorders. The cortex, the outermost layer of the brain, is divided into four lobes and is responsible for higher-level functions such as language and voluntary movements. Impacts to the frontal lobe, the largest of the four lobes, can cause **anosognosia**, or lack of insight/self-awareness, which can cause individuals with mental health disorders to be unaware they have or are exhibiting symptoms of a mental health disorder. When this condition is encountered, it is often misunderstood by others to be denial. Understanding that a patient's lack of insight is a part of the disease process can help inform EMS clinicians to provide nonjudgmental care.

The subcortical regions of the brain are where more basic functions occur, such as temperature regulation, body homeostasis, and memory and emotion processing. The cortical and subcortical regions are continuously communicating with each other (**Figure 9-1**). This communication allows us to determine how to express or suppress emotions or what to pay attention to. With alterations in either of these areas or in the communication between them, mental health disorders can develop.

In addition to neurologic and genetic factors, psychosocial, medical, and environmental factors (often referred to as **social determinants of health**) such as the following can contribute to triggering crises as well as the development of a mental health disorder:

- Home, school, relationship, or work stress
- Physical or emotional trauma
- Abuse/exploitation
- Poverty
- Alcohol and substance use
- Exposure to violence
- Loss/grief/relationship changes
- Medication changes or discontinuation
- Lack of access to medical and mental health care
- Nutrition and hydration deficits
- Recent infections
- Pregnancy and postpartum period
- Lack of case management/access to resources
- Lack of social, familial, and/or emotional support
- Lack of acceptance due to sexual orientation and/or gender identity

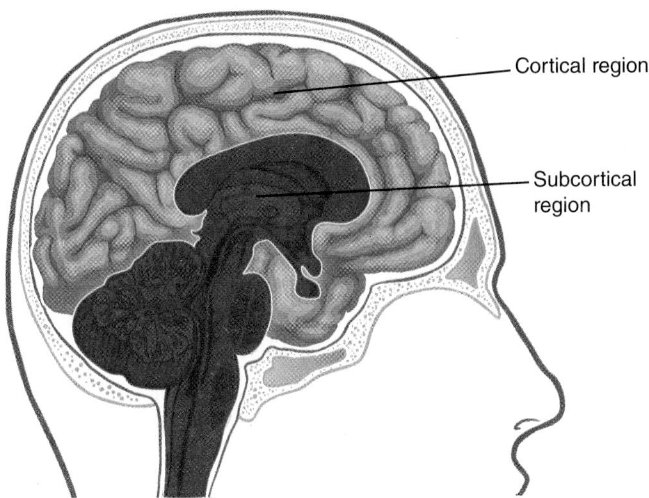

Figure 9-1 Cortical and subcortical regions of the brain.

- Other medical conditions/medical trauma
- Discrimination/disenfranchisement

Although these factors may be discussed as part of the patient history on scene, further discussion by EMS clinicians and medical social workers working within the EMS care system may be helpful in managing and mitigating these psychosocial and environmental challenges and help engage the patient in a plan of care within the health care continuum. Such a plan may lead to stabilization of symptoms, improved chronic disease management, increased safety, and improved quality of life.

Stigma in Mental Health Care and the Patient Experience

Stigma is a negative association based on a particular circumstance, trait, or condition the person has. Stigma in mental health often stems from the false belief that patients living with mental health disorders are to blame for their condition and for the behaviors attributable to their disorder. Many members of society believe individuals who have a mental health disorder could control their symptoms if they simply wanted to, or they could stop the behaviors causing issues in their lives if they were motivated to do so. This stigma often drives discriminatory and, at times, abusive treatment of patients who need medical intervention for their mental health disorder. In recent years, we have seen a shift in terminology to the use of "behavioral health" versus "mental health"; however, the term *behavioral* can reinforce the false notion that individuals with a mental health disorder—that is, a brain disorder—can simply control, or learn to control, their symptoms. For many people who live with a mental health diagnosis, this perception is further stigmatizing, as it suggests they do not have a medical issue, but rather a behavioral one. Fear of stigma, being labeled, being blamed for not controlling behavioral symptoms, and the impacts these factors have on a patient's life are critical reasons why many patients may not reach out for medical management and support of their mental health conditions. Mental health disorders can develop in anyone, including individuals who work within EMS. Stigma about mental health within the health care community can present a barrier to reaching out for treatment. The language used by prehospital clinicians when talking to and about patients experiencing a mental health crisis or emergency can lead to more fear and resistance to care, not only for the patient and family, but also for health care workers who may benefit from early intervention for their own mental health needs.

As an EMS clinician, suppose you were transporting a 42-year-old female with Graves disease for possible thyroid storm. The patient is exhibiting symptoms including agitation, disorientation, memory loss, and delusions. Now suppose you were transporting a 24-year-old male with schizophrenia in your ambulance. This patient is exhibiting the same symptoms of agitation, disorientation, memory loss, and delusions. How might you care differently for the patient with thyroid storm than for the patient with schizophrenia? Would your perceptions of the two patients be the same? Would you view the patient with thyroid storm as having a medical condition that is causing her behavior? Would you view the patient with schizophrenia as having a medical condition that is causing his behavior?

Understanding your own bias as it relates to stigma surrounding mental health is critical to the nonjudgmental and ethical care of this patient population. To eliminate stigma, consider the following points:

- Educate yourself and others about mental health disorders you commonly encounter at work.
- Understand mental health disorders as medical conditions, just as you would diabetes or epilepsy.
- Act with compassion when managing the needs of patients with mental health disorders, just as you would for patients with other medical conditions.

Interventions for Mental Health Emergencies

Upon their arrival on scene at any medical emergency, EMS clinicians must complete a scene assessment and general impression quickly to determine how they will respond to the patient and safely manage the scene itself. EMS clinicians combine their training, experience, protocols, and compassion to inform their approach to every patient care scenario. As mental health emergencies are indeed medical emergencies, the Advanced Medical Life Support (AMLS) Assessment Pathway approach should also be applied.

However, in the case of mental health emergencies, training and compassion become vital to successfully and safely navigating the patient's needs and ensuring the safety of both the patient and the patient's caregivers. Protocols and standard operating guidelines are a required element that the prehospital clinician brings to EMS calls, but any seasoned clinician also knows that at times best practices and protocols must be combined with the capacity to react to and manage unexpected events. On the scene of mental health emergencies, clinicians are often required to think outside the box and utilize their problem-solving skills to most effectively help the patient. The following section explores best practices, while acknowledging that you will be called upon to sometimes rely on medical direction, command staff experience, and your own problem-solving expertise to ensure the best outcome feasible on the scene of mental health emergencies.

Medical Assessment

Mental health emergencies may be triggered by myriad issues other than a mental health disorder. For example, changes in mental status and behavior can be seen in calls involving patients with any health issue, such as the following:

- Hypoxemia
- Electrolyte abnormalities
- Endocrine disorders (e.g., diabetes, hypo/hyperthyroidism)
- Traumatic brain injury (TBI)
- Brain tumors
- Respiratory diseases/distress
- Infection/sepsis
- Epilepsy
- Stroke
- Human immunodeficiency virus (HIV) infection
- Dehydration
- Medication side effects and toxicity
- Autoimmune disorders
- Toxicity
- Metabolic disorders

When a medical condition other than a mental health disorder causes a patient to have psychosis, this symptom is termed secondary psychosis. EMS clinicians should always consider a medical explanation for the presenting symptoms by using the AMLS Assessment Pathway, which includes patient history and both primary and secondary surveys. Clinicians should obtain vital signs, including oxygen saturation (SpO_2) and, when indicated, blood glucose. Even in patients who present with a known mental health disorder, an acute medical cause for the current symptoms, such as hypoxia or hypoglycemia, must be considered and ruled out or treated per agency protocol.

Several components of the prehospital clinician's assessment can help evaluate the possibility of a medical (not mental health) issue, which may aid in prehospital care decision making as well as provide hospital clinicians with important information to aid in their continuation of patient care. These components may include the following:

- The patient, or individuals known to patient, report no prior psychiatric history
- Vital signs abnormalities (e.g., fever, hypoxemia, hypotension, hypertension, tachycardia)
- Various physical complaints (e.g., headache, chest tightness)
- Sudden onset of symptoms
- Fluctuating attention and concentration as well as waxing/waning pattern of symptoms
- Altered mental status (patients with a psychiatric disorder will not present with a decreased level of consciousness)
- Focal neurologic deficit
- Patient has only visual hallucinations (rather than any auditory hallucinations)
- Recent initiation or cessation of any medications or substances, such as alcohol

Research shows that patients with mental health disorders are generally nonviolent and are themselves at increased risk of becoming victims of violence. Nevertheless, some specific risk factors for violence toward others may be observed when responding to calls for a mental health emergency. Specifically, intoxication, a prior history of violence, and impaired reality testing such that a patient feels that their life is being threatened by others (i.e., paranoia) could increase the risk of violence. The following risk factors or warning signs may be present in a patient who may become aggressive or violent:

- History of prior aggressive behaviors (e.g., striking, biting, or spitting)
- Evidence on scene of harm toward others
- Brandishing or threat of using a weapon
- Physical posturing—making fists, getting into a fighting stance, throwing items, engaging in property destruction
- Agitation—increased physical activity, restlessness
- Verbal aggression—raised voice, threats
- Delirium with agitated behavior
- Signs of acute substance intoxication
- Paranoia and persecutory delusions—beliefs that others are hurting them despite evidence or

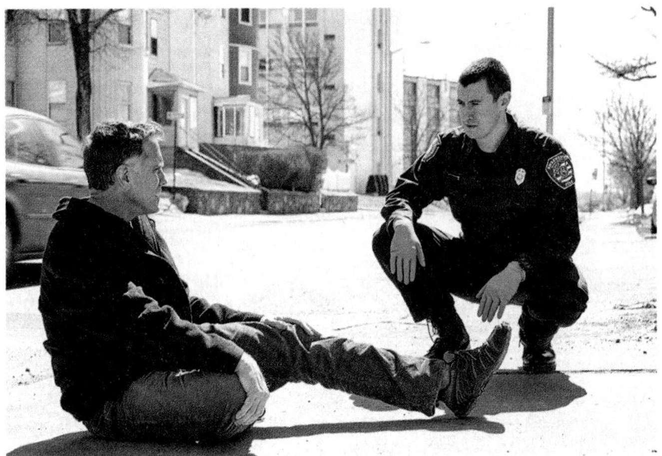

Figure 9-2 It is important to maintain situational awareness while engaging with a patient.

reassurance to the contrary (e.g., believing that clinicians are attempting to give them poison under the pretense that it is medication)

Scene assessment is a critical aspect during all phases of a mental health emergency call (**Figure 9-2**). Although every scene and every patient must be managed based on their unique circumstances, situational awareness must continue throughout the entire patient care contact. A scene deemed safe initially can quickly become unsafe, causing risk to both the patient and the EMS clinician (**Tip Box 9-1**). In such scenarios, you should recognize some important basic safety considerations:

- Request law enforcement on any scene that has the potential to become unsafe or is not deemed safe.
- If safe to do so, remove any potentially harmful objects or weapons, or prevent patient access to these items if feasible. Follow your agency's protocols regarding the handling of weapons on scene or on the patient.
- If you are in immediate danger, disengage safely from the patient and the scene, if able, until law enforcement arrives.
- If you are in immediate danger and cannot safely disengage from the patient and/or the scene, use verbal de-escalation techniques (see the discussion of de-escalation techniques in the "Communication" section) and other defensive tactics (e.g., create distance or place obstacles between you and any threat) until law enforcement arrives.
- In addition to engaging in skillful communication with patients, you should establish verbal and nonverbal cues with your partners to ensure safe practices and alert each other to potential dangers.
- Follow agency guidelines for use of distress signals if you believe your own life is in danger.

TIP BOX 9-1

Scene Safety

On-scene violence is real and can be a danger to responding clinicians. Having minimal information prior to arriving on scene, combined with environmental factors such as darkness, poor weather, and EMS clinician unfamiliarity with the building or property layout, can impact these concerns. All national EMS organizations advocate for the safety of their clinicians. Scene and transport safety should always be the highest priority. In urban settings, law enforcement may be readily available to assist EMS clinicians quickly. By comparison, in rural areas, a law enforcement response may take longer and may not be an option for immediate intervention to support you on scene or during a transport. The unavailability of immediate law enforcement support creates a dilemma for EMS systems and must be recognized and considered when crafting protocols and operating guidelines.

Providing on-scene safety education, strategies, and tools for response both with and without law enforcement support, and creating standard operating guidelines and policies to inform personnel of their responsibility in these situations, are essential. Operating guidelines should include methods to receive on-scene guidance from commanding officers and supervisors as well as a mechanism for reporting safety issues encountered on scene. Reporting scene safety incidents at the national, regional, state, and local levels is highly encouraged, as it can encourage development of additional guidance and support to address the need to protect patients, EMS clinicians, health workers, and the community. The EMS Voluntary Event Notification Tool (EVENT) is a national system that tracks anonymously reported safety events that affect EMS.

- Maintain a calm tone of voice, calm demeanor, and attitude of nonjudgment, respect, and compassion. How you are perceived by patients can have a significant positive impact on their behaviors and reactions to their surroundings and caregivers.
- Utilize personal protective equipment (PPE) when deemed appropriate per agency protocol—particularly when there is a risk of spitting, biting, contact with blood and body fluids, and other potential contaminants.

TIP BOX 9-2

Use of Restraints

Most patients with mental health disorders are nonviolent or can be managed with verbal de-escalation techniques. Verbal de-escalation should always be the first method of trying to calm a situation. Nevertheless, prehospital clinicians must be well versed in how and when to apply physical restraints and when to provide pharmacologic sedation. Restraints are sometimes essential for safety, especially if verbal de-escalation is infeasible (**Figure 9-3**). Physical restraints and pharmacologic treatments are employed to protect the patient from self-harm or from harming others; they are designed to restrict movement and to ensure patient safety while not inflicting pain on the patient. Restraints are not a form of punishment. If restraints are necessary, ongoing use of de-escalation techniques is recommended, as well as consideration of medications to treat acute agitation. Know your agency's specific policies and procedures regarding physical restraints and pharmacologic sedation.

While EMS agency protocols and training should identify appropriate physical restraint techniques and the use of pharmacologic interventions for agitated patients, some general principles are important for all EMS clinicians to recognize. EMS clinicians are encouraged to be familiar with the National Association of Emergency Medical Technicians (NAEMT)/ National Association of EMS Physicians (NAEMSP) position statement on the care and restraint of agitated patients. Generally, patients should not be restrained in a prone position, should not be restrained using hard restraints or techniques reserved for law enforcement, and should receive an assessment to identify medical conditions that may cause delirium. Although they should work in a coordinated way to ensure the safest care of a patient, law enforcement and EMS have different techniques and responsibilities that ideally are complementary in caring for a patient. It is the primary responsibility of EMS to assess the patient, provide medical interventions, and continuously monitor the patient for deterioration when medical interventions are being used. Law enforcement plays an important role in physical restraint and scene safety, but these personnel should not order interventions (such as requesting medication intervention by EMS).

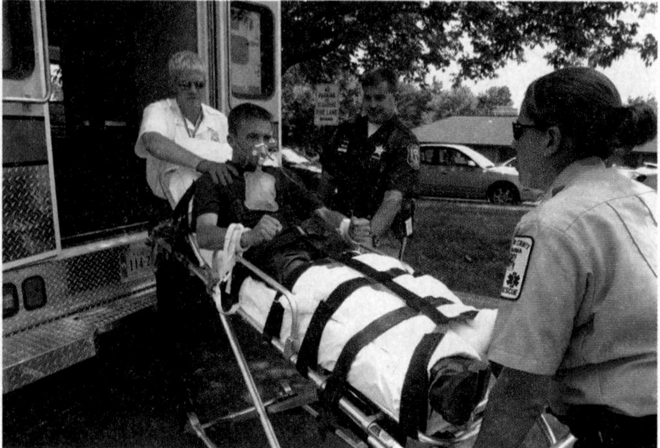

Figure 9-3 Restraints may be needed to protect patients from self-harm or from harming others.

- Reserve physical restraints and medication management of delirium with agitated behavior for patients with whom verbal de-escalation techniques are not effective in reducing unsafe behavior (**Tip Box 9-2**). Follow agency protocols for use of medications such as physical restraints and medications like ketamine, butyrophenones, or benzodiazepines. See the additional discussion of medication management of agitated patients in Chapter 2, *Clinical Approach to Pharmacology*.
- Appropriate patient care and use of restraints should help minimize the possibility of patient elopement, while the vehicle is either stationary or in transit. If a patient elopes from the transport vehicle, follow agency protocols to ensure the safety of the patient, those caring for the patient, and the community. In most agencies, this is a reportable event and would trigger immediate contact with law enforcement to notify them of a vulnerable person who is a risk to self or others and requires medical care. Elopement is a very dangerous scenario for all involved. Each EMS agency should have policies or protocols for responding to this situation.

Communication

When communicating with a patient who has a mental health crisis, your communication strategy is a vital component of de-escalating the patient's situation. In essence, communication is the first line of **intervention**, or treatment, which should be employed to help reduce the symptoms the patient is experiencing and mitigate the risks associated with escalation of behaviors to violence.

As with all communication, how we say things matters. Our tone of voice, our nonverbal cues, and which words

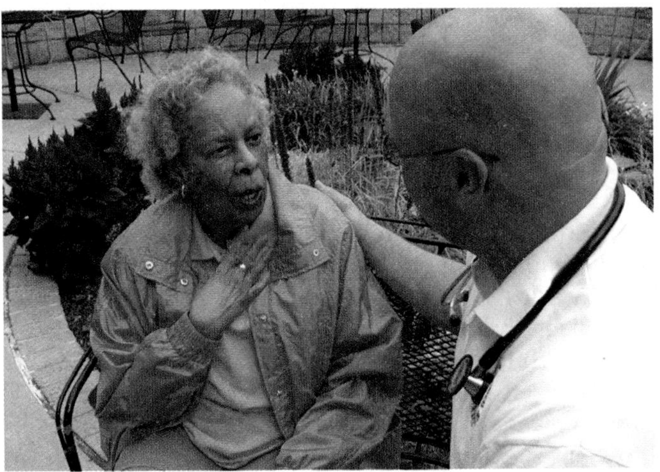

Figure 9-4 Communication with a patient can be employed to de-escalate the patient's crisis.

we use can all greatly influence the reaction of the person to whom we are speaking. With patients, families, and bystanders who are experiencing a crisis of any kind, communication is a critical element for promoting calm, getting the information needed to make decisions, and reducing risks to the patient and the patient's caregivers (**Figure 9-4**).

Verbal De-escalation Techniques

For all EMS calls, every scene and patient must be managed based on their unique circumstances. However, the following principles of verbal de-escalation can be applied to most all patient encounters:

- Respect personal space—remain two arm's-lengths away from the patient if they are acutely agitated. Avoid touching patients without their permission.
- Use a calm and nonaggressive tone of voice, and monitor your nonverbal communication (e.g., do not cross your arms, roll your eyes, smirk, laugh, or engage in other provocative communication; turn down your radio if possible to avoid further escalation).
- Identify yourself and let the patient know you are there to help.
- Build trust by asking how the patient wants to be identified (by name/nickname and by preferred pronouns [e.g., he/she/they]).
- Look at the patient, but avoid intense direct eye contact.
- Be concise. Use short, direct, clear statements.
- Identify what the patient needs/wants and feels. Listen closely and compassionately.
- Active listening is critical.
- Tell the patient you want to partner with them to help, and they can make decisions with you. In cases where patients do not have the capacity to make decisions, expressing that you want to partner with them to help is still appropriate.
- Avoid language that makes any patient feel forced or coerced. Offer choices where possible.
- Avoid abrupt physical movements.
- Do not argue with or challenge the patient. For example, if a patient has a different perception of reality due to memory issues or delusions/hallucinations, it is not recommended to challenge this perception directly. In these circumstances, identifying what emotion the patient is experiencing and reflecting it back can be validating. This technique also opens up a dialogue that allows the patient to share what usually helps when they are feeling this way.
- If a patient is experiencing evident hallucinations and/or delusions and asks if you are experiencing what they are, avoid confirming or denying what they see/hear/taste/smell/feel/believe. Instead, provide reassurance through active listening, focusing on the emotions the patient is having versus the experience itself, and attempting redirection to a topic that you believe the patient may have interest in.
- Do not tell patients to "calm down" or threaten them if their behavior does not stop. In general, agitated patients have a loss of behavioral control and do not want to be feeling/acting this way. This tactic may escalate agitation and promote further risk to patients and those caring for them.
- Be honest. If a patient asks a question, answer as directly as possible.
- Avoid judgmental and blaming words and statements, such as "If you didn't drink, this would not happen," or "You are crazy right now."
- Recognize that because communication is the treatment on scene, these calls take extra time. You might expect to be off scene in 10 minutes for a trauma alert, but for a mental health emergency you may be on scene for more than 30 minutes before you are able to stabilize the situation and transport the patient for further care.
- Consider how you would want to be communicated with if you were having a mental health emergency.
- If the patient is verbally abusive to you or your team, do not take it personally. Assume it is the disease talking and count it as a sign of illness. Redirect the patient back toward considering their own care.

The following communication techniques are important to practice:

- Paraphrase: Use fewer words to repeat back what you have heard the patient say.
- Summarize: Sum up what the patient has said to you after listening for a period of time.

- **Reflective listening**: Restate what you hear and see, with a focus on how the patient is feeling.
- Open-ended questions: Clarify what the patient is thinking or feeling by asking questions that require more than a yes-or-no answer.
- I statements: Start your sentences with "I" to take ownership of what you have said and avoid putting the patient on the defensive. Example: "I heard you say that you are scared of going to the hospital. I can understand why you would feel scared. I am here to help you feel less scared, and I am going to be with you in the ambulance the entire way there."

Mental Health Conditions and Disorders

Mental illness is defined as a disorder of the brain that makes it difficult for an individual to function from day to day. The causes of mental illness are still poorly understood. For the purposes of EMS response, a mental health crisis is any situation involving thoughts or behavior that puts the patient at risk of harming self or others or prevents them from being able to care for self or function independently.

Currently, there is not a specific set of tests that can be used to definitively diagnose mental illness. However, qualified health professionals such as psychiatrists, psychologists, emergency physicians, and clinical social workers can use symptoms, clinical observations, and response to treatment to help diagnose patients and manage their care.

Many mental health disorders and conditions exist (**Figure 9-5**), and the criteria for their diagnosis and treatment plan recommendations can be found in the American Psychiatric Association's *Diagnostic and Statistical Manual of Mental Disorders*, fifth edition text revision (DSM-5-TR). In this chapter, we will focus on some of the more common mental health disorders you may encounter as an EMS clinician.

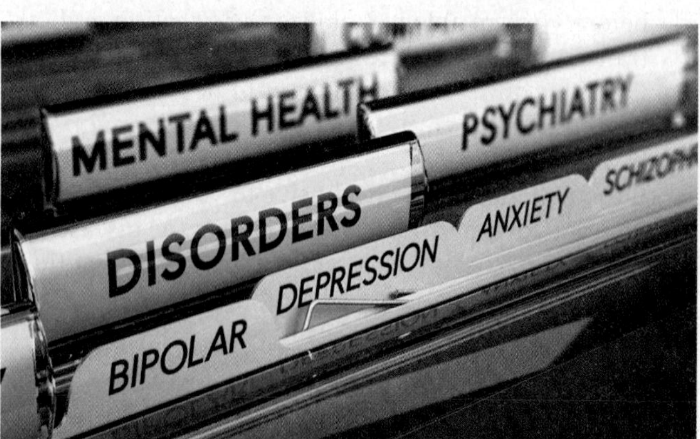

Figure 9-5 Many different mental health disorders can cause patients to have crises.

Depressive Disorder

Depression is one of the most common mood disorders, resulting in a wide range of disability. Some patients may exhibit signs of depression without having previously been diagnosed. Many individuals living with depression can be high functioning and well managed with medications and counseling. For other patients, depression leads to significant challenges that impact every aspect of their life. Forms of depressive disorder include major depressive disorder, persistent depressive disorder, postpartum depression, substance/medication-induced depressive disorder, seasonal affective disorder, and premenstrual dysphoric disorder. These are simply categories that help further define different temporal patterns in depression or apparent triggers, but these subclassifications are generally not important for EMS clinicians to learn.

Symptoms

Symptoms of depression include persistent feelings of sadness and/or loss of interest impairing activities of daily living. Symptoms (lasting for at least 2 weeks for diagnosis) may include significant changes to sleep and appetite, low energy level, difficulty with concentration, unusual behavior such as withdrawing from others, low self-esteem, restricted or flat affect (lack of expression of emotion through facial expressions, gestures, tone of voice, and other emotional signs such as laughter or crying), and changes in personality. Some patients with depression experience suicidal thoughts or even attempt suicide.

Common Treatments

Common treatments for depression include medication and outpatient counseling. Patients exhibiting suicidal or homicidal thoughts will often require inpatient stabilization prior to transitioning to an outpatient care plan.

Safety Considerations

Patients with depression may experience suicidal thoughts, may attempt suicide, and may self-harm (e.g., self-mutilation via cutting or burning). Patients who have attempted suicide, such as via overdose or hanging, or who have engaged in extensive self-injury should be transported per agency protocol for hospital-based medical evaluation. Patients who are actively experiencing suicidal thoughts or are in danger due to uncontrollable self-harm require immediate mental health care for stabilization and should be transported per agency protocol.

Some agencies have alternative-destination protocols that offer transport to patients who agree with voluntary assessment at a psychiatric facility, or the facilitation of involuntarily admission to a psychiatric facility when deemed necessary. State laws and regulations will dictate how involuntary transport can be achieved and what level of practitioner has the authority to determine whether a patient can be treated involuntarily.

Patients may self-medicate with alcohol or drugs to treat their depression, so clinicians should consider signs and symptoms in the context of possible intoxication. In addition, patients are at increased risk of death by suicide if they have a co-occurring substance use disorder and when intoxicated. So, when working with a patient who is intoxicated and expressing suicidal thoughts, it is important to recognize this risk and advocate for them to receive appropriate psychiatric help.

Bipolar Disorder

Bipolar disorder is another type of mood disorder that is marked by periods of extreme highs and lows in mood and energy and often brings challenges in many areas of a patient's life. The main subtypes of bipolar disorder include bipolar I disorder (both depressive and manic episodes) and bipolar II disorder (both depressive and hypomanic episodes).

Symptoms

Symptoms of bipolar disorder include discrete depressive episodes and discrete manic or hypomanic episodes. Depressive episodes are as outlined previously. Typically, manic or hypomanic episodes are characterized by a more elevated or extreme mood, an increase in goal-directed activity and energy, and a decreased need for sleep. Manic episodes are more disruptive to functioning than are hypomanic episodes. Patients with bipolar disorder may also experience psychotic symptoms, such as paranoia or grandiose delusions.

Common Treatments

Common treatments for bipolar disorder include medication and outpatient counseling. Affected individuals can have successful outcomes with these treatments; however, due to the neurobiology of this diagnosis, acute episodes or treatment adherence issues can be a challenge. Patients who present with suicidal or homicidal thoughts or are unable to care for themselves will require inpatient or intensive day program stabilization prior to transitioning to an outpatient care plan.

Safety Considerations

Patients with bipolar disorder may experience suicidal thoughts, may attempt suicide, and may have self-injurious thoughts or behaviors. Some may develop psychotic symptoms. Patients who are acutely manic often present with psychomotor agitation and are more impulsive, which can pose additional safety risks to clinicians. Patients who are actively experiencing suicidal thoughts or are in danger due to uncontrollable self-harm require immediate mental health care for stabilization and should be offered voluntary admission to a psychiatric facility, or if incapacitated, should be involuntarily admitted to a psychiatric facility, per local protocols.

Anxiety Disorder

Anxiety disorders are the most common mental health disorder in the United States and have varying severity. Many individuals living with anxiety experience both physical symptoms and cognitive effects. Individuals may be able to learn strategies to manage their anxiety, and symptoms can be managed with medications and counseling. However, as with depression, for some individuals, anxiety leads to significant challenges that impact every aspect of their life. Types of anxiety disorders include generalized anxiety disorder, panic disorder, social anxiety disorder, and specific phobia, among others.

Symptoms

Symptoms of generalized anxiety include persistent feelings of worry, anxiety, and/or fear that impact the individual's activities of daily living. Symptoms may also include worry or a stress response that seems out of proportion to the inciting event; inability to stop worrying; and feeling jumpy, irritable, and restless (**Figure 9-6**). Patients may complain of shortness of breath, chest tightness, palpitations, sweating, stomach issues, insomnia, and headaches. Panic attacks, which are feelings of sudden or intense anxiety that often cause physical

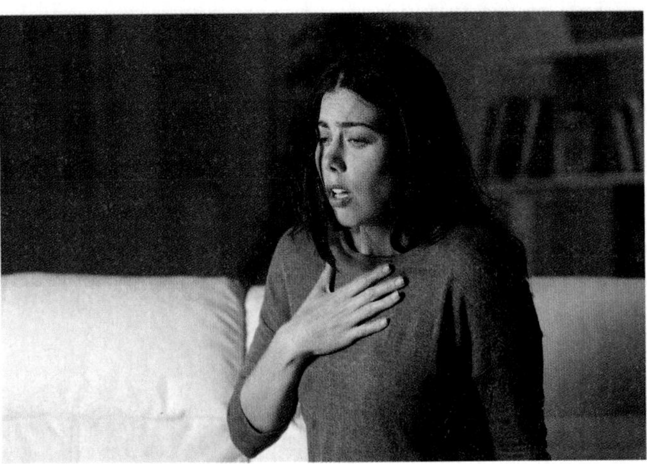

Figure 9-6 Anxiety disorder can cause patients to feel overwhelmed with worry or stress.

symptoms, may occur. Such panic attacks often present with physical or other behavioral complaints; the EMS clinician must consider those possible etiologies in their differential diagnoses as well. This consideration often complicates the evaluation of these patients.

Common Treatments

Common treatments for anxiety include medication and outpatient counseling.

Schizophrenia

Schizophrenia is an exceptionally complex disorder; however, with medication management and support, individuals living with this diagnosis can have great success with reducing or eliminating their symptoms and achieving independence and higher life quality. However, due to the nature of some aspects of schizophrenia, this disorder can lead to challenges that impact every area of life. Some symptoms of schizophrenia can also cause behavioral issues that, without treatment, could create safety risks for both affected individuals and the clinicians caring for them (**Figure 9-7**). For example, a patient having delusions about a family member and access to weapons may be a risk to that individual and EMS clinicians.

Symptoms

Symptoms of schizophrenia are often classified into three categories: positive, negative, and cognitive. Positive symptoms involve unusual behaviors or aberrations in thinking, such as delusions, hallucinations, heightened sensory sensitivity, changes in personality, inaccurate perceptions, and paranoia. Negative symptoms reflect the absence of something; they include apathy, flat affect, loss of motivation, poverty of speech, and anhedonia (lack of pleasure). Cognitive symptoms include impairment in memory, processing speed, attention, and ability to problem-solve. These symptoms can cause a withdrawal from the world that often leads to issues with relationships, such as a loss of interest in conversation or not wanting to leave the home.

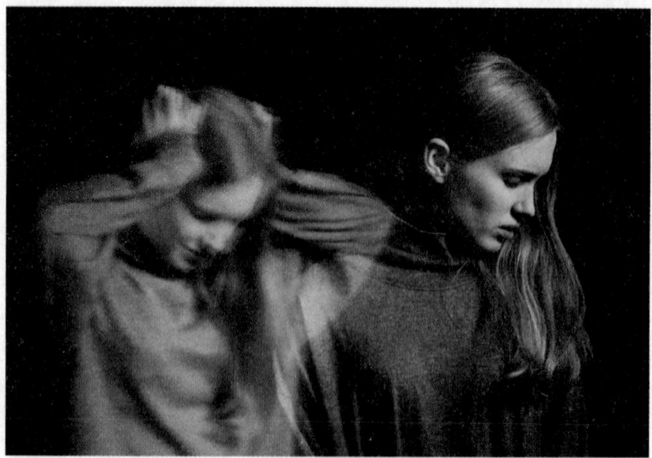

Figure 9-7 Schizophrenia is a complex mental health disorder that produces symptoms that can also cause behavioral issues.

Common Treatments

Common treatments for schizophrenia include medication, outpatient counseling, and case management. Patients who experiencing suicidal or homicidal thoughts, or who are gravely disabled, will require inpatient or intensive day program stabilization prior to transitioning to an outpatient care plan.

Safety Considerations

Patients with schizophrenia are often inaccurately portrayed as being universally violent. Patients who are experiencing acute psychotic symptoms, and specifically having persecutory delusions, may pose a safety risk to others due to the symptoms they are experiencing. Suicide is a major cause of death in patients with schizophrenia. Patients who are actively experiencing suicidal thoughts, experiencing homicidal thoughts, unable to attend to their basic needs (e.g., not eating/drinking), or engaging in significant self-injury due to their psychotic symptoms require immediate mental health care for stabilization; they should be offered voluntary transport or be transported involuntarily to an appropriate facility.

Autism Spectrum Disorder

Patients diagnosed with autism spectrum disorder (ASD) are becoming a more commonly encountered patient population in the EMS setting secondary to an improved screening process and greater community awareness. The most recent data suggest that the current prevalence is 1 in 68 children, with males being affected 4 times more often compared to females. Patients have varying degrees of communication difficulties. Those whose language and social engagement is more impaired can easily be overstimulated by sounds and examination attempts, sometimes leading to defensive, and occasionally aggressive, maneuvers.

Pathophysiology

The underlying cause of ASD is not well understood. There was a brief period of speculation that childhood vaccinations might be associated with ASD, but this notion has been irrefutably debunked. Both genetic and environmental factors are thought to influence brain development in patients with ASD. Patients must undergo a series of neurologic and behavioral assessments to be formally diagnosed with ASD.

Signs and Symptoms

There have been scant research and resources dedicated to the evaluation and management of patients with ASD in prehospital settings. As a result, in 2005, the Autism Society developed the Safe and Sound campaign to disseminate training materials to first responders and emergency department personnel to help them more appropriately interact with these patients. Older patients with ASD can seem intoxicated or intellectually disabled. Recognition of common characteristics among patients with moderate to severe ASD requires careful and meticulous observation for the following symptoms:

- Avoids eye contact
- Speech delays, repetitive speech, or mimicking; 30% to 50% of patients are nonverbal
- May not recognize EMS, fire, or police emblems
- Fixation on certain objects
- Sensory behaviors (can include self-stimulation behaviors such as rocking)
- May have flat affect and not respond to social interactions
- Violent or aggressive behaviors with overstimulation (e.g., lights and siren)
- May speak at inappropriate volumes

Evaluation and Treatment

Patients with ASD commonly have a health care proxy and caregiver who is very familiar with the patient's communication patterns and responses to outside stimuli. These individuals are invaluable resources in assisting with evaluation, management, communication, and transport. For patients with ASD, the clinician should determine a baseline level of function, competence, and communication abilities. Move slowly through the examination, working distally to proximally, and communicate slowly and with gentle gestures to keep the patient calm and cooperative. Patients may have ritualized patterns of speech or movement that they feel they need to follow. If the patient is fixated on a phone or similar device, do not interrupt the fixation, as the distraction may facilitate the physical examination, treatment, or transportation.

Many patients with ASD have either hypoactive or hyperactive tolerance to pain and have difficulty interpreting and displaying facial expressions consistent with pain. Treat pain as per local protocols. As many as 30% of patients with ASD will develop a seizure disorder; acute seizures should be treated in standard fashion with benzodiazepine administration and respiratory support as appropriate.

As a result of their inability to accurately interpret social cues, patients with ASD are frequently victims of criminal and sexual abuse. In many cases, they will be unable to communicate what has transpired. Such patients should undergo an initial trauma evaluation and stabilization with the assistance of caregivers. It is good practice to ask receiving facilities for a quiet area away from excessive stimuli upon arrival to prevent further anxiety and overstimulation.

Substance Use Disorders

Substance use disorders are widespread and have the potential to impact every aspect of an individual's life (**Figure 9-8**). The stigma surrounding substance use creates additional challenges for affected individuals, their support system, and the health professionals caring for them.

Symptoms

Key symptoms of substance use disorders include impaired control regarding how much, how often, or how long substance use is occurring, even with attempts to reduce use or with negative consequences of use. Intense urges to use, changes in behavior and personality due to substance use, difficulty maintaining activities of daily living or fulfilling role obligations (e.g., work, school, relationships), and physical withdrawal if substance use is discontinued are additional symptoms. Every substance can induce unique behavior changes, physical reactions, and withdrawal symptoms. For example, withdrawal from alcohol or benzodiazepines can lead to seizures, hallucinations, and delirium tremens. Additionally, substance use disorders often accompany and complicate baseline mental health disorders. Some common substances you may encounter a patient using are listed in **Table 9-1**. See also Chapter 14, *Toxicology*, for an in-depth discussion of substance use and abuse.

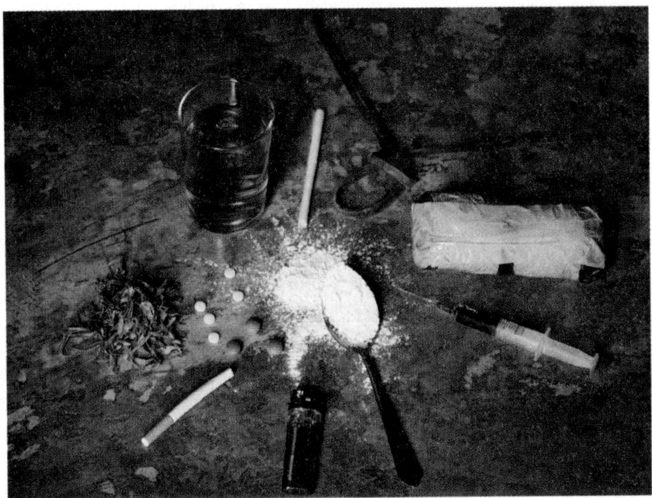

Figure 9-8 Substance use disorders affect a patient's ability to maintain activities of daily living.

Table 9-1 Characteristics of Commonly Used Drugs

Drug	Method of Administration	Signs of Recent Use
Alcohol	Most commonly ingested; can also be inhaled, snorted, and injected	■ A sense of euphoria ■ Smell of alcohol on breath ■ Confusion ■ Difficulty with gait and balance ■ Increased blood pressure and heart rate ■ Red eyes ■ Dry mouth ■ Decreased motor coordination ■ Difficulty focusing ■ Slow reaction time ■ Mood lability
Marijuana	Smoked, ingested, inhaled	■ A sense of euphoria ■ Heightened sense of visual, taste, and auditory perceptions ■ Increased blood pressure and heart rate ■ Red eyes ■ Dry mouth ■ Decreased motor coordination ■ Difficulty focusing ■ Slow reaction time ■ Anxiety/paranoia ■ Smell of marijuana on clothes or in environment ■ Food cravings ■ Cyclic vomiting is a common issue for marijuana users
K2/spice/synthetic cannabinoids	Smoked/vaped, ingested	■ A sense of euphoria ■ Elevated mood ■ Altered sense of visual, taste, and auditory perceptions ■ Increased blood pressure and heart rate, or onset of cardiac arrest ■ Hallucinations ■ Extreme anxiety/agitation ■ Paranoia ■ Vomiting ■ Confusion
Bath salts (synthetic cathinones)	Ingested, insufflated, inhaled, injected	■ Sense of euphoria ■ Increased sociability ■ Increased energy ■ Increased blood pressure and heart rate ■ Hallucinations ■ Loss of muscle control ■ Difficulty concentrating ■ Extreme anxiety/agitation ■ Paranoia ■ Panic attacks ■ Psychosis and violent behavior

Drug	Method of Administration	Signs of Recent Use
Barbiturates, benzodiazepines, and hypnotics	Ingested or injected	■ Sleepiness ■ Slurred speech ■ Lack of coordination ■ Irritability ■ Difficulty concentrating ■ Memory issues ■ Involuntary eye movements ■ Lack of inhibition ■ Slow breathing and decreased blood pressure ■ Falls ■ Dizziness
Methamphetamine, cocaine, and other stimulants	Smoked, injected, snorted, or ingested	■ Overconfidence ■ Increased alertness ■ Increased energy/restlessness ■ Rambling or rapid speech ■ Dilated pupils ■ Increased blood pressure and heart rate, or onset of cardiac arrest ■ Delusions/hallucinations ■ Irritability/agitation ■ Anxiety/paranoia ■ Vomiting ■ Impaired judgment ■ Nasal congestion (secondary to snorting) ■ Mouth sores/tooth decay (secondary to smoking) ■ Skin sores from picking behavior ■ Confusion ■ Depression coming off high ■ Insomnia
Ecstasy, MDMA (3,4-methylenedioxy-methamphetamine), GHB (gamma-hydroxybutyrate), Rohypnol (flunitrazepam)/roofies, and ketamine	Ingested, injected, snorted	■ Muscle cramps ■ Chills/sweats ■ Involuntary shaking ■ Behavior changes ■ Rambling or rapid speech ■ Dilated pupils ■ Increased or decreased blood pressure and heart rate ■ Reduced consciousness/sedation ■ Heightened senses ■ Poor judgment ■ Impaired judgment ■ Loss of memory ■ Reduced inhibitions ■ Seizures

(*continues*)

Table 9-1 Characteristics of Commonly Used Drugs (*continued*)

Drug	Method of Administration	Signs of Recent Use
Hallucinogens (e.g., psilocybin, lysergic acid diethylamide [LSD], phencyclidine [PCP])	Ingested, smoked, snorted, injected	▪ Hallucinations ▪ Reduced perception of reality ▪ Rapid mood changes ▪ Increased blood pressure and heart rate ▪ Impaired judgment ▪ Impulsive behavior ▪ Tremors ▪ Aggressive/violent behavior ▪ Involuntary eye movements ▪ Lack of pain sensation ▪ Difficulty thinking clearly ▪ Lack of coordination ▪ Problems speaking ▪ Seizure/coma ▪ Sensory sensitivity
Inhalants (e.g., glues, solvents, compressed gases)	Inhaled	▪ Intoxication ▪ Decreased inhibition ▪ Increased energy/restlessness ▪ Combativeness ▪ Dizziness ▪ Vomiting ▪ Involuntary eye movements ▪ Irregular heartbeat ▪ Tremors ▪ Rash around nose and/or mouth
Opioids	Ingested, injected, smoked, inhaled, snorted	▪ Reduced sense of pain ▪ Sedation/drowsiness ▪ Slurred speech ▪ Constricted pupils ▪ Decreased respiratory drive ▪ Lack of attention to surroundings ▪ Irritability/agitation ▪ Depression ▪ Constipation ▪ Impaired judgment ▪ Nasal congestion (secondary to snorting) ▪ Needle marks (secondary to injections)

Common Treatments

Common treatments for substance use disorders include medication-assisted treatment (MAT) and inpatient or outpatient drug/alcohol counseling. Patients exhibiting symptoms indicating a risk to self or others, or who have medical complications related to withdrawal, require inpatient detoxification or intensive day program stabilization prior to transitioning to an outpatient care plan.

With the increasing understanding of opioid overuse and available treatment options, EMS agencies and community paramedic programs have recently been engaging with community partners to establish MAT programs. Based on additional clinician training and available community resources, these programs are able to conduct assessments of appropriate patients and initiate treatment in the field (e.g., buprenorphine–naloxone) with referral of the patients for timely follow-up with community support services for additional care. To date, these programs have proved to be a successful part of community treatment programs and are effective in decreasing recidivism.

Safety Considerations

Patients living with substance use disorders often have a co-occurring mental health disorder. They may experience suicidal thoughts, may attempt suicide, and may self-harm. Patients with substance intoxication or withdrawal may be agitated and at increased risk of violence toward others. Patients who are actively experiencing suicidal or homicidal thoughts, engaged in significant self-harm, or experiencing physical symptoms related to withdrawal require immediate attention and/or mental health care for stabilization; they should be offered voluntary transport to an appropriate facility that manages co-occurring disorders, or if incapacitated, should be involuntarily transported to a facility with resources capable of managing their condition. During active use or overuse of some substances, patients may become agitated, delirious, or both. This could pose a potential danger to both patient and clinician. Pharmacologic management options for patients who are agitated are covered in more detail in Chapter 2, *Clinical Approach to Pharmacology*. Safe practices for patient restraint are covered in more detail in the NAEMT EMS Safety Course.

Personality Disorders

Personality disorders are common but often are not easy to treat and manage due to their impacts on an individual's insight, which make it difficult to recognize the disorder's symptoms. As medications cannot assist a person to gain insight, counseling is often encouraged. The U.S. Food and Drug Administration (FDA) has not approved any medications specifically for the treatment of personality disorders; however, medication management has proved successful in managing symptoms in some individuals, and recent research suggests new medication protocols may be on the horizon. Each personality disorder is associated with its own unique set of symptoms, but as a group they are often sorted into three separate clusters to connect disorders with similar characteristics.

Symptoms

- Cluster A (paranoid, schizoid, schizotypal): Odd and eccentric thinking and behavior that impacts the patient's relationships and activities of daily living. Distrustful, secretive, paranoid, angry/hostile, hold grudges, difficulty with social cues, flat affect, delusions, social anxiety.
- Cluster B (antisocial, borderline, histrionic, narcissistic): Dramatic, overly emotional, attention seeking, disregard for safety, risky/impulsive behavior, self-focus, rapid mood changes, unpredictable thinking and behavior.
- Cluster C (avoidant, dependent, obsessive–compulsive): Anxiety, fear-driven thoughts and behavior. Sensitive to criticism or rejection, dependence, shyness or clingy behavior, low self-esteem, rigid, need for order, desire for control.

Individuals with a personality disorder may exhibit multiple signs.

Common Treatments

Common treatments for personality disorders include outpatient counseling and possibly medication to target specific symptoms. Patients exhibiting symptoms indicating an immediate risk to self or others will require inpatient or intensive day program stabilization prior to transitioning to an outpatient care plan.

Safety Considerations

Patients with personality disorders may experience suicidal thoughts, attempt suicide, and have self-harm thoughts or behaviors. Some may have co-occurring substance use disorders or use substances to try to manage their symptoms. Patients who are acutely experiencing suicidal thoughts or are in danger due to uncontrollable self-harm require immediate mental health evaluation per agency protocol; they should be offered transport to an appropriate facility, or if incapacitated, involuntarily transported.

Special Considerations for Patients Experiencing Suicidal Thoughts

Suicide is the 12th leading cause of death overall in the United States; it is the second leading cause of death for people ages 10 to 14 and 25 to 34, the third leading cause of death for people ages 15 to 24, the fourth leading cause of death for people ages 35 to 44, the seventh leading cause of death for people ages 45 to 54, and the ninth leading cause of death for people ages 55 to 64. In 2020, there were almost 46,000 deaths by suicide. Firearms are used by more than half of the individuals who die by suicide. Many EMS calls also involve patients who have attempted suicide. Approximately 1.2 million people attempt suicide each year. Patients who attempt suicide always require transport for further care and evaluation; however, depending on the nature of their injuries, the main focus of this type of call may be treatment for trauma, overdose, or other associated clinical problems.

Some patients may not disclose that they have attempted suicide, so it is helpful to use nonjudgmental and compassionate interview techniques during the patient assessment. When possible, you can also utilize situational awareness and family or bystander observations to inform your decision making on the appropriate agency protocol to follow for your response. For patients who are experiencing suicidal thoughts but have not yet attempted suicide, it is critical that you employ communication to assist the patient until a voluntary or involuntary commitment can be facilitated by law enforcement or a qualified health professional. When communicating with a patient who is experiencing suicidal thoughts, consider these communication strategies:

- Be direct and ask patients if they are thinking of suicide.
- Ask patients if they have a plan to attempt suicide; if they state they do, ask what that plan is and if they have taken any steps toward acting on their plan.
- Ask patients if they have the means to carry out their plan in the home; if so, secure it and/or notify law enforcement if they arrive on scene. Similarly, ask about their access to firearms in the home and either recommend removal of these weapons and/or notify law enforcement if they arrive.
- Provide compassionate listening.
- Avoid trying to talk patients out of their plan to attempt suicide by making statements such as "You have so much to live for" or "How could you leave your children behind?"
- Avoid judgmental language.
- Offer validation. Example: "I am honored you feel comfortable sharing how you feel with me. We will get through this together."
- Explore patients' feelings by asking open-ended questions such as "Tell me about other times you may have felt this way" or "What have you tried to help yourself feel better in the past?"
- Keep patients talking until law enforcement or a qualified health clinician arrives to discuss voluntary or involuntary transport to an appropriate facility.

EMS clinicians are sometimes required to manage the initial evaluation and triage of a patient who may be experiencing suicidal thoughts. Many tools are available to assist with this process. The U.S. Department of Health and Human Services' Substance Abuse and Mental Health Services Administration (SAMHSA) has designed the SAFE-T (Suicide Assessment Five-step Evaluation and Triage), a tool that is appropriate for patients of all ages (**Figure 9-9**). SAFE-T allows you to:

1. Identify risk factors-.
2. Identify protective factors.
3. Conduct suicide inquiry.
4. Determine risk level/intervention.
5. Document.

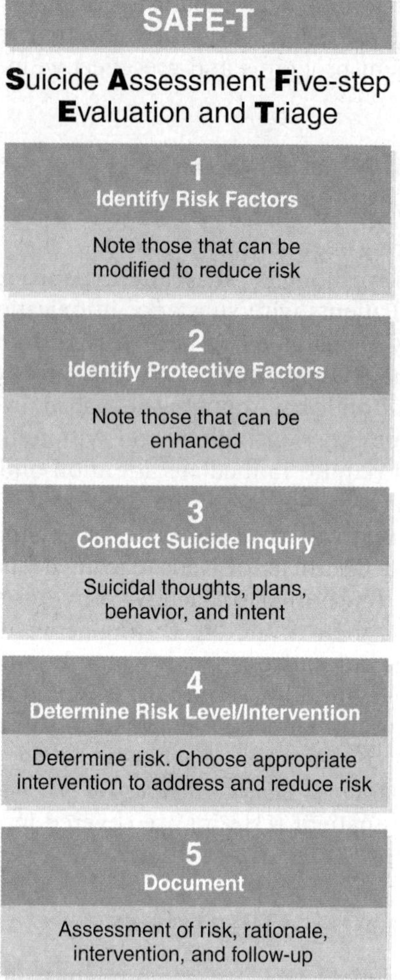

SAFE-T
Suicide Assessment Five-step Evaluation and Triage
1
Identify Risk Factors
Note those that can be modified to reduce risk
2
Identify Protective Factors
Note those that can be enhanced
3
Conduct Suicide Inquiry
Suicidal thoughts, plans, behavior, and intent
4
Determine Risk Level/Intervention
Determine risk. Choose appropriate intervention to address and reduce risk
5
Document
Assessment of risk, rationale, intervention, and follow-up

Figure 9-9 SAFE-T evaluation tool.

Courtesy of U.S. Department of Health and Human Services.

You can download the SAFE-T evaluation tool at www.sprc.org.

Management of Mental Health Emergencies

Decision-Making Capacity

Decision-making capacity is an important concept for EMS clinicians to understand. The framework used for determining decision-making capacity allows for patient autonomy when appropriate and provides medical care as needed. Capacity is not solely dependent on a preexisting diagnosis or substance or medication use, but rather reflects the patient's specific ability to understand the issues at the time the person is being evaluated. It is, in the end, a judgment made by the EMS clinician and other health care professionals.

The following is a simplified approach to determining decision-making capacity:

- The patient must be able to communicate their choice.
- The patient must understand and convey the medical condition or situation they are in as well as the proposed treatment options.
- The patient must appreciate and acknowledge their condition and the potential consequences of obtaining treatment/transport versus the risks of refusing treatment. Courts have recognized that patients who do not acknowledge their illness (lack of insight) may not be able to make valid decisions about treatment.
- The patient must be able to reason rationally through the treatment options.
- The patient is not actively experiencing suicidal or homicidal thoughts. Those factors presume a lack of decision-making capacity.
- When medically and situationally appropriate, alternative options such as in-home assessment/response teams, alternative-destination transport, or other innovative care programs may be offered to the patient if they are available in your system of care.

If the patient is determined to have decision-making capacity and refuses care, consultation with online medical oversight may be advisable—and is specifically required in some agency protocols. It is also a best practice to invite the patient to call again or for the EMS clinician to assist in obtaining alternative treatments or destinations as a good-faith effort. Obtaining witness information in the event that additional contact is required is recommended as well.

The concept of decision-making capacity is not always easy to apply in the real world. You should become familiar with your local policies, protocols, and ability to contact your supervisor or online medical direction to assist with these sometimes difficult decisions. Given the complexity of balancing the patient's civil rights with their risk of harm to self or others, when in doubt, do what you think is best for the safety and well-being of the patient. In general, the courts will look more favorably on well-intentioned attempts to care for a patient who seems to be in danger, even against their will, than on what can appear to be abandonment.

Prehospital Treatment

Patients who are experiencing a psychiatric emergency will almost always require transport for further assessment, stabilization, and care. Although transport to a hospital is common, the recent increase in options for care—including the national 988 mental health hotline, telehealth options, mental health response teams, and alternative destinations—gives some EMS agencies alternatives to transport for some patients. Treatment options in the prehospital realm are separated into three categories: voluntary, involuntary, and community care.

- *Voluntary treatment.* When individuals have the capacity to make their own decisions, and for those who have a mental health issue that does not pose an imminent risk to themselves or others, EMS clinicians should offer them the opportunity to be voluntarily transported to an emergency department or other appropriate facility for evaluation and psychiatric and/or addiction care. The transport of these patients should still be managed as a safety risk, as they may decompensate mentally or behaviorally at any time.

  If the patient is already receiving mental health care services, a call to the patient's mental health care team may be an alternative to transport. In these cases, patients should still be offered the option of voluntary transport for care or to remain in their environment and receive services from their usual provider. A community-based mobile crisis mental health response team, staffed by qualified health care professionals such as a clinical social worker, psychiatric nurse, psychologist, or psychiatrist, may also be an option. Sometimes a community paramedic is a valuable member of these response teams. All of these options must be considered according to local protocols.
- *Involuntary treatment.* In cases where there is an imminent safety risk to the patient or others, and/or when patients do not demonstrate the capacity to make their own health decisions and choices, an involuntary transport to a facility will be required. All U.S. states and the District of Columbia have involuntary commitment laws that allow law enforcement and/or qualified health professionals to involuntarily commit a patient for mental health and/or addiction care for a period of time that varies by state. Traditionally, EMS agencies called upon law enforcement to facilitate involuntary transports and mental health holds for patients. However, as EMS is evolving, so too are the types of health professionals who may be working within EMS agencies. Depending on the state laws, EMS clinicians, clinical social workers, advanced registered nurse practitioners, licensed psychologists, physicians, and some other health professionals may also have authority to facilitate involuntary transport of patients from the scene. Follow your agency protocol for initiating an

involuntary transport. and learn about your state's criteria for involuntary commitment.

- *Community care.* Today, an increasing number of EMS agencies have mobile integrated health and/or community paramedicine programs that may allow for continued involvement in the care needs of patients after their 911 call. Community paramedics and medical social workers on these teams may ensure a patient's discharge plan is in place after a crisis or may help a patient prevent a crisis by partnering with the patient and their mental health team to create and coordinate a mental health care plan within the community. Community care options may include the following:
  - Referral to outpatient mental health providers
  - Mental health education
  - Connections to peer support
  - Connections to mental health advocates and case managers
  - Referral to county and state programs
  - Creation of safety plans for future crisis events
  - Support and encouragement for the patient
  - Supportive guidance and services for the patient's family

Resources

Resources are an important element of supporting patients and families who are living with mental health disorders. As an EMS clinician, you may be called upon to contact or suggest resources for the patient. Additionally, mental health and substance use responses offer opportunities for agencies with community paramedic or mobile integrated health programs to be referred to patients who may benefit from additional follow-up after their 911 encounter. There is always help available for patients and families 365 days a year, on a 24/7 basis. The following resources are available nationwide:

- *988/Suicide and Crisis Lifeline:* Nationwide live emotional support, crisis care, suicide intervention, and resource database for mental health care and suicide intervention and prevention. Can provide guidance to professionals who are with a patient who is in crisis. Available 24/7 in 250 languages and TTY. Dial 988 or go to www.988lifeline.org for chat and online messaging options.
- *211:* Resource database for community resources and programs. Generally, this option does not have immediate resources for active counseling. Available 24/7 in 180 languages. Dial 211 or go to www.211.org for online, chat, and messaging options.
- *Veterans Crisis Line:* Nationwide live crisis care, emotional support, suicide intervention/prevention, and resource database for active-duty service members, veterans, and their families. Dial 988 and select option 1, or go to www.veteranscrisisline.net.
- *National Alliance on Mental Illness (NAMI):* Advocacy, resource provider, and direct-service organization for individuals and families living with mental health disorders. Offers a crisis line 24/7. Call 1-800-950-6264, text "NAMI" to 741741, or go to www.nami.org.
- *The Trevor Project:* Free and confidential crisis support for LGBTQ minors. Crisis line is available 24/7. Call 1-866-488-7386 or text "START" to 678-678. The website, thetrevorproject.org, also offers live chat crisis support.

Mental Health and Special Populations

Pediatric Patients

Caring for a child or teen during an emergency always brings an added layer of emotion for everyone involved. The compassion and care that EMS clinicians can offer on the scene of medical emergencies involving minors is unparalleled. Responding to mental health emergencies involving minors should inspire the same effort as any other pediatric medical emergency call.

Children and teens do present unique challenges on all types of EMS calls, and mental health emergencies are part of that spectrum (**Figure 9-10**). Children and teens may respond to environmental and organic stressors differently than adults, especially those young patients in whom mental health disorders are developing. Children and teens experiencing depression, anxiety, post-traumatic stress, adjustment disorder, conduct disorder, or other disorders may exhibit irritability, disruptive behaviors, anger, or emotional lability. In some situations, the minor may seem to be acting out to seek attention. Regardless of what is causing the current crisis, each encounter should be carefully assessed and managed.

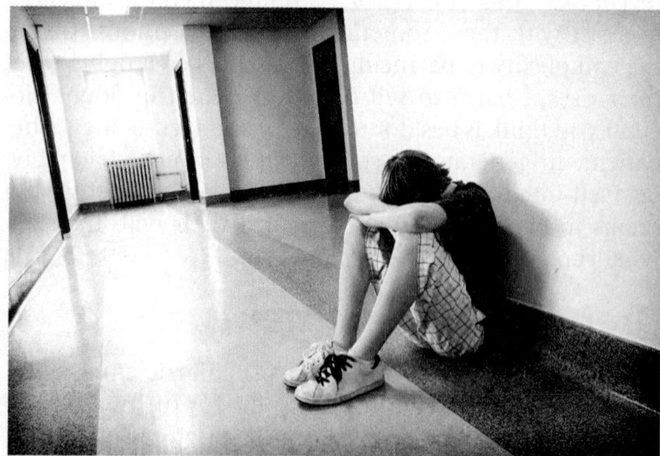

Figure 9-10 Responding to pediatric calls with compassion is an important part of patient care.

Remember that children who are enduring maltreatment from parents or other caregivers may have behavioral reactions without other means to convey what is happening within the home environment. Carefully evaluate these situations with an open mind.

An additional layer of challenge is presented by parents and siblings on scene, who may seem frantic, angry, frightened, or disconnected from the event. Families of minors living with mental health disorders are often overwhelmed and isolated, and they may lack social and family support.

Given that as many as 20% of minors may have a mental or developmental disorder, the need for emergency mental health care for minors continues to increase. Rates of emergency department visits have been on the rise over the last decade. Reports of adolescent mental health issues rose 31% between 2019 to 2020. Even more concerning is the 51% increase from 2019 to 2021 in the number of adolescent females presenting to the emergency department for a suicide attempt. Among the realities for this population are a lack of specialized pediatric mental health care and, even when it is available, a lack of affordable care; together, these factors often cause families to wait until a crisis occurs and then use EMS and the emergency care system to obtain help.

In minor patients, it can sometimes be a challenge to know what is causing behavior. The frontal lobe is still developing in children and teens, and they are not yet emotionally mature and often act to test boundaries. Look for the following signs in minors, which may indicate a mental health issue exists:

- Inability to manage daily tasks
- Rapid mood swings
- Increased agitation
- Aggressive behavior toward self or others
- Psychosis
- Isolation
- Physical symptoms/complaints that have been worked up and have no medical cause

In addition to obtaining a past psychiatric history, getting a separate history from the parents or guardian of the minor is helpful to determine whether the patient has any medical and/or neurologic issue, such as diabetes, epilepsy, or a TBI, that could be causing the child to behave in ways outside their day-to-day baseline. As part of the history, the EMS clinician should ask about any changes in the child's environment, any recent losses or changes (e.g., in the home, at school, or with peers), or other stressors that could trigger behavior changes in a pediatric patient.

For children and teens who are not in crisis, the family should be advised to call their primary care provider or mental health provider (if such a relationship exists) or community mental health resources immediately for guidance on care options. Any minor experiencing a mental health crisis should always be transported for a full assessment and mental health care. Likewise, any minor who is struggling with suicidal thoughts, self-injury, or homicidal thoughts should always be transported for evaluation.

As with adult mental health emergencies, the best treatment on scene and while transporting children with mental health emergencies is communication. In addition to the prior information covered on de-escalation techniques, consider the following unique elements when interacting with pediatric patients:

- Try to get on the same physical level as the patient.
- Introduce yourself to the child or teen and let them know you care and are there to help them.
- For younger children, it is helpful to build rapport by talking to them about their interests. For example, you can ask about the character on their shirt or a toy they are holding.
- Avoid touching the minor patient unless you ask permission and explain why the touch is needed. Example: "Doug, I would like to see how the blood is working in your body; I would like to put this cuff on your arm so we can take a measurement. Is it OK for me to touch your arm?" It can be helpful to demonstrate the action on yourself or someone else first.
- Be patient.
- Offer validation. Example: "Doug, thank you for sharing. I can understand why you would be scared to hear loud noises at night and have a hard time sleeping after what happened to your brother recently."
- Avoid threatening or ordering the minor; instead, as feasible, set a tone of working with the minor in partnership to help the patient feel better.
- If appropriate for your agency response, utilize the SAFE-T tool to initiate a discussion and evaluation of suicide risk if the minor patient is reporting suicidal thoughts or exhibiting symptoms that may indicate a risk of suicide.

Families of children and teens who are experiencing mental health issues and/or have mental health disorders are also in need of support and resources. On these scenes, consider providing families with the community resources listed earlier so they can connect to help and support after the EMS call.

If you suspect abuse, neglect, or exploitation or are concerned about the vulnerability of the family, you must report this issue to your local Child Protective Services (CPS) agency, as all EMS clinicians are mandated reporters. You do not need proof of your concerns if you are reporting in good faith. Reporting to CPS is not always punitive for the parents or guardians involved. CPS has the capacity and resources to connect families to care and services quickly. This agency's goal is to help families be self-sufficient and healthy, and for many families, your report to CPS will open access to needed support and services that may make a powerful difference in their health and lives. To find the contact number for your local CPS agency, visit www.childwelfare.gov.

Older Adult Patients

EMS clinicians often have vast experience managing the medical emergencies of older adults, as this population more frequently experiences common medical issues such as falls and cardiac events. Older adults are a heightened risk for presenting with medical issues that may cause psychiatric symptoms such as delusions, disorientation, memory loss, agitation, combativeness, and hallucinations. These medical conditions may include the following:

- Electrolyte abnormalities
- Diabetes
- TBI
- Brain tumors
- Respiratory diseases/distress
- Infection/sepsis
- Epilepsy
- Stroke
- HIV
- Dehydration
- Medication use, side effects, or toxicity

Gathering a history and completing the primary and secondary assessments are critical in all mental health emergencies, but in the case of seniors, who often have complex medical histories and comorbidities, these tasks are of vital importance to determine whether medical causes of the mental health symptoms other than a primary mental health disorder are likely. This may help determine the most appropriate transport and destination decisions. Remember that hypoglycemia may manifest as psychiatric symptoms, including agitation, confusion, and hallucinations.

Another important aspect of older adult mental health disorders is the high prevalence of dementia, or major neurocognitive disorder (MNCD), in the older population. The most common types of MNCDs include Alzheimer disease (AD), vascular dementia, Lewy body dementia (which includes Parkinson disease), mixed dementia (e.g., Alzheimer and vascular), and frontotemporal dementia. About one in nine adults age 65 or older are living with AD; for adults age 85 or older, the prevalence increases to one in three.

Symptoms of MNCDs include the following:

- Impairment in activities of daily living
- Memory impairment
- Disorientation
- Confusion
- Impaired speech
- Wandering
- Difficulty concentrating
- Sleep disturbances
- Delusions
- Hallucinations
- Agitation
- Combativeness
- Mood swings

Although the usual communication techniques for adults apply to this population, learning about MNCDs and how to manage behaviors associated with them is important for all prehospital clinicians.

Individuals with dementia or even mild cognitive impairment are at increased risk of developing acute encephalopathy, or delirium, as a result of acute medical issues. These individuals may present with fluctuating attention and orientation, confusion, increased or decreased level of activity, new-onset perceptual disturbances (such as visual hallucinations), and even combativeness.

Unlike patients in younger age categories, older adults are often assumed to have dementia or delirium even when an acute medical issue is causing their mental health symptoms. However, older adults can also present with a primary mental health disorder and are at risk for death by suicide. Indeed, older adults are a high-risk group for suicide both in the United States and internationally. Men age 85 and older have the highest rate of death by suicide of any age group in the United States. Some reasons for this especially high risk among older adults include the following:

- Higher rates of depression
- Isolation
- Grief
- Substance abuse or misuse (including prescription medications)
- Medical issues that cause pain and disability

This population is more likely to use a lethal method, such as a gun, to commit suicide, and is less likely to survive a suicide attempt. It is imperative to ask older adults who are exhibiting symptoms of a mental health emergency if they are thinking about attempting suicide as part of the AMLS assessment of the patient's needs. If the patient has no medical issues requiring transport other than suicidal ideation, then the patient should be managed using the same best practices and agency protocols as are used for adult patients experiencing suicidal thoughts. However, if the patient presents with other medical issues requiring transport, or with new-onset agitation, the priority should be to transport as appropriate for managing the primary medical issue; then, ensure that you communicate to the emergency department staff that the patient has voiced suicidal thoughts (**Figure 9-11**). On arrival at the hospital, reinforce the message that the patient has indicated they are experiencing suicidal thoughts. The emergency

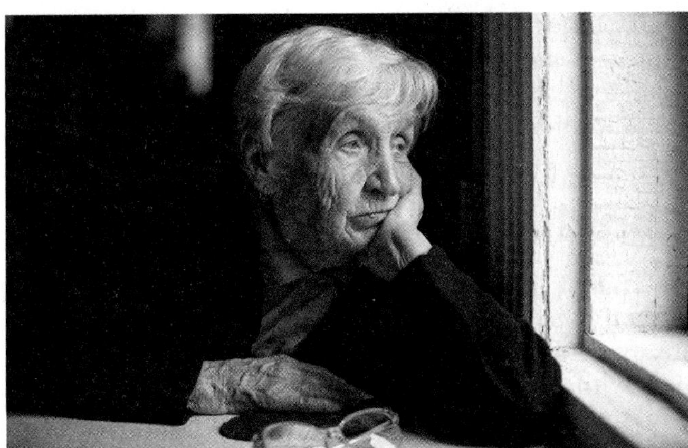

Figure 9-11 Older adults who experience a mental health emergency should be screened for suicidal thoughts and behaviors.

department staff should be asked to ensure the patient receives a mental health evaluation once the primary medical issue is stabilized to ensure the patient's safety and mental health care needs are met.

EMS Clinician Mental Health

EMS clinician mental health has come to the forefront of EMS agencies' attention in recent years: 85% of first responders report they have experienced symptoms of mental health issues, and 75% of rescue workers report mild symptoms of psychological trauma after working a disaster. This attention has resulted in better access to mental health and addiction care, as well as more robust programs to prevent issues commonly encountered among first responders, such as posttraumatic stress disorder (PTSD), moral injury, compassion fatigue, secondary trauma, and substance abuse. However, a sense of stigma—the perception that EMS clinicians seeking help is a sign of weakness—persists within the first responder community. In addition, 40% of first responders report a belief that they would face negative repercussions if they sought mental health support at work. EMS clinicians have the same risk of developing mental health disorders as any other people, but their exposure to constant trauma and stress heightens the potential of a disorder being triggered. This reality puts EMS clinicians at a higher risk of suicide and substance use disorders.

Many programs have been developed to end the stigma of seeking help and to bring attention to the signs and symptoms of PTSD and other mental health disorders among first responders. These programs include those offered through EMS advocacy groups such NAEMT, as well as the International Association of Fire Fighters (IAFF) and SAMHSA.

It is imperative to know the signs of stress and PTSD and to know where to access resources for support and care if these symptoms begin to impact day-to-day functioning. Signs to watch for include the following:

- Difficulty sleeping
- Aggressive behavior
- Overwhelming feelings of guilt or shame
- Abusing alcohol or drugs
- Irritability
- Difficulty concentrating
- Easily startled
- Chronic pain
- Digestive issues
- Headaches
- Nightmares/flashbacks
- Depression
- Anxiety/panic attacks
- Withdrawal from activities once enjoyed
- Relationship issues
- Dreading coming to work
- Emotional numbness
- Avoidance of situations or discussions that cause memories or stress

Many EMS agencies now offer employee assistance programs (EAP) and an identified Mental Health Resiliency Officer role to ensure EMS workers have confidential access to mental health care. Additionally, many EMS agencies participate in peer support programs and offer after-event stress management guidance through formal debriefings and/or critical incident stress management. EMS agencies also frequently offer chaplaincy services, and some have specially trained psychologists and/or clinical social workers on staff or available as consultants who provide EAP services, mental health education, and other supportive programming. Clinicians are encouraged to become familiar with their agency's access points for help, and to advocate for increased accessibility of mental health resources and wellness offerings. Even if they do not require these supports themselves, they may recognize fellow EMS clinicians who do and help guide their peers to the appropriate resources. NAEMT has developed courses to further knowledge on mental health in the field of EMS, including the Mental Health Resilience Officer course, which is intended to empower agencies to create an identified resilience officer role to offer a clear and confidential pathway to resources and care for personnel and their families.

In addition to the resources listed previously, many mental health and resilience resources have been specifically designed for EMS clinicians and other first responders:

- *CrewCare:* A mental health awareness and resource app offering education, resources, and information

on wellness and crisis support for first responders. Visit www.crewcarelife.com.
- *Fire/EMS Helpline:* Offered by the National Volunteer Fire Council to provide 24/7 support to first responders. Call 1-888-731-FIRE (3473).
- *Safe Call Now:* 24/7 Helpline staffed by first responders for first responders and their families. Call 1-206-459-3020.
- *IAFF Center of Excellence for Behavioral Health Treatment and Recovery:* Offers training in peer support and other mental health topics. Call 1-855-737-0949 or visit www.iaffrecoverycenter.com.
- *Code Green Campaign:* Offers connection to a resource database for first responder mental health care, educational initiatives, and financial assistance for first responders seeking mental health care. Go to www.codegreencampaign.org.

If you or someone you know is experiencing symptoms of a mental health disorder, please reach out for help. You can best care for others when you have cared for yourself first.

Conclusion

Prehospital clinicians are in the unique position of often being the first professionals to engage with patients who are experiencing mental health symptoms or emergencies. With appropriate knowledge, training, and compassion, those who work in EMS can not only save lives, but also bring significant positive changes that will empower patients living with mental health disorders and help them find stability to reduce their reliance on EMS and improve their quality of life.

SCENARIO SOLUTION

- Consider any other medical issues that could be causing the patient to have hyper motor activity and be experiencing paranoia, especially hypoglycemia and hypoxia. Other possibilities include medication side effects or toxicity, sepsis, neurologic disorders, and trauma.
- Issues to consider include whether the patient has the capacity to decide what care he may need, and if the patient does not appear to have decision-making capacity, whether law enforcement or a qualified health professional should be called to the scene to facilitate an involuntary admission to a psychiatric facility for further assessment, stabilization, and care. Also consider whether you could use communication techniques to de-escalate the mental health crisis and reduce the risk of agitation or combative behavior during the patient care episode, and which tools you may need to utilize during transport to ensure the patient and those caring for him are safe, including the potential need for pharmacologic sedation, physical restraint, and PPE.

SUMMARY

- Mental health disorders and conditions are, at their core, medical conditions requiring the same approach to assessment and treatment as any other chronic disease or medical condition.
- Although mental health disorders are the outcome of neurobiologic impacts in the brain, psychosocial, medical, and environmental factors can contribute to triggering episodes of crisis.
- Fear of stigma, being labeled, and being blamed for not controlling behavioral symptoms, and the impacts these factors have on a patient's life, may dissuade many patients from reaching out for medical management and support of their mental health conditions.
- On the scene of mental health emergencies, EMS clinicians are often required to think outside the box and utilize their problem-solving skills to most effectively help the patient.
- EMS clinicians should always rule out another medical explanation for the presenting mental health symptoms by using the AMLS Assessment Pathway, which includes a patient history and both primary and secondary surveys.
- Although patients with mental health disorders are generally nonviolent, when in a crisis, especially one involving a loss of reality (psychosis), both the patient and the clinicians caring for the patient are at risk.
- When communicating with a patient who has a mental health disorder, the clinician's communication strategy is a vital component of verbally de-escalating the patient's crisis.

- If verbal de-escalation is not effective, some patients will require physical restraint and possibly medication management. EMS clinicians must understand the principles related to this process to safely decrease the need for patient restraint interventions.
- Some specific mental health disorders include depression, bipolar disorder, anxiety, schizophrenia, substance use disorders, and personality disorders.
- Patients who are experiencing a psychiatric emergency—especially those who are experiencing suicidal thoughts—will almost always require transport for further assessment, stabilization, and care.
- With minor patients, it can sometimes be a challenge to know what is causing disturbed behavior. As with all mental health emergencies, your best treatment on scene and while transporting children is communication.
- Gathering a history and completing the primary and secondary assessments are critical with elderly patients, who often have complex medical histories and comorbidities, to rule out other medical causes of the mental health symptoms aside from a primary mental health disorder.

Key Terms

anosognosia Lack of insight caused by a neurologic condition such as a psychiatric disorder.

bipolar disorder A disorder with discrete episodes of both decreased mood (depressive episodes) and elevated mood (manic or hypomanic episodes).

decision-making capacity The ability to understand choices, the risks and rewards of choices, and alternatives available so as to make an informed decision for oneself.

intervention Action taken to improve something, such as administering medication for a medical issue.

personality disorders A group of mental disorders that cause an inflexible and unhealthy way of thinking, behaving, and functioning that impacts daily life and relationships.

reflective listening A communication technique in which you listen to a speaker, and then repeat back what you heard to confirm the speaker was understood.

schizophrenia A mental disorder that causes a breakdown between thoughts, emotions, and behavior that leads to faulty perceptions, loss of reality, inappropriate behavior, and difficulty with daily functioning and relationships.

social determinants of health Nonclinical factors that impact a person's health outcomes, including income, education, age, health literacy, racism, environment, housing, and social mobility, as well as access to health care, transportation, safe food and water.

stigma Viewing someone in a negative way due to a characteristic, trait, or condition the person has.

Bibliography

American Association for Marriage and Family Therapy. Suicide in the elderly. Accessed September 24, 2023. https://www.aamft.org/AAMFT/Consumer_Updates/Suicide_in_the_Elderly.aspx. Published 2019

American Psychiatric Association. *Diagnostic and Statistical Manual of Mental Disorders*. 5th ed. American Psychiatric Association; 2013.

DiNitto DM, Choi NG. Older adults and suicide. University of Texas at Austin, Steve Hicks School of Social Work. Published November 1, 2017. Accessed September 24, 2023. https://socialwork.utexas.edu/news/dinitto-and-choi-older-adults-and-suicide

Dunn T. Psych patient transport: 5 tips to make it safe for providers and patients. *EMS1*. Published August 4, 2015. Accessed September 24, 2023. https://www.ems1.com/ems-products/ambulances/articles/psych-patient-transport-5-tips-to-make-it-safe-for-providers-and-patients-8qnV2Ubq24jplq4r

Frankel C, Blaisch B, Hagen B. Meeting the challenges of pediatric behavioral emergencies. Published 2019. Accessed September 24, 2023. http://ems.acgov.org/ems-assets/docs/Clinical/meeting_challenges_pediatric_behavioral_emergencies.pdf

Friese G. Expert tips for EMS handling of behavioral emergencies. *EMS1*. Published February 4, 2016. Accessed September 24, 2023. https://www.ems1.com/assault/articles/expert-tips-for-ems-handling-of-behavioral-emergencies-FEB0mKmFYqBIiOWX

Grange K. Behavioral emergency: 6 EMS success tips. *EMS1*. Published January 28, 2016. Accessed September 24, 2023. https://www.ems1.com/violent-patient-management/articles/behavioral-emergency-6-ems-success-tips-TxYc8TglWWa6vme9

Keshavan MS, Kaneko Y. Secondary psychoses: an update. *World Psychiatr.* 2013;12(1):4-15. doi:10.1002/wps.20001.

Kupas DF, Wydro GC, Tan DK, et al. Clinical care and restraint of agitated or combative patients by emergency medical services practitioners. *Prehosp Emerg Care*. 2021;25:721-723.

Luthra S. Many children rely on emergency room for psychiatric care. *Kaiser Health News*. Published October 26, 2016. Accessed September 24, 2023. https://www.spectrumnews.org/news/many-children-rely-emergency-room-psychiatric-care

National Alliance on Mental Illness. Mental health by the numbers. Updated April 2023. Accessed September 24, 2023. https://www.nami.org/mhstats

National Alliance on Mental Illness. Navigating a mental health crisis. Published 2018. Accessed September 24, 2023. https://nami.org/About-NAMI/Publications-Reports/Guides/Navigating-a-Mental-Health-Crisis

National Alliance on Mental Illness, Minnesota Chapter. Mental health crisis planning for children. Published 2019. Accessed September 24, 2023. https://namimn.org/wp-content/uploads/sites/48/2021/12/104876_NAMI_MentalHealthCrisisChild2021_FINAL-1-1.pdf

National Association of Emergency Medical Technicians. When patients become attackers. *NAEMT News*. Published Winter 2016. Accessed September 24, 2023. http://www.naemt.org/docs/default-source/2017-publication-docs/2016-winter-naemt-news---patients-become-attackers.pdf

National Institute of Mental Health. Suicide. Updated May 2023. Accessed September 24, 2023. https://www.nimh.nih.gov/health/statistics/suicide

National Institute on Drug Abuse. Comorbidity: substance use and other mental disorders. Published August 15, 2018. Accessed September 24, 2023. https://nida.nih.gov/research-topics/trends-statistics/infographics/comorbidity-substance-use-other-mental-disorders

Oakland County Medical Control Authority. *Adult Treatment Protocols: Psychiatric Emergencies.* Oakland County Medical Control Authority; March 2018.

Palm Beach County Fire Rescue. *Patient Care Protocols.* Palm Beach County Fire Rescue; January 2019.

Rapaport L. More U.S. youth seeking help during psychiatric emergencies. *Reuters Health Online.* Published March 2019. Accessed September 24, 2023. https://www.reuters.com/article/us-health-youth-psych-emergency/more-u-s-youth-seeking-help-during-psychiatric-emergencies-idUSKCN1QZ2CR

Reinert M, Fritze D, Nguyen T. *The State of Mental Health in America 2022.* Mental Health America; 2021. Accessed September 24, 2023. https://mhanational.org/sites/default/files/2022%20State%20of%20Mental%20Health%20in%20America.pdf

Substance Abuse and Mental Health Services Administration. *Key Substance Use and Mental Health Indicators in the United States: Results from the 2020 National Survey on Drug Use and Health* (HHS Publication No. PEP21-07-01-003, NSDUH Series H-56). Center for Behavioral Health Statistics and Quality, Substance Abuse and Mental Health Services Administration; October 2021. Accessed September 24, 2023. https://www.samhsa.gov/data/sites/default/files/reports/rpt35325/NSDUHFFRPDFWHTMLFiles2020/2020NSDUHFFR1PDFW102121.pdf

Substance Abuse and Mental Health Services Administration. SAFE-T pocket card: suicide assessment five-step evaluation and triage for clinicians. Published September 2009. Accessed September 24, 2023. https://store.samhsa.gov/product/SAFE-T-Pocket-Card-Suicide-Assessment-Five-Step-Evaluation-and-Triage-for-Clinicians/sma09-4432

CHAPTER 10

Abdominal Disorders

Chapter Editor
W. Scott Gilmore, MD, FACEP, FAEMS

Abdominal discomfort can have its origins in any system of the human body. The severity of such illness can range from minor to life-threatening, yet only limited treatment is available in the field. Diagnosing and treating abdominal discomfort requires you to draw on all your skills as a clinician. It is essential to identify patients who are critically ill as soon as possible. Patients with abdominal complaints exhibit a wide range of signs and symptoms. Formulating a broad differential diagnosis and then arriving at a working diagnosis is challenging for even the most experienced clinicians. This chapter will increase your expertise by examining the clues that add up to an accurate diagnosis, beginning with a review of the gastrointestinal system and the functions of the digestive organs. The signs, symptoms, and treatment of various abdominal disorders you are likely to encounter most often in the field are discussed. Common causes of abdominal discomfort originating in body systems other than the gastrointestinal system are reviewed as well.

LEARNING OBJECTIVES

At the conclusion of this chapter, you will be able to:

- Describe the anatomy and physiology of the following systems as they relate to abdominal disorders: cardiovascular, respiratory, gastrointestinal, genitourinary, reproductive, neurologic, and endocrine.
- List effective ways of obtaining the SAMPLER history and determine how this information will affect patient care.
- Correlate the finding of pain as it relates to abdominal discomfort based on location, referral, and type—visceral or somatic—using the OPQRST mnemonic.
- Apply the AMLS Assessment Pathway to assist in formulating a differential diagnosis using sound clinical reasoning skills and advanced clinical decision making in caring for patients presenting with abdominal discomfort.
- Evaluate patients for life-threatening conditions during the primary, secondary, and ongoing assessments.
- Apply appropriate treatment modalities for the management, monitoring, and continuing care of patients with abdominal discomfort/disorders.

SCENARIO

You are dispatched to a local tavern for a sick call. When you arrive, you find a 40-year-old woman curled up in the fetal position on the floor. Chunky yellow vomitus is pooled beside her and has sprayed onto the nearby wall. Her medical history includes sickle cell disease, hypertension, and high cholesterol. The bartender and other patrons call her by name and say she was not herself this evening, but she hates to miss coming in each day. The patient tells you, "This is the worst pain I've ever had." As you roll her onto her back, she moans loudly

(continues)

SCENARIO (CONTINUED)

and holds her abdomen. Her vital signs include a blood pressure of 98/50 mm Hg; pulse rate, 124 beats/min; and respirations, 24 breaths/min. You note that she is pale, and small beads of sweat have welled up on her forehead.

- Which differential diagnoses are you considering based on the information you have now?
- Which additional information will you need to narrow your differential diagnosis?
- What are your initial treatment priorities as you continue your patient care?

Abdominal pain remains one of the most often-cited reasons for seeking medical care. In 2019, a report from the Centers for Disease Control and Prevention found abdominal complaints to be the most common reason for an emergency department (ED) visit in patients ages 15 years and older. In children younger than 15 years, abdominal complaints are less frequent. Given the varied anatomy and physiology of the **gastrointestinal (GI)** system, the causes of abdominal signs and symptoms are extremely diverse and difficult to diagnose in the field.

Anatomy and Physiology

The GI tract links organs involved in the breakdown of food, processing of nutrients, and elimination of waste. It begins at the mouth, moves to the esophagus as it travels through the chest cavity into the abdomen, and terminates in the pelvic girdle at the rectum. Along this lengthy path, many problems can arise. Patients' complaints are often nonspecific, so arriving at a diagnosis can be challenging even with advanced diagnostic tools at your disposal.

Upper Gastrointestinal Tract

The GI system begins in the mouth with the tongue and salivary glands (**Figure 10-1**). The process of digestion starts with mastication, or chewing. Mastication is the process by which the teeth and saliva break down solid food to facilitate its passage into the esophagus. Food passes from the mouth to the stomach through the esophagus,

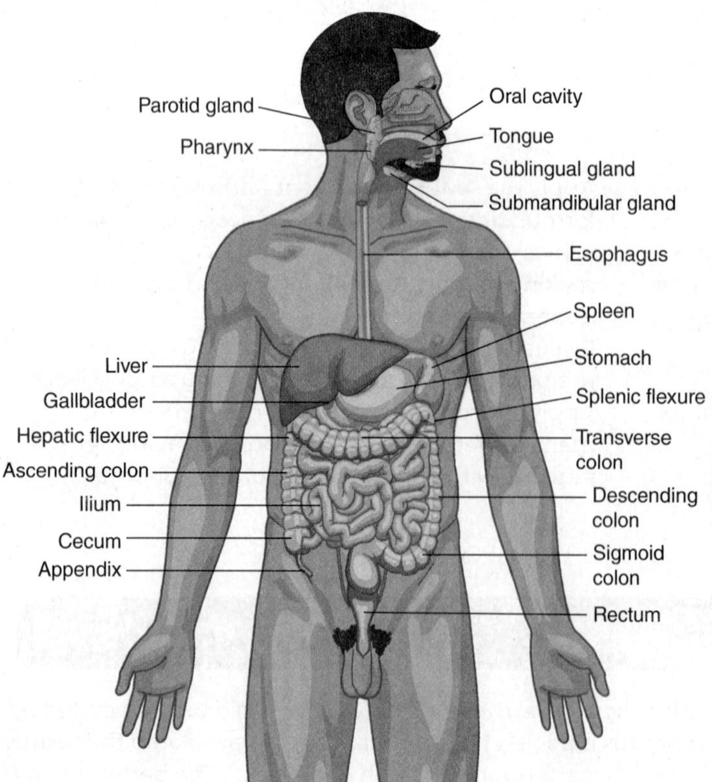

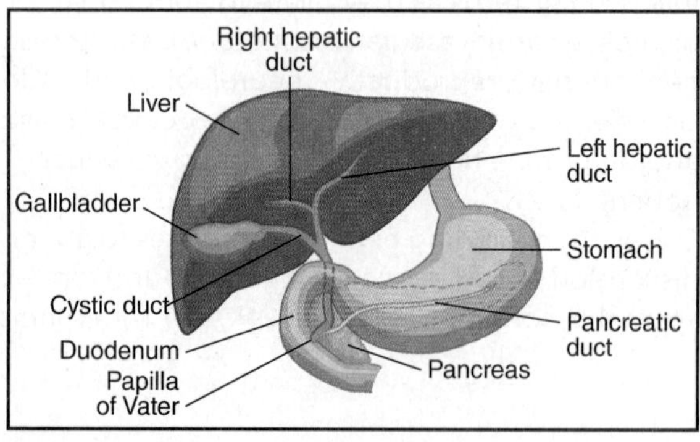

Figure 10-1 Digestive organs.

a hollow, muscular organ located posterior to the trachea that passes distally through the chest, progresses through the diaphragm, and terminates at the stomach. The muscular wall of the esophagus rhythmically contracts to propel food toward the stomach from the mouth, a process known as peristalsis. Because the esophagus lacks a rigid framework, it is easily compressible. At the termination of the esophagus is the lower esophageal sphincter, a muscular band preventing the reflux of gastric contents from the stomach into the esophagus.

The stomach lies inferior to the diaphragm, just below the left lobe of the liver, and is protected by the rib cage. When empty, the stomach has numerous folds, or rugae, allowing it to expand to accommodate 1 to 1.5 liters of food and fluid. Three layers of smooth muscle enhance its expansion and the processing of food. Glands within the stomach produce digestive enzymes to aid digestion and protect the body from the potentially harmful microorganisms that can enter with the food. The speed at which the stomach empties its contents into the lower digestive tract, known as the rate of gastric emptying, depends on the type and amount of food ingested and on other factors such as the person's age, medications, and medical condition.

Lower Gastrointestinal Tract

Digestion continues from the stomach into the small intestine, the first structure in the lower GI tract. When stretched out, the small intestine is about 22 feet (6.7 meters) long, but in the body it is looped tightly within the relatively small abdominal cavity. The duodenum, the jejunum, and the ileum are the three sections of the small intestine. The duodenum extends from the stomach. At just 1 foot (0.3 meters) in length, it is the shortest portion of the small intestine. The duodenum receives the semifluid, partially digested stomach contents, called chyme, as well as exocrine secretions from the liver and pancreas. The jejunum is about 8 feet (2.4 meters) long and is responsible for most of the chemical digestion and absorption of nutrients. The ileum, the final section of the small bowel, and is the longest portion at 13 feet (4 meters). It is responsible for nutrient absorption as well.

The large intestine includes the cecum, colon, and rectum. The cecum is a pouch that receives the products of digestion from the small intestine. The appendix attaches to the cecum. The large intestine is primarily responsible for the reabsorption of water and absorption of vitamins. The rectum is responsible for expelling stool.

Accessory Organs

Liver

The liver lies mostly in the right upper quadrant of the abdominal cavity below the diaphragm. The functions of the liver are broad and include bile production and metabolic and hematologic regulation. The liver performs more than 200 functions in the body, several of which are listed in Table 10-1.

Table 10-1 Functions of the Liver

Metabolic	Hematologic	Other Major Functions
Extraction of nutrients from blood	Removal of aged or damaged red blood cells	Secretion of bile
Extraction of toxins from blood	Synthesis of plasma proteins, including albumin	Absorption and breakdown of hormones
Removal and storage of excess nutrients such as glucose	Synthesis of clotting factors	
Maintenance of normal glucose levels by means of glycogenesis, glycogenolysis, and gluconeogenesis		
Storage of vitamins, including vitamin A, vitamin D, vitamin B_{12}, and vitamin K		

The liver is a dense, heavy organ, weighing approximately 3.3 lb (1.5 kg). It is divided into left and right lobes made up of lobules, masses of cells that form the basic structural units of the liver. The liver contains about 100,000 lobules and is an extremely vascular organ. In fact, because it is the largest reservoir of blood in the body, even a small laceration to the liver can cause extensive blood loss.

Gallbladder

The gallbladder is a pear-shaped organ located just below the liver. Its function is to modify and store bile. Excessive precipitation of bile salts can cause painful gallstones to form. Bile's primary function is to assist in digestion and absorption of fats and fat-soluble vitamins.

Pancreas

The pancreas lies posterior to the stomach between the first part of the duodenum and the spleen in the mid-epigastric area. The pancreatic duct joins the common bile duct and empties into the duodenum. It functions in digestion as an exocrine organ, secreting digestive enzymes, bicarbonate, electrolytes, and water. The pancreas also performs an endocrine function, which is not directly involved in digestion, by secreting the following substances:

- Glucagon, to raise glucose levels
- Insulin, to promote movement of glucose into the tissues
- Somatostatin, to regulate other endocrine cells in the pancreatic islets

Functions of the Gastrointestinal System

To process or digest nutrients effectively, the four chief functions of the GI system—motility, secretion, digestion, and absorption—must be intact. These functions require complex interactions among the nervous system, the endocrine system, the musculoskeletal system, and the cardiovascular system.

Motility

Food progresses through the GI tract by a process called *motility*. This process also mixes food components and reduces particle size so food can be digested and nutrients absorbed. A structured, coordinated muscular response known as peristalsis is required for the motility process to be successful. The neurologic system—specifically, the sympathetic and parasympathetic nervous systems—orchestrates this effort.

The vagus nerve, part of the parasympathetic nervous system, innervates the GI tract to the level of the transverse colon. This nerve plays a pivotal role in gastric emptying and the motility of the GI tract by controlling the contraction and dilation of sphincters and smooth muscle. In addition, the vagus nerve has a secretory function and helps stimulate vomiting. Bradycardia is often present when a person vomits because the vagus nerve also helps regulate the heart rate. The pelvic splanchnic nerves stimulate the descending colon, sigmoid colon, rectum, and anal canal. The vagus and pelvic nerves innervate the striated muscle in the upper third of the esophagus and the external anal sphincter, respectively.

The sympathetic nervous system includes the major ganglia (celiac, superior mesenteric, inferior mesenteric, and hypogastric), the secretory cells, and endocrine cells.

Secretion

The digestive tract is lined with cells that secrete fluids to aid in motility and digestion. These cells secrete as much as 9 liters of water, acids, buffers, electrolytes, and enzymes in a 24-hour period. A majority of this fluid is reabsorbed. However, when diarrhea occurs and is severe or extended, significant fluid loss can occur, and dehydration and shock may ensue.

Digestion

Digestion is the process of breaking down food into components to be used for nutrition by the body at the cellular level. Digestion involves the mechanical and chemical breakdown of the ingested food.

Absorption

The small intestine is the primary site for absorption of fluid and nutrients, and the large intestine is the primary site of absorption of water and salts.

Pain

The most common GI complaint is abdominal pain. Despite (or perhaps because of) the frequency of this complaint, determining its cause can challenge even a seasoned health care clinician. Often, the complaint of abdominal pain is vague and ill defined. To obtain the necessary information from the patient and arrive at a diagnosis, you must be familiar with GI system pathophysiology, understand how to take a history, and perform an assessment in a reassuring and supportive way. Because an accurate diagnosis is not always immediately apparent, patients can become frustrated and may feel as if you do not believe them. Establishing an environment of trust can allow you to acquire the needed information, including precipitating factors and a description of additional symptoms that may point to a probable diagnosis.

Both very young patients and elderly individuals may have difficulty relaying information about their pain to clinicians. These groups have different perceptions of pain, and they localize pain differently. Older adult patients may get confused about where pain originates and often live with chronic pain that may affect their perception. Pediatric patients poorly localize the exact pain location and may have difficulty verbalizing their pain.

One complicating factor in the diagnosis of abdominal pain is that the perception of discomfort varies widely, depending on its cause and the patient's individual level of tolerance. In addition, abdominal pain often evolves over time, becoming better defined as the disease process progresses. Abdominal pain can be divided into three categories: visceral pain, parietal pain, and referred pain.

Visceral Pain

Visceral pain occurs when the walls of the hollow organs are stretched, thereby activating the stretch receptors. This kind of pain is characterized by a deep, persistent ache, ranging from mild to intolerable. Common descriptors include cramping, burning, and gnawing.

Visceral pain is difficult to localize, as the abdominal organs transmit pain signals to both sides of the spinal cord, but is typically felt in the epigastric, periumbilical, or suprapubic region. Epigastric visceral pain typically comes from the stomach, gallbladder, liver, duodenum, or pancreas. Periumbilical pain tends to be related to the appendix, small bowel, or cecum, while suprapubic pain arises from the kidneys, ureters, bladder, colon, uterus, or ovaries (**Figure 10-2**).

The patient may have trouble finding a comfortable position and so will shift frequently; their positioning may need to be adjusted during transport as well. Depending on the cause, diaphoresis, nausea, vomiting, restlessness, or pallor may be present. Table 10-2 outlines a small number of the possible differential diagnoses of abdominal discomfort in patients with nausea and vomiting.

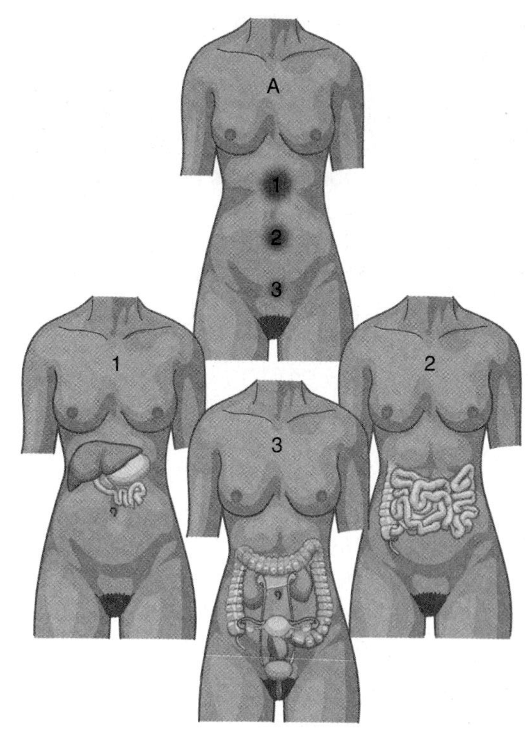

Figure 10-2 Localization of visceral pain. Pain arising from organ areas depicted in 1, 2, and 3 is felt in the epigastrium, mid-abdomen, and hypogastrium, respectively, as shown in A.

Somatic (Parietal) Pain

Somatic (parietal) pain is caused by an irritation of the nerve fibers in the parietal peritoneum or abdominal wall. The origin of somatic pain is easier to pinpoint than the source of visceral pain. Physical findings include sharp, discrete, localized pain accompanied by tenderness to palpation; guarding of the affected area; and rebound tenderness.

Table 10-2 Differential Diagnosis of Abdominal Discomfort with Nausea and Vomiting

Diagnosis	Definition	Causes/ Contributing Factors	Signs and Symptoms	Diagnostic Tests	Treatment
			Cardiac		
Acute coronary syndrome	Infarction or ischemia of the heart muscle	Coronary artery disease, smoking, high cholesterol, history of MI, diabetes, hypertension	Chest, epigastric, back, and neck pain Nausea Difficulty breathing	Serial 12-lead ECG, troponin	Administer oxygen if needed (goal: SpO_2 95–99%). Establish IV access. Administer ASA and nitroglycerin, if indicated. Transport to appropriate STEMI/ heart attack center capable of PCI if STEMI on ECG.
			Gastrointestinal		
Boerhaave syndrome	Rupture of the esophagus	Explosive vomiting, coughing, seizures, childbirth, status asthmaticus	Pain in the chest, neck, back, or abdomen Difficulty breathing, tachycardia, hematemesis, fever, subcutaneous emphysema	Chest x-ray and CT of chest/ abdomen/ pelvis	Treat airway compromise, hypoxia, and shock. Surgery will be performed at the receiving facility.

(continues)

Table 10-2 Differential Diagnosis of Abdominal Discomfort with Nausea and Vomiting (*continued*)

Diagnosis	Definition	Causes/ Contributing Factors	Signs and Symptoms	Diagnostic Tests	Treatment
Mallory-Weiss syndrome	Longitudinal tears in the esophageal mucosa, causing bleeding	Severe, protracted vomiting	Severe, protracted vomiting Hematemesis Chest/epigastric pain	Chest x-ray, chest CT, endoscopy	Treat airway compromise and shock Establish IV access Administer oxygen (goal: SpO_2 95–99%). Endoscopy and possibly surgery may be performed at the receiving facility.
Upper GI bleeding	Bleeding proximal to the junction of the duodenum and jejunum	Gastric or duodenal ulcers, use of NSAIDs or alcohol, liver disease, varices	Abdominal pain Hematemesis, red or coffee-colored vomitus or stool	Chest and abdominal x-rays, CTA, CBC, coagulation studies Endoscopy	Administer oxygen (goal: SpO_2 95–99%). Establish IV access. Treat shock, including administering blood products if indicated and available.
Ischemic bowel	Necrosis of the GI tract	Atrial fibrillation, hypercoagulability, severe vascular disease, recent surgery, shock	Abdominal pain (often out of proportion to tenderness), tachycardia, hypotension, fever, restlessness	CBC, lactate 12-lead ECG CTA of abdomen and pelvis	Administer oxygen (goal: SpO_2 95–99%). Establish IV access. Treat shock.
			Endocrine		
Diabetic ketoacidosis	Hyperglycemia, ketosis, and acidosis	Diabetes, especially type 1, but can occur in patients with type 2 diabetes who are ill	Nausea, vomiting, polydipsia, polyuria, polyphagia, abdominal pain, metabolic acidosis	Blood glucose, serum electrolytes, arterial or venous blood gas, ketones	Administer oxygen (goal: SpO_2 95–99%). Establish IV access. Administer isotonic fluids. Insulin is usually administered in hospital.

ASA, acetylsalicylic acid; CBC, complete blood count; CT, computed tomography; CTA, computed tomography angiography; ECG, electrocardiogram; GI, gastrointestinal; IV, intravenous; MI, myocardial infarction; NSAIDs, nonsteroidal anti-inflammatory drugs; PCI, percutaneous coronary intervention; SpO_2, oxygen saturation; STEMI, ST-elevation myocardial infarction.

Pain that originates from internal organs usually starts as vague visceral pain and then later becomes more localized and sharp somatic pain. Because the parietal peritoneum surrounds the organs involved, it takes longer for the affected structures to become irritated and painful. The dorsal root ganglia in the spine activate peritoneal pain, so the pain is typically experienced on the same side and in the same dermatome as the affected organ. Dermatomes identify the relationship between a spinal nerve and the skin over the portion of the body that nerve innervates.

Figure 10-3 shows the diseases and medical conditions that are associated with differential diagnoses for pain in various quadrants of the abdomen.

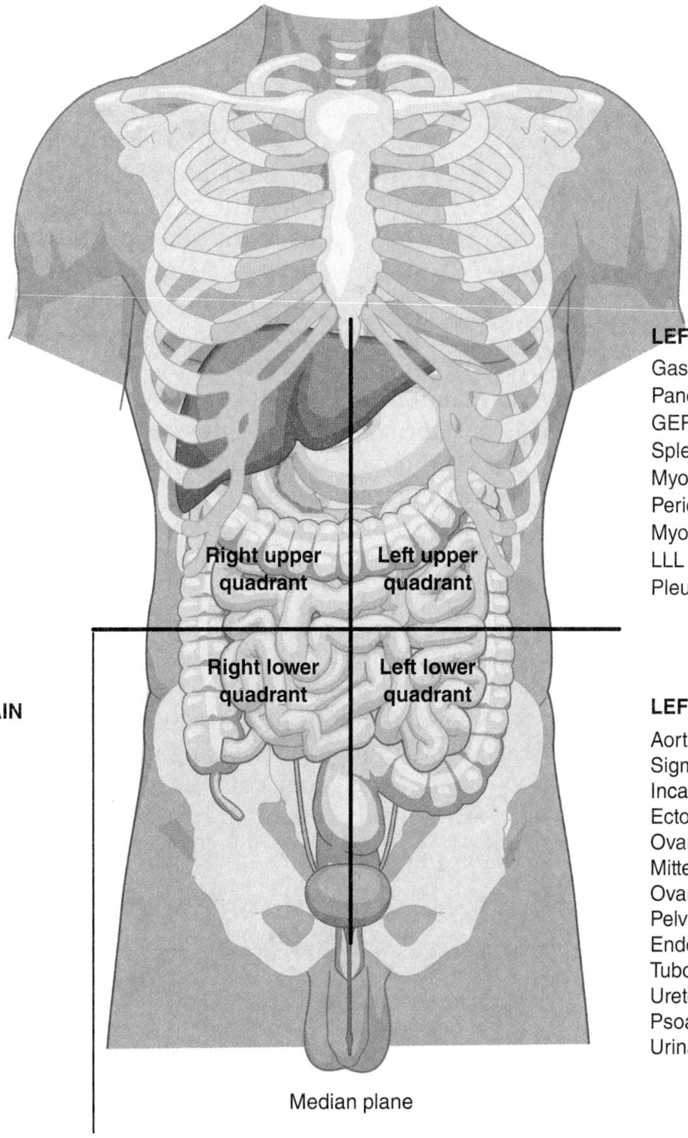

Figure 10-3 Differential diagnosis of acute abdominal pain. GERD, gastroesophageal reflux disease; HF, heart failure; LLL, left lower lobe; RLL, right lower lobe.

Data from Marx JA, Hockberger RS, Walls RM, et al. *Rosen's Emergency Medicine.* 7th ed. St. Louis, MO: Mosby; 2009.

Referred Pain

When pain is perceived as coming from a site other than its origin, it is said to be **referred pain**. In other words, the pain is "referred" from its origin to another location. Overlapping neural pathways are responsible for this phenomenon. For example, referred pain often accompanies cholecystitis, in which the patient usually feels pain in the right scapular area. Kehr sign is when pain from a ruptured spleen is referred to the left shoulder. Pain from myocardial infarction is often referred to the neck, jaw, or arm.

AMLS Assessment Pathway ▸▸▸▸

▾ Initial Observations

Scene Safety Considerations

Your field impression begins when you receive the dispatch information related to an abdominal complaint. When you arrive on scene, you will be able to determine how well your field impression agrees with your initial observations. Multiple patients are not a common occurrence with GI complaints. A call for assistance to an office building where several patients are reporting abdominal pain, for example, should lead you to consider a scene where a chemical or biologic agent has been released.

Follow standard precautions. Blood, emesis, and feces are hazards associated with abdominal disorders and require you to use personal protective equipment to shield yourself from exposure to body fluids. In addition to gloves, gowns, and masks, the following equipment is essential to ensuring good patient hygiene while maintaining personal safety:

- Eye protection
- Towels and wash rags
- Extra linens
- Absorbent pads
- Emesis bag (preferred) or basin
- Disposable basin
- Biohazard bags
- Water for irrigation

Immediately address any apparent life-threatening emergencies. The primary life threat associated with abdominal discomfort is shock caused by hemorrhage, dehydration, or sepsis, as in the following circumstances:

- Internal bleeding due to a ruptured aneurysm, GI bleeding, or ectopic pregnancy
- Dehydration caused by vomiting or diarrhea from a wide range of causes
- Sepsis secondary to conditions such as a ruptured appendix or perforated bowel, bacteremia from an indwelling catheter, or pyelonephritis

If no life threat is present, focus your assessment on identifying the cardinal presentation/chief complaint.

Patient Cardinal Presentation/ Chief Complaint

Signs and symptoms associated with a range of emergent and nonemergent abdominal disorders are summarized in Table 10-3. Gather clues during your assessment and combine them to build a differential diagnosis.

Primary Survey

Your main goals are maintenance of the ABCs and management of pain/nausea. Once you have addressed the patient's airway, breathing, and circulation, begin to narrow down your list of potential diagnoses and continue your assessment. The patient presentation will dictate your next actions. If you have the resources to perform a more detailed assessment as you stabilize the patient's condition, then do so—but further assessment should not be done before stabilization of the patient's ABCs has been achieved.

Level of Consciousness

Observing the patient's level of consciousness can help you gauge the severity of the problem. Patients who are confused, pale, and diaphoretic may be critically ill. Many GI conditions are associated with shock, which can diminish the patient's mentation. Someone who is talking is providing you with foundational physiologic information. Talking means an open airway. To talk, the patient must also be breathing, have adequate blood pressure to maintain brain activity, and have a sufficient blood glucose level.

Airway and Breathing

Airway obstruction and aspiration may occur in patients who are vomiting or are unresponsive. Closely inspect the airway for foreign bodies. Remove or suction obstructions. Note any unusual odors from the mouth. Patients who have bowel obstructions can have breath that smells of stool. Consider the most appropriate positioning of the patient: The head of the bed should be raised if the patient is not hypotensive.

Breathing is not usually affected by GI problems. However, irritation of the diaphragm from upper organ inflammation or peritonitis may cause pain with breathing and lead to hypoventilation. Severe ascites may also limit the depth of breathing. Tachypnea can be a sign of pain, anxiety, or acidosis, which can be caused by diseases such as diabetic ketoacidosis or sepsis.

Table 10-3 Emergent and Nonemergent Disorders with Abdominal Signs and Symptoms

Disorder	Signs and Symptoms
Life Threatening	
Gastrointestinal	
Boerhaave syndrome (rupture of esophagus)	Chest pain, hematemesis
Gastrointestinal tract bleeding	Upper: epigastric pain, hematemesis Lower: bright red, maroon, or blackish stools
Neurologic	
Intracerebral bleeding	Nausea/vomiting, headache
Meningitis	Nausea/vomiting, headache, and neck pain
Cardiovascular	
Acute myocardial infarction	Epigastric pain, nausea/vomiting
Aortic dissection	Pain, lower-extremity ischemia
Budd-Chiari syndrome (obstruction of hepatic veins)	Pain, nausea/vomiting, jaundice
Ruptured aortic aneurysm	Jaundice, lower-extremity ischemia
Severe heart failure	RUQ discomfort, edema, dyspnea
Endocrine	
Adrenal insufficiency	General weakness, nausea/vomiting, diarrhea, hypotension
Obstetric	
Placental abruption	Pain, vaginal bleeding
Placenta previa	Vaginal bleeding
Preeclampsia/HELLP	Elevated blood pressure, jaundice, nausea/vomiting, RUQ/epigastric pain
Immunologic	
Anaphylaxis	Pain, vomiting, diarrhea, hypotension
Emergent	
Gastrointestinal	
Gastric outlet obstruction	Postprandial vomiting
Intestinal obstruction	Colicky pain, nausea/vomiting, constipation, diarrhea
Acute appendicitis	RLQ or periumbilical pain, nausea/vomiting, fever
Acute cholecystitis	Constant RUQ pain, nausea/vomiting
Bowel perforation	Pain, nausea/vomiting, fever, constipation
Cholangitis (infection of biliary tract)	RUQ pain, nausea/vomiting, jaundice, fever
Crohn disease	Pain, nausea/vomiting, diarrhea (may be bloody)
Fulminant hepatic failure	RUQ pain, nausea/vomiting, jaundice, ascites/edema, altered mental status
Ischemic bowel/mesenteric ischemia	Severe pain, nausea/vomiting, diarrhea (may be bloody)
Mallory-Weiss syndrome (small tear of esophagus)	Pain, vomiting (blood streaks in emesis)
Pancreatitis	Epigastric pain, nausea/vomiting
Ulcerative colitis	Pain, nausea/vomiting, diarrhea (often bloody)
Neurologic	
Central nervous system tumor	Nausea/vomiting
Obstetric	
Hyperemesis gravidarum	Extreme nausea/vomiting
Endocrine	
Diabetic ketoacidosis	Diffuse abdominal pain, nausea/vomiting, polyuria, polydipsia
Genitourinary	
Testicular or ovarian torsion	Acute onset of pain, nausea/vomiting
Nonemergent	
Gastrointestinal	
Biliary colic	Postprandial pain, nausea/vomiting
Diverticulitis	Lower abdominal pain, constipation, diarrhea, fever possible
Gastroenteritis	Pain, nausea/vomiting, diarrhea
Hepatitis	Pain, nausea/vomiting, diarrhea, jaundice
Irritable bowel syndrome	Pain, nausea/vomiting, constipation and/or diarrhea

HELLP, hemolysis, elevated liver enzymes, low platelet count; RUQ, right upper quadrant.

Circulation/Perfusion

An assessment of the circulatory system is essential in understanding the impacts of GI disease on the body. As with all patients, assess skin color, temperature, and moisture. Note any findings indicating shock. Determine the patient's pulse rate, strength, regularity, and equality. Evaluate the peripheral pulses and compare them with the central pulses.

Many GI disorders involve pain or hemorrhage. As the patient's blood volume begins to drop, the body compensates by releasing catecholamines (epinephrine and norepinephrine) to vasoconstrict the periphery, increase the pulse rate, and increase the force of left ventricular contraction. Pain stimulates similar body responses. Either problem can leave the patient with tachycardia; diminished peripheral pulses; diaphoresis; and pale, cool, clammy skin.

▾ First Impression

The fundamental determination you must make in the field is whether the patient's condition is life threatening, as evidenced by abnormal vital signs or respiratory distress. Patients who exhibit either of these findings must be rapidly treated and transported to an appropriate facility.

The following list reviews the management of life-threatening abdominal complaints after the scene has been determined to be safe and personal protective equipment is donned:

- Manage the airway as necessary using appropriate basic life support (BLS) techniques. Maintain the patient's oxygen saturation (SpO_2) at > 94% by administering additional oxygen through an appropriate means (e.g., nasal cannula or nonrebreather mask) or by assisting ventilation as necessary.
- Control any obvious hemorrhage.
- Apply a cardiac monitor (consistent with your level of training) and consider acquiring a 12-lead electrocardiogram (ECG) if appropriate.
- Establish intravenous (IV) access and administer crystalloid fluid if there is concern for sepsis, dehydration, or hypovolemia. Use care, however, because aggressive fluid administration can dilute the concentration of red blood cells and impede clot formation if bleeding is present. Blood pressure should be maintained at just high enough a level to perfuse the vital organs. Generally, a systolic pressure of 80 to 90 mm Hg is adequate, but it is best to use the patient's mental status and other physiologic parameters as a gauge to assess whether perfusion is adequate.
- Administer medications per your local protocols. Analgesia is appropriate in most cases, but which medication is best will depend on the differential diagnosis and patient-specific factors. Antiemetics are appropriate for treatment of nausea and vomiting.
- Monitor the patient closely, and reassess frequently to determine the response.
- If uncontrolled bleeding or hemorrhagic shock is suspected, be prepared to administer blood products and/or tranexamic acid (TXA), if either is available and indicated.

If the situation is not life threatening, closely examine where the patient is found. The patient's body posture or position can give you hints as to what happened. Has the patient been in bed sick for several days? Was the patient at work when a sudden bout of pain caused doubling over and clutching the stomach? Look to the environment for clues as to the length and degree of illness the patient is experiencing.

One aspect of your first impression of the patient with an abdominal disorder is odor. Note the smell of the room. Foul-smelling stool may be present in these disorders. Also examine the patient's living conditions. This information can help you determine whether the problem is chronic or acute, and can suggest whether the patient's emergency is isolated to the GI system.

Many people with GI complaints have long-standing medical problems, so the information provided can assist you in generating an initial differential diagnosis.

▾ Detailed Assessment

History Taking

OPQRST and SAMPLER

Gathering an accurate, detailed history is essential with every patient. The SAMPLER and OPQRST mnemonics will help you remember to ask the right questions. Demonstrating patience and taking a genuine interest in the patient will improve your rapport. Table 10-4 points out involvement of body systems for patients with abdominal discomfort. Table 10-5 lists clinical signs associated with selected abdominal disorders. As you gather the patient's history, any abdominal complaint should also prompt you to ask about appetite, bowel regimen, urinary symptoms and output including amount and frequency, menstrual history and pregnancy status, and discharge from genital organs.

Secondary Survey

Pain Assessment

In evaluating GI complaints, your assessment must include a detailed appraisal of the patient's pain. Abdominal pain is often diffuse and difficult to categorize, and

Table 10-4 Selected System Considerations for Assessment of Abdominal Complaints

System	History, Differential Diagnosis, and Other Assessment Considerations
Neurologic	Ask about recent accidents or trauma, particularly if the patient has an altered level of consciousness or nausea and vomiting.
Respiratory	Explore any evidence of breathing problems. Pneumonia may be associated with upper abdominal discomfort. Esophageal ruptures may present with respiratory signs and symptoms.
Cardiovascular	Indigestion and upper abdominal discomfort should prompt you to evaluate the patient for acute coronary syndrome.
Gastrointestinal, genitourinary, and reproductive	Explore any history of chronic or acute diagnoses. Question the patient about any changes in eating, bowel, or urinary habits that may suggest a diagnosis. Vaginal discharge, bleeding, and menstrual changes suggest specific disease processes.
Musculoskeletal and skin	Observe the skin for pallor, jaundice, uremia, and other changes that may suggest the cause of abdominal pain. Look for any scars, ostomies, or external devices (such as drains, tubes, and pumps) that may indicate the cause of the patient's abdominal symptoms.
Endocrine, metabolic, and environmental	Collect any related past medical history. Assess the patient's blood glucose level. Assess the scene or thoroughly question the patient, family, and bystanders if you are unable to observe the patient's environment.
Infectious disease and hematologic	Is there a history of prolonged and severe vomiting and/or diarrhea? Has the patient recently engaged in foreign travel or camping? Has the patient been exposed to contaminated drinking water? These factors may indicate gastroenteritis from bacteria, viruses, protozoans, or other microbes. Is there a history of fever? Take the patient's temperature to evaluate for fever. The patient's history, a foul smell, and the presence of a Foley catheter or other invasive drain may point to an infectious process.
Toxicologic (nuclear, biologic, and chemical)	Inquire about and observe for signs of potential exposures. Many toxidromes have a gastrointestinal component and can present with vomiting or diarrhea.

documenting it methodically can help you refine your diagnosis. The initial task is to ascertain the origin of the pain and determine its referral sites (see Figure 10-2, Figure 10-3, and **Figure 10-4**). Knowing the time of onset will help you assess how the pain has evolved, which may indicate the severity of the illness. Be alert for any signs that typically accompany pain, such as vomiting.

Document pain in the patient's own words because they may be more revealing than the words a health care professional might use. Ask open-ended questions: What does your pain feel like? Can you describe your pain? Encourage candid responses, which may range from "It hurts" to "It feels like I'm being shredded apart." If the person is unable to describe the pain, offer a few helpful descriptions. Ask, is it sharp, tearing, hot, burning, dull? Ask which activities or movements worsen or improve the pain, and note if any home remedies or corrective measures were attempted, even if they were ineffective.

Using a pain scale allows you to compare the patient's pain over time. People have widely different levels of pain tolerance depending on cultural norms and their own pain thresholds. The best use of a pain scale, therefore, is not in determining the severity of pain, which is largely subjective, but in tracking any improvements or worrisome trends. Ask the patient frequently to reassess the pain, taking care to document the response, and trust the patient's statements about the severity of their symptoms.

Table 10-5 Clinical Signs Associated with Selected Abdominal Disorders

Sign	Description	Differential Diagnosis
Hematemesis	Blood in vomitus	Upper GI bleeding
Coffee-ground emesis	Vomiting of partially digested blood	Upper GI bleeding
Feculent vomiting	Emesis that smells like feces	Bowel obstruction
Hematochezia	Bright red blood passed through the rectum	Lower GI bleeding
Melena	Black, tarry stool that contains digested blood	Upper GI bleeding
Very light-colored stools	Very light or light yellow, chalky stool	Liver or gallbladder disease
Hematuria	Blood in the urine	Bladder infection Kidney disease Trauma Tumor

GI, gastrointestinal.

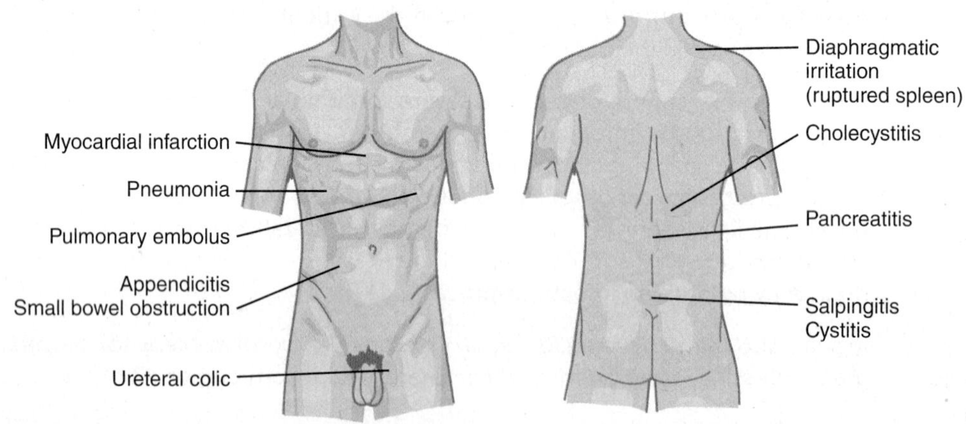

Figure 10-4 Referred pain patterns. Pain or discomfort in these areas often provides clues to underlying disease processes.

Vital Signs

Analysis of the patient's vital signs is critical to making a reliable diagnosis. Fever, for example, indicates an infection may be present; typically, a temperature ≥ 100.5°F (38°C) is considered significant. However, this rule does not apply to older adults or to patients with compromised immune systems. In such patients, a serious infection may be present even if the patient's body temperature is normal. A temperature < 96.8°F (36°C) is also a significant finding. Low blood pressure and a rapid heart rate can point to hypovolemia. The heart rate may accelerate as body temperature rises, except in patients who take beta blockers, because such agents reduce the heart rate. An elevated respiratory rate can be a red flag portending serious illness such as pneumonia, myocardial infarction, sepsis, metabolic acidosis, or hypoperfusion.

Physical Assessment

Perform a systematic, thorough physical examination. Be sensitive to the possibility that this examination might be a difficult experience for the patient. No one likes to be poked and prodded, but discomfort or unpleasantness is magnified in the face of the anxiety often associated with illness and injury. An already uncomfortable patient may worry that the exam will be painful. Preparing the patient by explaining the procedure first may diminish uncertainty and improve cooperation.

Physical examination skills include inspection, auscultation, percussion, and palpation.

Inspection

Examination of the abdomen should always begin with inspection, because any palpation can alter the abdomen's general appearance and may provoke the patient's pain, after which further palpation may be hampered by guarding. Look for distention, pulsation, ecchymosis, asymmetry, pregnancy, scars, masses, and anything else unusual.

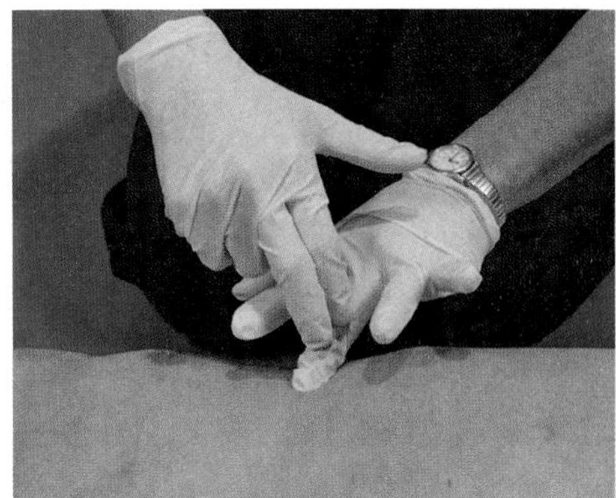

Figure 10-5 Abdominal percussion.

Auscultation

Auscultation is the second step in the general physical examination. Auscultate before palpating, as palpating the abdomen before listening to it can alter the findings by artificially increasing bowel sounds. If time and circumstances allow, auscultate each quadrant of the abdomen for about 30 seconds. Normal bowel sounds sound like water gurgling. Without experience, it is difficult to tell whether bowel sounds are normal or abnormal. Hyperactive bowel sounds may signal gastroenteritis or early bowel obstruction. Hypoactive or silent bowel sounds in one quadrant can indicate an ileus. It may be impossible, however, to hear abdominal sounds in a noisy environment like the back of an ambulance. To thoroughly assess bowel sounds, an extended auscultation time of up to 5 minutes in each quadrant is required. A shortened time is often used in the field, however, or the sounds are not auscultated because it is impractical. If a shortened auscultation time is used, it does not mean bowel sounds are absent; it means the bowel sounds may not have been heard at that time.

In addition to bowel sounds, vascular sounds may help in making a diagnosis. A bruit, or harsh sound that matches the patient's pulse rate, may indicate an aneurysm or stenotic occlusion of an artery.

Prehospital clinicians should not extend scene time to perform auscultation, as this component of the exam has limited usefulness.

Percussion

Percussion is performed by placing your nondominant hand on the abdomen and tapping a finger with the dominant hand (**Figure 10-5**). Abdominal percussion helps to identify areas of gas or liquid. Borders of organs and masses may also be determined using percussion. Before you perform any palpation or percussion of the abdomen, make sure the patient understands what you are doing. The procedure is easier for the patient to tolerate and produces less anxiety if you begin with the unaffected side and then progress to the areas of discomfort. Percuss the abdomen lightly in all four quadrants to assess the distribution of tympany (hollow sound) and dullness. Tympany usually predominates because of gas in the GI tract. Pain and tenderness present with percussion should be noted. Like auscultation, percussion requires practice.

Palpation

It is important that the patient be relaxed during palpation because abdominal rigidity and guarding caused by anxiety can make the findings less reliable. During palpation of each quadrant, watch the reaction on the patient's face and ask how the patient feels. Grimacing or tears may reveal more than verbal complaints. Attempt to elicit differences in pain before, during, and after palpation. Pain when the palpation pressure is quickly released, known as rebound tenderness, is a classic sign of peritoneal irritation, but it is present in as many as 25% of patients with nonspecific abdominal complaints. Gently shaking the pelvis, tapping on the heel, or asking the patient to cough are other ways to elicit peritoneal irritation. Each of these activities causes the inflamed visceral peritoneum to irritate the parietal peritoneum, causing local pain.

Diagnostics

With the growing availability of point-of-care testing, some emergency medical services (EMS) clinicians may be able to determine some laboratory findings in the field. These laboratory findings can assist with the differential diagnosis and help guide treatment. Laboratory parameters often measured in patients with abdominal complaints are summarized in Table 10-6. Radiologic studies used to diagnose abdominal disorders are summarized in Table 10-7.

At the hospital, specific laboratory tests performed may include a complete blood count, comprehensive

Table 10-6 Laboratory Studies for the Diagnosis of Abdominal Complaints

Component or Parameter	Normal Values	Interpretation	Indications
Alkaline phosphatase	50–120 units/L	Above normal level can indicate cirrhosis, biliary obstruction, liver tumor, hyperparathyroidism Below normal level can indicate hypothyroidism, malnutrition, pernicious anemia, celiac disease, hypophosphatemia	Abdominal pain
Ammonia	15–45 µg/dL (11–32 µmol/L)	Above normal level indicates hepatocellular disease, Reye syndrome, portal hypertension, GI bleeding or obstruction with mild liver disease, hepatic encephalopathy or coma, genetic metabolic disorder; with hepatic failure, an altered mental status may occur, which is often misdiagnosed as hypoglycemia or an acute cerebral event	Altered mental status
Amylase	25–80 units/L	Above normal level can indicate pancreatitis, penetrating or perforated peptic ulcer, necrotic or perforated bowel, acute cholecystitis, ectopic pregnancy, DKA, duodenal obstruction Usually not measured due to false elevations caused by salivary amylase; has been replaced by lipase	Abdominal pain
Bilirubin	Total: 0.3 mg/dL (5.1–17 µmol/L) Indirect: 0.2–0.8 mg/dL (3.4–12 µmol/L) Direct: 0.1–0.3 mg/dL (1.7–5.1 µmol/L)	Above normal level may indicate liver disease, biliary obstruction, liver metastases, large-volume transfusion, hemolysis, sickle cell anemia. Can also be caused by certain drugs, such as allopurinol, anabolic steroids, dextran, diuretics, and many others.	Septic shock
Blood/urine cultures	Negative	Positive result indicates infection	Septic shock
Lipase	Adults younger than 60 years: 10–140 units/L Older than 60 years: 18–180 units/L	High levels may be caused by diseases of the pancreas and gallbladder, chronic kidney disease, intestinal problems, peptic ulcer disease, hepatic disease, alcohol or drug abuse	Abdominal pain

DKA, diabetic ketoacidosis; GI, gastrointestinal.

metabolic profile, blood typing, and cross-match. Imaging studies may include computed tomography (CT) and possibly endoscopy. For a critically ill patient, however, resuscitation takes precedence.

Point-of-care ultrasound (POCUS) is a tool that is increasingly being utilized in the prehospital setting. The two greatest barriers to widespread implementation of this technology are the equipment cost and the availability of training. POCUS can be used to assess for causes of abdominal pain such as abdominal aortic aneurysm and ruptured ectopic pregnancy. Its primary role in the prehospital environment currently is to assist in resuscitation. POCUS has been adopted more widely in the critical care transport setting.

Table 10-7 Radiologic Studies for the Diagnosis of Abdominal Disorders

Test	Description	Indications	Advantages and Disadvantages
Abdominal x-rays (plain films)	An upright abdominal film displays air–fluid levels and free air A supine abdominal film detects radiopaque foreign bodies and gas in bowel	Can show free air, small-bowel obstruction, bowel ischemia, and foreign bodies	Inexpensive Easy to perform Causes minimal discomfort Provides limited information compared to CT
Computed tomography (CT)	Images the body cross-sectionally in thin slices, which allows detailed visualization of body tissues	Commonly performed if concern for acute intra-abdominal inflammatory or obstructive condition, renal colic or urinary obstruction, hemorrhage, or pelvic emergencies	Unlike radiography, a good image can be obtained no matter what the level of air or gas in the bowel Much more radiation than x-ray and may or may not involve IV contrast administration Causes minimal discomfort Not available 24 hours a day at some hospitals
Computed tomography angiography (CTA)	Images vascular structures	Preferred test for abdominal aortic aneurysm, aortic dissection, mesenteric ischemia	Involves radiation and IV contrast administration
Ultrasonography	Reflects and refracts sound waves as they strike fluid, air, and solid tissues in the body, allowing imaging of organs, tissues, and body cavities	Useful for evaluation of right upper quadrant pain, pelvic pain and pregnancy Can detect cholelithiasis, cholecystitis, pancreatic masses, and biliary duct dilation Used to detect ovarian or testicular torsion and assess for intrauterine and ectopic pregnancy	Noninvasive Can be performed at the bedside Accurate reading depends on operator skill Not available 24 hours a day at some hospitals

Refine the Differential Diagnosis

The components of the primary and secondary surveys will help you refine your differential diagnosis and determine the severity of the patient's condition. Manage any life threats as they appear during the assessment process. Remember that most diseases or conditions are caused by more than one factor. Considering the specific conditions described later and in Table 10-8 is an approach that can help you determine the differential diagnosis and recognize key findings.

Ongoing Management

Monitor the patient for changes in their condition. Routine monitoring should include the pulse rate, ECG, blood pressure, respiratory rate, and pulse oximetry.

Table 10-8 Abdominal Disorders with Potential Emergent Presentations

Disorder	Causes	History	Findings	Prehospital Treatment	Hospital Testing/ Treatment
Acute pancreatitis	Alcohol, cholelithiasis, trauma, infection, inflammation, tumor, hypertriglyceridemia	Alcohol use, use of certain drugs, recent trauma, cholelithiasis	Mid-epigastric abdominal pain, with possible radiation to back, low-grade fever, nausea, vomiting	Place patient in position of comfort. Establish IV access. Administer nothing by mouth. Administer analgesia, antiemetics, and IVF as needed.	Lipase level CT of abdomen/ pelvis
Intestinal obstruction	Can be due to stool, foreign body, intussusception, adhesions, polyps, volvulus, tumors, ulcerative colitis, or diverticulitis	Abrupt onset: suspect small-bowel obstruction Onset over 1–2 days: suspect distal obstruction History of bowel obstruction, abdominal surgery, cancer, radiation therapy, chemotherapy, hernia, or abdominal illness	Crampy abdominal pain, vomiting, no or minimal stool output, inability to pass flatus, distended abdomen Absent or high-pitched hyperactive bowel sounds	Place patient in position of comfort. Establish IV access. Administer nothing by mouth. Administer analgesia, antiemetics, and IVF as needed.	Laboratory studies X-ray and/ or CT to determine location and extent of obstruction
Mesenteric ischemia	Shock, valvular heart disease, arrhythmia, peripheral vascular disease, hypercoagulability, oral contraceptive use, aortic dissection, trauma, smoking, diabetes, hypercholesterolemia	Acute onset of severe midabdominal pain, nausea, vomiting, and diarrhea	Severe midabdominal pain, nausea, vomiting, diarrhea Pain out of proportion to tenderness	Administer oxygen. Place patient in position of comfort. Establish IV access. Administer nothing by mouth. Administer analgesia and antiemetics as needed.	CTA Surgical consult

Disorder	Causes	History	Findings	Prehospital Treatment	Hospital Testing/ Treatment
Perforated viscus	Peptic ulcer disease, diverticula, trauma, use of NSAIDs, advancing age, alcohol use	Acute progressively worsening pain	Localized or generalized pain, vomiting, fever, shock, sepsis Elevated WBCs and amylase	Place patient in position of comfort. Establish IV access. Administer nothing by mouth. Administer analgesia, antiemetics, and IVF as needed.	Laboratory studies X-ray and CT
Ruptured appendix	Obstruction, infection	Initially patient feels diffuse pain, especially in umbilical area. Later, pain settles in the right lower quadrant or lower back. If rupture occurs, pain may initially improve, then return as more severe and diffuse.	Nausea, vomiting, fever, positive Rovsing sign	Place patient in position of comfort. Establish IV access. Administer nothing by mouth. Administer analgesia and antiemetics as needed.	Laboratory, CT/ ultrasound, antibiotics, and surgical consult

CT, computed tomography; CTA, computed tomography angiography; IV, intravenous; IVF, intravenous fluids; NSAIDs, nonsteroidal anti-inflammatory drugs; WBCs, white blood cells.

If the patient has GI bleeding, continue to assess for signs of shock. Document the patient's response to treatment.

Choosing the appropriate method of transport for a patient with a GI complaint can be complicated. First, you must decide whether the patient is critically ill and determine which modes of transportation the patient can tolerate. Altitude changes during flight can cause severe pain unless the pressure is relieved. The GI system contains a large amount of air. Under normal circumstances, the pressure in the GI system is equal to the pressure in the external environment. At altitude, gases will expand and may possibly cause discomfort or complications for patients with GI-related issues. Typically, a medical patient can be safely transported via aeromedical fixed- and rotary-wing aircraft. Most helicopters and pressurized fixed-wing aircraft can safely transport these patients.

Patients who had recent laparoscopic surgery will likely have air in their abdomen typically for several days, but sometimes for as long as 7 to 10 days. These individuals and patients with known bowel obstruction or ileus may experience increased distention at altitude. Empty any ostomy bags, and monitor the patient closely so the new bag does not rupture from an excessive buildup of gas.

Gastrointestinal Causes of Abdominal Disorders

Upper Gastrointestinal or Esophageal Bleeding

Pathophysiology

Acute upper GI bleeding affects 50 to 150 people per 100,000 population, leading to 250,000 hospital admissions per year. Men and elderly persons are at much higher risk for this disorder. Lower GI bleeding is less common overall but has a higher incidence among women. The list of possible causes of an upper GI bleed is quite extensive. Observations indicating a higher risk of mortality include hemodynamic instability; repeated **hematemesis** or **hematochezia**; age older than 60 years; and existence of an additional organ system disease, such as cardiovascular or pulmonary disease.

Signs and Symptoms

Each of the many conditions that can cause GI bleeding has its own pattern of disease progression. For example, esophageal diverticular disease has a rather gradual onset, whereas Mallory-Weiss syndrome (a small partial tear of esophagus) has a sudden onset. Many patients do report bleeding, but others have more ambiguous initial signs and symptoms such as tachycardia, syncope, hypotension, angina, weakness, confusion, or cardiac arrest. Taking a thorough history may be the only way to determine the cause of such complaints (see Table 10-3).

Differential Diagnosis

To refine your diagnosis, in addition to finding out the patient's past medical history, determine if the patient is taking any anticoagulant or antiplatelet medications. Try to ascertain whether the bleeding is an acute or chronic condition, and if the bleeding was preceded by pain. Acute-onset GI bleeding is characterized by massive sudden hemorrhage and signs of hypovolemic shock. Chronic bleeding may present with progressive weakness and fatigue, and the patient may note melena or blackish stools. There are several questions specific to GI bleeding complaints: When was the onset of the bleeding? Was it gradual or sudden? Does anything make it better or worse? Has anything caused an increase—for example, vomiting? What does the stool or vomitus look like? What color is it? How much are you bleeding? From where are you bleeding? Are you prescribed blood thinners or taking an aspirin daily?

Question the patient about upper and lower GI bleeds. For example, you might ask: Is the bleeding increasing or decreasing in severity? How long have the symptoms been present? Are they continuous or intermittent? Even if the patient does not complain of pain, the OPQRST mnemonic is helpful.

Treatment

Treatment for the patient with GI bleeding follows several general management guidelines. Fluid resuscitation is common. In most patients, even those with stable vital signs, it is prudent to establish an IV line and fluid resuscitate the patient. However, titrate crystalloid fluids and use blood products as soon as available if the patient in shock or has had significant blood loss or is severely anemic. Tranexamic acid may be considered in some cases of GI bleeding (**Tip Box 10-1**).

Peptic Ulcer Disease

Pathophysiology

Peptic ulcer disease is the most common cause of GI bleeding in the United States. Because *Helicobacter pylori* has been found to be the cause of most peptic ulcers, this condition is no longer considered to be a chronic disease.

Duodenal, gastric, and stomal ulcers are all types of peptic ulcer disease. Because the gastric mucosa secretes hydrochloric acid and pepsinogen, the stomach is

TIP BOX 10-1

GI Bleeding, Tranexamic Acid, and Blood Products

Current resuscitation of many GI bleeding disorders may benefit from modern resuscitation methods. After all, hemorrhagic shock is hemorrhagic shock, no matter its source. Although not approved specifically for GI bleeding, the use of tranexamic acid (TXA) in upper GI bleeding appears to have a beneficial effect in terms of decreasing the risk of rebleeding and decreasing the need for surgery. TXA has no effect on the need for blood transfusion, risk of thromboembolic events, or mortality in upper GI bleeding. The effectiveness of TXA in lower GI bleeding has yet to be determined.

The use of whole blood in the prehospital field is also growing in popularity, although logistics challenges currently prevent its widespread use. Patients with moderate to severe GI bleeding conditions may benefit from infusions of whole blood, packed red blood cells, plasma, and platelets. In fact, ground agencies using whole blood have reported more utilization in patients with medical causes of hemorrhagic shock than in trauma patients.

an acidic environment. This acidity is necessary for the proper digestion of protein. A delicate balance is maintained by secretion of sodium bicarbonate in the duodenum. Peptic ulcers form when this balance is upset and the acidic environment is allowed to predominate. A few of the factors that may irritate or contribute to ulcers include nonsteroidal anti-inflammatory drugs (NSAIDs), smoking, excessive alcohol ingestion, and stress.

Signs and Symptoms

Patients typically experience a classic sequence of pain in the stomach that subsides or diminishes immediately after eating and then reemerges 2 to 3 hours later. The pain will be described as burning or gnawing. Nausea, vomiting, belching, and heartburn are common. If erosion is severe, gastric bleeding can occur, resulting in hematemesis and **melena**. Bleeding in peptic ulcer disease can be severe. The patient may show signs of shock, pallor, hypotension, and tachycardia, which should be quickly documented and treated. Ulcers may perforate (erode through the lining of the stomach or bowel), causing pancreatitis and/or peritonitis. Swelling of the ulcerated tissue may cause an acute obstruction.

Differential Diagnosis

The patient's past medical history is important for narrowing down the possible diagnoses. Ask the patient about previous ulcers, whether the pain occurs prior to or after eating, whether the patient regularly consumes alcohol, and previous episodes of bleeding. The patient's answers will help you accurately assess the degree of blood loss and prepare to manage any hypotension that is present. The differential diagnosis may include other diseases that cause epigastric pain, including cholecystitis and pancreatitis.

Treatment

After the patient's condition is stabilized, proton-pump inhibitors (PPIs) may be initiated if the patient is not already taking them, but controversy exists as to the efficacy of PPIs as emergency treatment and stabilization therapies. PPIs diminish bleeding by reducing the amount of acid in the stomach. These medications can be given as an IV bolus followed by an IV drip. Antiulcer medications are used to suppress acid secretion and to form a barrier over the ulcer. These medications are summarized in Table 10-9.

Table 10-9 Antiulcer Medications

Antisecretory Agents	Specific Drugs	Mechanism of Action
H_2 receptor antagonists	Cimetidine Famotidine Nizatidine	Suppresses acid secretion by blocking H_2 receptors on parietal cells
Proton-pump inhibitors	Esomeprazole Lansoprazole Omeprazole Pantoprazole RABEprazole	Suppresses acid secretion by inhibiting H,K-ATPase
Muscarinic antagonists	Pirenzepine	Suppresses acid secretion by blocking muscarinic cholinergic receptors
Mucosal protectants	Sucralfate	Forms a barrier over ulcer

H,K-ATPase, hydrogen, potassium, adenosine triphosphatase; H_2, histamine-2.

Erosive Gastritis and Esophagitis

Pathophysiology

Erosive gastritis and esophagitis, as the name suggests, is due to erosion and inflammation of the gastric and esophageal mucosa. This condition can have an acute or chronic onset, and has numerous potential causes. Nonspecific causes include alcohol, NSAIDs, corrosives, and radiation exposure. Erosive gastritis and esophagitis typically causes less bleeding than peptic ulcer disease, and the condition is self-limiting.

Signs and Symptoms

The chief signs and symptoms include indigestion, heartburn, dyspepsia, and belching. A few patients may also have nausea and vomiting or a chronic cough. The severity of symptoms does not accurately indicate the severity of the lesions.

Differential Diagnosis

Making a diagnosis in the field is typically difficult because of the myriad signs and symptoms.

Treatment

Little can be done for this condition in the prehospital setting. Maintain the patient's airway, breathing, and circulation, and offer comfort measures such as proper positioning, analgesics, and **antiemetics**. If the patient has no active bleeding, a mixture of viscous lidocaine and an oral antacid may provide relief. For long-term care, as with peptic ulcer disease, the patient may be placed on a PPI and should be advised to avoid NSAIDs, caffeine, and alcohol. Although taking low-dose aspirin increases the risk of upper GI bleeding, its preventive benefits for cardiovascular disease may outweigh that risk for some patients.

Esophageal and Gastric Varices

Pathophysiology

Esophageal and gastric varices are dilated veins that form as a result of mounting pressure damaging the vessels walls and weakening the venous structure. Varices occur when blood flow through the liver is restricted by cirrhosis, leading to portal hypertension. This causes the blood to back up into the veins in the wall of the esophagus, causing the vessels to dilate. Varices are typically asymptomatic until they rupture and bleed, causing massive blood loss. Patients who have bled from their varices have a 70% chance of bleeding again. If they do bleed a second time, 30% of the cases result in death.

Signs and Symptoms

A patient with esophageal and gastric varices exhibits signs of liver disease, including fatigue, weight loss, jaundice, anorexia, ascites, pruritus, abdominal pain, nausea, and vomiting. Severe dysphagia, vomiting of bright red blood, hypotension, and signs of shock may also occur. The disease process is gradual, taking months to years to reach a state of extreme discomfort.

Differential Diagnosis

The differential diagnosis may include peptic ulcer disease.

Treatment

In the prehospital setting, treat the patient according to the general guidelines, just as you would any patient with a GI bleeding disorder. Accurate assessment of the degree of blood loss is critical. Be prepared for a hemodynamically unstable patient needing volume resuscitation and aggressive suctioning of the airway. If the patient's level of consciousness begins to decrease, consider securing the airway to prevent aspiration.

If the hemorrhage is uncontrolled, balloon tamponade may be performed in the hospital using a Sengstaken-Blakemore or similar tube to apply pressure directly to the bleeding varices. This is a temporary solution that requires frequent monitoring (**Figure 10-6**). If transportation to another facility is necessary, special precautions should be taken to protect the patient from changes in barometric pressure at higher elevations or during flight.

Standard medical therapy includes administration of a PPI and an antibiotic. Octreotide may be administered, but has limited effectiveness as a treatment for variceal

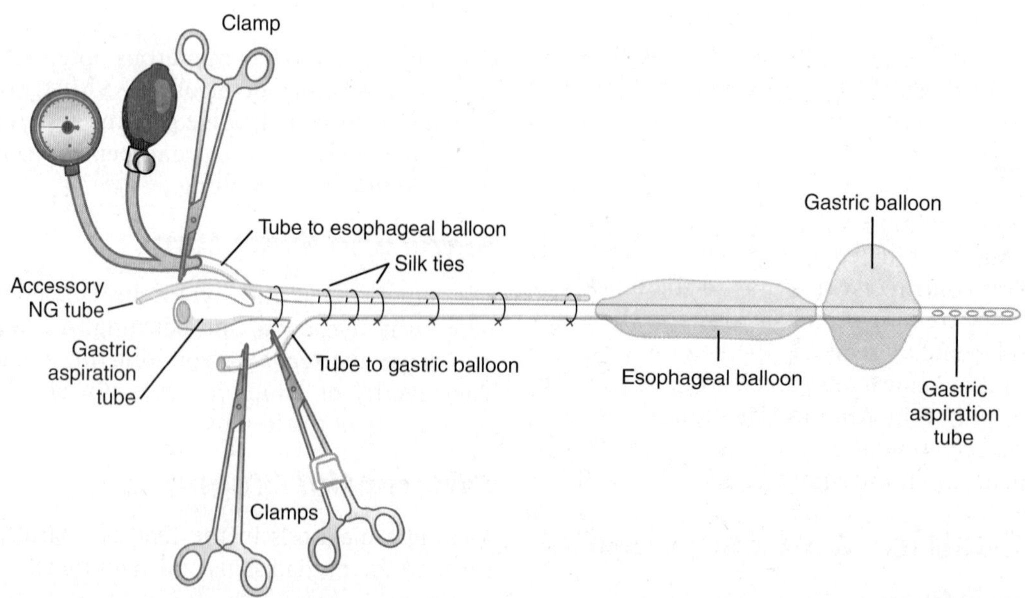

Figure 10-6 Modified Sengstaken-Blakemore tube. Note the accessory nasogastric (NG) tube for suctioning of secretions above the esophageal balloon, and the use of two clamps (one secured with tape) to prevent inadvertent decompression of the gastric balloon.

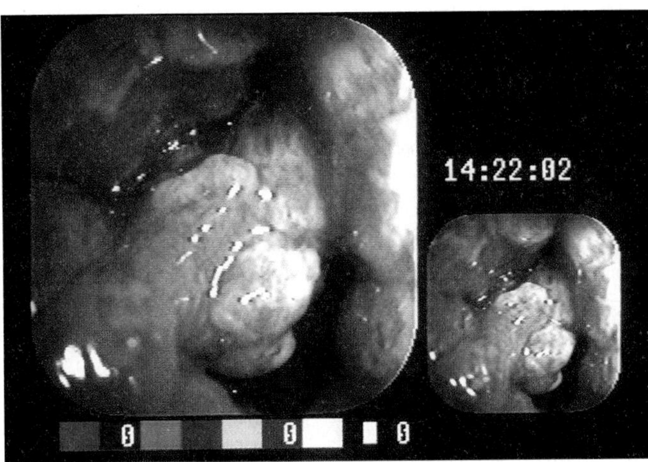

A

B

Figure 10-7 Endoscopic view of variceal ligation–related ulcers. **A.** Gastroesophageal junction is seen on a retroflexed view following ligation of multiple gastric varices, which resemble polyps. **B.** Upper endoscopy in the same patient 4 weeks later demonstrates multiple ulcers at sites of prior ligation.

bleeding. Vasopressin infusion is an additional pharmacologic option. Endoscopy may be performed to inject a sclerosing agent (a strong irritating solution) that promotes clot formation, a procedure known as sclerotherapy. Another option to promote clot formation is band therapy using rubber bands on the varices. Varices resemble polyps, and banding can prevent bleeding (**Figure 10-7**).

Mallory-Weiss Syndrome

Pathophysiology

Mallory-Weiss syndrome is a condition in which severe hemorrhage occurs from longitudinal tears of the esophageal and gastric mucosa, usually near the gastroesophageal junction. Severe, protracted vomiting or retching is the most common cause. Mallory-Weiss syndrome affects both men and women equally. It tends to occur in patients younger than 40 years. The mortality rate is less than 10%.

Signs and Symptoms

This syndrome can range in severity from mild and self-limited to severe and life threatening. Vomiting usually precedes the onset of bleeding; hematemesis occurs in 85% of patients with Mallory-Weiss syndrome. Aspirin use, excessive alcohol use, and bulimia (an eating disorder associated with episodes of binge eating followed by self-induced vomiting) are associated with the syndrome as well.

Differential Diagnosis

The differential diagnosis includes esophageal and gastric varices and Boerhaave syndrome.

Treatment

Primary management is supportive because the bleeding usually resolves spontaneously. If it continues, endoscopy may be necessary. If the patient is still nauseated or vomiting, antiemetics should be considered.

Perforated Viscus

Pathophysiology

A perforated or ruptured **viscus (pl. viscera)**—that is, any part of the GI tract—is an emergent event. A common cause is a duodenal ulcer eroding through the full thickness of the bowel wall. Peritonitis ensues when the intestinal contents spill into the abdominal cavity. As the time between perforation and diagnosis lengthens, the mortality rate climbs. Risk factors include advanced age, diverticular disease, use of NSAIDs, and a history of peptic ulcer disease.

Signs and Symptoms

Perforation usually causes an acute onset of abdominal pain; however, older adult patients may not have significant pain. The pain may be diffuse, with guarding and rebound tenderness. A rigid abdomen is a late sign. Approximately half of affected patients experience vomiting. A low-grade fever, attributable to the peritonitis, may also be a late sign. Bowel sounds are diminished, tachycardia is common, and septic shock may develop. Massive bleeding may occur but is uncommon.

Differential Diagnosis

The differential diagnosis includes appendicitis, pancreatitis, colitis, enteritis, and mesenteric ischemia, which are discussed later in this chapter.

Treatment

In prehospital care, establishment of IV access and support of the patient's airway, breathing, and circulation are essential.

In the ED, diagnostic lab tests and imaging should be performed. An elevated white blood cell count may be seen due to the peritonitis. In 70% to 80% of patients, an upright radiograph will show free air under the diaphragm if an ulcer perforates. CT will reveal more information about the extent of the perforation.

Boerhaave Syndrome

Pathophysiology

Boerhaave syndrome is a rupture of the esophagus as a consequence of hyperemesis gravidarum, childbirth, violent coughing, seizures, status asthmaticus, weightlifting, certain neurologic disorders, or explosive vomiting after an excessive intake of food and drink.

Signs and Symptoms

The patient typically has severe, distracting pain in the chest, neck, back, and abdomen, as well as difficulty breathing, tachycardia, hematemesis, and fever. If the rupture occurs in the neck, subcutaneous emphysema may be present.

Differential Diagnosis

Differential diagnoses may include a Mallory-Weiss syndrome, myocardial infarction, aortic dissection, and peptic ulcer disease.

Treatment

Provide supplemental oxygen and rapidly transport the patient to the hospital. Resuscitate as needed. The mortality rate for Boerhaave syndrome is as high as 50% without early surgical intervention.

Acute Pancreatitis

Pathophysiology

Diabetes is the most common disorder related to the pancreas, but pancreatitis is also common. Acute pancreatitis is an inflammatory process in which premature activation of pancreatic enzymes causes the pancreas to begin to digest itself, resulting in pain and necrosis as the inflammation spreads. This disease is thought to be caused by cholelithiasis or alcohol abuse in more than 90% of cases. Alcoholic pancreatitis is more common in men between the ages of 35 and 45 years. Hypertriglyceridemia and, rarely, certain medications can also cause pancreatitis.

Signs and Symptoms

The patient with acute pancreatitis experiences constant, severe mid-epigastric pain that radiates to the back. Anorexia, nausea, and vomiting are usually present and exacerbated by oral intake. Cullen sign, an ecchymotic discoloration around the umbilicus, and Grey Turner sign, a similar ecchymotic discoloration around the flanks, may be present in the hemorrhagic form of this condition. Fever may also be present. A systemic inflammatory response can develop, leading to shock and multiorgan failure.

Differential Diagnosis

The differential diagnosis for acute pancreatitis includes other causes of epigastric abdominal pain, such as peptic ulcer disease, cholecystitis, perforated viscus, acute mesenteric ischemia, and intestinal obstruction. Diagnostic testing includes serum lipase, bilirubin and liver enzymes, and possibly CT of the abdomen. Lipase is more sensitive and specific than amylase; the lipase level is more specific to the pancreas and stays elevated for several days.

Treatment

Treat patients with suspected pancreatitis by establishing IV access, giving nothing by mouth, providing fluid resuscitation, and administering analgesics and antiemetics. Complications can include pancreatic hemorrhage or necrosis. The treatment of chronic pancreatitis is similar and is generally supportive.

Gastroparesis

Gastroparesis, also called delayed gastric emptying, is a medical condition characterized by paresis (partial paralysis) of the stomach, resulting in food remaining in the stomach for an abnormally long time. Normally, the stomach contracts to move food down into the small intestine for additional digestion. The vagus nerve controls these contractions. Gastroparesis may occur when the vagus nerve is damaged and the muscles of the stomach and intestines do not function properly. Food then moves slowly or stops moving through the digestive tract. Transient gastroparesis may arise in acute illness of any kind, as a consequence of certain cancer treatments or other drugs affecting digestive action, or due to abnormal eating patterns. Patients with gastroparesis are disproportionately female. One possible explanation for this finding is that females have an inherently slower stomach-emptying time compared to males. A hormonal link has also been suggested, as gastroparesis symptoms tend to worsen the week before menstruation when progesterone levels are highest. Neither theory has been proven definitively.

Gastroparesis is frequently caused by autonomic neuropathy involving the vagus nerve. This condition may occur in people with type 1 or type 2 diabetes. In fact, diabetes mellitus is considered the most common cause of gastroparesis, as high levels of blood glucose may cause chemical changes in the nerves. Other possible causes include anorexia nervosa and bulimia nervosa. Gastroparesis has also been associated with connective tissue diseases such as scleroderma and Ehlers-Danlos syndrome, and with neurologic conditions such as Parkinson disease. It may also occur as part of a mitochondrial disorder.

Chronic gastroparesis can be caused by other types of damage to the vagus nerve, such as abdominal surgery. Heavy cigarette smoking is also a plausible cause because smoking causes damage to the stomach lining.

Idiopathic gastroparesis (gastroparesis with no known cause) accounts for one-third of all chronic cases. It is thought that many of these cases are due to an autoimmune response triggered by an acute viral infection. "Stomach flu," mononucleosis, and other ailments have been anecdotally linked to the onset of the condition, but no systematic study has proven a link.

Gastroparesis can also be connected to hypochlorhydria and can be caused by chloride, sodium, and/or zinc deficiency. These minerals are needed for the stomach to produce adequate levels of gastric acid to properly empty itself of a meal.

Signs and Symptoms

The most common symptoms of gastroparesis include chronic nausea, vomiting (especially of undigested food), and abdominal pain. Other symptoms include palpitations, heartburn, abdominal bloating, erratic blood glucose levels, loss of appetite, gastroesophageal reflux, spasms of the stomach wall, weight loss, and malnutrition. Morning nausea may also indicate gastroparesis. Vomiting may not occur in all cases, as patients may adjust their diets to include only small amounts of food.

Differential Diagnosis

Gastroparesis can be diagnosed with tests such as radiographs and gastric emptying scans. The clinical definition of gastroparesis is based solely on the emptying time of the stomach (and not on other symptoms), and the severity of symptoms does not necessarily correlate with the severity of gastroparesis. Some patients with gastroparesis have a jejunostomy tube or implanted gastric neurostimulators ("stomach pacemakers").

Treatment

To treat a patient with gastroparesis, establish IV access, administer analgesics and antiemetics, and transport the patient to the hospital in a position of comfort.

Appendicitis

Pathophysiology

Appendicitis is typically caused by an infection or the buildup of fluid in the appendix. As the appendix becomes distended and inflamed, it may rupture, spilling toxins into the abdomen, and cause peritonitis. Bacteria can also enter the bloodstream, causing sepsis. Even if the appendix does not rupture, gangrene is a possibility and constitutes a surgical emergency. Despite a 7% incidence among the general population, there is no way of predicting when appendicitis will develop, although the condition is most common in persons ages 5 to 45 years.

Signs and Symptoms

Patients with appendicitis have pain localized to the right lower quadrant or right lower back. The pain classically begins in the periumbilical region, then becomes more localized in the right lower quadrant as inflammation worsens. Other signs and symptoms include fever, nausea and vomiting, and a positive psoas sign, which is quite specific to appendicitis. To assess for this sign, place the patient in the left lateral decubitus position and extend the right leg at the hip. Exacerbation of pain in the right lower quadrant is a positive psoas sign.

Young children, older adult patients, pregnant women, and patients who have human immunodeficiency virus/acquired immunodeficiency syndrome (HIV/AIDS) may have an abnormal presentation of appendicitis and be at higher risk of complications. In young children, the onset of appendicitis may be delayed and nonspecific. Misdiagnosis is common because of the limitations in communicating with preverbal patients and because of the atypical presentation. As you might expect, misdiagnosis elevates the risk of perforation. In patients older than 70 years, the rate of misdiagnosis is as high as 50%, and rupture is common. Appendicitis is the most common cause of extrauterine abdominal pain during pregnancy and should be suspected with GI complaints in pregnant women. Patients with HIV/AIDS have the same symptoms as other patients, but they have a much higher risk of complications. They are also more likely to delay seeking treatment for appendicitis because of the frequency of other GI problems.

Differential Diagnosis

The differential diagnosis of appendicitis is difficult because the signs and symptoms may be attributed to many conditions. Notably, pancreatitis, Crohn disease, cecal diverticulitis, and endometriosis often present with similar symptoms.

At the receiving facility, a definitive diagnosis will be made using ultrasound or CT. Laboratory studies such as a complete blood cell count and a urinalysis will be evaluated. CT is the most useful study because it can also reveal an alternative diagnosis if the patient does not have appendicitis. In fact, use of CT has been shown to reduce the number of unnecessary appendectomies in women. However, a gravid uterus makes appendicitis difficult to diagnose. To avoid radiation exposure with CT, ultrasound or magnetic resonance imaging can aid in the diagnosis.

If appendicitis is confirmed, surgery to remove the appendix has been the traditional treatment. In recent years, the literature has shown some cases may respond to IV antibiotics without surgical intervention.

Treatment

To treat a patient with suspected appendicitis, establish IV access and fluids, administer analgesics and antiemetics, and transport the patient to the hospital in a position of comfort.

Mesenteric Ischemia

Pathophysiology

Mesenteric ischemia is caused by an occlusion of a mesenteric artery or vein. Symptoms typically include an acute onset of nausea, vomiting, diarrhea, and severe midabdominal pain that may be out of proportion to abdominal tenderness. This condition is more common in older adult patients and in individuals with a history of atrial fibrillation, myocardial infarction, valvular heart disease, or peripheral vascular disease. Smoking, hypertension, and hypercholesterolemia are also risk factors for mesenteric ischemia. In addition, use of oral contraceptives, hypercoagulability, aortic dissection, and trauma can precipitate an ischemic event. It is a rare but serious condition, with a high mortality rate.

Signs and Symptoms

Depending on the exact cause, pain may have a gradual or sudden onset. The location of the pain tends to be ill defined and its level is severe. Nausea, vomiting, and diarrhea are also common. Blood may be present in the stool.

Differential Diagnosis

Mesenteric ischemia is difficult to diagnose. Its cardinal presentation includes severe abdominal pain with only mild or minimal abdominal tenderness. A thorough history is needed. No laboratory studies are specifically diagnostic, although the finding of an elevated serum lactate can aid in clinical diagnosis. Abnormal radiologic findings are a late sign. You should suspect mesenteric ischemia in patients with other risk factors and no other cause for the abdominal pain.

Treatment

Mesenteric ischemia can progress to infarction if not identified early and may result in gangrenous bowel, perforation, and death. Treatment for these patients requires rapid transport. Monitor the patient closely, checking vital signs for evidence of sepsis. If shock is present, initiate fluid resuscitation. Analgesics may be indicated. In-hospital treatment will include imaging studies (angiogram or computed tomography angiography) and antibiotics. Depending on the cause, surgery, anticoagulants, or vasodilators will be used.

Intestinal Obstruction

Pathophysiology

Intestinal obstruction is an emergent event in which stool, a foreign body, or a mechanical process obstructs passage of intestinal contents. Mounting pressure in the intestine proximal to the obstruction diminishes blood flow, leading to septicemia and intestinal necrosis. The mortality rate rises dramatically as shock develops. Patients with a history of bowel obstruction, abdominal surgery, recent abdominal illness, cancer, radiation, chemotherapy, or hernia are at greater risk of experiencing an intestinal obstruction.

Compression or twisting of the bowel by scar tissue from prior surgery is the most common cause. Other mechanical causes of small-bowel obstruction include intussusception, polyps, volvulus, and tumors.

Gastric **volvulus**, a condition in which the stomach rotates more than 180 degrees, is a rare event that has been documented in only 400 cases in the United States. This twisting seals the stomach on both ends, blocking the flow of blood and the passage of fluid and food. The condition is characterized by an acute onset of abdominal pain, severe vomiting, and shock. The patient is likely to die in the absence of timely intervention.

Intussusception occurs when a portion of the bowel telescopes into an adjacent portion of the intestine, thereby occluding passage of intestinal contents and diminishing blood flow to the area. Intussusception accounts for 7% of all intestinal obstructions. This condition is more common in children than among adults. Approximately 80% of intussusceptions in adults occur in the small intestine.

Large-bowel obstruction is less common than small-bowel obstruction because of the greater diameter of the colon. When such an obstruction does develop, it is usually caused by cancer, fecal impaction, ulcerative colitis, sigmoid or cecal volvulus, diverticulitis, or intussusception.

Signs and Symptoms

Patients with intestinal obstruction have nausea, vomiting, and abdominal pain. In addition, they may be unable to pass flatus (bowel gas) and may have constipation or a distended abdomen. The natural peristalsis of the intestines continues despite the obstruction, causing intermittent pain that the patient may describe as being crampy or feeling like a knot.

Any abdominal complaint should prompt you to ask the patient about appetite and bowel regimen as you gather the patient's history. In a patient with an obstruction, auscultation of the bowel will reveal high-pitched or absent sounds. The sounds can be difficult to hear because sound may be referred from one portion of the abdomen to the other, so be sure to auscultate each quadrant for several minutes. Percussion may reveal a hollow sound. Palpation may provoke the pain, and a distended, firm abdomen indicates a severe obstruction.

Differential Diagnosis

It is impossible to make a definitive diagnosis of intestinal obstruction in the field, but you can still treat the patient if you suspect the condition.

Treatment

Begin treatment by addressing any life threats. Next, establish IV access and administer medications for nausea and pain per local protocol. Give nothing by mouth because the patient may need to undergo immediate surgery. Transport the patient in a position of comfort.

In the ED, a CT scan or both flat and upright x-rays of the abdomen and chest will be taken to confirm the obstruction. A complete blood count and electrolyte analysis will be performed. An elevated white blood cell count and lactate level may indicate ischemia and impending bowel necrosis. A nasogastric tube may be placed to decompress the GI tract proximal to the obstruction pending surgical intervention.

Abdominal Compartment Syndrome

Pathophysiology

Abdominal compartment syndrome is caused by severe elevation of hydrostatic pressure within the abdominal cavity and is a critical presentation for patients with abdominal discomfort. This condition is rare but must be detected as early as possible.

Signs and Symptoms

The patient may have a tense, tender, distended abdomen; respiratory distress; metabolic acidosis; declining urine output; and dwindling cardiac output. The drop in cardiac output occurs as the pressure builds up in the abdomen, restricting venous return to the heart.

This condition is more common among trauma patients, but may be seen in medical patients as well. Because its signs and symptoms are often associated with other critical events such as hypovolemia, compartment syndrome may be missed. Awareness is essential.

Differential Diagnosis

The differential diagnosis may include appendicitis, heart failure, mesenteric ischemia, and urinary obstruction.

Treatment

Treatment in the field for this condition is limited to loosening restrictive clothing, placing the patient in supine position, avoiding excessive fluid administration, and assuring adequate pain control. Avoid external pressure or weight on the abdomen. In the ED, removing fluid may decompress the abdomen. Surgical intervention for decompression is often required.

Acute Gastroenteritis

Pathophysiology

Acute gastroenteritis, the second leading cause of illness in the United States, is characterized by watery diarrhea, nausea and vomiting, mild abdominal pain, and low-grade fever. Many viruses cause acute gastroenteritis. These agents typically enter the body via the fecal–oral route through contaminated food or water. The norovirus is responsible for most cases of acute viral gastroenteritis in adults, whereas rotavirus causes the same condition in children. Various parasites may be contracted by swimming in water contaminated with them. Viral gastroenteritis is easily transmissible and can cause large outbreaks, which are usually sporadic and tend to flourish in the winter months.

Signs and Symptoms

Depending on the organism involved, patients may begin to experience GI upset and diarrhea in as soon as several hours or as long as multiple days after contact with the contaminated food or water. The disease can run its course in 2 to 3 days or continue for several weeks.

Patients can experience various types of diarrhea—large dumping type or frequent small, liquid stools. The diarrhea can contain blood and/or pus, and it may have a foul odor or be odorless. Abdominal cramping is frequent as hyperperistalsis continues. Nausea and vomiting, fever, and anorexia are also present.

If the diarrhea continues, dehydration and hemodynamic instability will result. As the volume of fluid loss increases, the likelihood of potassium and sodium imbalance also increases. Watch for changes in level of consciousness and other profound signs of shock, which clearly indicate a critical volume loss.

Differential Diagnosis

The possible diagnoses include appendicitis, hepatitis, colitis, and food poisoning.

Treatment

Treatment is symptomatic and consists of administering antiemetics and providing IV fluid replacement.

Cannabinoid Hyperemesis Syndrome

Pathophysiology

As of 2022, 38 U.S. states and the District of Columbia had laws legalizing cannabis in some form, with 21 states and the District of Columbia allowing for some form of recreational use. Adverse effects from cannabis, from both recreational and medicinal use, have been reported for decades. More recently, reporting has increased with greater access to cannabis. Among the more commonly cited adverse effects is cannabinoid hyperemesis syndrome (CHS). CHS is a syndrome of cyclic vomiting in the setting of chronic, high-dose cannabis use that is frequently associated with compulsive hot baths/showers, used in an attempt to control symptoms.

The exact pathophysiology of CHS is unclear, but one suggested mechanism is dysregulation of the endocannabinoid system, a group of endogenous cannabinoid receptors located in the brain, GI tract, peripheral nervous system, and immune system. The endocannabinoid system is thought to play a role in GI motility, appetite, nausea/vomiting, inflammation, mood, sleep, pain, and more. Additionally, it is thought that cannabinoids interact directly with receptors in the GI tract and alter GI motility.

Signs and Symptoms

Severe nausea and vomiting in a cyclical pattern is the predominant symptom reported by patients with CHS. It is frequently accompanied by diffuse abdominal pain, which can be severe. Dehydration and hemodynamic instability may occur due to vomiting and decreased oral intake. Symptom onset is preceded by daily to weekly cannabis use.

Differential Diagnosis

CHS is a diagnosis of exclusion. Thus, other causes of nausea and vomiting have to be considered before diagnosing CHS.

Treatment

Cannabis cessation is the best treatment. Supportive care in the form of IV hydration and antiemetics may be necessary secondary to profound dehydration and acute renal failure. Very limited evidence suggests that sedatives such as benzodiazepines, dopamine antagonist medications such as droPERidol, and the application of capsaicin cream to the abdomen may be helpful strategies to manage acute symptoms.

Sepsis

Abdominal pain is not a typical presentation of sepsis, but some patients do have nausea and vomiting. Sepsis is discussed further in Chapter 5, *Shock*, and in Chapter 6, *Sepsis*.

Abdominal Disorders Associated with Liver Disease

A number of disorders and diseases affect the liver. One sign of liver disease is jaundice, or a distinct yellow discoloration of the eyes (scleral icterus), mucous membranes, and skin. Jaundice is caused by the presence of excessive bilirubin in the bloodstream. To be eliminated from the body, bilirubin must be conjugated by the liver. As the excess unconjugated bilirubin crosses the blood–brain barrier, encephalopathy and death can occur. Obstruction of the biliary ducts (from tumor or stones) can lead to accumulation of conjugated bilirubin and is another cause of jaundice. Jaundice is often associated with prematurity in infants due to insufficiency of bilirubin clearance; this is typically a benign condition. Patients with jaundice may show no symptoms or a wide variety of symptoms, depending on the underlying cause, which range in severity from mild to life threatening. Patients with acute illness may have a fever, chills, abdominal pain, and flulike symptoms.

During the early stages of liver disease, patients may be diagnosed with influenza or gastroenteritis. In-hospital diagnostic tests include CT or ultrasound and laboratory studies such as a complete blood count, serum bilirubin, alkaline phosphatase, prothrombin time/partial thromboplastin time (PT/PTT), serum amylase, ammonia level, a pregnancy test, and toxicology screening. Hepatic encephalopathy is a specific form of liver disease that presents with elevated ammonia levels and altered mental status. Asterixis (discussed later in this section) is present. These patients will have confusion and often try to refuse transport. It is essential to determine medical decision-making capacity in these patients.

Hepatitis

Pathophysiology

Hepatitis simply means an inflammation of the liver. Despite its simple name, the etiology of hepatitis is often complex. Causes include viral, bacterial, fungal, and parasitic infections; exposure to toxic substances; adverse drug reactions; and immunologic disorders.

Alcohol is one of the toxic substances causing severe liver disease and hepatitis, because the liver is responsible for degrading alcohol. Chronic alcohol abuse leads to liver disease, malnutrition, accumulation of toxic metabolites, and enzyme alteration. The interaction of these mechanisms is thought to cause hepatitis, although researchers do not yet understand precisely how.

Acetaminophen overdose is one of the most common causes of acute liver injury.

Viruses are among the most frequent causes of hepatitis. Viral hepatitis is typically classified as either type A, B, C, D, E, or G. After declining for many years, the incidence of both hepatitis B and C is increasing due to the opioid epidemic. Approximately 67% of persons living with hepatitis B and 51% of persons living with hepatitis C infection do not know that they have the virus, according to recent reports from the Centers for Disease Control and Prevention. The progression of hepatitis leads to fulminant hepatic failure and liver cancer.

Hepatitis A

Hepatitis A virus (HAV) is typically spread from person to person through the fecal–oral route. It thrives in areas with poor sanitation, particularly in unsanitary cooking facilities. HAV exposure is widespread. In fact, in some regions of the world, 100% of the population has been exposed to this virus. In the United States, the rate of exposure is as high as 50%. However, very few people who have been exposed to HAV actually become ill. A vaccination can be given to prevent HAV. HAV is not a chronic illness.

Hepatitis B

In infected people, hepatitis B virus (HBV) is most prevalent in blood, wound discharge, and semen and vaginal fluid, but can be found in most bodily secretions, including saliva, stool, tears, and urine. This virus is usually spread through exposure to infected blood or by sexual activity. The highest rates, then, are among IV drug users and men who have sex with men. Historically, blood transfusions were a frequent cause of HBV, but careful screening of blood products has virtually eliminated the risk of exposure through this route. Unlike with HAV, once infected with HBV, a person is always a carrier and can always transmit the disease. A vaccine for HBV, which is required for most health care workers, has led to significant decrease in the spread of this virus among members of the health care professions.

Hepatitis C

Hepatitis C has a prevalence of about 3 million persons in the United States and is linked to blood transfusions, unsafe needle-sharing practices, and accidental exposure of health care workers to the blood of infected patients. The cause of infection is not found in 40% to 57% of cases. Many cases persist in chronic form.

Hepatitis D

The hepatitis D virus (HDV) is structurally unrelated to the hepatitis A, B, and C viruses. HDV causes a unique infection that requires the assistance of viral particles from HBV to replicate and infect other hepatocytes. Its clinical course varies, ranging from acute self-limited infection to acute fulminant liver failure. Chronic liver infection can lead to end-stage liver disease and associated complications. HDV infection occurs more commonly among adults than among children. It is more commonly observed among patients with a history of IV drug use. Hepatitis B vaccines also provide protection from hepatitis D.

Hepatitis E

Hepatitis E, also called enteric hepatitis (*enteric* means "related to the intestines"), is similar to hepatitis A, and is more prevalent in Asia and Africa. It is transmitted through the fecal–oral route. Although generally not fatal, it is considered more serious in women during pregnancy and can cause fetal complications. Most patients with hepatitis E recover completely.

Hepatitis G

Hepatitis G is the newest strain of hepatitis; very little is known about it. Transmission is believed to occur through blood and is most commonly seen in IV drug users, individuals with clotting disorders such as hemophilia, and individuals who require hemodialysis for renal failure. Often, hepatitis G shows no clinical symptoms.

Fulminant Hepatic Failure

Fulminant hepatic failure sets in when hepatitis progresses to hepatic necrosis (death of the liver cells). Extensive hepatic necrosis is irreversible and can be treated only with a liver transplant. Hepatitis B and C are most often responsible for this condition, but drug toxicity (acetaminophen overdose) and metabolic disorders can also be the cause. Liver function test results will be elevated in a patient with fulminant hepatic failure.

Signs and Symptoms

The symptoms of hepatitis vary but tend to be nonspecific. They include malaise, fever, and anorexia, followed by nausea and vomiting, abdominal pain, diarrhea, and jaundice later in the course of the disease. Classic symptoms of fulminant hepatic failure include anorexia, vomiting, jaundice, abdominal pain, and asterixis, or "flapping." The mechanism causing asterixis is unknown.

To test for it, ask the patient to extend the arms, dorsiflex the wrists, and spread the fingers, and then observe for slow rhythmic flapping of the hands.

Differential Diagnosis

The possible differential diagnoses include acute gastroenteritis, acute cholangitis, hemolytic anemia syndromes, and colitis.

Treatment

Prehospital treatment of patients with hepatitis focuses on supportive care. In the case of acetaminophen overdose, if the patient is seen soon after ingestion, the antidote *N*-acetylcysteine can be given with excellent results. Time of ingestion of the acetaminophen is key to determining whether the patient meets the treatment criteria. First, support the patient's airway, breathing, and circulation; then establish IV access and administer antiemetics and pain medication as necessary. Consider transport to a hospital that offers toxicology services if one is available within a reasonable distance.

Hepatic Encephalopathy

Hepatic encephalopathy is a brain dysfunction caused by liver insufficiency and/or portosystemic shunting. It manifests as a wide spectrum of neurologic/psychiatric abnormalities, ranging from subclinical alterations to coma.

Pathophysiology

Despite years of research, the exact mechanism of hepatic encephalopathy remains elusive; it likely involves a complicated interplay of many factors instead of a single process. Abnormality of ammonia metabolism is the primary mechanism associated with this disease. Excessive plasma ammonia can accumulate in the central nervous system because of the damaged liver's inability to metabolize it—a by-product of protein digestion in the gut. This high level of ammonia can cause alterations in neurotransmission and is likely one cause of the motor dysfunction exhibited by individuals with hepatic encephalopathy. Gamma aminobutyric acid (GABA), the principal neuroinhibitory neurotransmitter, is increased in the cerebrospinal fluid (CSF) of patients with hepatic encephalopathy. Other toxins associated with hepatic encephalopathy that are found in the CSF include benzodiazepine-like compounds, oxygen free radicals, and inflammatory cytokines.

Common precipitants of hepatic encephalopathy include medications such as diuretics and benzodiazepines, noncompliance with medications, GI bleeding, constipation, hypokalemia, alkalosis, volume depletion, and sepsis. Cerebral edema is the most common cause of death in patients with hepatic encephalopathy due to the rapid accumulation of ammonia. Cerebral edema may be clinically subtle.

Signs and Symptoms

Detecting hepatic encephalopathy early can be critically important to patients' prognosis. Some of the first early clinical signs include mild personality changes such as irritability, disinhibition, and apathy. Sleep disturbances can often be detected with excessive daytime sleepiness and yawning. Minor impairments can lead to falls, impaired driving, and overall decreased quality of life. Motor disturbances typically begin after this early symptomatic period. Asterixis of the hands (a "flapping" of the wrists when held in hyperextension) is common, but asterixis of other body parts can be detected as well, including the feet, legs, arms, tongue, and eyelids. Extrapyramidal symptoms and Parkinsonian-like features may also occur. Although rare, focal neurologic deficits—most commonly hemiplegia—can occur. Nearly 70% of patients with cirrhosis will have episodes of hepatic encephalopathy. In general, the more altered the patient's condition, the more severe their disease is.

Differential Diagnosis

The differential diagnosis of hepatic encephalopathy includes thiamine deficiency, sepsis, renal failure, alcohol withdrawal, intracranial bleeding, and disorders of the central nervous system. In the hospital, the serum ammonia level is helpful but not definitive in making the diagnosis.

Treatment

In patients with suspected hepatic encephalopathy, rule out other causes of altered mental status such as hypoglycemia, hypoxia, and seizure. Replace fluid and glucose deficits. Normal saline is the fluid of choice in hepatic encephalopathy. One bolus of dextrose may not be adequate therapy for hypoglycemia because of the patient's depleted glycogen stores. Maintenance infusions of $D_{10}W$ should also be administered after the initial dextrose bolus. If cerebral edema is suspected, keep the head of the bed elevated at 45 degrees.

In the hospital, the goal of hepatic encephalopathy treatment is to reduce the amount of ammonia. Current therapies are aimed at changing the gut biome to reduce the amount of intestinal ammonia production using medications such as lactulose, lactitol, rifaximin, and probiotics.

Abdominal Disorders Associated with Inflammatory Conditions

Irritable Bowel Syndrome

Pathophysiology

Irritable bowel syndrome (IBS) is a chronic disorder affecting 10% to 15% of the U.S. population. Although not life threatening, it causes abdominal pain, diarrhea, constipation, and nausea that can greatly impair patients' quality of life. Because lab findings and radiologic studies are normal in patients with IBS, the disorder was originally thought to be psychiatric in origin. Current physiologic research, however, suggests this condition is due to an error of gut motility and sensation. IBS occurs more often in persons with a history of depression or anxiety and worsens when patients are under stress. It also appears to be more prevalent among women.

Signs and Symptoms

IBS is a chronic condition. Prehospital presentations will typically involve a flare-up of the condition. Patients may be initially seen with abdominal pain or discomfort, which is relieved by a bowel movement. When the pain starts, there is usually a change in the frequency and consistency of bowel movements. Patients may experience diarrhea, constipation, and bloating.

Differential Diagnosis

The differential diagnosis includes food allergies, gastroenteritis, endometriosis, and mesenteric ischemia. IBS may be associated with a coexisting psychiatric disorder such as depression or anxiety.

Treatment

Treatment is mainly supportive. Assess the patient's mood and thoughts. Be compassionate. If depression and/or suicidal thoughts are noted, treat those accordingly. Analgesia may be needed. A confirmed diagnosis may indicate the need for dietary modification, behavioral therapy, and supportive care.

Diverticular Disease

Pathophysiology

Diverticulosis is characterized by small, saclike appendages called *diverticula* that form when the lining of the colon herniates through the mucosal wall. This disease is far more likely to appear in individuals older than 50 years than in younger adults.

Signs and Symptoms

Diverticulosis is often asymptomatic. When the disorder does generate symptoms, they include abdominal bloating, crampy pain, and changes in bowel habits. Diverticulitis is inflammation and/or infection of the diverticula causing persistent left lower quadrant pain, diffuse tenderness, vomiting, and abdominal distention. Patients can have either diarrhea or constipation. Abscesses and perforation may form in more severe cases. The other common complication of diverticulosis is bleeding, which may be painless.

Differential Diagnosis

The differential diagnosis includes appendicitis, bowel obstruction, mesenteric ischemia, colitis, and inflammatory bowel disease.

Treatment

Treatment is mainly focused on making the patient comfortable. Potential complications include bowel perforation and consequent peritonitis and sepsis. Patients should be monitored closely to ensure severe infection is not present. They may need large amounts of fluids and/or vasopressors to maintain blood pressure. In-hospital treatment will include antibiotics, IV hydration, and GI tract rest (by giving the patient a liquid diet). Patients with severe diverticulitis may require surgical colectomy or abscess drainage.

Cholecystitis and Biliary Tract Disorders

Pathophysiology

Biliary tract disorders are a group of conditions involving inflammation of the gallbladder and/or bile ducts. The gallbladder is an organ that stores bile to aid digestion of fats and fat-soluble nutrients. The bile ducts conduct bile from the liver to the gallbladder and small intestine. Cholangitis, an inflammation of the bile ducts, is typically a severe infectious process. Cholelithiasis refers to the presence of gallstones in the gallbladder. This condition is more prevalent among older adults, women, people with morbid obesity, individuals who have lost weight rapidly, those with a familial predisposition to the disorder, and those who have taken certain drugs. Cholecystitis, acute inflammation of the gallbladder, is usually due to complete obstruction of the biliary duct caused by gallstones, a stricture, or a malignancy.

Signs and Symptoms

Gallstones are asymptomatic in some people. In others, they provoke severe pain in the right upper quadrant, sometimes referred to the right shoulder, accompanied by nausea and vomiting. This pain, called *biliary colic*, is typically cyclic and tends to be aggravated by eating fatty foods. By definition, the pain subsides within hours of onset.

Signs and symptoms of cholecystitis include persistent right upper quadrant pain, nausea, vomiting, and fever. Murphy sign may be present and can be elicited by pressing firmly upward into the right upper quadrant and asking the patient to take a deep breath. Arrest of inspiration because of pain is a positive finding. Cholecystitis will be treated urgently with antibiotics and usually cholecystectomy (gallbladder removal).

Cholangitis has the same symptoms as cholecystitis, but often with jaundice. Sepsis will develop if this condition is left untreated.

Differential Diagnosis

Differential diagnoses include appendicitis, mesenteric ischemia, abdominal aortic aneurysm, gastroenteritis, colitis, pyelonephritis, and peptic ulcer disease.

Treatment

Prehospital treatment is directed at making the patient comfortable. Biliary colic can be treated with outpatient elective cholecystectomy. Treatment of cholangitis centers on maintaining hemodynamic stability, controlling pain and nausea, administering antibiotics, and decompressing the biliary tract.

Ulcerative Colitis

Pathophysiology

Ulcerative colitis is an autoimmune disease that causes inflammation of the colon. The inflammation is generalized and does not occur in patches, as in Crohn disease. In ulcerative colitis, the inflammation causes bleeding from the colonic mucosa and over time may lead to a thinning and bulging of the wall of the colon. This condition affects only the large intestine portion of the GI tract.

Signs and Symptoms

The onset of ulcerative colitis is usually gradual, and is associated with bloody diarrhea, hematochezia, and mild to severe abdominal pain. Other signs and symptoms can include joint pain and skin lesions. These effects lend credence to the idea that this condition has an autoimmune component. Patients can also experience fever, fatigue, and loss of appetite from infection.

Differential Diagnosis

Differential diagnoses may include gastroenteritis, Crohn disease, and irritable bowel syndrome.

Treatment

Treatment of patients with ulcerative colitis is mainly supportive. Determine the degree of hemodynamic instability. Look for signs of shock. If the diarrhea and bleeding have caused sufficient volume loss to make the patient's condition unstable, administer fluids to return the patient to a near-normal volume balance. Patients are often treated with long-term predniSONE or other immunosuppressive therapy. Complications include severe bleeding and toxic megacolon.

Crohn Disease

Pathophysiology

Crohn disease is similar to ulcerative colitis; however, the entire GI tract can be involved. The main part of the GI tract that tends to be involved is the ileum, which is the last portion of the small intestine before it joins the large intestine. There are several theories about the etiology of Crohn disease, but no definitive cause has been identified. Regardless of the cause, the result is a series of attacks by the immune system on the GI tract. This inflammatory activity damages all layers of the portion of the GI tract involved. The result is most often a scarred, narrowed, stiff, and weakened portion of the small intestine. This patch of damage is found among areas of intestine that are normal, and the resulting narrowing can cause bowel obstruction.

Signs and Symptoms

Of interest with Crohn disease and ulcerative colitis is the presence of signs and symptoms outside the GI system. This evidence helps support the theory that an autoimmune component is operating within the disease. Patients with Crohn disease experience chronic abdominal pain, often in the lower right area of the abdomen. This pain corresponds to the location of the ileum. Rectal bleeding, weight loss, diarrhea, arthritis, skin problems, and fever may also be present. Bleeding tends to occur in small amounts over a long period of time. Acute, severe hemorrhage is rare, but chronic bleeding resulting in anemia and hypotension does occur. Crohn disease may be complicated by development of fistulae and bowel obstructions. Patients often have recurrent episodes of mild to severe signs and symptoms.

Differential Diagnosis

The distinction between Crohn disease and ulcerative colitis is hard to determine clinically. Laboratory studies and imaging studies may help narrow down the diagnosis, but definitive diagnosis involves upper and lower endoscopy and biopsy.

Treatment

Patients with diarrhea and chronic hemorrhaging may require volume resuscitation. Control of nausea and pain are commonly required.

Cardiovascular and Pulmonary Causes of Abdominal Disorders

Disorders of organs adjacent to the diaphragm often cause symptoms in the neighboring body cavity. Pulmonary and cardiac diseases can give rise to symptoms in the epigastrium; conversely, disorders within the spleen or gallbladder can cause pain to be referred to the chest or scapular areas. When patients complain of upper abdominal discomfort or have nausea and vomiting, you should consider cardiovascular and pulmonary conditions, including acute myocardial infarction. Pulmonary embolism and pneumonia are other possible causes of abdominal pain, particularly when associated with shortness of breath. Consider acquiring a 12-lead ECG if you suspect the patient's signs and symptoms have a cardiopulmonary cause.

Abdominal Aortic Aneurysm

Abdominal aortic aneurysm is an enlargement of part of the aorta caused by a weakness in the vascular wall. These bulges in the arterial wall typically begin small and become larger over the course of several months to years. Most such aneurysms do not rupture, leak, or dissect. Fewer than one-half of all patients with an abdominal aortic aneurysm exhibit the classic triad of symptoms: hypotension, abdominal or back pain, and a pulsatile abdominal mass. Be sure to consider this diagnosis in patients with syncope or any one of the triad of symptoms.

Because of the large size of the aorta, its rupture causes massive blood loss, and survival depends primarily on the body's ability to spontaneously contain the bleeding. Any patient suspected of having a ruptured abdominal aortic aneurysm should be treated as having a life-threatening condition. Fluid resuscitation should be provided carefully, maintaining blood pressure just high enough to ensure adequate perfusion of the vital organs. Transport the patient to a hospital with immediate emergency surgical capability. Interfacility transfers may go directly to the operating room if the patient has a known ruptured aneurysm. If the patient is older than 50 years and is complaining of abdominal or back pain, an abdominal aneurysm should be considered, even if hypotension and a pulsatile mass are not present. Remember that even with a patient in stable condition, deterioration can happen suddenly at any time. Even patients who have had a repair are at risk for an aneurysm rupture.

See Chapter 4, *Cardiovascular Disorders and Conditions Presenting as Chest Pain*, for more information on aortic aneurysm. Other vascular causes of abdominal pain are also covered in Chapter 4.

Acute Coronary Syndrome

Myocardial infarction and angina can be accompanied by mid-epigastric pain and nausea, causing it to mimic an abdominal complaint such as peptic ulcer disease or gastritis. Because it may be difficult to distinguish between GI and cardiac causes, assess the patient for acute coronary syndrome and initiate care as appropriate. Review Chapter 4, *Cardiovascular Disorders and Conditions Presenting as Chest Pain*, for the diagnosis and treatment of acute coronary syndrome and myocardial infarction.

Pulmonary Embolism

As with acute coronary syndrome, pulmonary embolism should be suspected in patients who have upper abdominal pain. A pulmonary embolism is a potentially life-threatening condition that occurs when a thrombus (a blood clot, cholesterol plaque, or air bubble) travels through the bloodstream and becomes lodged in a pulmonary artery. At that point, the area of the lung perfused by that portion of the pulmonary artery no longer receives oxygenated blood, causing pain and shortness of breath.

You should suspect pulmonary embolism in patients with hip or long-bone fractures; people who are sedentary or have recently taken a long flight or car trip; those who smoke, use oral contraceptives, or have a history of deep vein thrombosis or cancer; and patients who are pregnant or were recently pregnant. See Chapter 3, *Respiratory Disorders*, for more information about pulmonary embolism.

Budd-Chiari Syndrome

Budd-Chiari syndrome is an extremely rare vascular disorder resulting from occlusion of the major hepatic veins or inferior vena cava. The venous thrombosis that characterizes this syndrome can be due to hematologic disease, coagulopathy, pregnancy, use of oral contraceptives, abdominal trauma, or a congenital disorder. Signs and symptoms include acute or chronic fulminant liver failure, emergent abdominal pain, hepatomegaly, ascites, and jaundice. Diagnosis is usually made by ultrasound. The treatment selected depends on the cause of the occlusion, but anticoagulants and supportive therapy are typically given.

Pneumonia

Pneumonia in the lower lobes of the lungs causes upper abdominal pain in some patients. Pneumonia is usually accompanied by a fever, chest pain, and respiratory distress. Chapter 3, *Respiratory Disorders*, addresses pneumonia at greater length.

Obstetric Causes of Abdominal Disorders

When you assess any female patient of childbearing age for an abdominal complaint, you should assume the patient is pregnant until proven otherwise. Many complications of pregnancy can be mistaken for abdominal conditions, and abdominal conditions can be exacerbated by pregnancy. Keep in mind that medications administered to treat abdominal symptoms may potentially be harmful to the fetus.

While caring for a pregnant patient, you must recognize the survival of two patients depends on maintaining adequate perfusion in the mother. As the fetus grows, it places increasing pressure on the internal organs, diaphragm, and inferior vena cava. Because of the boost in cardiac output and expansion of intravascular volume that occurs during pregnancy, signs of hypoperfusion may be delayed. During the second half of pregnancy, you should position the patient carefully to avoid triggering hypotension by putting pressure on the vena cava. Tilt or wedge the patient onto the left side, and transport. Consider transport to a facility that cares for high-risk obstetric patients as appropriate.

Abruptio Placentae

Pathophysiology

During the second half of pregnancy, approximately 4% of patients have vaginal bleeding. Bleeding during the second trimester signals imminent fetal distress and should be considered an emergency. Placental abruption, the premature separation of the placenta from the uterine wall, is responsible for approximately 30% of all cases of bleeding during the second half of pregnancy. Trauma, maternal hypertension, or preeclampsia typically precipitates abruption. Other risk factors include patients younger than 20 years, advanced maternal age, multiparity, a history of smoking, prior miscarriage, prior placental abruption, and cocaine use.

Signs and Symptoms

Placental abruption should be considered in patients who are greater than 20 weeks' pregnant with vaginal bleeding and abdominal pain. Contractions and uterine pain, or abdominal tenderness, and a decrease in fetal movement may be present. The majority (80%) of patients with placental abruption report vaginal bleeding. The blood is usually dark. With small abruptions, bleeding may not be noted until delivery. The volume of blood loss can vary from minimal to life threatening. The condition of these patients can progress from stable to unstable in a short period of time. Fetal distress or death occurs in approximately 15% of patients.

Differential Diagnosis

Possible diagnoses include appendicitis, placenta previa, preeclampsia, preterm labor, and ectopic pregnancy.

Treatment

Assessment should include evaluation of vaginal bleeding, contractions, and uterine tenderness and assessment of fundal height and fetal heart tones. Fetal heart tones may vary from absent to fetal bradycardia to decelerations. Short-term variability may be decreased as well if the fetus is compromised. Vaginal exams should not be performed until an ultrasound can be completed to rule out placenta previa.

Management is based on the severity of the blood loss. The following interventions may be indicated: supplemental oxygen, fluid support with two large-bore IVs, blood administration, and administering Rh globulin if the patient is Rh negative.

Placenta Previa

Pathophysiology

In some pregnancies, the placenta becomes implanted over the cervical os (opening). This anomaly is one of the leading causes of vaginal bleeding in the second and third trimesters. It may be identified early in the pregnancy but may resolve as the uterus expands. The patient is at risk of significant bleeding, however, if the condition does not resolve and the placenta completely occludes the cervix. Ultrasound is used to localize the placenta. Advanced maternal age, multiparity, and a history of smoking and prior cesarean section predispose individuals to placenta previa.

Signs and Symptoms

The patient will usually present with bright red bleeding. The bleeding is usually painless, but some patients (20%) will have uterine irritability as well. Many patients have an initial episode of bleeding that spontaneously stops and then have additional episodes of bleeding later in the pregnancy.

Differential Diagnosis

Possible diagnoses include placental abruption, disseminated intravascular coagulopathy, and preterm labor.

Treatment

In addition to monitoring the patient's bleeding, monitor the patient for signs and symptoms of shock, uterine tone (usually soft and nontender), and fetal heart tones. Do not perform vaginal or rectal examinations. Speculum exam can trigger hemorrhage if the condition is present. Monitor for disseminated intravascular coagulopathy, as maternal deaths with placenta previa are associated with blood loss or disseminated intravascular coagulopathy. Care is directed at supporting the patient's hemodynamic status, with interventions including supplemental oxygen, two large-bore IVs, fluids, and administration of blood as needed.

Preeclampsia/HELLP

Pathophysiology

Preeclampsia with HELLP syndrome (*H*, hemolysis; *EL*, elevated liver enzymes; *LP*, low platelet count) is a life-threatening complication of pregnancy thought to be a variant or complication of preeclampsia. Preeclampsia, which occurs in 6% to 8% of pregnancies, is characterized by hypertension and protein in the urine. The risk of preeclampsia is higher among individuals younger than age 20 years and in those with first or multifetal pregnancies, gestational diabetes, obesity, or a family history of gestational hypertension. Gestational hypertension typically resolves within 6 weeks postpartum. HELLP and preeclampsia usually occur during the last trimester of pregnancy or soon after delivery. Preeclampsia may progress to eclampsia with central nervous system involvement, including altered mental status and seizures.

HELLP syndrome is considered by some sources to be a severe and rare form of preeclampsia; others suggest it may be a syndrome of its own. Its precise cause has not been established. HELLP is a multisystem disease resulting in vasospasm, thrombi formation, and coagulation issues. It is often misdiagnosed or found late in the course of the syndrome, so your awareness of the signs and symptoms is vitally important. HELLP syndrome usually occurs antepartum, but may also present during the postpartum period (approximately one-third of cases appear postpartum). Left untreated, HELLP syndrome can lead to maternal end-organ failure as well as fetal demise.

Signs and Symptoms

Right upper quadrant pain, mid-epigastric pain, nausea and vomiting, and visual disturbances are the chief symptoms of preeclampsia. Patients should also be monitored for hyperreflexia or clonus. Seizures occur in eclampsia.

Most patients with HELLP syndrome complain of feeling generally unwell or fatigued; abdominal pain, especially in the upper quadrant; nausea; vomiting; and headache. The key to identification is a low platelet count. An elevated D-dimer may also help identify HELLP syndrome.

Differential Diagnosis

The diagnosis of preeclampsia may be difficult in the field, especially if no previous blood pressure readings are available. You will need to rely on a thorough history and examination to refine the diagnosis.

Treatment

Prehospital treatment is supportive and focuses on blood pressure control, fluid replacement, blood product replacement, and monitoring for disseminated intravascular coagulopathy. Pharmacologic interventions may include corticosteroids (for fetal lung development), magnesium sulfate, and hydralazine or labetalol (to address hypertension). Delivery may have to be induced to protect both the fetus and the mother. Transport the pregnant patient on the left side to prevent the gravid uterus from compressing the vena cava.

Ectopic Pregnancy

Pathophysiology

Ectopic pregnancy is implantation of the fertilized ovum (egg) outside of the uterus. The characteristic site of implantation is the fallopian tube, but the ovum may also implant in the abdominal cavity or elsewhere. If the fertilized ovum implants in the fallopian tube, the tube will begin to stretch as the embryo divides, causing pain and bleeding. The bleeding may be internal or vaginal. Rupture may lead to life-threatening hemorrhage, so early recognition is critical.

Risk factors for ectopic pregnancy include scarring or inflammation of the pelvis from previous surgeries or ectopic pregnancies, pelvic inflammatory disease, tubal ligation, and placement of an intrauterine device. Because symptoms become apparent within 5 to 10 weeks of implantation, many people are not yet aware that they are pregnant.

Signs and Symptoms

Consider ectopic pregnancy in any female patient of childbearing age who has either vaginal bleeding or lower abdominal pain. Syncope is a common presenting sign. Bleeding can be severe, especially after an ectopic rupture, placing the patient at risk of shock.

Differential Diagnosis

Possible diagnoses include appendicitis, abruptio placentae (placental abruption), placenta previa, threatened abortion, and complications from an abortion.

Treatment

Your initial goals for the patient will be to ensure that the airway and breathing are secure and to establish IV access. In the ED, a urine or serum pregnancy test will be obtained to establish whether the patient is pregnant. If a pregnancy is confirmed, a quantitative beta-hCG (human chorionic gonadotropin) level will be obtained to help determine the stage of the pregnancy. The level of beta-hCG rises as the pregnancy progresses through the early stages. The next step will be transvaginal ultrasound to determine whether the pregnancy has been established in the uterus or in an extrauterine location. If the latter is confirmed, obstetric consultation will be required.

Hyperemesis Gravidarum

Hyperemesis occurs early in pregnancy, usually in the first trimester, and can result in dehydration and fluid and electrolyte imbalance. It is defined by weight loss, starvation metabolism, and ketosis. Once other causes of vomiting are ruled out, management includes fluid therapy, electrolyte replacement, and antiemetics.

Renal Causes of Abdominal Disorders

Pyelonephritis

Pyelonephritis is a bacterial infection of the kidneys. It can be acute or chronic, and is most often due to the ascent of bacteria from the bladder up the ureters to infect the kidneys. Symptoms include dysuria (pain or burning during urination), flank (side) pain, fever, shaking chills, and sometimes foul-smelling urine, frequent and/or urgent need to urinate, and general malaise. Tenderness is elicited by gently tapping over the kidney with a fist (percussion). Diagnosis is made via urinalysis, which will reveal white blood cells and bacteria in the urine, and urine culture. Usually there is also an increase in circulating white cells in the blood. Treatment involves IV fluids, antipyretics, pain medications, and use of appropriate antibiotics.

Nontraumatic Kidney Injury

Pathophysiology

Nontraumatic kidney injury (meaning dysfunction) can be acute or chronic. Acute kidney injury (AKI) indicates new onset or worsening of kidney function, whereas chronic kidney disease (CKD) is defined as dysfunction present for 3 months or more.

In-hospital laboratory tests that indicate renal function include the glomerular filtration rate (GFR), blood urea nitrogen (BUN), and serum creatinine (Cr). Normal GFR in young adults is ≥ 125 mL/min/1.73 m^2 and decreases with age. The criterion for CKD is persistent GFR < 60 mL/min/1.73 m^2. The BUN and Cr levels typically rise in the setting of both AKI and CKD. The normal ratio of serum urea nitrogen to creatinine is $< 15:1$. A ratio $> 20:1$ suggests a prerenal cause of the failure. A ratio $< 15:1$ suggests intrinsic renal failure.

Acute Kidney Injury

Acute kidney injury can have prerenal, intrinsic, or postrenal causes. In prerenal failure, poor perfusion of the kidney leads to dysfunction, as measured by BUN and Cr levels and decreased GFR. Common causes of prerenal AKI include hypovolemia, hypotension, and decompensated heart failure. This process is usually reversible if the causative condition is corrected within the first day or two.

Intrinsic acute renal injury is commonly caused by autoimmune disease, chronic uncontrolled hypertension, or diabetes mellitus. Heavy metals, poisons, and nephrotoxic medications may also be responsible for intrinsic acute renal injury. Under certain conditions, a heat emergency or crush injury may lead to rhabdomyolysis, in which myoglobin released from damaged muscles obstructs the tubular portion of the nephrons, causing permanent damage if not caught early. Myoglobin in the urine turns it tea colored, which may be an early clue to the presence of the renal injury.

Postrenal injury occurs when urine flow is obstructed, causing a backflow of urine into the ureters and kidneys and causing the kidneys to dilate (hydronephrosis). This process disrupts kidney function, ultimately causing necrosis. If the obstruction is not resolved, chronic renal failure may be the result. Prolonged urinary retention and bilateral ureteral obstruction from retroperitoneal fibrosis are potential causes of this condition.

Chronic Kidney Disease

Chronic kidney disease is the permanent loss of some degree of renal function. End-stage renal disease is defined as GFR < 15 mL/min/1.73 m^2, which is reached when approximately 80% of the estimated 1 million nephrons in the kidney are damaged or destroyed. At that point, dialysis or a kidney transplant is required for survival. When caring for a patient with CKD, you must know how the disease is typically managed and be aware of the complications associated with the disease and its treatment, especially dialysis.

Signs and Symptoms

A patient with renal dysfunction may have complaints of weakness, changes in urinary habits, edema, rash/itching, nausea, vomiting, dyspnea, and chest discomfort. It is important to remember that many patients with kidney disease have diabetes, so symptoms of acute coronary syndrome may be masked or silent. Initially, patients with kidney injury may have no symptoms.

Differential Diagnosis

Kidney disease can have a variety of presentations, including urinary obstruction and volume overload, depending on the stage of disease and the cause. The diagnosis of kidney injury is made by laboratory tests that measure serum urea nitrogen, Cr, and GFR, as well as radiologic studies.

Treatment

Assessment to identify any life-threatening symptoms should be performed immediately. Warning signals include altered level of consciousness, signs of heart failure, dysrhythmia, and electrolyte imbalance.

If you are called to treat a patient who might have AKI or CKD, you must know how to identify the most serious complications of acute renal injury: pulmonary edema and hyperkalemia. Patients should be treated with supplemental oxygen and noninvasive positive-pressure ventilation (NIPPV) as needed for hypoxia and respiratory distress and with calcium IV if cardiac conduction changes are present. Aggressive treatment of any likely identifiable cause of AKI—hemorrhage, sepsis, heart failure, or shock of any kind—is also important.

Patients with chronic renal failure are some of the most challenging patients you will encounter. These patients usually have multiple medical problems, including complications that are unique to CKD and end-stage renal disease. It is impossible to cover all the presentations you might potentially see in these patients. Vascular overload caused by retention of fluid and sodium may be responsible for severe hypertension, acute pulmonary edema, or decompensated heart failure. Treatments for these conditions include nitroglycerin, angiotensin-converting enzyme (ACE) inhibitors, and NIPPV as indicated.

Some myths and misconceptions regarding patients in renal failure are as follows:

- *Fluid administration*. Fluids should not be withheld from a patient with renal injury in need of fluid resuscitation, but consult with medical direction before initiating aggressive fluid resuscitation. Hypovolemic or hypotensive patients should receive a fluid bolus when indicated. Be careful to limit fluids in patients who do not need fluids. Typically, IV access is difficult to obtain in patients with renal injury. If IV access is indicated, it should not be deferred simply because a patient is in renal failure.
- *Diuretic administration*. Some patients with end-stage renal failure continue to have some degree of residual kidney function. These patients may retain as much as 20% of normal renal function, so a patient who presents in pulmonary edema may respond to a large dose of a loop diuretic such as furosemide. Patients will be able to tell you whether they still make urine, which will indicate whether diuretics will be effective in increasing urine output. Patients in renal failure often require large doses of diuretics, so consult with medical direction if necessary. In addition to decreasing fluid volume through increased renal excretion, furosemide causes venodilation and has a secondary therapeutic effect in patients with acute heart failure.
- *Analgesia*. Pain is undertreated in 75% of the population with renal failure, yet pain medication administration in renal patients is extremely controversial. Codeine, meperidine, propoxyphene, and morphine are renally excreted. The metabolites build up in patients with chronic kidney disease and can cause neurotoxicity. According to the World Health Organization, the preferred pain medication is fentaNYL, as it has been proven safe and effective in patients with chronic kidney disease. HYDROmorphone may also be used, albeit with caution. The World Health Organization recommends codeine, meperidine, propoxyphene, and morphine not be used. When in doubt, always consult with your local medical direction.

Special Considerations for Patients on Dialysis

When you are assessing and evaluating a patient on dialysis, the following information may be crucial to your treatment:

- All patients on dialysis require special consideration regarding administration of any medication because of their altered pharmacokinetic and pharmacodynamic issues and increased potential for adverse reactions. They are at high risk for medication-related problems.
- Be sure to obtain a 12-lead ECG and initiate cardiac monitoring to look for myocardial infarction or ischemia and for cardiac conduction changes and dysrhythmias. Administer supplemental oxygen if the oxygen saturation is $< 94\%$. Consider administering nitroglycerin for chest pain or severe hypertension with pulmonary edema. Severe respiratory distress should be treated with NIPPV (continuous positive airway pressure [CPAP] or bilevel positive airway pressure [BiPAP]). Administration of antiarrhythmics may also be required. Consult medical direction when administering medications to renal patients because of the complexity of their fluid and electrolyte imbalances and the potential for multisystem involvement.
- Do not overlook the possibility of hyperkalemia, which is a life threat. It can develop rapidly in a renal patient, and weakness may be the only sign or symptom present. Patients may remain asymptomatic until a fatal arrhythmia occurs. Cardiac monitoring and early lab studies will help

you identify this complication in time to treat it. If you detect ECG changes that appear concerning for hyperkalemia, administer calcium by the IV route. These changes include prolonged PR and QT intervals, a widened QRS, and large T waves. Consider administering nebulized albuterol and furosemide, if available. Insulin (with dextrose, unless the patient's blood glucose level is elevated) is used in both the critical care and hospital settings. Calcium stabilizes cardiac conduction, insulin and albuterol shift potassium into the cells, and furosemide increases renal excretion of potassium. If acidosis is present, sodium bicarbonate may be used as well. Hyperkalemia is discussed in more detail in Chapter 11, *Endocrine and Metabolic Disorders*.

Acidosis stemming from an electrolyte imbalance, hypoperfusion, or diabetic complications may be identified if the patient exhibits an altered level of consciousness, Kussmaul respirations, or abnormal arterial blood gas levels. Management may include support of ventilation, fluid administration, and perhaps administration of sodium bicarbonate to address the electrolyte imbalance.

- Anticoagulant administration during dialysis may cause hemorrhage. This bleeding is complicated by anemia caused by dwindling erythropoietin secretion, which reduces production of red blood cells. You should have a high index of suspicion for bleeding and severe anemia if the patient has shortness of breath or angina. Blood loss may be obvious, as in trauma to a vascular access site, or not so obvious, as in a patient with occult blood loss through GI bleeding. Prehospital priorities should be to control bleeding, ensure adequate oxygenation, and administer whole blood or packed red blood cells if available. If a dialysis fistula is the site of external hemorrhage, a tourniquet may be necessary to stop the severe bleeding.
- Sudden onset of respiratory distress, chest pain, cyanosis, hypotension, and change in mental status during or immediately after dialysis may indicate an air embolism. If the cardinal presentation is respiratory distress (suggestive of venous air embolism), administer high-flow oxygen and place the patient in the left lateral recumbent position. If the patient has acute change in mental status or other neurologic or cardiac symptoms (suggestive of arterial air embolism), place the patient in supine position. Maintain IV access and be prepared to support blood pressure.
- Disequilibrium syndrome is a neurologic condition that patients sometimes experience during or immediately after hemodialysis. Researchers believe this syndrome is caused by cerebral edema that develops when the serum urea nitrogen is lowered too quickly. In mild cases, patients may complain of headache, restlessness, nausea, muscle twitching, and fatigue. In severe cases, signs and symptoms include hypertension, confusion, seizures, and coma. Disequilibrium syndrome can be fatal. In most cases, however, the episode is self-limiting and will resolve over a few hours. If the patient does have a seizure, consider administering anticonvulsant medications. Prevention is the priority in these patients: Disequilibrium syndrome can be prevented by slowing the rate at which urea is removed from the body during hemodialysis.

Kidney Stones

Pathophysiology

Kidney stones, or renal calculi, form as a result of metabolic abnormalities, primarily calcium buildup. Individuals at greater risk of developing this condition include males; individuals with a family history of kidney stones; those who abuse laxatives; and patients with primary hyperparathyroidism, Crohn disease, renal tubular acidosis, or recurrent urinary tract infection.

Kidney stones typically cause symptoms when they migrate out of the renal pelvis into the ureter (acute renal colic). Partial—or, less commonly, complete—obstruction of the ureter may lead to hydronephrosis and injury of the involved kidney. The size and location of the stone determine its ability to pass through the ureter.

Signs and Symptoms

Patients typically have constant dull flank pain radiating to the abdomen, punctuated by bouts of severe, sharp, colicky pain during hyperperistalsis of the smooth muscle of the ureter. Patients often feel the need to walk around, bending and twisting in an attempt to relieve the pain. Nausea, vomiting, and hematuria may be present. Fever indicates an infection but is an infrequent finding.

Differential Diagnosis

The differential diagnosis includes urinary tract infection, appendicitis, gallstones, inflammatory bowel disease, bowel obstruction, retroperitoneal hemorrhage, and abdominal aortic aneurysm.

Treatment

Prehospital treatment is supportive. Transport the patient in a position of comfort, establish IV access, and administer pain medications and antiemetics. At the hospital, a urinalysis will be ordered to look for blood in the urine. BUN and Cr levels may be checked, and CT or ultrasound studies may be performed. These patients may require significant amounts of parenteral medications for pain relief. Intravenous ketorolac alleviates the prostaglandin-mediated pain process.

Endocrine Causes of Abdominal Disorders

Diabetic Ketoacidosis

Diabetic ketoacidosis is a life-threatening complication of diabetes. It is often characterized by nausea, vomiting, and abdominal pain in addition to polyuria, polydipsia, hyperglycemia, polyphagia, and metabolic acidosis. Although it is possible for diabetic ketoacidosis to develop in people with type 2 diabetes, especially in the presence of an infection, the condition is far more characteristic of type 1 diabetes. More information is available in Chapter 11, *Endocrine and Metabolic Disorders*. Additional endocrine causes of abdominal discomfort are addressed in Chapter 11 as well.

Special Considerations

Home Medical Devices

As medical technology advances, prehospital medical clinicians are encountering in the home environment a wider variety of medical devices used by patients with abdominal disorders. The devices that you are most likely to see are as follows:

- *Nasogastric and nasointestinal feeding tubes*. Nasogastric and nasointestinal feeding tubes are typically small-diameter, flexible tubes that travel through the nose to the stomach or intestines. They are used for food intake or fluid administration in patients who cannot consume sufficient amounts of food or water by mouth, as well as for medication infusion. Patients who use such devices might include those with a history of cancer, gastric bypass surgery, or stroke. Many complications can occur, including the following:
    - The tube can become displaced, causing the patient to aspirate fluid into the lungs. A dislodged tube can actually go into the lungs. Suspect either of these if the patient begins coughing or choking, the patient is unable to speak, or air bubbles appear when the proximal end of the tube is placed in water.
    - The walls of the tube are typically thin and can easily develop a small leak.
    - An occlusion can form if the tube is not irrigated sufficiently after food or medication administration.

  If any abnormalities occur, use of the tube should be discontinued.
- *Transabdominal feeding tubes*. Transabdominal feeding tubes are placed surgically to provide a route for direct feeding into the stomach (gastrostomy tube; **Figure 10-8** and **Figure 10-9**), the jejunum (jejunostomy tube), or both (gastrojejunostomy tube). They are used when food, fluid, or

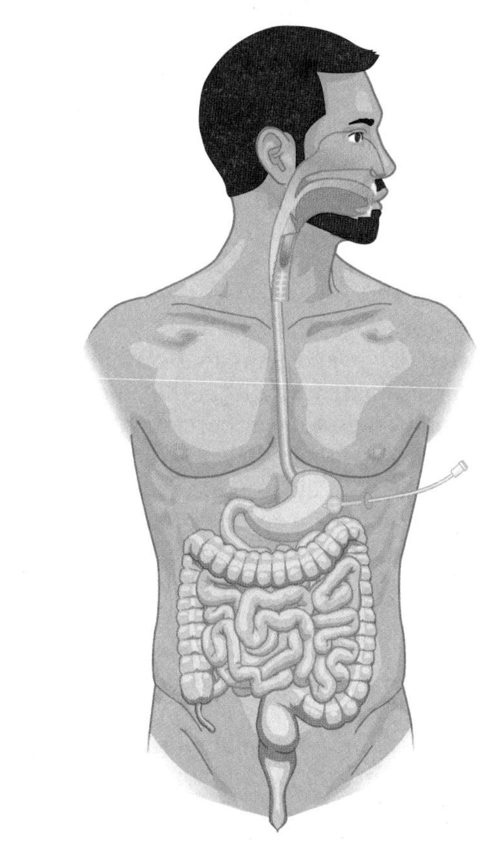

Figure 10-8 A gastrostomy tube is surgically placed into the stomach through the abdominal wall.

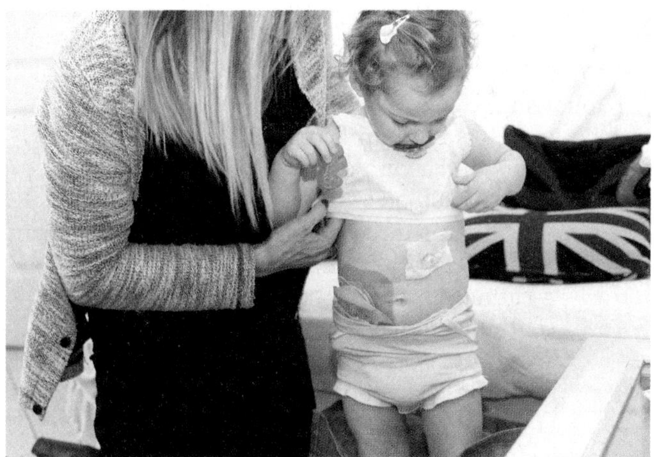

Figure 10-9 Gastrostomy button.

medication must be administered for a longer term than would be suitable for a nasally placed tube.

Transabdominal feeding tubes are often used in patients who have difficulty swallowing, esophageal atresia, esophageal burns or strictures, chronic malabsorption, or severe failure to thrive. Potential complications include the following:

- The stoma site can become infected. Look for drainage at the site and redness and inflammation of the surrounding skin. Ulcerations and bleeding can also occur.
- Leakage from the stoma can occur if the tube is too small.
- The feeding tube can become occluded or dislodged.
- The patient can develop peritonitis or gastric or intestinal perforation.

If any abnormalities are apparent, feedings should be discontinued.

- *Bowel ostomy*. A bowel ostomy is a surgically created opening to eliminate waste from the bowel. It can be placed temporarily or permanently in patients with congenital bowel abnormalities, cancer, severe Crohn disease, ulcerative colitis, or abdominal trauma. Any portion of the intestine can be rerouted through the abdominal wall. If the intestinal opening is closer to the stomach in the ileum, the patient is likely to have diarrhea, as stools cannot be formed. A bag placed over the ostomy to collect waste must be emptied regularly to minimize tissue degradation caused by prolonged contact with stool. This mucosa should typically be pink and should glisten. If it is dusky or cyanotic, this is a concerning sign.
- *Hemodialysis access devices*. Hemodialysis is the process of passing the patient's blood through a machine called a *dialyzer* to remove waste products and stabilize the patient's fluid and electrolyte balance. Multiple sites and devices are used to gain vascular access so the blood can be cleaned and returned to the body during dialysis. These include the following:
  - A graft is a surgical connection between an artery and a vein using synthetic tubing or a cadaveric blood vessel.
  - A fistula is a direct surgical connection between an artery and a vein.
  - A catheter placed in the subclavian or other central vein may also be used to gain vascular access.
  - A button-shaped port (Hemasite) may be placed at the entry site.

  Assess for a thrill (palpable vibration) or bruit (whooshing sound on auscultation) to verify the patency of a graft or fistula, which is usually found in the arm but may be located in the leg. It is important not to take blood pressure or attempt IV access in an extremity with a graft or fistula.
- *Peritoneal dialysis access devices*. A peritoneal dialysis access device is a catheter placed through the abdominal wall into the peritoneal cavity that allows fluids to be infused into and then drained out of the abdomen. This process removes waste products and temporarily stabilizes the electrolyte and fluid balance.

Older Adult Patients

Caring for the older adult population presents special challenges for prehospital clinicians. Because of diminishing cardiac and pulmonary reserves, altered gastric motility, and inadequate nutrition, older adult patients may become ill more quickly and be more vulnerable to conditions such as abdominal aortic aneurysm, ischemic colitis, pancreatitis, cholecystitis, and large-bowel obstruction.

Many abdominal complaints become more common with advanced age and have ambiguous symptoms. In fact, in diagnosing the cause of abdominal pain in patients older than age 50 years, the rate of accuracy is less than 50%. This rate drops to less than 30% in patients older than age 80 years. Further confounding the diagnostic challenge is the fact that many medications frequently prescribed to older adults can mask signs of critical illness. Finally, obtaining a reliable and complete history may be complicated by memory deficits, dementia, hearing impairment, or anxiety in the patient.

Bariatric Patients

Morbid obesity is defined as having a body mass index ≥ 40 or, alternatively, being ≥ 100 lb (45 kg) overweight. In recent years, this condition has become more prevalent in the United States. Abdominal assessments in these patients can be very challenging. Surgical options are available to facilitate weight loss in patients with morbid obesity. Restrictive procedures shrink the size of the stomach or the bowel circumference. Gastric banding, for example, reduces the amount of food the patient can eat by restricting the size of the opening from the esophagus to the stomach. These bands are sometimes adjustable, allowing the bariatric surgeon to enlarge or reduce the capacity of the stomach as indicated. Another option is gastric bypass surgery, in which food is diverted around the stomach and upper small bowel through a pouch about the size of an egg. Unlike gastric banding, this procedure is not reversible.

The problems in bariatric patients with which clinicians should be concerned depend on when the procedures were performed. Like all surgeries, both gastric banding and gastric bypass surgery carry the risk of complications, including infection, bleeding, abdominal pain, abdominal hernia, and lower-extremity deep vein thrombosis secondary to inactivity during recovery from surgery. Potential complications specific to patients who have undergone bariatric surgery include ulcers; bowel obstruction; and short gut syndrome, which causes diarrhea, electrolyte imbalance, and malnutrition, especially if the patient does not take vitamins as advised. These complications are ongoing and not solely associated with the surgery itself. Typically, patients with a history of bariatric surgery and abdominal pain should be transported and evaluated in the ED.

Putting It All Together

Assessment of a patient with abdominal discomfort begins with the initial observation to determine whether the patient is sick or not sick. Let this initial impression tell you whether to intervene immediately or proceed to a more detailed assessment. Assess the patient for critical or emergent diagnoses first, and then consider less-menacing conditions. The rule of thumb is to consider the more common or likely diagnosis and work toward the less common. To confirm or rule out the conditions that make up your differential diagnosis, use tools such as SAMPLER, OPQRST, physical examination findings, and lab results. If the patient becomes unstable, support of their airway, breathing, and circulation always takes precedence. Once the patient has been stabilized, return to your assessment. Because the possible causes of abdominal discomfort are so numerous and advanced diagnostic testing is often needed, it is important to recognize that you usually will not be able to make a definitive diagnosis in the field. Offering supportive care, managing signs and symptoms, and providing quick transport is the best strategy for many patients with abdominal discomfort.

SCENARIO SOLUTION

- There are many possible causes of this patient's abdominal pain. She is still of childbearing age, so it is possible she has an obstetric problem such as ectopic pregnancy. She is the right age for cholecystitis. If she is a frequent drinker, she could have pancreatitis. It is also possible that she is having a sickle cell crisis, or has an ulcer.
- To narrow your differential diagnosis, you will need to obtain a past history as well as the history of the present illness. Perform a physical examination of her abdomen. Assess her oxygen saturation. Consider acquiring a 12-lead ECG. Palpate for tenderness, masses, guarding, or pulsatile mass.
- The patient has signs of impending shock. You should administer supplemental oxygen. Prepare to suction her airway if she vomits again. Establish vascular access and deliver IV fluids. Consider medication for nausea or pain if her blood pressure improves. Transport her to the closest appropriate hospital for further diagnostic tests and definitive intervention.

SUMMARY

- The causes of abdominal discomfort are innumerable and may seem overwhelming when you try to make a diagnosis.
- Identify life threats first and then progress toward generating a differential diagnosis as time and the patient's condition allow.
- The patient's presentation, history, physical examination, and lab results are the keys to arriving at an accurate differential diagnosis of abdominal discomfort.
- The abdomen contains multiple systems, each of which—alone or in combination—may be responsible for abdominal discomfort.
- Abdominal discomfort may be associated with other cardinal symptoms, such as nausea and vomiting, constipation, diarrhea, GI bleeding, jaundice, and vaginal bleeding. Taking into account these cardinal symptoms/chief complaints may assist pinpointing a diagnosis.
- Making a diagnosis should not take precedence over intervention in a patient with abdominal discomfort.

Key Terms

antiemetics Substances that prevent or alleviate nausea and vomiting.

gastrointestinal (GI) Pertaining to the organs of the gastrointestinal tract. The GI tract links the organs involved in consumption, processing, and elimination of nutrients. Components include the mouth, pharynx, esophagus, stomach, small and large intestines, and rectum/anus.

gastroparesis A medical condition characterized by paresis (partial paralysis) of the stomach, resulting in food remaining in the stomach for an abnormally long time.

hematemesis Vomiting of bright red blood, indicating upper gastrointestinal bleeding.

hematochezia Passage of red blood through the rectum.

intussusception Prolapse of one segment of the bowel into the lumen of adjacent bowel. This kind of intestinal obstruction may involve segments of the small intestine, colon, or terminal ileum and cecum.

melena Abnormal black, tarry stool that has a distinctive odor and contains digested blood; results from an upper gastrointestinal source of bleeding.

referred pain Pain felt at a site different from that of an injured or diseased organ or body part.

somatic (parietal) pain Generally well-localized pain caused by an irritation of the nerve fibers in the parietal peritoneum or other tissues (e.g., musculoskeletal system). Physical findings include sharp, discrete, localized pain accompanied by tenderness to palpation, guarding of the affected area, and rebound tenderness.

visceral pain Poorly localized pain that occurs when the walls of the hollow organs are stretched, thereby activating the stretch receptors. This kind of pain is characterized by a deep, persistent ache ranging from mild to intolerable and commonly described as cramping, burning, and gnawing.

viscus (pl. viscera) An organ enclosed within a body cavity. Typically used to refer to hollow organs such as esophagus, stomach, and intestines.

volvulus A condition in which a segment of the gastrointestinal tract twists on itself, causing a closed loop bowel obstruction. Often the feeding blood vessels also become twisted, blocking the flow of blood and leading to ischemia and eventually infarction of the involved loop of bowel. This most commonly occurs in the cecum and sigmoid regions of the large intestine but may involve the stomach and small intestine.

Bibliography

Aehlert B. *Paramedic Practice Today: Above and Beyond.* Mosby; 2009.

American Academy of Orthopaedic Surgeons. *Nancy Caroline's Emergency Care in the Streets.* 8th ed. Jones & Bartlett Learning; 2018.

Bakker R. Placenta previa. Medscape. Updated January 23, 2023. Accessed September 24, 2023. https://emedicine.medscape.com/article/262063-overview

Becker S, Dietrich TR, McDevitt MJ, et al. *Advanced Skills: Providing Expert Care for the Acutely Ill.* Springhouse; 1994.

Bucurescu G. Neurologic manifestations of uremic encephalopathy. Medscape. Updated June 27, 2023. Accessed September 24, 2023. https://www.medscapecrm.com/article/1135651-overview

Burke E, Harkins P, Ahmed I. Is there a role for tranexamic acid in upper GI bleeding? A systematic review and meta-analysis. *Surg Res Pract.* 2021;8876991:2021.

Cairns C, Kang K. National Hospital Ambulatory Medical Care Survey: 2019 emergency department summary tables. National Center for Health Statistics. Updated July 29, 2022. Accessed September 24, 2023. https://www.cdc.gov/nchs/data/nhamcs/web_tables/2019-nhamcs-ed-web-tables-508.pdf

Carale J, Azer A, Mekaroonkamol P. Portal hypertension. Medscape. Updated November 30, 2017. Accessed September 24, 2023. https://emedicine.medscape.com/article/175248-overview

Dean M. Opioids in renal failure and dialysis patients. *J Pain Symptom Manage.* 2004;28:497-504.

Deering SH. Abruptio placentae. Medscape. Updated November 30, 2018. Accessed September 24, 2023. https://emedicine.medscape.com/article/252810-overview

Gould BE. *Pathophysiology for Health Care Professionals.* 3rd ed. Saunders; 2006.

Hamilton GC. *Emergency Medicine: An Approach to Clinical Problem-Solving.* 2nd ed. Saunders; 2003.

Haram K, Svendsen E, Abildgaard U. The HELLP syndrome: clinical issues and management: a review. *BMC Pregn Childbirth.* 2009;9:8. doi:10.1186/1471-2393-9-8.

Holander-Rodriguez JC, Calvert JF Jr. Hyperkalemia. *Am Fam Physician*. 2006;73:283-290.

Holleran RS. *Air and Surface Patient Transport: Principles and Practice*. 3rd ed. Mosby; 2003.

Johnson LR, Byrne JH. *Essential Medical Physiology*. 3rd ed. Elsevier Academic Press; 2003.

Krause R. Dialysis complications of chronic renal failure. Medscape. Updated November 18, 2019. Accessed September 24, 2023. https://emedicine.medscape.com/article/777957-media

Lehne RA. *Pharmacology for Nursing Care*. 6th ed. Saunders; 2007.

Mayo Clinic Staff. Acute kidney failure. Published July 30, 2022. Accessed September 24, 2023. https://www.mayoclinic.org/diseases-conditions/kidney-failure/symptoms-causes/syc-20369048

McCance KL, Huether SE. *Pathophysiology: The Biologic Basis for Disease in Adults and Children*. 6th ed. Mosby; 2009.

Mosby's Dictionary of Medicine, Nursing and Health Professions. 8th ed. Mosby; 2009.

National Institute of Diabetes and Digestive and Kidney Diseases. Anemia in chronic kidney disease. Last reviewed September 2020. Accessed September 24, 2023. https://www.niddk.nih.gov/health-information/kidney-disease/anemia

Padden MO. HELLP syndrome: recognition and perinatal management. *Am Fam Physician*. 1999;30:829-836.

Paula R. Abdominal compartment syndrome. Medscape. Updated January 30, 2023. Accessed September 24, 2023. https://emedicine.medscape.com/article/829008-diagnosis

Rosen P, Marx JA, Hockberger RS, et al. *Rosen's Emergency Medicine: Concepts and Clinical Practice*. 6th ed. Mosby; 2006.

Sanders M. *Mosby's Paramedic Textbook*. 3rd ed. Mosby; 2007.

Sharma K, Akre S, Wanjari M. Hepatic encephalopathy and treatment modalities: a review article. *Cureus*. 2002;14(8):e28016.

Silen W, Cope Z. *Cope's Early Diagnosis of the Acute Abdomen*. Oxford University Press; 2000.

Song L-M, Wong KS. Mallory-Weiss tear: overview of Mallory-Weiss syndrome. Medscape. Updated October 2, 2019. Accessed September 24, 2023. https://emedicine.medscape.com/article/187134-overview.

Sorensen CJ, DeSantos K, Borgelt L, et al. Cannabinoid hyperemesis syndrome: diagnosis, pathophysiology, and treatment: a systematic review. *J Med Toxicol*. 2017;13:71-87.

Taylor MB. *Gastrointestinal Emergencies*. 2nd ed. Williams & Wilkins; 1997.

Wagner J, McKinney WP, Carpenter JL. Does this patient have appendicitis? *JAMA*. 1996;276:1589.

Wakim-Fleming J. Liver disease in pregnancy. In: Carey WD, ed. *Cleveland Clinic: Current Clinical Medicine*. 2nd ed. Elsevier Saunders; 2010.

Wingfield WE. *ACE SAT: The Aeromedical Certification Examinations Self-Assessment Test*. ResQ Shop Publishers; 2008.

CHAPTER 11

Endocrine and Metabolic Disorders

Chapter Editors
Vincent N. Mosesso, Jr., MD, FACEP, FAEMS
Douglas F. Kupas, MD, EMT-P, FAEMS, FACEP
Erica Carney, MD, FAEMS

This chapter will give you a fundamental understanding of endocrine and metabolic disorders. You will learn to integrate your knowledge of anatomy, physiology, and pathophysiology with the Advanced Medical Life Support (AMLS) Assessment Pathway to formulate differential diagnoses for life-threatening, emergent, and nonemergent conditions. You will also learn how to implement and adapt management strategies for a variety of endocrine and metabolic disorders in prehospital and in-hospital settings.

LEARNING OBJECTIVES

At the conclusion of this chapter, you will be able to:

- Describe the anatomy, physiology, and pathophysiology of common endocrine disorders.
- Outline primary, secondary, and ongoing assessment strategies for the patient with an endocrine disorder using the AMLS Assessment Pathway.
- Identify the cardinal presentations/chief complaints of a broad range of endocrine disorders.
- List and recognize the signs and symptoms of acid-base imbalances, electrolyte derangements, and endocrine disorders.
- Formulate provisional diagnoses based on assessment findings for a variety of endocrine disorders.
- List the causes, diagnostic techniques, and treatment strategies for diseases of glucose metabolism and thyroid, parathyroid, and adrenal disorders.
- Use clinical reasoning skills to formulate and refine a differential diagnosis based on a systematic, thorough secondary survey of a patient with an endocrine disorder.
- Implement effective treatment plans consistent with your assessment findings, and determine whether to continue the treatment on the basis of your ongoing assessment.
- Describe the pathophysiologic processes responsible for electrolyte and acid–base derangements, explain their causes, and discuss common modalities used to treat them.
- Compare and contrast normal and abnormal electrocardiogram (ECG) findings in the patient with an electrolyte derangement.

SCENARIO

You are caring for a 58-year-old woman who presents with severe fatigue and weakness. She has a history of type 2 diabetes, polymyalgia rheumatica, hypertension, and heart failure. Her medications include metformin, predniSONE, lisinopril, furosemide, and digoxin. Her vital signs include blood pressure, 88/52 mm Hg; pulse rate, 58 beats/min; respirations, 20 breaths/min; and oxygen saturation (SpO_2), 97%.

- Which differential diagnoses are you considering based on the information you have now?
- Which additional information will you need to narrow your differential diagnosis?
- What are your initial treatment priorities as you continue your patient care?

The endocrine system regulates metabolic processes of the body. The primary functions of the endocrine glands include the following:

- Regulating metabolism
- Regulating reproduction
- Controlling the balance of extracellular fluid and electrolytes (sodium, potassium, calcium, and phosphates)
- Maintaining an optimal internal environment (e.g., regulation of blood glucose)
- Stimulating growth and development during childhood and adolescence

Performing an assessment of a patient's endocrine system is challenging because the locations of most of these glands (with the exceptions of the thyroid gland and testes) make it impossible to physically examine them. It is also difficult to assess this system because of the different effects the hormones have on various systems throughout the body. Hormones are substances produced by various organs and tissues that signal actions to be done by other organs and tissues that have target receptors. For example, thyroid-stimulating hormone released from the pituitary gland signals the thyroid gland to release thyroid hormone, which then leads to various responses in other organs and tissues. Assessment of endocrine function depends on gathering data and recognizing the underlying pattern of an endocrine disorder.

Anatomy and Physiology

Glands are organs that manufacture and secrete chemical substances. Glands may be endocrine or exocrine. Exocrine glands secrete chemicals to the outer surface of the body (e.g., sweat and tears) or into a body cavity (e.g., saliva and pancreatic digestive enzymes). Endocrine glands secrete hormones into the bloodstream. The network of endocrine glands that secrete hormones throughout the body is collectively referred to as the endocrine system.

The major components of the endocrine system include the pituitary gland, thyroid gland, parathyroid glands, adrenal glands, pancreas (both an endocrine and exocrine gland), and the reproductive organs (ovaries in females and testes in males) (**Figure 11-1**). Hormones released by these glands regulate homeostasis, reproduction, growth, development, and metabolism by transmitting messages directly to receptors located on their respective target organs. A complex system of feedback loops work together to maintain balanced levels of all hormones. As part of the management of this balancing act, levels of hormone secretion are regulated by positive and negative feedback mechanisms: Increased levels of a

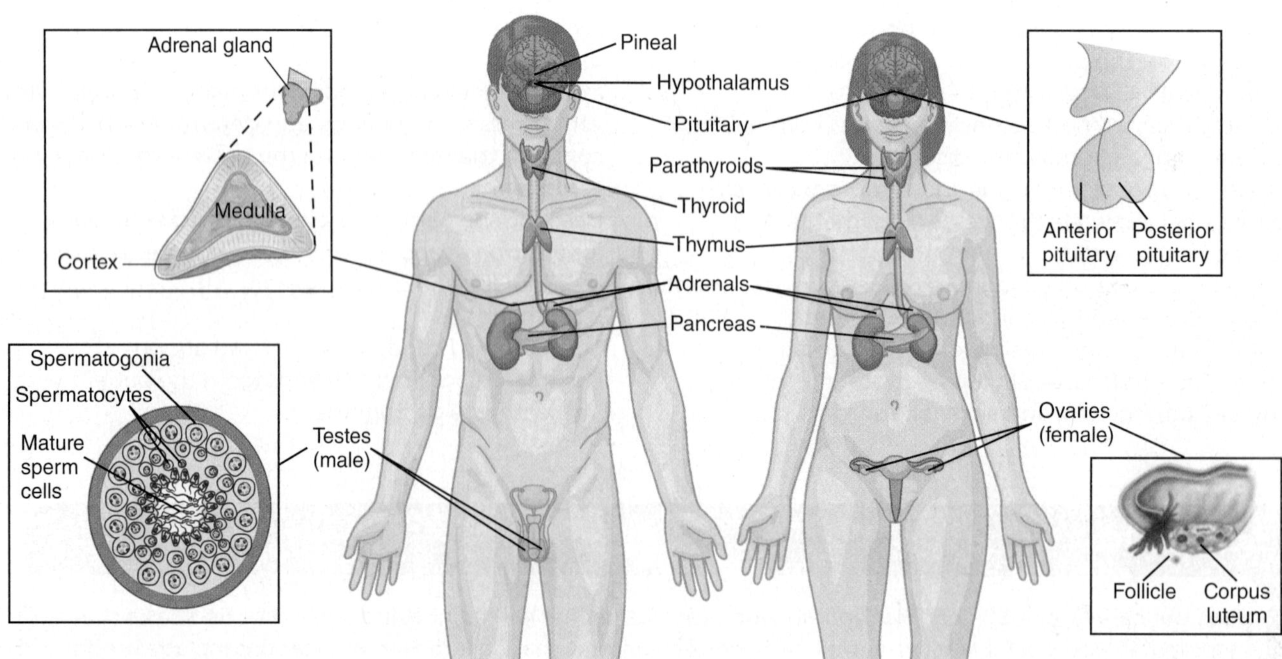

Figure 11-1 The endocrine system uses the various glands within the system to deliver chemical messages to organ systems throughout the body.

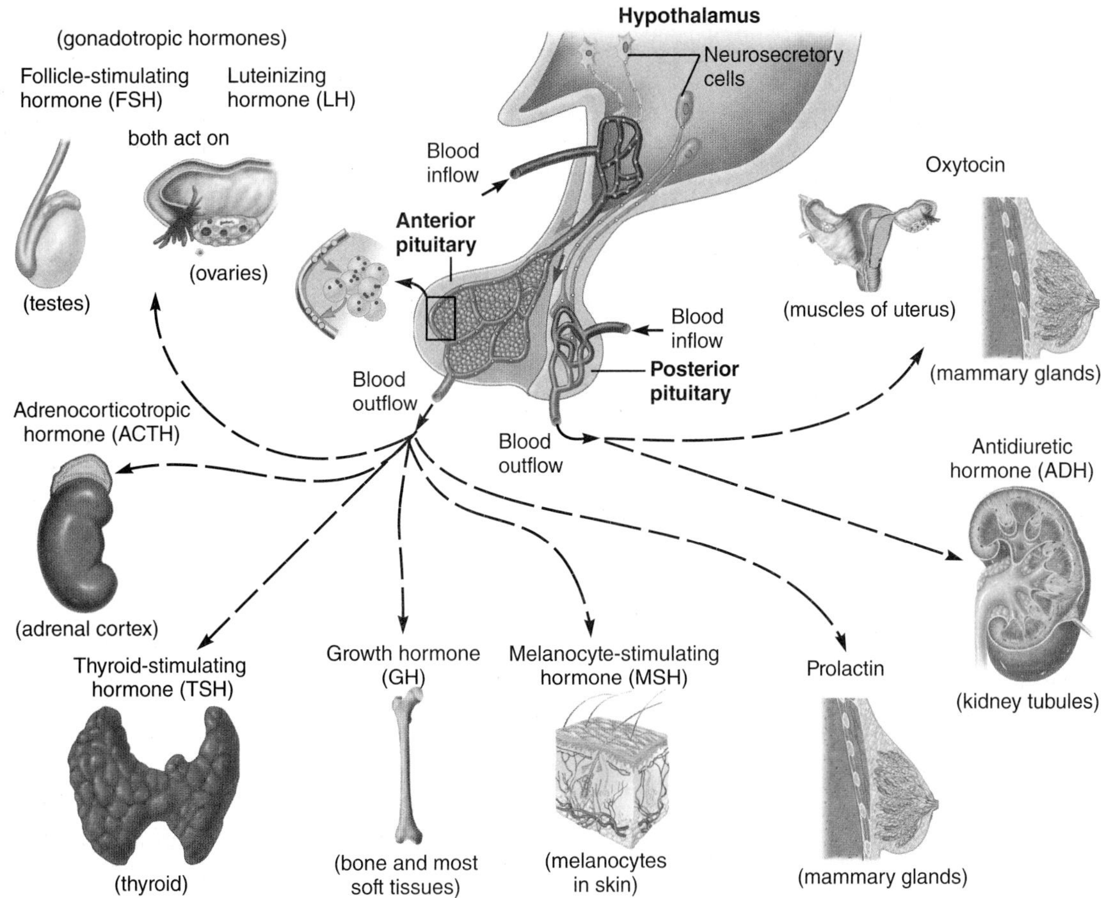

Figure 11-2 The pituitary gland secretes hormones from its two regions: the anterior pituitary lobe and the posterior pituitary lobe.

particular hormone will inhibit secretion, and decreased levels of a particular hormone will stimulate secretion.

The pituitary gland (**Figure 11-2**) is often referred to as the *master gland* because its secretions orchestrate the activity of other endocrine glands. The hypothalamus, which is located directly superior to the pituitary gland, is the part of the brain responsible for monitoring body conditions and maintaining homeostasis in the body. The hypothalamus contains several control centers for body functions and emotions. It is the primary link between the endocrine system and the nervous system.

The thyroid gland is a good example of the interdependent nature of endocrine gland function and the feedback loops that work to maintain homeostasis. The thyroid gland lies in the anterior part of the neck below the larynx, at the level between the fifth cervical and first thoracic vertebrae. It is located inferior to the thyroid cartilage, the rigid cartilage that is palpable in the anterior part of the neck. Its two lobes straddle the midline, and are joined by a narrow isthmus. Histologically, the thyroid gland is composed of secretory cells, follicular cells, and C cells (parafollicular cells). The hormones secreted by this gland (triiodothyronine [T_3] and thyroxine [T_4]) affect many tissues and organs in the human body, including the heart, musculoskeletal and nervous systems, and adipose tissue. Thyrotropin-releasing hormone (TRH), which is secreted by the hypothalamus, causes the release of thyroid-stimulating hormone (TSH, or thyrotropin) from the pituitary. The TSH then travels to and activates receptors in the thyroid gland, triggering a biochemical cascade that results in the secretion of T_3 and T_4 by follicular cells. T_3 and T_4 travel through the bloodstream to affect many tissues, but also inhibit synthesis of TRH in the hypothalamus, closing the feedback loop. Like many substances in the body, thyroid hormones are largely bound by carrier proteins while they are circulating in the bloodstream. The terms "free T_3" and "free T_4" refer to thyroid hormones that are present in the circulation but not bound to proteins. Only these free hormones are able to act on target tissues. TSH secretion can also be affected by factors such as stress, glucocorticoids, and warmth. Parafollicular cells, which are less numerous than follicular cells, are responsible for secreting calcitonin hormone, which controls calcium metabolism. Calcitonin release is determined by the serum level of calcium.

The parathyroid glands lie posterior to the thyroid gland and are composed of three types of cells, each of which has a particular function. Chief cells are responsible for producing parathyroid hormone (PTH), which stimulates the production of the active form of vitamin D in the kidneys, encourages the reabsorption of calcium by the renal tubules, and inhibits phosphate reabsorption in the kidneys. PTH also liberates calcium from bone to increase calcium levels. A low calcium concentration stimulates PTH secretion, whereas an increase in calcium inhibits the production and release of PTH.

At the apex of each kidney is a triangular adrenal gland about 3.8 cm (1.5 inches) tall and 7.6 cm (3 inches) long. These two glands lie retroperitoneal and lateral to the inferior vena cava and abdominal aorta. Their venous and arterial blood supplies are derived from the upper and lower branches of the inferior vena cava and aorta, respectively. The cortex, or surface, of each adrenal gland secretes glucocorticoids such as cortisol, mineralocorticoids such as aldosterone, and small amounts of sex hormones. The medulla, or body, of each adrenal gland produces epinephrine and norepinephrine.

The hypothalamus secretes corticotropin-releasing factor (CRF), which stimulates the pituitary to produce adrenocorticotropin hormone (ACTH) and melanocyte-stimulating hormone (MSH). The adrenal gland reacts to ACTH by producing cortisol and aldosterone. The level of cortisol in the blood regulates the production of ACTH from the pituitary and CRF from the hypothalamus.

Glucose Metabolism and Control

Glucose is a vital fuel for key metabolic processes in organs, especially those controlled by the central nervous system (CNS). The CNS is particularly dependent on glucose metabolism and relatively intolerant to changes in blood glucose levels. This explains why acute episodes of hypoglycemia manifest as mental status changes, and persistent episodes of hypoglycemia can lead to irreversible brain damage.

Cellular survival depends on the body's ability to maintain a balanced serum glucose concentration. Under normal circumstances, the body is able to keep serum glucose within a relatively tight range, 70 to 150 mg/dL (3.9 to 8.3 mmol/L), before and after meals. This control essentially derives from three metabolic processes:

- *Gastrointestinal (GI) absorption*: direct intestinal absorption of glucose through the intestine
- *Glycogenolysis*: glucose produced as glycogen breakdown occurs in the liver
- *Gluconeogenesis*: the formation of new glucose from precursors including pyruvate, glycerol, lactate, and amino acids

A series of complex interactions among regulatory mediators, including neural (autonomic nervous system) and humoral (hormones and other substances circulating in the blood) factors, ensures maintenance of a normal serum glucose concentration. When the level of glucose in the blood is insufficient, glucagon is released from alpha cells in the pancreas and increases glucose production through gluconeogenesis. Glucagon release can also be triggered by exercise, trauma, and infection. These mechanisms increase glucose levels within minutes, though the increase is only a transient effect. Epinephrine and norepinephrine increase glucose levels even more rapidly by enabling gluconeogenesis and hepatic glycogenolysis. Insulin, which is secreted by the pancreatic islet cells, is essential for efficient cellular glucose utilization and drives glucose into the cells.

AMLS Assessment Pathway ▸▸▸▸

▾ Initial Observations

Scene Safety Considerations

As in any patient encounter, make sure that all potential hazards are addressed and follow standard precautions when responding to a patient with a suspected endocrine emergency. Your observation of the scene can give you important clues about the patient's underlying illness. Look for medications in the patient's sleeping area, inside the refrigerator or other cooling device (for insulin), inside the medicine cabinet in the bathroom, or any other place where medication might be stored. Take note of any insulin pumps or other medical devices that may be present. Bring any medication bottles to the hospital with the patient.

Patient Cardinal Presentation/ Chief Complaint

Investigate the patient's cardinal presentation/chief complaint. Consider the patient's signs and symptoms. Remember that endocrine disorders present with signs and symptoms that indicate hormone secretion or production is affected. With many endocrine disorders and in case of altered metabolic functioning, patients may experience restlessness, agitation, and a short attention span. In patients who have an altered mental status, check for a medical identification bracelet or necklace, which may list the patient's known conditions. Patients who are unresponsive need their ABCs assessed immediately.

Primary Survey

The primary survey begins with the ABCs. Manage any life threats immediately.

Level of Consciousness

A patient who is experiencing an endocrine emergency will often be in serious distress. The patient's position may give you an indication of the severity of their condition. A patient who is unresponsive is in a critical state and may be experiencing an endocrine crisis such as hypoglycemia or hyperglycemia.

Airway and Breathing

Patients with endocrine emergencies may present with a variety of breathing levels. You should immediately assess the patient's effort of breathing. Increased work of breathing, an abnormal respiratory rate, and hypoxia may all be indications that oxygen administration is necessary. Be alert for abnormal respiratory patterns such as Kussmaul respirations, which are often present in patients with diabetic ketoacidosis. This compensatory mechanism acts to "blow off" excess acid by increasing both respiratory rate and volume; thus, it is a respiratory compensation for a metabolic acidosis.

Circulation/Perfusion

Assess the patient's skin color, moisture, and temperature, and obtain the patient's blood pressure. A patient with pale or ashen, cool, moist skin may be in shock or have hypoglycemia, whereas a patient with hot, dry skin may have a fever or hyperglycemia.

▼ First Impression

The difficult part of assessing patients with endocrine emergencies is that their problems tend to affect many organ systems and the seriousness of their presentations varies greatly. Many of these patients will have had their conditions for some time and may already be receiving treatment from their primary care provider or a specialist. The patient or their family members will likely share information about the endocrine problem as part of the patient history. This information, along with the common signs and symptoms associated with each endocrine emergency described in this chapter, should help you determine possible causes of the current problem and generate an initial differential diagnosis.

▼ Detailed Assessment

History Taking

Collecting a complete history is critical to identifying endocrine emergencies. The signs and symptoms of endocrine disorders are often vague, and a complete history may give clues to endocrine disorders. The OPQRST and SAMPLER mnemonics can provide valuable additional information. Likewise, other parts of a complete history, such as the patient's past medical history, family history, and social history, may help to identify possible endocrine etiologies.

OPQRST and SAMPLER

The OPQRST and SAMPLER mnemonics should be used to obtain the patient's complete history using a systematic approach. Look for any signs that may assist you in confirming the patient's reported symptoms. Additional symptoms that may be noted include polyphagia, polyuria, and polydipsia in patients with undiagnosed or poorly managed diabetes. Tachycardias, atrial fibrillation, premature ventricular contractions (PVCs), premature atrial contractions (PACs), and other atrial dysrhythmias may occur in patients with hyperthyroidism or thyrotoxicosis.

Patients experiencing an endocrine emergency may have a previously diagnosed condition and can often provide useful information about their situation. Document all medications the patient is currently taking and whether the patient has been compliant with the regimen. The medications list often provides another clue to the patient's condition.

Ask females of childbearing age about their last menstrual period; some patients with hypothyroidism may have a history of light or absent periods. Also ask if female patients have been pregnant in the past 12 months. A history of gestational diabetes is important because it increases the risk that a female patient will develop diabetes mellitus following her pregnancy.

Secondary Survey

Vital Signs

Once you have determined that the ABCs are intact and the patient has no life threats, careful evaluation of the patient's vital signs can provide clues about the underlying endocrine and metabolic conditions that you might consider. Patients with hypothyroidism and hypoadrenalism may be bradycardic, whereas patients with diabetic ketoacidosis (DKA) or hyperglycemic hyperosmolar syndrome will likely be tachycardic; hypotension is likely in all of those cases. Patients with Cushing syndrome or hyperthyroidism may be hypertensive. As mentioned earlier, patients with DKA will likely demonstrate deep, rapid respirations as compensation for the associated metabolic acidosis. As you read through the descriptions of the various endocrine conditions in this chapter, think about how they would affect a person's vital signs.

Physical Exam

Start the physical examination by noting the patient's appearance and the position in which the patient was found.

During the physical examination, be alert for specific findings that might indicate an endocrine or metabolic condition. These include unexpected hair thinning or loss (hypothyroidism), fruity or acetone breath odor (DKA), fatty hump across the upper back (Cushing syndrome), and other findings associated with specific conditions (and described later in this chapter). Unless the patient had an endocrine emergency that caused some sort of trauma, a focused trauma assessment is usually not necessary. As always, a full-body exam should be completed after any life threats are managed.

The secondary survey may reveal finer abnormalities that will help you determine your treatment. For example, if the patient's skin is cold and clammy, this may signal severe hypoglycemia, such as might occur from an insulin reaction and the body's response to catecholamine release. Hypothermia may be related to hypothyroidism, and hyperthermia to a hyperthyroid crisis. The goal of the secondary survey is to systematically examine the patient's whole body to look for specific abnormalities that may help to determine the cause of the patient's symptoms or condition.

Diagnostics

If your local protocol recommends obtaining blood samples for later analysis, it is important to obtain them early during patient care, before administration of glucose or other medications that might affect the analysis. In cases involving an altered level of consciousness, emergency medical services (EMS) clinicians should assess the patient's blood glucose level and begin treatment as indicated. The nuances of treatment for hypoglycemia and hyperglycemia are covered in specific sections later in this chapter.

Refine the Differential Diagnosis

The components of the primary and secondary survey, history of present illness, and past medical history will help you refine your differential diagnosis and determine the severity of the patient's condition. Manage any life threats as they appear during the assessment process. Remember that most diseases or conditions, including endocrine disorders, are caused by more than one factor. The descriptions of the specific conditions found later in this chapter offer an approach that can help you determine the differential diagnosis and recognize key findings.

Ongoing Management

Frequent reassessment of patients is important. A typical approach is to recheck vital signs and level of consciousness every 5 minutes in unstable patients and at least every 15 minutes in stable patients. Every patient should have at least two sets of vital signs documented.

Electrolyte Disturbances

Electrolyte imbalances are common findings in patients with medical emergencies. A healthy electrolyte balance is fundamental to carrying out cellular functions. Electrolyte disturbances generally cannot be diagnosed based on clinical examination alone, but a thorough history and exam may point to a likely diagnosis. Severe electrolyte disturbances can be fatal. Most patients have only nonspecific chief complaints until life-threatening manifestations appear. In the following section, the most important electrolyte problems you are likely to encounter in the field are discussed.

Hyponatremia

Sodium is the most important electrolyte in maintaining water balance in the body. As the principal cation in the extracellular fluid, sodium, together with the anions chloride and bicarbonate, regulates osmotic forces (the flow of water in and out of cells). Water balance is maintained by hormonal regulation controlled by the brain and kidneys.

Hyponatremia is defined as a serum sodium concentration < 135 mEq/L. To guide management, hyponatremia is classified into three categories (hypervolemic, hypovolemic, and euvolemic), depending on the patient's volume status:

- *Hypervolemic hyponatremia* occurs when an excessive amount of water is retained relative to the amount of sodium. This condition classically occurs in a patient with an edematous condition such as decompensated heart failure. It may also occur in patients who have excessive water intake, such as with psychogenic polydipsia, or when large amounts of water are ingested over a short period of time.
- *Hypovolemic hyponatremia* is caused by the loss of water and sodium, with a higher degree of sodium loss relative to the amount of water loss. Common precipitants include vomiting, diarrhea, GI problems, nasogastric tubes, and third spacing of fluids. Third spacing (movement of intravascular and intracellular water into interstitial spaces) is a phenomenon that may occur in patients with burns, pancreatitis, and sepsis, and in those who take certain medications, such as diuretics.

- *Euvolemic hyponatremia* occurs when the serum sodium is low in a patient with normal volume status. A common cause is the syndrome of inappropriate antidiuretic hormone.

Signs and Symptoms

The clinical presentation of hyponatremia depends on how quickly the sodium concentration declines. Patients who experience a rapid drop in serum sodium level often begin to show symptoms when the concentration is in the range of 125 to 130 mEq/L; however, a patient with chronic hyponatremia may tolerate a level < 120 mEq/L without symptoms.

Most signs and symptoms of hyponatremia are related to CNS manifestations, such as agitation, hallucinations, weakness, lethargy, and seizures. Abdominal pain, cramps, and headache may also occur. Patients with severe hyponatremia appear to be very ill and may have seizures or exhibit an altered mental status.

Athletic events such as marathons and triathlons can precipitate exercise-induced hyponatremia. Although the mechanisms that cause this condition are not completely understood, it can be largely avoided by titration of free-water intake based on thirst rather than forcing intake based on a formula. Exercise-induced hyponatremia can cause loss of coordination, pulmonary edema, and changes in intracranial pressure that result in seizure and coma.

Patients with very high glucose levels (or excessive lipids or proteins in the blood) will exhibit pseudohyponatremia with a measured sodium level that appears quite low. This low sodium measurement must be corrected by using a formula to ascertain the true sodium level.

Differential Diagnosis

Determining the differential diagnosis for hyponatremia and identifying the underlying cause are often complex and may be difficult tasks even for specialists in the hospital. In the prehospital environment, the history and exam should help guide you to consideration of hyponatremia.

Treatment

On the basis of the patient's history and physical exam, determine if the patient might be suffering from hyponatremia, and if so, the most likely cause. In patients who are hemodynamically unstable, initiate fluid resuscitation with isotonic crystalloids or 0.9% normal saline. But be careful: All fluids—and particularly those given to patients who are hemodynamically stable—should be administered with extreme caution in patients with hyponatremia. Until a serum sodium level is known and a total body water deficit has been calculated, aggressive hydration runs the risk of correcting the sodium too quickly and leading to severe complications (pontine myelinolysis).

You will rarely have serum sodium measurements to guide management of patients in the prehospital environment, although point-of-care testing is available in some circumstances. As a general rule, hyponatremia should be corrected extremely slowly. The recommended rate of correction is no faster than 1 to 2 mEq/L per hour. The exception to this rule is patients with severe neurologic symptoms such as altered mental status or seizures. In these patients, a rapid correction may be needed to alleviate the symptoms. This may be done with a 100-mL bolus of 3% sodium chloride (hypertonic saline). Correcting the sodium level too aggressively (either with normal saline or hypertonic saline) can cause severe neurologic complications as a result of osmotic demyelination.

Hypokalemia

Potassium is responsible for the following vital functions in the body:

- Maintaining a normal electrical and osmotic gradient in all cells
- Facilitating neuronal transmission and cardiac impulse conduction
- Serving as a buffering mechanism in the cell membranes to help maintain acid–base homeostasis

Normal serum potassium levels range from 3.5 to 5 mEq/L, but do not accurately reflect total body stores of this cation because most potassium is stored within cells. Hypokalemia is an abnormally low serum level of potassium, usually < 3.5 mEq/L. Hypokalemia is fairly common and usually occurs secondary to decreased intake or increased excretion.

Signs and Symptoms

Hypokalemia often manifests with no signs or symptoms initially. As it progresses and the potassium level falls to < 2.5 mEq/L, signs and symptoms of hypokalemia become apparent in multiple organ systems, including the neurologic, GI, and cardiovascular systems. Common symptoms include weakness, nausea, vomiting, lethargy, confusion, and paresthesia of the extremities.

A patient with severe hypokalemia (< 2 mEq/L) will appear to be very ill and may have cardiac dysrhythmias and muscular paralysis. Frequent cardiovascular manifestations include palpitations; low blood pressure; and cardiac electrical disturbances such as heart blocks, PVCs, and supraventricular tachycardia. Fatal types of dysrhythmia, such as ventricular fibrillation and asystole, can also occur. Signs of hypokalemia apparent on a 12-lead electrocardiogram (ECG) include flattened

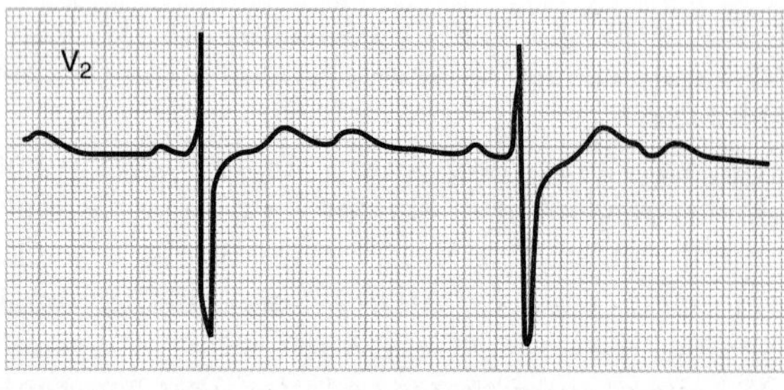

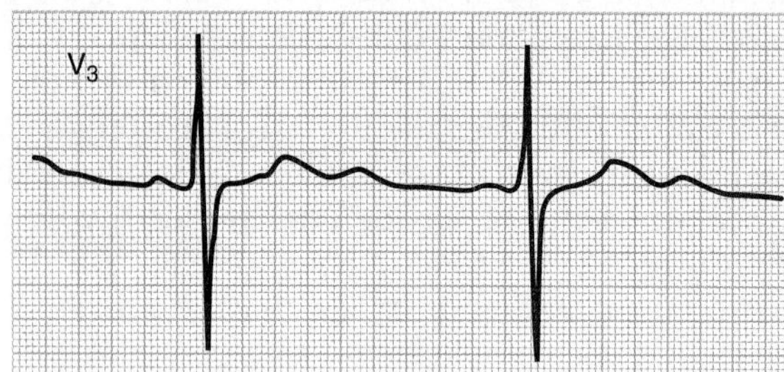

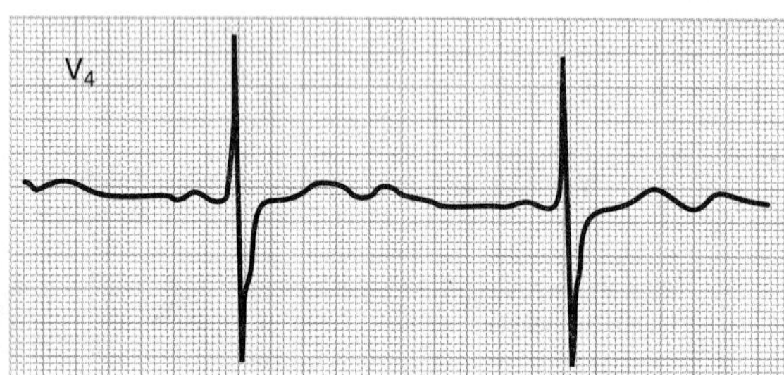

Figure 11-3 Electrocardiographic manifestations of hypokalemia. Serum potassium concentration was 2.2 mEq/L. The ST segment is prolonged, the U wave is following the T wave, and the T wave is flattened.

Goldman L, Ausiello DA, Arend W, et al., eds. Cecil Medicine. 23rd ed. Elsevier; 2007

T waves, the presence of U waves, and ST-segment depression (**Figure 11-3**).

Differential Diagnosis

The differential diagnosis will depend on the signs and symptoms with which the patient presents. These are often nonspecific, so a broad differential diagnosis should be considered during the initial evaluation.

Treatment

Treatment of hypokalemia may require intravenous (IV) fluids for dehydration. Oral potassium replacement (20 to 40 mEq per dose) is preferred over IV administration because of the potential side effects of IV potassium. Patients who are unable to take oral replacement or are critically ill will require IV potassium administered at a rate of 10 to 20 mEq per hour. Critically ill patients (those with respiratory muscle weakness) can receive higher doses, but they should be given through a central venous catheter. Overly rapid infusion of IV potassium can result in cardiac arrest. A common complaint during IV administration is burning at the site of infusion, which can usually be resolved by slowing the rate of infusion.

Hyperkalemia is a potential complication of potassium administration, which is especially likely to manifest in patients with kidney disease. It is therefore critical to know the patient's renal function status before you administer potassium.

Hyperkalemia

Hyperkalemia, a level of serum potassium > 5.5 mEq/L, is an electrolyte disorder that can be caused by ingestion of potassium supplements, acute or chronic renal failure, blood transfusion, sepsis, Addison disease, acidosis, and crush syndrome (from rhabdomyolysis).

Signs and Symptoms

Hyperkalemia manifests primarily as neurologic and cardiovascular dysfunction. The patient may have generalized weakness, muscle cramps, tetany, paralysis, or cardiac palpitations or arrhythmias.

Differential Diagnosis

In the prehospital setting, the only diagnostic study available to guide you toward a diagnosis of hyperkalemia is the ECG, which can help you determine whether the patient has an associated arrhythmia. Classically, the first change detected on the ECG of a patient with hyperkalemia is the development of peaked T waves. As serum potassium continues to increase, P waves disappear, and the QRS complex widens. If hyperkalemia is not corrected, the ECG will progress to bradycardia and then terminate in a sine wave pattern or asystole (**Figure 11-4**).

Treatment

Assess and treat the underlying cause of hyperkalemia, institute rapid and appropriate treatment, and transport the patient to a hospital facility. Treatment of hyperkalemia has three goals:

- *Cellular membrane stabilization and decreased cardiac irritability.* Maintain the patient on a cardiac monitor at all times. If the patient has signs of hyperkalemia on ECG, hypotension, or arrhythmias, administer 1 g (5 mL of 10% solution) of calcium chloride by slow IV push or short-duration infusion. The equivalent dose of calcium gluconate is 3 g. In many systems, this treatment may require consultation with online medical direction unless the patient is already in cardiac arrest.
- *Potassium shift into cells.* The combined administration of 5 units of regular insulin produces a shift of potassium into the cells and is the primary treatment in the emergency department

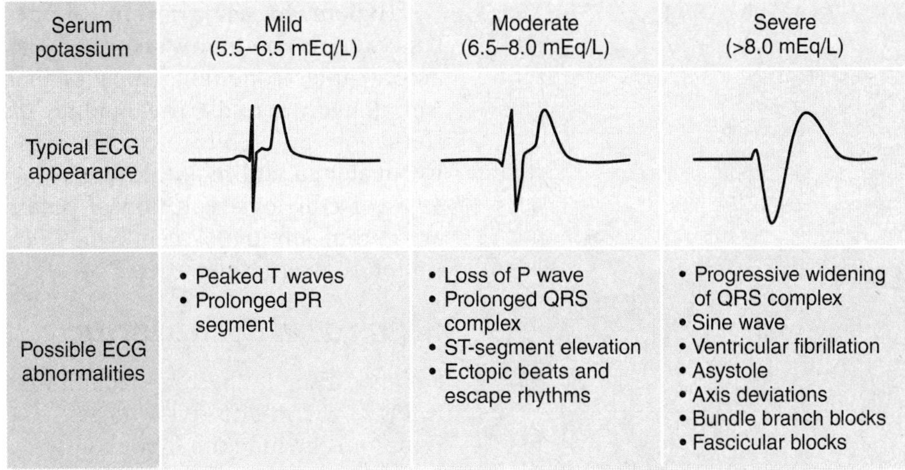

Serum potassium	Mild (5.5–6.5 mEq/L)	Moderate (6.5–8.0 mEq/L)	Severe (>8.0 mEq/L)
Typical ECG appearance			
Possible ECG abnormalities	• Peaked T waves • Prolonged PR segment	• Loss of P wave • Prolonged QRS complex • ST-segment elevation • Ectopic beats and escape rhythms	• Progressive widening of QRS complex • Sine wave • Ventricular fibrillation • Asystole • Axis deviations • Bundle branch blocks • Fascicular blocks

Figure 11-4 ECG findings associated with hyperkalemia.

(ED)/hospital setting. This treatment with insulin is usually given with concomitant IV dextrose to prevent hypoglycemia. Nebulized albuterol, 5 to 20 mg, will lower the serum potassium level by shifting potassium into cells. Albuterol has a minimal effect overall, so it should have a lower priority for administration. Sodium bicarbonate was historically suggested to drive potassium into cells and out of the serum, but this practice is not strongly supported by evidence. This intervention has been removed from guidelines or reserved only for cases of renal failure and acidosis, and it is no longer suggested for routine use.

- *Elimination of potassium from the body.* To help eliminate potassium from the body, treatments may include loop diuretics such as furosemide IV and exchange resins such as sodium zirconium cyclosilicate administered by the oral or rectal route. Be careful when administering exchange resins in a cardiac patient, however, as they can produce fluid overload.

Hypocalcemia

Calcium is essential for a number of body functions, including muscular contraction, neuronal transmission, hormone secretion, organ growth, and immunologic and hematologic responses. Most of the calcium in an adult is stored as a mineral component of bone. Hypocalcemia occurs when ionized calcium levels fall to < 4 mEq/L. This condition occurs because of increased losses or decreased intake of calcium. Hypocalcemia is also seen in patients who receive blood transfusions due to the citrate preservative found in stored blood components.

Signs and Symptoms

Patients with symptomatic hypocalcemia may have seizures, hypotension, tetany, or cardiac dysrhythmias. Two specific signs may be present—Trousseau (**Figure 11-5**) and Chvostek (**Figure 11-6**) signs—and can help you narrow down the possible diagnosis.

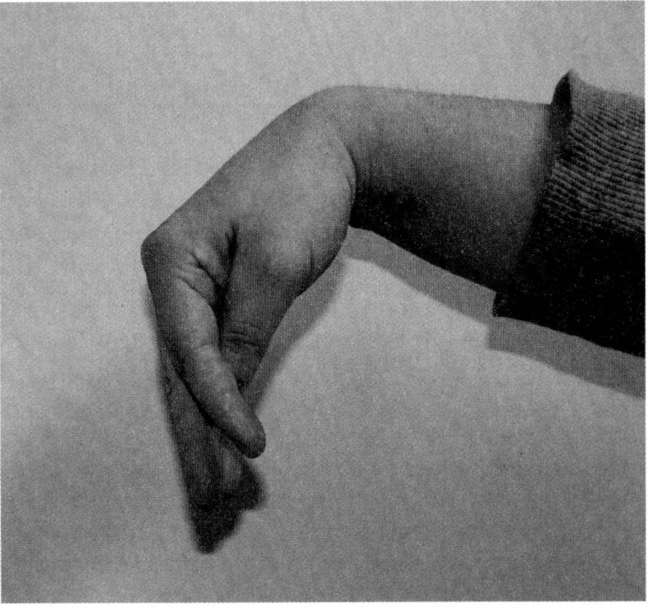

Figure 11-5 Trousseau sign.

Differential Diagnosis

These patients with hypocalcemia often present with nonspecific findings, so a broad range of metabolic conditions should be considered in the differential diagnosis.

Treatment

Treatment of hypocalcemia is guided principally by laboratory results. However, when hypocalcemia is presumed to be the cause of the patient's symptoms, it may be reasonable to begin empiric treatment. Parenteral calcium

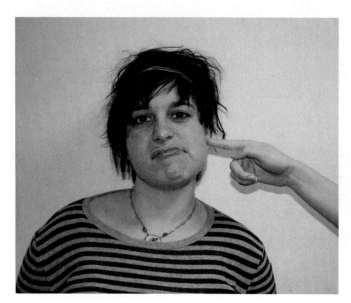

Figure 11-6 Chvostek sign.

is the primary treatment in patients with symptomatic hypocalcemia. Use one of the following two options:

- 10 mL 10% calcium chloride, which contains about 270 mg elemental calcium
- 20 to 30 mL 10% calcium gluconate, which contains about 90 mg elemental calcium per 10 mL

In an adult patient, the recommended dose is 100 to 300 mg elemental calcium. In a pediatric patient, administer 0.5 to 1 mL/kg of a 10% calcium gluconate solution over 5 minutes. To avoid significant side effects, dilution in normal saline or D_5W is highly recommended. Care must be taken to ensure the peripheral catheter is working properly before administering calcium, because extravasation may cause tissue necrosis. Calcium administration will increase the serum concentration of calcium for only a short period of time, so repeated doses may be necessary, especially during a long transport or interfacility transfer.

Patients whose signs and symptoms persist after adequate treatment may have concomitant electrolyte problems such as hypomagnesemia.

Hypomagnesemia

Magnesium is the second most abundant intracellular bivalent cation in the human body. It is a cofactor in the activation of numerous enzymatic reactions. Its physiologic effects on the CNS are similar to those of calcium. Magnesium is distributed throughout the body in a unique way. One-half of the total amount of magnesium (2,000 mEq/L) is stored as a mineral component of bone, and 40% to 50% is intracellular. Only 1% to 2% of magnesium in the body is found in the extracellular fluid; thus, the serum magnesium level is a poor reflection of the body's total magnesium content.

Hypomagnesemia is one of the electrolyte disturbances most commonly seen in clinical practice. It often accompanies conditions such as malnutrition, alcoholism, dehydration, diarrhea, kidney disease, diuresis, and starvation, and tends to coexist with diseases that cause hypokalemia and hypocalcemia. Magnesium also serves as a cofactor for absorption of potassium. Patients who are chronically hypokalemic may benefit from administration of magnesium.

Signs and Symptoms

Patients usually become symptomatic at magnesium levels ≤ 1.2 mg/dL (0.06 mmol/L). Common signs and symptoms include the following:

- Tremors
- Hyperreflexia
- Tetany
- Nausea or vomiting
- Altered mental status and confusion
- Seizures
- Cardiac dysrhythmias, including torsades de pointes, polymorphic ventricular tachycardia, and cardiac arrest

Treatment

Take immediate steps to maintain the patient's airway, breathing, and circulation. It is reasonable to start magnesium replacement therapy when you suspect a diagnosis of hypomagnesemia. In patients with no history of renal problems, administer 2 g of 50% magnesium sulfate. This dose must be given with normal saline or dextrose, ideally administered over 30 to 60 minutes per gram. However, in a patient with severe signs and symptoms, including dysrhythmias, you may need to give a rapid infusion over the course of 2 to 10 minutes. Do not give magnesium sulfate as a rapid IV push because this been associated with severe side effects, including bradycardia, heart block, and hypotension.

Rhabdomyolysis

Rhabdomyolysis is a breakdown of muscle tissue that causes myoglobin to be released into the bloodstream, leading to kidney damage. This muscle injury usually results from prolonged periods of immobilization, certain metabolic insults, or pressure or crush force on the tissue. Examples of situations that may result in rhabdomyolysis include someone who has experienced an opioid overdose, a person pinned under an industrial machine, a marathon runner, or an elderly person who has spent several hours on the floor after falling. Regardless of the cause, the end result in each of these cases is the release of intracellular contents as the individual muscle cells rupture and die. Subsequently, myoglobin—one of the main proteins found in skeletal muscle cells—travels to the kidneys and causes injury and even renal failure. Electrolytes that are normally sequestered within the cell, particularly potassium, may also be released, resulting in metabolic disturbances that are only exacerbated by the concurrent renal injury. In extreme cases, patients may have massive hyperkalemia, resulting in fatal cardiac arrhythmias.

Pathophysiology

Common precipitants of rhabdomyolysis include the following conditions:

- Metabolic problems
- Heatstroke and other severe heat-related emergencies
- Trauma
- Crush injuries
- Cocaine or other stimulant use
- Toxic ingestion/overdose
- Infections (rarely)
- Electrolyte abnormalities
- Various medications

Dysfunction of the sodium–potassium–ATPase pump allows uncontrolled calcium influx into skeletal muscle cells. The increased intracellular calcium content leads to cellular necrosis and release of myoglobin, potassium, and intracellular enzymes, such as creatinine phosphokinase. Once myoglobin enters the plasma, it is filtered and excreted through the kidneys. An excess of myoglobin can be directly toxic to the renal tubules; alternatively, it can obstruct them, especially if the patient is hypovolemic or acidotic as a result of the primary problem. If not treated aggressively with IV fluids, rhabdomyolysis can cause severe kidney damage and renal failure.

Signs and Symptoms

Patients with rhabdomyolysis report diffuse or localized weakness and muscle pain. Once the process of rhabdomyolysis has begun, patients may have dark-colored urine. If the patient develops hyperkalemia, the aforementioned signs and symptoms may also occur.

Differential Diagnosis

Rhabdomyolysis is diagnosed in the ED by noting myoglobinuria (the presence of myoglobin, a protein released in muscle breakdown, in the urine) and an elevated creatine kinase level in the blood. However, you should suspect this diagnosis based on a comprehensive history (including the history of the primary condition) and physical exam findings. The patient may not have rhabdomyolysis initially, but an emergent condition may induce its development later. A thorough physical exam is the key to identifying potential causes. For example, you may discover dark or cola-colored urine, which is an indicator of the presence of rhabdomyolysis.

Treatment

Aggressive fluid hydration is crucial for patients with rhabdomyolysis. IV fluids should be given (while taking care to avoid hypothermia) to mitigate the complications of this condition. In addition to standard supportive care, consider the following measures:

- Aggressive saline infusion early, especially in patients with trauma or crush injuries. Saline infusion is vital in the treatment of rhabdomyolysis.
- Titration of saline infusions to obtain a urine output of 200 to 300 mL per hour. Be aware of potential electrolyte complications (such as hyperkalemia with hypocalcemia) that may elicit malignant cardiac dysrhythmias. If they occur, you must treat them aggressively.

Parathyroid, Thyroid, and Adrenal Gland Disorders

Hypoparathyroidism

Hypoparathyroidism is a rare condition characterized by low serum levels of parathyroid hormone (PTH) or resistance to its action. Congenital, autoimmune, and acquired diseases are among its many causes. Regardless of the etiology, the hallmark of the condition is hypocalcemia (which will be discussed later).

Pathophysiology

The most common cause of acquired hypoparathyroidism is iatrogenic damage or inadvertent removal of the glands during thyroidectomy. Such damage can be transitory or permanent.

Signs and Symptoms

Patients with acute hypoparathyroidism report muscle spasms, paresthesias, and tetany. Some may even have seizures. These signs and symptoms are directly due to hypocalcemia (**Figure 11-7**).

Differential Diagnosis

In the prehospital setting, no laboratory studies are immediately available to confirm hypoparathyroidism. Thus, you must have a high index of suspicion for this condition based on the patient's history and physical examination findings. Recent anterior neck surgery is a risk factor for iatrogenic hypoparathyroidism.

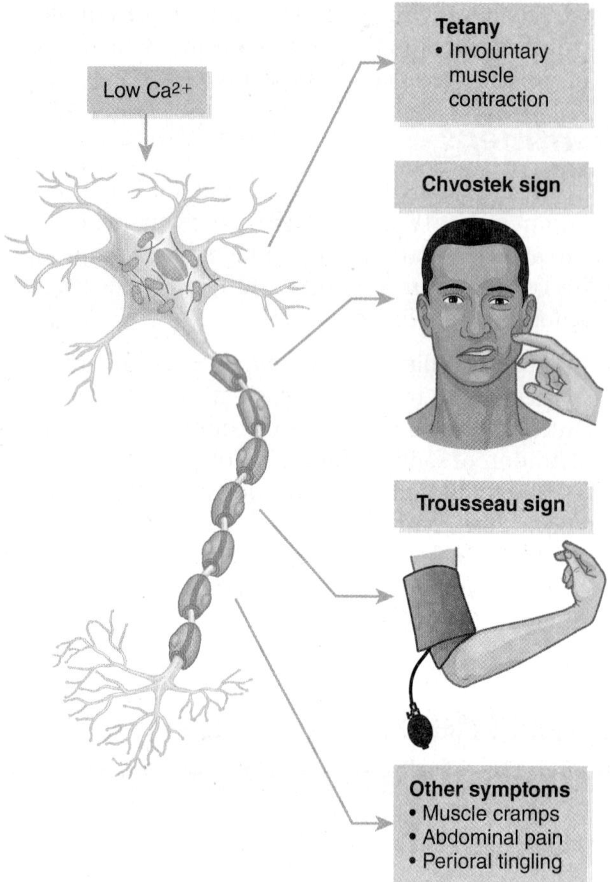

Figure 11-7 Signs and symptoms of hypocalcemia.

It is helpful to be aware of Trousseau sign (Figure 11-5) and Chvostek sign (Figure 11-6), both of which can help you detect muscular irritability caused by hypocalcemia. To elicit a positive Trousseau sign, place a blood pressure cuff around the patient's arm, inflate it to 30 mm Hg above the systolic blood pressure, and hold it in place for 3 minutes. This will induce spasm of the muscles of the hand and forearm. The wrist and metacarpophalangeal joints will flex, the distal and proximal interphalangeal joints will extend, and the fingers will adduct. You can elicit a positive Chvostek sign by tapping the patient's facial nerve against the mandibular bone just anterior to the ear, which produces a spasm of the facial muscles. Note that this sign is not as sensitive as Trousseau sign.

Another tool available is the ECG. In patients with hypocalcemia, the QT interval is prolonged (**Figure 11-8**).

Treatment

As in any emergent condition, you must assess and stabilize the patient's airway, breathing/ventilation, and hemodynamic status. Obtain IV access and provide supportive treatment. If the patient is having seizures, administer benzodiazepines. When you have a strong clinical suspicion or laboratory analysis confirms hypocalcemia, the patient may be given IV calcium. In emergent situations, administer calcium chloride 1 g or calcium gluconate 2 g IV bolus. In nonemergent situations, administer calcium chloride 10% solution, 500 to 1,000 mg IV, over

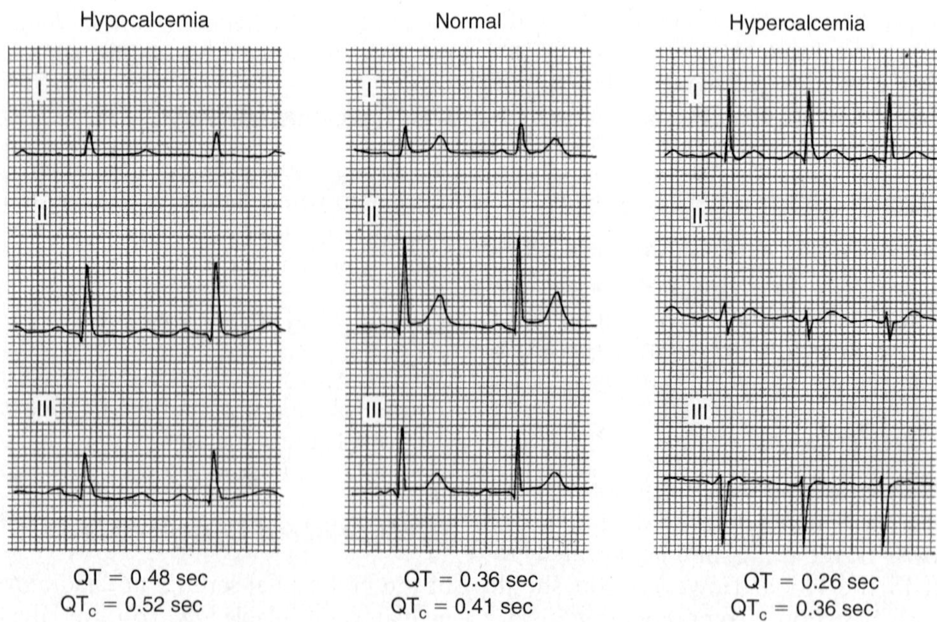

Figure 11-8 Hypocalcemia prolongs the QT interval by stretching out the ST segment. Hypercalcemia decreases the QT interval by shortening the ST segment so that the T wave seems to take off directly from the end of the QRS complex.

5 to 10 minutes, or calcium gluconate 10% solution, 1,500 to 3,000 mg IV, diluted in normal saline or 5% dextrose in water (D_5W), over 2 to 5 minutes.

Hyperthyroidism

Hyperactivity of the thyroid gland, or hyperthyroidism, is a common ailment that results in a hypermetabolic state called **thyrotoxicosis**. Contrast this with **thyroid storm**, a rarer complication of hyperthyroidism that occurs in only 1% to 2% of patients. Thyroid storm is a life-threatening condition characterized by hemodynamic instability, altered mental status, GI dysfunction, and fever.

Pathophysiology

Graves disease, also known as *diffuse toxic goiter*, is the most common form of hyperthyroidism. In this autoimmune disorder, antibodies mimic the role of TSH, which leads to increased secretion of thyroid hormones. Graves disease most often occurs in females of middle age, but can arise at any age and can also affect males. Other causes of hyperthyroidism include acute intoxication with exogenous thyroid hormones and (less commonly) use of drugs with high iodine loads such as amiodarone or iodinated IV contrast, which may precipitate sudden release of excess thyroid hormones in susceptible individuals. In cases of autoimmune destruction of the gland, a temporary hyperthyroidism may precede the more chronic hypothyroidism.

Thyroid storm typically occurs when the body is stressed by an emergent condition, such as a diabetic emergency, an adverse drug reaction, or an infection. You should suspect thyroid storm if the patient experiences cardiac decompensation after taking amiodarone. Table 11-1 provides a comprehensive list of triggers that cause thyroid storm.

Signs and Symptoms

The characteristic clinical presentation of a patient with hyperthyroidism includes apprehension, agitation, edginess, heart palpitations, and weight loss of as much as 18 kg (40 lb) over a few months. Heat intolerance and increased sweating caused by this hypermetabolic state are frequently reported symptoms.

A complete physical exam will reveal signs and symptoms of thyrotoxicosis, including the exophthalmos that is characteristic of the condition (**Figure 11-9**). Signs and symptoms of hyperthyroidism include the following:

- Apprehension/agitation
- Palpitations
- Tachycardia
- Atrial fibrillation or other tachydysrhythmias
- Weight loss
- Exophthalmos
- Shortness of breath
- Disorientation
- Abdominal pain
- Diarrhea
- Chest pain
- Enlarged thyroid gland (palpable goiter)
- High-output cardiac failure
- Fever
- Drug interactions
- Altered mental status
- Jaundice
- Weakness

Differential Diagnosis

In the prehospital setting, no laboratory studies are immediately available to confirm hyperthyroidism or thyroid storm, so you must have a high index of suspicion based on the patient's history and physical examination

Table 11-1 Triggers of Thyroid Storm

Medical Triggers	Endocrine Triggers	Pharmacologic Triggers
Infectious disease	Hypoglycemia	Iodine therapy
Cardiac ischemia	Diabetic ketoacidosis	Amiodarone ingestion
Serious burns	Nonketotic hyperosmolar state	Administration of contrast medium
Thromboembolism		Drug interactions
Major surgery		
Trauma		

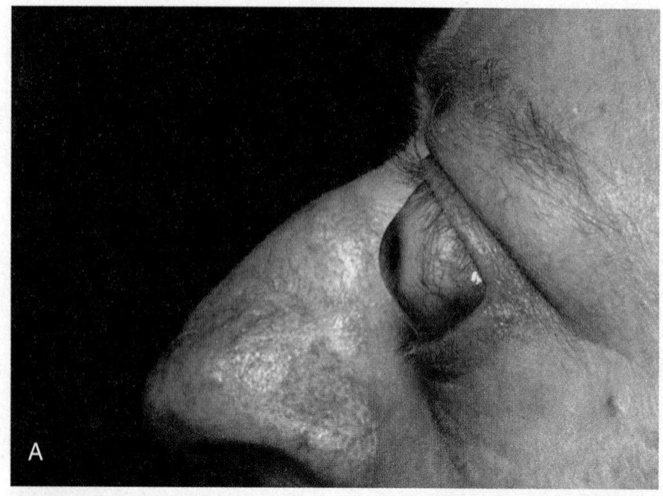

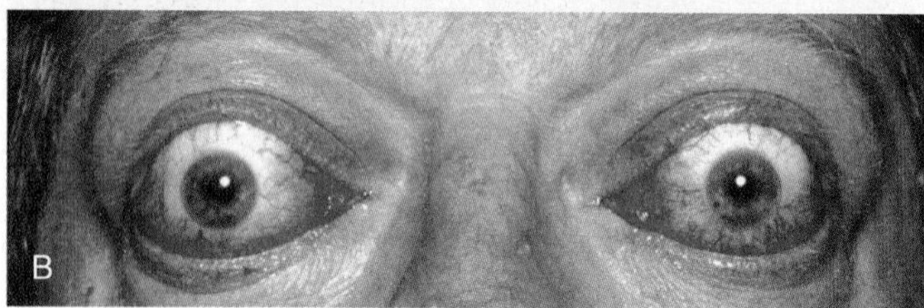

Figure 11-9 Person with hyperthyroidism (**A** and **B**). Exophthalmos—a wide-eyed, staring gaze caused by overactivity of the sympathetic nervous system—is one feature of this disorder. The accumulation of loose connective tissue behind the eyeballs also adds to the protuberant appearance of the eyes.

A: © Science Photo Library/Science Source; **B:** ©SPL/Science Source

findings. You can begin to stabilize the patient and initiate early treatment on the strength of clinical judgment alone.

In the hospital, the most rapid and useful test for hyperthyroidism is a serum TSH level; if it is low and the patient has clinical signs and symptoms of hyperthyroidism, the test is essentially diagnostic. To confirm this presumptive diagnosis, the levels of the actual thyroid hormones, usually T_4 and T_3, may be obtained. Imaging studies and biopsy can help determine the specific cause of the disorder.

As part of the differential diagnosis, consider stroke, diabetic emergencies, heart failure, toxic ingestion (particularly ingestion of a sympathomimetic agent), and sepsis.

Treatment

The key to providing optimal patient care is to differentiate among the various hypermetabolic states induced by thyroid disorders. These include subacute (chronic) hyperthyroidism, acute severe hyperthyroidism, and its most critical complication, thyroid storm. A patient with chronic hyperthyroidism generally requires only supportive care and early management of symptoms. If severe hyperthyroidism or thyroid storm is detected, however, it is imperative to stabilize the patient's condition. As in any acute emergency, begin with the ABCs. Patients experiencing acute severe hyperthyroidism or thyroid storm may exhibit altered mental status, which can potentially progress to coma.

Patients with thyroid storm often have moderate to severe dehydration because of excessive diarrhea and sweating. These patients should be treated with aggressive IV hydration. Although aggressive hydration is indicated, care must be taken to avoid inducing acute pulmonary edema, as these patients may experience cardiac instability.

Patients with hyperthyroidism are also prone to dysrhythmias such as sinus tachycardia, atrial fibrillation, atrial flutter, and PVCs. For this reason, you should begin continuous cardiac monitoring as soon as you suspect this diagnosis.

Patients with thyroid storm may have fever associated with the pathophysiologic process itself or with an infection that precipitated the thyroid storm. Assess body temperature and treat hyperpyrexia in thyroid storm with acetaminophen and external cooling. *Do not* use aspirin: It is associated with decreased protein binding of thyroid hormones and correspondingly increased levels of unbound or free T_3 and T_4, which will exacerbate symptoms.

The goals of pharmacologic treatment in the prehospital setting are to block the peripheral adrenergic hyperactivity that the thyroid hormones elicit (tachycardia, fever, anxiety, and tremors) and to inhibit the conversion of T_4 to T_3 in the peripheral tissues. Both objectives can be achieved by administering beta blockers, such as propranolol. Beta blockers should be administered with extreme caution in patients with bronchial asthma, chronic obstructive pulmonary disease (COPD), atrioventricular blocks, hypersensitivity, and severe heart failure. A patient with thyroid storm and concomitant heart failure most likely has a high-output cardiac failure. This is not considered a contraindication to the use of propranolol unless the patient also has significant cardiomyopathy with systolic dysfunction. Adjunctive corticosteroid therapy—typically hydrocortisone, 100 mg IV, or dexAMETHasone, 10 mg IV—may be given to slow the conversion of T_4 to T_3. In most agencies, these treatments should be administered only after consultation with physician online medical oversight.

Hypothyroidism

Hypothyroidism is an endocrine dysfunction characterized by decreased or absent secretion of thyroid hormones. Its incidence in the United States is 4.6% to

Table 11-2 Causes of Hypothyroidism

Primary	Secondary
Chronic autoimmune thyroiditis	Pituitary tumor
Iodine deficiency (or excess)	Congenital hypothyroidism
Thyroidectomy	Hypothalamic lesions
Radiation therapy (external or radioiodine therapy	Pituitary apoplexy
Sarcoid infiltration	
Medications/drugs (e.g., lithium, interferon alfa, amiodarone, certain tyrosine kinase inhibitors)	

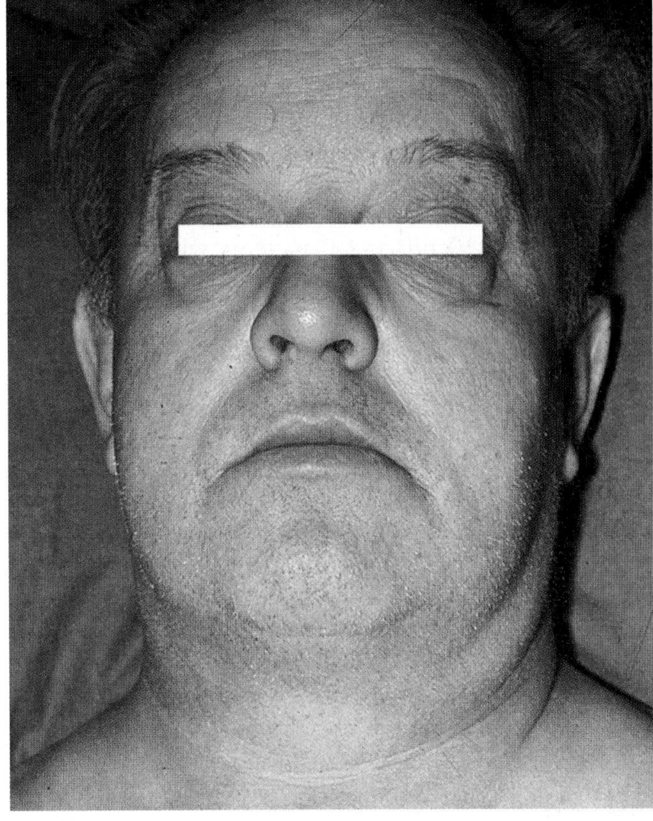

Figure 11-10 Localized accumulations of mucinous material in the neck of a hypothyroid patient (myxedema facies).

5.8%, but half of all individuals with this condition are asymptomatic. Hypothyroidism is most common among white females between the ages of 40 and 50 years. It is highly associated with autoimmune conditions.

Pathophysiology

Defective thyroid hormone secretion is classified as either primary or secondary hypothyroidism. The causes of each are summarized in Table 11-2. Primary hypothyroidism involves direct thyroid injury caused by an autoimmune disorder or an adverse drug reaction. Patients who have undergone surgical thyroidectomy or radiofrequency ablation therapy (use of radiation to decrease the amount of functional glandular tissue) for a hyperthyroid state may have resultant hypothyroidism. In secondary, or central, hypothyroidism, damage to the hypothalamus or pituitary gland results in decreased stimulation of the thyroid gland (specifically, a decline in the production and release of TSH). Many complications result from clinical hypothyroidism, including hypoxia, hypothermia, hypoglycemia, sepsis, and narcosis.

Signs and Symptoms

Hypothyroidism has a deleterious effect on many body systems, including the integumentary, metabolic, nervous, and cardiovascular systems. The skin of a patient with this condition is cool, dry, coarse, and often doughy due to nonpitting edema. The patient typically has thinning of the eyebrows; coarse hair; intolerance to cold temperatures; and neurologic changes such as altered mental status, ataxia, and delayed relaxation of deep tendon reflexes.

When hypothyroidism becomes chronic and extreme, it may evolve into a life-threatening condition called **myxedema coma** (Figure 11-10), which is characterized by hypotension, bradycardia, hypoglycemia, and low serum sodium (hyponatremia). Precipitants of myxedema coma include the following conditions:

- Lung infection
- Cold exposure
- Heart failure
- Stroke
- GI bleeding
- Trauma
- Stress
- Hypoxia
- Electrolytic disturbances
- Low serum glucose levels

Differential Diagnosis

In the prehospital setting, no laboratory studies are immediately available to confirm hypothyroidism or myxedema coma. The patient's history and physical examination findings will suggest the diagnosis. Stabilization and early treatment must be initiated solely on the basis of clinical judgment.

In the hospital, TSH levels will be elevated, generally > 10 μU/mL (10 mU/L), in patients with primary hypothyroidism. In addition, total and free thyroxine (FT_4) levels may be ordered to determine the thyroid hormone level in the serum and evaluate for abnormal protein levels that may in turn affect the level of functional T_4. A T_4 level < 0.8 ng/dL (10 pmol/L) indicates that the thyroid gland is not producing adequate levels of the hormone. Ultrasound imaging can be performed to reveal the size, shape, and position of the thyroid gland and to identify cysts or tumors that may contribute to thyroid dysfunction.

Treatment

Patients with hypothyroidism require supportive care and early management of symptoms. EMS clinicians must have a high index of suspicion for this disorder. If severe hypothyroidism or myxedema coma is detected in the prehospital environment, it is imperative to stabilize the patient's condition by providing supportive care as needed. Consider transport to a tertiary care center if one is located within a reasonable distance.

As in any acute emergency, begin with the ABCs. Patients with hypothyroidism, similar to those with acute hyperthyroidism and thyroid storm, may show evidence of altered mental status or be comatose. Airway management and ventilatory support may be needed. Particular attention must be paid to assessing the patient for heart failure. Initiate a peripheral IV line early during prehospital management to provide medications as needed.

If the patient has altered mental status, determine the serum glucose level. If the value is < 60 mg/dL (3.3 mmol/L), administer IV dextrose.

The hypothyroid patient is prone to experiencing heart arrhythmias, especially bradycardia, so begin continuous cardiac monitoring as soon as possible. Be aware that standard treatments for bradycardia may be ineffective until the thyroid hormone deficiency has been remedied.

A patient in myxedema coma may be hypothermic because of either the pathophysiologic process itself or a triggering infection. Always assess body temperature and treat hypothermia with blankets and other warming techniques. Rapidly transport the patient to a well-equipped hospital facility for definitive treatment, which may include L-triiodothyronine IV, hydrocortisone IV, and subsequent daily oral replacement therapy if the condition proves irreversible.

Chronic Adrenal Insufficiency

Adrenal insufficiency, defined as the failure of the adrenal cortex to produce a sufficient amount of cortisol, is classified as primary, secondary, or tertiary, depending on whether the cortex is damaged directly or indirectly. Primary adrenal insufficiency, known as **Addison disease**, is a metabolic and endocrine ailment caused by a direct insult to, or malfunction of, the adrenal cortex. This chronic disease has a protracted onset. Almost any condition that directly harms the adrenal cortex can cause primary adrenal insufficiency, including autoimmune disorders; adrenal hemorrhage; and infectious diseases such as acquired immunodeficiency syndrome (AIDS), tuberculosis, and meningococcemia.

Pathophysiology

As noted previously, the adrenal cortex produces the corticosteroid hormones aldosterone and cortisol. Aldosterone is responsible for keeping serum levels of sodium and potassium in balance. When the body experiences any type of stress—trauma, infection, cardiac ischemia, or a severe illness, to name a few possibilities—the adrenal glands may become unable to produce sufficient amounts of corticosteroid hormones to supply the body's demands, triggering an acute exacerbation of adrenal insufficiency.

In secondary adrenal insufficiency, although the cortex itself is intact, it fails to receive a signal to produce cortisol because the pituitary gland fails to release ACTH, which normally stimulates the adrenal cortex. Thus, the adrenal insufficiency is one step removed from its origin. Tertiary (third-level) adrenal insufficiency, in which the pituitary's failure to release ACTH stems from a disorder of the hypothalamus, is even less direct.

In primary adrenal insufficiency, patients may develop hyperpigmentation of the skin due to overproduction of MSH. This overproduction results from the fact that MSH and ACTH are produced from the same precursor protein (pro-opiomelanocortin) in the pituitary. MSH stimulates melanocytes in the skin to produce the skin pigment melanin. Secondary and tertiary adrenal insufficiency are not associated with hyperpigmentation of the skin because they involve low levels of MSH rather than high levels.

Signs and Symptoms

The clinical presentation of patients with Addison disease is consistent with the endocrine and electrolyte disorders brought on by the disease. These individuals will have

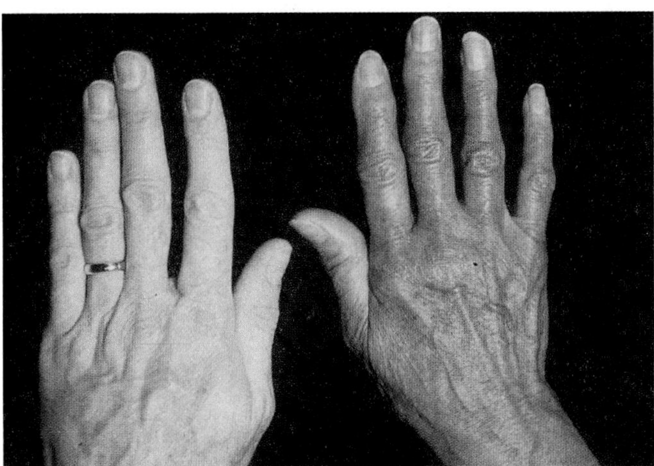

Figure 11-11 The hand of a patient with Addison disease (right) compared with the hand of a healthy person (left).

chronic fatigue and weakness, loss of appetite and consequent weight loss, and hyperpigmentation of the skin and mucous membranes (**Figure 11-11**). Patients will also have hypotension; electrolyte disturbances including hyponatremia and hyperkalemia; and (sometimes) GI disturbances such as abdominal pain, nausea, vomiting, and diarrhea. Delirium and altered mental status are other symptoms associated with Addison disease. Additionally, patients with this disease process often follow the same pattern: They feel better after taking their medications, believe that they are "cured," and then stop the medications, which results in an exacerbation of an acute adrenal crisis. Patients with known Addison disease should be encouraged to wear a bracelet or neck tag indicating they have this condition.

Differential Diagnosis

Diagnostic tools to identify adrenal insufficiency are not available in the prehospital setting. It is important that you ask the patient for any prior diagnostic laboratory reports that might be readily available. Past abnormal electrolyte findings that correlate with the patient's current clinical presentation, such as metabolic acidosis, hyponatremia, hyperkalemia, and hypoglycemia, should raise a red flag. Definitive diagnosis of this condition is made by measuring the patient's baseline serum cortisol level and then conducting stimulation testing, in which synthetic ACTH (called *cosyntropin*) is administered. If the cortisol level fails to rise shortly afterward, the patient can be diagnosed as having primary adrenal insufficiency.

Treatment

The prehospital management of an acute exacerbation of adrenal insufficiency, known as an "Addisonian crisis," includes supportive care and administration of steroids. If the patient has tachycardia and hypotension, administer an IV fluid bolus of normal saline solution. Continual reevaluation of the patient's hemodynamic state, early administration of hydrocortisone per local EMS protocol to supplement the failing adrenal function, and rapid transport to the ED are paramount in treating this condition. Provide correction of hypoglycemia, as well as symptomatic medical treatment of nausea and vomiting.

In the hospital, diagnostic testing will be carried out to identify electrolyte abnormalities such as hyponatremia and hyperkalemia. Management includes correction of electrolyte abnormalities, restoration of metabolic balance (e.g., by replacing glucocorticoids), and volume replacement for hypovolemia.

Acute Adrenal Insufficiency

Acute adrenal insufficiency is a condition in which the body's need for glucocorticoids and mineralocorticoids exceeds the delivery of these hormones by the adrenal glands. The most common cause is abrupt discontinuation of pharmacologic steroid therapy after prolonged use. This condition can also occur when such a patient fails to receive an adjusted dosage during times of stress, such as during illness or after major surgery or trauma.

Pathophysiology

Like chronic adrenal insufficiency, acute insufficiency is classified as primary, secondary, or tertiary, depending on the dysfunctional endocrine gland. *Primary adrenal insufficiency* refers to dysfunction of the adrenal glands, *secondary adrenal insufficiency* refers to dysfunction of the pituitary gland, and *tertiary insufficiency* is linked to hypothalamic dysfunction.

Signs and Symptoms

The clinical picture of acute adrenal insufficiency will include nausea, vomiting, dehydration, abdominal pain, and weakness. Clues from the patient history, such as tan skin on a patient who denies sun exposure, may alert the clinician to the possibility of chronic adrenal insufficiency. Ask the patient about recent medication changes that may have precipitated the symptoms. When adrenal insufficiency is accompanied by hypotension, the condition is called **adrenal crisis** and constitutes a true life-threatening emergency.

Differential Diagnosis

Diagnosing acute adrenal insufficiency in the prehospital setting can be challenging. The definitive confirmatory laboratory test is not available in the field, and the presentation can easily be confused with more common conditions causing hypotension. EMS clinicians must use the various tools available to them to find indirect evidence of an adrenal disorder. Assess for hypoglycemia with a glucometer, and look for evidence of hyperkalemia on the ECG. Assess for signs and symptoms of other abnormalities such as anemia, hyponatremia, and metabolic acidosis. Classic findings include the combination of hyponatremia, hyperkalemia, and hypoglycemia.

Vital signs can also provide key clues. For example, in patients with adrenal crisis, hypotension is likely to respond poorly to administration of IV fluids. The diagnosis can be confirmed in the hospital, using the cosyntropin stimulation test.

Treatment

As with any life-threatening emergency, first evaluate the patient's ability to maintain a patent airway, breathing, and circulation. For patients with hypotension, immediate resuscitation with normal saline is warranted. Administer dextrose if hypoglycemia is present. Address a deficit of glucocorticoids with hydrocortisone, which must be administered under online medical oversight in some systems. If a cosyntropin stimulation test will be performed at a later time, dexAMETHaxone is preferable to hydrocortisone because hydrocortisone can create a false-positive test result.

Hyperadrenalism

Hyperadrenalism, or Cushing syndrome, is caused by long-standing exposure to excessive circulating serum levels of glucocorticoids, particularly cortisol, as a result of overproduction in the adrenal cortex. This condition is more common in females, especially those aged 20 to 50 years. Cushing syndrome can be brought on by an adrenal or pituitary tumor or by long-term corticosteroid use.

Pathophysiology

Regardless of the cause, excess cortisol causes characteristic changes in many body systems. Metabolism of carbohydrate, protein, and fat is disturbed, such that the blood glucose level rises. Protein synthesis is impaired so that body proteins are broken down, which leads to loss of muscle fibers and muscle weakness. Bones become weaker and more susceptible to fracture.

Signs and Symptoms

Patients with Cushing syndrome have a distinct presentation that includes the following characteristics:

- Chronic weakness
- Increased body and facial hair
- Full, puffy face (moon facies) (**Figure 11-12**)
- Fatty "buffalo hump" at the back of the neck
- Central body obesity
- Purple striae on the abdomen, buttocks, breasts, or arms
- Atrophied proximal muscles
- Thin, fragile skin
- Amenorrhea
- Decreased fertility or diminished sex drive
- Diabetes mellitus
- Hypertension

Differential Diagnosis

Definitive diagnostic testing for Cushing syndrome is not available in the prehospital setting, but many patients will have been diagnosed prior to their encounter with the EMS system. If not, ask the patient for any old diagnostic laboratory reports readily available as a part of recent discharge paperwork. Past abnormal electrolyte

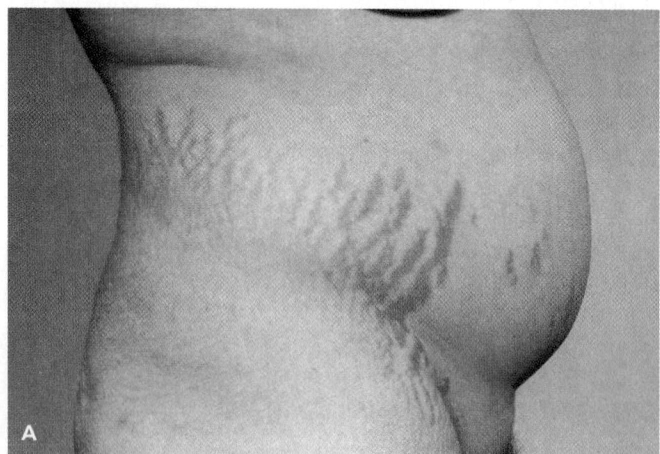

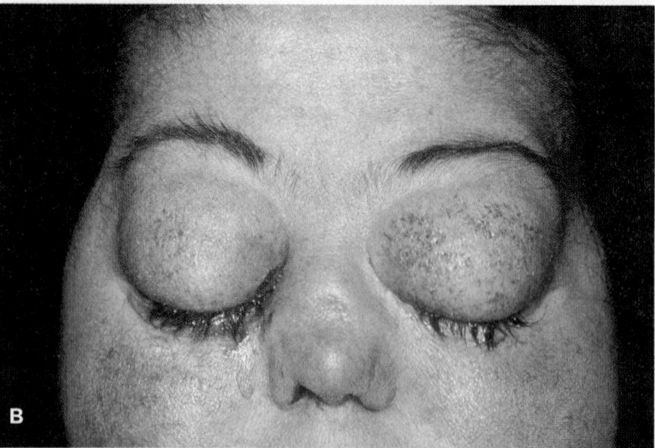

Figure 11-12 Patient with Cushing syndrome **A.** Central obesity. **B.** "Moon facies."

findings that correlate with the patient's current clinical presentation, such as metabolic alkalosis, hypernatremia, hypokalemia, and hyperglycemia, should raise suspicion for the disease.

Treatment

Patients with Cushing syndrome often have chronic or subacute symptoms. Management is guided by the clinical presentation. Affected patients may have fluid retention or, because of the osmotic diuresis brought on by hyperglycemia, may be dehydrated. Thus, fluid replacement should be dictated by the patient's volume status. Hypertension does not require specific therapy unless it is causing end-organ dysfunction or symptoms (e.g., acute heart failure, cardiac ischemia, encephalopathy, acute renal failure). If such a condition is present, administer antihypertensive treatment. Monitor the patient's vital signs, mental status, and cardiac rhythm closely.

Glucose Metabolism Disorders

Glucose metabolism disorders play a role in many clinical conditions and are associated with nonspecific symptoms, causing a potential delay in treatment. The following sections discuss some of the fundamental clinical principles to consider to promptly arrive at a diagnosis and begin appropriate treatment.

Diabetes Mellitus

Diabetes mellitus, the most common endocrine disorder, is characterized by hyperglycemia (high blood glucose levels) resulting from defects in insulin production, insulin action, or both. Glucose is a vital energy source for the body, but insulin is required for glucose to travel into the cell, where it can be used. In essence, insulin acts like a key that unlocks the cell membrane and allows the glucose to enter.

Pathophysiology

Clinically, diabetes manifests as a high level of blood glucose (hyperglycemia). A random plasma glucose level > 200 mg/dL (> 11.1 mmol/L) or a fasting serum glucose > 140 mg/dL (> 7.7 mmol/L) meets the threshold for a diagnosis of diabetes. The percentage of glycated hemoglobin (also called glycosylated hemoglobin or Hb_{A1c}) is often used as a measure of a patient's diabetes control because this percentage correlates to the average blood glucose levels over a 3-month period. Chronically poor glucose control tends to cause microvascular problems in multiple organ systems, including the heart, blood vessels, kidneys, eyes, and neurologic system. Patients with diabetes should be considered as being at high risk for coronary disease and complications from infections.

The classification of diabetes is based on the underlying pathologic process related to insulin production and insulin resistance. This classification system includes three main categories:

- *Type 1 diabetes mellitus:* characterized by inability to produce any insulin due to pancreatic beta cell destruction. This type of diabetes is typically diagnosed during childhood or adolescence and accounts for 5% to 10% of all cases of diabetes mellitus. It is believed to be due to autoimmune destruction of beta cells. Acquired type 1 diabetes is associated with pancreatectomy or severe chronic pancreatitis. Patients with type 1 diabetes usually require daily insulin administration, and so are described as "insulin-dependent."
- *Type 2 diabetes mellitus:* characterized by progressive cellular insulin resistance and a gradual failure of pancreatic beta cell insulin production. Type 2 diabetes accounts for 90% to 95% of all diagnoses of diabetes, is most common among older adults, and is associated with physical inactivity and obesity. Patients with type 2 diabetes often remain asymptomatic for years before they begin to show signs and symptoms. Type 2 diabetes is often treated initially with oral hypoglycemic medications but may eventually require newer parenteral non-insulin therapies and/or insulin therapy to maintain adequate glucose control. There has been a significant increase in the number of pediatric patients who are being diagnosed with type 2 diabetes. Increasing rates of childhood obesity and decreasing levels of physical exercise appear to be contributing factors.
- *Gestational diabetes:* characterized by glucose intolerance in pregnant persons. It typically has the same clinical presentation as type 2 diabetes. Patients usually have hyperglycemia but no acidosis. Gestational diabetes predisposes patients to future development of type 2 diabetes.

Hypoglycemia in people with diabetes tends to be the result of overdose—usually inadvertent—of insulin or less commonly oral hypoglycemic agents, or inadequate oral intake of glucose (relative to activity and medication dose). Because glucose levels must be maintained within a narrow range, diabetes is a difficult disease to control. Hypoglycemia is the most common endocrine emergency, accounting for 1% to 2% of all EMS responses. Diabetic medication overdoses may be intentional, in which cases the clinician must attend to both conditions—the hypoglycemia and the mental health condition related to intentional overdose. This also underscores the need for blood glucose measurement in all patients with altered mental status.

Other commonly seen complications of diabetes are hyperglycemia, diabetic ketoacidosis (DKA), and hyperosmolar hyperglycemic syndrome (HHS).

Signs and Symptoms

The classic clinical manifestations of diabetes mellitus are referred to as the three *P*s: polyuria, polydipsia, and polyphagia. As the levels of glucose increase in the bloodstream, the kidneys' ability to reabsorb glucose may be overwhelmed, causing glucose to "spill" into the urine and inducing an osmotic diuresis. Normally, glucose is not found in the urine, so the presence of any glucose in the urine is an abnormal finding. Weight loss, thirst, blurred vision, and fatigue may also be present.

Differential Diagnosis

Hyperglycemia can be caused by hormonal tumors, pharmacologic agents, liver disease, and muscle disorders. It can also be precipitated by an infectious process, trauma, or coronary event. Diagnostic procedures for diabetes are complex and include a thorough history, physical exam, urinalysis, and blood analysis.

Treatment

Use of a glucometer to quantify serum glucose at the patient's side has become a common practice in modern EMS. In the past, dextrose was given empirically to all patients with altered mental status without first quantifying their serum glucose. Later, researchers found that few patients benefited from such an approach. A glucometer gives rapid point-of-care glucose results, and its use in the prehospital setting has been found to be safe and accurate. Glucose levels in capillary blood are usually slightly higher than those in venous blood, and may be inaccurate in the setting of hypotension, so this possibility needs to be taken into consideration. Many glucose strips are required to be stored in temperature-controlled, airtight compartments in the ambulance to ensure their accuracy and reliability.

Hypoglycemia

Hypoglycemia, a frequent complication of diabetes, is the most common endocrine emergency. **Hypoglycemia** is generally defined as a blood glucose level < 70 mg/dL (3.3 mmol/L), although many EMS protocols use a lower target of < 60 mg/dL. Keep in mind that individual responses to blood glucose levels vary, and the levels discussed here represent averages; patients with diabetes may become symptomatic at higher glucose levels. Generally, as the plasma glucose level falls, the following sequence of events occurs in quick succession:

- First, the body decreases insulin secretion in an effort to arrest the decline in blood glucose levels.
- Next, there is an increase in the secretion of counter-regulatory hormones, primarily epinephrine and norepinephrine.
- Finally, signs and symptoms, including impaired cognition, become apparent. Once the glucose level falls to < 50 mg/dL (2.8 mmol/L), significant mental status changes occur.

Untreated hypoglycemia is associated with significant morbidity and mortality. To decrease these risks, you should be able recognize the signs and symptoms and be prepared to initiate treatment quickly and effectively.

Pathophysiology

Hypoglycemia in persons with insulin-dependent diabetes often is the result of having taken too much insulin, too little food, or both. Unlike other tissues, which can usually metabolize fat or protein in addition to sugar, the tissues of the CNS (including the brain) depend entirely on glucose as their source of energy. If the level of glucose in the blood drops dramatically, the brain is literally starved. Triggers of hypoglycemia include the following:

- Exogenous insulin administration (intentional and unintentional)
- Medications
  - Oral hypoglycemic agents
  - Beta blockers
  - Antimalarial drugs
- Alcohol ingestion
- Aggressive treatment of hyperglycemia
- Malnutrition
- Medication adjustments
- Insulin pump failure
- Sepsis
- Kidney disease
- Liver disease
- Pancreatic tumors
- Thyroid disease
  - Hypothyroidism
  - Hyperthyroidism
- Adrenal disease
  - Addison disease

Hypoglycemia in patients who have no history of diabetes is called *fasting* or *postprandial hypoglycemia*. Fasting hypoglycemia is usually the result of an imbalance between glucose utilization and production. Postprandial hypoglycemia is characterized by alimentary hyperinsulinism and is commonly seen in patients who have undergone gastric surgery. A number of conditions may elicit fasting hypoglycemia, including severe liver disease, pancreatic tumors (e.g., insulinomas), enzyme defects, drug overdoses (e.g., insulin, sulfonylureas), and severe infection. The clinical characteristics are similar to those of diabetic hypoglycemia.

Signs and Symptoms

Clinical manifestations of hypoglycemia usually evolve rapidly. The patient will seek treatment for myriad signs and symptoms directly related to the release of endogenous stress hormones, including diaphoresis; tachycardia; tremors; and pale, cold, clammy skin. If hypoglycemia is not treated, the patient may experience an altered mental status and generalized seizures. When treating patients who are actively seizing or have an altered mental status after a seizure, EMS clinicians should obtain a blood glucose level. Given that only 1.2% of these patients will have hypoglycemia, therefore, administration of an anticonvulsant should not be delayed by efforts to measure the blood glucose. While the definition of hypoglycemia is a blood glucose level < 70 mg/dL, the absolute level at which signs and symptoms appear may be altered by the patient's medical history, age, sex, and overall health. For example, an older adult with a complex medical history may have signs of severe hypoglycemia at a glucose level > 50 mg/dL (> 2.8 mmol/L). By comparison, a young adult may not show signs of severe hypoglycemia until the level falls to < 50 mg/dL (< 2.8 mmol/L).

Most clinical manifestations of hypoglycemia are generated by counter-regulatory hormones (e.g., epinephrine), which are secreted in response to a low glucose concentration. Signs and symptoms may include the following:

- Sweating
- Tremors
- Nervousness
- Tachycardia
- Altered level of consciousness or behavior
- Seizures
- Coma

Some patients may be taking a medication, such as a beta blocker, whose effects initially mask the signs of hypoglycemia. They can rapidly lose consciousness or begin having seizures in the absence of any early symptoms of hypoglycemia.

Differential Diagnosis

Differential diagnoses may include adrenal insufficiency/crisis, anxiety disorders, severe hypothyroidism/myxedema coma, and other causes of altered mental status. If the comprehensive history and physical exam are suspicious for hypoglycemia, the diagnosis can be confirmed with a serum glucose test.

Treatment

Long-term management of diabetes emphasizes tight plasma glucose control, which means getting the blood glucose level as close to normal (nondiabetic) as possible by safely using subcutaneous insulin injections, oral antihyperglycemics, or a combination of both. This tight control helps to decrease the risks for long-term complications such as renal failure and heart disease. However, patients on such regimens are at increased risk of hypoglycemic episodes.

To prevent further complications, such as seizures or permanent brain damage, begin providing glucose immediately when a patient is symptomatically hypoglycemic. The simplest option is to give oral glucose in the form of a small snack, a sugar-containing beverage, or a sugar gel. This option should always be considered in awake and alert patients who are able to swallow. For patients who have altered mentation or cannot safely swallow due to risk of aspiration, administration of 10% dextrose (250 mL of $D_{10}W$) by rapid IV infusion is the treatment of choice. In the past, 50% dextrose or $D_{50}W$ had been the standard, but this option is now deemphasized because administering such a high concentration of glucose is associated with more serious complications (such as tissue damage if extravasation occurs). Studies have found no difference in the amount of time necessary for a hypoglycemic patient to regain consciousness when the 10% and 50% options are compared. When patients are given $D_{10}W$, they may receive a considerably smaller amount of glucose while achieving the same therapeutic response and are less likely to have a high glucose level after treatment.

If rapid IV access proves difficult, intramuscular (IM) or intranasal administration of glucagon can be an effective alternative. Be aware that glucagon may not have the intended effect in patients with chronic illness who have depleted glycogen stores (e.g., those with alcohol use disorder and chronic liver disease). Recovery time with glucagon is significantly longer than with IV dextrose, and glucagon may cause side effects such as nausea and vomiting. If this medication is used, the standard dose is 1 to 2 mg IM. Glucagon autoinjectors and nasal powder injectors are available to appropriately trained lower-level EMS clinicians and laypersons, but the current cost of these glucagon devices limits their use in some EMS agencies. After regaining consciousness, patients treated with glucagon should be provided with oral food intake, preferably complex carbohydrates, to replete their glycogen stores.

Management of hypoglycemia in patients without diabetes is similar to management of the condition in patients with diabetes. However, hypoglycemia may recur in patients without diabetes, especially in those with drug overdose. Such patients may require more than one dose of dextrose or even a continuous infusion.

Patients may wish to refuse transportation to the hospital after successful treatment of hypoglycemia by EMS clinicians, and some agencies have protocols for treatment-in-place without transport for many of these patients. While some of the literature supports this practice, caution is warranted when the patient is taking any long-acting antihyperglycemic medications (insulin or oral medications) due to the risk of recurrent hypoglycemia. Protocols should differentiate conditions in which patients can be treated without transport and those in which online medical oversight is necessary before considering nontransport. Online medical oversight is particularly warranted with patients who are minors, those on oral hypoglycemic medications, those unable to tolerate taking food, and those living alone.

Additionally, a careful search for the cause of the hypoglycemic episode should be undertaken. Some patients may have an obvious cause, such as a change in their medication regimen or a lack of oral intake, that can be readily addressed. In contrast, unexplained episodes of hypoglycemia may be the first manifestation of other conditions that are increasing the body's metabolic needs (e.g., infection, trauma).

Diabetic Ketoacidosis

Diabetic ketoacidosis (DKA) is an acute endocrine emergency in which insulin deficiency and an excessive glucagon level combine to create a hyperglycemic, acidotic, volume-depleted state. This condition is often associated with electrolyte imbalances. It is characterized by a plasma glucose concentration > 350 mg/dL (> 19.4 mmol/L), ketone production, a serum bicarbonate level < 15 mEq/L, and anion gap metabolic acidosis. The mortality rate for DKA ranges from 9% to 14%.

Pathophysiology

DKA may be elicited by certain metabolic stressors such as infection, myocardial infarction, trauma, and sometimes pregnancy. One frequently encountered trigger is an interruption of the insulin regimen of a person with diabetes. Lack of insulin prevents glucose from entering cells; consequently, the cells become starved of the glucose necessary for cellular metabolism and turn to other sources of energy such as fat. As a result, glucose begins to accumulate in the bloodstream.

Overflow of glucose into the renal tubules draws water, sodium, potassium, magnesium, and other ions into the urine, creating a significant osmotic diuresis. This diuresis, combined with vomiting, produces volume depletion, electrolyte imbalances, and subsequently shock. These osmotic changes are largely responsible for the declining mental status of a patient with DKA and are particularly dangerous in children. The clinical hallmark of DKA is metabolic acidosis, which is discussed later. Physiologically, the body attempts to compensate and eliminate acids by breathing faster and deeper (Kussmaul respiration) and retaining more bicarbonate renally. Acidosis encourages the shift of potassium into the blood, from where it is then lost via the osmotic diuresis occurring in the kidneys. This process results in a pseudohyperkalemia—that is, an initially high blood level that rapidly changes to hypokalemia with the treatment of DKA.

Signs and Symptoms

Patients with DKA are dehydrated and appear ill. They usually report polydipsia, polyphagia, and polyuria. Patients with severe DKA will exhibit altered mental status. In addition, tachycardia, rapid breathing, and orthostatic changes are likely to be present. End-tidal carbon dioxide ($ETCO_2$) will be low, reflecting the metabolic acidosis and compensatory respiratory alkalosis present in DKA. Signs and symptoms of DKA include the following:

- Nausea and vomiting
- Abdominal pain (especially common in children)
- Tachypnea/hyperpnea
- Fruity breath odor
- Fatigue and weakness
- Increased diuresis
- Altered level of consciousness
- Orthostatic hypotension
- Cardiac dysrhythmia
- Seizures
- Hypovolemic shock in severe cases

Differential Diagnosis

Several conditions bear a clinical resemblance to DKA, and distinguishing among them may be difficult in the field without the diagnostic testing used in hospitals. Conditions that produce acidosis—sepsis, for example—may mimic DKA. Prolonged fasting in a third-trimester pregnant patient or nursing mother who is not eating properly can also resemble DKA. People who abuse alcohol may have a fruity breath odor and a rapid respiratory rate due to alcoholic ketoacidosis. In any case, rapid breathing should raise the clinician's suspicion that the patient's body is trying to compensate for metabolic acidosis. It is critical to check the patient's blood glucose level to try to narrow the differential diagnosis.

Make sure to perform a 12-lead ECG if you suspect DKA. The information it provides could change the management strategy (e.g., if the ECG reveals a myocardial infarction). In addition, electrolyte abnormalities often accompany diabetic emergencies, and a 12-lead ECG could reveal worrisome anomalies. Although many conditions can present similarly to DKA, the initial treatment steps are often the same.

Treatment

Patients with severe DKA look critically ill and require immediate treatment. A patient with an altered level of consciousness may be actively vomiting and, therefore, at risk of aspiration. If intubation is necessary to protect the airway, remember that patients with DKA breathe rapidly to compensate for their metabolic acidosis; therefore, if you intubate such a patient, you must maintain hyperventilation to prevent deterioration of their acid–base status.

Initiate aggressive fluid resuscitation using 0.9% normal saline. Adult patients with DKA usually require 3 to 6 L of fluid during initial resuscitation. Children may have similar fluid deficits but must be managed much more cautiously to prevent severe complications resulting from rapid electrolyte shifts. Monitor patients with DKA closely because their condition can decompensate rapidly. Patients with a history of heart failure can easily go into fluid overload; therefore, be cautious when administering IV fluids to these patients. Consider triggering causes of DKA, such as myocardial infarction, and provide appropriate treatment.

Insulin therapy is a mainstay of treatment for DKA, along with fluid resuscitation and electrolyte correction. Generally, however, insulin is not administered in the prehospital setting. EMS services that transport patients on insulin infusions (i.e., interfacility services) should have a protocol in place to guide management of such patients during transport. You must be able to recognize potential for, and emergence of, side effects of continuous insulin therapy. High-dose insulin is associated with iatrogenic hypoglycemia and hypokalemia, for example. This effect results from the shift of glucose and potassium into the cells after insulin administration. Although patients with DKA may initially appear to have hyperkalemia, this condition reflects a temporary shift of potassium out of the cells into the bloodstream caused by the acidosis. In reality, they typically have a total-body deficiency in potassium. Abnormal potassium levels can result in life-threatening cardiac arrhythmias, so you should confirm the patient's most recent potassium level before beginning transport.

Key treatment considerations for patients with DKA or HHS include the following points:

- If the patient is intubated, maintain hyperventilation to prevent worsening of the acidosis. This is one of the most critical steps in managing critically ill patients with DKA. If you do not hyperventilate these patients and monitor $ETCO_2$, they may not be able to compensate for their acidosis and can die quickly.
- Provide fluid rehydration. You may need to rapidly administer 1 to 2 L of normal saline. Monitor glucose levels regularly because fluid resuscitation will decrease glucose levels.
- Evaluate the ECG for signs of hyperkalemia (peaked T waves, widened QRS complex, loss of P waves, bradycardia, or sine wave morphology), and treat accordingly.
- In pediatric patients, administer initial fluid resuscitation of 20 mL/kg. Additional fluids should be administered only with expert consultation through online medical oversight.
- Antiemetics are often needed.

For extended critical care transports, consider the following treatments:

- Change the IV solution to D_5W in 0.45% normal saline when glucose levels fall to < 300 mg/dL (< 16.6 mmol/L).
- Correct electrolytes when indicated, using the following guidelines:
  - *Potassium.* If the potassium level is low, first ensure that the patient's renal functioning is adequate, and then add 20 to 40 mEq/L of potassium chloride for each liter of fluid administered. If the patient is able to swallow and is not vomiting, oral potassium is preferred.
  - *Magnesium.* If the magnesium level is low, correct the level with 1 to 2 g of magnesium sulfate in the first 2 L of fluid administered.
  - *Acidosis.* If the pH < 7, correct it by adding 44 to 100 mEq of sodium bicarbonate to a liter of IV fluid.
  - *Complications.* Be aware of the potential complications of insulin infusions, such as hypokalemia and hypoglycemia.
- In cases of suspected DKA, constant monitoring is essential. Treat underlying causes if possible, and transport the patient to a hospital with intensive care unit capabilities.

An important consideration in DKA treatment relates to fluid administration in pediatric patients. Rapid shifts in fluid and electrolyte balances may cause potentially fatal cerebral edema in a small percentage of children with DKA. Although the specific risk factors for development of cerebral edema have not been definitively identified, consensus guidelines recommend a measured approach to fluid resuscitation in pediatric patients with DKA. While these patients are most certainly volume depleted, they are rarely in hypovolemic shock, and the initial bolus should not exceed 10 to 20 mL/kg over 1 to 2 hours unless the patient demonstrates hemodynamic instability. Research is investigating this issue, but the current body of knowledge remains uncertain about the care of such patients.

Complications of Treatment of DKA

The treatment of DKA is difficult and complex, requiring the participation of a multidisciplinary group of medical professionals. Even then, complications may develop in some patients. Five major complications increase morbidity and mortality in the setting of DKA:

- *Hypokalemia* can occur as a result of inadequate potassium replacement during treatment because aggressive insulin treatment shifts potassium into the cells.
- *Hypoglycemia* can be attributed to aggressive treatment and failure to closely observe glucose levels. It is important to begin administering a D_5W solution when glucose levels fall to < 300 mg/dL.
- *Fluid overload* can be caused by aggressive fluid resuscitation in patients with chronic heart failure.
- *Alkalosis* can be caused by overly aggressive treatment with bicarbonate. It can further complicate electrolyte imbalances, specifically by increasing potassium requirements as potassium is displaced into body cells.
- *Cerebral edema*, the most feared complication of DKA treatment, occurs as a result of rapid osmolar shifts. Cerebral edema generally appears 6 to 10 hours after the initiation of therapy and carries a mortality rate of 90%. You should suspect this complication in a patient who becomes comatose after acidosis is reversed during treatment of DKA.

Hyperosmolar Hyperglycemic Syndrome

Hyperosmolar hyperglycemic syndrome (HHS), previously referred to as hyperosmolar hyperglycemic nonketotic coma (HHNC), is a serious diabetic emergency, carrying a mortality rate of 10% to 50%. Clinicians may not be able to differentiate DKA from HHS in the field, but they should suspect the latter diagnosis based on the patient's history, extremely elevated glucose level, and absence of low $ETCO_2$. HHS is more common in patients with type 2 diabetes mellitus and is triggered by the same stressors that cause DKA. This condition is characterized by the following findings:

- Elevated plasma glucose concentration, often > 600 mg/dL (> 33.3 mmol/L)
- Absent ketone production
- Increased serum osmolality, usually > 315 mOsm/kg, due to severe dehydration

HHS is associated with significant dehydration and a decline in mental status. Occasionally, it progresses to full coma. In contrast to DKA, acidosis and ketosis are usually absent, so $ETCO_2$ will not be decreased. It is important to realize that other factors, such as underlying sepsis or respiratory dysfunction, may still alter the $ETCO_2$.

Pathophysiology

The pathophysiology of HHS is complex but similar to that of DKA. This condition does not usually develop suddenly, but rather evolves over a period of several days; the time frame varies, depending on the patient's overall health. HHS usually occurs in older adults and in patients debilitated by comorbid conditions. As in DKA, the hallmark is decreased insulin action, which triggers a volley of counter-regulatory mechanisms that increase serum glucose. Once insulin function decreases, gluconeogenesis (the body's internal manufacture of glucose), glycogenolysis (the release of glucose stored as glycogen), and decreased glucose uptake in the periphery begin to dominate. Hyperglycemia then pulls fluid into the intravascular space, triggering osmotic diuresis, which in turn causes hypotension and volume deficit. Patients are initially able to maintain their intravascular volume with constant fluid intake, but the diuresis eventually overtakes the system. Keep in mind that other conditions such as sepsis may be causing further volume depletion.

Common causes of HHS include the following:

- Infection, particularly of the respiratory, GI, or genitourinary system
- Myocardial infarction
- Stroke
- Medications that decrease insulin effect (e.g., thiazide diuretics, beta blockers, glucocorticoids, some antipsychotics)
- Medications that cause fluid loss
- Not taking medications to treat diabetes
- Undiagnosed diabetes

Signs and Symptoms

Patients with HHS are usually acutely ill, with marked volume depletion, altered mental status, nausea, vomiting, abdominal pain, tachypnea, and tachycardia. Many of these patients have at least a 25% fluid deficit. In addition, they may have focal neurologic deficits and seizures or signs of stroke. Signs and symptoms of HHS include the following:

- Fever
- Dehydration
- Vomiting and abdominal pain
- Hypotension
- Tachycardia
- Rapid breathing
- Thirst (polydipsia)
- Polyuria, then oliguria
- Focal seizures
- Altered level of consciousness
- Focal neurologic deficits

Differential Diagnosis

Many conditions have signs and symptoms similar to those of DKA (see the earlier discussion) and HHS. In most cases, the EMS clinician's initial intervention will be similar for all of these possible illnesses, but be alert for time-sensitive underlying conditions that can cause DKA and HHS, such as myocardial infarction and sepsis.

To differentiate HHS from DKA, remember that the former is usually accompanied by a more profound decrease in mental status. Additionally, $ETCO_2$ may help distinguish the presence or lack of a metabolic acidosis. Signs and symptoms of HHS can be confusing, because they may resemble those associated with hypoglycemia. If blood glucose cannot be rapidly evaluated, hypoglycemia must be assumed until proven otherwise.

Treatment

The initial management of a patient with HHS is the same as that for a patient with DKA. Take immediate steps to stabilize the patient's airway, breathing, and circulation. The patient may have significant volume depletion; begin IV fluid resuscitation immediately. The initial fluid of choice is an isotonic crystalloid or 0.9% normal saline. Early boluses may be necessary to stabilize the patient hemodynamically. Use caution, however, when the patient has comorbidities such as heart failure. Remember that fluid administration alone will correct much of the hyperglycemia. Be aware that the management controversies linked to DKA apply to HHS as well. For example, rapid correction of serum osmolality can predispose patients—especially children—to the development of cerebral edema.

Acid–Base Disorders

As previously discussed, endocrine disorders involve the body's overproduction or underproduction of certain hormones. In contrast, acid–base disorders affect the body's ability to process certain nutrients and vitamins.

Acid–Base Balance

The body requires the ongoing maintenance of a delicate balance, or homeostasis, to function optimally. Fluid, electrolytes, and pH all play critical roles in maintaining homeostasis. Acid–base stability is crucial to sustain life and maintain health. Acid–base balance is achieved through a variety of buffer systems and compensatory mechanisms. Body fluids, the kidneys, and the lungs play a pivotal role in maintaining this balance.

Acid–base balance is measured by examining pH (the concentration of hydrogen ions) and is associated with a narrow safety margin (normal serum pH is 7.35–7.45). Acid–base imbalances can vary in severity based on the degree of pH change. A pH < 7.35 constitutes acidosis; a pH level > 7.45 constitutes alkalosis. These pH derangements are classified according to their primary cause as either metabolic or respiratory. Death can occur if serum pH levels fall to < 6.8 or rise to > 7.8. Changes in pH can result from a variety of conditions, including infections, organ failure, and trauma. In many cases, the acid–base fluctuations will cause more negative effects than the causative condition; in consequence, the resulting acid–base imbalance is often corrected before treating the underlying condition.

Two body systems can compensate for pH imbalances—the renal and respiratory systems. If the cause of the imbalance originates within one of those systems, the other system will have to act as the primary compensatory mechanism. Thus, if the problem originates in the lungs, the kidneys will manage it. If the problem originates outside the lungs, the lungs will manage it (Table 11-3).

Buffers

Buffers are the chemicals that combine with an acid or base to resist changes in pH. Buffering is an immediate reaction to counteract pH variations until longer-term compensation is established. The body has four major buffer mechanisms: the bicarbonate–carbonic acid system, the phosphate system, the hemoglobin system, and the protein system.

Respiratory Regulation

The respiratory system manages pH deviations by changing the amount of expired CO_2 (acid excretion). Increased minute ventilation will lead to excretion of more CO_2, thereby decreasing acidity. Decreased minute ventilation will lead to excretion of less CO_2, increasing acidity. Chemoreceptors that sense pH changes trigger this change in breathing pattern. The only way the lungs can remove acids is through the elimination of CO_2—the lungs cannot remove other acids. The respiratory system is also a mechanism that can respond quickly to pH imbalances, but its quick action is short lived. It reaches its maximum compensatory response in 12 to 24 hours, but can maintain the changes in breathing pattern for only a limited time before becoming fatigued. A patient cannot hyperventilate for long.

Renal Regulation

The renal system is the slowest mechanism to react to pH changes, taking hours to days to achieve its buffering effect, but it is the longest lasting. The kidneys respond by changing the excretion or retention of hydrogen (acid) or bicarbonate (base). The renal system acts to balance

Table 11-3 Acid-Base Disorders

Acid-Base Disturbance	pH	Partial Pressure of Carbon Dioxide (PCO_2)	Bicarbonate (HCO_3)	Body's Compensatory Response	Timing of Compensation
Metabolic acidosis	Decreased	Normal, then decreased	Decreased	Respiratory compensation with hyperventilation and decreased PCO_2	Immediate
Respiratory acidosis	Decreased	Increased	Increased or neutral	Kidneys compensate by retaining HCO_3	Delayed
Metabolic alkalosis	Increased	Normal, then increased	Increased	Respiratory compensation with hypoventilation and increased PCO_2	Immediate
Respiratory alkalosis	Increased	Decreased	Decreased or neutral	Kidneys compensate by releasing HCO_3	Delayed

pH levels by permanently removing hydrogen from the body. Additionally, the kidneys can reabsorb acids or bases and produce bicarbonate to correct pH imbalances.

Compensation

To maintain homeostasis, the body will take actions to compensate for the pH changes. The body never overcompensates; instead, the pH is adjusted so that it remains just within the normal range. The cause of the imbalance often determines the compensatory change. For example, if pH is becoming more acidic because of lung disease that limits gas exchange (e.g., emphysema), the renal system will kick in to compensate for the problem by retaining more bicarbonate and excreting more hydrogen. If a lung disease is increasing CO_2 excretion (e.g., hyperventilation), which increases the pH, the kidneys will compensate by decreasing bicarbonate production and hydrogen excretion. In contrast, if the problem originates outside the lungs, the lungs can compensate for it. For example, if a condition increases the loss of an acid (e.g., vomiting), the lungs will decrease the rate and depth of respirations to retain more CO_2. If a condition increases the loss of a base (e.g., diarrhea), the lungs will increase the rate and depth of respirations to excrete more CO_2. If the kidneys and lungs cannot compensate to restore the pH levels to the normal range, cellular activities will be affected, leading to disease states. Various mathematical formulas exist to calculate expected levels of compensatory responses and help determine if a condition is acute or chronic.

Respiratory Acidosis

Respiratory acidosis is one of the most common acid–base problems encountered in the prehospital setting. This condition is characterized by a decline in pH as a result of CO_2 retention. Hypoventilation is the classic example of a clinical problem that leads to CO_2 retention.

Respiratory acidosis may be classified as acute or chronic. The only way to distinguish between these states is to determine whether the body has begun to retain bicarbonate to compensate for the acidosis, which is possible only through lab analysis and trending of these values over time. During the acute phase, the serum bicarbonate level is normal. Once the body begins to retain bicarbonate, it has made the transition to chronic status.

Pathophysiology

Any disorder that results in hypoventilation (e.g., primary pulmonary problems, airway obstruction, illnesses that depress the respiratory drive) will cause respiratory acidosis. Precipitants of respiratory acidosis are summarized in Table 11-4.

Signs and Symptoms

EMS clinicians may encounter different clinical scenarios involving respiratory acidosis, depending on the severity of the primary problem. Common signs and symptoms include weakness, breathing difficulty, and altered level of consciousness. Noting the level of consciousness is

Table 11-4 Precipitants of Respiratory Acidosis

Acute	Chronic
Pharmacologic CNS Depression	***Lung Diseases***
■ Opioids ■ Benzodiazepines ■ Alcohol ingestion ■ Gamma-hydroxybutyrate (GHB) toxicity	■ Chronic bronchitis ■ Emphysema ■ Pulmonary fibrosis
Lung Diseases	***Neuromuscular Diseases***
■ Interstitial edema ■ Pneumonia ■ Pneumothorax ■ Flail chest	■ Muscular dystrophy ■ Myasthenia gravis
Airway Problems	***Obesity***
■ Foreign body ■ Aspiration ■ Bronchospasm ■ Apnea	■ Obesity hypoventilation syndrome ■ Sleep apnea
CNS-Induced Hypoventilation	
■ Guillain-Barré syndrome ■ Primary CNS disorders ■ Brain injury	

CNS, central nervous system.

critical when evaluating a patient with suspected respiratory acidosis because it may indicate the severity of the process and signal the need for advanced airway management. For example, in a patient with COPD who has a diminished mental status, a high level of CO_2 is most likely responsible for the altered level of consciousness. Such a patient has a higher risk of complications such as aspiration and, therefore, requires more aggressive intervention.

Differential Diagnosis

Many conditions can cause hypoventilation and/or impair gas exchange, resulting in respiratory acidosis (see Table 11-3).

Treatment

Standard monitoring equipment should be used according to the clinician's scope of practice, including an ECG monitor, SpO_2, and $ETCO_2$. The $ETCO_2$ measurement is an approximate measure of partial pressure of arterial carbon dioxide ($PaCO_2$) and is typically accurate to within 5 to 10 mm Hg. Keep in mind that $ETCO_2$ is always lower than $PaCO_2$, and its measurement may be erroneous in patients without an advanced airway or who have significant ventilation–perfusion (V-Q) mismatching. After the initial evaluation and stabilization of the patient's airway, breathing, and circulation, therapy should focus on correcting the patient's minute ventilation to decrease the CO_2 level and thereby correct the acidosis. Depending on the etiology, this may be accomplished either by assisting ventilation or by providing pharmacologic intervention. Ventilatory assistance can range from airway positioning to bag-valve mask ventilation with a nasopharyngeal airway or oropharyngeal airway, continuous positive airway pressure (CPAP) or bilevel positive airway pressure (BiPAP), or endotracheal intubation with ventilator support. Naloxone administration can reverse respiratory depression related to the toxic effects of opioid overdose. Albuterol, ipratropium, and other medications may improve hypoventilation in patients with COPD.

All newly hypoxic patients should be treated with supplemental oxygen—but use caution when attempting aggressive correction of oxygen saturation in patients with COPD or emphysema. Patients with chronically elevated CO_2 levels (e.g., patients with COPD who chronically retain CO_2) may have switched from relying on the normal hypercapnic respiratory drive to relying on the hypoxic drive. Thus, they must be monitored for decreased respiratory effort when supplemental oxygen is administered. Chapter 3, *Respiratory Disorders*, discusses the hypercapnic and hypoxic drives in more detail.

Respiratory Alkalosis

Respiratory alkalosis is caused by an increase in ventilations per minute, tidal volume, or both. It is characterized by a decreased $PaCO_2$ level and increased pH. The only way to differentiate between acute and chronic respiratory alkalosis is to measure the patient's serum bicarbonate. A patient with acute respiratory alkalosis will have a normal serum bicarbonate level; a patient with chronic respiratory alkalosis will have a decreased serum bicarbonate level.

Pathophysiology

Respiratory alkalosis usually emerges as a secondary compensatory mechanism for a primary metabolic problem, but it can be a primary derangement as well. Some of the causes of primary respiratory alkalosis include aspirin overdose, anxiety reaction, and pulmonary embolism. On occasion, this condition may be a normal physiologic response. The classic example is alkalemia of pregnancy, in which the pH is 7.46 to 7.5. This condition is primarily respiratory in origin and is characterized by a partial pressure

Table 11-5 Precipitants of Respiratory Alkalosis

Pulmonary
■ Pulmonary embolism ■ Pneumonia (bacterial or viral) ■ Acute pulmonary edema ■ Assisted hyperventilation
Infections
■ Septicemia
Drug Induced
■ Sympathomimetic and stimulant drugs ■ Thyroxine ■ Aspirin or caffeine toxicity
Hypoxia
■ Ventilation–perfusion mismatch ■ Altitude changes ■ Severe anemia
Hyperventilation
■ Hysteria/anxiety ■ Psychogenic disorders ■ Central nervous system tumor ■ Stroke
Metabolic and Electrolyte Disturbances
■ Diabetic ketoacidosis ■ Alcoholic ketoacidosis ■ Hepatic insufficiency ■ Encephalopathy ■ Hyponatremia ■ Metabolic acidosis

of carbon dioxide (PCO_2) of 31 to 35 mm Hg. Precipitants of respiratory alkalosis are summarized in Table 11-5.

Signs and Symptoms

The patient's clinical presentation depends on whether the respiratory alkalosis is chronic or acute. Most signs and symptoms are nonspecific and are related to peripheral or CNS complaints, such as paresthesia of the face or distal extremities, lightheadedness, dizziness, and muscular pain or cramps.

Differential Diagnosis

The diagnosis of respiratory alkalosis may not be obvious because some of its signs and symptoms are almost identical to those of certain electrolyte emergencies, such as hypocalcemia. A thorough history and physical exam will yield clues as to the underlying cause of the respiratory alkalosis, which may guide the clinician's management strategies. Be careful not to overlook life-threatening toxicologic causes such as aspirin overdose.

Treatment

Administer oxygen to patients with hypoxemia without delay, and take steps to stabilize and support the airway, breathing, and circulation. For hyperventilation caused by anxiety, use coaching techniques to calm the patient. Instruct the patient to use pursed-lip breathing. To avoid precipitating hypoxia, do not use a paper bag or a nonrebreather mask (NRB) without oxygen attached.

Metabolic Acidosis

Metabolic acidosis is caused by a deficiency of bicarbonate ion (base) and an excess of hydrogen ion (acid). In the acute state, the body's physiologic response is to hyperventilate and compensate by reducing $PaCO_2$. This is sometimes referred to as "blowing off CO_2." Chronic metabolic acidosis is considered to be present when the renal system begins to reabsorb bicarbonate in an effort to compensate for the acidosis.

Pathophysiology

Metabolic acidosis is generated by three mechanisms: decreased renal excretion of acids, increased production or ingestion of acids, and loss of buffering mechanisms in the body.

Signs and Symptoms

The clinical manifestations of metabolic acidosis are related to the underlying condition and the body's compensatory mechanisms. Most patients have nausea, vomiting, abdominal pain, a rapid and deep respiratory pattern (Kussmaul respirations), and, in more severe cases, an altered level of consciousness and shock.

Differential Diagnosis

Metabolic acidosis is classified as either non–anion-gap acidosis or anion-gap acidosis. The anion gap is calculated using the following formula:

$$\mathbf{AG = Na^+ - (Cl^- + HCO_3)}$$

This information gives the clinician an estimate of the concentration of unmeasured anions in the plasma. An anion gap of 12 to 15 is considered normal. An elevated gap points to conditions that may cause acidosis. The mnemonic CAT MUDPILES can help you remember the precipitants of high-anion-gap metabolic acidosis

RAPID RECALL BOX 11-1

CAT MUDPILES

Mnemonic for precipitants of high-anion-gap metabolic acidosis:

- **C**arbon monoxide or **C**yanide intoxication
- **A**lcohol intoxication or alcoholic ketoacidosis, **A**cetaminophen overdose
- **T**oluene exposure
- **M**ethanol exposure, **M**etformin
- **U**remia
- **D**iabetic ketoacidosis
- **P**araldehyde ingestion, **P**henformin
- **I**soniazid or iron intoxication, **I**buprofen overdose
- **L**actic acidosis
- **E**thylene glycol intoxication
- **S**alicylate/acetylsalicylic acid (ASA) intoxication

RAPID RECALL BOX 11-2

F-USED CARS

Mnemonic for precipitants of normal-anion-gap metabolic acidosis:

- **F**istulae, pancreatic
- **U**reteroenteric conduits
- **S**aline administration (0.9% normal saline)
- **E**ndocrine dysfunction
- **D**iarrhea
- **C**arbonic anhydrase inhibitor ingestion
- **A**rginine, lysine (parenteral nutrition)
- **R**enal tubular acidosis
- **S**pironolactone (diuretic) ingestion

(**Rapid Recall Box 11-1**). The mnemonic F-USED CARS will help bring to mind the causes of normal-anion-gap metabolic acidosis (**Rapid Recall Box 11-2**).

Prehospital clinicians may not have access to the laboratory information necessary to calculate the anion gap. Management decisions, therefore, are often made on the basis of sound clinical judgment, a thorough history, and physical exam findings. A critical care transport clinician conducting a hospital transfer may have laboratory values available for calculating the anion gap and can adjust the differential diagnosis accordingly. Capnography can also provide key information, but it seldom changes prehospital treatment in the endocrine cases listed in this chapter. A patient with tachypnea and a low PCO_2 should be suspected to have metabolic acidosis or a primary respiratory alkalosis, as previously discussed.

When patients present with clinical signs of acidosis, the following five conditions must be considered:

- *Diabetic ketoacidosis*. As discussed earlier in the chapter, DKA is caused by inadequate insulin as a result of poor compliance or increased need. Patients with diabetes sometimes require higher insulin doses during periods of infection, after trauma, or in other circumstances that increase metabolic demands. DKA sets in when glucose utilization is impaired and fatty acids are metabolized, causing the formation of ketone bodies that generate hydrogen ions. If more acids are produced than the body's buffering system is able to tolerate, acidosis ensues.
- *Renal failure*. The kidneys are vital in maintaining an optimal acid–base balance. The renal tubules have the primary responsibility for eliminating hydrogen ions. This function is directly related to the filtration rate of the kidneys, known as the glomerular filtration rate. Any pathology that alters this process will increase the concentration of hydrogen ions, especially in the form of hydrogen sulfate (HSO_4) and hydrogen phosphate (HPO_4) increasing the anion gap. Patients with chronic renal failure will have some degree of anion gap acidosis, though the gap rarely exceeds 25. Patients with acute renal failure, however, more often have hyperchloremic non–anion-gap acidosis.
- *Lactic acidosis*. Lactic acid is largely generated when a significant number of cells in the body are inadequately perfused. Hypoperfusion shifts the cellular metabolism from aerobic (with oxygen) to anaerobic (without oxygen). Anaerobic metabolism produces lactic acid. This reaction occurs in medical conditions associated with hypoperfusion (e.g., sepsis, ischemia, extreme physical exertion states, prolonged seizures, circulatory shock). Lactic acidosis occurs when lactic acid accumulates in larger amounts than the body can buffer.
- *Toxin ingestion*. Toxic metabolites that cause metabolic acidosis may be a by-product of ingestion of toxins such as acetylsalicylic acid (ASA), ethylene glycol, methanol, and isoniazid. Patients with toxin-induced metabolic acidosis show some degree of respiratory compensation. The toxin must be identified as soon as possible because an antidote may be available to prevent further adverse effects.
- *Alcohol ketoacidosis*. This condition is caused by abrupt cessation of intake after a prolonged period of ingesting a considerable amount of alcohol. The main problem—accumulation of keto acids—is precipitated by dehydration, hormone imbalance,

and chronic malnutrition. Although alcohol ketoacidosis is similar in presentation to DKA, blood glucose levels are normal or low. Patients with alcohol ketoacidosis often have mixed acid–base disorders associated with the vomiting that accompanies alcohol withdrawal.

Treatment

Most patients with metabolic acidosis will require a significant amount of volume resuscitation. Rapidly establish IV access to replenish volume status. Support the patient's airway, breathing, and circulation with supplemental oxygen as appropriate, and ensure adequate ventilation. In patients with a history of renal failure or heart failure, use caution to avoid causing pulmonary edema when administering IV fluids. If the patient needs ventilatory support, be sure to maintain hyperventilation. Patients with metabolic acidosis are hyperventilating as a respiratory compensatory mechanism, and if they are sedated or paralyzed for intubation, their metabolic acidosis will worsen. Initiate adjunct treatments based on the primary etiology. For example, patients with high-anion-gap metabolic acidosis due to DKA can be started on insulin.

The use of sodium bicarbonate may be necessary for patients with certain conditions that elicit acute metabolic acidosis, but administration of bicarbonate can be fraught with complications, including hypocalcemia, volume overload, CNS acidosis, hypokalemia, and impaired oxygen delivery. Nevertheless, despite the controversy that surrounds its use, administration of sodium bicarbonate may be useful in treating certain life-threatening conditions. A dilute bicarbonate infusion rather than a rapid push of concentrated solution is preferred in most cases. Clinicians use blood gas and plasma electrolyte values to guide the decision of whether to administer bicarbonate. Although such information is unlikely to be available in the prehospital setting, administering bicarbonate is warranted in the following circumstances:

- Cardiac arrest with suspected metabolic acidosis (e.g., an arteriovenous fistula is visible)
- Crush injury prior to release of the involved body part
- Overdose with tricyclic antidepressants (ECG shows QRS complex widening > 0.10 second)
- Severe metabolic acidosis, particularly in patients with kidney injury)

Metabolic Alkalosis

Metabolic alkalosis is produced by illnesses that raise the level of serum bicarbonate or reduce the level of hydrogen in the body, such as those that cause volume, potassium, and chloride loss.

Table 11-6 Precipitants of Metabolic Alkalosis

Normal Saline-Responsive Metabolic Alkalosis	Normal Saline-Unresponsive Metabolic Alkalosis
Volume depletion ▪ Vomiting ▪ Nasogastric suction ▪ Diuretic use ▪ Low chloride ingestion	Mineralocorticoid excess
	Exogenous ingestions ▪ Chewing tobacco ▪ Licorice
	Primary aldosteronism
	Cushing syndrome
	Bartter syndrome

Pathophysiology

Metabolic alkalosis occurs by one of two mechanisms: retention of bases or loss of acids. Table 11-6 provides a list of specific conditions that may precipitate metabolic alkalosis.

Signs and Symptoms

Common signs and symptoms in patients affected by metabolic alkalosis are anorexia, nausea, vomiting, confusion, hypotension, paresthesia, and weakness. A thorough assessment may reveal the use of antacids (e.g., sodium and calcium bicarbonates), loop diuretics such as furosemide, and corticosteroids. Underlying medical illnesses such as Cushing syndrome and renal disease are also commonly reported.

Patients with metabolic alkalosis will present with slow, shallow respirations. ECG changes with depressed T waves that merge with P waves indicate hypocalcemia and hypokalemia. Hypotension is also present. Many patients present with muscle twitching and loss of reflexes and numbness and tingling in the extremities; a thorough neurologic exam should be performed. Blood gas analysis reveals a blood pH > 7.45 and elevated base excess and bicarbonate levels.

If respiratory compensation is occurring, the $PaCO_2$ level may be > 45 mm Hg.

Differential Diagnosis

To make a definitive diagnosis of metabolic alkalosis, the clinician needs to know the serum bicarbonate level and the arterial or venous PCO_2 level. A rise in the serum bicarbonate level may be a renal compensatory response to chronic respiratory acidosis. This information can be obtained only by blood gas testing.

Treatment

Management of metabolic alkalosis is directed toward correcting the underlying cause. A comprehensive history and physical exam are vital. Administration of IV fluids is essential if the primary cause is volume depletion, and isotonic solutions are the fluids of choice. Hypokalemia may need to be corrected with potassium replacement.

Mixed Disorders

Patients often have mixed acid–base disturbances, the diagnosis of which may be difficult even for an experienced ED physician or intensivist. Mixed disturbances are identified on the basis of clinical history combined with blood gas analysis. The initial clinical impression of whether the patient is sick or not sick is especially important. As always, take any immediate steps necessary to support the patient's airway, breathing, and circulation.

Putting It All Together

Patients with endocrine and metabolic disorders can be some of the most challenging a health care clinician faces. Similarities and differences in the chief complaint/cardinal presentation are sometimes subtle, and your ability to determine the underlying diagnosis can be obscured, delaying appropriate interventions. Following the AMLS Assessment Pathway will assist you in obtaining a comprehensive history and focused physical exam. This assessment-based approach supports putting your knowledge of anatomy, physiology, and pathophysiology to work to figure out both the common and uncommon causes of these diverse disease processes. The use of pattern recognition can help you compare the patient's clinical presentation to the chief complaint and formulate a working diagnosis. Becoming proficient in analyzing and synthesizing information to safely, efficiently, and effectively care for these patients will be well worth the effort it takes. Your contributions as an EMS clinician are always a vital link in helping improve patient outcomes.

SCENARIO SOLUTION

- Differential diagnoses may include an electrolyte imbalance such as hypokalemia or hypernatremia, metabolic alkalosis (related to Cushing syndrome) or metabolic acidosis (related to treatment with metformin); hyperglycemia or hypoglycemia; digoxin toxicity; sepsis; and heart failure.
- To narrow the differential diagnosis, you will need to obtain the history of past and present illness. Perform a physical examination that includes assessment for dehydration, assessment of heart and breath sounds, and mental status. Diagnostic testing should include blood glucose, ECG monitoring and 12-lead ECG, SpO_2, $ETCO_2$, and blood chemistry if available.
- This patient has signs that may indicate shock, infection, or electrolyte imbalance. Signs of shock may be masked by prednisone treatment, and the presence of digoxin will prevent an increase in heart rate to compensate for shock. Administer oxygen, establish vascular access, and administer IV fluids. Continue to monitor the ECG, and transport the patient to the closest appropriate hospital.

SUMMARY

- The endocrine system is responsible for hormone regulation, including regulating the functions of homeostasis, reproduction, growth, development, and metabolism. It is composed of the pituitary, thyroid, parathyroid, and adrenal glands, as well as the pancreas, ovaries, and testes.
- Hormones stimulate growth and development throughout the body, regulate the flow of water in and out of cells, help muscles contract, control blood pressure and appetite, modulate the sleep cycle, and influence many other functions.
- Endocrine glands are interdependent on one another.
- Parathyroid glands are composed of three types of cells and are responsible for producing parathyroid hormone (PTH), detecting changes in extracellular calcium concentration, and inhibiting calcitonin secretion.

(continues)

SUMMARY (CONTINUED)

- Hypoparathyroidism is characterized by low serum levels of PTH, with the hallmark of this condition being hypocalcemia.
- The thyroid gland is composed of secretory cells, follicular cells, and C cells.
- Hyperthyroidism can result in thyrotoxicosis and, potentially, thyroid storm.
- The adrenal gland secretes glucocorticoids, mineralocorticoids, and supplemental sex hormones.
- Addison disease, or primary adrenal insufficiency, is a metabolic and endocrine ailment caused by direct insult to or malfunction of the adrenal cortex.
- Acute adrenal insufficiency is a condition in which the body's need for glucocorticoids and mineralocorticoids exceeds the delivery of these hormones by the adrenal glands.
- Hyperadrenalism, or Cushing syndrome, is caused by long-standing exposure to excessive circulating serum levels of glucocorticoids, particularly cortisol, as a result of overproduction in the adrenal cortex.
- Glucose is a vital fuel for key metabolic processes in organs, especially those in the central nervous system.
- Cellular survival depends on preserving a balanced serum glucose concentration.
- Diabetes is the most common endocrine disorder; in turn, hypoglycemia, a frequent complication of the treatment of diabetes, is the most common endocrine emergency.
- Diabetes mellitus is characterized by defective insulin production or utilization, a high level of blood glucose, and unbalanced lipid and carbohydrate metabolism. Left untreated, it results in hyperglycemia.
- Hypoglycemia in patients with diabetes results from the disruption of the delicate balance among the interdependent factors of exogenously administered insulin, glucose metabolism, and glucose intake.
- Hypoglycemia may occur in patients taking only oral hypoglycemic agents, but it should alert the health care clinician to the potential presence of an underlying pathophysiologic state such as new-onset renal failure.
- Type 1 diabetes is characterized by pancreatic beta cell destruction, which renders the body incapable of producing the insulin necessary to carry out cell metabolism.
- Type 2 diabetes is characterized by cellular insulin resistance and a gradual failure of pancreatic insulin production.
- Gestational diabetes is a form of glucose intolerance that occurs during pregnancy.
- Hypoglycemia results in a decrease in insulin secretion and an increase in secretion of counter-regulatory hormones such as epinephrine. Symptoms include impaired cognition. If untreated, hypoglycemia can lead to significant morbidity and mortality.
- Hypoglycemia in patients who do not have diabetes is characterized by alimentary hyperinsulinism; it is commonly seen in patients who have undergone gastric surgery or as the result of an imbalance between glucose utilization and production.
- Diabetic ketoacidosis is an acute endocrine emergency in which insulin deficiency and an excessive glucagon level combine to create a hyperglycemic, acidotic, volume-depleted state.
- Hyperosmolar hyperglycemic syndrome (HHS) is a serious diabetic emergency that typically occurs in patients with type 2 diabetes mellitus, and carries a mortality rate of 10% to 50%.
- Healthy cellular function is directly related to the maintenance of a precise acid-base balance in the body. The kidneys and lungs manage this balance, which is measured by pH.
- Respiratory acidosis is characterized by a decrease in pH as a result of CO_2 retention. Respiratory alkalosis, which is caused an increase in ventilation per minute, is characterized by a decreased $PaCO_2$ and increased pH.
- Metabolic acidosis is caused by the accumulation of acids in excess of the body's buffering capabilities. The most common serious causes of metabolic acidosis are diabetic ketoacidosis, renal failure, lactic acidosis, toxic ingestion, and alcoholic ketoacidosis.
- Metabolic alkalosis is produced by illnesses that raise the level of serum bicarbonate or reduce the level of hydrogen in the body, such as those that cause volume, potassium, and chloride loss.
- A healthy electrolyte balance is fundamental to carrying out cellular functions; electrolyte imbalances include hyponatremia, hypokalemia, hyperkalemia, hypocalcemia, and hypomagnesemia.
- Rhabdomyolysis is a skeletal muscle injury characterized by release of cellular contents, specifically myoglobin and potassium, potentially leading to acute renal failure and hyperkalemia.

Key Terms

Addison disease An endocrine disease caused by a deficiency of corticosteroid hormones produced by the adrenal cortex. The disease is characterized by nausea, vomiting, abdominal pain, and tanning of the skin.

adrenal crisis An endocrine emergency caused by a deficiency of corticosteroid hormones produced by the adrenal cortex. The disease is characterized by nausea, vomiting, abdominal pain, hypotension, hyperkalemia, and hyponatremia.

diabetic ketoacidosis (DKA) An acute endocrine emergency caused by a lack of insulin. The condition is characterized by an elevated blood glucose level, ketone production, metabolic acidosis, dehydration, nausea, vomiting, abdominal pain, and tachypnea.

hyperosmolar hyperglycemic syndrome (HHS) An endocrine emergency characterized by a high plasma glucose concentration, absent ketone production, and increased serum osmolality (> 315 mOsm/kg). The syndrome causes severe dehydration, nausea, vomiting, abdominal pain, and tachypnea.

hypoglycemia A plasma glucose concentration of < 70 mg/dL. This condition is often associated with signs and symptoms such as sweating, cold skin, tachycardia, and altered mental status.

myxedema coma Severe hypothyroidism associated with cold intolerance, weight gain, weakness, and declining mental status.

thyroid storm An endocrine emergency characterized by hyperfunction of the thyroid gland. This disorder is associated with fever, tachycardia, nervousness, altered mental status, and hemodynamic instability.

thyrotoxicosis A condition of elevated thyroid hormone levels, which often leads to signs and symptoms of tachycardia, tremor, weight loss, and high-output heart failure.

Bibliography

American Academy of Orthopaedic Surgeons. *Nancy Caroline's Emergency Care in the Streets.* 8th ed. Burlington, MA: Jones & Bartlett Learning; 2018.

Beskind DL, Rhodes SM, Stolz U, et al. When should you test for and treat hypoglycemia in prehospital seizure patients? *Prehosp Emerg Care.* 2014;18(3):433-441. doi:10.3109/10903127.2013.864358.

Hamilton GC, Sanders AB, Strange GR. *Emergency Medicine.* 2nd ed. St. Louis, MO: Saunders; 2003.

Higgins C. Measurement of circulating blood glucose: the problem of inconsistent sample and methodology. *Acute Care Testing.* https://acutecaretesting.org/en/articles/measurement-of-circulating-glucose-the-problem-of-inconsistent-sample-and-methodology. Published January 2008. Accessed October 9, 2023.

Hong H, Lee J. Thyroid-stimulating hormone as a biomarker for stress after thyroid surgery: a prospective cohort study. *Med Sci Monit.* 2022;28:e937957. doi:10.12659/MSM.937957.

Kumar G, Sng BL, Kumar S. Correlation of capillary and venous blood glucometry with laboratory determination. *Prehosp Emerg Care.* 2004;8(4):378.

Marx JA, Hockberger RS, Walls RM. *Rosen's Emergency Medicine.* 7th ed. St. Louis, MO: Mosby; 2009.

Mistovich JJ, Krost WS, Limmer DD. Beyond the basics: endocrine emergencies. *EMS Mag.* 2007;36(10):123-127.

Mistovich JJ, Krost WS, Limmer DD. Beyond the basics: endocrine emergencies, Part II. *EMS Mag.* 2007;36(11):66-69.

Pagan KD, Pagana TJ. *Mosby's Manual of Diagnostic and Laboratory Tests.* 4th ed. St. Louis, MO: Mosby; 2010.

Sanders MJ. *Mosby's Paramedic Textbook.* 3rd ed. St. Louis, MO: Mosby; 2005.

Schwerin DL, Svancarek B. EMS diabetic protocols for treat and release. In: *StatPearls.* Treasure Island, FL: StatPearls Publishing. July 17, 2023. PMID:32809447.

Stárka L, Dušková M. What is a hormone? *Physiol Res.* 2020; 69(suppl 2):S183-S185. doi:10.33549/physiolres.934509.

Story L. *Pathophysiology: A Practical Approach.* 4th ed. Burlington, MA: Jones & Bartlett Learning; 2022.

U.S. Department of Transportation, National Highway Traffic Safety Administration. *EMT-Paramedic National Standard Curriculum.* Washington, DC: U.S. Department of Transportation; 1998.

U.S. Department of Transportation, National Highway Traffic Safety Administration. *National EMS Education Standards, Draft 3.0.* Washington, DC: U.S. Department of Transportation; 2008.

CHAPTER 12

Women's Health Emergencies

Chapter Editors
Emily Nichols, MD
Rickquel Tripp, MD, MPH, CDR USN
Carolina C. Pereira, MD, FACEP, FAEMS

This chapter will present health care issues of concern to women. The influence of physiologic differences between males and females on disease presentations will be discussed, with a focus on cardiovascular, respiratory, and neurologic diseases. Various gynecologic and obstetric emergency presentations and treatments will be presented. Additionally, human trafficking, sexual assault, and domestic violence will be discussed.

LEARNING OBJECTIVES

At the conclusion of this chapter, you will be able to:

- Discuss the influence of the physiologic differences between the male and female sexes on disease presentation.
- Identify how female physiology affects the presentation of cardiovascular, respiratory, and neurologic diseases.
- Describe the presentations for various gynecologic and obstetric emergencies.
- Recognize the characteristics and warning signs of human trafficking and intimate partner violence.

SCENARIO

You are dispatched to a 41-year-old woman who complains of chest pain, shortness of breath, and dizziness. You immediately notice that the patient appears pale and unwell.

Your patient states that she began experiencing abdominal pain and bloating 3 days ago. She has associated nausea and vomiting and has been urinating only small amounts of dark yellow urine since yesterday. Last night, she noticed swelling in her legs that progressively worsened and extended into her abdomen. Her past medical history includes transient high blood pressure during her most recent doctor's visit and depression. Medications include escitalopram, a multivitamin, and multiple "hormone medications [she] can't remember the name of" that were taken for her recent IVF egg retrieval.

Initial vital signs include blood pressure 97/53 mm Hg, pulse rate 106 beats/min, respirations 24 breaths/min, and temperature 37.2°C (99.0°F). You hear normal heart sounds and diminished breath sounds in the lower lung fields upon auscultation. You also notice distended jugular veins.

- What differential diagnoses are you considering based on the information that you have now?
- What additional information will you need to narrow your differential diagnosis?
- What are your initial treatment priorities as you continue your patient care?

Sex Differences in Physiology

The male and female sexes have many important differences in physiology. Rather than focus on secondary sex characteristics, this chapter will focus on the differences that result from chromosomal and hormonal differences between sexes.

The comparisons made in this section are generalizations based on a broad swath of the population who are of the female sex compared to the male sex. However, it is not possible to apply population statistics to an individual patient. Additionally, these comparisons are based on the presumption of male sex as a single copy of an X chromosome and a single copy of a Y chromosome and female sex as two X chromosomes. This section does not delve into but wants to acknowledge that patients who have sex-linked chromosomal differences are not well addressed by this construct. Therefore, it is of the utmost importance to consider each individual patient and their particular circumstances when applying these concepts to patient care. Demonstrating care and concern for each individual is far more impactful than understanding the differences in physiology that come with having XX chromosomes.

The nidus of these differences is based on hormonal differences between sexes. The main sex hormones include estrogens; progestogens, including progesterone; and androgens, including testosterone. The primary male sex hormone is testosterone; progestogens and estrogens are the primary female sex hormones. Although both sexes have all of these hormones, they are present in varying amounts. Female sex hormones also vary over the lifetime, affecting the risk for certain pathologies as a person ages. This section presents two examples of body systems that demonstrate this difference: the cardiovascular and immune systems.

Cardiovascular System

In females in their reproductive years, the regularity of menses, especially when heavy vaginal bleeding is present, increases the risk for anemia, which is contrary to their male counterparts, whose androgens increase red blood cell counts by comparison. Hemoglobin levels will be similar when comparing males to females before age 10 or after age 50, but differences do exist during the expected reproductive years when estrogen and progesterone production are at their highest.

Estrogen offers some protection from the progression of cardiovascular heart disease. The risk for females for cardiovascular disease prior to menopause is significantly lower than males of similar age and risk profile. However, this risk becomes higher than that of males once the protective effects of endogenous estrogen are decreased. This increasing risk for vascular disease becomes more pronounced as females go on to live longer than males. The same holds true for other atherosclerotic processes such as strokes.

Immune System

The female immune system is more active than the male immune system. Although the reason for this is not fully understood, some theories suggest that estrogens are hormonal mediators that bolster natural immune responses, whereas testosterone serves a modulatory role. This hormonal mediation can be both adaptive and pathologic. From an adaptive perspective, females have shown lower rates of severe urinary tract infections and significantly lower infectivity rates of contracting COVID-19 than their male cohorts. However, from a pathologic perspective, they are much more likely to have autoimmune conditions, as 85% of patients with autoimmune diseases are female. Further, some autoimmune conditions flare during pregnancy and remit during menopause, implying an estrogen-mediated response.

Gender Differences in Interactions with the Health Care System

In addition to the physiologic differences that affect health care, there are personal, behavioral, and systemic aspects that also influence how different genders interact with the health care system.

Women are more likely to seek out health care earlier in their disease processes than men. As a result, women have a greater number of visits to primary and preventative care clinicians than men. Women self-report their own health status as worse than men's even when controlling for the same underlying health conditions. This same pattern of increased use of health care resources in women is true for mental health care as well. Along the same vein, women are less likely to require emergency care than men. This is partially due to the increased likelihood of being seen in primary care and preventative settings, but also attributable to the decreased likelihood of engaging in risky behaviors.

When women interact with emergency care services, they are more likely to have the clinicians who evaluate them attribute their symptoms and concerns to less serious presentations with lower acuity. In a simulated patient presentation of coronary health disease using "typical" presentation descriptions, clinicians were more likely to attribute women's chest pain to a gastrointestinal or mental health etiology even when presented in the same fashion as men. This effect was further magnified when the patient was of a younger age and had a lower socioeconomic status.

As previously noted, as women age their risk profile for atherosclerotic processes, including acute coronary syndrome (ACS) and stroke, surpasses men's. This is further compounded by the fact that women have worse clinical outcomes from those conditions.

Considerations in Health Care Delivery to Women

Women's health extends beyond sexual and reproductive health. Countries and health care systems benefit socially and economically when they consider and attend to the leading causes of death and disability for women. EMS agencies should study and teach the acute presentations of noncommunicable illness and the disparate symptoms of women and men that clinicians may encounter.

Clinicians should never assume a patient's sex or gender based on presentation and should ask patients regarding this information when medically indicated. Also, clinicians should maintain a high index of suspicion for conditions with sex-specific signs/symptoms in gender-diverse patients, as these may not present in the manner expected for a patient's gender presentation. [See Chapter 1, *Advanced Medical Life Support Assessment for the Medical Patient*, for a discussion about clinical considerations related to assessing and communicating with patients while considering a patient's gender.]

Prevalence and Presentation of Noncommunicable Diseases

Noncommunicable diseases are chronic conditions that often require long-term treatment and primarily impact morbidity and mortality within communities. By taking a gender-inclusive approach to assessments, clinicians are more likely to recognize the unique presentations of these common conditions when they occur in women.

Cardiovascular Disorders

Cardiovascular diseases are the leading cause of death for women and men of all ages globally. Well-known risk factors for ischemic heart disease (e.g., hypertension, diabetes, dyslipidemia, smoking) are present in people of any gender. Less recognized risk factors are usually psychological, economic, and/or cultural—these have been found to disproportionately affect women (**Figure 12-1**). Depression and intimate partner violence are just two of the social conditions now understood to increase one's risk of cardiovascular disease. Ongoing research is identifying additional sex-specific and psychosocial associations.

Despite an increased awareness of cardiovascular disease in women over the last 30 years, many health care clinicians continue to underestimate its prevalence. Cardiovascular disease in women rises substantially after menopause. Additionally, women who experience premature menopause (age < 40 years) have an increased cardiovascular risk. Underestimation of disease risk has

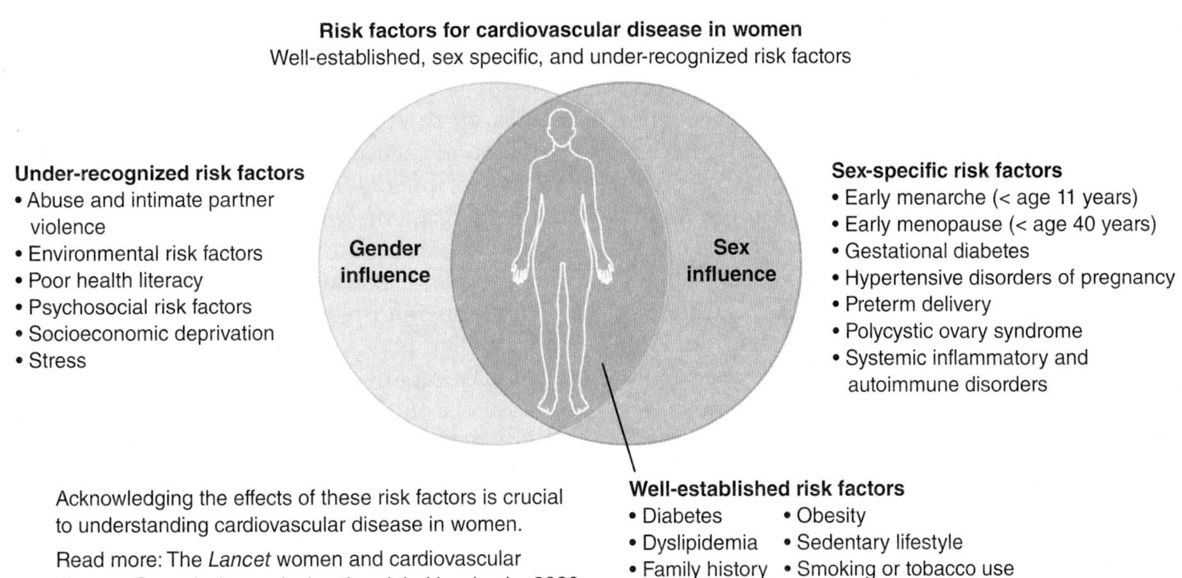

Figure 12-1 Risk factors for cardiovascular disease in women.

historically led to more missed diagnoses of ST-elevation myocardial infarction (STEMI) among women than men in the prehospital setting, resulting in delayed reperfusion therapy.

Acute Coronary Syndrome

Women with STEMI more commonly present with symptoms other than chest pain. Patients may describe pain in the jaw, neck, or shoulder; they also may complain solely of nausea or fatigue. Clinicians should also consider spontaneous coronary artery dissection as a possible cause of acute myocardial infarction (AMI) in women younger than 50 years and inquire about conditions that lead to increased intracoronary shear stress. Known causes of spontaneous coronary artery dissection include but are not limited to systemic inflammatory disease, hormonal therapy use, extreme physical or emotional stress, and multiple previous pregnancies. At least 10% to 15% of patients with these dissections will not have ECG changes consistent with a STEMI, though many will have transient ST- or T-wave changes. A high index of suspicion is frequently necessary to make this diagnosis.

Studies have found that women are more susceptible than men to cardiogenic shock after ACS. Clinicians should monitor patients with ACS closely to identify and treat hemodynamic compromise during transport to the appropriate receiving facility.

Sudden Cardiac Death

Rate estimates vary, but sudden cardiac death is believed to occur more often in women than men. Women have fewer ventricular dysrhythmias (ventricular fibrillation or ventricular tachycardia) documented as the first identified rhythm during cardiac arrest. Women also have a lower incidence of receiving bystander resuscitation in public places compared to men. A recent small-scale study by Hussain et al. (2023) found that paramedics continue to report hesitancy with 12-lead ECG acquisition in female patients, expressing concerns for patient discomfort and privacy in addition to clinician liability and risk. A survey of 50 healthy women volunteers found that all respondents would allow an ECG to be performed by any clinician—regardless of clinician gender—if they understood it would reduce the time to definitive treatment. Clinicians should identify opportunities to appropriately communicate the urgency of this procedure early during a patient encounter as they are building rapport and while they are articulating their clinical impression to the patient.

Respiratory Disorders

Chronic Obstructive Pulmonary Disease

Chronic obstructive pulmonary disease (COPD) was the fourth leading cause of death among women globally in 2019. A massive uptake in tobacco consumption; greater exposure to indoor air pollution (e.g., smoke from cooking and heating); and anatomic, hormonal, and behavioral differences all have led to this increase in pulmonary disease in the last 20 years. However, women are less likely to be diagnosed with COPD if they are younger, have milder symptoms, have a shorter smoking history, or if they report that they have a high quality of life. Because this condition is underdiagnosed in the primary care setting, prehospital clinicians may miss the signs of an acute COPD exacerbation when it is not part of a patient's past medical history. Clinicians should consider COPD in anyone with shortness of breath or cough, especially if there is any reported history of tobacco consumption. Additionally, the incidence of depression is higher in both male and female COPD patients compared to the general population, and women are more likely than men to have anxiety or depression during an acute COPD exacerbation. Clinicians should not mistake anxiety as the primary cause of a patient's subjective dyspnea but instead should consider it a component of one's inability to oxygenate and/or ventilate.

Pulmonary Artery Hypertension

As noted in Chapter 3, *Respiratory Disorders*, women are 5 to 10 times more likely to have pulmonary artery hypertension (PAH) than men. The role of estrogen is hypothesized but uncertain in efforts to explain this imbalance. Early recognition of PAH and right ventricular failure is critical to appropriately resuscitating patients. Although many cases of PAH will have a chief complaint of dyspnea, clinicians should consider the diagnosis in any individual with syncope or signs of right ventricular dysfunction (e.g., jugular vein distention [JVD], abdominal distention, edema). Identification of PAH in the prehospital setting is dependent on gathering details as part of the patient's history of present illness and past medical history to raise suspicion for the diagnosis. Primary resuscitation measures focus on preventing hypoxemia and hypercapnia. Judicious volume resuscitation is imperative in patients who are fluid overloaded, and early use of vasopressors and/or pulmonary vessel dilators may be appropriate. Prehospital clinicians should be aware of common phosphodiesterase inhibitors—frequently infused in-hospital via a pump—and recognize that patients may rapidly decompensate when these medications are discontinued.

Pregnant women with PAH have a very high risk of both maternal and fetal mortality. Physiologic changes in oxygen consumption and pulmonary blood flow place a large cardiovascular burden on the mother while pregnant, and there is a high chance of premature birth. Elective termination of pregnancy was historically recommended for women with PAH, but more individuals are now delivering children when intensive monitoring is utilized during the entire pregnancy. Clinicians should recognize the risk for death among pregnant women with PAH, especially during the third trimester and the first few days following delivery.

Venous Thromboembolism

Although published data do not support any consistent sex difference in the incidence of venous thromboembolism (VTE), several known risk factors for VTE are sex specific. It has been postulated that sex hormones (e.g., estrogen, progesterone, and androgens) have a direct effect on platelet function and an indirect effect on pulmonary vasculature. As a result, women experience fluctuation of prothrombotic activity related to menstrual cycles, the use of oral contraceptives, pregnancy, menopause, and hormone replacement therapy. These associations should be considered during acute presentations of dyspnea, chest pain, and/or leg swelling in women. Though most research on the relationship between sex hormones and VTE has been done in cisgender women, prior studies found an association between oral ethinyl estradiol and VTE in transgender women. As a result, this hormone is no longer recommended for gender-affirming hormone therapy. Further research of cardiovascular health in transgender individuals is needed to develop better guidelines for future care.

Neurologic

Women have historically had poor stroke-related outcomes compared to men and are less likely to report typical symptoms of weakness, numbness, or language disturbance. Chief complaints of headache or dizziness are common symptoms of missed strokes, and women with a medical history of migraines or anxiety are more likely to be misdiagnosed. Young women aged 25 to 34 years have a higher stroke incidence than similarly aged men; a near sevenfold risk of misdiagnosis has been reported in certain clinical trials. Additionally, numerous studies have found that complaints of "nonspecific" or "atypical" symptoms commonly reported by women are not just stroke mimics and instead are ultimately diagnosed as minor ischemic events. With a corresponding medical history of cardiovascular risk factors, clinicians should consider transient ischemic attack and cerebrovascular accident in patients even when the symptoms and exam findings are subtle.

Psychiatric

Sex differences in mental health can be explained by sex hormones and dysregulations in the hypothalamic-pituitary-adrenal axis, especially for stress-related psychiatric disorders. Even so, there is no consistent body of literature that identifies a sex or gender difference in the acute presentation of mental illness. A growing body of research indicates that psychiatric disorders are largely caused by a combination of stress and environmental, neurobiologic, and genetic factors. Comprehensive analysis of gender differences would require a consensus on the diagnostic categories of mental health and elimination of the historical tendency to pathologize mental health in women.

In the prehospital setting, clinicians should consider and evaluate for psychiatric emergencies in individuals who present as victims of power inequity. Women who have experienced intimate partner violence, sexual assault, or human trafficking all have an increased risk of stress-related mental health disorders.

Gynecologic/Obstetric Emergencies

Although women's health is not limited to gynecologic and obstetric disease, many disparities in illness are hormone related and will manifest during a woman's childbearing years. Even beyond menopause, women will have unique urologic considerations and health care emergencies. The following sections briefly review commonly encountered gynecological emergencies in nonpregnant pediatric and adolescent patients along with the most frequent obstetrical emergencies in pregnant and postpartum patients, including less-than-typical complaints and clinical considerations.

Sexually Transmitted Infections

Sexually transmitted infections (STIs) (formerly called sexually transmitted diseases [STDs]) are caused by the transmission of bacteria, viruses, or parasites through sexual contact involving the exchange of bodily fluids or skin contact via vaginal, oral, and anal sex. STIs are a major health problem around the world among individuals of every age, race, and sexual orientation, but they disproportionately affect young people, racial and ethnic minorities, and men who have sex with men (MSM). Youth aged 15 to 24 years account for half of the 20 million new cases of STIs in the United States each year. Factors contributing to this increased risk for youth include variation in biological maturation; age of sexual debut; type and number of sexual partners; patterns of condom use; access to and quality of health care services, along with economic means; education; and employment.

According to the Centers for Disease Control and Prevention (CDC), roughly 2 million cases of chlamydia, gonorrhea, and syphilis are reported in the United States annually, and chlamydia and gonorrhea are the most common bacterial STIs. Human papillomavirus (HPV) is the most common STI overall in the United States, with more than 40 distinct HPV types infecting the anogenital tract. HPV types 16 and 18 are predominant in anogenital carcinoma and are involved in more than 99% of all cervical cancers; more than 90% of all anal cancers; and up to 70% of all carcinomas of the penis, vulva, and vagina. HPV types 6 and 11 account for 90% of anogenital warts. Other common infections in the United States include herpes simplex virus and trichomoniasis.

Chlamydia trachomatis infections are asymptomatic, with only 10% of men and 5% to 30% of women developing symptoms that include dysuria, pelvic pain, vaginal discharge, rectal pain, or sore throat, depending on the extent of the infection and route of exposure. Most *Neisseria gonorrhea* infections are symptomatic in men, with up to 95% of women being asymptomatic. Symptoms include mucopurulent vaginal and penile discharge (referred to in males as the "drip"). Double infections with both gonorrhea and chlamydia occur in up to 20% of patients. Complications of chlamydia and gonorrhea include pelvic inflammatory disease (PID); infertility; ectopic pregnancy; chronic pelvic pain; increased human immunodeficiency virus (HIV) transmission; adverse pregnancy and neonatal outcomes; epididymitis; reactive arthritis; gonococcal hepatitis (Fitz-Hugh-Curtis syndrome); and, rarely, disseminated gonococcal infection.

Syphilis is a systemic STI that consists of four stages: primary, secondary, latent, and tertiary. The primary stage consists of a chancre, which is a painless, indurated ulcer at the site of inoculation that heals spontaneously. The secondary stage has symptoms of fever, fatigue, sore throat, myalgia, arthralgia, lymphadenopathy, polymorphous maculopapular rash (palms and soles), and condyloma lata (hypertrophic papular lesions affecting moist areas around the vulva or anus). Latent syphilis demonstrates no signs or symptoms. The tertiary stage involves cardiovascular syphilis (aortitis), gummatous syphilis (soft, noncancerous but destructive growths), and neurosyphilis (meningitis, uveitis, seizures, optic atrophy, dementia, and posterior spinal cord degeneration).

Herpes simplex virus (HSV) has two types: HSV type 2 (HSV-2), which causes most genital infections, and HSV type 1 (HSV-1), which is typically associated with orolabial infections and is often acquired during childhood. Classic HSV presentation consists of a cluster of painful vesicles or ulcers.

Trichomoniasis is a protozoal infection caused by *Trichomonas vaginalis* and is frequently asymptomatic in 70% to 85% of cases. Typical symptoms include copious, malodorous, watery, yellow-green vaginal discharge and cervical punctate hemorrhages in women and urethritis, epididymitis, and prostatitis in men. Complications involve increased risk of HIV transmission and PID along with adverse pregnancy outcomes.

The major focus on management of STIs is early detection, accurate identification, treatment, and prevention in order to ameliorate the public health threat to high-risk patient populations and to the sex partners of those recently diagnosed. Most STIs are asymptomatic and, therefore, it is difficult for people to be aware they are infected. However, some STIs have distinctive symptomatology and physical exam findings allowing for a rapid diagnosis with clear treatment options, which helps to deter transmission and decrease overall STI occurrence.

Unfortunately, the consequences of contracting STIs may lead to severe health outcomes, especially for young women. If chlamydia and gonorrhea are left untreated or there is a delay in diagnosis, the infection may ascend to the upper reproductive tract, resulting in PID. PID leads to inflammation and damage to the fallopian tubes, which increase a woman's risk of tubal-factor infertility and ectopic pregnancy. Results from recent studies show declining rates of PID cases caused by chlamydia or gonorrhea (< 50% testing positive) in hospital and ambulatory settings. Contributing factors to declining PID diagnoses include increases in chlamydia and gonorrhea screening, more sensitive diagnostic technologies, and the availability of single-dose therapies that increase adherence to treatment. PID can be present with a wide variety of nonspecific, subtle symptoms, but the most common ones are abnormal vaginal bleeding, lower abdominal/pelvic pain, dyspareunia, and abnormal vaginal discharge. On pelvic exam done in the health care setting, common findings are cervical motion tenderness, uterine tenderness, or adnexal tenderness along with mucopurulent uterine or vaginal discharge and white blood cells on microscopy of vaginal fluid. Due to the potential for severe illness or complications from PID, clinicians should maintain a low threshold for PID diagnosis. Although most PID cases are treated in an outpatient setting with cefTRIAXone intramuscular (IM) injection and oral doxycycline and metroNIDAZOLE, hospitalization should be considered for suspected tubo-ovarian abscess, pregnancy, severe illness, high fever, inability to tolerate or failure to respond to oral therapy, or concern for alternative surgical emergency (i.e., appendicitis).

Tubo-Ovarian Abscess

Tubo-ovarian abscess (TOA) is a rare but high-risk, serious inflammatory infectious mass located in the fallopian tube, ovary, or other pelvic organs (i.e., bladder and bowel). It is associated with a high rate of morbidity and mortality. TOA most commonly arises from a gynecologic infection or PID but is also associated with gastrointestinal sources, intrauterine devices, uterine procedures such as hysteroscopy, multiple sexual partners, diabetes, and immunocompromised states. Fifty percent of patients diagnosed with TOA on transvaginal ultrasound or computerized tomography (CT) scan with contrast imaging exhibited symptoms of systemic illness such as fever, nausea, and vomiting. Other symptoms associated with TOA include abdominal or pelvic pain and tenderness, chills, and abnormal vaginal discharge. Failure to provide early treatment with antibiotics could lead to peritonitis and sepsis.

Abnormal Uterine Bleeding

Abnormal uterine bleeding can occur from a number of causes, both infectious and noninfectious. (Abnormal uterine bleeding as a result of menopause is discussed later.) Genital warts can produce vaginal bleeding if located on the mucosa of the introitus or just inside the hymenal ring. They are caused by HPV infection due to vertical transmission (birth via mother's infected lower genital tract), autoinoculation of common warts, nonabusive contact, or sexual contact. Infectious vaginitis associated with *Streptococcus pyogenes* (group A beta-hemolytic streptococci) and *Shigella* species occasionally produces bloody vaginal discharge along with other symptoms of pruritus, dysuria, pain, or inflammation. Treatment consists of metroNIDAZOLE, clindamycin, tinidazole, and secnidazole.

When evaluating irregular menstrual bleeding in adolescents (who have passed **menarche** and are in the state of puberty) and premenopausal adults, the clinician should first inquire about the date of the patient's last menstrual period. Most common etiologies of irregular menstrual bleeding besides pregnancy include polycystic ovarian syndrome (PCOS), hemorrhagic cysts, delayed pubertal maturation, hormonal contraception, malignancy, and bleeding disorders (i.e., platelet dysfunction, von Willebrand disease, or coagulation factor deficiency).

PCOS is diagnosed by the classic features of hirsutism, acne, or male-pattern hair loss due to androgen excess; irregular menstrual cycles; and polycystic ovarian morphology on transvaginal ultrasound. Women with PCOS are at an increased risk for cardiovascular disease and type 2 diabetes related to the increased rates of overweight/obesity (seen in 40% to 85% of patients) and insulin resistance in these patients.

Sepsis Following Abortion

A **septic abortion** is a clinical diagnosis that refers to any abortion (spontaneous or induced with medication or procedures/surgery) complicated by upper genital tract or uterine infection, including endometritis or parametritis. Even though the data are limited due to varying definitions of infection following both spontaneous pregnancy loss and pregnancy termination (medical and surgical), the incidence of septic abortion varies based on the type of abortion: 0% to 0.4% of surgical procedures, 0.92% following medical abortion using miFEPRIStone and miSOPROStol, and 5% following nonmedical abortion. Fourteen percent of pregnancy-related deaths are due to induced and spontaneous abortions worldwide. Miscarriage (spontaneous abortion) causing a natural pregnancy loss can lead to an intrauterine infection involving fetal demise, a partially passed demised pregnancy (i.e., incomplete abortion), or completed pregnancy loss with an infected uterus, often related to retained products of conception. Surgical (including vacuum-assisted, dilation and evacuation, and dilation and curettage) and medication-induced elective abortions can result in intrauterine infections from retained products of conception involving the fetus and placenta. Abortion practices incorporating the expertise of health care clinicians, adherence to standard sterile practices for infection prevention and control, and routine use of preoperative antibiotics have reduced infection rates significantly.

Nonmedical abortion methods include insertion of unclean objects such as coat hangers or knitting needles into the cervix and uterus; ingestion of toxic substances such as bleach, turpentine, or quinine; injecting caustic substances into the uterine cavity; physical violence to the abdomen with the intention of disrupting the placenta; and placement of harmful chemicals into the vagina, which may cause chemical burns and erode through the vagina into the rectum.

Pelvic and/or abdominal pain, uterine tenderness (on lower abdominal exam), cervical motion tenderness (on pelvic exam done in hospital or office), purulent or foul-smelling vaginal discharge, prolonged vaginal bleeding, and/or fever are typical signs and symptoms of septic abortion. If left untreated, it will rapidly progress to worsening fever, hypothermia, tachypnea, tachycardia, elevated inflammatory markers, and leukocytosis, along with bacteremia, life-threatening organ dysfunction, septic shock, and mortality. Women at highest risk for septic abortion include those with a history of nonmedical abortion, uterine instrumentation, or prolonged vaginal bleeding. Infections are mostly polymicrobial, arising from the vagina and lower genital tract and ascending to the uterine cavity, with a mix of anaerobic *Peptostreptococcus*, antibiotic-resistant and toxin-producing *Staphylococcus aureus*, strains of clostridia such *Clostridium perfringens*, Group A and B *Streptococcus*, *Escherichia coli*, and *Bacteroides*, and untreated STIs, such as chlamydia or gonorrhea. Severe and significant medical outcomes of septic abortion are acute—sepsis, coagulopathy such as disseminated intravascular coagulation (DIC), multiple organ failure, and death—and chronic—persistent pelvic pain, chronic PID, and infertility (due to obstructed fallopian tubes). Treatment consists of early broad-spectrum antibiotics and necessary removal of retained products of conception with prompt engagement of OB/GYN specialists since any delay could be fatal.

Family Planning and Pregnancy

The human body undergoes numerous hormonal and physiologic changes during pregnancy. In addition, more and more people are using **assisted reproductive technology (ART)** to achieve pregnancy, which comes with additional risks and potential complications. ART is now utilized in over 100 countries worldwide and is associated with increased maternal and neonatal morbidity and mortality—its practice, outcomes, and safety vary significantly among populations. Both assisted and natural conception can result in potentially fatal pregnancy-related complications that prehospital clinicians may encounter.

Ovarian Hyperstimulation Syndrome

Ovarian hyperstimulation syndrome (OHSS) is a well-known complication that affects 20% to 30% of patients who use ART. Exogenous hormones are used to induce the growth of a large number of ovarian follicles through "controlled ovarian hyperstimulation." This increased follicular growth causes the release of proinflammatory cytokines and molecules that increase capillary permeability; the result is a fluid shift from within the vessels into the extravascular space, leading to pulmonary and peripheral edema (**Figure 12-2**). Patients experiencing OHSS frequently become hypovolemic as intravascular fluid is third-spaced into the interstitium. Risk factors for OHSS include age younger than 35 years and a history of PCOS.

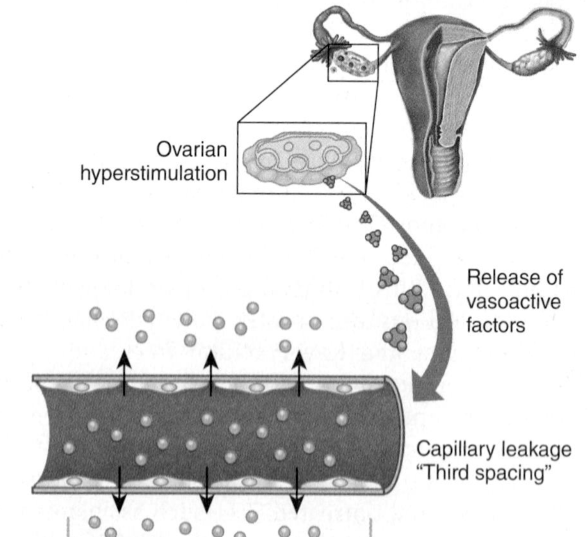

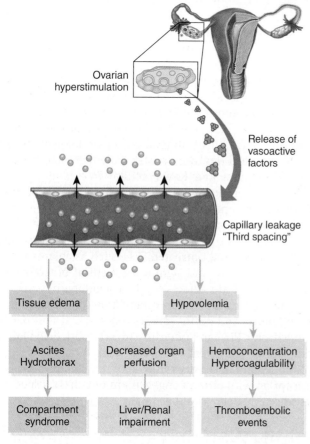

Figure 12-2 Physiologic changes associated with ovarian hyperstimulation syndrome.

Severe OHSS is rare but may be life threatening. Patients usually present with shortness of breath, chest pain, or dizziness. They also may report gastrointestinal symptoms, abdominal distension, swelling, and/or decreased urine output. The physical examination may reveal edema and hemodynamic instability. The clinical presentation of OHSS may resemble that of acute heart failure or pulmonary embolism.

Recognition of acute OHSS often occurs when one obtains a history of recent fertility treatment. Clinicians should ensure that their history taking includes appropriate questioning to gather this information. Management of OHSS requires mobilizing fluid from the interstitium (third space) back into the vessels while symptomatically treating pulmonary edema. Initial fluid resuscitation with a balanced crystalloid is often required in severe OHSS until the patient is hemodynamically stable. Clinicians should simultaneously provide oxygen and consider progressive ventilatory support (e.g., positive-pressure ventilation or intubation).

Hyperemesis Gravidarum

Although nausea and vomiting are common in the first trimester, hyperemesis gravidarum (HG) is a severe form that can lead to maternal and fetal adverse events (e.g., Wernicke encephalopathy, acute kidney injury, vitamin K deficiency). As noted in Chapter 10, *Abdominal Disorders*, HG includes weight loss, starvation metabolism, and prolonged ketosis. Management includes fluid and electrolyte repletion in addition to antiemetics.

Diabetic Ketoacidosis

Clinicians should consider diabetic ketoacidosis (DKA) in women who experience nausea and vomiting during the second or third trimester of pregnancy. The metabolic changes that accompany pregnancy predispose the body to DKA; specifically, the fetus and the placenta use large amounts of maternal glucose as a major source of energy. Additionally, the pregnant body produces insulin-antagonistic hormones that create insulin resistance. These factors create a period of relative insulin deficiency, to which the body responds by increasing its free fatty acids and developing ketosis, similar to nonpregnancy cases of DKA.

DKA during pregnancy is more common in patients with type 1 diabetes, but it has also been recognized in patients with type 2 diabetes and isolated gestational diabetes. A new diagnosis of diabetes may also occur when the pregnant patient is found in DKA. The symptoms of DKA in pregnancy are no different from those seen in women who are not pregnant, except that they tend to develop more rapidly in pregnancy. Treatment with corticosteroids to support fetal lung maturity or beta$_2$ agonists (e.g., albuterol, terbutaline) to prevent preterm labor also increases the risk of this disease. It is common for a pregnant patient in DKA to have a normal or minimally elevated blood glucose level due to the increased fetal metabolic demands as outlined previously. Prehospital clinicians should maintain DKA in their differential diagnosis even when pregnant patients are found to be euglycemic. Treatment of DKA in pregnancy is the same as in nonpregnant patients; this is discussed in detail in Chapter 11, *Endocrine and Metabolic Disorders*.

Hemorrhagic Shock

The physiologic changes of pregnancy make the detection of shock more complicated than in the nonpregnant patient. During pregnancy, there is an increase in maternal blood volume and blood flow to the uterus; this leads to increased cardiac output that continues to rise until the end of the second trimester. Pregnant patients frequently have a heart rate that is about 120% above their baseline, yet the normal maternal heart rate still is frequently between 80 and 100 beats/min. Pregnant patients also experience decreased systemic vascular resistance due to progesterone, which results in a blood pressure that is 5 to 15 mm Hg less than the patient's baseline measurement.

These changes in baseline vital signs may confound the diagnosis of hemorrhagic shock in pregnant patients. Recent studies suggest that the use of the shock index (SI) is better at detecting peripartum hemorrhage than either heart rate or blood pressure. A shock index greater than 0.9 is associated with an increased risk of adverse outcomes in pregnancy. It is important to understand that hemorrhagic shock in pregnant and immediately postpartum patients must be quickly recognized and addressed. Recognition and management of hemorrhagic shock is discussed at length in Chapter 5, *Shock*.

Gestational Hypertension/Eclampsia/Preeclampsia

As discussed in Chapter 10, *Abdominal Disorders*, preeclampsia and eclampsia are extensions of gestational hypertension. Up to 50% of women with gestational hypertension will develop preeclampsia. Despite hypertensive disorders of pregnancy being a leading cause of maternal morbidity and mortality, most emergency department (ED) visits by pregnant women are related to causes other than blood pressure. Even though gestational hypertension is not routinely treated in the prehospital setting, clinicians can support their patients through early recognition of this condition. Clinicians may translate a diagnosis of hypertension into the coordination of acute ED and obstetrics care plus prompt follow-up for chronic management. Although preeclampsia and the risk of eclampsia are generally thought of as prepartum conditions, it has been found that the risk of both continues for 1 to 2 months postpartum; thus, these complications must be considered when responding to patients in the recent postpartum period.

Peri- and Postmenopausal Conditions

Menopause is the period of time following cessation of menstruation. This is typically defined as starting 12 months from the last menstrual period, and on average starts at 51 years of age. Perimenopause refers to the time just prior to menopause. Perimenopause is often defined by a period of irregular menstrual cycles prior to ceasing completely. The woman may still have some menstrual cycles that may become increasingly irregular.

Dysfunctional Uterine Bleeding

Dysfunctional (abnormal) uterine bleeding is the irregularity of menstrual cycles or even heavy vaginal bleeding. It is important to ask the patient about the timing of their last menstrual cycle to attempt to differentiate perimenopause from menopause in determining if the vaginal bleeding is tied to a menstrual cycle or rather is dysfunctional. As this bleeding is abnormal, it can also be much heavier than a normal menstrual cycle. Determining the amount of vaginal bleeding will help in the determination of what emergent treatments are warranted, up to and including treatment for life-threatening bleeding. Life-threatening vaginal bleeding should be treated much like any other form of hemorrhage in a noncompressible area of the body. Intravenous (IV) fluid resuscitation should be judicious and based on the severity and timing of symptom onset. Vaginal bleeding has shown to have a good response to treatment with tranexamic acid if bleeding is severe. Any amount of vaginal bleeding for women who have already progressed into menopause is always considered dysfunctional and may be indicative of further pathology such as cancer. These patients warrant further evaluation by an OB-GYN specialist.

Fibroids, or leiomyomas, are benign tumors of the myometrium of the uterus. They are reported in 70% to 80% of women in the United States. The majority of fibroids are asymptomatic. As fibroids are so common and so often asymptomatic, it is debated whether fibroids should be considered a pathologic finding. However, they can also be debilitating depending on their location, size, and the effects they cause. Fibroids are intrinsically linked to increased estrogen and progesterone levels, making them more common during the years that women menstruate, but they can become symptomatic in peri- and postmenopausal women. In addition to causing an increase in vaginal bleeding, they may cause a sensation of pelvic fullness or cramping. Gynecologic cancers can also cause vaginal bleeding post menopause.

Pelvic Organ Prolapse

Pelvic organ prolapse is defined as the herniation of the internal pelvic organs within or beyond the vaginal canal. This condition happens as a result of a weakening of the muscles and connective tissues of the pelvic floor that connect to the pelvic bones. Pelvic organ prolapse becomes a medical emergency as organs move external to the vagina or cause obstructions in urination or defecation. Risk factors include advancing age, multiparity, and obesity. Although pelvic organ prolapse can happen to women prior to menopause, its connection to advancing age gives it much higher prevalence in menopause. Should the cervix, uterus, or other organs have prolapsed beyond the vaginal opening, these organs should be kept moist by applying sterile gauze moistened in saline during transport to definitive care.

Special Considerations

Trauma-Informed Care

Trauma-informed care recognizes the impact of any form of trauma throughout the life of the patient and the signs and symptoms of trauma in order to respond appropriately while minimizing retraumatization. The steps of culturally sensitive trauma-informed care are (1) recognizing variations in the subjective perception of trauma; (2) restoring safety and reestablishing trust; (3) attending to distress while highlighting survivors' strengths and supporting their resiliency; and (4) working within and through the family to address stressors such as housing, physical and mental health, and legal issues. This approach builds better understanding of the effects of trauma on behavior, improves interactions between health care clinicians and patients, and enhances healing and recovery.

Although it is important for clinicians to be respectful of and sensitive to the life histories of all patients, utilizing trauma-informed care can be especially helpful when caring for those who have been victims of personal and/or sexual violence, as discussed next.

Human Trafficking

Human trafficking (also known as "trafficking in persons" or "modern slavery") is emerging as a health care priority and public health issue worldwide, Per the Trafficking Victims Protection Act (TVPA) of 2000, which criminalizes trafficking by making it illegal to use force, fraud, or coercion to exploit a person for profit or for personal services, human trafficking is defined as "(a) the recruitment, harboring, transporting, supplying, or obtaining a person for labor or services through the use of force, fraud, or coercion for the purpose of involuntary servitude or slavery; or (b) sex trafficking in which a commercial sex act is induced by force, fraud, or coercion, or in which the person induced to perform sex acts is under 18 years of age." Persons of all ages and genders can be trafficked, but due to the inequalities that women face in societies and cultures worldwide, they are particularly vulnerable, and children are the most vulnerable (due to ease of kidnapping and long-term value for those purchasing them). According to the U.S. Department of State, 14,500 to 17,500 people are trafficked in the United States each year and an estimated 27 million people are enslaved worldwide. Research estimates about 100,000 to 300,000 children younger than 18 years of age are at risk for commercial sexual exploitation, with the average age of entry into sex work in the United States being 12 to 14 years for girls and 11 to 13 years for boys.

Trafficking victims may frequently experience physical and psychological abuse, including beatings, sexual abuse, food and sleep deprivation, extreme stress, shame, intimidation, deportation, threats to themselves and their family members, and isolation from the outside world. Common health problems of victims trafficked into prostitution or sex slavery include STIs, unintended pregnancies, vaginal or rectal trauma, infertility, and frequent urinary tract infections. Therefore, it is crucial that clinicians develop interviewing techniques focused on identifying at-risk patients and practicing culturally sensitive patient-centered and trauma-informed care that acknowledges, respects, and integrates patients' and families' cultural values, beliefs, and customs.

Common red flags that should raise suspicion of human trafficking include the following:

- An individual who accompanies the patient and is reluctant to let them speak to health care clinicians alone
- Inconsistent or nonsensical history
- Adolescents who do not know their address or how to get home
- Falsified identifying information
- Unfamiliarity with the city or town in which they are located
- Unexplained absences from school, work, or other social activities
- Work-related injuries
- Sexually expressive behavior
- Untreated chronic illnesses
- Sexually transmitted infection
- Trauma to the vagina or rectum
- Cigarette, iron, or acid burns
- History of abortions or miscarriages
- Tattoo or "brand" with an individual or organization's insignia

Studies report that up to 88% of trafficked persons see a health care clinician during their time in captivity, and one study surveyed over 100 survivors of domestic sex trafficking and found 63% reported being seen in the ED while being trafficked. Survivors of human trafficking commonly seek medical care for severe health issues focusing on psychological and physical abuse. Therefore, the medical community must be vigilant in reporting human trafficking to law enforcement along with recognizing and responding to the complex health care needs and necessary comprehensive care for this vulnerable and underserved patient population.

Intimate Partner Violence

The World Health Organization defines **intimate partner violence (IPV)** as "behavior within an intimate relationship that causes physical, sexual or psychological harm, including acts of physical aggression, sexual coercion, psychological abuse and controlling behaviors." IPV is ubiquitous to all ages, races, genders, and socioeconomic classes: 26% of women and 11% of men have experienced severe IPV. It accounts for 15% of all violent crime in the United States. IPV includes violence inflicted by both current and former intimate partners.

Despite being so prevalent, IPV may be difficult to identify because individuals who experience it may feel culpable and ashamed in the violence that has been done to them. We often equate IPV with physical and sexual violence and abuse. However, the psychological, emotional, and economic abuse that may accompany the physical violence help perpetuate the cycle and place some of the greatest barriers to recovery and to those well-meaning health care clinicians hoping to help end this cycle.

The abuser will often slowly and systematically discourage the abused from interacting with friends and family, particularly those who are apt to point out the controlling behaviors. This isolation gives the relationship with the abuser greater importance and exerts more control over the life of the abused. This control also can manifest as financial control over the relationship, which makes leaving the relationship even more challenging, particularly if there are children involved. Abusers frequently tell their partners that the partners are not capable of functioning independently or that they wouldn't be desired by anyone else. These statements make the victim feel that even if they were capable of leaving, it isn't in their best interest.

The cycle of violence moves through three phases and often escalates over time and with increased stressors on the perpetrator. These three phases are the tension-building phase, the crisis phase, and the honeymoon phase. During the tension-building phase, the abused will feel increasingly like they have to take great care in their actions to not provoke the abuser. This is frequently described as having to "walk on eggshells," furthering the idea that the partner experiencing abuse can prevent the abusive behavior if they only are careful enough. The crisis phase is when the abuse and tension lead to actual physical or sexual violence. This phase is short-lived, usually lasting only a few minutes to a few hours, but is of great threat to the patient. Lastly, the honeymoon phase consists of the abuser apologizing for their actions, often promising to change in the future. Those experiencing IPV will, on average, attempt to leave that partner 7 to 12 times before they are able to permanently leave the relationship because the power and control exerted upon them by the cycle of violence is so strong.

Clinicians can most help those experiencing IPV primarily by recognizing it. Some research suggests that only 5% of women experiencing IPV are identified by health care professionals when presenting to an emergency department setting. Clinicians need to become familiar with possible indicators of IPV. Patients who are experiencing IPV frequently have a hard time keeping scheduled medical appointments or may have their partner with them dominating the conversation or refusing to leave the patient's side. These patients often present in the emergency setting with unexplained injuries or injuries inconsistent with the history given. They may present more frequently than their peers. They may have a history of recurrent urinary tract infections, STIs, pelvic or lower back pain, headaches, repeat pregnancies, repeat abortions, or recurrent miscarriages.

Clinicians should have a low threshold for inquiry of IPV when caring for all patients. Clinicians should also be prepared to report this information to a receiving facility.

Next, health care clinicians can address the abuse. Remind the patient that abuse is not a consequence of their actions, but rather an unacceptable response on the part of the abuser. Indicate the patient is not alone. Addressing violence in a straightforward and nonjudgmental manner is of the utmost importance in establishing rapport with the patient and helping them feel supported.

Clinicians can help end the cycle of violence by avoiding behaviors that revictimize the patient and by emphasizing empowerment through choice. Revictimization can happen when forcing the patient into actions and decisions or by imparting shame on the patient for their situation. This is similar to the power-and-control imbalance that the victim experiences with the perpetrator of violence. Further, this will contribute to feelings of helplessness and dissuade patients from seeking help in the future. How you talk to a patient experiencing IPV is important. Table 12-1 provides some examples of how to phrase statements or questions to show support to the patient.

Empower patients by giving them choices about their care, and support their decisions regardless of what they

Table 12-1 Communication Awareness for Patients Experiencing IPV

Unhelpful Phrases in Addressing IPV	Why This Is Counterproductive	Say This Instead	Why This Is Different and Can Help
"I would never let someone treat me that way."	This is an isolating statement that creates a difference between the clinician and the patient by making the patient seem less rational or less capable than the clinician.	"No one deserves to be treated that way."	This builds the patient into a bigger community and takes the blame for stopping or preventing the violence from the victim.
"I don't understand why anyone would go back to a relationship like that."	This ignores the power that a perpetrator may be exerting over that person's life while placing blame for that patient's situation on themselves.	"I understand that it can be difficult to leave a relationship. What are some things that keep you in this relationship?"	This acknowledges the role that isolation and coercion can play in a relationship. This also allows the patient to discuss some of the barriers to leaving the relationship giving the clinician a way to address those specific concerns.
"You need to leave them."	This is a forced choice. Empower the patient through options and support in those options.	"We are able to offer you resources that can help in the transition should you want to leave the relationship."	This places the decision making under the patient's control, doesn't imply a correct choice, and offers support in that process.

are. Know what resources are available in your community to support those experiencing IPV, and ask the patient if it is safe to share those resources with them. Support for patients may need to come from multiple sources (e.g., health care, law enforcement, legal), and know that as an EMS clinician you are part of the patient's safety net.

It can be frustrating for health care clinicians to see patients elect to go back into the situation that has just caused them harm. Although the patient may not be able or ready to leave their partner during this cycle, by providing compassionate care and support the clinician can set the groundwork to help them leave during the next cycle. This care indicates that the clinician has a deep understanding of the pathology of IPV and how to help treat it.

Sexual Assault

Sexual assault is defined as any nonconsensual sexual act. Although sexual violence may be a component of IPV, it doesn't have to occur within the confines of an intimate partner relationship. Sexual assault is common, particularly for women. Sexual assaults are most often perpetrated by someone known to the survivor; 8 out of 10 rapes are committed by someone the survivor knows. Forty-three percent of women report some form of sexual contact violence in their lifetime, with 4.7% reporting forced sexual contact in the previous 12 months.

The approach to sexual assault survivors is similar to those of IPV. Less than half of sexual assault survivors report their sexual assault; those who do report likely do not report it immediately. Those who are less likely to report include members of the LGBTQIA community, those whose sexual assault is perpetrated by a partner, and those for whom the power differential between the perpetrator and the victim is greater.

Avoiding retraumatization is of immense importance in the assessment of a patient who has been sexually assaulted. This is accomplished by, again, empowering the patient through choice. Obtain express consent for any patient assessment. Sexual assault assessments are often performed by clinicians who are specially trained to do so. However, building a rapport with the patient based on empowerment and choice can be done by any prehospital clinician. Discuss reporting options with the patient and ask if the patient would like law enforcement contacted (if not already present). Patients may feel more comfortable with a same-gendered clinician performing the assessment or at least present. Keep in mind that evidence preservation will assist with potential prosecution.

Putting It All Together

Although physiologic and hormonal differences may contribute to varying presentations and incidences of diseases between males and females, patient health has been proven to be impacted by one's lifestyle and social position. As such, clinicians must take into consideration the physical, mental, and socioeconomic status of patients, particularly women and gender-diverse patients, to provide the best possible care.

Prehospital clinicians can best contribute to the advancement of women's health through enhanced education and implementation of more sensitive and inclusive clinical policies. More focus on cultural understanding and social and structural health determinants will enable clinicians to meet their patients' cultural, social, and linguistic needs most effectively.

Diminishing biases and disparities in the diagnosis and treatment of acute disease ensures improved patient outcomes—this applies to patients of any race, ethnicity, gender, sexual orientation, or socioeconomic status.

SCENARIO SOLUTION

- The differential diagnosis may include acute coronary syndrome, ranging from unstable angina to STEMI; pulmonary embolism; COPD; and acute pulmonary edema secondary to heart failure or pulmonary artery hypertension. A thorough review of the patient's medical history—including recent procedures and medications—helps to expand the differential diagnosis to include conditions such as peripartum cardiomyopathy and OHSS.
- Additional information includes obtaining details within the history of present illness to understand the timing of recent births, medications, and procedures. The secondary survey plus ECG monitoring and SpO_2 are also vital to narrowing the cause for emergent disease.
- This patient has signs of acute pulmonary edema. With the history of recent fertility treatment, OHSS should be considered as a likely diagnosis. In severe cases of OHSS, patients are frequently hypovolemic; initial stabilization includes fluid resuscitation to maintain adequate circulation. EMS also must provide sufficient respiratory support. Administer oxygen and consider noninvasive ventilation if needed. Transport to the appropriate facility, and note that a clear and concise handoff is equally as important as direct patient intervention in this case. By informing receiving clinicians of the primary impression of OHSS, a bedside ultrasound in the emergency department can help to rapidly confirm the diagnosis and expedite OB/GYN consultation and intervention.

SUMMARY

- Women's health should highlight sex-based differences in physiology. Clinicians should also recognize the unique life experiences that impact disease morbidity and mortality. Using this approach helps to narrow gender bias and broaden differential diagnoses.
- Hormonal and other sex-based changes alter the presentation of various diseases for women. The effects of these hormonal changes are different during the childbearing years and the peri- and postmenopausal periods. These sex-based differences in patient presentation of various disorders are apparent in cardiovascular, respiratory, neurologic, and mental health disorders.
- Human trafficking, sexual assault, and interpersonal violence can occur to both women and men. A sensitive and caring approach can prepare a patient to change their situation and helps to relieve the inappropriate feelings of guilt that patients may have.

Key Terms

assisted reproductive technology (ART) Fertility treatments that help women become pregnant.

human trafficking Using force, fraud, or coercion to obtain some type of forced labor or commercial sex act (sexual slavery).

intimate partner violence (IPV) Violence by a spouse or partner (current or former) in an intimate domestic relationship against the other spouse or partner.

menarche Onset of menstruation and fertility.

menopause End of menstruation and fertility.

septic abortion A severe infection of the uterus associated with an induced or spontaneous abortion.

sexual assault Nonconsensual sexual contact.

sexually transmitted infections (STIs) Infections transmitted through sexual contact.

trauma-informed care Clinical approach acknowledging that a patient's previous experiences affect their responses to subsequent health care issues and encounters.

Bibliography

Adamson GD, Zegers-Hochschild F, Dyer S. Global fertility care with assisted reproductive technology. *Fertil Steril.* 2023;120 (3 Pt 1):473–482. doi:10.1016/j.fertnstert.2023.01.013

Ali P, McGarry J, Dhingra K. Identifying signs of intimate partner violence. *Emerg Nurse.* 2016;23(9):25–29. doi:10.7748/en.23.9.25.s25

American Academy of Pediatrics & Society for Adolescent Health and Medicine. Screening for nonviral sexually transmitted infections in adolescents and young adults. *Pediatrics.* 2014;134(1):e302.

American Civil Liberties Union. Human trafficking: modern enslavement of immigrant women in the United States. May 31, 2007. https://www.aclu.org/other/human-trafficking-modern-enslavement-immigrant-women-united-states

Bridwell RE, Koyfman A, Long B. High risk and low prevalence diseases: tubo-ovarian abscess. *Am J Emerg Med.* 2022;57: 70–75. doi:10.1016/j.ajem.2022.04.026

Burnett AM, Anderson CP, Zwank MD. Laboratory-confirmed gonorrhea and/or chlamydia rates in clinically diagnosed pelvic inflammatory disease and cervicitis. *Am J Emerg Med.* 2012;30(7):1114–1117.

Centers for Disease Control and Prevention. *Sexually transmitted disease surveillance 2017.* U.S. Department of Health and Human Services; 2018.

Connelly PJ, Freel EM, Perry C, et al. Gender-affirming hormone therapy, vascular health and cardiovascular disease in transgender adults. *Hypertension.* 2019;74:1266–1274. doi:10.1161/HYPERTENSIONAHA.119.13080

Costa CB, McCoy KT, Early GJ, Deckers CM. Evidence-based care of the human trafficking patient. *Nurs Clin North Am.* 2019;54(4):569–584. doi:10.1016/j.cnur.2019.08.007

EMS World. Prehospital management of the pregnant patient. Updated March 2004. https://www.hmpgloballearningnetwork.com/site/emsworld/article/10324831/prehospital-management-pregnant-patient

Eschenbach DA. Treating spontaneous and induced septic abortions. *Obstetr Gynecol.* 2015;125:1042–1048.

Eshkoli T, Barski L, Faingelernt Y, et al. Diabetic ketoacidosis in pregnancy—case series, pathophysiology, and review of the literature. *Eur J Obstet Gynecol.* 2022;269:41–46.

Estes RJ, Weiner NA. *The Commercial Sexual Exploitation of Children in the US, Canada and Mexico.* University of Pennsylvania School of Social Work; 2021.

Fuchs W, Brockmeyer NH. Sexually transmitted infections. *J Dtsch Dermatol Ges.* 2014;12(6):451–463. doi:10.1111/ddg.12310

Grimes DA, Benson J, Singh S, et al. Sexual and reproductive health 4: unsafe abortion—the preventable pandemic. *Lancet.* 2006;368:1908–1919.

Gut-Gobert C, Cavaillès A, Dixmier A, et al. Women and COPD: do we need more evidence? *Eur Respir Rev.* 2019;28(151):180055. doi:10.1183/16000617.0055-2018

Hill TD, Needham BL. Rethinking gender and mental health: a critical analysis of three propositions. *Soc Sci Med.* 2013;92: 83–91. doi:10.1016/j.socscimed.2013.05.025

Hussain A, McDonald N, Little N, et al. Paramedic perspectives on sex and gender equity in prehospital electrocardiogram acquisition. *Australas J Paramed.* 2023;20(1):23–34. doi:10.1177/27536386221150947

Kamalakannan D, Baskar V, Barton DM, et al. Diabetic ketoacidosis in pregnancy. *Postgrad Med J.* 2003;79:454–457.

Kassebaum N, Bertozzi-Villa A, Coggeshall M, et al. Global, regional, and national levels and causes of maternal mortality during 1990–2013: a systematic analysis for the Global Burden of Disease Study 2013. *Lancet.* 2014;384:980–1004.

Kent M, Blickley Z. Resuscitation of acute decompensated pulmonary hypertension: a prehospital perspective. *JEMS.* Updated March 10, 2020. https://www.jems.com/exclusives/acute-decompensated-pulmonary-hypertension/

Lang T. Estrogen as an immunomodulator. *Clin Immunol.* 2004;113(3):224–230.

McCormack D, Koons K. Sexually transmitted infections. *Emerg Med Clin North Am*. 2019;37(4):725–738. doi:10.1016/j.emc.2019.07.009

Lederer L, Wetzel C. The health consequences of sex trafficking and their implications for identifying victims in healthcare facilities. *Ann Health Law*. 2014;23:61–91.

Logan TK, Walker R, Hunt G. Understanding human trafficking in the United States. *Trauma Violence Abuse*. 2009;10(1):3–30. doi:10.1177/1524838008327262

Moores L, Bilello KL, Murin S. Sex and gender issues and venous thromboembolism. *Clin Chest Med*. 2004;25(2):281–297.

Morrow M, Hankivsky O, Varcoe C. *Women's Health in Canada: Challenges of Intersectionality*, 2nd ed. University of Toronto Press; 2022.

Nobelius AM, Wainer J. *Gender and Medicine: A Conceptual Guide for Medical Educators*. Monash University School of Rural Health; 2004.

Owusu-Edusei K, Bohm MK, Chesson HW, et al. Chlamydia screening and pelvic inflammatory disease: insights from exploratory time–series analyses. *Am J Prev Med*. 2010;38(6):652–657.

Pyra M, Casimiro I, Rusie L, et al. An observational study of hypertension and thromboembolism among transgender patients using gender-affirming hormone therapy. *Transgender Health*. 2020;5(1):1–9.

Ranney ML, Locci N, Adams EJ, et al. Gender-specific research on mental illness in the emergency department: current knowledge and future directions. *Acad Emerg Med*. 2014;21:1395–1402.

Renda G, Patti G, Lang IM, et al. Thrombotic and hemorrhagic burden in women: gender-related issues in the response to antithrombotic therapies. *Int J Cardiol*. 2019;286:198–207. doi:10.1016/j.ijcard.2019.02.004

Riecher-Rössler A. Comment: Sex and gender differences in mental disorders. *Lancet Psychiatr*. 2016;4(1):8–9. doi:10.1016/S2215-0366(16)30348-0

Rodriguez-Arias JJ, García-Álvarez A. Sex differences in pulmonary hypertension. *Front Aging*. 2021;2:727558. doi:10.3389/fragi.2021.727558

Sabella D. The role of the nurse in combating human trafficking. *Am J Nurs*. 2011;111(2):28–37; quiz 38–39. doi:10.1097/01.NAJ.0000394289.55577.b6

Schon SB, Kelley AS, Jiang C, et al. Emergency department utilization for ovarian hyperstimulation syndrome. *Am J Emerg Med*. 2022;60:134–139. doi:10.1016/j.ajem.2022.08.014

Shannon C, Brothers LP, Philip NM, Winikoff B. Infection after medical abortion: a review of the literature. *Contraception*. 2004;70(3):183–190. doi:10.1016/j.contraception.2004.04.009

Sieving RE, Gewirtz O'Brien JR, Saftner MA, Argo TA. Sexually transmitted diseases among US adolescents and young adults: patterns, clinical considerations, and prevention. *Nurs Clin North Am*. 2019;54(2):207–225. doi:10.1016/j.cnur.2019.02.002

Stubblefield PG, Grimes DA. Septic abortion. *New Engl J Med*. 1994;331(5):310–314.

Substance Abuse and Mental Health Services Administration. *SAMHSA's Concept of Trauma and Guidance for a Trauma-Informed Approach*. HHS Publication No. (SMA) 14-4884. Substance Abuse and Mental Health Services Administration; 2014.

Tarnutzer AA, Lee SH, Robinson KA, et al. ED misdiagnosis of cerebrovascular events in the era of modern neuroimaging: ameta-analysis. *Neurology*. 2007;88(15):1468–1477. doi:10.1212/WNL.0000000000003814

Tiller J, Reynolds S. Human trafficking in the emergency department: improving our response to a vulnerable population. *West J Emerg Med*. 2020;21(3):549–554. doi:10.5811/westjem.2020.1.41690

Timmons D, Montrief T, Koyfman A, et al. Ovarian hyperstimulation syndrome: a review for emergency clinicians. *J Emerg Med*. 2019;37(8):1577–1584. doi:10.1016/j.ajem.2019.05.018

United Nations. Integrating a gender perspective into statistics. Updated January 5, 2021. https://unstats.un.org/wiki/display/genderstatmanual/Mortality+and+causes+of+death.

Vicard-Olagne M, Pereira B, Rougé L, et al. Signs and symptoms of intimate partner violence in women attending primary care in Europe, North America and Australia: a systematic review and meta-analysis. *Fam Pract*. 2022;39(1):190–199. doi:10.1093/fampra/cmab097

Vogel B Acevedo M, Appelman Y, et al. The Lancet Women and Cardiovascular Disease Commission: reducing the global burden by 2030. *Lancet*. 2021;397:2385–2438.

Vousden N, Nathan HL, Shennan AH. Innovations in vital signs measurement for the detection of hypertension and shock in pregnancy. *Reprod Health*. 2018;15(Suppl 1):92. doi:10.1186/s12978-018-0533-4

Warriner IK, Shah IH, eds. *Preventing Unsafe Abortion and Its Consequences: Priorities for Research and Action*. Guttmacher Institute; 2006.

White K, Carroll E, Grossman D. Complications from first-trimester aspiration abortion: a systematic review of the literature. *Contraception*. 2015;92(5):422–438. doi:10.1016/j.contraception.2015.07.013

Wilcox SR, Kabrhel C, Channick RN. Pulmonary hypertension and right ventricular failure in emergency medicine. *Ann Emerg Med*. 2015;66(6):619–628. doi:10.1016/j.annemergmed.2015.07.525

Wilkerson G, Ogunbodede AC. Hypertensive disorders of pregnancy. *Emerg Med Clin N Am*. 2019;37(2):301–316.

Willging C, Gunderson L, Shattuck D, et al. Structural competency in emergency medicine services for transgender and gender non-conforming patients. *Soc Sci Med*. 2019;222:67–75. doi:10.1016/j.socscimed.2018.12.031

Wittels KA, Mayes KD, Eyre A. Ovarian hyperstimulation syndrome: a simulation case for emergency medicine residents. *MedEd PORTAL*. 2022;18:11271. doi:10.15766/mep_2374-8265.11271

World Health Organization. Intimate partner violence. 2022. https://apps.who.int/violence-info/intimate-partner-violence/#:~:text=Intimate%20partner%20violence%20refers%20to,and%20former%20spouses%20and%20partner

Yu AY, Penn AM, Lesperance ML, et al. Sex differences in presentation and outcome after an acute transient or minor neurologic event. *JAMA Neurol*. 2019;76(8):962–968. doi:10.1001/jamaneurol.2019.1305

Yu S. Uncovering the hidden impacts of inequality on mental health: a global study. *Transl Psychiatr*. 2018;8:98. doi:10.1038/s41398-018-0148-0

Zachow R. Applied and integrative endocrinology case: a 31-year-old woman with shortness of breath, chest pain, nausea, and dizziness. *MedEdPORTAL*. 2012;8:9121.

CHAPTER 13

Environmental Disorders

Chapter Editor
B. Craig Ellis, MBChB, Dip IMC (RCSEd), FACEM

In this chapter, illnesses and injuries related to cold, heat, and atmospheric pressure are discussed. Unique to environmental emergencies are the conditions that directly cause harm or complicate treatment and transport considerations. Wind, rain, snow, temperature extremes, and humidity may all affect the body's ability to adapt to its environment. The AMLS Assessment Pathway will guide your decisions and help you recognize and effectively treat patients with environmental emergencies in various settings.

LEARNING OBJECTIVES

At the conclusion of this chapter, you will be able to:

- Describe the pathophysiology, assessment, and management of environmental emergencies.
- Formulate provisional diagnoses based on assessment findings for various environmental disorders.
- Describe cold injuries and their underlying causes.
- Describe the process of providing emergency care to a person who has experienced an emergency related to cold using the AMLS Assessment Pathway.
- Describe the spectrum of illnesses caused by heat exposure, including their signs and symptoms.
- Describe the process of providing emergency care to a person who has experienced an emergency related to heat using the AMLS Assessment Pathway.
- Define drowning, diving, and altitude emergencies, and explain how they may be treated.

SCENARIO

You are caring for a 30-year-old man who fell through the ice while riding his snowmobile. He was able to walk home from the incident and wrap himself in a blanket. He was lying on the floor conscious and shivering when you arrived. His vital signs include a blood pressure of 80/40 mm Hg; pulse rate, 104 beats/min, weak and irregular; and respirations, 10 breaths/min, slow and shallow.

- How do you begin assessment of this patient?
- What clinical conditions and injuries might this patient be suffering from? What information do you need to determine which of these are present?
- What are your initial treatment priorities as you continue your patient care?

You may not expect to encounter environmental emergencies frequently in your practice, particularly if you are in an urban setting. However, environmental emergencies are more common than expected. Socioeconomic factors contribute to a surprisingly high number of environmental emergencies even in urban areas. For example, on average, 1,301 deaths from hypothermia occurred annually in the United States during the years 1999–2011.

Environmental emergencies (Table 13-1) include medical conditions caused or worsened by the weather, terrain, or unique atmospheric conditions present at high altitude or underwater.

Anatomy and Physiology

Temperature Regulation and Related Disorders

Most heat- and cold-related emergencies occur during seasonal exposure to significant temperature changes. You may associate environmental emergencies with outdoor activities, but such problems are also common among special populations. Deaths from heat illness and hypothermia have consistently been shown to occur more in the homeless and elderly populations. The importance of this for EMS lies in the need to consider these causes both as a primary diagnosis and as a contributing factor in wider presentations in those at risk. Both hypo- and hyperthermia can cause an altered mental state. It is important to consider this in your differential diagnosis in appropriate populations and situations.

Table 13-1 Causes of Environmental Emergencies

Environmental Condition	Resulting Disease States
Cold	Hypothermia: nonfreezing injuries (immersion foot, frostnip); freezing injuries (frostbite)
Heat	Hyperthermia: heat-related dehydration and mild electrolyte disturbance; heat exhaustion (physiologically unwell but retained temperature regulation); heatstroke (physiologically unwell with loss of temperature regulation)
Pressure change	Diving related: barotrauma, decompression sickness Altitude related: HACE, HAPE
Submersion	Drowning (the term "near-drowning" is no longer used)

HACE, High-altitude cerebral edema; HAPE, high-altitude pulmonary edema.

Many medical conditions and medications also impair the body's ability to thermoregulate and make people more susceptible to insults from changes in environmental temperature.

The process by which the body compensates for temperature changes is called **thermoregulation**. Normal body temperature has a diurnal fluctuation between 36°C and 37.5°C (96.8°F and 99.5°F), and the body uses both behavioral (avoidance of temperature discomfort) and physiologic mechanisms to maintain precise control within approximately 1.8°C (1°F) of this range. Physiologic control is centered in the hypothalamus, which contains not only the control mechanisms (selecting a temperature set point like a thermostat) but also the sensory mechanisms necessary to detect temperature changes. The body responds to differences between the set point and actual temperature using both hormones and neural control to cause changes in heat production, dissipation, and retention. For example, sweating begins almost precisely at a skin temperature of 37°C (98.6°F) and increases quickly as skin temperature rises.

Temperature measurements may be obtained via the oral, axillary, forehead surface, tympanic, rectal, or esophageal routes using either a digital or analog thermometer. The core body temperature—the temperature in the part of the body that contains the heart, lungs, brain, and abdominal viscera—is considered the best representation of actual body temperature. Historically, rectal temperature has been considered the best representation of core body temperature. However, because the rectal temperature lags behind actual core body temperature, esophageal temperature is considered the gold standard, and some EMS monitors are equipped to be able to obtain continuous esophageal temperatures.

If the body temperature falls below the set point determined in the hypothalamus, the body attempts to retain heat using a range of mechanisms, including the following:

- Vasoconstriction to decrease radiant heat loss from the skin
- Cessation of sweating
- Shivering to increase heat production in the muscles
- Secretion of norepinephrine, epinephrine, and thyroxine to increase heat production

If the body temperature rises above the set point determined in the hypothalamus, the body attempts to shed excess heat through vasodilation and sweating. Even when people are faced with extreme environmental heat, the heat production in the body from basal metabolic processes remains nearly constant.

In cases of infection, the temperature set point in the hypothalamus is adjusted temporarily to increase body temperature and make the body less hospitable to invading pathogens. This results in a transient increase in heat generation to achieve the new set point. As the body makes these adjustments, patients may be seen to shiver or have rigors during heat production and sweat to lose heat as the fever subsides. Many drugs and toxins may also alter this temperature set point, as reviewed in Chapter 14, *Toxicology*.

AMLS Assessment Pathway ▸▸▸▸

▾ Initial Observations

Environmental conditions should be noted as you prepare for the problems your patient may experience—wind chill, air temperature, and whether the conditions are wet or dry. Although your dispatch information may indicate a medical or trauma emergency, cold- or heat-related illness may be part of the picture. The environment, especially when it is hot outside, may have an impact on your patient's condition. You must also remember to protect yourself from the cold and heat; this includes ensuring that your agency has appropriate summer and winter uniforms and that personal protective equipment (PPE) such as ballistic vests or bunker coats are only worn when there is a strong operational reason to do so in a hot or very humid environment. Even in hot weather, it may be more appropriate to wear long sleeves to help you from being splashed with blood and other body fluids.

Scene Safety Considerations

On arrival, assess scene safety. Consider potential safety hazards, such as icy streets or extremely hot pavement. Cold weather may present special problems for you and your patients, especially if a hazard such as an avalanche exists. Use appropriate standard precautions, and note the number of patients at the scene. Identify whether you need additional help, such as a search and rescue team, and request assistance as soon as possible. When an injured patient is exposed to cold or heat or has an extended extraction time, it is important to be alert for patient heat loss to the environment and take steps to prevent the development of hypothermia or heat illness.

Patient Cardinal Presentation/Chief Complaint

In a cold emergency, the patient's cardinal presentation/chief complaint may be that of being cold, or the cold may be a complication of an existing medical or trauma condition. The National Institutes of Health has initiated a public awareness campaign informing the public to watch for "umbles"—stumbles, mumbles, bumbles, and grumbles. These behaviors are good indicators of how the environment affects the cerebral and cognitive functioning of patients in the early stages of hypothermia or hyperthermia.

In a heat emergency, the patient's cardinal presentation/chief complaint may indicate heat illness as the primary problem, or heat may be an aggravating factor in a medical or trauma condition. The patient may report specific signs and symptoms such as a decreased level of consciousness, muscle cramping, nausea, vomiting, and the absence of perspiration.

Primary Survey

Level of Consciousness

Evaluate the patient's mental status. The patient's level of consciousness diminishes as alterations in body temperature become more severe.

Airway and Breathing

Assess your patient's airway and breathing, and address any immediate life threats. With a suspected cold- or heat-related illness, your patient assessment should consider the physiologic changes that occur. Remove the patient from the altered environment and into a controlled environment as soon as possible to minimize further heat loss or heat exposure. Providing warm, humidified oxygen if possible in hypothermic cases may assist in rewarming as well.

Nausea and vomiting may occur with heat-related illness and in patients who cannot protect their airway, so place the patient in a position that protects the airway. Breathing may be fast because of elevated core temperature (the tachypnea is a direct response to the raised temperature and is also a cooling mechanism). In unresponsive patients, secure the airway and provide manual ventilation if indicated.

Circulation/Perfusion

Palpate the patient's pulse to assess circulation. Remember that patients suffering from hypothermia may have extreme bradycardia. In more severe hyper- or hypothermia, the patient's perfusion may be compromised, and there may be marked hemodynamic instability. These are late signs in both.

If the patient's pulse rate is adequate, assess the patient for perfusion and bleeding. The patient's skin condition may provide helpful clues to an environmental condition.

Once all immediate life threats have been addressed, a more comprehensive exam should be done to uncover any injuries or information that may not have been found during the primary survey.

First Impression

After you have stabilized the patient and treated any life threats, form a general impression of the patient's status and develop a list of differential diagnoses. Determine whether the patient is "sick" or "not sick," and build on this as you obtain more information in the detailed assessment. Be sure to consider less obvious conditions as well as underlying conditions that may have contributed to the patient's cardinal presentation/chief complaint.

Detailed Assessment

History Taking

It may be difficult to obtain the patient's history during an environmental emergency, but you should make an attempt to find out how long the patient has been exposed to the cold or heat and whether there are other medical conditions of consideration. You may need to talk with the patient's family members or bystanders to obtain the patient's history and the history of the present event.

OPQRST and SAMPLER

The OPQRST and SAMPLER mnemonics should be used to obtain the patient's complete history using a systematic approach. If possible, find out whether the patient has any underlying medical conditions that could affect treatment. It is also important to identify any medications the patient may be taking and the time the patient was last known to be well. Find out what the patient was doing prior to the exposure to help you determine the cause of the problem. Remember, older people typically do not adjust well to heat—they perspire less, feel less thirsty in response to dehydration, and acclimatize more slowly. They are also more likely to have chronic conditions such as cardiovascular disease. Among young and healthy people, infants and young children are most vulnerable to heat stress when exposed to a hot environment. Tailor your questions to help rule in and rule out conditions in your differential diagnosis.

Secondary Survey

Vital Signs

A patient's vital signs can be affected by cold or heat exposure. Vital signs are a good indicator of the severity of the condition. If the respirations are slow and shallow, low levels of oxygen in the body will be found. Low blood pressure and a slow pulse may indicate moderate to severe hypothermia. With heat exposure, the patient may be tachycardic and tachypneic. When heat-related illness becomes severe, the patient's blood pressure begins to fall, and the patient may go into shock. Monitor the patient's vital signs closely.

Physical Exam

If time permits in the ambulance, the detailed assessment should focus on assessing any areas of the body that have been directly affected by the exposure, especially cold. Determine the degree of damage. Is the entire body involved, or have only parts been exposed to the cold? If the patient is shivering, heat is being produced. When shivering stops and the patient remains exposed to the cold, the injury is more severe. Pay particular attention to the patient's mental status and cardiovascular status.

With heat exposure, the physical exam should focus on the patient's metabolism, muscles (e.g., muscle cramps), and cardiovascular system. Continue to monitor the patient's mental status, skin temperature, and wetness. Perform a neurologic exam if time permits.

Diagnostics

A thermometer can be used to determine the patient's body temperature (**Tip Box 13-1**). A low-temperature thermometer is required to take the temperature of a patient with hypothermia, generally done through the

TIP BOX 13-1

Measuring Temperature

Variations in a patient's measured temperature will occur depending on the measurement location and the type of thermometer used. The ideal measurement of a patient's temperature is to measure core body temperature. Accurate readings from esophageal probes (as used in emergency departments and critical care units) or rectal thermometers are not practical for many patients in the field. Less accurate modalities for field use are electronic oral thermometers and infrared tympanic monitors (**Figure 13-1**). Electronic thermometers are common and inexpensive. Disposable probes are available for sublingual or rectal use. Tympanic infrared temperature monitors are relatively inexpensive, not overly intrusive, and efficient. Less ideal are temporal artery scan thermometers and distant infrared scan monitors. Temporal skin monitoring strips are not reliable.

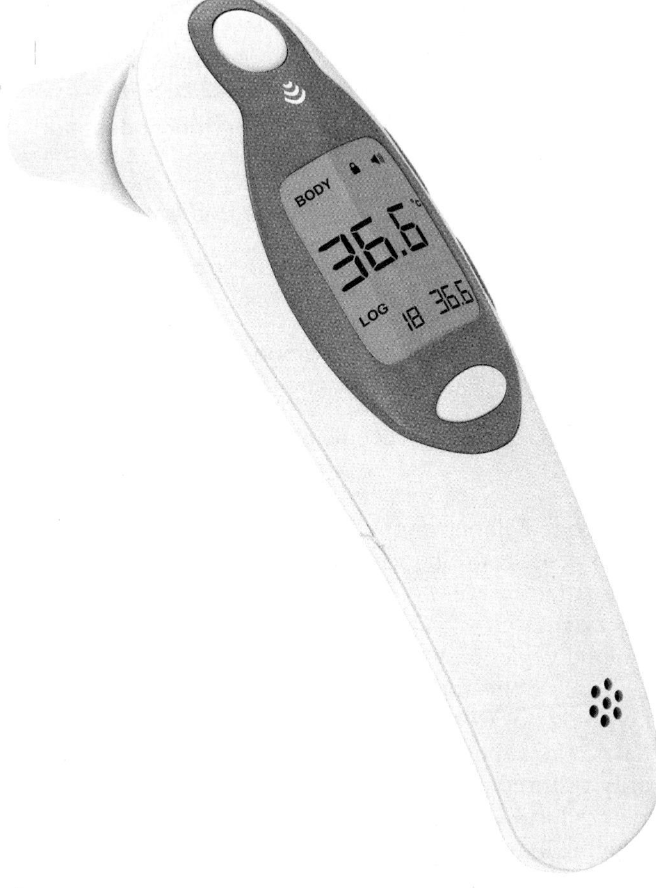

A

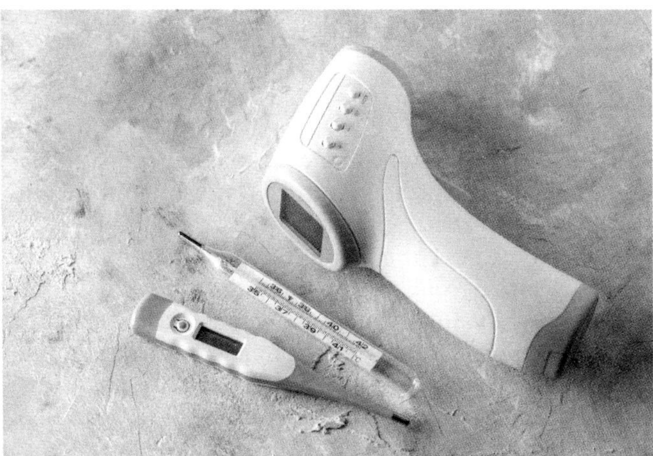

B

Figure 13-1 Thermometers. **A.** Tympanic membrane. **B.** Oral, glass mercury, rectal.

rectum or, when available, the esophagus. Pulse oximetry readings are often inaccurate because of the lack of perfusion to the extremities. The electrocardiogram (ECG) may show signs of hypothermia, such as bradycardia or Osborn waves, and electrolyte abnormalities.

Refine the Differential Diagnosis

Use the information gained during the secondary survey to refine your list of differential diagnoses. Prioritize these by classifying them by severity (life-threatening, emergent, and nonemergent) and by likelihood. Be sure to consider less obvious conditions as well as underlying conditions that may have contributed to the patient's cardinal presentation/chief complaint.

Remember that both heat and cold injuries, regardless of the severity of the exposure, require you to look for indicators of the underlying medical condition to enable you to provide the appropriate treatment. If you are unsure about the cause of the patient's elevated temperature and suspect a heat-related illness, treat the patient for heatstroke and consult with medical direction, if necessary, to assist you in your treatment plan.

Ongoing Management

All patients with cold injuries, even mild degrees of hypothermia, require transport for evaluation and treatment. Handle the patient gently to avoid causing any pain or further injury to the skin. If the patient is alert and shivering, you may begin active rewarming by moving the patient into an area of warmth and using radiant heat to assist in recovering body temperature. Continue oxygen administration if applied during the primary survey, or consider administering oxygen if the patient is hypoxic (oxygen saturation [SpO_2] $< 94\%$) or has signs of respiratory distress. Monitor vital signs frequently.

If the patient has moderate or severe hypothermia, passive rewarming is insufficient and active rewarming should be started. Bumps and rough handling can precipitate ventricular fibrillation in a hypothermic patient. These patients should be moved as smoothly and gently as possible. Active rewarming can be provided in the prehospital setting by heating the ambulance, placing hot packs in the axillae and groin, using a warming blanket, and warming intravenous fluids (IVF). The focus should be on warming the core before extremities due to the concern for the afterdrop phenomenon that results from cold peripheral blood returning to the central circulation from warmed extremities, further dropping the patient's core temperature.

Patients with heat-related illness need to be removed from the hot environment, if not already done earlier during the primary survey. Reassess the patient's condition by monitoring vital signs at least every 5 minutes and noting any deterioration. Avoid inducing shivering in the patient during cooling because shivering generates more heat. Patients with heatstroke should receive immediate cooling, including ice bath immersion if available on scene, and then be transported with ongoing cooling efforts.

Cold-Related Illness and Injury

Hypothermia related to wilderness cold exposure is considered primary hypothermia, whereas hypothermia related to socioeconomic (e.g., homelessness, inability to heat home) or concurrent medical factors, medications, or substance use disorder is considered secondary hypothermia. Cold-related illness includes injuries due to decreased temperature (e.g., frostbite). Cold weather injuries can also occur when the weather is warmer but the person is wet as a result of water immersion. As a health-care clinician, you are also at risk if you work in a cold environment. If cold weather search and rescue operations are conducted in the areas you serve, you need to receive specialized training to both protect yourself and provide appropriate care.

Frostbite

Local cold injury sets in at frigid temperatures, usually below the freezing point. **Frostbite** is the formation of ice crystals within local tissue in exposed areas. It commonly occurs in distal body areas, particularly the toes, feet, and nose, but it can affect the both upper and lower extremities and other areas as well. Factors that increase an individual's chance of developing a cold injury include central hypothermia, prolonged time of exposure, exposure to wind, wearing wet clothing, inactivity or immobility, alcohol consumption, and preexisting medical conditions and medications resulting in decreased peripheral circulation. The areas of the body most at risk are the extremities and the nose and ears.

Frostbite injury can be divided into several clinical stages. **Frostnip** is the first and least severe manifestation of frostbite and is characterized by the skin becoming pale or ashen and cold, with a tingling sensation.

For the purposes of management, frostbite is classified as either superficial (first and second degrees) or deep (third and fourth degrees). However, like burns, frostbite has been classified into degrees of injury *after* rewarming, because most frostbite injuries initially appear similar (Table 13-2).

Table 13-2 Classification of Frostbite

Degree	Characteristics After Rewarming
First	No blisters or erythema; numbness and tingling
Second	Clear blisters, edema, and erythema
Third	Hemorrhagic blisters, subcutaneous involvement, dead skin, and tissue loss
Fourth	Full-thickness (bone and muscle) tissue loss, necrosis, and deformity

Pathophysiology

The pathophysiology of frostbite is complex and involves several stages of cold injury. The amount of tissue destruction is directly related to the extent of cold exposure. Systemic hypothermia predisposes patients to more severe injury, because the body is unable to oppose the cold temperatures at the extremities. The formation of ice crystals in vulnerable tissues triggers an inflammatory reaction that culminates in cellular death. The crystals tend to form in extracellular areas, altering the local electrolyte balance as the crystals draw water out of adjacent cells, resulting in cellular dysfunction and death. If the affected areas continue to be exposed to cold, the crystals may grow, causing a local mechanical obstruction of blood vessels.

One of the most important concepts in the pathophysiology of frostbite is thawing. When a frozen tissue thaws, the supply of blood to local capillaries is temporarily restored. The blood supply rapidly dwindles, however, as local arterioles and venules release small emboli, inducing hypoxia and thrombosis within the local vasculature. Starved of nutrients, local tissues begin to die, releasing further inflammatory substances and electrolytes. The process of thawing and refreezing is more dangerous and damaging than the initial cold insult.

Signs and Symptoms

Frostbite can initially have a deceptively benign appearance, but it is important not to confuse frostbite with frostnip, a superficial cold insult. The patient may complain of clumsiness or heaviness in an extremity and will probably report coldness and numbness of the affected area, with pain and sensitivity to light touch. The patient may also report tingling, throbbing, and transient numbness that resolves fairly rapidly with rewarming. This is because nerves and blood vessels are most susceptible to cold injury. Complete anesthesia in a cold extremity is a red flag for severe injury. These injuries can become very painful during rewarming.

The initial clinical examination will help you determine the extent and severity of the frostbite, but it is important to note that it may take weeks or even months for the full extent of tissue damage to be visible. Frostbitten tissue will look white or blue-white, will be cool to the touch, and may be hard if still frozen. The skin may lack sensation. Signs and symptoms of superficial (**Figure 13-2**) and deep frostbite (**Figure 13-3**) are provided in Table 13-3.

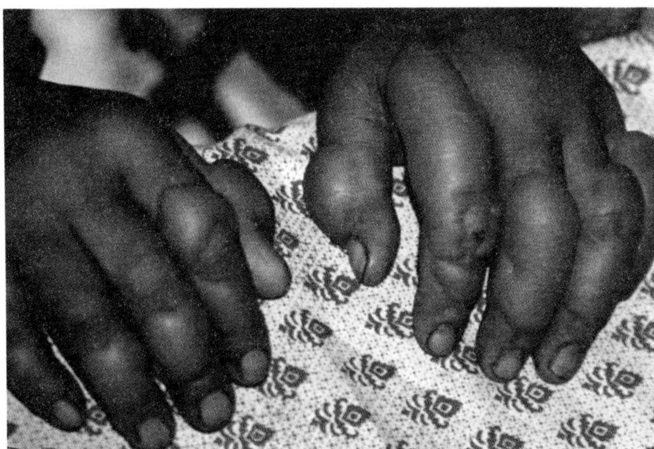

Figure 13-2 Blister formation associated with cold exposure and frostbite.

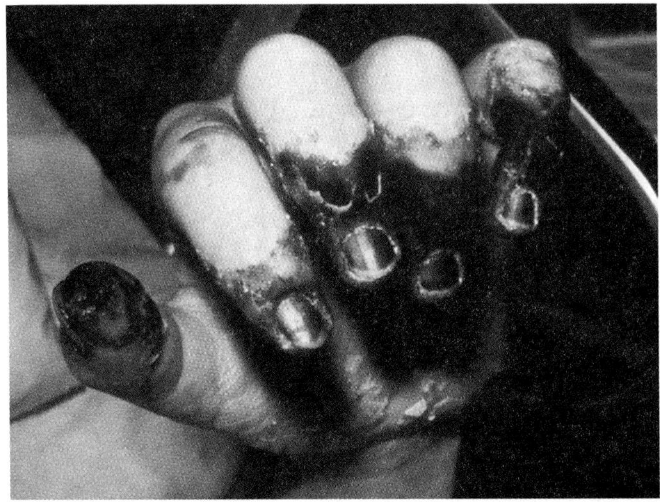

Figure 13-3 An example of third- and fourth-degree frostbite.

Treatment

Prehospital intervention is primarily limited to supporting vital functions and protecting affected extremities. Always search for and treat any systemic hypothermia or trauma first. If frostbite involves the lower extremities, do not allow the person to walk. Remove any jewelry or clothing that may compress the tissue, and remove wet or cold clothing. Apply constant warmth with blankets or towels but avoid using solid objects that make limited contact with the body surface. Friction or massage is ineffective and can damage injured tissue. The most effective therapy is rapid rewarming of the frozen area by immersion in warm (40°C [104°F]) water for 30–40 minutes. This treatment is not recommended, however, if there is *any* risk of refreezing (**Tip Box 13-2**). Rewarming can be extremely painful and opiate analgesia is often required. Transport the patient to an appropriate facility. Patients may require tetanus boosters, antibiotics, specialized wound care, and in some cases, amputation.

Table 13-3 Comparison of Superficial and Deep Frostbite Initial Presentations

Superficial Frostbite	Deep Frostbite
Numbness	Hemorrhagic blisters
Paresthesia (extreme pain during rewarming)	Diminished range of motion
Poor fine motor control (clumsiness)	Necrosis, gangrene
Pruritus	Cold, mottled, gray area (after rewarming)
Edema (usually after rewarming)	Immobile tissue (lost elasticity)
Coldness	

TIP BOX 13-2

Rewarming

Do not start rewarming an injured extremity until you are certain you are in an environment in which you can maintain a rewarming environment. Freezing temperatures create vasoconstriction and lead to ice crystal formations in the tissues. Microcirculatory clots may form as well. If a frozen extremity has been partially thawed and then refreezing occurs, this can worsen the outcome for the patient's extremities. It is best to ensure you are in a location where you can definitively warm the patient's extremity without the risk of re-exposure and refreezing.

Immersion Foot

Pathophysiology

Immersion foot, also known as "trench foot" or a "nonfreezing cold injury," was most famously described in soldiers who spent many hours standing in the wet trenches during World War I. The condition results from prolonged periods of wetness of the feet, particularly in cool water. This prolonged cold and wet exposure is thought to result in vasoconstriction and ischemia of the tissues of the foot, which eventually lead to necrosis. Today, this condition may be seen in builders, hikers, extreme-sports enthusiasts, security guards, campers, and aid workers during natural disasters.

Signs and Symptoms

Immersion foot begins with local discomfort in the affected foot. A tingling or heavy sensation is sometimes described. The foot will be blotchy, cold, and devitalized and will have a wrinkled appearance. The discomfort will increase with rewarming, and the tissue will become erythematous. Blisters eventually form, and the skin may slough off.

Treatment

Prehospital management of immersion foot should be centered around removing the patient from the cold and wet conditions. Dry and warm the feet. Pain control may be needed. Longer-term care involves strict hygiene, antibiotics if infection occurs, and keeping the feet warm and dry.

Systemic Hypothermia

Systemic **hypothermia**, defined as a core body temperature below 35°C (95°F), is a common environmental emergency. Hypothermia is caused by heat loss, decreased heat production, or a combination of the two. The condition can be attributed to a range of metabolic, traumatic, environmental, and infectious causes, but it occurs most often in patients who are exposed to cold environments. It is important to remember that in the presence of certain risk factors (prolonged time of exposure, exposure to wind, wearing wet clothing, inactivity or immobility, alcohol consumption), hypothermia can be precipitated at temperatures well above freezing. It is also more common in the very young, the elderly, and those who are homeless. EMS clinicians must be able to recognize the signs and symptoms of systemic hypothermia.

Pathophysiology

Heat loss occurs via four mechanisms: radiation (direct loss from the body into the atmosphere by emission of electromagnetic energy—heat waves), conduction (direct loss from skin into another solid object, e.g., a cold rock), evaporation (loss via the state change of liquid water to vapor), and convection (direct transfer of heat from the body to air or liquid in contact with the body) (**Figure 13-4**). Any time the body's heat production ability is overwhelmed by heat loss the patient is at risk of hypothermia. The pathophysiology of hypothermia is complex and involves the cardiovascular, renal, neurologic, and respiratory systems. As the body's core temperature drops, each of these systems responds with the aim of preserving heat via the following mechanisms:

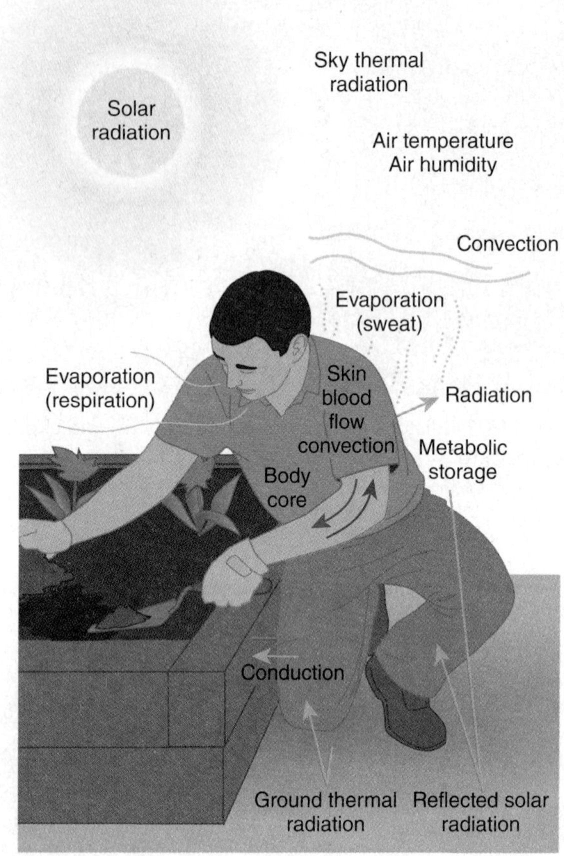

Figure 13-4 How humans exchange thermal energy with the environment.

- *Vasoconstriction*. First, peripheral blood vessels constrict in an effort to shift more blood to vital organs. The other consequence is it reduces the amount of warm blood in the peripheries from which heat can be lost. Later, in severe hypothermia, blood flow to entire organs such as the kidneys drops by up to 50%, threatening renal function and upsetting electrolyte balance.
- *Diuresis*. Vasoconstriction increases urinary output. Urinary output is up to 3.5 times higher if the patient is immersed in cold water. Alcohol consumption further increases diuresis.
- *Respiratory acidosis*. Respiratory rate decreases, followed by a drop in minute ventilation as a result of diminished metabolism. This results in less heat loss via respiration, although it is not the primary driver. In severe hypothermia, carbon dioxide retention causes respiratory acidosis.

- *Tachycardia and bradycardia.* Sinus tachycardia predominates during the initial phases of hypothermia. Later, as hypothermia becomes more severe, bradycardia ensues as a result of diminished depolarization in the pacemaker cells. In this type of bradydysrhythmia, administration of atropine is often ineffective and is not needed because overall metabolism is diminished.
- *Atrial or ventricular fibrillation and asystole.* In mild to moderate hypothermia, atrial or ventricular dysrhythmias can develop because of conduction changes that decrease transmembrane resting potential. As hypothermia worsens, the risk of ventricular fibrillation and asystole increases. Although it can vary, the threshold for ventricular fibrillation is below 28°C (82.4°F).
- *Electrocardiographic anomalies.* Several unique ECG manifestations are seen in patients with a diagnosis of hypothermia. The classic Osborn (J) wave appears at the junction between the QRS complex and the ST segment (**Figure 13-5**). Osborn waves usually become evident at temperatures below 33°C (91.4°F). Osborn waves are largely of academic interest, because the clinical diagnosis of hypothermia is made by measuring the temperature, not by findings on an ECG. As the condition worsens, all intervals—particularly the QT interval—become prolonged. You may have trouble analyzing the ECG because of artifact generated by the patient's shivering.

Signs and Symptoms

EMS clinicians must maintain a high degree of suspicion for hypothermia. In some cases, when the patient has been exposed to cold elements, the diagnosis is obvious. In other cases, the clinical findings may be subtle. Nonspecific symptoms—chills, nausea, hunger, vomiting, dyspnea, or dizziness—may be early signs of hypothermia.

A rapid determination of accurate body temperature is often difficult in the prehospital environment. Normal household thermometers will not be able to accurately measure extremely low temperatures. Available methods such as tympanic, rectal, and esophageal all pose difficulties with accuracy and availability. Because of this, it is often necessary to diagnose systemic hypothermia in the prehospital environment based on history and presentation rather than discrete body temperature measurement. Systemic hypothermia is classified as mild, moderate, or severe based on temperature. Certain clinical findings and core temperatures are characteristic of each stage, although signs and symptoms are variable, and the stages often overlap.

Mild Hypothermia

In mild hypothermia (32°C to 35°C [89.6°F to 95°F]), most people will shiver vigorously. This can be accompanied by nonspecific symptoms such as dizziness, lethargy, nausea, and weakness. An increased metabolic rate occurs in this temperature range as the body tries to produce more heat. More severe neurologic signs such

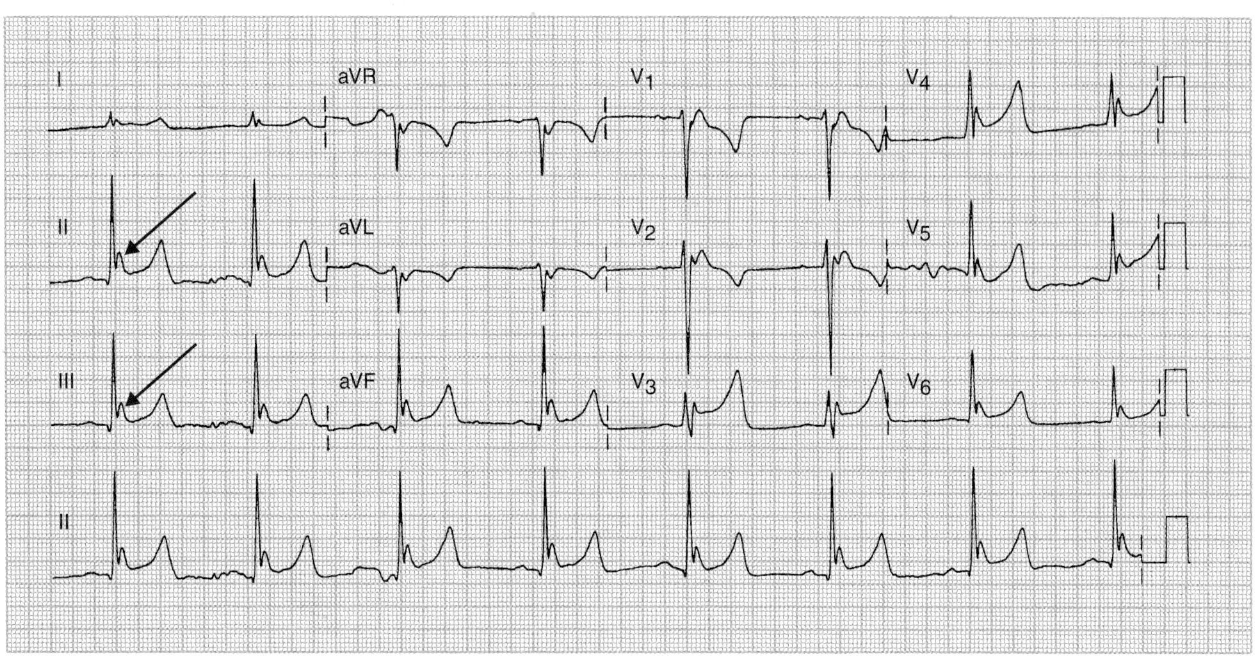

Figure 13-5 Systemic hypothermia is associated with distinctive bulging of the J point (very beginning of the ST segment). Prominent J waves (arrows) with hypothermia are referred to as Osborn waves.

as ataxia (uncoordinated movement) appear once a person's temperature drops to 33°C (91.4°F). Other signs include the following:

- Hyperventilation
- Tachypnea
- Tachycardia

In this stage, the body is generally able to rewarm itself if removed from the cold stress quickly and adequate energy reserves are still available. Shivering generates significant heat from muscular activity.

Moderate Hypothermia

As moderate hypothermia (28°C to 32°C [82.4°F to 89.6°F]) develops, clinical signs of deterioration become apparent. Breathing and heart rate slow, and mental status declines. At 32°C (89.6°F), the patient may become stuporous. As core temperature approaches 31°C (87.8°F), the patient will lose the shivering reflex. Other signs and symptoms of moderate hypothermia include the following:

- Poor judgment
- Atrial fibrillation
- Bradycardia, bradypnea
- Diuresis (increased urinary output)
- J waves may be seen on ECG

In this stage, the body has very little ability to generate heat for self-rewarming.

Severe Hypothermia

Life-threatening cardiovascular problems appear during severe hypothermia (< 28°C [82.4°F]). Hypotension and ventricular arrhythmias become apparent, and an Osborn wave (J wave) is commonly seen on the patient's ECG. The patient is usually unconscious, with dilated and minimally responsive pupils. At this stage, the patient is near cardiac arrest and very susceptible to ventricular fibrillation from even minimal physical manipulation. In this stage, the body has no ability to self-rewarm. Extracorporeal rewarming by cardiopulmonary bypass or extracorporeal membrane oxygenation (ECMO) are the fastest methods of rewarming, and they are the most efficient ways to warm a patient with severe hypothermia.

Differential Diagnosis

Other causes of hypothermia include metabolic disorders linked to a decreased basal metabolic rate and can be related to dysfunction of the thyroid, adrenal, or pituitary glands. Toxicologic emergencies are another common reason for hypothermia.

Treatment

Prehospital management must be guided by the severity of the hypothermia and by the methods available to rewarm the patient. The number one priority should be to stop further heat loss, usually by removing the patient from the cold environment and removing any wet clothing. A patient in a cold, remote setting needs immediate evacuation to a warm environment. Rewarm the patient, prevent further heat loss, and avoid actions that may precipitate complications. For example, rough handling of a severely hypothermic patient has been reported to precipitate a cardiac arrhythmia.

Regardless of the severity of the hypothermia, you must focus on supporting airway, breathing, and circulation as needed and remove any cold, wet clothing to prevent a further drop in core temperature. In addition, nearly all hypothermic patients experience volume depletion. Before administering fluids, warm the fluids to 40°C to 42°C (104°F to 107.6°F). EMS systems that regularly respond to patients with hypothermia should have access to fluid warmers.

Mild Hypothermia

Most cases of mild hypothermia (32°C to 35°C [89.6°F to 95°F]) will resolve with passive rewarming techniques (e.g., using blankets to help contain the patient's own body heat). In addition to the aforementioned general management instructions, provide warm oral fluids (preferably containing sugar) assuming the patient can safely swallow and there are no airway concerns. Warm drinks such as hot chocolate provide heat and sugar, and they can lift a patient's spirit. Avoid caffeinated beverages, however, because they can encourage diuresis. Alcohol and tobacco should also be avoided. If appropriate, encourage gentle exercise. Reassess the patient frequently to evaluate for improvement or decline. Mildly hypothermic patients can quickly deteriorate to become moderately or severely hypothermic.

Moderate Hypothermia

Mental status changes become more apparent in patients with moderate hypothermia (28°C to 32°C [82.4°F to 89.6°F]). Management begins with immediate stabilization of airway, breathing, circulation, and core temperature. Keep the patient supine, and minimize unnecessary movement, because this could precipitate a cardiac arrhythmia. Prevent further cooling by wrapping the patient in a hypothermic wrap with a heat source (e.g., a heating pad/pack) against the torso. Establish IV access and initiate warmed IVF resuscitation. Transport the patient rapidly and gently to an emergency department for continuous rewarming and observation.

Severe Hypothermia

Patients with severe hypothermia (< 28°C [82.4°F]) are usually unconscious. Stabilization of airway, breathing, and circulation is essential to prevent further deterioration. If there is a palpable pulse, handle the patient gently

Table 13-4 Key Considerations in the Management of Severe Hypothermia

Dependent lividity and fixed, dilated pupils are not dependable criteria for withholding CPR in a hypothermic patient.
Evaluation of vital signs may be difficult because the patient may have an undetectable pulse. Spend a longer time than usual (up to 60 seconds) to check for signs of circulation. If there is any doubt or you are unable to detect a pulse, start CPR immediately.
Patients with severe hypothermia often have bradycardia. This may be a protective mechanism because a slow heart rhythm can deliver sufficient oxygen under hypothermic conditions. The use of pacing is rarely indicated.
Consider early endotracheal intubation for ventilation with warm humidified oxygen when available.
Defibrillation is less likely to be effective at core temperatures < 30°C (86°F).
Gastric dilation and decreased gastric motility can occur in severe hypothermia. Physical examination of the abdomen is unreliable because of rectus muscle rigidity, so after endotracheal intubation, you should place a nasogastric tube in patients with moderate or severe hypothermia if allowed by local protocols.

CPR, cardiopulmonary resuscitation.

and avoid abrupt movements. If available, the patient should be transported to a facility that can provide extracorporeal rewarming with cardiac bypass or ECMO. Key considerations in managing severe hypothermia are described in Table 13-4.

Cardiac Arrest in Hypothermia

If the patient is in cardiac arrest, begin CPR immediately. The priority will be to provide quality chest compressions during active rewarming. The resuscitation is likely to be prolonged, and consideration should be given to using a mechanical CPR device if available. IV medications and defibrillation may have limited benefits at these temperatures. Active rewarming techniques include warming blankets, warm IVF, and bladder irrigation. More invasive active rewarming techniques include warm fluid irrigation of the thoracic and peritoneal cavities. ECMO or bypass rewarming is the ultimate modality for both warming the patient and providing circulatory and respiratory support. In some remote regions, resuscitation efforts for hypothermic patients who are found in cardiac arrest are terminated in the field if allowed by local protocols. However, in most jurisdictions, hypothermia is a contraindication to field termination of resuscitation.

Heat Illness

Heat illness constitutes a spectrum of conditions related to heat exposure. The most severe form of heat illness, known as heatstroke, occurs when the body's thermoregulatory mechanisms are overwhelmed, resulting in **hyperthermia**. This can occur in response to excessive exposure to heat, excessive heat production, or impaired heat loss. Patients at increased risk of developing heat illness include those who are elderly, frail, intellectually impaired, immobile, intoxicated, malnourished, injured, or young children. Although there are a number of medical conditions and drug overdoses that can cause hyperthermia, this section relates specifically to environmental hyperthermia.

Hyperthermia may be classified as either classic or exertional. Although it is not critical to differentiate these conditions in the field because treatment is similar, they will be discussed separately here. It is important to remember that heat illness is a spectrum of disorders with a crossover of some signs and symptoms between each type, and classification is somewhat arbitrary.

Classic hyperthermia (nonexertional heat stroke) is associated with prolonged exposure to even a moderately high environmental temperature and humidity level. It is usually associated with the chronically ill, bedridden, elderly, or psychiatric patient who lacks air conditioning or is using medications that impair tolerance to heat stress, such as diuretic, anticholinergic, and neuroleptic agents. Anhidrosis (lack of perspiration) is caused by extreme dehydration, skin disorders, or medication side effects.

In contrast, exertional heat illness is associated with young people, such as athletes who train in conditions of high temperature and humidity, during which the core temperature rises faster than the body can dissipate heat. Many of these patients will continue to sweat even as they develop severe hyperthermia.

Pathophysiology

The human body can tolerate lower body temperatures much more so than higher temperatures, with organ dysfunction developing as temperatures rise as little as 4.5°C (9°F) above normal. The mechanisms described previously that result in hypothermia also serve to prevent hyperthermia. These include evaporation, which is the most effective mechanism for heat dissipation; radiation; convection; and conduction. As heat generation increases, blood vessels in the extremities and near the body surface dilate to promote greater blood flow to these regions to facilitate heat transfer to the environment. But when ambient temperature is higher than body temperature, the latter three mechanisms are not functional, and when relative humidity goes above about 75%, evaporation becomes ineffective.

As body temperature rises, metabolism increases, and thus oxygen consumption rises, leading to tachycardia and increased minute ventilation. Evaporation leads to dehydration and electrolyte loss. Cellular respiration and enzyme function are impaired as body temperature reaches 42°C (108°F), leading to organ failure. Cells in the liver, blood vessels, and nervous system are affected first, but eventually, all tissues suffer damage, leading also to kidney damage and muscle breakdown (rhabdomyolysis). Dysfunction of clotting factors leads to disseminated intravascular coagulation, and central nervous system (CNS) hypoxia and damage often lead to seizures and severe alteration of mental status.

Forms of Exertional Heat Illness

Heat Cramps (Exercise-Associated Muscle Cramping)

Muscle cramps are common among people who work or exercise vigorously in not only hot but also cool temperatures. The physiologic mechanism leading to muscle cramps is not well understood but may include dehydration, electrolyte changes, neurogenic fatigue, extreme environmental conditions, and performance of new exercises. These painful muscle contractions occur during or shortly after physical activity.

Signs and Symptoms

Patients present with severe muscle pain and spasms, particularly in the muscles being exercised, but without significant elevation of body temperature or signs and symptoms of more severe forms of heat illness.

Treatment

Treatment consists of hydration with salt-containing solutions (oral is as effective as IV) and local therapy of involved muscles, including passive stretching and massage. Some clinicians will administer a benzodiazepine, such as diazepam, or magnesium for their muscle relaxant effects in severe cases. Other causes such as hyponatremia and rhabdomyolysis should be considered if symptoms do not respond to initial measures described previously.

Heat Syncope and Exercise-Associated Collapse

Heat syncope is fainting or light-headedness associated with exposure to a high-heat environment, typically in nonacclimatized individuals. This most often occurs after a period of prolonged standing or upon standing after prolonged sitting or lying. The physiologic mechanism involves the body's effort to dissipate heat through vasodilation, thus increasing the intravascular space. As such, standing leads to blood pooling in the lower body, a decrease in venous return, and insufficient perfusion to the brain and vital organs.

In athletes, a similar phenomenon related to vigorous exertion or endurance events (such as running a marathon) is termed *exercise-associated collapse* (EAC). This typically occurs immediately after cessation of exercise, particularly if the individual remains quiet in an upright position, with the same mechanism responsible as for heat syncope.

In both heat syncope and EAC, there should be rapid return of consciousness once the person collapses or is assisted to supine position as venous return and cardiac output are restored. Persistent altered mental status or significant elevation of body temperature should trigger concern for heatstroke.

Signs and Symptoms

Patients with heat syncope and EAC will note onset of light-headedness, particularly upon standing or after prolonged standing. This may be accompanied by tunnel vision or darkening of vision and subsequent collapse to the ground. Some body twitches (myoclonus) may occur, but true seizure is rare. The patient's color will be pale and skin is usually sweaty. Heart rate may be bradycardic or tachycardic. Core temperature should be normal or only minimally elevated (typically not above 39°C [102°F]). Symptoms should improve, and consciousness should return very soon after assuming a recumbent position.

Treatment

Supportive care includes cooling as needed; allowing the patient to rest in a recumbent or semirecumbent position; and administering fluids, preferably those containing glucose and electrolytes, by the oral route if tolerated. Guidance for many endurance athletic events recommends determining sodium levels prior to starting IVF.

Heat Exhaustion

Heat exhaustion is a continuation on the spectrum of heat-related illness. People who work in hot environments, such as laborers, athletes, and military personnel, are at risk if they do not drink enough fluid and are unable to shade themselves. If left untreated, heat exhaustion can progress to heatstroke.

Signs and Symptoms

The clinical manifestations of heat exhaustion are nonspecific. Body temperature may be mildly elevated (up to 40°C [104°F]), but not severely so. Mild CNS abnormalities such as mild confusion may develop, but resolve quickly with treatment. The most common signs and symptoms are as follows:

- Weakness and malaise
- Headache
- Light-headedness and syncope
- Nausea and vomiting
- Ataxia or clumsiness
- Tachycardia and hypotension
- Sweating, often profuse, and pallor
- Nonspecific abdominal pain/cramps
- Muscle cramps

Treatment

The patient should be moved to a cool, shady location or air-conditioned indoor environment and placed in supine position with legs elevated. The patient should be actively cooled—excess clothing should be removed and cold water should be applied to the head and body by using a spray bottle or covering with a wet sheet. Ensure that there is airflow over the patient. Cooling should be guided by rectal (or esophageal) temperature with a goal of 38.3°C (101°F).

Most patients with heat exhaustion have dehydration with both water and electrolyte depletion. In patients with normal consciousness and who are not vomiting, oral rehydration is appropriate and preferred. Dilute glucose-electrolyte solutions should be used. If the patient cannot tolerate oral fluids or has any decreased consciousness, then crystalloid IV fluids (such as lactated Ringer's or normal saline solution) should be administered. Ongoing interventions should be based on patient response to treatment with close monitoring of vital signs, including temperature. Patients who do not have rapid recovery within an hour or so should be transported to the emergency department.

Heatstroke

Heatstroke is the most severe form of heat illness and develops when the body loses its ability to regulate temperature, resulting in CNS dysfunction, elevated core body temperature, and multiorgan failure. Core body temperature is > 40°C (104°F). Consequent damage will depend on how high the body temperature is and how long it stays elevated.

Pathophysiology

An almost universal finding in patients with severe hyperthermia is neurologic dysfunction, including altered mental status, headache, seizures, and coma. Markedly increased demands are made on the cardiovascular system, which can be a principal contributor to the ultimate collapse of bodily functions. Continued heat exposure produces peripheral vasodilatation with subsequent splanchnic and renal circulatory vasoconstriction, sometimes accompanied by hepatic dysfunction. Continued heat exposure will cause hemodynamic instability; poor skin perfusion; a further elevation of core temperature; and multiorgan failure, including acute kidney injury, liver failure, rhabdomyolysis, and disseminated intravascular coagulation.

Signs and Symptoms

The primary distinguishing feature of heatstroke from other forms of heat illness is CNS dysfunction. This can manifest in a number of ways, including headache, disorientation/confusion, behavioral and emotional irritability, altered alertness/responsiveness, and seizure. It is important to know most of these patients will still be sweaty, *not* dry, as some texts describe. The most common signs and symptoms include the following:

- Altered mental status/syncope/seizures/coma
- Hyperventilation
- Tachycardia/hypotension
- Nausea/vomiting/diarrhea
- Dehydration/dry mouth
- Muscle cramps
- Sweating, possibly profuse

Differential Diagnosis

Heatstroke is often suspected due to the setting and environmental conditions. These patients typically present with sudden collapse. Other conditions that must be considered include sudden cardiac arrest, exercise-associated hyponatremia, and malignant hyperthermia. The latter condition is most commonly associated with anesthetic agents but has been described with extreme exercise. Malignant hyperthermia may be distinguished by the presence of muscle rigidity, rather than flaccid weakness as seen in exertional heat stroke.

Treatment

The first step in management is to recognize this potentially lethal condition. Maintain airway, ventilation, and circulation; initiate immediate cooling measures; and transport the patient rapidly to the emergency department. Place the patient on a cardiac monitor, establish two peripheral IV lines, and initiate supplemental oxygen therapy if the patient is hypoxic ($SpO_2 < 94\%$) or shows signs of respiratory distress.

Recognizing the need for and initiating cooling measures immediately can be lifesaving. Do not delay active cooling measures to start an IV, move to another area, transport, etc.; start cooling at once.

The patient's clothes must be removed. Immediate cooling should begin on scene. The most effective method is immersion in ice water or some type of ice water bath. At sporting events where there is a risk of heatstroke, such as marathons, tubs of ice are often prearranged. In the EMS setting, one method of providing an ice bath is to place ice and water into a body bag. If this is not possible, apply cold water with a hose or place towels soaked in ice water on the patient. Fanning and air conditioning are also beneficial. Check and record core temperature, preferably with a rectal or esophageal probe, every 5 minutes. Once core body temperature drops to < 39°C (102.2°F), active cooling measures should be stopped and preparation for transport initiated. If evidence of hypovolemic shock is present, resuscitate the patient with fluid boluses as needed. Cold IV fluids can be used. Reassess hemodynamic stability, and maintain a mean arterial pressure (MAP) of > 60 mm Hg or systolic blood pressure of > 90 mm Hg. Avoid fluid overload, because the patient is at risk of developing high-output cardiac failure and pulmonary edema. If seizures are present, administer a benzodiazepine according to local protocol. Continue close monitoring of mental status, respiratory status, cardiac rhythm, and vital signs during transport.

Exercise-Associated Hyponatremia

A disorder closely related to the sodium depletion seen in moderate to severe hyperthermia is **exercise-associated hyponatremia**. This is one of the most common causes of death in young, healthy athletes who are involved in endurance sports such as marathon running.

Pathophysiology

The most common cause of exercise-associated hyponatremia is overhydration with hypotonic fluids. Athletes lose both water and sodium through perspiration at a significant rate during exercise. If water is used as a replacement without an adequate sodium ingestion, the patient's serum sodium level is driven down. This can lead to CNS edema, neurologic symptoms, and death. Risk factors shown to increase the risk of exercise-associated hyponatremia in the setting of marathons include excessive hydration, nonsteroidal anti-inflammatory drug (NSAID) use, female sex, finishing time over 4 hours, and low body mass index. A similar disorder known as psychogenic polydipsia occurs in some patients with mental health disorders who drink excessive volumes of free water, resulting in fluid overload and hyponatremia.

Signs and Symptoms

Patients should be categorized based on symptoms rather than measured serum sodium concentrations, but relative values are given in parentheses:

- *Mild*: Dizziness, nausea, vomiting, headache (sodium 135–130 mmol/L)
- *Moderate*: Mental status changes (confusion, disorientation) (sodium 130–125 mmol/L)
- *Severe*: Altered consciousness, lethargy, pulmonary edema, seizures, coma (sodium < 125 mmol/L)

Differential Diagnosis

Symptoms of exercise-associated hyponatremia can be nonspecific, as previously discussed. A diagnosis of this type of heat illness can be challenging because there is a great deal of overlap with the signs and symptoms of heatstroke. To help differentiate between the two conditions, heatstroke always involves an altered mental status with an elevated temperature, whereas exercise-associated hyponatremia may occur without significant hyperthermia.

Treatment

As with most conditions, prevention through education of persons at risk is the best course. Athletes should be instructed to avoid excessive ingestion of hypotonic fluids during exercise. Even commercially available sports drinks do not contain enough sodium to prevent hyponatremia. Salty snacks should be eaten along with fluids.

For patients with mild to moderate symptoms, fluid restriction should be initiated, and salty snacks or broth should be administered while a sodium level is obtained. IV fluids are generally contraindicated. For patients with severe symptoms, prehospital treatment begins as usual with the ABCs. Treatment with hypertonic (3%) saline may be indicated but is extremely dangerous without appropriate expertise and the ability to monitor serum sodium levels. Treatment with hypertonic saline must be done under extremely controlled conditions and only with medical direction, because rapid correction of serum sodium concentration may result in central pontine myelinolysis, an irreversible injury to the CNS. Patients with severe symptoms should be transported to a facility with intensive care unit capabilities.

Other Common Environmental Emergencies

Drowning

Drowning is the process of experiencing respiratory impairment from submersion or immersion in liquid. Drowning outcomes include death, morbidity, and near morbidity. Terminology describing these patients continues to evolve. Terms such as *near-drowning* and *wet, dry,* and *secondary drowning* are confusing and, while previously popular, are no longer useful.

Pathophysiology

The drowning continuum progresses from breath holding, to laryngospasm (severe constriction of the larynx), to the accumulation of carbon dioxide and the inability to oxygenate the lungs, to subsequent respiratory and cardiac arrest from multiple-organ failure due to tissue hypoxia, resulting in the accumulation of metabolic and respiratory acids. The patient can be resuscitated at any point along this continuum, and, generally, the earlier the resuscitation takes place, the better the success rate.

Signs and Symptoms

Most drownings are not witnessed, and therefore the person's body is found submerged or floating in water. Toddlers typically drown in bathtubs, school-age children in pools, and teens in lakes or rivers. Comorbidities such as a seizure disorder or medical or physical disabilities may also contribute to drowning in an apparently safe environment such as a bathtub. In teens or adults, alcohol use also may contribute to the risk of drowning.

Treatment

The resuscitation of a victim of a drowning incident is the same as for any other patient in respiratory or cardiac arrest, but the victim first must be reached. Clinicians who have specialized training and experience in water rescue are the best able to accomplish the rescue. Rescuers should not put themselves or other rescuers in danger when attempting a rescue. The treatment of drowning is provided in Table 13-5.

In patients who are in cardiac arrest due to drowning, the focus needs to be on high-quality CPR with early attention given to optimizing ventilations. In drowning, standard CPR with ventilations is preferred, and chest compression–only CPR is not advised. An endotracheal tube should be placed as early as possible in the resuscitation (supraglottic airways and bag-valve mask ventilation may be ineffective due to high airway pressures). Drug therapy should be a low priority. Survivors tend to come from the group of patients for whom return of spontaneous circulation occurs within 10–15 minutes, usually with good CPR and oxygenation alone.

Table 13-5 Treatment of Drowning
Rescuers trained and practiced in performing water rescue should participate in the rescue.
Consider a cervical spine injury in cases of obvious trauma, diving, waterslides, or alcohol intoxication. Placing a collar is not a priority and should not interfere with resuscitation or initial care.
Ensure that basic life support measures are being carried out with an emphasis on airway and oxygenation.
Anticipate vomiting; have suction immediately available.
Anticipate pulmonary edema; suction is generally unhelpful. Assisted ventilation via a BVM with peak expiratory pressure support (PEEP) of 2.5–5 cm H_2O if the edema is interfering with oxygenation.
Administer supplemental oxygen, and intubate if needed.
Establish IV access.
Measure core temperature; prevent or treat hypothermia.
Administer a beta-2 adrenergic agent for wheezing.
Monitor pulse oximetry and end-tidal carbon dioxide, as indicated.
Insert an advanced airway per protocol if indicated. Insert a nasogastric tube in intubated patients if local protocols allow.
Every drowning patient requires a period of observation and monitoring. Transport to hospital usually is the most appropriate option, including for patients who seem to recover at the scene.

BVM, bag-valve mask; IV, intravenous.

Diving Emergencies

Diving and altitude emergencies can arise from extremes of pressure at altitude or water depth. Divers have long feared "the bends," the colloquial name for **decompression sickness**. Decompression sickness; direct **barotrauma**, such as sinus or middle ear injury; and arterial gas emboli are the major illnesses associated with extreme high-pressure environments such as SCUBA diving.

All divers, irrespective of the type of diving they do, are subject to the increased pressures that occur under water. Injury results from the physical effect of these pressures on the body. In order to understand these changes, it is important to review how gases act under certain physical conditions.

Pathophysiology

Diving barotrauma is explained by the laws of physics that govern the behavior of gases under pressure. Pressure changes affect the volume in air-filled spaces—in the case of the mostly fluid-filled human body, these spaces are the lungs, bowel, sinuses, and middle ear. According to **Boyle's law**, these spaces compress on descent and expand on ascent because as pressure increases, the gas volume is reduced; conversely, as pressure eases, gas volume increases (**Figure 13-6**).

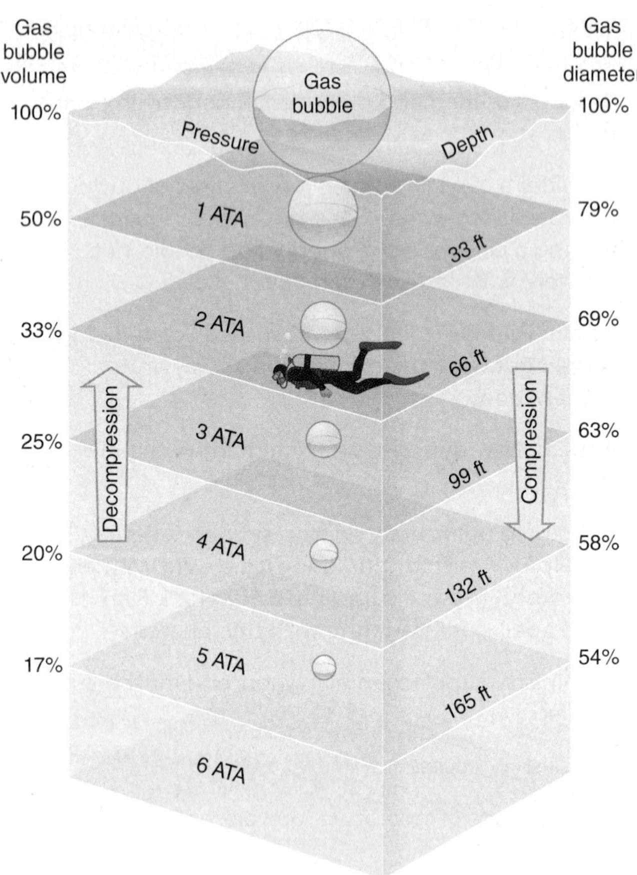

Figure 13-6 Boyle's law. The volume of a given quantity of gas at constant temperature varies inversely with pressure.

In addition, the solubility of a gas in liquid is governed by the amount of pressure exerted on that gas, so a gas will become increasingly dissolved with increasing pressure at depth and less dissolved (more gas in the liquid [i.e., blood]) as the body ascends while diving. The body can tolerate this if the amount of gas separating from the blood is small enough to be exhaled. If the ascent is rapid, large amounts of gas are liberated, and life-threatening gas bubbles (air emboli) can block circulation—the phenomenon known as decompression sickness.

The location and size of the gas bubbles will determine their clinical effects. Bubbles trapped in the muscles or joints cause pain in corresponding areas. In fact, the source of the nickname "the bends" is that this condition leaves the afflicted person doubled over for long periods of time. Gas bubbles in the spinal cord can cause paralysis, paresthesia, and anesthesia. Gas emboli in the arterial circulation can cause limb ischemia, in the pulmonary arteries can cause pulmonary gas embolism, and in the cerebral arteries can cause stroke. Decompression sickness typically occurs with too rapid return to surface, not allowing the gases to equilibrate. This is the reason for periodic rest stops at various depths when surfacing from deep dives.

Nitrogen narcosis, a change in mental status while diving, is a different clinical entity. Its effect is similar to alcohol or benzodiazepine intoxication. The condition may occur at shallow depths, but it typically does not set in unless the dive is more than 98 feet (30 meters). The effect is explained by the increased solubility of nitrogen under higher pressure, with the increased nitrogen causing consequent impairment of cognition, motor function, and sensory perception. Nitrogen narcosis also impairs judgment and coordination, potentially causing serious errors that can jeopardize underwater safety. The condition, however, is reversible and resolves over several minutes once the diver has ascended.

Signs and Symptoms

The average risk of severe decompression sickness is slightly more than 2 cases per 10,000 (1 per 5,000) dives. Asthma, pulmonary blebs, and patent foramen ovale increase the risk and severity of symptoms. Decompression sickness can present as late as 24 hours after diving and may begin with sinus and ear pressure, pressure in the back, and joint pain and aches that worsen with motion. More severe decompression sickness may be characterized by dyspnea, chest pain, altered mental status, or shock. The most severe illness is seen with arterial gas embolism. Gas emboli often occur a few minutes after surfacing. Acute-onset dyspnea and severe chest pain are common in people with acute gas emboli, and the condition can be fatal.

Treatment

The physical exam should focus on detecting emergent symptoms, including gas emboli. Pay particular attention to performing a complete cardiovascular exam, listening for decreased breath sounds, muffled heart sounds, and heart murmurs. Jugular venous distention or petechiae on the head or neck can indicate more severe decompression sickness. Palpate the skin to detect crepitus (from subcutaneous gas) and palpate all pulses.

Emergency care for decompression sickness includes paying careful attention to maintaining the airway with supplemental oxygen. IV hydration should be given to maintain systolic blood pressure. Chest decompression is indicated if pneumothorax occurs. Consider hyperbaric therapy in symptomatic patients, especially those having neurologic symptoms, unstable blood pressure, respiratory compromise, or altered mental status. Arrange for transport per protocol to a hyperbaric facility. If you do not know where the facility is, contact the Divers Alert Network for assistance at 919-684-9111.

High-Altitude Illnesses

Pathophysiology

The illnesses associated with ascent to high altitudes are precipitated by a combination of low atmospheric pressure and the resultant low partial pressure of oxygen. That is, although oxygen makes up 21% of atmospheric gas at all altitudes, as you ascend the total pressure of atmospheric gas decreases according to Boyle's law and the air becomes "thinner," with fewer molecules of oxygen in each liter of air. This condition is sometimes referred to as **hypobaric hypoxia**, which results in hypoxemia. The body attempts to compensate for this decreasing availability of oxygen by increasing respiratory rate, cardiac output, and cerebral vasodilatation. Low atmospheric pressure causes capillary leaking in both the lungs and brain. Hypoxia causes a diffuse pulmonary vasoconstriction (as the body tries to overcome a perceived ventilation-perfusion mismatch), which results in pulmonary hypertension and edema. Together, these adaptive and maladaptive responses may result in the development of acute mountain sickness, high-altitude cerebral edema, and high-altitude pulmonary edema. These illnesses may overlap and coexist.

Rapid rate of ascent, lack of preacclimatization, poor physical fitness levels, history of prior altitude illness, and many medications and intoxicants may increase the risk for high-altitude emergencies. Surprisingly, people younger than 50 years are at higher risk of experiencing high-altitude illnesses.

Signs and Symptoms

Acute Mountain Sickness

Acute mountain sickness (AMS) is a nonspecific syndrome that may be confused with general fatigue, dehydration, hangover, or influenza-like illness. The single most common complaint is mild to severe protracted headache. Symptoms generally begin within 24–48 hours following ascent and resolve in 3–5 days without further ascent. There are no definitive physical exam findings, making a high index of suspicion critically important.

High-Altitude Cerebral Edema

High-altitude cerebral edema (HACE) represents a more severe illness that is often preceded by AMS, and the signs and symptoms are likewise more severe and include nausea and vomiting, ataxia, altered mental status, seizures, and paralysis. HACE often does not develop until the third day after ascent but may occur much earlier, most commonly at altitudes above 12,000 ft (2,750 m). HACE may be fatal if not appropriately treated. Even though delayed in onset, symptoms can develop rapidly.

High-Altitude Pulmonary Edema

High-altitude pulmonary edema (HAPE) most commonly occurs on the second night following ascent. In mild cases, a dry cough and decreased tolerance to exercise may be noted. In more severe cases, dyspnea on exertion, hypoxia, and cyanosis may all develop. The rate of HAPE progression may be hastened by cold exposure, vigorous exertion, and continued ascent. Of the three high-altitude illnesses, HAPE accounts for the most fatalities.

Treatment

For all high-altitude illnesses beyond mild AMS, the mainstay of treatment is supplemental oxygen and immediate descent (see Table 13-6). If descent or evacuation

Table 13-6 High-Altitude Illnesses

	Signs/Symptoms	Treatment	Duration
AMS	Mild to severe protracted headache; no physical exam findings	NSAIDs, acetazolamide for symptom control (if mild) Supplemental oxygen, immediate descent if severe	Resolves in 3–5 days
HACE	Nausea and vomiting, headache, ataxia, altered mental status, seizures, and paralysis	Dexamethasone, diuretics, supplemental oxygen, immediate descent; portable hyperbaric chamber/bag treatment when immediate descent is not possible	May be fatal if not appropriately treated.
HAPE	Mild: dry cough, decreased tolerance to exercise Severe: dyspnea on exertion, hypoxia, cyanosis	Continuous positive airway pressure, diuretics, calcium channel blockers, supplemental oxygen, immediate descent; portable hyperbaric chamber/bag treatment when immediate descent is not possible	Rate of progression may be hastened by cold exposure, vigorous exertion, and continued ascent; may be fatal if not treated

AMS, acute mountain sickness; HACE, high-altitude cerebral edema; HAPE, high-altitude pulmonary edema; NSAIDs, nonsteroidal anti-inflammatory drugs.

cannot be accomplished expeditiously, a portable hyperbaric chamber may be employed if available. Other therapies may be employed as follows:

- Continuous positive airway pressure, diuretics, and calcium channel blockers may all be used in the treatment of HAPE.
- Dexamethasone and diuretics are used in treating HACE.
- NSAIDs and acetazolamide may be used for symptom control in mild AMS.

Expert consultation should be sought in all cases of high-altitude–related illnesses.

Putting It All Together

Assisting patients with environmental emergencies can be among some of the most challenging problems a healthcare clinician faces. Similarities and differences in cardinal presentations/chief complaints are sometimes subtle, and the underlying diagnosis can be obscured, delaying appropriate interventions. Utilizing the AMLS Assessment Pathway will assist in generating an appropriate differential diagnosis, obtaining a comprehensive history and focused physical exam, and refining that differential diagnosis.

SCENARIO SOLUTION

- Differential diagnoses may include mild, moderate, or severe hypothermia.
- To narrow your differential diagnosis, you will need to perform a physical examination that includes assessing for trauma injuries. The patient has hypotension and a weak and rapid radial pulse; therefore, treatment priorities will focus on the treatment of any trauma injuries and passive rewarming.
- The patient has signs that may indicate hypothermia because he is shivering, but retaining the ability to shiver indicates a milder form of hypothermia; as such, the patient can generate heat, so passive rewarming may be all that is required.

SUMMARY

- Body temperature is regulated by neural feedback mechanisms that operate primarily through the hypothalamus; the hypothalamus contains not only the control mechanisms (that maintain a temperature set point), but also the sensory mechanisms necessary to detect and respond to body temperature changes.
- Cold emergencies include frostnip, frostbite, and systemic hypothermia.
- Heat emergencies include a spectrum of presentations from mild heat-related fluid and electrolyte disturbances (which can present as cramps or fainting) to physiologic instability with loss of the ability to regulate body temperature.
- Drowning is the process of experiencing respiratory impairment from submersion or immersion in liquid. Drowning progresses from breath holding, to laryngospasm, to respiratory and cardiac arrest.
- Barotrauma can result from too rapid ascent after a dive, owing to a barometric pressure imbalance between the inside of the body and the outside atmosphere.
- High-altitude illnesses result from hypobaric hypoxia.

Key Terms

acute mountain sickness (AMS) Illness from exposure to a high-altitude environment that presents with a variety of mild to moderate symptoms, including headache, weakness, fatigue, and body aches.

barotrauma Injury resulting from severe changes in barometric pressure, typically from rapid ascent after diving.

Boyle's law At a constant temperature, the volume of a gas is inversely proportional to its pressure (if you double the pressure of gas, you halve its volume; written as PV = K, where P = pressure, V = volume, and K = a constant).

decompression sickness A broad range of signs and symptoms caused by nitrogen bubbles in blood and tissues coming out of solution on ascent.

drowning The process of experiencing respiratory impairment from submersion or immersion in liquid.

exercise-associated hyponatremia A condition due to prolonged exertion in a hot environment coupled with excessive hypotonic fluid intake that leads to nausea; vomiting; and, in severe cases, mental status changes and seizures (also known as exertional hyponatremia).

frostbite Localized damage to tissues resulting from prolonged exposure to extreme cold.

frostnip Early frostbite, characterized by numbness and pallor without significant tissue damage.

heat illness A spectrum of illnesses related to excessive heat exposure or heat generation, ranging from rash and cramps to heat exhaustion and heatstroke.

high-altitude cerebral edema (HACE) Brain swelling and dysfunction associated with exposure to high altitudes.

high-altitude pulmonary edema (HAPE) A noncardiogenic form of pulmonary edema (fluid accumulation in the lungs) that occurs in high altitudes.

hyperthermia Unusually elevated body temperature above 38.5°C (101.3°F).

hypobaric hypoxia Low oxygen content caused by low atmospheric pressure.

hypothermia Core body temperature below 35°C (95°F); at lower temperatures, it may induce cardiac arrhythmia and precipitate a decline in mental status.

nitrogen narcosis A state resembling alcohol intoxication produced by nitrogen gas dissolved in the blood at high ambient pressure.

thermoregulation The process by which the body compensates for environmental extremes.

Bibliography

American Academy of Orthopaedic Surgeons. *Nancy Caroline's Emergency Care in the Streets*, 8th ed. Jones & Bartlett Learning; 2018.

Centers for Disease Control and Prevention. *Trench foot or immersion foot. Disaster recovery fact sheet.* Last reviewed September 8, 2005. https://www.cdc.gov/disasters/trenchfoot.html

Cone D, Brice JH, Delbridge TR, et al. *Emergency Medical Services: Clinical Practice and Systems Oversight*. Wiley; 2015.

DiCorpo JE, Harris M, Merlin MA. Evaluating temperature is essential in the prehospital setting. *JEMS*. November 2, 2017. https://www.jems.com/patient-care/evaluating-temperature-is-essential-in-the-prehospital-setting/

Hamilton GC, Sanders AB, Strange GR. *Emergency Medicine*, 2nd ed. Saunders; 2003.

Kumar G, Sng BL, Kumar S. Correlation of capillary and venous blood glucometry with laboratory determination. *Prehosp Emerg Care*. 2004;8(4):378.

Mallet ML. Pathophysiology of accidental hypothermia. *QJ Med.* 2002;95:775–785.

Marx JA, Hockberger RS, Walls RM. *Rosen's Emergency Medicine*, 7th ed. Mosby; 2009.

Mistovich JJ, Krost WS, Limmer DD. Beyond the basics: endocrine emergencies, part I. *EMS Mag*. 2007;36(10):123–127.

Mistovich JJ, Krost WS, Limmer DD. Beyond the basics: endocrine emergencies, part II. *EMS Mag*. 2007;36(11):66–69.

Pagan KD, Pagana TJ. *Mosby's Manual of Diagnostic and Laboratory Tests*, 4th ed. Mosby; 2010.

Plaisier BR. Thoracic lavage in accidental hypothermia with cardiac arrest—report of a case and review of the literature. *Resuscitation*. 2005;66:95–104.

Sanders MJ, McKenna K, American Academy of Orthopaedic Surgeons. *Sanders' Paramedic Textbook*, 5th ed. Public Safety Group; 2019.

Thomas R, Cahill CJ. Case report: successful defibrillation in profound hypothermia (core body temperature 25.6°C). *Resuscitation*. 2000;47:317–320.

U.S. Department of Transportation National Highway Traffic Safety Administration. *EMT-Paramedic National Standard Curriculum*. U.S. Department of Transportation National Highway Traffic Safety Administration; 1998.

U.S. Department of Transportation National Highway Traffic Safety Administration. *National EMS Education Standards, Draft 3.0*. U.S. Department of Transportation National Highway Traffic Safety Administration; 2008.

Walpoth BH, Walpoth-Aslan BN, Mattle HP, et al. Outcome of survivors of accidental deep hypothermia and circulatory arrest treated with extracorporeal blood warming, *N Engl J Med*. 1997;337:1500–1505.

Xu J. Number of hypothermia-related deaths—by sex: National Vital Statistics System, United States, 1999–2011. *MMWR*. 2013;61:1050.

CHAPTER 14

Toxicology

Chapter Editors
Austin W. Gay, MD
Benjamin D. Pilkey, MD
Ratna M. Malkan, DO
Bryan A. Everitt, MD, NRP, FAAEM
Shawn M. Varney, MD, FACEP, FAACT, FACMT

This chapter explores the devastating effects of natural toxins on the human body. As always, when responding to a patient with presumed toxin exposure, follow the methodical AMLS Assessment Pathway approach, including a thorough scene survey, pertinent and complete assessment, and rapid stabilization of life threats. Medications and drugs of abuse are examined in detail. The chapter covers toxins in the home, streets, and workplace. The chapter also discusses land and marine environmental toxicology, which includes arthropod, snake envenomation, and plant toxins.

LEARNING OBJECTIVES

At the conclusion of this chapter, you will be able to:

- Understand the basic approach to an intoxicated/poisoned patient.
- Identify and describe common toxidromes.
- Recognize which patients are at risk of respiratory depression and cardiac dysrhythmias from poisoning.
- Discuss the cardinal presentation/chief complaint, assessment, differential diagnoses, and treatment of patients with toxicologic emergencies using the AMLS Assessment Pathway.
- Describe the value of poison centers in treating patients with toxicologic emergencies.
- Understand the treatment of toxin-induced dysrhythmias.

SCENARIO

A 24-year-old man with quadraplegia is anxious and slightly combative. His vital signs include a blood pressure of 188/104 mm Hg, pulse rate of 136 beats/min, and respirations of 28 breaths/min. He was found this way when his roommate returned home from work.

- What diagnoses are you considering based on the information you have now? (Include any toxidrome or specific drugs you may be considering.)
- What additional information will you need to narrow your differential diagnosis?
- What treatments would you consider for this patient?

Toxicologic emergencies caused by accidental and intentional exposures are a principal cause of morbidity and mortality in the United States. Poisoning has surpassed motor vehicle collisions as the leading cause of unintentional injury death in the United States. In 2021, an estimated 107,622 drug overdose deaths (approximately 295 per day) occurred, more than 75% of which were unintentional. The remaining deaths were the result of suicide attempts or unknown intent. According to the Centers for Disease Control and Prevention (CDC), approximately 1,500 patients were treated each day in 2021 in U.S. emergency departments for the misuse or abuse of drugs. This number has continued to rise. The 2020 Annual Report of the American Association of Poison Control Centers' National Poison Data System reported a total of 2,128,198 human poison exposures, as well as a continued increase in cases with serious outcomes.

EMS clinicians and other health care professionals frequently encounter toxicologic emergencies such as intentional overdose, inadvertent poisoning, occupational exposure, environmental hazards, and envenomation. Early recognition of toxicity and identification of the causative agent can help you initiate appropriate management; maintain safe conditions for yourself, the patient, and the public; and provide essential information to your colleagues at all levels.

Early recognition and management of dangerous environments and life-threatening patient presentations necessitate following an orderly, unwavering set of fundamental principles. Identifying and treating toxicologic disorders requires a solid grasp of nervous system, cardiovascular, and respiratory physiology. This chapter focuses on the body's response to classes of drugs and toxins (toxidromes) but does not analyze numerous specific agents. The following topics are emphasized:

- Obtaining historical information
- Identifying toxins
- Understanding the pathophysiology of toxicity
- Making a preliminary evaluation
- Applying general treatment concepts
- Selecting specific therapies

The AMLS Assessment Pathway guides you through an efficient and comprehensive assessment of the poisoned patient. After first verifying scene safety, preventing life-threatening sequelae may mean immediately initiating therapy, such as stabilizing the airway or administering cardioactive drugs. Then performing a more detailed history and examination often narrows the differential diagnosis significantly, allowing you to institute potentially lifesaving treatment measures without delay.

AMLS Assessment Pathway ▸▸▸▸▸

▾ Initial Observations

Carefully observing the scene upon arrival can help you quickly gather useful information about potential poisoning and prognosis. For example, finding an altered patient in a house where opioid overuse has been known to occur can guide appropriate evaluation and management. Observing pill bottles in the room can provide helpful information even before you begin your examination.

Scene Safety Considerations

Verify the scene is safe. Toxicologic emergencies may be unsafe in two primary ways. First, patients who have been poisoned can rapidly become dangerous. Do not hesitate to call for law enforcement assistance, especially in the case of a patient who is altered and combative. Second, the offending toxin may still be present and active. Although ingested substances are unlikely to harm others directly, several gases and toxins may cause injury or incapacity to medical personnel. The presence of more than one patient suggests that the toxicity may be related to a gas, which can rapidly induce symptoms, be difficult to detect, not be appreciated until it is too late, and directly affect clinicians. Toxins that harm patients by skin or mucosal contact may still be present on the patient; medical personnel should first avoid direct contact with such substances and subsequently attempt to decontaminate the patient to reduce ongoing damage. Note that fentaNYL powder is not toxic through the skin and will not induce opioid toxicity symptoms unless inhaled, ingested, or injected.

If the involvement of a venomous animal is suspected, do not pursue the animal. If it has already been killed, a picture will usually suffice for identification. Do not bring the animal in transport, as some may still be harmful. For example, contact with the fangs of a dead snake may still cause envenomation.

Dispatchers should obtain and relay sufficient information about scene safety to all responding clinicians, particularly when multiple patients are affected. The causative agent in an exposure is often unknown. When a hazardous material is suspected, consider requesting a hazardous materials (hazmat) response team.

Patient Cardinal Presentation/ Chief Complaint

Patients who are experiencing a toxicologic emergency may experience various symptoms, including altered mental status, nausea and vomiting, difficulty breathing, seizures, and many others. Common signs and symptoms of poisoning are given in Table 14-1.

Primary Survey

As in any emergency situation, evaluating the patient's airway, breathing, and circulation forms the backbone of your assessment.

In addition to checking the ABCs, be sure to check for disability, or D, which includes altered mental status. In

Table 14-1 Common Signs and Symptoms of Poisoning

Sign or Affected Body System	Type	Possible Causative Agents
Odor (could be detected in breath or environmental odor)	Bitter almonds	Cyanide
	Garlic	Thallium, arsenic, organophosphates, phosphorus
	Sulfur	Hydrogen sulfide, mercaptans, sulfur dioxide
	Acetone	Acetone, aspirin, isopropyl alcohol, methanol
	Wintergreen	Methyl salicylate
	Pears	Chloral hydrate
	Violets	Turpentine
	Alcohol	Alcohol (ethanol)
Pupils	Constricted (miosis)	CloNIDine, nicotine, nutmeg, opioids, organophosphates
	Dilated (mydriasis)	Anticholinergics (antimuscarinics) including atropine, jimson weed, barbiturates, carbon monoxide, cocaine, cyanide, ethanol, lysergic acid diethylamide (LSD), sympathomimetics*
Mouth	Salivation	Arsenic, mercury, organophosphates, strychnine, thallium
	Dry mouth	Atropine (belladonna), amphetamines, diphenhydrAMINE
	Burns in mouth	Acids, alkalis, formaldehyde, iodine, lye, phenols, phosphorous, pine oil, silver nitrate
Skin	Pruritus	Belladonna, boric acid, methamphetamines, poison ivy/oak
	Dry, hot skin	Anticholinergics/antimuscarinics, antihistamines, atropine (in belladonna or eye drops)
	Sweating	Arsenic, aspirin, barbiturates, mushrooms, naphthalene, organophosphates, sympathomimetics*
Respiratory	Depressed respirations	Barbiturates, botulism, cloNIDine, ethanol, gamma hydroxybutyrate (GHB), opioids
	Increased respirations	Amphetamines, aspirin, boric acid, kerosene, methanol, nicotine
	Pulmonary edema	Beta blockers, calcium channel blockers, chlorine, organophosphates, petroleum products, opioids
Cardiovascular	Tachycardia	Albuterol, arsenic, aspirin, atropine, bupropion, caffeine, dextromethorphan, ethanol/sedative-hypnotic withdrawal, ketamine, phencyclidine (PCP), sympathomimetics*
	Bradycardia	Beta blockers, calcium channel blockers, cloNIDine, cyanide, digoxin, mushrooms, nicotine, opioids, mistletoe
	Hypertension	Ketamine, lead, nicotine, PCP, sympathomimetics*, ethanol/sedative-hypnotic withdrawal
	Hypotension	Barbiturates, beta blockers, calcium channel blockers, cloNIDine, nitroglycerin, opioids, tricyclic antidepressants, mistletoe

(*continues*)

Table 14-1 Common Signs and Symptoms of Poisoning (*continued*)

Sign or Affected Body System	Type	Possible Causative Agents
Central nervous system	Seizures	Bupropion, camphor, isoniazid (INH), PCP, sedative-hypnotic withdrawal, strychnine, sympathomimetics*, traMADol, tricyclic antidepressants
	Coma	All central nervous system (CNS) depressant drugs (anticonvulsants, antidepressants, barbiturates, benzodiazepines, ethanol, muscle relaxants, opioids), carbon monoxide, cyanide
	Hallucinations	Atropine, LSD, mushrooms, organic solvents, PCP, nutmeg
	Headache	Carbon monoxide, disulfiram, ethanol, nitroglycerin
	Tremors	Albuterol, carbon monoxide, organophosphates, sympathomimetics*
	Weakness or paralysis	Botulism, poison hemlock, nerve agents (sarin), organophosphates, puffer fish
Gastrointestinal	Cramps, nausea, vomiting, and/or diarrhea	Many, if not most, ingested poisons, metals, mushrooms from yard

*Sympathomimetics = amphetamines and derivatives such as methamphetamine and MDMA (methylenedioxymethamphetamine), synthetic cannabinoids (spice), synthetic cathinones (bath salts), cocaine.

the setting of acute intoxication, the list of causes of mental status changes is long. Perhaps the most important, however, is serum glucose derangement. It is vitally important to take a serum glucose measurement in patients who exhibit neurologic symptoms. Also keep in mind E for exposure. Fully expose the patient, decontaminating as appropriate, and thoroughly examining as you go. Possible significant findings include rashes, bumps, needle marks, bites, or sting sites. Exposure may help identify medication patches, which could be located on the back or along the axilla. In addition, E should prompt you to ensure that the environment is not making your patient too cold (hypothermic) or too hot (hyperthermic). The next section will further discuss the ABCDE pathway in conjunction with vital sign abnormalities you may find during your assessment.

First Impression

Determine whether the patient's condition is life threatening or emergent, as opposed to stable and nonemergent. Weak or erratic vital signs and poor mental status generally contribute to this impression. In patients with toxicologic emergencies, mental status changes can range from mild confusion to agitation or delirium to coma. Agitation and **delirium** may indicate significant metabolic derangements and can be associated with agitated behavior or trigger acute, severe cardiovascular disorders that may be fatal. Coma is associated with respiratory depression and an inability to protect the airway.

The adage "vital signs are vital" holds true in toxicologic emergencies. Identifying and stabilizing abnormal vital signs is critical in early management. Frequent ongoing evaluation can help you gauge the nature and severity of toxicity in a poisoned patient. General toxidromes and specific toxins will be discussed later in this chapter. Vital sign abnormalities will often provide the most reliable clues for identifying which toxins may be involved. Using the AMLS Assessment Pathway, the information obtained from the history, the secondary survey, and vital signs can be used to expand and focus the differential diagnosis in toxicologic cases.

Detailed Assessment

History Taking

As an on-scene clinician, you are often in the best position to gather the most accurate information. Historical information, however, is often untrustworthy. In an unconscious patient, reports from bystanders or family, along with physical examination, may provide the only data for arriving at a prehospital diagnosis. Therefore, it is essential that you become proficient in recognizing environmental variables, mechanisms of injury, patient posturing, and odors that may offer insight regarding the cause of the patient's condition. A thorough accounting of possible ingestants is critical—immediately search through available medications if overdose is suspected and bring bottles with you during transport.

OPQRST and SAMPLER

Most poisoning and overdose cases involve patients with medical conditions, so you will need to elaborate on their chief complaint using the OPQRST questions and SAMPLER history from the patient or bystanders. Historical information is often critical in the diagnosis and treatment of toxicity. Note that people who intentionally try to harm themselves may not tell you what they have ingested. Therefore, interviewing family members and witnesses, particularly when treating a child or a patient with altered mental status, can be crucial. When the offending agent has been identified (including formulation if possible—immediate release vs. extended or sustained release), ask about coingestions and verify the following:

- Time of ingestion
- Suspected dose/amount
- Patient's access to the drug or chemical
- Situational information such as the patient's position and location and the presence or absence of nearby drug paraphernalia or other intoxicated patients
- Potential access to other medications or substances

Secondary Survey

The primary and secondary surveys focus on identifying and managing potential life-threatening emergencies related to the specific toxin exposure. As with all other patients, the secondary survey includes assessment of vital signs and appropriate physical examination. Interventions are aimed at treating the patient's mental status changes and perfusion abnormalities. If the patient's medical condition may also be complicated by trauma, for example after a fall in an overdose patient, the secondary survey should include appropriate assessment for traumatic injuries, too.

If the patient is not transported, or if EMS clinicians need additional information about the treatment of an overdose or poisoning, your regional poison center should be contacted as allowed by local protocols. Not only will diagnostic and treatment recommendations optimize patient care, but notification will also allow for near real-time surveillance of poisonings both locally and nationally as well as continued patient follow-up in the emergency department and afterward when necessary (**Rapid Recall Box 14-1**).

RAPID RECALL BOX 14-1

The Role of Poison Centers and EMS Clinicians

The 55 poison centers in the United States are staffed 24/7 with pharmacists, physicians, nurse practitioners, and nurses who are nationally certified as Specialists in Poison Information. They provide professional clinical recommendations and treatment advice to EMS clinicians and all callers from home or health care facilities. In 2021, poison centers received 36,351 calls from EMS clinicians. Poison centers fall under "covered entities" in the HIPAA Privacy Rule regulations and are considered part of the health care team. The National Poison Center hotline number is (800) 222-1222; calls and patient information are kept confidential. Calls to poison centers are entered into a database and then uploaded and analyzed approximately every 8 minutes to detect events, trends, and threats that may be of public health significance.

Poison centers can give valuable, real-time information to EMS clinicians, including the following:

- Toxic dose ranges
- Overdose, poisoning, exposure, and envenomation signs and symptoms
- Toxidrome identification
- Specific treatment and decontamination recommendations
- Assistance locating antidotes and antivenom
- Pill identification
- Information on drug interactions
- Identification of chemicals that may be hazardous to EMS clinicians

Refine the Differential Diagnosis

A **toxidrome** (an abridgement of *toxic* and *syndrome*) is the constellation of symptoms, vital signs, and exam findings typically associated with exposure to a particular toxin. Taken together, a patient's history and toxidrome can often help you identify the class of drug or, in some instances, the specific toxin responsible for the patient's illness. In general, if the class of toxin is known, the specific agent is unimportant because the treatment will be the same. Descriptions of various toxidromes are given in Table 14-2. The classic toxidromes will be featured later in this chapter.

Table 14-2 Major Toxidromes and Symptom Complexes of Toxicology

Toxidrome	Drug Examples	Signs and Symptoms
Stimulant/ sympathomimetic	Amphetamines, methamphetamine, cocaine, diet aids, nasal decongestants, phenylephrine, pseudoephedrine, synthetic cannabinoids, synthetic cathinones (bath salts, bupropion)	Tachycardia, tachypnea, hypertension, hyperthermia, anorexia, dilated pupils, restlessness, incessant talking, insomnia, paranoia, agitation, seizures, cardiac arrest
Opiate and opioid	Buprenorphine, fentaNYL, heroin, HYDROcodone, HYDROmorphone, methadone, morphine, opium, oxyCODONE	Miosis, marked respiratory depression, needle tracks (IV users), drowsiness, stupor, coma
Sedative-hypnotic	Barbiturates (PHENObarbital, thiopental), benzodiazepines (diazePAM, LORazepam, midazolam), ethanol, skeletal muscle relaxants	Drowsiness, disinhibition, ataxia, slurred speech, mental confusion, hypotension, respiratory depression, progressive CNS depression
Sedative-hypnotic withdrawal		Tachycardia, tachypnea, hypertension, hyperthermia, diaphoresis, mydriasis, agitation, seizures
Cholinergic	Chlorpyrifos, diazinon, dichlorvos, malathion, parathion, sarin, VX	Increased salivation, lacrimation, urination, diarrhea, diaphoresis, vomiting, bronchorrhea, bronchospasm, bradycardia, apnea, seizures, coma
Anticholinergic (antimuscarinic)	Antihistamines (diphenhydrAMINE), antipsychotics, atropine, scopolamine	Dry, flushed skin; hyperthermia, tachycardia, dilated pupils, blurred vision, mild hallucinations, delirium, urinary retention, seizures

Airway Security

Beyond ensuring scene safety both for you and the patient, evaluating and managing the patient's airway is the top priority in a toxicologic emergency. The two primary indications for inserting an advanced airway (either endotracheal or supraglottic) in an intoxicated patient are altered mental status and aspiration risk. Many toxins affect the central nervous system (CNS) and may lead to depressed mental status. Coma, a state of unconsciousness or deep sedation from which the patient cannot be aroused by any external stimulus, is a common presentation after intoxication. Of note, although the term **intoxication** refers to the presence of a poison or toxin in the body, with no specific implication of altered consciousness, it is often used to describe patients who have an impaired or depressed mental status. The Glasgow Coma Scale (GCS) may be used to evaluate the mental status of intoxicated patients. If a patient is known to have ingested a drug or medication that is short-acting, you may attempt less invasive airway measures initially (examples include nasopharyngeal airway, bag-valve mask ventilation, and jaw-thrust maneuvers) in the hopes of rapid recovery.

The other primary indication for obtaining an advanced airway is risk of aspiration. Intoxicated patients may vomit due to toxin effects or because of toxin-induced seizures. They may also produce copious oral secretions. In these cases, consider intubation if needed to protect the airway from aspiration.

Breathing Problems

Respiratory Rate Abnormalities

One vital sign often overlooked or inaccurately recorded is respiratory rate. This can be an important clue in diagnosing intoxicated patients and guiding therapy. Both under- or overbreathing can be problematic. Bradypnea (decreased respiratory rate) and hypopnea (decreased tidal volume) are associated with opioid use, but can result from multiple toxic exposures, including beta blockers, sedative-hypnotics, and others.

Early recognition of hypoventilation by physical examination or capnography is critical in the appropriate treatment of an intoxicated patient. Capnography, which is often available in the prehospital environment, may be helpful for patients at risk of hypoventilation from poisoning or overdose. Opioid overdose should be suspected in all patients with bradypnea, and administration of naloxone should be considered. In addition, supportive care such as ventilatory assistance or advanced airway insertion may be necessary.

Tachypnea (fast breathing) may be an indicator of acute respiratory disease such as pneumonia or pneumonitis, or it may reflect an underlying metabolic acidosis, which occurs with many toxic exposures. In the setting of metabolic acidosis, the exaggerated respiratory rate is a compensatory mechanism that allows the body to decrease the partial pressure of carbon dioxide (PCO_2), thereby raising systemic pH. In some patients, the actual rate of respiration may not accelerate significantly, but an uptick in tidal volume and minute ventilation has the same effect. Arterial or venous blood gas measurements can be used in the hospital setting to further differentiate acid–base disturbances. Toxin-induced metabolic acidosis has a broad differential diagnosis that can typically be narrowed rapidly by careful history taking and further laboratory testing. A mnemonic for possible causes is CAT MUDPILES (**Rapid Recall Box 14-2**).

An increase in the depth of breathing (hyperpnea) may also be secondary to a metabolic acidosis. Another cause of hyperventilation is direct activation of the brain's respiratory center. Classically, salicylate toxicity may cause an initial tachypnea or hyperpnea without metabolic acidosis. In fact, early salicylate toxicity is accompanied by an isolated respiratory alkalosis. It is critical to account for a patient's native respiratory rate prior to performing airway interventions. If the patient is tachypneic or hyperpneic, they are likely compensating for an acidosis. If intubated, provide breaths at a faster rate than usual. Also be aware that patients who breathe fast and/or deeply may tire out and require mechanical ventilation.

RAPID RECALL BOX 14-2

Causes of Toxin-Induced Metabolic Acidosis

C	Carbon monoxide, Cyanide
A	Alcoholic ketoacidosis, Acetaminophen (massive overdose)
T	Toluene
M	Methanol, Metformin
U	Uremia
D	Diabetic (or starvation) ketosis
P	Phenformin, valProic acid, Propylene glycol
I	Iron, Isoniazid (INH), Ibuprofen (massive overdose)
L	Lactic acidosis
E	Ethanol, Ethylene glycol
S	Salicylates

Oxygen Saturation Abnormalities

Measure oxygen saturation in any acutely ill patient. A normal oxygen saturation is reassuring but does not rule out the possibility of lung disease, hemoglobin dysfunction, or impaired oxygen delivery to body tissues. For example, oxygen saturation measured by noninvasive pulse oximetry may remain normal despite severe carbon monoxide toxicity that prevents delivery of oxygen to tissues. Toxic emergencies related to ingestion can be accompanied by a high incidence of vomiting, which is a risk factor for aspiration. Noncardiogenic pulmonary edema and pneumonitis can also complicate the course of opioid toxicity and withdrawal, salicylate toxicity, and toxin inhalation, all of which may cause hypoxemia and diffuse alveolar disease. Pneumothorax has also been reported in patients who smoke or inhale toxins.

Pulse oximetry in carbon monoxide poisoning may be falsely elevated, and abnormal pulse oximetry readings sometimes accompany hemoglobinopathies such as methemoglobinemia and sulfhemoglobinemia as well. Methemoglobinemia results in poor oxygen delivery to tissues, and the pulse oximetry reading may falsely be maintained around 85% even when supplemental oxygen is delivered. Cyanosis is a common finding and may present as a bluish discoloration of the skin in lighter-skinned patients or as gray or whitish skin in those with darker skin tones. Treatment with the reducing agent, methylene blue, allows reduction of ferric iron to ferrous iron and consequent restoration of the tissues' capability to deliver oxygen.

Uncouplers and inhibitors of oxidative phosphorylation impede the proper functioning of the mitochondrial electron transport chain, which is responsible for using oxygen during adenosine triphosphate (ATP) synthesis. The result is diminished energy production and cellular injury. Salicylates (aspirin) and cyanide are examples of these toxicities that affect the production of ATP from oxygen. Both classes of toxins cause metabolic acidosis, altered mental status, seizures, and eventual cardiovascular collapse. In either scenario, treating patients with sodium bicarbonate buffers acidosis and, in the case of salicylates, decreases tissue distribution and toxicity. Cyanide toxicity may be treated with a cyanide antidote kit.

Arterial and venous oxygen content, measured by conventional pulse oximetry and blood gas evaluation, can be altered by various anatomic and physiologic changes in intoxicated patients. Recognizing and identifying the underlying cause and rapidly reversing decreased blood oxygen content and tissue oxygen delivery are critical to treat toxicity effectively. Administer high-flow oxygen to any patient with respiratory compromise and abnormal oxygen saturation.

Cardiovascular Compromise

Toxins affecting the circulatory system may cause issues in two primary categories: rate/rhythm and blood pressure. Both heart rate and blood pressure may be low or high. Toxin-induced dysrhythmias may also occur.

Cardiac Rate Abnormalities

In a toxicologic emergency, tachycardia may result directly from the drug effect. A variety of pharmacologic mechanisms may accelerate the heart rate, including sympathomimetic toxicity; dopamine receptor agonism; and calcium channel blockade, which may cause vasodilation and reflex tachycardia (Table 14-3). Many toxins are active at more than one receptor site, which may complicate treatment algorithms. In addition to these pharmacologic effects, toxicity from drugs, plants, or chemicals can cause volume depletion as a result of reduced oral intake, prolonged immobilization, vomiting, diarrhea, or a combination of such factors. Regardless of the etiology, initial treatment with isotonic intravenous (IV) fluids is indicated and may be all that is required. In many patients, agitation and tremulousness may accompany tachycardia. Administering **benzodiazepines** to these patients provides sympatholysis, helping to moderate vital signs and quell agitation. A degree of tachycardia is acceptable if the patient's blood pressure is controlled and intensive supportive care has been initiated, but give special consideration to patients with underlying coronary artery disease or evidence of myocardial ischemia.

Table 14-3 Mechanisms of Toxin-Induced Tachycardia

Mechanism of Toxicity	Examples	Treatment
Sympathomimetic toxicity	Amphetamines, synthetic cannabinoids, cathinones, cocaine, ePHEDrine, phencyclidine	IV fluids, benzodiazepines
Peripheral alpha blockade	Tricyclic antidepressants, antipsychotics, doxazosin	IV fluids, phenylephrine
Peripheral calcium channel blockade	Dihydropyridine calcium channel blockers (amLODIPine, NIFEdipine)	IV fluids, phenylephrine
Muscarinic receptor blockade	Tricyclic antidepressants, antipsychotics, cyclobenzaprine, diphenhydrAMINE	IV fluids, benzodiazepines, +/− PHYSostigmine
Nicotinic receptor activation	Carbamates, organophosphates, poison hemlock, tobacco	IV fluids, benzodiazepines
Serotonin receptor stimulation	Tricyclic antidepressants, cocaine, meperidine, selective serotonin/norepinephrine reuptake inhibitors, traMADol	IV fluids, benzodiazepines
Dopamine receptor agonism	Amantadine, amphetamine, bromocriptine, bupropion, cocaine	IV fluids, benzodiazepines, +/− haloperidol
Gamma-aminobutyric acid (GABA) agonist withdrawal/GABA antagonism	Benzodiazepine or ethanol withdrawal, flumazenil, water hemlock	IV fluids, benzodiazepines, barbiturates
Adenosine receptor antagonism	Methylxanthines (e.g., caffeine, theophylline)	IV fluids, benzodiazepines, esmolol
Beta receptor agonism	Albuterol, clenbuterol, terbutaline	IV fluids, esmolol

Table 14-4 Mechanisms of Toxin-Induced Bradycardia

Mechanism of Toxicity	Examples	Treatment
Cardiac sodium channel opening	Veratrum alkaloids, aconite, grayanotoxin, ciguatera	Atropine
Cardiac sodium channel blockade	Tricyclic antidepressants, carBAMazepine, diphenhydrAMINE, hydroxychloroquine, propranolol, traMADol, yew plant	Sodium bicarbonate, hypertonic saline, vasopressors
Beta adrenergic receptor blockade	Atenolol, metoprolol, propranolol	Glucagon, EPINEPHrine, high-dose insulin and glucose, atropine
Calcium channel antagonism	DilTIAZem, verapamil	Calcium, EPINEPHrine, high-dose insulin and glucose, atropine
Na^+/K^+-ATPase inactivation	Digoxin, foxglove, lily of the valley, oleander	Digoxin-specific antibody fragments (Fab), atropine
Muscarinic and nicotinic activation	Carbamates, *Clitocybe* (mushrooms), nerve agents, organophosphates, tobacco (late)	Atropine, vasopressors, +/− pralidoxime, +/− benzodiazepines
Peripheral alpha receptor agonists	Imidazolines (e.g., cloNIDine initial activity)	Supportive care, +/− phentolamine
Central alpha receptor agonists	Imidazolines (e.g., cloNIDine secondary activity)	Atropine, DOPamine when associated with hypotension

ATPase, adenosine triphosphatase; K^+, potassium; Na^+, sodium.

More aggressive control of heart rate and blood pressure is required in this patient population.

A variety of plant and drug toxicities and chemical exposures can cause bradycardia (low heart rate) (Table 14-4). Many patients require no treatment. In those who do, the goal is to maintain end-organ perfusion. Monitor patients closely for blood pressure, urine output, mental status, renal function, and acid–base status. Prior to hospital arrival, the first-line intervention may be atropine, which has little downside but inconsistent success, depending on the toxin, and its effects are often transient. Glucagon is a reasonable option, particularly when treating known beta blocker toxicity, but its effectiveness is limited, and it may cause nausea and vomiting. Cardioactive vasopressors such as DOPamine and EPINEPHrine are often required. Remember that the goal is to maintain perfusion; normalizing the heart rate itself is not necessary if the patient is maintaining an appropriate blood pressure and/or mental status.

Dysrhythmia

In addition to monitoring the patient's heart rate, recognizing electrocardiogram (ECG) rhythm and interval changes is also critically important to accurately diagnose and stabilize intoxicated patients. Toxin-induced ventricular dysrhythmias can result from excess sympathetic activation, increased myocardial sensitivity, or alterations in myocardial action potential and ion channel activity.

Fast-acting sodium channel influx is responsible for rapid depolarization of myocardial cells and corresponds to the QRS interval on an ECG. Sodium channel blockade results in QRS widening, which can eventually progress to bradycardia, hypotension, ventricular dysrhythmia, and death. A number of drugs and toxins, including cyclic antidepressants, anticholinergics, and traMADol, may induce sodium channel blockade.

Treatment indications include a widened QRS complex (> 120 ms, new right bundle branch block) or evidence of significant cardiovascular toxicity. Identifying a terminal or dominant R wave in lead aVR may suggest sodium channel blockade (**Figure 14-1**). Treatment consists of serum alkalinization by administering a bolus of sodium bicarbonate solution (1–2 mEq/kg) over several minutes, followed by a continuous infusion. Monitor strips often then show a decrease in QRS duration, but repeat boluses may be necessary. If adequate alkalinization has occurred without symptom resolution, or if clinical deterioration continues, hypertonic saline (3%)

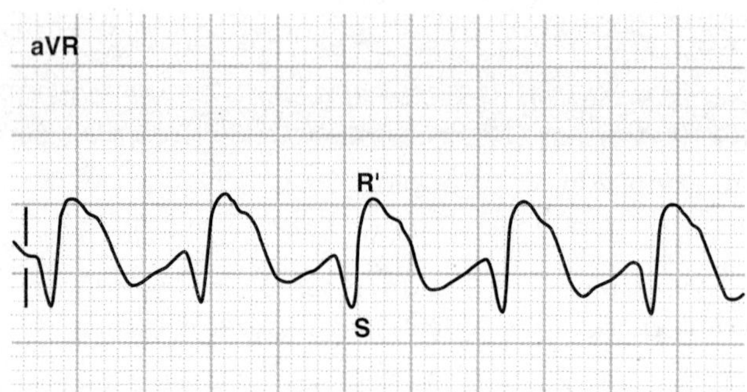

Figure 14-1 The terminal R wave in lead aVR indicates sodium channel toxicity.

Courtesy of LITFL.

0.5–1 mL/kg/hr may be required. Note that potassium supplementation may also be required to counter the effects of intracellular potassium shifts caused by alkalinization. However, it is rare to infuse potassium in the prehospital environment as incorrect administration can quickly become lethal.

Many drugs and toxins have potassium channel–blocking properties. The opening of potassium channels allows potassium efflux and repolarization, which is represented on the ECG by T waves. Inhibition causes prolongation of the QT interval corrected for heart rate (the QTc interval), eventually leading to polymorphic ventricular tachycardia (torsades de pointes). Consider preventive treatment with IV magnesium sulfate when the QTc interval is > 500 ms. If the patient has unstable torsades de pointes, perform defibrillation. The routine use of magnesium sulfate for ventricular fibrillation or pulseless ventricular tachycardia is no longer recommended. In patients with recurrent torsades de pointes, overdrive pacing with a mechanical pacemaker (transvenous or transcutaneous) is indicated, because the QTc interval shortens as heart rate accelerates.

A notable exception to Advanced Cardiac Life Support (ACLS) guidelines within the scope of toxicology is the avoidance of EPINEPHrine in patients suspected of **huffing** (abusing inhalants). Inhaled halogenated hydrocarbons enhance myocardial sensitivity to catecholamines and can provoke sudden sniffing death syndrome. Typically, the patient is suddenly startled while huffing, which releases a surge of epinephrine and norepinephrine, resulting in a ventricular dysrhythmia or even death. Administration of additional EPINEPHrine could worsen the dysrhythmia. The patient may benefit from a beta blocker such as esmolol. However, accurately diagnosing this cause of cardiovascular toxicity is fraught with difficulty. Unless you have evidence of inhalant use, follow standard ACLS protocols.

Hypertension

Because of significant baseline variation in normal blood pressure, as well as the possibility of underlying hypertension, blood pressure variation can be a misleading parameter to judge acute toxicity. Nevertheless, blood pressure extremes are important in identifying intoxication and guiding management. Depending on the agent, a toxic exposure may induce extreme hypotension or hypertension. In some cases (e.g., alpha-2 agonists), both hypertension and hypotension may be seen, depending on the time since ingestion. The degree of blood pressure derangement dictates care.

Many agents cause toxin-induced hypertension (i.e., sympathomimetics such as cocaine or amphetamines). These agents induce hypertension by increasing systemic vascular resistance (through stimulating peripheral alpha-1 and alpha-2 adrenergic receptors) and by increasing cardiac output via beta adrenergic effects. Toxins with isolated alpha receptor stimulation can cause hypertension and reflex bradycardia, as may be seen with medications such as cloNIDine and oxymetazoline. Other agents, such as anticholinergic agents and hallucinogens, can cause mild hypertension but are rarely responsible for severe hypertension.

The treatment of toxin-induced hypertension depends on both the severity and the mechanism of hypertension. Mild hypertension frequently responds to supportive care, which includes benzodiazepines for agitated patients with sympathomimetic toxicity. However, if the patient has significantly increased blood pressure, vasoactive drugs may be necessary.

In general, beta adrenergic antagonists are a poor choice to treat toxin-induced hypertension, because these medications can generate unopposed alpha adrenergic stimulation, worsen hypertension, and result in coronary artery vasospasm or other end-organ injury. In particular, avoid beta blockers when suspecting cocaine use. Dihydropyridine calcium channel blockers (e.g., nicardipine) or direct vasodilators (e.g., nitroglycerin or nitroprusside) are typically preferred if supportive care and benzodiazepines fail to control severe hypertension.

Deciding when to treat toxin-induced hypertension is an art rather than exact science and depends on the patient and context. Remember that hypotension kills faster than hypertension, as rapid reduction of hypertension may lead to organ hypoperfusion and worsening neurologic function. However, evidence of end-organ damage (vision changes, chest pain, etc.) in the setting of severe hypertension should prompt treatment. Table 14-5 lists toxins that may precipitate hypertension. As always, when in doubt, contact online medical consultation resources.

Hypotension

Treating toxin-induced hypotension is often complicated, as it may have several discrete toxicologic mechanisms or a combination (Table 14-6). Although toxin-directed antidotal therapy is often the preferred approach to treating toxin-induced hypotension, general therapeutic principles apply as well.

Table 14-5 Toxin-Induced Hypertension

Drug Class	Examples	Clinical Presentation	Treatment
Sympathomimetics	Amphetamines and derivatives, cocaine, ePHEDrine, monoamine oxidase inhibitors (MAOIs), methylphenidate, phentermine	Tachycardia, mydriasis, diaphoresis, hypertension, agitation, tremors, seizure, delirium	Benzodiazepines; for MAOIs: phentolamine, labetalol, nitroprusside
Alpha-1 agonists	Ergot alkaloids, phenylephrine	Hypertension, reflex tachycardia, limb ischemia	Phentolamine nitrates, calcium channel blockers
Alpha-2 agonists	CloNIDine, oxymetazoline, tetrahydrozoline	Mental status depression, pinpoint pupils, bradycardia with hypertension initially, followed by bradycardia and hypotension	Nitroprusside or nitroglycerin for initial hypertension if needed; for cloNIDine, high-dose naloxone
Alpha-2 antagonists	Yohimbine	Tachycardia, hypertension, mydriasis, diaphoresis, lacrimation, salivation, nausea, vomiting, and flushing	Benzodiazepines, cloNIDine nitrates
Anticholinergic (antimuscarinic)	Benztropine, cyclobenzaprine, diphenhydrAMINE, doxylamine	Tachycardia, flushing, dry skin, mydriasis, urinary retention, delirium	Supportive care; vasodilators rarely required
Hallucinogens	Dextromethorphan, LSD, mescaline	Mydriasis, tachycardia, mild hypertension, hallucinations	Supportive care

A common cause of hypotension in intoxicated patients is volume depletion. A variety of mechanisms may lead to hypovolemia, including decreased oral intake; gastrointestinal (GI) losses from vomiting and diarrhea; excessive insensible losses from diaphoresis or tachypnea; or osmotic diuresis, as is seen in alcohol toxicity. Before resorting to vasopressor administration, aggressively resuscitate with isotonic fluids (such as lactated Ringer's or normal saline). Even in patients with toxin-induced heart failure, an initial trial of crystalloids is reasonable. However, carefully consider the total volume administered and the associated risk of pulmonary edema, particularly in patients with bradycardia and hypotension. Tachycardic patients with hypotension can generally tolerate a much larger fluid volume.

Norepinephrine and phenylephrine are the agents of choice to treat toxin-induced hypotension. Due to its selective alpha action increasing systemic vascular resistance, phenylephrine is preferable in patients with significant tachycardia and hypotension. Norepinephrine is first-line treatment for patients with low to normal heart rates. In cases of significant bradycardia, depressed ejection fraction, and associated hypotension, consider EPINEPHrine (adrenalin). A common pitfall with vasopressors is underdosing. In toxin-induced hypotension, high doses of vasopressors are often required to compete with the toxic effects of the overdosed drug.

Another common pitfall is the use of DOPamine monotherapy. DOPamine is a mixed-acting sympathomimetic agent, and its vasopressor activity depends primarily on presynaptic uptake and subsequent release of endogenous norepinephrine. At low doses, dopamine receptor activation boosts heart rate and contractility but may result in splanchnic vasodilation and worsening hypotension. This is particularly true in the setting of overdose, in which many drugs (e.g., tricyclic antidepressants) block presynaptic uptake channels. DOPamine may be effective in the setting of mild hypotension and bradycardia associated with a sodium channel opener

Table 14-6 Toxin-Induced Hypotension

Drug Class	Examples	Clinical Presentation	Treatment
Sodium channel openers	Veratrum alkaloids	Nausea, vomiting, bradycardia, hypotension, paresthesias, dysesthesias, mental status depression, paralysis, seizures	IV fluids, atropine, EPINEPHrine, norepinephrine
Sodium channel blockers	Tricyclic antidepressants, carbamazepine, diphenhydrAMINE, quinine, taxine	Nausea, vomiting, bradycardia, QRS prolongation, hypotension, coma, seizures (many are also antimuscarinic)	IV fluids; sodium bicarbonate; hypertonic saline; EPINEPHrine, norepinephrine, or phenylephrine
Alpha-1 antagonists	Doxazosin, prazosin, tricyclic antidepressants, antipsychotics	Mental status depression, hypotension, reflex tachycardia	IV fluids, norepinephrine or phenylephrine
Alpha-2 agonists	CloNIDine, oxymetazoline, tetrahydrozoline	Mental status depression, pinpoint pupils, bradycardia with hypertension initially followed by bradycardia and hypotension	IV fluids; atropine; DOPamine, EPINEPHrine, or norepinephrine; for cloNIDine: high-dose naloxone
Beta blockers	Atenolol, labetalol, metoprolol, propranolol, sotalol	Bradycardia, hypotension, mental status depression	Atropine, glucagon, EPINEPHrine, or high-dose insulin
Beta 2 agonists	Albuterol, clenbuterol, terbutaline	Supraventricular tachycardia, hypotension	Esmolol +/− phenylephrine
Adenosine antagonists	Caffeine, theophylline	Supraventricular tachycardia, hypotension, altered mental status, tremor, seizure	Benzodiazepines, esmolol +/− phenylephrine, hemodialysis
Calcium channel blockers	DilTIAZem, verapamil, amLODIPine, felodipine, NIFEdipine	Hypotension with bradycardia (dilTIAZem; verapamil; high-dose amlodipine, felodipine, and NIFEdipines) or reflex tachycardia (amLODIPine, felodipine, and NIFEdipine)	IV fluids, atropine, calcium salts, EPINEPHrine, norepinephrine, high-dose insulin
Sedative-hypnotics and opioids	Ethanol, barbiturates, benzodiazepines, heroin, morphine	Sedation, pinpoint pupils and respiratory depression (with opioids)	IV fluids, supportive care; vasopressors rarely required
Na^+/K^+-ATPase inhibitors	Digoxin, foxglove, lily of the valley, oleander, *Bufo* toads, Chan su	Nausea, vomiting, atrioventricular node block, premature ventricular contractions, ventricular dysrhythmias	Digoxin-specific antibody fragments (Fab), atropine

Drug Class	Examples	Clinical Presentation	Treatment
Electron transport chain toxins	CN, cyanogenic glycosides (e.g., amygdalin), carbon monoxide, HS, salicylates	Hypotension, reflex tachycardia, severe metabolic acidosis, hyperthermia (uncouplers), altered mental status, seizures	Dextrose, IV fluids, sodium bicarbonate, hydroxocobalamin (CN, HS), hyperbaric oxygen (carbon monoxide), EPINEPHrine vs. norepinephrine vs. phenylephrine, sodium thiosulfate (CN)

ATPase, adenosine triphosphatase; CN, cyanide; HS, hydrogen sulfide; K^+, potassium; Na^+, sodium.

and alpha-2 agonist toxicity or as an adjunctive treatment in combination with a more potent vasopressor after beta blocker– or calcium channel blocker–induced heart failure.

Disability: Altered Mental Status

Many toxins may cause altered mental status through a multitude of mechanisms. Toxin-induced mentation changes range from excitation to severe agitation to coma. Prehospital care should focus on three steps in this regard. First, ensure responder and patient safety. This may often include sedating the patient to control agitation. Also, if the patient is obtunded, consider intubation to protect the airway and prevent aspiration. Second, obtain a serum glucose level. Hypoglycemia is an easily reversible cause of altered mentation. Third, use your knowledge of the major toxidromes (discussed later in this chapter) in conjunction with history and physical exam to attempt to diagnose the toxin exposure. If appropriate, provide antidotal therapy, which may resolve the altered mental status.

Blood Glucose Derangements

Hypoglycemia is a rapidly reversible, life-threatening cause of altered mental status. It may result from a number of toxins, including antidiabetic agents, excessive alcohol intake, and beta blockers. Availability of bedside glucose testing allows quick testing for hypoglycemia before administering glucose. IV administration of a dextrose solution ($D_{10}W$ or D_{25}) is safe and advisable.

Hyperglycemia is unusual in toxic exposures. Calcium channel blockers may lead to elevated glucose; however, this is unlikely to be of clinical significance. Altered mental status in the setting of severe hyperglycemia should prompt you to consider diabetic ketoacidosis (DKA) and hyperosmolar hyperglycemic state (HHS). Although these conditions could occur in the setting of toxic exposure, they are unlikely to be direct effects of the toxin and should be managed per usual protocols (administration of fluids and insulin, along with electrolyte monitoring and repletion).

Pupillary Exam

An abnormal pupillary exam may provide clues to the class of toxins to which the patient was exposed. Miosis (abnormally constricted pupils) may result from opioid intoxication or organophosphate exposure. Mydriasis (dilated pupils) is a sign of sympathomimetic use, anticholinergic toxicity, as well as opioid withdrawal. Specific treatments for these intoxications will be discussed later.

Seizures

Toxin-induced CNS excitation can lead to seizures, which are most often generalized tonic-clonic seizures. Such seizures rarely progress to status epilepticus, although exceptions do occur (e.g., isoniazid toxicity). Chapter 8, *Neurologic Disorders*, provides additional information on seizure management. Seizure activity should always prompt you to evaluate the patient's blood glucose level or to administer dextrose empirically. Otherwise, benzodiazepines are the mainstay in both preventing and treating seizures acutely. If a patient shows tremor activity, especially if accompanied by tachycardia and anxiety, administer benzodiazepines to prevent seizure activity. Once a seizure occurs, administer high-dose benzodiazepines.

If benzodiazepines do not stop the seizure activity, then consider hypoglycemia, isoniazid toxicity, and hypoxemia as potential causes. These respond to glucose, pyridoxine (vitamin B_6), and oxygen, respectively. If benzodiazepines are still ineffective, additional treatment options may include levETIRAcetam (or other antiepileptics except phenytoin), barbiturates, or propofol (a GABA agonist and N-methyl-D-aspartate [NMDA] antagonist). These options are generally outside the scope of EMS clinicians. Note that propofol administration may necessitate intubation, and barbiturates mandate close monitoring of airway and breathing status. Consider continuous electroencephalogram (EEG) monitoring during hospitalization if seizures are prolonged or if the patient fails to return to baseline.

Agitation

Many drugs and toxins can cause CNS excitation, delirium, agitation, or psychosis. Regardless of the cause, initial management is the same. The goal of treatment is to decrease CNS excitability to protect the patient from metabolic derangements associated with agitation, tissue injury from cardiovascular toxicity, and self-injury. Delirium with agitated behavior from a drug or toxin can be accompanied by marked sympathetic stimulation (tachycardia, hypertension, hyperthermia). This is a life-threatening condition and requires immediate sedation for the safety of both clinician and patient. The mainstays of pharmacologic treatment for agitation are benzodiazepines, antipsychotics (haloperidol, droPERidol), and ketamine. For delirium with agitated behavior (sometimes called hyperactive delirium), emergency clinicians will typically administer intramuscular (IM) ketamine or an IM combination of a benzodiazepine with an antipsychotic agent (e.g., midazolam 5 mg and droPERidol 5 mg).

Benzodiazepines depress the CNS by increasing the release of GABA, an inhibitory neurotransmitter. Benzodiazepines' large safety profile and wide therapeutic index make this medication class the first-line agent to prevent injury to intoxicated patients and the clinicians who care for them. Benzodiazepines also have the benefit of preventing seizure activity, attenuating sympathetic hyperactivity, and reducing other causes of morbidity often associated with severe agitation (e.g., rhabdomyolysis). The benzodiazepines most commonly used to sedate the acutely agitated patient in the emergency care setting are diazePAM, LORazepam, and midazolam. DiazePAM is available in IV, intraosseous (IO), oral, and rectal forms; LORazepam is available IV and IM; and midazolam is available in IV, IM, intranasal (IN), IO, and oral forms. The dose required to sedate a patient adequately varies significantly with body size, degree of agitation, history of benzodiazepine tolerance, and amount of stimulant ingested. Although benzodiazepines are associated with sedation and potential loss of airway protective reflexes, they do not, on their own, suppress respiratory drive. When combined with other sedative agents, such as opioids, ethanol, and barbiturates, benzodiazepines do synergistically contribute to respiratory depression.

Antipsychotic medications, especially haloperidol and droPERidol, are commonly used in emergency care to treat agitated patients. Both antipsychotic agents potently antagonize dopamine D_2 receptors. A desired side effect is sedation. Ziprasidone, a second-generation antipsychotic, is approved for acute agitation in schizophrenic patients. The antipsychotic activity of ziprasidone, like haloperidol, is mediated primarily by antagonism at dopamine D_2 receptors. OLANZapine is also commonly used to treat the acutely agitated patient. It is effective when given IM, but should not be administered via IV. An oral dissolving tablet is available for patients who are cooperative enough to take this formulation. The newer atypical antipsychotics have less-potent dopamine antagonist effects as well as enhanced effects at alternative receptors such as muscarinic blockade. Haloperidol and droPERidol, however, remain the preferred antipsychotics of choice when use becomes necessary.

Despite the potential for adverse effects, using antipsychotics after or with benzodiazepines plays a central role in treating agitated patients. Adverse effects associated with antipsychotic use include extrapyramidal symptoms and QT prolongation. Consider obtaining a baseline ECG prior to giving antipsychotics, although this can be difficult in the acutely agitated patient. Intoxicated patients with excess dopaminergic stimulation exhibit acute psychosis, often manifested by visual and tactile hallucinations or abnormal repetitive involuntary movements. Antipsychotic agents can be effective in treating these specific toxic effects.

Ketamine is a dissociative anesthetic that quickly and safely calms agitated patients, especially those experiencing delirium with agitated behavior who are at increased risk of serious adverse outcomes (acidosis, rhabdomyolysis, respiratory failure, and death). Ketamine is an NMDA receptor antagonist that also inhibits uptake of norepinephrine, dopamine, and serotonin. It calms the patient rapidly without typically affecting airway patency or ventilation control. It is becoming more common in the prehospital setting, can be given IM, and prevents the severely agitated patient from continued CNS stimulation and physical exertion. Although respiratory depression is less common with the use of ketamine, other depressants/sedatives used in conjunction could lead to apnea. Note that ketamine is typically faster-acting than both benzodiazepines and antipsychotics, and so is often preferred for delirium with severe agitation.

Regardless of the situation, any patient receiving sedative therapy requires immediate close and constant cardiorespiratory monitoring as well as frequent airway evaluation. All classes of sedating medications, especially when given in combination or in the setting of possible toxic coingestants, have the potential to cause airway loss and respiratory depression. Continuous pulse oximetry and end-tidal CO_2 ($ETCO_2$) monitoring can help ensure that the patient is oxygenating and ventilating adequately.

During administration of these medications, brief physical restraint by law enforcement or medical personnel may be necessary. Patients should never be restrained in the prone position. If continuing physical restraint is necessary, pharmacologic options should also be used if the patient is aggressively struggling against restraints and may be a harm to themselves or others. Physically restrained patients require frequent monitoring for adverse physiologic effects.

Coma

The extreme of altered mental status is coma, a state of unconsciousness or deep sedation from which the patient cannot be aroused by any external stimulus. Many toxins may precipitate a comatose state.

Treatment is primarily supportive and may include advanced airway support. Most current recommendations suggest positioning the patient to protect the airway, supporting breathing and circulation, and then considering drug therapy. Therapeutic agents used to reverse coma include glucose and naloxone. Thiamine and flumazenil (a benzodiazepine-reversal agent) are only of historical interest and do not play a role in EMS care today.

Exposure: Temperature Alteration

As discussed earlier, the patient should be completely exposed, examined, and decontaminated if necessary. Pay special attention to substances, patches, or wounds (from stings, bites, punctures, etc.) that may offer an explanation for the patient's symptoms or may be causing ongoing toxin exposure.

Although often overlooked, particularly in the prehospital setting, obtaining an accurate body temperature is crucial in managing toxicologic emergencies. Temperature alteration is a cardinal feature of some toxicologic diagnoses, such as serotonin syndrome, neuroleptic malignant syndrome, malignant hyperthermia, and sympathomimetic/stimulant use/overdose. Stimulant intoxication or poisoning is associated with increased mortality when accompanied by hyperthermia. The therapeutic goal for such patients is rapid normalization of temperature through discontinuation of offending agents, external cooling techniques, and medication administration. Patients with altered mental status and temperatures greater than 38°C (100.4°F) must be cooled as rapidly as possible, because severe hyperthermia may be lethal. The best method for doing so is cold water immersion. Place the patient in a body bag or tub and fill the container halfway with ice water. While the patient is immersed, continue to monitor temperature. Once the core temperature has been reduced to an appropriate level (typically a target temperature of 38–39°C [100.4–102.2°F]), the patient may be removed from the ice water.

Hypothermia can also occur after ingestion of sedative-hypnotic agents or opioids. Whether the patient's temperature has climbed or fallen, initiate treatment of any severe temperature alteration as soon as the condition is discovered. Treatment before transport may be indicated and lifesaving.

▼ Ongoing Management

Ongoing management focuses on monitoring the patient's condition, limiting further toxin exposure, providing antidotes if possible, and providing supportive care.

Patient Monitoring

Enroute to the hospital, monitoring the patient's response to therapy is essential, and, as always, early communication with the receiving facility can ensure a fluid continuum of care. The patient's vital signs should be continuously monitored during transport. Consider continuous pulse oximetry and capnography on patients who may have been exposed to CNS depressants, whether ingested or given by responders for agitation. If the patient's vital signs deteriorate, restart the primary survey. Intoxications are often progressive, and the patient's condition may worsen over time. For example, an initially secure airway may fail during transport, leading to the need for intubation after the initial survey is complete. Continuously monitor these patients and never hesitate to reassess.

Gastrointestinal Decontamination

After completing your initial patient evaluation and stabilization, consider treatment strategies to attempt to limit GI absorption of an ingested toxin. **Gastrointestinal decontamination** with syrup of ipecac and activated charcoal has been studied and debated for decades. The current standard of care does *not* call for administration of ipecac in any patient and rarely indicates administration of activated charcoal. Activated charcoal, if allowed by local protocol, is recommended only when less than 1 hour has elapsed between the confirmed time of potentially toxic exposure and the time of administration. Even then, activated charcoal is contraindicated in patients with any alteration in mental status or with nausea or vomiting because of the significant documented risk of aspiration of the activated charcoal.

"Body stuffers" represent one notable exception to these contraindications to the use of activated charcoal. Stuffers will attempt to dispose of a toxin by quickly swallowing the substance to avoid the discovery of the substance by law enforcement or other interested party. If good mentation exists after ingestion of a poorly wrapped packet of drugs, administration of single-dose activated charcoal is recommended. If the patient's mental status is altered, a dose of activated charcoal may be attempted enterally (through a nasogastric tube) only with close monitoring and suction capabilities present. Consult online medical oversight for discussion in that case.

Activated charcoal also continues to play a role in treating some ingestions (e.g., salicylates), but the risks associated with its use may outweigh the benefits.

Antidotes

Antidotes are medications that directly counteract specific toxic agents. When available, these should almost always be given according to protocol or online consultation. Certain antidotes may be given only in cases of severe disease, as they may be resource limited (e.g., rare, exceedingly expensive) or have significant side effects (e.g., possible anaphylactic reaction). Patients who have been exposed to dangerous toxins may also have only minimal symptoms and may have good outcomes with supportive care alone. When in doubt, contact online medical control or local poison center for guidance. See Table 14-7 for antidotes that EMS carries.

Table 14-7 Common Poisoning Antidotes

Medication	Poisoning
Activated charcoal	Various ingested poisons
Atropine	Organophosphate overdose
Benzodiazepines (LORazepam, midazolam)	Sympathomimetic/ stimulant overdose
Calcium chloride	Calcium channel blocker overdose Beta blocker overdose Hydrofluoric acid burns
Calcium gluconate	Calcium channel blocker overdose Beta blocker overdose Hydrofluoric acid burns
CyanoKit (hydroxocobalamin)	Cyanide poisoning
Dextrose	Sulfonylurea overdose Insulin overdose
Glucagon	Beta blocker overdose
Magnesium sulfate	Hydrofluoric acid exposure
Naloxone	Opioid overdose
Sodium bicarbonate	Tricyclic antidepressant overdose Salicylate overdose

Key Supportive Management Recap

No antidotes exist or are readily available for many toxins. For patients with such exposures, supportive care is critical. For airway, remember positioning and adjuncts (e.g., jaw thrust and nasopharyngeal airways), as well as suctioning as needed. Many patients may require supplemental oxygen or positive-pressure ventilation. Initiate IV fluid resuscitation in any tachycardic patient unless they have specific contraindications. In such cases (e.g., known heart failure, renal failure), give a smaller bolus and reassess. Treat agitation as discussed previously, with benzodiazepines, antipsychotic agents, and/or ketamine. In cases of seizures, always check a glucose level or provide dextrose, and then administer benzodiazepines as necessary. Antiemetics or other treatments to reduce nausea (e.g., having patient sniff an alcohol prep) may be indicated, as many toxins cause nausea and vomiting.

Toxidromes

Many toxins result in similar symptoms and require similar treatments. This section discusses the classic toxidromes (or "toxic syndromes"). Refer back to Table 14-2 for a summary of each. Specific drugs are discussed later. Understanding the basic principles of each toxidrome will allow you to better recognize patterns of toxicity and more rapidly treat toxicologic emergencies.

Cholinergic

Case Presentation: A 43-year-old male farmer presents with diaphoresis, salivation, lacrimation, urinary and bowel incontinence, emesis, bronchorrhea, and fasciculations. He is noted to have the following vital signs: blood pressure 130/80 mm Hg, pulse 50 beats/min, respirations 36 breaths/min, temperature 36.7°C (98°), and SpO_2 84%.

Pathophysiology

The term **cholinergic** refers to toxins that increase the neurotransmitter acetylcholine (ACh), which plays an important role within both the central and peripheral nervous systems. Of special significance, ACh is the primary neurotransmitter at the neuromuscular junction, which connects neurons to muscle fibers. ACh acts on two types of receptors: muscarinic and nicotinic.

The most important toxins that act cholinergically are the organophosphates and carbamates. These chemicals are widely used as insecticides and are typically responsible for over 100,000 deaths annually worldwide. Although less commonly fatal in the United States, over 10,000 cases of insecticide toxicity were reported in the

United States in 2020. Organophosphates and carbamates are readily absorbed through the skin and mucous membranes, including through inhalation or ingestion. These toxins bind to and inhibit acetylcholinesterase (AChE), which normally reduces the concentration of ACh. This creates a "double-negative," in which the insecticides inhibit an inhibitor and raise the concentration of ACh.

Of note, organophosphates and carbamates inhibit AChE in slightly different ways. Organophosphates and nerve agents contain an organic phosphate group that binds to AChE. Over a variable period of time, these two molecules form a permanent bond, a process referred to as aging, which permanently inactivates the enzyme. Aging does not occur with carbamates, nor does the irreversible binding. Carbamates also have less CNS penetration compared to organophosphates and are generally less toxic.

Signs and Symptoms

The hallmark symptom of cholinergic toxicity is diffuse "wetness." Any gland or body part that can produce fluid does so when ACh is toxically elevated. The classic mnemonic for cholinergic toxicity is "SLUDGE and the Killer Bs" (Rapid Recall Box 14-3). SLUDGE represents the general state of wetness of these patients. You will recognize a cholinergic intoxication by the constellation of **s**weating, **l**acrimation (crying), excessive **u**rination, **d**iarrhea, **G**I upset, and vomiting (**e**mesis). However, these symptoms are not fatal if the patient is given basic supportive care. Monitor closely for the Killer Bs, which can lead to a fatal outcome: **b**radycardia, **b**ronchorrhea, and **b**ronchospasm. Bronchorrhea, specifically, is the most important symptom to monitor when treating these patients.

AChE inhibitors (organophosphates and carbamates) are widely used in pesticides. Examples are given in Table 14-8. They are found in insect sprays as a liquid, in rose-dusting formulations as a solid, and in mist preparations for application over larger areas. Pesticides intended for commercial use can be highly concentrated and deadly. The dangers these agents pose vary widely, depending on the chemical structure of the pesticide and the carrier in which the pesticide is dissolved. Household formulations are typically more dilute, and the chemical agents they contain are often less potent. Of note, organophosphates were originally developed in pre–World War II Germany as chemical weapons. Only later were they used as agricultural products. Nerve agents may act as AChE inhibitors and possess lethal cholinergic toxicity. Some mushrooms also have similar effects through direct receptor stimulation rather than enzyme inhibition.

Differential Diagnosis

Any drug, agent, or condition that can cause or mimic excessive cholinergic stimulation could be considered in this situation. These can include gastroenteritis, nicotine toxicity, myasthenia gravis, mushroom toxicity, Guillain-Barré syndrome, or botulism.

RAPID RECALL BOX 14-3

SLUDGE and the Killer Bs:

S Salivation
L Lacrimation
U Urination
D Defecation
G Gastrointestinal distress
E Emesis
B Bradycardia
B Bronchorrhea
B Bronchospasm

Table 14-8 Selected Organophosphates and Carbamates

Organophosphates	Carbamates
Acephate	Aldicarb
Azinphos-methyl	Carbaryl
Chlorpyrifos	Carbofuran
Diazinon	Ethinenocarb
Dichlorvos	Methomyl
Malathion	Propoxur
Phosmet	Sevin
Parathion	Trimethacarb

Treatment

When treating a patient with pesticide (organophosphate/carbamate) poisoning, you must take great care to avoid self-contamination or contamination of others from the victim (Tip Box 14-1). The patient's clothing must be removed and isolated (bagged or removed from the immediate area). Wear personal protective clothing, including gloves, a gown, and eye protection, while treating the patient. In addition, some organophosphates and carbamates are volatile, and respiratory protection may be required. Emesis may also contain significant amounts of poison and must be isolated and handled carefully.

TIP BOX 14-1

Treatment of Pesticide (Organophosphate/Carbamate) Exposure

- Don appropriate PPE (including neoprene or nitrile gloves, a gown, mask, and face shield).
- Decontaminate the patient prior to performing primary survey.
- Remove and isolate the patient's clothing.
- Identify agent of exposure.
- Open the patient's airway. Ensure adequate ventilation and oxygenation.
- Orotracheal or nasotracheal intubation may be indicated if the patient is unconscious, has severe pulmonary edema, or is in severe respiratory distress.
- Consider positive-pressure ventilation with a bag-valve mask.
- Monitor for and treat noncardiogenic pulmonary edema.
- Monitor cardiac rhythm and treat dysrhythmias.
- Establish an IV line and start a saline infusion at 30 mL/hr.
- For hypotension:
  - If the patient has signs of hypovolemia, administer fluid cautiously.
  - Consider vasopressors if the patient is hypotensive with a normal fluid volume. Watch for signs of fluid overload.
- Correct hypoxia and then administer atropine per local protocol. The goal of atropine administration is the drying of pulmonary secretions, not correcting mydriasis or tachycardia.
- Administer pralidoxime chloride per local protocol.
- Treat seizures with benzodiazepines (diazePAM, LORazepam, or midazolam) per local protocol.
- If patient's eyes are contaminated, immediately flush with water. Continuously irrigate each eye with normal saline during transport.
- Patients must be transported to an appropriate medical treatment facility for further evaluation and management.
- Continuously monitor during transport.
- Contraindications: Succinylcholine and other cholinergic agents

Supportive care, including management of airway, breathing, and circulation, is of paramount importance. Airway management is a priority because of the increased bronchial secretions and muscle paralysis associated with the cholinergic effects of these agents. Cardiac monitoring is also necessary. Activated charcoal may be indicated if less than 1 hour has elapsed since the exposure, although the patient will likely already be vomiting. The antidotes for organophosphate poisoning are atropine and pralidoxime (2-PAM). Atropine treats the wet symptoms, and pralidoxime reactivates acetylcholinesterase.

Atropine binds to the muscarinic acetylcholine receptor, inhibiting the parasympathetic stimulation caused by the organophosphate or carbamate. The end point of atropine administration is drying of the secretions and improved respiratory function. There is no maximum dose. Note that these doses are significantly higher than those used for cardiac conditions, and cholinergic toxicity may require relatively large amounts of atropine.

Adequate amounts of atropine may be difficult to obtain rapidly for a single pesticide exposure, let alone an intentional event. A typical hospital may go through its entire supply of atropine for a single patient exposure. Obtaining Strategic National Stockpile medications may not be rapid enough to have a clinical effect, although many states have ChemPacks, which can be obtained more quickly. Alternative routes of atropine administration include dry powder inhalation, nebulized, and sublingual. National stockpiles of the powder formulation may be the most readily available for mass casualty exposures.

The binding of organophosphates and nerve agents to AChE becomes permanent over time. To be most effective, pralidoxime should be administered before the aging process occurs. If given prior to this occurring, pralidoxime can prevent structural change to the enzyme and dramatically reduce the duration of symptoms and of hospitalization. Of note, known isolated carbamate toxicity does not require administration of pralidoxime.

Glycopyrrolate and possibly diphenhydrAMINE are alternative anticholinergic agents that may benefit these patients as well. Unfortunately, these agents do not cross the blood–brain barrier, and, therefore, may not alleviate central effects.

Anticholinergic

Case Presentation: A 17-year-old female presents with delirium, dry and flushed skin, mydriasis, and urinary retention. She is hot to the touch. Her friends report they have been drinking "tea" to get high. She is noted to have the following vital signs: blood pressure 150/85 mm Hg, pulse 128 beats/min, respirations 16 breaths/min, temperature 39.4°C (103°F), and SpO_2 98%.

Pathophysiology

Anticholinergic toxicity may perhaps be best understood as the opposite of cholinergic toxicity. Most anticholinergic toxins act as antagonists to acetylcholine at muscarinic receptors; these are specifically referred to as antimuscarinics, as they do not affect nicotinic receptors. Although there are multiple mechanisms of action, all drugs or chemicals that lead to decreased ACh transmission at these receptors will produce the same syndrome.

Signs and Symptoms

In opposition to the "wet" symptoms of cholinergic toxicity, anticholinergics cause "hot and dry" symptoms. The classic mnemonic begins "hot as a hare, red as a beet, dry as a bone, mad as a hatter." Symptoms include elevated temperature, dry and flushed skin/mucous membranes, mydriasis, altered mental status, and tachycardia. Altered mentation may include hallucinations.

Differential Diagnosis

Many drugs and other chemicals possess anticholinergic effects. The classic examples are atropine (used to treat bradycardia), scopolamine (an antiemetic), and glycopyrrolate (used to treat excessive secretions). Naturally occurring anticholinergics include *Atropa belladonna* (deadly nightshade) and jimson weed. Nightshade is an alkaloid-containing plant that causes lethal anticholinergic toxicity. Jimson weed is typically smoked or made into tea for its hallucinogenic effects. Many other drugs have anticholinergic effects (either primarily or as part of mixed effects), including benztropine, diphenhydrAMINE and other antihistamines, cyclic antidepressants, and some antipsychotics.

Anticholinergic toxicity should be high on your differential diagnosis when considering an altered patient with elevated temperature. Other considerations include heatstroke, serotonin syndrome (serotonergic toxicity), neuroleptic malignant syndrome (antipsychotic toxicity), malignant hyperthermia (usually in the setting of surgery and anesthesia), and stimulant/sympathomimetic toxicity. The key clue will often be that the patient is dry and is not sweating. Context, including nearby pill bottles, will also assist with making the correct diagnosis.

Treatment

Treatment of anticholinergic toxicity is largely supportive, including active cooling if necessary. Give benzodiazepines for agitation, tachycardia, or hypertension. The antidote for anticholinergic is physostigmine, which inhibits acetylcholinesterase and thereby increases ACh transmission (cholinergic effect). Give physostigmine to patients with anticholinergic toxicity who have altered mental status, signs of end-organ damage, or are a danger to themselves or others. Side effects of physostigmine are muscarinic (SLUDGE) symptoms.

Sedative-Hypnotic

Case Presentation: A 37-year-old male is found down with altered mental status. He smells of alcohol, and an empty bottle of muscle relaxants is found next to him. He is noted to have the following vital signs: blood pressure 90/60 mm Hg, pulse 50 beats/min, respirations 12 breaths/min, temperature 35°C (95°F), and SpO_2 88%.

Pathophysiology

Sedative-hypnotics are a class of medications that primarily affect the gamma-aminobutyric acid (GABA) receptor, specifically $GABA_A$. These include ethanol (alcohol), benzodiazepines, and barbiturates.

Ethanol is readily absorbed into the bloodstream through the GI tract. Most of the alcohol consumed is absorbed within 1 hour. Ethanol then passes easily through the blood–brain barrier, leading to intoxicating effects through central $GABA_A$ agonism and NMDA receptor antagonism.

Benzodiazepines affect $GABA_A$ receptors by allowing increased frequency of chloride channel opening. Barbiturates primarily cause prolonged opening of the chloride channel (in addition to inhibition of the excitatory neurotransmitter glutamate at the NMDA receptor). Both mechanisms cause CNS depression and sedation at both therapeutic and toxic levels. More recently, nonbenzodiazepine sleep aids such as zolpidem, zaleplon, and eszopiclone have surpassed benzodiazepines in popularity for treating sleep disorders. The primary activity of these drugs is also $GABA_A$ agonism, although they are typically less potent.

Signs and Symptoms

Sedation is the primary clinical effect of sedative-hypnotic intoxication. Symptoms of CNS depression will be seen with intoxications of all drugs of this class.

Signs and symptoms of ethanol intoxication vary by blood alcohol concentration (Table 14-9) and may include euphoria, confusion, lethargy, ataxia (and associated injuries from falls), stupor, respiratory depression, hypothermia, hypotension, coma, and cardiovascular collapse. Extreme intoxication can lead to severely decreased levels of consciousness, severe respiratory difficulties, or death. Preexisting conditions are often exacerbated by the effects of ethanol. Vasodilation from ethanol may lead to hypotension and hypothermia.

Patients with benzodiazepine overdose exhibit a variable clinical picture. Most notable is that respiratory rate depression typically does *not* occur after benzodiazepine ingestion alone, even with massive overdoses. Some patients display mild bradycardia, but clinically significant hypotension rarely develops. Hypoxemia may be present, however, when there is concomitant ingestion of another sedative or opioid or in cases of aspiration pneumonitis. Underlying respiratory disease, such as chronic obstructive pulmonary disease (COPD), may also cause respiratory complications. Pressure ulcers may occur after protracted immobilization but are not specific to benzodiazepines.

Table 14-9 Effects of Ethanol Related to Blood Alcohol Concentration

Concentration (%)	Effects
0.02	Few obvious effects, slight intensification of mood
0.05	Loss of emotional restraint, feeling of warmth, flushing of skin, mild impairment of judgment
0.10	Slight slurring of speech, loss of fine motor control, unstable emotions, inappropriate laughter
0.12	Coordination and balance difficult, distinct impairment of mentation and judgment
0.20	Responsive to verbal stimuli, very slurred speech, staggering gait, diplopia, difficulty standing upright, memory loss
0.30	Briefly aroused by painful stimuli; deep, snoring respirations
0.40	Unresponsiveness, incontinence, hypotension, irregular respirations
0.50	Death possible from apnea, hypotension, or aspiration of vomitus

Data from Aehlert B. *Paramedic Practice Today: Above and Beyond*. Mosby; 2009.

Neurologic signs and symptoms vary with the degree of sedation. Mild benzodiazepine intoxication causes ataxia, slurred speech, somnolence, and nystagmus. Severe toxicity induces deep sedation. Patients may display hyporeflexia and sluggish cranial nerve reflexes. Patients often respond to noxious stimuli, but some have no response.

Toxicity of older nonbenzodiazepine sedative-hypnotics may have unusual features. For example, carisoprodol is prescribed as a centrally acting muscle relaxant, which may produce sinus tachycardia and myoclonic jerking. Zolpidem, zaleplon, and eszopiclone are GABA agonists but not benzodiazepines. Nevertheless, their toxic effects are similar; they do not cause respiratory depression and are likewise reversible with flumazenil. Overall, these drugs are associated with less severe toxicity and withdrawal.

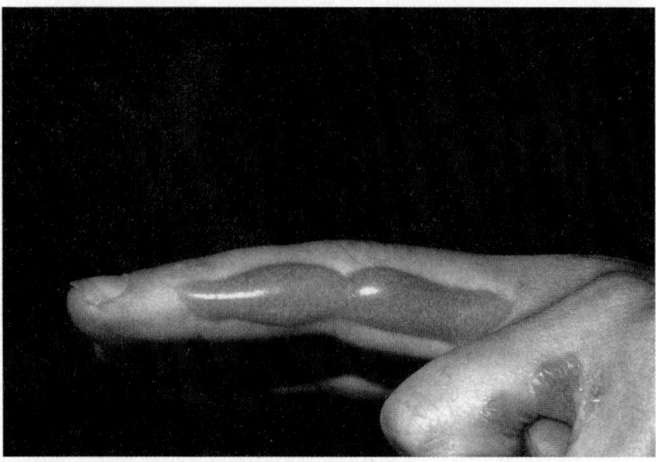

Figure 14-2 A "barb blister." Skin changes due to immobilization can be seen in patients with barbiturate overdose.

Signs of significant barbiturate overdose may include hypothermia, bradycardia, hypotension, and coma. Unlike benzodiazepines, barbiturates alone will induce hypoventilation, respiratory depression, and apnea. Coingestion of other sedative-hypnotic agents, including alcohol and opioids, synergistically inhibits the respiratory drive.

Secondary injury after barbiturate ingestion, including renal and hypoxic brain injuries, often occurs as a result of hypoxemia, hypotension, and tissue hypoperfusion. Severe CNS depression may lead to loss of airway reflexes and aspiration pneumonia. In addition, prolonged immobilization while comatose can lead to skin breakdown, rhabdomyolysis, and compartment syndrome, depending on the patient's position. Pressure ulcers found in comatose patients are often still referred to as "barb blisters" because of this complication's historical prevalence among barbiturate-overdose patients. These fluid-filled bullae (**Figure 14-2**) are the direct effect of protracted pressure on skin during immobilization and can occur in patients immobilized for any reason; they are not a direct result of barbiturate toxicity.

Differential Diagnosis

Any medication with the potential to cause altered mental status should also be considered in the differential diagnosis of possible sedative-hypnotic intoxications.

Differentiation of Agents

Ethanol is not a particularly toxic chemical at low doses, as evidenced by its legal use in beer, wine, and distilled spirits, but chronic overuse causes significant morbidity, including cirrhosis and different types of cancers. Because of its wide availability and classification as a food, ethanol causes more toxicologic emergencies than any other kind of alcohol. Most cases are classified as intentional because they involve alcoholic beverages; however, ethanol is also used in industrial solvents. Inhaling powdered ethanol is a dangerous trend. When powdered ethanol is poured over dry ice and the vapors are inhaled, ethanol bypasses the stomach and enters directly into the lungs, which is more likely to lead to lethal poisoning than typical ingestion.

Benzodiazepines were introduced in the 1960s, largely replacing barbiturates because of their improved safety profile and lower potential for addiction. As a group, these medications are frequently prescribed, and overdose is common. However, significant morbidity or death due to benzodiazepine ingestion alone is rare. The risk of morbidity and mortality is greater when a benzodiazepine is coingested with another CNS depressant, such as alcohol, an opioid, or a barbiturate. Benzodiazepines are differentiated from one another by half-life of the parent compound, estimated duration of action, and presence of active metabolites. Table 14-10 lists this information for selected common benzodiazepines, as well as for the benzodiazepine-like drug zolpidem.

Barbiturates have been commercially available since the early 1900s. PHENObarbital was used extensively to treat seizure disorders before the advent of newer anticonvulsants, and it is still used to treat uncontrolled seizure disorders. Some patients are treated successfully with PHENObarbital for years. Primidone, which is metabolized to PHENObarbital, is also used as an anticonvulsant. Butalbital combined with caffeine and either aspirin or acetaminophen is a barbiturate that was used as a pain reliever, primarily for migraine headaches. Other barbiturates, or "barbs" as commonly known, are available but rarely prescribed. Barbiturates have a narrow therapeutic window and are responsible for the highest risk of morbidity and mortality of all sedative-hypnotic agents.

Table 14-10 Duration and Half-Life of Selected Benzodiazepines

Estimated Duration	Benzodiazepine/ Benzodiazepine-Like Drug	Half-Life (hours)
Short	Zolpidem	1.4-4.5
	Triazolam	1.5-5.5
Intermediate	Oxazepam	3-25
	Temazepam	5-20
	ALPRAZolam	6.3-26.9
	LORazepam	10-20
Long	Chlordiazepoxide	5-48
	ClonazePAM	18-50
	DiazePAM	20-80

Evaluation

With any sedative-hypnotic intoxication, associated mental status depression often makes an accurate history difficult to obtain. In unresponsive patients, the position of the patient on discovery and an estimate of the duration of toxicity may help guide treatment and predict outcome. This information can usually be obtained from friends or family members. After the initial airway, breathing, and vital signs evaluation, conduct a thorough neurologic exam, including cranial nerves and deep tendon reflexes. The absence of these reflexes indicates severe toxicity. The patient may also have decreased bowel sounds and abdominal distention. Pulmonary exam may reveal bradypnea with or without crackles (also known as rales), but may be normal in patients with only mild toxicity. Pay special attention to skin bullae during the musculoskeletal exam, and palpate the muscle compartments of the upper and lower extremities. Early identification of compartment syndrome can significantly improve the patient's overall outcome.

Treatment

Treatment of sedative-hypnotic intoxication typically begins and ends with supportive care. Follow the AMLS Assessment Pathway with special emphasis placed on airway and respiratory management.

Airway management, including endotracheal intubation, is often required in significant toxicity. Mild to moderate toxicity may only necessitate supplemental oxygen and continuous pulse oximetry and possibly $ETCO_2$ monitoring. Treat hypotension initially with IV fluid boluses; refractory hypotension warrants vasopressor administration, typically norepinephrine. General supportive care (hydration, elevation of the head, wound care, prevention of recurrence) is indicated. Take care to prevent aspiration as possible; activated charcoal is not recommended for these patients. Monitor core temperature and prevent hypothermia. Hypoglycemia should be ruled out by performing a serum glucose test. If the patient is unresponsive or demonstrates respiratory depression, a trial dose of naloxone should be considered to evaluate for potential opioid toxicity.

Flumazenil, a GABA antagonist, is the antidote to benzodiazepines. However, its routine use is not recommended. Unless the benzodiazepine toxicity is iatrogenic (clearly caused by excessive administration by a health care clinician), do not give flumazenil unless directed to do so by online medical consultation or a poison center. In patients with chronic benzodiazepine use, flumazenil can cause severe acute withdrawal, seizures refractory to treatment, and death.

The end point of treatment is mental status improvement rather than a specific serum drug level. In severe cases that fail to respond sufficiently to standard therapy, hemodialysis effectively hastens recovery.

Opioids and Opiates

Case Presentation: A 40-year-old female presents comatose. Physical exam is remarkable for IV track marks in her arms bilaterally, decreased respiratory rate, and pinpoint pupils. She is noted to have the following vital signs: blood pressure 90/60 mm Hg, pulse 50 beats/min, respirations 4 breaths/min, temperature 35°C (95°F), and SpO_2 85%.

Pathophysiology

Opiates and opioids (synthetic opiates) are CNS and respiratory depressants that act on the opiate receptors in the brain. Their effects can be agonistic or antagonistic, depending on the opioid in question.

Opioids may be administered by oral, nasal (snorting), dermal (skin-popping), IV (mainlining), or inhalational (smoking) routes. A speedball is a bolus of heroin and cocaine injected intravenously. Injection track marks can often be seen in patients who mainline (**Figure 14-3**), but the absence of obvious injection sites does not rule out a possible heroin, fentaNYL, or opioid overdose.

In today's opioid epidemic, fentaNYL and potent fentaNYL analogs are commonly encountered in illicit lab and drug seizures. Proper personal protective equipment (PPE) will provide protection as you care for opioid-intoxicated patients. Although fentaNYL can be absorbed dermally when prepared appropriately, as in medication patches, simply contacting fentaNYL on your skin will not produce an opioid intoxication or toxidrome.

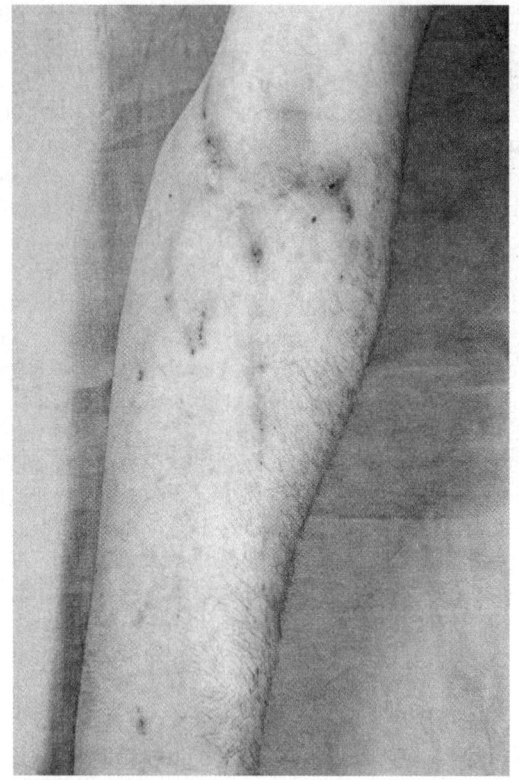

A

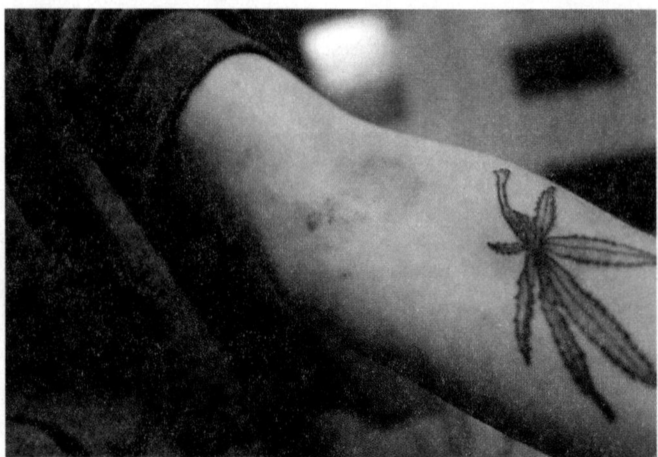

B

Figure 14-3 Injection track marks.

A: © St Mary's Hospital Medical School/Science Source; B: © Spencer Platt/Getty Images

Signs and Symptoms

Signs and symptoms of opioid overdose may include the following:

- Euphoria or irritability
- Diaphoresis
- Miosis (pupil constriction)
- Abdominal cramps
- Nausea and vomiting
- CNS depression
- Respiratory depression
- Hypotension
- Bradycardia or tachycardia
- Pulmonary edema

These signs and symptoms can generally be treated with supportive care. CNS depression, pinpoint pupils, and respiratory depression—the "opioid triad"—are classic signs. Severe intoxication can cause respiratory arrest, seizures, and coma. Opioid intoxication is distinguished from other causes of toxicity by euphoria, pinpoint pupils, and hypotension.

Differential Diagnosis

Any medication with the potential to cause altered mental status should also be considered in the differential diagnosis of possible opioid intoxication.

Differentiation of Agents

A thorough physical exam and patient history are necessary to narrow the possible diagnoses. If possible, it is especially important to determine the type of opiate, the formulation (short- or long-acting), the quantity ingested, the time of ingestion, and whether any other toxins were coingested.

FentaNYL, morphine, methadone, oxyCODONE, HYDROcodone, meperidine, propoxyphene, heroin, codeine, and opium are included in this drug class. Heroin is a bitter-tasting, white or off-white powder that is usually adulterated, or cut, with various substances, including sugar, baking soda, or starch. Recently, fentaNYL and various potent fentaNYL analogs have been found as adulterants in heroin, or even replaced it completely. FentaNYL is also found in illicit HYDROcodone and oxyCODONE tablets. The opioids' depressant effect increases the risk of respiratory failure when an overdose occurs.

Treatment

Opioid overdose treatment consists of supportive care and administration of naloxone. Naloxone is structurally similar to opioids but has only antagonistic properties. Due to its stronger attraction for the mu-opioid receptor, naloxone displaces the opioid molecules from the opiate receptors, reversing the toxic opioid effects. Clinical response to naloxone indicates opioid or similar poisoning. Users sometimes become agitated or violent when their "high" wears off unexpectedly and they are faced with people in uniform. Abrupt opioid withdrawal/reversal may cause seizures, so reserve naloxone for patients experiencing respiratory depression. Although naloxone is the most common opioid reversal medication in the prehospital environment, other agents are available, such as naltrexone and nalmefene (longer-acting versions), but these are not typically used in the prehospital setting.

Supportive care, including management of airway, breathing, and circulation, is of primary importance. Administer naloxone early if significant CNS and respiratory depression are evident, but be cautious when doing so. Start with a low dose according to your local EMS protocol to avoid prompting opioid withdrawal. Respiratory and cardiac monitoring are important, especially for severe intoxication. Patients requiring additional doses of naloxone can receive a continuous naloxone infusion, typically at two-thirds the initial dose required to achieve improved respiratory status given per hour, while appropriately monitored.

Naloxone acts for 45 to 90 minutes, whereas opioids sometimes act for 3 to 6 hours. Thus, although the patient may have a normalized respiratory and mental status immediately after receiving naloxone, it will wear off, and the potentially lethal opioid effects will return. This has implications for protocols involving reversal of opiate-induced intoxication with naloxone and subsequent patient-initiated refusal for transport to a health care facility. However, multiple studies have systematically reviewed these protocols, comparing information with medical examiner reports, and found no deaths related to this practice.

Buprenorphine is a potent opioid, strongly attracted to the mu-opioid receptor, that can displace fentaNYL and heroin but produces only a limited effect on respiratory rate. Because respiratory depression is less likely than with other opioids, buprenorphine and combination medications are currently administered to treat opioid dependency. This is accompanied with referral and counseling to enhance success. A few EMS agencies and mobile integrated health programs initiate this therapy in the field as part of a comprehensive treatment plan. This is typically coordinated with additional treatment resources and follow-up.

Sympathomimetic/Stimulant

Case Presentation: A 24-year-old male presents with agitation, diaphoresis, altered mental status, and tremors. He subsequently has a seizure. He is noted to have the following vital signs: blood pressure 180/100 mm Hg, pulse 120 beats/min, respirations 28 breaths/min, temperature 39.4°C (103°F), and SpO_2 99%.

Pathophysiology

Sympathomimetic toxicity is defined by a toxin-induced excess of catecholamines that leads to overstimulation of the sympathetic nervous system. Various drugs and compounds affect this system in different ways producing the same effect.

Amphetamines are structurally similar to endogenous catecholamines (epinephrine and norepinephrine), acting at presynaptic nerve terminals to promote the release of biogenic amines (norepinephrine, dopamine, and serotonin) and to prevent reuptake from the synaptic cleft. This leads to the clinical manifestations of toxicity as well as to euphoria. Chemical molecular substitutions alter the potency of amphetamines and confer slight alterations in toxicity. For example, methylenedioxymethamphetamine (MDMA) has predominantly serotonergic properties, which are responsible for the drug's characteristic clinical effects.

Cocaine is a strong CNS stimulant, causing robust sympathetic discharge resulting in increased catecholamine release. It also acts as a sodium channel blocker, leading to anesthetic properties and cardiac toxicity. Most fatalities occur from cardiac dysrhythmia.

The following two forms of cocaine are in common use today:

1. Powdered cocaine, a fine white crystalline substance that is cocaine in its pure form. It is typically inhaled, or snorted, through the nose.
2. Freebase ("crack") cocaine, which takes the form of solid white or off-white lumps, crystals, or rocks. Freebase cocaine is much more potent than the powdered form. The rocks of cocaine are heated in a metal or glass pipe, and the fumes are inhaled.

Synthetic cannabinoids and cathinones (bath salts) have mixed effects. These drugs may lead to sympathetic hyperstimulation as well as to hallucinogenic effects, which are discussed later in this chapter.

Signs and Symptoms

Sympathomimetic toxicity results in tachycardia, hypertension, agitation, and tremor. Severe toxicity may cause seizures, intracranial hemorrhage, myocardial infarction, ventricular dysrhythmia, or death. Patients may show a marked increase in strength as well as blunted pain perception. Because of excessive dopamine release, amphetamine toxicity may induce psychosis and involuntary movements.

Cocaine has a wide variety of effects on the body. In addition to the common symptoms of excessive catecholamines, it acts as a local anesthetic by blocking nerve conduction. In the myocardium, it decreases the rate of depolarization and the amplitude of the action potential. By inhibiting the reuptake of norepinephrine and dopamine, cocaine activates the brain's pleasure center. This produces a high that users say makes them feel euphoric and energetic. Because cocaine is a CNS stimulant, people high on cocaine often appear mentally alert and talkative. Unlike opiates, cocaine causes dilated (although sluggish) pupils.

Sympathomimetic vasoconstriction and increased motor activity may cause life-threatening hyperthermia. Because dopamine reuptake is limited, seizures may occur. The risk of stroke is significantly increased. For many reasons, chief among them cardiac stimulation and hypertension, sudden death is common among people who use cocaine, especially on hot days and nights. Be aware that patients with underlying cardiac and vascular conditions (hypertension, prior myocardial infarction/stroke, aneurysms, etc.) are at particularly high risk for complications.

Sympathomimetics may also precipitate hyperactive delirium with severe agitation and serotonin syndrome, which are discussed elsewhere in this chapter. These are life-threatening conditions, which you must be able to recognize.

Differentiation of Agents

Cocaine is derived from the coca plant, which is native to South America. It has been used in its natural form for thousands of years and in medicinal form since the 1800s.

Amphetamines are a diverse class of commonly abused legal and illicit drugs. These medications are commonly used to treat attention deficit hyperactivity disorder (ADHD) and are prescribed to an increasing number of adolescents and adults. Prescription amphetamines include methylphenidate, amphetamine/dextroamphetamine, phentermine, atomoxetine, dexmethylphenidate, and lisdexamfetamine. Amphetamines are used in some cases as diet pills (either by prescription or illicitly). In addition, selegiline, an agent used to treat Parkinson disease, is metabolized to L-methamphetamine.

A wide variety of illicit amphetamines has been produced, including amphetamine, methamphetamine, MDMA ("Ecstasy"), and methcathinone ("cat," "bathtub speed," "m-kat," or "Jeff"). Most users are simply trying to get high, but others take the drugs as physical performance enhancers. Methamphetamine abuse is particularly dangerous because of the drug's astonishing potency. According to the Drug Abuse Warning Network, emergency department visits related to methamphetamine use rose from 102,961 in 2011 to almost 800,000 in 2021. People abuse both prescription and illicit amphetamines in many ways. They can be taken orally, or they can be crushed and then snorted, injected, or smoked if sufficiently pure.

Cathinone is the active compound in khat leaves, which people in Eastern Africa commonly chew for their stimulant effects. The chemical structure of cathinone has been altered to create multiple newer and stronger stimulants such as methylmethcathinone and methylenedioxypyrovalerone (MDPV), the constituents in the abused stimulants referred to as "bath salts." Additionally, newer stimulant hallucinogens with amphetamine properties referred to as 2C, 2C-I, 25I, and 25C-NBOMe compounds based on their chemical structure are commonly called acid or N-bombs and are gaining popularity.

Use of a dangerous synthetic cathinone drug called alpha-pyrrolidinopentiophenone (alpha-PVP), popularly known as "flakka," has surged in Florida and other parts of the country. Alpha-PVP is chemically similar to other synthetic cathinone drugs popularly called "bath salts" and takes the form of a white or pink, foul-smelling crystal that can be eaten, snorted, injected, or vaporized in an e-cigarette or similar device. Vaporizing, which sends the drug quickly into the bloodstream, makes it particularly easy to overdose. The drug has been linked to deaths by suicide as well as heart attack.

Evaluation

Although obtaining a history of the dose or time of ingestion may be helpful, this information probably will not significantly affect your management. Drug identification is the most important component of the patient's history. Knowing the street names of drugs may help you identify them (Table 14-11). Gathering additional information about past medical history of cardiovascular disease, seizure disorder, or stroke also aids in management.

Physical examination often reveals mydriasis and diaphoresis, which result from sympathetic overstimulation. In patients who have taken MDMA, you may observe bruxism (jaw clenching or chewing). MDMA use, especially in the setting of rave parties, has also been associated with hyponatremia, which can manifest as altered mental status or seizures. With any amphetamine overdose, hyperreflexia and excessive motor activity can cause muscle breakdown and rhabdomyolysis, raising the specter of possible myoglobinuric renal failure. Hyperthermia is a late and ominous sign. In fact, of all the vital signs, hyperthermia is the most predictive of significant morbidity and mortality in patients with amphetamine overdose.

Table 14-11 Names of Common Street Drugs

Drug	Street Name (not inclusive)
Amphetamine	Amped, bennie, blue or black mollies, cartwheels, dexies/dexy, eye poppers/eye openers, footballs, jelly beans, lid poppers/lid openers, pep pills, speed, uppers, wake ups
Cocaine	*Powder:* blow, bump, C or big C, coca, coke, crack, dust, flake, line, snow *Crack:* black rock, candy, dice, hail, hard rock, moon rock, nuggets, rock, sleet, snow coke, tornado
Methamphetamine	*Oral or injected form:* crank, speed *Smoked form:* ice, crystal meth
Methcathinone	Cat, khat, Jeff, ephedrine, flakka
Methylenedioxy-methamphet-amine (MDMA)	Ecstasy, E, X, XTC, Molly, Adam, 007, B-bomb, care bear, Deb, go Jerry Garcia, love pill, playboy, wafer, white diamond

Treatment

Supportive care, including support of airway, breathing, and circulation, is the primary treatment for sympathomimetic intoxication. Supplemental oxygen, establishing IV access, cardiac monitoring, and pulse oximetry are usually indicated.

EPINEPHrine should be avoided, if possible, because its cardiovascular effects are similar to those of sympathomimetics. Vasopressin is often a better alternative if pressors are required. Some evidence also indicates nonselective beta blockers should be avoided in these patients, as the unopposed alpha stimulation they lead to can result in worsening hypertension.

Sympathomimetic drug users, especially after consuming large doses, can exhibit erratic or violent behavior. Your safety is of paramount importance. Summon help from law enforcement early, and monitor the patient's body language and behavior carefully.

When able, initiate cardiac monitoring with a 12-lead ECG to look for cardiac ischemia due to coronary vasospasm. Use benzodiazepines as necessary to calm the patient, reduce CNS stimulation, and treat seizures.

Hyperpyrexia that accompanies delirium with agitated behavior must be treated aggressively; treatments for these conditions are discussed at length in the AMLS Assessment Pathway portion of this chapter. Hypoglycemia, cardiac symptoms, and trauma should be treated per standard protocols. Benzodiazepine administration, IV fluid hydration, and rapid aggressive external cooling are the mainstays of treatment in any sympathomimetic toxicity. For all intents and purposes, benzodiazepines may be thought of as the antidote to these drugs.

Withdrawal

Case Presentation: A 40-year-old male presents with agitation, confusion, diaphoresis, and postictal state. He smells of urine and alcohol. He is noted to have the following vital signs: blood pressure 170/100 mm Hg, pulse 130 beats/min, respirations 24 breaths/min, temperature 38.8°C (102°F), SpO_2 92%.

Pathophysiology

Withdrawal may occur as a result of the absence of any number of drugs to which the body has become dependent. Derangement of neurotransmitters (either too little GABA or too little glutamate) leads to over- or understimulation of the nervous system and causes a variety of symptoms. Typically, withdrawal will present as the "opposite" of the specific drug intoxication. Withdrawal ranges from mild to life-threatening depending on the drug(s) involved and on the patient's context.

Signs and Symptoms

Sedative-hypnotic withdrawal is an important syndrome for prehospital clinicians to recognize. Signs and symptoms include tachycardia, hypertension, diaphoresis, tremor, seizure, and delirium. This syndrome is most often seen in patients who are chronically dependent on alcohol or on short- or intermediate-acting benzodiazepines, especially ALPRAZolam. Opioid withdrawal is marked by mydriasis (dilated pupils), GI symptoms (cramping, nausea/vomiting, diarrhea), agitation, diaphoresis, and severe muscle aches. Sympathomimetic withdrawal symptoms may include depression/anxiety, sleep disturbance, and general feelings of malaise.

Differential Diagnosis

One of the challenges in recognizing withdrawal lies in distinguishing it from active intoxication with other drugs. For example, opioid withdrawal symptoms overlap significantly with sympathomimetic toxicity. Knowing key symptoms will allow you to discriminate. Opioid withdrawal may be recognized by GI upset and pain. Sympathomimetic withdrawal is particularly marked by sleep and psychiatric disturbance. However, when in doubt, obtain more history from the patient, friends, and family, as well as by making observations on scene.

With any patient in withdrawal, consider why the patient is no longer taking the drug. In some cases, an underlying medical condition may have caused the patient to be unable to acquire their substance of choice. In such cases, both problems should be managed simultaneously.

Treatment

The general principle of treating withdrawal is to safely and appropriately replace the missing drug. First, always perform the AMLS Assessment Pathway and assess for ABCDE. You may then administer specific medications. Supportive care is indicated as well. This will likely include IV fluids, antiemetics, and analgesia.

Sedative-hypnotic withdrawal is treated primarily with benzodiazepines. PHENObarbital and ketamine are increasingly being used to treat severe alcohol withdrawal. For opioid withdrawal, no specific treatment is indicated in the prehospital setting, although some programs are starting buprenorphine in the field and referring directly to detoxification programs. Manage the patient's symptoms and transport to the hospital, where the patient may then receive cloNIDine and/or buprenorphine. Finally, sympathomimetic withdrawal is rarely life threatening. Usually, supportive care is all that is needed. If the patient has severe symptoms, including bradycardia or hypotension, pressors may rarely be required.

Special Considerations

Individuals who ingest packets of drugs, known commonly as **stuffers**, may experience severe toxicity because of the relatively large amount of drug ingested and because the packaging was not designed to traverse the GI tract. They are often identified early by police, who may see them swallow the packets. Administer activated charcoal to attenuate potential toxicity according to local protocol. Toxic effects do not always develop, but these patients must undergo observation in the emergency department because of the risk of delayed absorption and toxicity. Otherwise, evaluation and treatment remain the same as for any toxic ingestion.

Packers, people who smuggle large amounts of drugs by ingesting them, require admission to the intensive care unit when identified. Although the risk of packaging failure is relatively low, such a large amount of drug is present in the GI tract that its release would unleash a torrent of severe toxicity, GI ischemia, and death regardless of treatment. In fact, surgical removal of drug packages may be indicated after any sign of toxicity in such patients.

Another concern with any illicit drug trafficking, but particularly amphetamine trafficking, is the possibility of drug contamination. Many amphetamines are produced by generating chemical reactions that may in themselves cause injury. For example, outbreaks of lead and mercury toxicity have been traced to methamphetamine contamination. Amphetamines are also used in combination with other drugs, such as cocaine, heroin, fentaNYL, and marijuana, which may alter their toxicity and clinical presentation.

Illicit methamphetamine laboratories pose a particular danger to EMS clinicians. The chemicals used to manufacture methamphetamine are extremely volatile, and toxic gases such as phosphine can be generated as a by-product of methamphetamine production. Exposure to such chemicals can cause mucous membrane irritation, headaches, burns, and death. Of even greater concern is the risk of detonation of improvised explosive devices (IEDs). Methamphetamine manufacturers often place IED booby traps in and around their makeshift labs to deter thieves and law enforcement personnel from entering. Never enter such a facility without law enforcement support. If you inadvertently enter a meth lab, exit immediately using the same route by which you entered. If you should come upon a patient while exiting, remove the patient as quickly as possible.

Medications and Drugs of Abuse as Toxins

A number of prescription medications and over-the-counter (OTC) products can have toxic effects if used improperly, especially by vulnerable individuals such as the very young (see **Rapid Recall Box 14-4**), the older patient, and those with reduced drug clearance due to renal or liver impairment (Table 14-12).

Acetaminophen

Acetaminophen (N-acetyl-p-aminophenol [APAP]) is a commonly used OTC antipyretic and analgesic. The drug's benign safety profile at therapeutic doses has led to its inclusion in a variety of combination medications, including prescription and OTC pain relievers, cough and cold preparations, and allergy medications. You may recognize some of these medications by brand name, along with prescription medications, such as oxyCODONE with acetaminophen and HYDROcodone with acetaminophen, though this is not an exhaustive list. The drug is widely available and easy to obtain.

Although acetaminophen is safe at therapeutic levels, overdose ingestions carry significant risk and are one of the most common intentional and unintentional overdoses in the United States. The primary threat is hepatotoxicity/liver injury. In fact, acetaminophen-related liver injury is the leading cause of acute liver failure in the United States, making it a far more common cause of liver failure than acute viral hepatitis. Questions about possible acetaminophen toxicity, alone or in combination with other agents, accounted for approximately 111,926 calls to poison control centers in 2020.

Pathophysiology

Acetaminophen is metabolized through several pathways, and most of its metabolites are nontoxic. However, after supratherapeutic dosing, the major metabolic pathways become saturated, causing secondary metabolic pathways to predominate, resulting in excessive formation of the toxic metabolite N-acetyl-p-benzoquinone imine (NAPQI). Glutathione, a substrate utilized in the further metabolism of NAPQI to a nontoxic form, is a very important substrate in overdose. When insufficient glutathione is present, NAPQI causes a series of reactions that lead to cell death. The primary treatment for overdose involves increasing glutathione stores, as will be discussed later in this chapter. Cytochrome P450 enzyme systems seen in hepatic and renal cells are primarily affected, resulting in hepatic centrilobular necrosis and renal proximal tubular necrosis, or in general terms, cellular death of the liver and kidney, leading to possible organ failure. This failure can increase the risk for bleeding, fluid retention, and hepatic encephalopathy (confusion due to buildup of toxins that the liver typically metabolizes), among many other clinical problems.

Signs and Symptoms

The clinical presentation of APAP toxicity can vary significantly, depending on the dose and timing of ingestion. Single doses of over 150 mg/kg are considered toxic, but dosage history in overdose scenarios is notoriously unreliable, and the dosage threshold fails to account for unintentional repeated supratherapeutic ingestions. In a 70-kg (154-lb) person, ingestion of 10.5 g (70 kg × 150 mg/kg = 10.5 g) of acetaminophen, roughly equivalent to 21 extra-strength tablets (500 mg each), may be enough to cause toxicity. The ingestion time is also critical, both for evaluation of symptoms and interpretation of serum acetaminophen levels. Clinical manifestations can be loosely divided into stages based on the amount of time since a single toxic ingestion, as follows:

- *Stage I (< 24 hours).* Symptoms are nonspecific and may include nausea, vomiting, and malaise. In massive overdose, patients may have an altered level of consciousness and acidosis. It is also quite common for patients to have very mild or no symptoms whatsoever in this time frame, even after toxic ingestions.
- *Stage II (24 to 36 hours).* This stage is marked by the onset of hepatic injury, which is characterized by abdominal pain, worsening nausea and vomiting, and elevated liver enzymes and coagulation studies.
- *Stage III (48 to 96 hours).* Peak liver injury, perhaps progressing to fulminant hepatic failure, occurs during this period. Liver enzyme tests typically become significantly elevated, but of greater clinical relevance are the patient's coagulation studies, mental status, acidosis, and renal function. A systemic inflammatory response syndrome resembling septic shock can occur. Death may occur in this stage due to multiorgan failure, acute respiratory distress syndrome, sepsis, or cerebral edema.
- *Stage IV (> 96 hours).* If the patient survives, the liver regenerates quickly and is unlikely to evidence any chronic damage.

Nephrotoxicity (kidney damage) may occur with or without liver injury. Renal failure requiring hemodialysis generally occurs only in patients who have also suffered significant hepatotoxicity (liver damage), but otherwise, renal injury improves commonly to preingestion baseline with IV fluids and time. Long-term renal dysfunction is not an expected sequela of acute APAP toxicity.

Another variable confounding the clinical picture is the presence of a coingestion. APAP is often combined

Table 14-12 Toxic Effects of Drugs and Other Toxins

Drug or Toxin	Clinical Presentation of Intoxication	Specific Collaborative Management
Acetaminophen	*Mild/early stage* ▪ May be asymptomatic ▪ Anorexia, nausea, vomiting ▪ Pallor *12 hours to 4 days later* ▪ Signs of hepatotoxicity may occur: liver enzymes, bilirubin, prothrombin time increased; right upper quadrant pain. ▪ Gradual return to normal may occur. *Late: indications of hepatic failure* ▪ Anorexia, nausea, vomiting ▪ Jaundice ▪ Hepatosplenomegaly ▪ Clinical indications of hepatic encephalopathy: confusion to coma ▪ Bleeding ▪ Hypoglycemia ▪ Acute renal failure may develop. ▪ Dysrhythmias and shock may occur.	Consider single-dose activated charcoal up to 4 hours after a potentially liver-toxic amount of acetaminophen is ingested. N-Acetylcysteine (NAC) effectively decreases hepatotoxicity if administered within 8 hours of ingestion. One regimen is three-bag NAC: IV NAC (Acetadote) 150 mg/kg loading dose over 1 hour, then 50 mg/kg over 4 hours, then 100 mg/kg over 16 hours (21 hours and 300 mg/kg total). A 16-hour bag should be repeated until end points of therapy are met. Oral NAC 140 mg/kg initially, then 70 mg/kg every 4 hours × 17 doses to total of 1,330 mg/kg, or tailored to the patient's case. ▪ If given PO, dilute in juice or carbonated beverage. May cause anorexia, nausea, vomiting; repeat dose if vomiting occurs within 1 hour. Dextrose (e.g., 10%) may be needed. Antidysrhythmics may be needed.
Amphetamines	Hypertension Tachycardia Tachypnea Dysrhythmias Hyperthermia, diaphoresis Dilated but reactive pupils Dry mouth Urinary retention Headache Paranoid-type psychotic behavior Hallucinations Hyperactivity, anxiety Hyperactive deep tendon reflexes, tremor, seizures Confusion, stupor, coma	Calm, quiet environment Avoid overstimulation of patient. Do not speak loudly or move quickly. Do not approach from behind. Avoid touching the patient unless you speak to the patient first or are sure it is safe. DiazePAM, LORazepam, or midazolam for agitation Anticonvulsants (e.g., diazePAM, midazolam, PHENObarbital) for seizures Antidysrhythmics (e.g., lidocaine) for ventricular dysrhythmias Haloperidol, droPERidol, or risperidone for acute psychotic reactions Hypothermia blanket, ice packs, ice water sponge baths for hyperthermia

Drug or Toxin	Clinical Presentation of Intoxication	Specific Collaborative Management
Barbiturates, sedatives, hypnotics, anxiolytics	Bradycardia, cardiac dysrhythmias Hypotension Hypothermia Respiratory depression to respiratory arrest Headache Nystagmus, disconjugate eye movements Dysarthria Ataxia Depressed deep tendon reflexes Confusion, stupor, coma Hemorrhagic blisters Gastric irritation (chloral hydrate) Pulmonary edema (meprobamate)	PHENObarbital: sodium bicarbonate to alkalinize the urine and increase rate of barbiturate excretion; multidose activated charcoal; hemodialysis (in hospital) Monitor electrolyte levels if point-of-care testing available. Anticonvulsants (e.g., diazePAM, PHENObarbital) for withdrawal seizures Hemodialysis or hemoperfusion may be required.
Benzodiazepines	Hypotension Loss of airway protective reflexes (but will not depress respiratory drive) Decreased deep tendon reflexes Confusion, drowsiness, stupor, coma	Flumazenil, a benzodiazepine receptor antagonist, may be given in extremely rare cases (e.g., pediatric or iatrogenic exposure). Otherwise, its use is contraindicated. Monitor for seizures, agitation, flushing, nausea, and vomiting as side effects of flumazenil. Intubation and mechanical ventilation may be necessary.
Beta blockers	Sinus bradycardia, arrest, block Junctional escape rhythm, AV nodal block Bundle branch block (usually right) Hypotension Heart failure Cardiogenic shock Cardiac arrest Decreased level of consciousness Seizures Bronchospasm Possible hypoglycemia	May consider activated charcoal within 1 hour of ingestion Glucagon 5–10 mg IV, IM, or SQ, followed by infusion of 5 mg/hr EPINEPHrine, DOPamine, or atropine for bradycardia and hypotension; temporary pacing may be required. Dextrose (e.g., 10%) for hypoglycemia Anticonvulsants (e.g., diazePAM, PHENObarbital) for seizures; phenytoin is contraindicated.
Calcium channel blockers	Sinus bradycardia, arrest, block SA blocks (dilTIAZem) AV blocks (verapamil) Hypotension Heart failure Confusion, dizziness Seizures Nausea, vomiting	Activated charcoal within 1 hour of ingestion may be considered Calcium chloride 10 mL of 10% solution (1 g) or calcium gluconate 10% (1–3 g) Vasopressor therapy with EPINEPHrine, norepinephrine, and/or phenylephrine

(continues)

Table 14-12 Toxic Effects of Drugs and Other Toxins (*continued*)

Drug or Toxin	Clinical Presentation of Intoxication	Specific Collaborative Management
	Paralytic ileus Hyperglycemia Metabolic acidosis	Hyperinsulinemia-euglycemia therapy Glucagon 5–10 mg IV, IM, or SQ, followed by infusion of 5 mg/hr Anticonvulsants (e.g., diazePAM, PHENObarbital) for seizures Atropine, temporary external cardiac pacing for symptomatic bradycardia
Carbon monoxide (CO) Note: The affinity between carbon monoxide and hemoglobin is approximately 200 times greater than the affinity between oxygen and hemoglobin.	10% to 20%: mild headache, dyspnea or angina on vigorous exertion, nausea, dizziness 20% to 30%: throbbing headache, nausea, vomiting, weakness, dyspnea on moderate exertion, difficulty concentrating, ST-segment depression 30% to 40%: severe headache, vomiting, visual disturbances, collapse 40% to 50%: tachypnea, tachycardia, chest pain, syncope 50% to 60%: chest pain, respiratory failure, shock, seizures, coma 60% to 70%: respiratory failure, shock, seizure, coma, death Dysrhythmias Impaired hearing or vision Pallor; cherry-red skin coloring may be seen (late)	Remove from contaminated area. Oxygenate: 100% oxygen via mask initially; CPAP by mask as needed. Note: Remember that pulse oximetry is inaccurate in setting of CO poisoning. Provide high-concentration oxygen even if pulse oximetry is 100%. Intubation and mechanical ventilation if patient is unresponsive; PEEP as needed Fluids, diuretics, urine alkalinization to treat myoglobinuria if present Anticonvulsants (e.g., diazePAM or other benzodiazepine, PHENObarbital) Hyperbaric oxygen (at 2–3 atmospheres) as soon as available if: ▪ COHb > 25% (relative indication) ▪ CO-induced acute ECG changes or persistent CNS symptoms (altered mental status, coma) ▪ Pregnant with COHb > 15%
Caustic poisoning Acids (e.g., battery acid, drain cleaners, hydrochloric acid) Alkalis (e.g., drain cleaners, refrigerants, fertilizers, photographic developers)	Burning sensation in the oral cavity, pharynx, esophageal area Dysphagia Respiratory distress: dyspnea, stridor, tachypnea, hoarseness Soapy-white mucous membrane Acid: ▪ Oral ulcerations and/or blisters ▪ May have signs of shock Alkali: ▪ May have signs of esophageal perforation (e.g., chest pain, subcutaneous emphysema)	Dilute: flush mouth with copious volumes of water; drink water or milk (approximately 250 mL). Do not induce vomiting or perform gastric lavage. Do not give agents to neutralize acid or alkali (may produce exothermic reaction).

Drug or Toxin	Clinical Presentation of Intoxication	Specific Collaborative Management
Cocaine	Tachycardia, dysrhythmias Hypertension or hypotension (late) Tachypnea or hyperpnea Hyperthermia, diaphoresis Hyperexcitability, anxiety Cocaine-induced MI Pallor or cyanosis Headache Nausea, vomiting, abdominal pain Dilated but reactive pupils Confusion, delirium, hallucinations Seizures Coma Respiratory arrest	Swabbing of inside of nose to remove any residual drug if cocaine was snorted Single-dose activated charcoal for body stuffers (per local protocol) Bowel irrigation in hospital for body packers Anticonvulsants (e.g., diazePAM, PHENObarbital) for seizures Antidysrhythmics, usually lidocaine; calcium channel blockers (for coronary artery spasm) Antihypertensives: alpha blockers (e.g., phentolamine) or vasodilators (e.g., nitroprusside) Rapid cooling to include ice water immersion, hypothermia blanket, ice packs, ice water sponge baths for hyperthermia Fluids, diuretics, possibly urine alkalinization to treat myoglobinuria if present
Cyanide	Anxiety, restlessness, dyspnea, hyperventilation initially Tachycardia followed by bradycardia Hypotension Dysrhythmias Bitter almond odor to breath Cherry-red mucous membranes Nausea Headache Dizziness Pupil dilation Confusion Stupor, seizures, coma, death	100% oxygen initially by mask Intubation and mechanical ventilation are frequently necessary. Supportive care if only signs/symptoms are anxiety, restlessness, hyperventilation Discontinuance of causative agent (e.g., nitroprusside) Antidotes for more serious symptoms Hydroxocobalamin IV. If not available, consider amyl nitrite by inhalation, sodium nitrite IV, sodium thiosulfate IV. Flushing of eyes and/or skin with water if dermal contamination; removal and isolation of clothing Fluids, vasopressors as needed Anticonvulsants (e.g., diazePAM or other benzodiazepine, PHENObarbital) for seizures Antidysrhythmics (e.g., lidocaine) for ventricular dysrhythmia, atropine for bradydysrhythmias

(*continues*)

Table 14-12 Toxic Effects of Drugs and Other Toxins (*continued*)

Drug or Toxin	Clinical Presentation of Intoxication	Specific Collaborative Management
Digitalis preparations	Anorexia Nausea Vomiting Abdominal pain Headache Restlessness Visual changes Sinus bradycardia, block, or arrest PAT with AV block Junctional tachycardia AV blocks: first, second type I, third PVCs: bigeminy, trigeminy, quadrigeminy Ventricular tachycardia: especially bidirectional Ventricular fibrillation	Activated charcoal if less than 1 hour from ingestion Correction of hypoxia, electrolyte imbalance (hyperkalemia) Digoxin immune Fab (DigiFab) if hypoperfusion or life-threatening dysrhythmia. Indications include $>$ 10 mg ingested (adult), serum digoxin $>$ 10 ng/mL (6 hours post ingestion) or serum potassium $>$ 5.0 mEq/L. Monitor closely for exacerbation of underlying condition (e.g., increase in heart rate, worsened heart failure). Treatment of dysrhythmias: For symptomatic bradydysrhythmias and blocks: ▪ Atropine ▪ External pacemaker For symptomatic tachydysrhythmias: ▪ Lidocaine ▪ Phenytoin Magnesium if hypomagnesemia or hyperkalemia present Cardioversion at lowest effective voltage and only if life-threatening dysrhythmias exist Defibrillation for ventricular fibrillation
Ethanol	Ethanol concentration (mg/dL) ▪ $<$ 25: sense of warmth and well-being, talkativeness, self-confidence, mild incoordination ▪ 25–50: euphoria, decreased judgment and control ▪ 50–100: decreased sensorium, worsened coordination, ataxia, decreased reflexes and slowed reaction time ▪ 100–250: nausea, vomiting, ataxia, diplopia, slurred speech, visual impairment, nystagmus, emotional lability, confusion, stupor ▪ 250–400: stupor or coma, incontinence, respiratory depression ▪ $>$ 400: respiratory paralysis, loss of protective reflexes, hypothermia, death	Fluid and electrolyte replacement (potassium, magnesium, calcium may be needed) Note: Thiamine is necessary for the brain to utilize glucose; thiamine deficiency in patients with alcoholism may cause Wernicke encephalopathy. This is a very rare event and typically does not need to be addressed in the prehospital care of patients. Anticonvulsants (e.g., diazePAM or other benzodiazepine, PHENObarbital) for seizures

Drug or Toxin	Clinical Presentation of Intoxication	Specific Collaborative Management
	Note: These signs/symptoms and blood ethanol levels vary widely; these signs/symptoms are for a non-alcohol-dependent person Also: ▪ Alcohol odor to breath ▪ Hypoglycemia ▪ Seizures ▪ Metabolic acidosis	
Ethylene glycol	*First 12 hours after ingestion* ▪ Appears drunk without the odor of ethanol on breath ▪ Nausea, vomiting ▪ Focal seizures, coma ▪ Nystagmus, depressed reflexes, tetany ▪ Early: High osmolar gap, metabolic acidosis; later: Low osmolar gap; metabolic acidosis *12–24 hours after ingestion* ▪ Tachycardia ▪ Mild hypertension ▪ Pulmonary edema Heart failure 24–72 hours after ingestion Acute renal failure	Fomepizole 10% ethanol in D_5W IV to maintain serum ethanol level at 100–200 mg/dL Sodium bicarbonate for severe metabolic acidosis Hemodialysis Note: Thiamine is necessary for the brain to utilize glucose; thiamine deficiency in patients with alcoholism may cause Wernicke encephalopathy. This is a very rare event and typically does not need to be addressed in the prehospital care of patients. Anticonvulsants (e.g., diazePAM, or other benzodiazepine, PHENObarbital) for seizures
Hallucinogens (e.g., d-lysergic acid diethylamide [LSD])	Tachycardia, hypertension Hyperthermia Anorexia, nausea Headaches Dilated pupils Rambling speech Polyuria Dizziness Agitation, anxiety Impaired judgment Distortion and intensification of sensory perception Toxic psychosis	Reassurance Quiet environment with soft lighting Benzodiazepines (e.g., diazePAM, LORazepam, midazolam) for anxiety and agitation Anticonvulsants (e.g., diazePAM, PHENObarbital) for seizures
Isopropyl alcohol	GI distress (e.g., nausea, vomiting, abdominal pain) Hemorrhagic gastritis Headache CNS depression, areflexia, ataxia Respiratory depression Hypothermia, hypotension	Fluids and vasopressors for hypoperfusion Hemodialysis

(continues)

Table 14-12 Toxic Effects of Drugs and Other Toxins (*continued*)

Drug or Toxin	Clinical Presentation of Intoxication	Specific Collaborative Management
Lithium	*Mild* ▪ Vomiting, diarrhea ▪ Lethargy, weakness ▪ Polyuria, polydipsia ▪ Nystagmus ▪ Fine tremors *Severe* ▪ Hypotension, heart failure ▪ Severe thirst, dilute urine, renal failure ▪ Tinnitus ▪ Hyperreflexia, coarse tremors, ataxia, seizures ▪ Confusion, coma	Hydration Free water replacement to maintain sodium concentration Anticonvulsants (e.g., diazePAM, or other benzodiazepine, PHENObarbital) for seizures, which are rare Hemodialysis may uncommonly be necessary.
Methanol	Nausea and vomiting Hyperpnea, dyspnea Headache Visual disturbances (blurring to blindness) Speech difficulty CNS depression Motor dysfunction with rigidity, spasticity, and hypokinesis Metabolic acidosis	Gastric lavage (especially helpful if shortly after ingestion) Fomepizole 15 mg/kg IV loading dose followed by maintenance dosing is preferred to ethanol where available. 10% ethanol in D_5W IV to maintain serum ethanol level at 100–200 mg/dL. Sodium bicarbonate for severe metabolic acidosis Hemodialysis if visual impairment, metabolic acidosis, renal insufficiency, or blood methanol concentration > 30 mmol/L
Methemoglobinemia (caused by nitrites, nitrates, sulfa drugs, and others)	Tachycardia Fatigue Nausea Dizziness Cyanosis in the presence of a normal PaO_2; failure of cyanosis to resolve with oxygen therapy Dark red or brown blood Elevated methemoglobin levels Headache, weakness, dyspnea (30% to 40%) Stupor, respiratory depression (60%)	Oxygen Remove from exposure. Stop nitroglycerin, nitroprusside, sulfa drugs, anesthetic agents, or other causative agent. Methylene blue If stupor, coma, angina, or respiratory depression or if level 30% to 40% or more: administer methylene blue at 2 mg/kg over 5 min; repeated at 1 mg/kg if patient still symptomatic after 30–60 min. Exchange transfusion if methylene blue is contraindicated.
Opioids and opiates	Respiratory depression to respiratory arrest Bradycardia Hypotension Decreased level of consciousness Hypothermia	Bowel irrigation for body packers Naloxone (Narcan) 0.4–2 mg IV, IM, IO, IN, or transtracheal, or nalmefene 0.5 mg IV Naloxone lasts 45–60 minutes, whereas nalmefene lasts 4–8 hours (heroin and morphine last 4–6 hours).

Drug or Toxin	Clinical Presentation of Intoxication	Specific Collaborative Management
	Miosis Diminished bowel sounds Needle tracks, abscesses Seizures Pulmonary edema (especially with heroin)	Anticonvulsants (e.g., diazePAM, or other benzodiazepine, PHENObarbital) for seizures Intubation and mechanical ventilation may be required; PEEP may be needed for pulmonary edema.
Organophosphates and carbamates (cholinesterase inhibitors)	Nausea, vomiting, diarrhea Abdominal pain and cramping Increased secretions (GI, GU, pulmonary, integumentary) Urinary incontinence Bradycardia Bronchospasm, dyspnea Slurred speech Constricted pupils, visual changes Unsteady gait, poor motor control, twitching Change in level of consciousness Seizures	Consider gastric lavage, if ingested (according to local protocol). Remove and isolate clothing. Wash skin with soap and water. Atropine 1–5 mg IV or IM; repeat as required every 3–5 min. Pralidoxime chloride (2-PAM) 1–2 g IV over 15–30 min followed by infusion of 10 mg/kg/hr for organophosphates Anticonvulsants (e.g., diazePAM or other benzodiazepine, PHENObarbital) for seizures
Petroleum distillates	Tachypnea, dyspnea, coughing, cyanosis Breath sound changes: crackles, rhonchi, diminished breath sounds Hyperthermia Flushed skin Vomiting, diarrhea, abdominal pain Staggering gait Confusion, CNS depression or excitation	Wash skin with soap and water; remove and isolate clothing. Oxygen, bronchodilators, mechanical ventilation as required Potassium supplementation for toluene-associated hypokalemia Consider beta blockade for ventricular dysrhythmias presumed secondary to halogenated hydrocarbon toxicity
Phencyclidine (PCP)	Tachycardia Hypertensive crisis Hyperthermia Agitation, hyperactivity, violent, psychotic behavior Nystagmus, blank stare Hypoglycemia Ataxia Myoglobinuria, renal failure Seizures Lethargy, coma Cardiac arrest	Quiet environment Benzodiazepines (e.g., diazePAM) for anxiety and agitation Beta blockers for dysrhythmias Antihypertensives: vasodilators (e.g., nitroprusside) Hypothermia blanket, ice packs, ice water sponge baths for hyperthermia Anticonvulsants (e.g., diazePAM, PHENObarbital) for seizures Haloperidol/droPERidol for acute psychotic reactions Fluids and diuretics for myoglobinuria; urinary alkalinization interferes with urinary elimination of PCP, therefore sodium bicarbonate is contraindicated.

(*continues*)

Table 14-12 Toxic Effects of Drugs and Other Toxins (*continued*)

Drug or Toxin	Clinical Presentation of Intoxication	Specific Collaborative Management
Salicylates	*Early* ■ Hyperthermia ■ Hyperventilation (respiratory alkalosis) ■ Nausea, vomiting ■ Diaphoresis ■ Tinnitus ■ Thirst *Late* ■ Metabolic acidosis ■ Motor weakness ■ Vasodilation and hypotension ■ Respiratory depression to respiratory arrest ■ Respiratory acidosis ■ Altered mental status, seizure, coma ■ Death	Multidose activated charcoal (according to local protocol) Fluids with dextrose (e.g., D_5W) Hypothermia blanket, ice packs, ice water sponge baths for hyperthermia Sodium bicarbonate to alkalinize the serum/urine to prevent tissue distribution and to increase salicylate excretion rate Add potassium to bicarbonate infusion. Monitor electrolyte levels if point of care testing available. Anticonvulsants (e.g., diazePAM or other benzodiazepine, PHENObarbital) for seizures Hemodialysis may be necessary.
Cyclic antidepressants	*Antimuscarinic (anticholinergic)* ■ Tachycardia, palpitations ■ Hyperthermia ■ Flushed, dry skin ■ Dry mouth ■ Mydriasis ■ Hallucinations, restlessness, euphoria ■ Decreased bowel sounds ■ Urinary retention ■ Dysrhythmias ■ Headache ■ Decreased DTR ■ Seizures, coma *Anti-alpha adrenergic* ■ Hypotension ■ AV and bundle branch blocks ■ QT prolongation and quinidine-like dysrhythmias (including torsades de pointes)	Consider activated charcoal if within 1 hour post ingestion and patient is oriented and willing. Sodium bicarbonate to reduce tissue distribution and toxicity Monitor electrolyte levels if point-of-care testing available. Hyperventilation may be used to augment alkalosis. Avoid physostigmine due to risk of seizure in TCA toxicity. Sodium bicarbonate +/− hypertonic saline should be given for QRS prolongation (QRS > 110 ms) and ventricular dysrhythmias. Refractory wide complex ventricular dysrhythmia may be treated with lidocaine. Cardioversion, defibrillation, pacemaker as needed for dysrhythmias Magnesium sulfate and overdrive pacing for torsades de pointes Fluids and vasopressors for hypotension Anticonvulsants (e.g., diazePAM or other benzodiazepine, PHENObarbital) for seizures

AV, atrioventricular; CNS, central nervous system; COHb, carboxyhemoglobin; CPAP, continuous positive airway pressure; DTR, deep tendon reflexes; ECG, electrocardiogram; G6PD, glucose-6-phosphate deficiency; GI, gastrointestinal; GU, genitourinary; HIE, hyperinsulinemia euglycemia; IM, intramuscular; IN, intranasal; IO, intraosseous; IV, intravenous; MI, myocardial infarction; NAC, N-acetylcysteine; PaO_2, partial pressure of oxygen; PAT, paroxysmal atrial tachycardia; PEEP, positive end-expiratory pressure; PO, per os; PVCs, premature ventricular contractions; SA, sinoatrial; SQ, subcutaneous; TCA, tricyclic antidepressant.

Modified from Dennison RD. *Pass CCRN®*! 5th ed. Elsevier; 2018.

RAPID RECALL BOX 14-4

One Pill Can Ill or Kill

Young children are curious and frequently place objects in their mouths, putting them at high risk of accidental overdoses/ingestions. In 2020, more than 886,000 unintentional case exposures involving children younger than 6 years of age were reported to U.S. poison centers, accounting for 41.7% of all exposures reported. Despite the high exposure rate, these children accounted for approximately 1.8% of all exposure-related fatalities. Many medications may be dangerous and even lethal in small children (under 10 kg [22 lb]) when ingested. Table 14-13 presents common medications that may be fatal if one or two pills are ingested.

Table 14-13 Agents That May Cause Death in a 10-kg Child if One or Two Pills Are Ingested

Drug Class	Examples	Mechanism of Toxicity	Signs/Symptoms of Toxicity
Antidysrhythmics	Flecainide, quinidine	Sodium channel blockade	Prolonged PR/QRS, QT (Class 1A agents), headache, nausea/vomiting
Antimalarials	Chloroquine, quinine	Sodium channel blockade, direct retinal damage	Prolonged QRS/QT, torsades, hypotension, tinnitus, vision loss, headache, vertigo
Calcium channel blockers	DilTIAZem, verapamil	Myocardial suppression	Bradydysrhythmias, hypotension, HF
Opioids	Codeine, methadone, morphine, HYDROcodone	Respiratory depression	CNS depression, respiratory depression, miosis
Oral sulfonylureas (antihyperglycemics)	Glipizide glyburide	Activates insulin release	Hypoglycemia, irritability, lethargy, seizures, coma
Salicylates	Oil of wintergreen, aspirin	Acidosis, crosses BBB and interferes with cellular metabolism	Mixed respiratory alkalosis/metabolic acidosis, tinnitus, altered mental status, coma, pulmonary edema
Tricyclic antidepressants	Amitriptyline, imipramine	Sodium channel blockade, alpha-1 blockade	Tachycardia, coma, and seizures, then hypotension, bradydysrhythmias, ventricular dysrhythmias
Caution with these medications			
Alpha agonists (1 and 2)	CloNIDine, oxymetazoline, tetrahydrozoline	Mostly centrally acting alpha-2 agonists	Transient hypertension, then CNS depression, coma, bradycardia, hypotension
Liquid nicotine	e-Cigarette vaping solution	Nicotinic acetylcholine receptor (AChR) agonism at low doses; muscarinic AChR agonism at high doses	Biphasic pattern: vomiting, tachycardia, hypertension, then autonomic ganglionic blockade, bradycardia, hypotension, coma

BBB, blood-brain barrier; HF, heart failure; CNS, central nervous system.

Reproduced from Koren G, Nachmani A. Drugs that can kill a toddler with one tablet or teaspoonful: A 2018 updated list. *Clin Drug Investig*. 2019;39(2):217-220. doi:10.1007/s40261-018-0726-1; Bar-Oz B, Levichek Z, Koren G. Medications that can be fatal for a toddler with one tablet or teaspoonful: A 2004 update. *Pediatr Drugs*. 2004;6(2):123-126. doi:10.2165/00148581-200406020-00005 with anticholinergic and opioid medications (e.g., HYDROcodone). The toxicity of the other drug may obscure signs of acetaminophen-induced toxicity. Moreover, in an overdose scenario, acetaminophen ingestion must always be considered and specifically queried because of its wide availability and the relative absence of early symptoms. In cases of unintentional overdose, the patient may have taken repeated supratherapeutic doses to relieve unremitting pain (most commonly dental pain, headache, or abdominal pain). Additionally, patients may have unknowingly taken an acetaminophen-containing medication along with regular acetaminophen to treat pain, resulting in unintentional overdose. Obtaining a thorough, accurate history is vitally important in preventing advanced hepatotoxicity.

Differential Diagnosis

The differential diagnosis for acetaminophen toxicity includes hepatitis, liver failure, acute kidney injury, renal failure, coagulopathy, and hepatic encephalopathy. Given the common nature of including acetaminophen in many varied medication formulations, consider other toxicologic problems; for example, if a patient overdoses on oxyCODONE with acetaminophen, also consider possible opiate/opioid overdose, which would manifest as pinpoint pupils, stupor, respiratory depression, and abdominal pain.

Treatment

Treatment decisions center primarily on the time of ingestion and obtaining a thorough, accurate history, including coingestion, past medical history, vital signs, and patient mentation. The primary treatment is N-acetylcysteine, also known as NAC, in order to encourage the metabolism of acetaminophen into nontoxic compounds. Always provide supportive measures as well.

Prehospital Setting

Offer intensive supportive care, including airway management as needed based on mental and respiratory status. Provide IV fluid resuscitation and activated charcoal if the patient is cooperative. An IV antiemetic, such as ondansetron, may help with symptomatic management.

In-Hospital Setting

On arrival to the emergency department, diagnostic tests include an acetaminophen level 4 hours after the reported/believed time of ingestion; liver function tests; coagulation studies (international normalized ratio [INR]/activated partial thromboplastin time [aPTT]); and electrolytes, blood urea nitrogen, and creatinine. For severe toxicity, obtain an arterial or venous blood gas with lactic acid levels, as metabolic acidosis reliably predicts morbidity and mortality.

Interpretation of serum acetaminophen levels hinges on the ingestion time. The Rumack-Matthew nomogram, also known as the acetaminophen nomogram, can be used to predict which patients are likely to develop serious hepatic injury, defined as an aspartate aminotransferase (AST) level > 1,000 IU/L (**Figure 14-4**). The nomogram has an established treatment line that stretches from 150 μg/mL at 4 hours to about 5 μg/mL at 24 hours. Based on time since ingestion and serum level, you can plot an individual patient's data on the graph to evaluate the risk of toxicity. If the patient's mark is on or above the line, treat with NAC; if it falls below this threshold, no NAC is required. The gold standard is to initiate treatment at a 4-hour level above 150 μg/mL. Note, however, that this boundary is valid only for assessment of a single ingestion over a short period. It is not valid for chronic or multiple-dose ingestions—in such cases, more thorough evaluation is required to determine the patient's risk and the appropriate treatment plan. Consult the regional poison center at 1-800-222-1222.

Treatment of acetaminophen toxicity consists of administering either IV or oral NAC. NAC acts in a variety of ways, including the indirect replenishment of glutathione to detoxify NAPQI, while also decreasing inflammation and supporting the metabolism of acetaminophen to nontoxic metabolites. If given within 8 hours of ingestion, before glutathione stores have been depleted, severe hepatic injury can be avoided, preventing the progression of toxicity beyond stage I as described previously; this further emphasizes the importance of knowing the time of ingestion. Notably, regardless of how much time has elapsed, NAC benefits the patient compared with placebo. Continue NAC until one of three end points is reached:

1. Symptomatic and laboratory (AST/alanine transaminase [ALT], INR, creatinine, lactic acidosis) improvement occurs.
2. A liver transplant is performed.
3. The patient dies.

In patients without progression of toxicity, treatment protocols generally unfold over a minimum of 20 hours. Side effects of NAC therapy are generally minor, uncommon, and easily treated. Oral NAC is associated with nausea and vomiting due to its sulfur bond, causing a strong odor of rotten eggs. Intravenous NAC has been associated with anaphylactoid reactions, which are not true allergic reactions, but strongly resemble them. Symptoms generally include rash, pruritus, and occasionally wheezing and upper airway irritation/edema. If these symptoms occur, temporarily stop treatment while the patient is treated with antihistamines (e.g., diphenhydrAMINE, hydroxyzine), bronchodilators (e.g., albuterol), and EPINEPHrine, as necessary. Infusion may then be continued at a slower rate. If symptoms recur, switch to the oral NAC formulation.

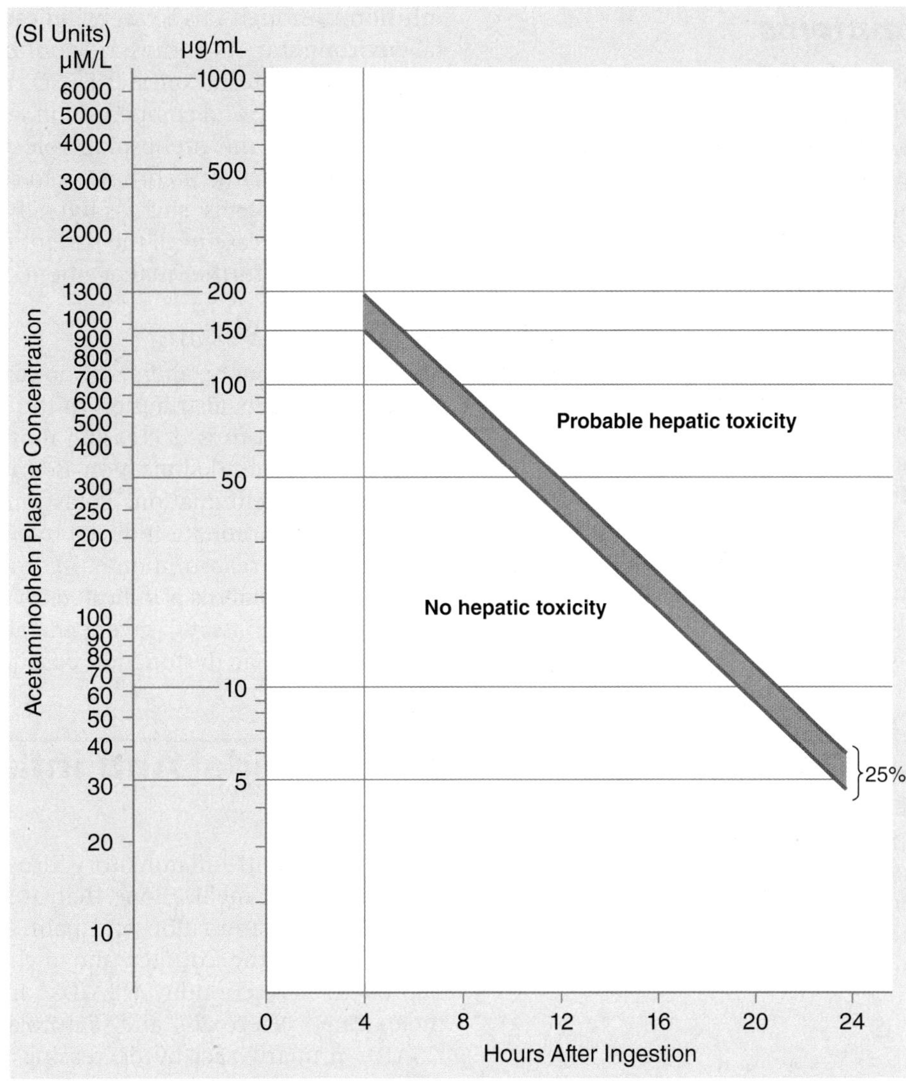

Figure 14-4 Rumack-Matthew nomogram.

Data from Rumack BH, Matthew H. Acetaminophen poisoning and toxicity. *Pediatrics.* 1975;55(6):871-876. doi:10.1542/peds.55.6.871

Pediatric patients are somewhat protected from acetaminophen toxicity compared with adults because they have an increased capacity for nontoxic metabolism of acetaminophen. Diagnosis and treatment of pregnant women does not differ from standard treatment. Patients with chronic alcohol overuse or malnutrition (who probably have decreased glutathione stores) may be at increased risk of hepatotoxicity. Nevertheless, the Rumack-Matthew nomogram and NAC therapy remain the same in these groups of patients, as no evidence exists to support alteration of treatment.

Salicylates

Salicylates, such as aspirin (acetylsalicylic acid), are common OTC analgesics and are involved in many toxicologic emergencies. Salicylate overdose is complicated because other medications are often coingested. Furthermore, patients frequently confuse OTC analgesic classes and mistakenly group them together as aspirin or ibuprofen, when they actually overdosed on acetaminophen, and vice versa.

Pathophysiology

Salicylates act therapeutically by inhibiting prostaglandin synthesis by acetylating cyclooxygenases (COX-1 and COX-2), enzymes that are dominant players in our body's inflammation pathways in the mitochondria, the cells' powerhouses. In larger doses, salicylates uncouple oxidative phosphorylation, which leads to decreased ATP production and the development of metabolic acidosis. Stimulation of the medullary respiratory center also causes a primary respiratory alkalosis from hyperpnea and/or tachypnea, which can make salicylate toxicity confusing due to complex changes to acid–base balance.

Signs and Symptoms

Early symptoms of acute salicylate poisoning include gastric irritation, vomiting, and pain. Symptoms may progress to include tinnitus (ringing ears) or diminished hearing, hyperpnea (deep breathing), tachypnea (rapid breathing), hyperthermia, altered mental status, and seizures. Chronic poisoning can occur with aspirin, because it is an extremely effective analgesic and is now being prescribed at low doses as a daily preventive agent for cardiac care. Symptoms of chronic poisoning, such as gastric irritation and pain, are similar to the early symptoms of acute poisoning, although mental status alteration is more commonly seen at the time of presentation in chronic exposure. Salicylate poisoning should be considered in all undifferentiated altered mental status patients, even those with psychiatric complaints, as this may be the only clue initially to the possibility of a toxic overdose. As a result, emergency department clinicians routinely obtain salicylate levels in all overdose patients to screen for salicylate toxicity.

Differential Diagnosis

Many conditions should be considered in the differential diagnosis when considering salicylate intoxication, including acute respiratory distress syndrome, sepsis and septic shock, pulmonary embolism, other medication intoxications (caffeine, iron, ethylene glycol, theophylline), toxic exposures (chlorine, hydrocarbons/organophosphates), schizophrenia, or multiple withdrawal syndromes.

Treatment

Salicylate poisoning has no direct antidote. The primary treatment is alkalinization of the blood and urine with sodium bicarbonate; doing so increases salicylate excretion in the urine, thus decreasing the actual level of salicylates in the patient's brain and blood.

Prehospital Setting

Give activated charcoal to alert, cooperative patients according to local protocol in the setting of early acute overdose (within 1 hour of ingestion). Administer IV fluids unless the patient is fluid overloaded or has heart or renal failure. Supportive care and airway management are of primary importance. Avoid intubating aspirin overdose patients if possible; it is very difficult for a mechanical ventilator to compensate for the acid–base disturbance the patient may be experiencing compared to the natural ability of the patient to do so. If necessary, match the preintubation respiratory rate to avoid removing the patient's respiratory compensation for the inherent metabolic acidosis. If metabolic acidosis develops, aggressively treat the condition with sodium bicarbonate bolus and infusion, although this is rarely indicated in the prehospital environment. As always, rule out hypoglycemia using a blood glucose test. Consider $ETCO_2$ monitoring to track respiratory drive and compensation.

In general, the prehospital role for salicylate overdose, whether acute or chronic, is to rule out other easily correctable problems, such as hypoglycemia, and to provide supportive care until the patient is in the emergency department for further management.

In-Hospital Setting

Sodium bicarbonate alters the ionized state of salicylate and affects its distribution in the body, limiting CNS penetration and thus decreasing mortality. A secondary benefit of serum alkalinization is urinary alkalinization and enhanced elimination. Potassium supplementation is critical as bicarbonate-induced hypokalemia allows for enhanced renal reabsorption of hydrogen and worsening acidosis. Hemodialysis is indicated for renal failure, rising serum salicylate assays, severe metabolic acidosis, CNS toxicity, or cardiac dysfunction despite maximal alkalinization efforts.

Nonsteroidal Anti-inflammatory Drugs

Nonsteroidal anti-inflammatory drugs (NSAIDs) are a broad group of medications that are primarily utilized to decrease inflammation and pain. Many of these are available over the counter and include ibuprofen and naproxen. Prescription NSAIDs include diclofenac, meloxicam, celecoxib, and ketorolac, among others. NSAIDs primarily act by decreasing prostaglandin production, a substance that mediates inflammation by blocking the COX enzymes. Most NSAIDs are not specific and simply block the actions of both COX-1 (found in the stomach) and COX-2 (found peripherally), though newer versions may exhibit some selectivity for one or the other. The benefit of not blocking COX-1 is that COX-1 produces a protective layer that lines the stomach to reduce the risk of gastric irritation for stomach acid. Thus, COX-1 blockade increases the risk for gastritis and gastric ulcers.

Pathophysiology

NSAIDs are rapidly absorbed in the GI tract with peak serum levels occurring generally within 2 hours of ingestion, although large ingestions may have a delayed peak serum level of 3 to 4 hours. Large ingestions cause excessive COX-1 blockade, which inhibits thromboxane A2 and may lead to decreased platelet aggregation and increased bleeding risk. Adverse effects also include gastric ulcers with risk for perforation, hepatic injury, hemorrhage, acute renal failure with subsequent fluid retention, asthma exacerbation, pneumonitis, hallucinations, delirium, and aseptic meningitis.

At excessively high doses, COX-2 inhibitor NSAIDs may lose their selectivity and inhibit COX-1 as well. Thus, in large overdoses of selective or nonselective NSAIDs, the clinical manifestations are similar.

Signs and Symptoms

The most common symptoms of acute overdose are GI distress, including nausea, vomiting, and epigastric pain, though in severe cases GI hemorrhage may occur. CNS depression may occur and present with changes in cognition, hallucinations, and even seizures. Chronic NSAID use, such as daily ibuprofen for osteoarthritis, headaches, or back pain, may cause gastritis and present as constant, gnawing abdominal pain with possible melena (digested blood in stool) from chronic, irritative bleeding within the stomach.

Differential Diagnosis

History and physical exam may direct your differential diagnosis—in particular, ask patients presenting with epigastric pain if they take ibuprofen or naproxen on a regular basis. For those who present primarily due to a known/reported overdose, knowing the time of ingestion, amount taken, other medical problems, and possible coingestants is important for formulating your differential diagnosis. For example, patients with known chronic gastritis (e.g., from chronic NSAID use or *Helicobacter pylori* infection) who present with sudden, severe worsening of their abdominal pain may have a perforated gastric ulcer causing their stomach acid to leak out of the stomach into the peritoneum. Other GI pathology must also be considered. Overdose patients presenting with altered mental status or seizures should be evaluated for hypoglycemia as well as other problems, such as meningitis, urinary tract infection, other medication overdose, hypothermia, or a primary seizure disorder. Assessment of fluid status in known chronic NSAID use or intentional overdose may reveal fluid overload such as pulmonary crackles, hypoxia on pulse oximetry, or lower extremity edema from NSAID-induced acute kidney injury and fluid retention.

Treatment

The majority of NSAID toxic ingestions require only supportive care with symptomatic management. If there are indications of fluid overload from renal injury, use IV fluids judiciously.

Prehospital Setting

Supportive care is vital; start with the ABCDEs. Massive NSAID overdose may cause coma and require airway intervention. Note that NSAIDs may induce acid–base imbalances primarily through kidney and hepatic injury. Therefore, if intubation is required, attempt to match the patient's own respiratory rate as that is their way to compensate for the acid–base derangement. Give supplemental oxygen if hypoxemic. Apply direct pressure to any external bleeding.

In-Hospital Setting

Management is like that in the prehospital setting, focusing primarily on supportive care as described. It is possible to obtain serum NSAID levels, but this is unnecessary as they do not correlate with clinical presentation. Give activated charcoal per local protocols for a single large ingestion or coingestions within 1 hour of presentation to decontaminate the GI tract. Consider the downstream effects of NSAIDs, such as bleeding, seizures, and cardiovascular toxicity. For example, assess patients with acute or chronic ingestion for clinically relevant gastric ulcers by monitoring for melena, hematemesis, and decreased hemoglobin levels. These findings may indicate rapid GI hemorrhage requiring endoscopy or possible surgical intervention if a perforated ulcer is suspected. Of note, NSAIDs are highly bound to proteins in the bloodstream, so hemodialysis is not useful in removing the NSAIDs from circulation, but it might be used if the patient develops clinically significant renal injury.

Beta Blockers

Beta blockers are frequently prescribed to treat hypertension, coronary artery disease, heart failure, dysrhythmias, migraine headaches, and anxiety disorders. Commonly prescribed beta blockers include metoprolol, carvedilol, propranolol, and atenolol; in general, medications that end in "-lol" are typically beta blockers. Topical ophthalmic preparations, including timolol, may be prescribed for glaucoma. Systemic toxicity has been reported with all types of beta blockers.

Both intentional and unintentional ingestions leading to beta blocker toxicity are frequently reported. In 2020, beta blocker ingestions accounted for 27,836 calls to U.S. poison centers resulting in health care facility visits. Despite this large number of ingestions, only 12 deaths were attributed to single-substance beta blocker exposures in 2020. Nevertheless, beta blocker ingestion is a dangerous condition seen frequently in the prehospital setting.

Pathophysiology

Beta blockers are classified as beta-1 receptor specific (primarily affecting the heart) or nonspecific (blocking both beta-1 and beta-2 receptors). Beta-1–specific drugs include atenolol and metoprolol, whereas propranolol is a nonspecific beta blocker. In general, beta-1 receptor inhibition decreases chronotropy and inotropy, thus decreasing heart rate and ventricular contraction, respectively. Nonspecific beta blockers also block the actions of beta-2 receptors found peripherally on blood vessels and smooth muscles. Normally, beta-2 receptor stimulation causes smooth muscle relaxation and vasodilation, whereas blockade causes the opposite effects—bronchoconstriction and respiratory distress—particularly in patients with asthma or COPD.

Signs and Symptoms

Patients experiencing beta blocker overdose typically present with bradycardia and hypotension. The bradycardia may be a sinus bradycardia or, uncommonly, a first-, second-, or third-degree heart block. Altered mental status may be present, depending on the specific drug ingested, and may result from cerebral hypoperfusion, hypoglycemia, or direct CNS depressive effects of the drug. Notably, lipophilic drugs such as propranolol cross the blood–brain barrier and enter the CNS more easily than nonlipophilic drugs. Seizures occur in some patients, particularly with propranolol toxicity. Patients with CNS depression may present with respiratory depression.

Differential Diagnosis

In patients with suspected beta blocker toxicity, obtain a detailed history of drug exposure, formulation (immediate vs. sustained release), approximate dose, and time of ingestion, as well as possible coingestants. In patients who have ingested prescribed beta blockers, knowing the diagnosis that required the prescription may aid in determining treatment. A history of severe coronary artery disease, heart failure, or dysrhythmia, for example, can affect decisions about the patient's long-term management. Remember to ask about previous pulmonary diseases such as asthma and COPD. Any other medication that can cause bradycardia and hypotension should also be considered in the differential (e.g., calcium channel blockers).

In a patient with suspected beta blocker toxicity, a focused physical examination of the cardiovascular system may reveal a decreased respiratory rate, pulmonary crackles secondary to acute pulmonary edema, or wheezes. Evaluating capillary refill may help estimate tissue perfusion. Beta blocker toxicity can also cause metabolic derangements such as mild hypoglycemia or slightly elevated potassium levels, which may be clinically significant in children. The presence of either mild *hypo*glycemia or *normo*glycemia can help differentiate beta blocker toxicity from calcium channel blocker toxicity (usually *hyper*glycemia), which has an otherwise similar presentation.

Evaluation of patients with suspected beta blocker toxicity focuses on identifying end-organ dysfunction and hypoperfusion. Beyond physical examination as detailed in this chapter, ancillary tests are often performed in the health care facility, including blood gas analysis, ECG, and troponin (cardiac enzymes) to evaluate the degree of toxicity and end-organ dysfunction.

Treatment

Prehospital Setting

After managing the patient's airway and establishing IV access, administer inhaled beta agonists such as albuterol to wheezing patients. Use caution when giving IV fluid boluses in hypotensive patients because the negative inotropic effects of beta blockers can cause pulmonary edema. If the patient remains underperfused, as indicated by altered mental status, decreased capillary refill, or evidence of ischemia, provide pharmacologic support. Atropine is an option for bradycardia associated with hypoperfusion; however, further support is typically required with pressors.

Glucagon is often considered the antidote for beta blocker toxicity; however, it is a vasodilator and might not increase the patient's blood pressure. Human data regarding glucagon efficacy in these situations are limited to case reports and a case series.

If these therapies fail, administer vasopressors, preferably EPINEPHrine. Cardiac pacing is rarely effective in patients in whom pharmacologic therapy has failed.

In-Hospital Setting

Initial emergency department treatment of patients with beta blocker toxicity is the same as prehospital management, including possible vasopressors. EPINEPHrine (adrenalin) infusions can improve cardiac function and peripheral vasopressor effects. Primary vasoconstrictors such as norepinephrine and phenylephrine may be less beneficial because they increase afterload but produce little improvement in cardiac function. This intervention poses a risk of worsening heart failure and pulmonary edema. Regardless of the catecholamine used, very high doses—often higher than the recommended maximum dosage—may be required to have an effect as they typically act on the same beta receptors that are being blocked.

Decreased serum bicarbonate levels and elevated serum urea nitrogen and creatinine are markers of poor tissue perfusion. Accurate measurement of urine output with a Foley catheter often yields the best real-time measurement of perfusion. Close hemodynamic monitoring with arterial lines and possibly central venous pressure monitors may also assist with management.

A newer, preferred, and more effective therapy is high-dose insulin and glucose (hyperinsulinemia-euglycemia [HIE] therapy). A bolus dose of 1 unit/kg of insulin, followed by an infusion of 1–10 units/kg/hr, improves blood pressure, cardiac output, and myocardial blood flow in patients with hypotension from beta blocker toxicity. HIE therapy increases energy production by the poisoned myocardium, improves cardiac contraction, and enhances blood flow in the heart, lungs, and periphery. Monitor serum glucose levels closely while administering the insulin infusion to prevent hypoglycemia.

Although the basic therapeutic concepts in managing beta blocker toxicity can be generalized to all beta blockers, several agents have special properties and thus require customized management strategies. Propranolol, for example, may lead to sodium channel blockade, QRS prolongation, and ventricular dysrhythmias. (Sodium channel blockade is discussed later in more detail in the Cyclic Antidepressants section.) In addition to standard therapy, sodium bicarbonate administration may be required to treat propranolol toxicity. In addition, propranolol causes more significant CNS toxicity than other beta blockers and may cause seizures. Benzodiazepines are the first-line treatment for propranolol-induced seizures.

Calcium Channel Blockers

Calcium channel blockers are another common class of medications for cardiac pathologies and present similarly to beta blocker overdose. In 2020, there were 15,987 calls to U.S. poison centers for calcium channel blocker overdose. The three commonly prescribed classes of calcium channel blockers in the United States are:

1. Phenylalkylamines (e.g., verapamil)
2. Benzothiazepines (e.g., dilTIAZem)
3. Dihydropyridines (e.g., amLODIPine and felodipine)

Verapamil and dilTIAZem are often referred to as nondihydropyridines because their characteristic cardiovascular activity differs from that of dihydropyridines and they primarily affect the heart's contractile function.

Pathophysiology

Calcium channels are found on cardiac cells, vascular smooth muscle, and pancreatic beta islet cells. Calcium channel opening enhances myocardial contractility, vascular smooth muscle constriction, and pancreatic insulin release. Following that logic, calcium channel blockade may decrease chronotropy (heart rate) and inotropy (myocardial contraction strength), while causing vasodilation (hypotension) and hyperglycemia (due to decreased insulin). Dihydropyridine calcium channel blockers act preferentially on peripheral vascular calcium channels and decrease peripheral vascular resistance, resulting in hypotension with a reflex tachycardia at toxic doses.

Signs and Symptoms

Signs and symptoms of calcium channel blocker–induced toxicity may include chest pain, shortness of breath, light-headedness, syncope, hypotension, and bradycardia or tachycardia, depending on the class of calcium channel blocker ingested. First-, second-, or third-degree heart block may also be present. As discussed in the previous section, hyperglycemia typically accompanies calcium channel blocker toxicity, differentiating it from beta blocker toxicity.

Differential Diagnosis

The history obtained and physical examination performed after calcium channel blocker ingestion are like that of beta blocker ingestion, including a detailed medical history, particularly regarding cardiovascular disease, and a detailed history of dose, type and formulation, time of ingestion, and possible coingestions. Similar agents such as beta blocker intoxication must be considered in the differential diagnosis.

Acute pulmonary edema may cause bilateral crackles on auscultation and a decreased pulse oximetry measurement on room air. Calcium channel blockers generally do not affect mental status unless cerebral hypoperfusion from the cardiovascular effects occurs. Capillary refill examination, as in beta blocker toxicity, provides a clue to perfusion status. Obtain an ECG to evaluate for rhythm abnormalities and evidence of ischemia. Patients who are found unresponsive or are known to have been immobile for prolonged periods are evaluated for rhabdomyolysis by serum creatine phosphokinase studies and muscle compartment examination.

Treatment

Prehospital Setting

As with beta blocker poisoning, initial management of calcium channel blocker toxicity centers on controlling the patient's airway and breathing. You may administer IV boluses of normal saline for hypotension; however, the same concern as beta blockers for inducing pulmonary edema exists. Administer atropine in patients with symptomatic bradycardia, but note that it is often ineffective or only transiently effective in these cases. IV glucagon at doses like those studied in beta blocker toxicity has been used but with less consistent effects. Administering IV calcium gluconate poses little risk to the patient and may be beneficial, especially when given in doses of several grams. Calcium chloride contains more than three times as much elemental calcium as calcium gluconate, but it may provoke more peripheral venous irritation and other adverse effects. Therefore, calcium chloride must be given through a central venous line.

In-Hospital Setting

Like beta blockers, initial management is similar to prehospital management. After administering IV fluid boluses, give calcium gluconate or calcium chloride boluses. HIE therapy is started as soon as possible. As in beta blocker toxicity, the choice of vasopressor has been widely debated, with reports of success and failure of multiple agents. Norepinephrine is direct acting and is the first-line agent, whereas DOPamine remains a poor choice because of its indirect sympathomimetic activity.

Although *severe* dihydropyridine calcium channel blocker toxicity can cause bradycardia and hypotension, as with nondihydropyridine calcium channel blockers, toxic ingestions typically lead to hypotension with reflex tachycardia. As a result, after IV fluids, administer a peripheral vasoconstrictor such as norepinephrine or phenylephrine.

When standard therapies fail, consider invasive options such as left ventricular assist devices, extracorporeal membrane oxygenation (ECMO), intra-aortic balloon pump, or cardiopulmonary bypass, though limited success has been reported.

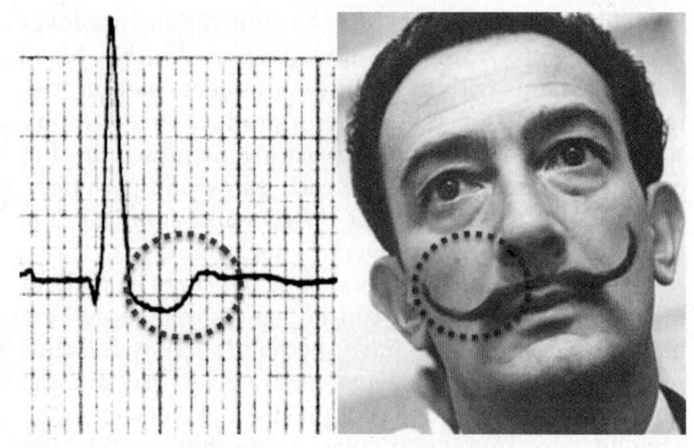

Figure 14-5 Digoxin effect on ECG, resembling Salvador Dali's mustache.

Courtesy of LITFL.

Digoxin

Digoxin (also known as digitalis) belongs to a class of medications called cardioactive steroids and is commonly used to treat heart failure and to control heart rate in atrial tachydysrhythmias (atrial fibrillation or atrial flutter). Digoxin has a very narrow therapeutic window with high risk for reaching toxic doses, whether accidental or intentional.

Pathophysiology

Digoxin acts by indirectly increasing intracellular calcium concentrations within the myocardium, primarily by inhibiting the sodium-potassium-ATPase, leading to increased myocardial contraction strength. The increased cardiac ejection fraction and improved (slowed) rate of ventricular depolarization optimize cardiac function and reduce ventricular response in atrial fibrillation and flutter. Notably, digoxin causes a characteristic ECG finding called the "digitalis effect": PR interval prolongation, QTc shortening, and "scooping" of the ST segments. This characteristic ST segment finding is often referred to as the "Salvador Dali" appearance, harkening to the artist's characteristic mustache (**Figure 14-5**).

Digoxin toxicity is categorized into acute toxicity from single-event overdoses in a digoxin-naive individual or chronic toxicity in those who have taken digoxin for an extended period. Toxicity may be intentional or inadvertent from interactions with other medications or due to other medical problems.

Acute toxicity is characterized by nausea, vomiting, abdominal pain, lethargy, confusion, and weakness; notably, these symptoms are primarily caused by the toxic effects of the medication itself rather than due to hemodynamic changes from the medication.

Chronic toxicity is much more difficult to identify and is typically insidious in nature; symptoms may resemble acute toxicity but are typically less obvious. Patients with chronic toxicity may also develop delirium, confusion, disorientation, headaches, or hallucinations. Patients may report a characteristic visual finding of yellow halos around objects. Bradydysrhthmias may occur in both acute and chronic toxicity.

Notably, digoxin-toxic patients may develop hyperkalemia (potassium > 5.0 mEq/mL), which is the best predictor of mortality if not treated with digoxin-specific antibody (Fab) fragments. Correcting the hyperkalemia through usual means does not affect mortality, but is only a marker for severe toxicity.

Signs and Symptoms

As noted previously, signs and symptoms of digoxin toxicity are nonspecific and can mimic many other pathologies; notably, patients may develop nausea, vomiting, abdominal pain, confusion, weakness, and headaches, which may result from other disease processes. The presence of the digitalis effect on an ECG does not indicate toxicity, but is only characteristic of those who take digoxin at baseline.

One ECG finding highly suggestive of digoxin toxicity is bidirectional ventricular tachycardia: the presence of atrial tachycardia with a high-degree AV block.

Differential Diagnosis

If the patient does not state that they purposefully overdosed on their digoxin, the differential is broad and includes electrolyte imbalance, acute coronary syndrome, sepsis, and other medication toxicity, such as beta blockers and calcium channel blockers.

Treatment

Prehospital Setting

Intensive supportive care and prevention of further digoxin ingestion or absorption are key management principles. Administer activated charcoal if the ingestion occurred within 1 hour of presentation. Obtain IV access for fluid resuscitation if hypotension develops. Obtain an ECG to assess the underlying rate and rhythm (bradycardia, AV blocks). Digoxin-toxic hearts are highly sensitive to stimulation (e.g., transcutaneous pacing) due to excess calcium and may develop dysrhythmias. Atropine 0.5 mg in adults (0.02 mg/kg with a minimum dose of 0.1 mg in children) may improve heart rate in bradydysrhythmias.

If possible, obtain the patient's medication list and past medical history to assist with further management in the emergency department.

In-Hospital Setting

Supportive care and symptomatic management continue in the hospital. Transcutaneous pacing has little to no benefit in bradydysrhythmias, and a transvenous pacemaker is contraindicated as it may induce lethal dysrhythmias. Check the patient's medical record if the diagnosis of digoxin toxicity has not been established to find other possible etiologies for the patient's presentation. Once there is high suspicion of toxicity, obtain serum digoxin levels. Check serum electrolytes (i.e., potassium and magnesium), a complete blood count, renal function, cardiac enzymes, and possibly blood gas analysis to guide treatment. The definitive treatment is digoxin-specific Fab fragments, more commonly known as digoxin immune Fab or DigiFab. These specially prepared antibodies strongly bind free digoxin and attract it away from the sodium-potassium-ATPase receptor, thus increasing urinary excretion of digoxin and decreasing overall serum digoxin concentrations. In cases where digoxin-specific Fab fragments are not readily available, continue supportive care by treating toxicity-induced hyperkalemia with insulin and glucose/albuterol/EPINEPHrine (induces flux of potassium from serum to intracellular spaces) and diuretics. Hemodialysis can treat hyperkalemia but it does not remove digoxin from the blood.

Diabetic Medications: Insulin and Sulfonylureas

Diabetes mellitus is one of the most common chronic medical diagnoses in the United States, affecting about 10% of the population. There are two variants of diabetes mellitus: type 1 and type 2.

Diabetes mellitus type 1 is characterized by insufficient insulin production and release from the pancreas. This disorder is either congenital or autoimmune, leading to dysfunction of the pancreatic beta islet cells that produce insulin. Medical management of type 1 diabetes involves subcutaneous insulin injections at home with close patient monitoring of their blood sugar. Historically, patients had to check their blood sugar with needles and glucometers, but insulin pumps can now administer insulin based on continuous blood sugar readings.

Diabetes mellitus type 2 is characterized by decreased sensitivity of peripheral tissues to insulin, meaning that different tissues and organs no longer respond adequately to insulin despite the amount present. Type 2 diabetes is typically managed with different types of medications; patients with type 2 diabetes may also require insulin administration in severe cases if their body does not make enough to overcome their decreased sensitivity despite oral medications.

This section will focus on the management of insulin and sulfonylurea overdoses.

Pathophysiology

Insulin is a peptide, or a short protein, produced and released by the beta cells of the pancreas in response to elevated blood sugar levels. Notably, the beta cells are also able to sense when blood sugar is low or normal and will stop releasing insulin to prevent hypoglycemia. Insulin primarily acts by binding to insulin receptors on cell membranes, inducing a series of intracellular changes that insert glucose transporters into the cell membrane to allow glucose entry into the cell. In type 1 diabetes, placement of these glucose transporters is severely limited, leading to hyperglycemia. A rare insulin-secreting tumor (insulinoma) may resemble insulin overdose because the tumor has lost its ability to respond to hypoglycemia, and thus continuously secretes insulin, even when blood sugar becomes low. It is possible to differentiate between insulinoma and exogenous insulin overdose by measuring c-peptide, a remnant produced during the body's own insulin production but not present in prescribed insulin formulations.

Sulfonylureas (e.g., glimepiride, glipizide, glyburide) are a class of medications commonly used to treat type 2 diabetes. Sulfonylureas act by increasing the pancreatic beta cell excretion of insulin into the bloodstream independent of the blood sugar level. The mechanism of action is through closing ATP-sensitive potassium channels located on the beta cells, which decreases potassium efflux from the cells. This process leads to electrical depolarization of the beta cells, which opens voltage-gated calcium channels, leading to insulin release. In sulfonylurea overdose, the beta cells continue to release insulin regardless of the hypoglycemia that would normally inhibit further insulin release. Profound, transient, treatment-resistant hypoglycemia may occur due to continued insulin release. Like insulinoma, c-peptide levels will be elevated as the insulin in question is being made from within the patient's own pancreas.

Signs and Symptoms

Whether the presentation is due to exogenous insulin overdose, insulinoma, or sulfonylurea overdose, the signs and symptoms are similar, including tremors, diaphoresis, and tachycardia. With progressively worsening hypoglycemia, the patient may develop stupor, lethargy, seizures, and, ultimately, cardiovascular collapse and death.

Differential Diagnosis

The differential diagnosis depends on the patient's known medical history and medication list. In the setting of unexplained hypoglycemia, consider insulin, sulfonylurea overdose, and insulinoma, particularly if recurrent hypoglycemia occurs despite dextrose administration. Other etiologies for hypoglycemia may include sepsis, malnutrition, and poor oral intake; however, these typically do not exhibit recurrent hypoglycemia following dextrose administration like the overdoses listed earlier.

Treatment

Prehospital Setting

Obtain a thorough history and physical examination, including a full medical history and list of medications. If able, assess when the patient most recently had their diabetic medications filled; excessive missing pills may suggest overdose. In particular, children presenting with recurrent hypoglycemia (findings suggestive of insulin/sulfonylurea exposure) should prompt investigation into medications at home.

Obtain IV access and give dextrose once hypoglycemia is identified. If the patient can tolerate oral intake without altered mental status, consider oral dextrose, but administer IV dextrose if hypoglycemia recurs. Although 50% dextrose historically has been used for treatment of hypoglycemia, this concentration is not recommended for pediatric patients and can lead to serious tissue damage if the IV extravasates. Many EMS agencies have switched to using 10% dextrose instead. A 250-mL infusion of D_{10} is equivalent to 25 g of dextrose and leads to resolution of altered mental status just as quickly as D_{50}.

Give IV fluids as needed. If the patient becomes symptomatic with recurrent hypoglycemia, initiate a dextrose infusion, initially in the range of 0.5–1.0 g of dextrose per kilogram.

In the rare case that IV access is not possible, glucagon can be administered; however, the onset time is long, so continue attempting IV access.

In-Hospital Setting

When the cause of persistent hypoglycemia is not clearly due to overdose, consider obtaining a c-peptide level for possible insulinoma or to differentiate overdose of prescribed insulin (low c-peptide level) versus sulfonylureas (high c-peptide level). Management in the hospital is primarily supportive with IV fluid resuscitation for hemodynamics and dextrose-containing fluids as detailed under Prehospital Setting. Consider further evaluation for possible sources of infection. Notably, patients receiving dextrose-containing fluids that have normal beta cell function may develop secondary hypoglycemia following initial resuscitation due to the dextrose-containing resuscitation fluid inducing further insulin release.

Serotonin Syndrome, Neuroleptic Malignant Syndrome, and Dystonic Reactions

Selective serotonin reuptake inhibitors (SSRIs; e.g., fluoxetine, paroxetine), other serotonergic medications (e.g., traMADol), antipsychotics (e.g., OLANZapine, haloperidol, risperidone), and other dopamine receptor antagonist medications (e.g., metoclopramide as an antiemetic) generally produce minimal life-threatening adverse effects; however, they all raise the risk of serious, potentially life-threatening syndromes. SSRIs and serotonergic medications may induce a life-threatening serotonin syndrome, whereas antipsychotics and dopamine receptor antagonists may cause life-threatening neuroleptic malignant syndrome (NMS) or the less severe spectrum of dystonic reactions. Serotonin syndrome and NMS are similar in presentation but have different treatment options, whereas dystonic reactions, while typically frustrating for patients, are not acutely life threatening.

Pathophysiology

Classically, serotonin syndrome is caused by SSRIs or serotonin norepinephrine reuptake inhibitors (SNRIs), though it may also result from medications that increase serotonin release, decrease serotonin metabolism (e.g., monoamine oxidase inhibitors), or directly stimulate serotonin receptors. These mechanisms stimulate different subsets of serotonin receptors, leading to a myriad of problems as discussed in the Signs and Symptoms section.

NMS most often results from the chronic treatment of psychotic disorders (e.g., schizophrenia) with antipsychotic medications that act as dopamine receptor antagonists or long-term use of dopamine antagonists such as metoclopramide for nausea or diabetic gastroparesis. Notably, patients with a history of Parkinson disease are treated with dopamine *agonists*, and withdrawal from these medications may cause a similar syndrome/presentation. Dopamine deficiency in the CNS, whether from blockade or withdrawal, may lead to an imbalance of heat production and heat dissipation, ultimately resulting in hyperthermia. Further signs and symptoms of NMS are listed in the next section.

Dystonic reactions exist on a spectrum, primarily resulting from dopamine receptor antagonism or withdrawal of dopamine agonists, like NMS. Possible dystonic reactions and their anticipated time course include the following:

- *Acute dystonia (hours to days)*: Presence of sustained, involuntary muscle contraction, such as torticollis. Recommended treatment includes discontinuing the offending medication and administering benzodiazepines or anticholinergics, such as benztropine or diphenhydrAMINE.
- *Akathisia (hours to days)*: A feeling of restlessness or uneasiness wherein the patient feels as if they must move. Recommended treatment includes discontinuing the offending medication and administering benzodiazepines, anticholinergics, or propranolol (a beta blocker).
- *Tardive dyskinesia (3 months to years)*: A rare, typically late presentation wherein the patient develops involuntary movements, classically of the face, including lip smacking and involuntary tongue movements. Recommended treatment is discontinuing the offending medication and changing to a different antipsychotic, plus the addition of cholinergic medications.

Signs and Symptoms

Dystonic reaction signs and symptoms were detailed in the previous section and are typically well managed as described.

As mentioned, serotonin syndrome and NMS have similar presentations with subtle differences and are easily confused with each other. Italicized items that follow are typically not seen in the other syndrome.

Serotonin syndrome typically develops over a short period of time (hours to 1 day) and returns to baseline quickly with appropriate treatment (classically in 24 to 48 hours). Symptoms and signs include altered mental status (confusion, depression, *agitation*, and *hyperactivity*), neuromuscular abnormalities (*tremors, shivering, hyperreflexia*, and *clonus*), autonomic instability (hypertension, tachycardia), and hyperthermia.

NMS typically develops over a longer period (days to 1 to 2 weeks) and resolves over the same time with appropriate management. Patient presentation may include altered mental status (depression and confusion), neuromuscular abnormalities (***bradykinesia*** [slow movements], *lead pipe rigidity*), autonomic instability (hypertension, tachycardia), and hyperthermia (Table 14-14).

Differential Diagnosis

The differential diagnosis is contingent upon knowing the patient's medical history, their medication list, and how long they have been taking their medications. When considering NMS or dystonic reactions, if the patient has a history of Parkinson disease, it is important to know if the patient has missed any of their medications. The different timelines of symptom/sign onset, along with reviewing the medication list and noting subtle neuromuscular findings, will help differentiate the two syndromes. The differential diagnosis may also include metabolic derangement, infection, allergic reactions, hypoglycemia, thyroid storm, sympathomimetic use, sepsis, and more.

Treatment

The treatment for both syndromes, along with dystonic reactions, is contingent on making the correct diagnosis. In general, these conditions require supportive management along with appropriately ruling out easily correctable pathologies, such as hypoglycemia.

Serotonin syndrome benefits from stopping the offending medication; addressing airway, breathing, and circulation; rapidly cooling the patient (external or invasive measures); and administering benzodiazepines. In severe cases, paralytics may be warranted for cooling as some evidence shows that the hyperthermia may be caused by persistent muscle contractions. Cyproheptadine, an antihistamine medication with serotonin receptor antagonism properties, has also shown some benefit.

NMS also benefits from stopping the offending medication; addressing airway, breathing, and circulation; and rapidly cooling the patient with ice packs to the groin/axilla and cooling blankets. A controversial pharmacologic intervention is dantrolene, a muscle relaxant, to decrease rigidity. Bromocriptine, a dopamine agonist, is useful in Parkinson patients withdrawing from their medications. Intubation is rarely indicated.

Prehospital Setting

Regardless of syndrome or dystonic reaction, obtain a thorough history and physical examination, particularly concerning the duration of symptom onset, past medical history, and the medication list and compliance. Obtain

Table 14-14 Neuroleptic Malignant Syndrome vs. Serotonin Syndrome

	NMS	Serotonin Syndrome
Cause	Dopamine antagonism or dopamine agonist withdrawal	Serotonin agonism
Time frame	Days to weeks	Hours to days
Duration of symptoms following treatment	Days to weeks	24–48 hours
Autonomic instability	+++	+++
Fever/hyperthermia	+++	+++
Depressed mental status/confusion	+++	+++
Agitation/hyperactivity	+	+++
Lead pipe rigidity	+++	+
Tremor/hyperreflexia	+	+++
Shivering	–	+++
Bradykinesia	+++	–

+++ = very common and severe; + = uncommon/mild presentation; – = typically not observed.

IV access and provide fluid resuscitation as needed. If the patient is hyperthermic, initiate external cooling with ice packs to the groin and axilla. Notably, the hyperthermia seen is not a fever, so antipyretic medications such as acetaminophen and ibuprofen provide no benefit for temperature control. Benzodiazepines are effective for serotonin syndrome and NMS and may be administered under the direction of medical direction.

In-Hospital Setting

Once in the hospital, if the diagnosis is still unknown, perform a thorough history, physical examination, and medical chart review to confirm or rule out these syndromes. Treat both conditions with active external cooling and benzodiazepines, along with bromocriptine for NMS if in a patient with Parkinson disease. Patients with serotonin syndrome or NMS require hospital admission.

As noted, dystonic reactions are relatively more straightforward to diagnose and manage and, outside of severe cases, do not generally require hospital admission.

Cyclic Antidepressants

Cyclic antidepressants have historically been a leading cause of toxicologic emergencies, especially intentional overdoses. These medications have a narrow therapeutic index, meaning there is a narrow dosing window that is effective and safe. Cyclic antidepressant use is much less common due to newer, safer antidepressant medications.

Pathophysiology

Tricyclic antidepressants (TCAs) act therapeutically by increasing the amount of norepinephrine and serotonin in the nerve synapses by blocking their reuptake in the CNS, thus prolonging their action. Additionally, TCAs block ion channels and alpha adrenergic, muscarinic, $GABA_A$, and histaminergic receptors. Cyclic antidepressant toxicity results from blocking sodium influx and inhibiting potassium efflux in the myocardium, inducing cardiac toxicity.

Signs and Symptoms

Early signs and symptoms include classic anticholinergic toxidrome effects such as dry mouth, tachycardia, urinary retention, constipation, mydriasis, and blurred vision. Late signs and symptoms include respiratory depression, confusion, hallucinations, coma, hyperthermia, ventricular dysrhythmias (such as wide QRS complexes, torsades de pointes and tachycardia and bradycardia), and seizures.

Differential Diagnosis

Serum levels of cyclic antidepressants do not correlate well with the severity of intoxication. Evaluate for

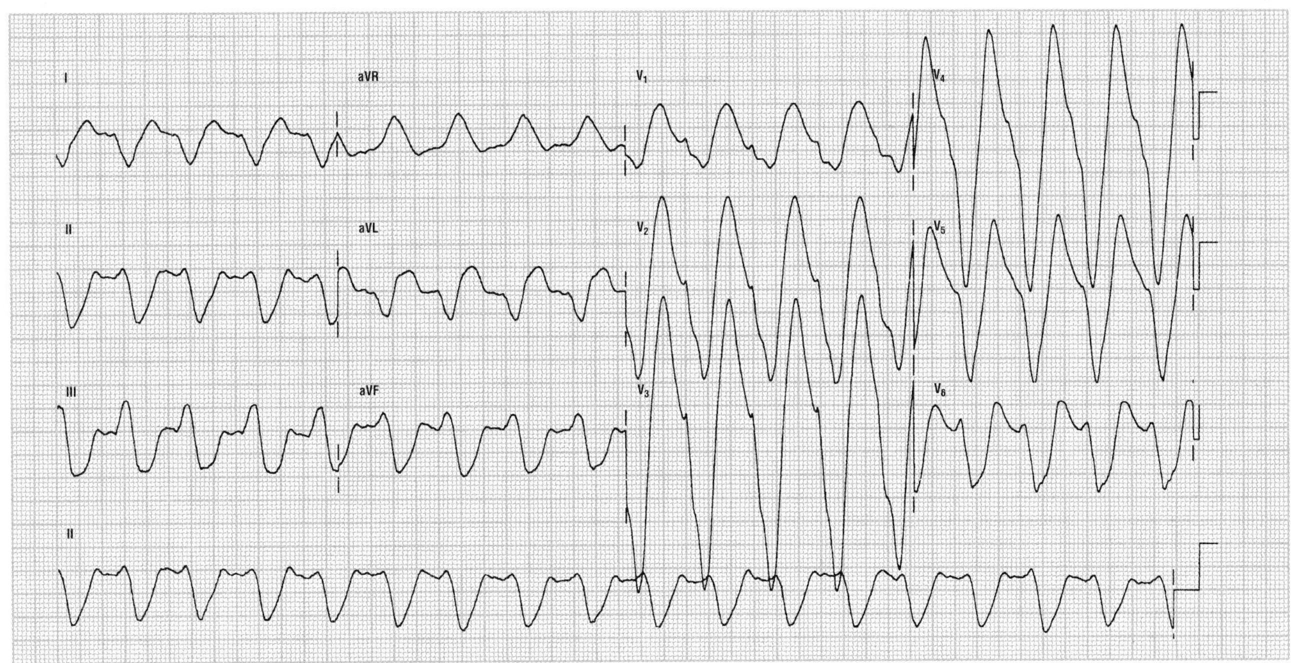

Figure 14-6 ECG demonstrating tachycardia, prolonged QRS (> 110 ms), and R wave in aVR. These findings are highly suggestive of cyclic antidepressant toxicity/overdose.

Reproduced from *12-Lead ECG: The Art of Interpretation*, Second Edition, courtesy of Tomas B. Garcia, MD.

coingestion of acetaminophen and salicylates. Obtain laboratory studies once at the hospital. Clinical and ECG evaluation should direct your differential diagnosis and treatment. Other considerations include hyperkalemia, hypocalcemia, heatstroke, and other medication intoxications. As always, if the patient has altered mental status, obtain a point-of-care blood glucose to rule out hypoglycemia.

Treatment

Cardiac monitoring is critical in patients with suspected cyclic antidepressant overdose because cardiac complications are the primary cause of death. Sudden cardiac arrest may occur days after the overdose. There is no direct antidote for tricyclic antidepressant poisoning, but bicarbonate is key, and supportive care is paramount. Activated charcoal administered in appropriate patients within 1 hour of ingestion may have benefit, if allowed by local protocols.

Prehospital Setting

Provide supportive care, especially cardiac monitoring. Establish IV access and administer sodium bicarbonate bolus and infusion if there is evidence of QRS widening (**Figure 14-6**) or seizures. Anticipate the potential for administering a large amount of sodium bicarbonate, often more than 4 ampules (e.g., 50 mEq per ampule), to maintain a QRS < 110 ms. Agitation, tremor, and seizures should be treated with escalating doses of benzodiazepines.

In-Hospital Setting

Observe asymptomatic patients for at least 6 hours to manage possible deterioration. Maintaining alkaline serum (pH 7.50–7.55) by bicarbonate infusion counteracts cardiac conduction effects. This treatment should be given if QRS widening (> 120 ms) or ventricular ectopy occurs. Tachycardia commonly occurs due to the anticholinergic effects of TCAs. Slowing of the rate indicates overwhelming sodium channel blockade, worsening cardiotoxicity, and the need for sodium bicarbonate.

Obtain the following labs studies: serum electrolytes, blood urea nitrogen, creatinine (kidney function), a complete blood cell count (CBC), and blood gas analysis. Qualitative urine immunoassays can test for TCAs but are unreliable. Chest imaging may show if aspiration has occurred.

Lithium

Lithium is used to treat bipolar disorder, also known as manic-depressive illness. Although lithium is an effective treatment, it has a narrow therapeutic index, increasing the likelihood of both accidental and intentional poisonings. To avoid accidental therapeutic poisoning, patients' lithium levels should be routinely monitored.

Several variables affect the drug's toxicity, including acute versus chronic ingestion, dose relative to existing serum levels, and overdose amount. In addition, dehydration, diuretic use, and renal dysfunction exacerbate lithium toxicity.

Pathophysiology

Lithium is a small cation (positively charged ion). It is similar to sodium and acts in place of it in cellular function; however, it has different effects compared to sodium. The precise mechanism by which lithium produces its medicinal benefit is still unknown, although the drug is thought to alter neuronal cell membrane function, cellular sodium and energy balance, and hormonal response. These effects may cause permanent CNS damage. Lithium decreases kidney function and is eliminated almost entirely by the kidneys. These drug properties sometimes cause inadvertent lithium reabsorption within the kidneys as renal function declines, thus inducing toxicity.

Signs and Symptoms

Signs and symptoms of lithium poisoning depend on the dose and whether toxicity is related to an acute, acute-on-chronic, or chronic ingestion. Serum levels can be misleading in predicting toxicity. Patients who have not previously been exposed to lithium would be expected to have higher serum levels and fewer symptoms because they do not have saturated tissue distribution. However, with chronic ingestion, more significant toxicity can be seen with lower levels due to preexisting CNS lithium levels. Minor symptoms include nausea, vomiting, excessive thirst, and muscle cramping. Progressive toxicity can result in tremor, myoclonus, diabetes insipidus with resulting hypernatremia, confusion, delirium, coma, and, in rare but serious cases, hypotension, electrocardiographic abnormalities, and dysrhythmias.

Differential Diagnosis

Consider alternative causes of symptoms, including thyroid dysfunction, other toxic ingestion, and possible meningitis or other CNS disturbance. Initiate cardiac monitoring to evaluate for dysrhythmias. To yield accurate results, the blood sample must be collected in a lithium-free tube.

Treatment

Prehospital Setting

In the field, treatment is mainly supportive. Maintain airway, breathing, and circulation. Establish IV access. Fluid administration is especially important in patients with lithium poisoning because of the effects of volume depletion on the cardiovascular and renal systems. Some reports indicate that sodium therapy enhances lithium elimination by the kidneys.

In-Hospital Setting

Hospital management centers on restoring euvolemia and maintaining a normal sodium level. Chronic lithium toxicity typically results from dehydration and associated kidney injury. Most patients with lithium toxicity can be treated with volume replacement alone. Acute lithium toxicity is often associated with predominantly GI toxicity and should be treated symptomatically. Hemodialysis is indicated in the rare cases of severe intoxication associated with persistent renal failure, severe cardiovascular effects, or severe neurologic symptoms, including altered mental status. The lab workup of a patient with suspected lithium toxicity includes a urinalysis and serial monitoring of serum lithium and sodium levels until symptoms resolve.

Hallucinogens

Hallucinogens cause visual disturbances (hallucinations) and alter the user's perception of reality. They include substances such as d-lysergic acid diethylamide (LSD), peyote, mescaline, and psychedelic mushrooms. Hallucinogens can be grouped into four major classes:

1. Indole alkaloids (e.g., LSD, lysergic acid amide [LSA], psilocin, and psilocybin)
2. Piperidines (e.g., PCP and ketamine)
3. Phenylethylamines (e.g., mescaline, MDMA, methylenedioxyamphetamine [MDA], and methoxy-methylenedioxyamphetamine [MMDA])
4. Cannabinoids (e.g., marijuana or tetrahydrocannabinol [THC])

Synthetic cannabinoids, or "spice," encompass a wide variety of herbal mixtures that produce experiences sometimes similar to marijuana (cannabis) and are marketed as "safe" alternatives. Continued experience with synthetic cannabinoids shows they are dangerous. Sold under many names, including K2, fake weed, Yucatan fire, skunk, moon rocks, and others—and labeled "not for human consumption"—these products contain dried, shredded plant material and chemical additives responsible for their psychoactive (mind-altering) effects. They do not contain marijuana, but rather experimental chemicals that cause a spectrum of clinical findings from severe agitation, combativeness, and hallucinations to somnolence and coma. Motor activities range from excessive to zombielike. The chemical additives change frequently to elude legal restrictions.

The synthetic cannabinoid compounds found in these products act as full agonists on the same cannabinoid 1 and 2 receptors (found throughout the body, but especially in the brain) as THC, the primary psychoactive component of marijuana. Some of the compounds found in synthetic cannabinoids (spice), however, bind more strongly to those receptors, which can lead to a much more powerful and unpredictable effect. Because the chemical composition of many products sold as spice vary, it is likely to contain substances that cause dramatically different effects.

Patients suspected of abusing synthetic cannabinoids typically present with rapid heart rate, vomiting, agitation, confusion, and hallucinations. These agents can also raise blood pressure and reduce blood supply to the heart (myocardial ischemia), and in a few cases they have been associated with heart attacks. Regular users may experience withdrawal and addiction symptoms.

Pathophysiology

The pathophysiology of hallucinogenic drugs as a class of agents is imperfectly understood, but they primarily affect the CNS. Hallucinogens may alter serotonin and norepinephrine concentrations in the brain. Indole amine derivatives act on serotonin receptors, whereas piperidine derivatives block serotonin, dopamine, and norepinephrine reuptake. Phenylethylamine derivatives block serotonin and norepinephrine reuptake and even increase their presynaptic release.

In the case of cannabinoids, the component delta (9)-THC is the source of pharmacologic effects at cannabinoid receptors. The chemical causes maximum plasma concentration within minutes and psychotropic effects in 2 to 3 hours.

Signs and Symptoms

Patients who have ingested hallucinogens can exhibit dangerous and sometimes bizarre behavior. They have altered mental status, which may include behavioral disturbances such as aggressiveness, delusional or paranoid thinking, and visual illusions (hallucinations). CNS effects can include stimulation or depression, depending on the causative agent, the dose, and the time elapsed since poisoning. Other possible effects include hypertension and tachycardia. Hallucinogen toxicity is distinguished from other possible causes on the basis of behavioral abnormalities and hallucinations.

Differential Diagnosis

The differential diagnosis of hallucinogen intoxication is very wide—essentially anything that can cause an altered mental status and altered perceptions. A lab workup is not particularly helpful for hallucinogen intoxication. Selected studies may be needed to differentiate it from other etiologies. A comprehensive drug screen can rule out coingestion or confirm a questionable diagnosis, but it is not clinically helpful due to the delay in getting results. Imaging studies are useful only to assess other possible causes of the patient's symptoms.

Treatment

Remember, patients under the influence of hallucinogens pose a threat to themselves and others, including the clinicians on scene. People who use hallucinogens may seek medical attention to treat traumatic injuries associated with hallucinogen use or to alleviate unpleasant or distressing psychotropic effects of the drug—a so-called bad trip. Hallucinogens typically have minimal acute side effects. Some patients become violent, and physical or chemical restraints may be needed. LSD is skin absorptive, and every effort should be made to avoid cross contamination. Primary treatment consists of calming the patient and providing reassurance that the drug's effects are temporary.

Prehospital Setting

Acquire a thorough patient history to help determine the correct etiology and ultimately to identify the hallucinogen. Determine if delirium with agitated behavior exists and, if so, treat aggressively. As possible, patients intoxicated with LSD should be isolated to help them remain calm. Administer benzodiazepines for agitation. In severe psychotic episodes, consider haloperidol or droPERidol.

In-Hospital Setting

Hospital treatment of these patients is similar to the prehospital phase. Note that although LSD intoxication lasts about 8 to 12 hours, the psychotic effects of the drug may persist for days and may require prolonged treatment.

Phencyclidine

The most common historical hallucinogen is PCP, which was originally developed as a general anesthetic and later used as a veterinary tranquilizer. PCP is notably similar to ketamine in chemical structure but is more potent. When its potential for abuse was discovered, it was replaced with safer alternatives. It is available as a white crystalline powder ("angel dust"), a liquid ("dippers"), or a tablet.

Pathophysiology

PCP is a dissociative anesthetic with hallucinogenic properties. It has both stimulant and depressant effects on the CNS. Its sympathomimetic effects are probably due to dopamine and norepinephrine reuptake inhibition. The drug also acts at nicotinic and opioid receptors, has cholinergic and anticholinergic effects, is a glutamate antagonist at NMDA receptors, and affects the dopamine pathway. Clearly, PCP produces some very complicated interactions. PCP is metabolized in the liver and has a half-life of about 15 to 20 hours.

Signs and Symptoms

At low doses (≤ 10 mg), PCP produces a combination of psychoactive effects, including euphoria, disorientation and confusion, and sudden mood swings (such as rage). Signs of PCP use may include flushing, diaphoresis, hypersalivation, and vomiting. The pupils generally remain reactive. Facial grimacing and rotatory nystagmus (involuntary eye movement), are identifiable effects of low-dose PCP use.

Persons who use PCP are much less sensitive to pain, which may give them the appearance of having superhuman strength as they overexert themselves. In fact, at low doses, mortality is associated with self-destructive behavior related to the analgesic and CNS depressant effects of PCP.

High doses of PCP (> 10 mg) may produce extreme CNS depression, including coma. Respiratory depression, hypertension, and tachycardia are common. The hypertension may cause cardiac difficulties, encephalopathy, intracerebral hemorrhage, and seizure. High-dose overdoses may require management of respiratory arrest, cardiac arrest, and status epilepticus.

Acute onset of PCP psychosis may occur even at low doses. This condition is a true psychiatric emergency that may persist for days or weeks after the exposure. Behavior can range from unresponsiveness (a catatonic state) to violent and enraged. Such patients can be extremely dangerous, and law enforcement should be called to help transport the patient to an appropriate medical facility.

Differential Diagnosis

As with other hallucinogens, the differential diagnosis of these patients can include any medical conditions or medications that cause altered mental status, hyperactivity, or aggressiveness and multiple vital signs abnormalities—it is wide. Patient history is critical to considering PCP intoxication.

Treatment

Primary treatment consists of calming the patient and providing reassurance that the drug's effects are temporary, although patients experiencing PCP intoxication rarely respond to verbal de-escalation. Obtain a thorough history from the patient, if able, or from bystanders to determine the etiology of the patient's signs and symptoms and to identify the hallucinogen ingested. Include the type and amount of drug ingested and the time of ingestion.

Prehospital Setting

Treatment is mainly supportive, including maintaining airway, breathing, and circulation and establishing IV access. Treat agitation with escalating doses of benzodiazepines. Treat delirium aggressively, as described elsewhere.

In-Hospital Setting

Cardiac monitoring is indicated in any patient with a suspected PCP overdose who has a preexisting heart condition. Keep the patient calm, and avoid abrupt movements, bright lights, and noise. Physical or chemical restraints may be necessary if the patient becomes erratic or violent. Benzodiazepines work well for this purpose. Avoid ketamine as it is a PCP derivative and may exacerbate PCP's effects. Antipsychotic agents such as haloperidol should not be given to patients with PCP intoxication because they may increase the risk of cardiac dysrhythmia or seizure. Rule out opioid use and hypoglycemia. The lab workup should include urine toxicology screening, a metabolic panel, measurement of serum glucose level, a CBC, and venous blood gas analysis. An elevated white blood cell count and increased serum urea nitrogen and creatinine levels are often seen in patients with PCP intoxication. Monitor serum creatine kinase and urine myoglobin for rhabdomyolysis. Clinicians should be aware that dextromethorphan, diphenhydrAMINE, ibuprofen, methadone, traMADol, and venlafaxine are common causes of positive results on qualitative urine drug screening for PCP. Notably, PCP is lipophilic, meaning that effects may be prolonged for several days if large amounts are ingested due to the drug accumulating within the patient's fat stores.

Ketamine

Ketamine is structurally related to PCP and has many similar clinical effects when used in an uncontrolled environment (e.g., illicitly). Medical personnel frequently administer ketamine for many reasons, including pain control, sedation for intubation, as well as chemical restraint. New research and practice styles are using small doses of ketamine to manage treatment-resistant depression, though the mechanism is not clear. Ketamine is believed to be psychologically addictive and is a known party drug going by the names "special K" and "vitamin K."

Pathophysiology

Ketamine works primarily by NMDA receptor antagonism, leading to anesthetic, analgesic, and psychogenic effects. Ketamine does interact with a multitude of other receptors within the body, including dopamine, catecholamine (alpha and beta), and others.

Signs and Symptoms

Ketamine may induce a multitude of symptoms, including anxiety, palpitations, chest pain, altered mental status, somnolence, and hallucinations. Chronic ketamine abuse may induce GI toxicity presenting as epigastric pain, hepatic injury, and impaired gallbladder activity. Rarely, it may even induce urinary symptoms known as ketamine cystitis. When used for medical management, it may provide analgesia at low doses and unresponsiveness at higher doses, such as during chemical restraint or when utilized for sedation during a procedure or mechanical ventilation.

Differential Diagnosis

Obtaining a thorough history and physical examination is paramount to developing the differential diagnosis. Given the multitude of symptoms that ketamine may cause, the differential diagnosis may also include other toxic/hallucinogenic ingestion, acute coronary syndrome, pneumonia, pancreatitis, hepatitis, cholecystitis, hypoglycemia, sepsis, and urinary tract infections. Utilizing tools such as point-of-care glucose, ECG, and a thorough physical examination may help parse through these differentials.

Treatment

Treatment of ketamine intoxication/toxicity is primarily supportive, including fluid resuscitation, symptomatic control, and keeping the patient calm. Although ketamine does not typically induce respiratory distress, closely monitor respiratory drive and airway patency. If intubation is indicated in an intoxication setting, use a different induction agent. Notably, when using ketamine medically for sedation/intubation, push the medication slowly, because rapid IV infusion may induce laryngospasm where the vocal cords close, making it difficult to pass the endotracheal tube. If this occurs, positive pressure with a bag-valve mask may open the cords prior to intubation; otherwise, quickly give a paralytic, such as succinylcholine or rocuronium, to break the laryngospasm.

Prehospital Setting

Treatment for intoxication is mainly supportive, including maintaining airway, breathing, and circulation and establishing IV access with IV fluid resuscitation. Keep the environment as calm as possible; benzodiazepines may help if the patient becomes aggressive. Cardiac monitoring should be continued as possible. Consider monitoring $ETCO_2$ to assess respiratory adequacy if benzodiazepines are used.

In-Hospital Setting

Cardiac monitoring and $ETCO_2$ monitoring are indicated in any patient with a ketamine overdose who has a preexisting heart condition. Place the patient in a calm environment with close monitoring. If they become agitated, give benzodiazepines, and have a low threshold for intubation and mechanical ventilation if concerned for airway compromise. In general, monitor the patient and provide supportive management until they metabolize their ingestion and recover.

Dextromethorphan

Dextromethorphan is a widely available OTC cough suppressant and has become a common drug of abuse, particularly in adolescents. Large doses must be ingested to experience its possible hallucinogenic effects. Because of its ease of access, many states have enacted age restrictions on its retail purchase. Many dextromethorphan formulations include other medications, such as antihistamines and acetaminophen, so consider toxicity from these other medications as well.

Pathophysiology

Dextromethorphan is a prodrug, meaning that it is metabolized into active molecules that cause its effects. In this case, it is converted into dextrorphan, which acts as a potent NMDA antagonist. It also acts as a SNRI inhibitor, among several other mechanisms of action.

Signs and Symptoms

Overdose symptoms typically require a minimum of more than three times the recommended dose for cough suppression. Overdose may induce nausea, insomnia, pressured speech, mydriasis, and dizziness. At escalating doses, particularly more than 10 times the recommended dose, hallucinations, dissociation, respiratory depression, diaphoresis, and vomiting may develop, among other symptoms. Contact dermatitis/mucositis may also be seen from chemical irritation of exposure sites.

Differential Diagnosis

As always, a thorough history and physical examination may help develop the differential diagnosis. Consider hypoglycemia as a simple cause of altered mental status or hallucinations. Presentation may also suggest alcohol intoxication/withdrawal, other hallucinogenic ingestion, sepsis, acute coronary syndrome, and meningitis. Remember, dextromethorphan is classically sold as a mixture with other medications, so consider acetaminophen and antihistamine toxicity.

Treatment

Primary treatment consists of calming the patient and providing reassurance that the drug's effects are temporary. Obtain a thorough patient history to determine the etiology of the patient's signs and symptoms and to identify the hallucinogen ingested. The history should include the type and amount of drug ingested and the time of ingestion. Endotracheal intubation is rarely needed, but monitor the airway in severely intoxicated patients.

Prehospital Setting

Obtain as much information as possible; if the patient is hallucinating or altered, gather collateral information from bystanders and scene evaluation. Supportive care is paramount, including symptom control, IV fluid resuscitation, and keeping a calm space. If severe agitation occurs, administer benzodiazepines. Avoid ketamine; it may worsen the patient's presentation due to its similar mechanism of action.

In-Hospital Setting

Perform cardiac monitoring in any suspected/known patient with dextromethorphan overdose who has a preexisting heart condition. Keep the patient calm, and avoid abrupt movements, bright lights, and noise. Give benzodiazepines if the patient becomes erratic or violent. Rule out possible acetaminophen coingestion with an acetaminophen level, ideally 4 hours post ingestion. A CBC, electrolytes, liver function tests, coagulation studies, and urinalysis may be indicated to assess for other possible etiologies. Provide supportive care until the patient has adequately metabolized their ingestion.

Inhalants

Inhalants are a broad group of typically nonpharmacologic molecules known as hydrocarbons found within household/industrial cleaners, including keyboard cleaner and aerosols. These compounds may also be found in gasoline, kerosene, butane, mineral oil, and paint. Most of these products are easily accessible and are a common drug of abuse in the adolescent population. Classically, when used as a substance of abuse, the inhalant is breathed in deeply and absorbed by the pulmonary capillary beds in the lungs. However, they are also a common source of accidental ingestion, such as children who drink them.

Pathophysiology

The pathophysiology is variable and depends on the chemical structure of the substance, as well as the route of exposure, concentration, and exposure dose. Notably, many of these substances are volatile, meaning that they readily turn from a liquid to a gaseous state. When swallowed, the more volatile compounds are known to vaporize into their gas form and can be inadvertently inhaled into the pulmonary system. The hydrocarbon may cause gastric/GI irritation as well as pulmonary inflammation known as pneumonitis.

Hydrocarbons are highly lipophilic molecules, leading to their rapid absorption and movement across cell membranes, particularly into the CNS, causing euphoria. Interaction with GABA and NMDA receptors accounts for their clinical effects. Most inhalants are removed from the body by exhalation without being metabolized, though a subset of inhalants is metabolized in the liver.

One acutely dangerous presentation from inhalant use involves myocardial sensitization by potassium channel blockade, leading to prolonged repolarization, exhibited as QTc prolongation on ECG. Classically, myocardial sensitization increases the risk of sudden-onset, lethal ventricular dysrhythmias, particularly if the patient is startled, and may cause death.

Signs and Symptoms

The action of inhalants is typically rapid onset and short-lived. Physical findings may suggest inhalant abuse, including discoloration around the nose and mouth, along with mucous membrane irritation, coughing, sneezing, and tearing. Patients may exhibit some degree of euphoria and hallucinations; with larger doses, patients may develop tremors, nausea, vomiting, abdominal pain, and worsening altered mental status.

Differential Diagnosis

A thorough history and physical examination may help determine the differential diagnosis. Consider possible coingestions, as well as sequelae due to the ingestion/inhalation of hydrocarbons. Other respiratory and GI irritants should be considered. Development of pneumonitis is highly possible in most cases and generally requires supportive care with oxygen supplementation. Check the blood sugar to assess for hypoglycemia in altered mental status. QTc prolongation induced by potassium channel blockade may also be witnessed.

Treatment

Primary treatment of inhalant toxicity is supportive care in a calm environment to mitigate the risk of inducing cardiac dysrhythmia. The typical timeline to return to baseline after isolated intentional inhalant abuse is generally short, about 1 to 3 hours.

Prehospital Setting

Wear proper PPE, and check the scene for safety before entering. Clinician exposure must be considered. Treatment is mainly supportive, including maintaining airway, breathing, and circulation. Obtain an ECG to assess for QTc interval prolongation; if present, keep acute disturbances to a minimum and place cardiac pads early in case the patient develops a life-threatening dysrhythmia to allow for rapid defibrillation/cardioversion. Provide oxygen supplementation in cases of desaturation indicating possible pneumonitis.

In-Hospital Setting

Symptomatic management and supportive care are the continued course of action in the emergency department. Monitor pulse oximetry to evaluate for possible pneumonitis. A chest x-ray may reveal pneumonitis, but note that initially it may appear normal because of the time it takes for radiographic changes to become evident. Lab work is rarely indicated; however, if the patient develops indications of arrhythmia, electrolytes, brain natriuretic peptide (BNP), troponin, and ECG are warranted to assess for other possible causes of dysrhythmia. Most patients with inhalant toxicity are monitored for several hours and discharged, though a small subset may require admission depending on their cardiac and respiratory status following initial management.

Toxins in the Home and Workplace

In the following sections, common causes of toxic exposure in the home and workplace are discussed. Some poisons, such as carbon monoxide, are inhaled. Others, such as antifreeze, are swallowed. Toxins such as pesticides and corrosives can be ingested, inhaled, or absorbed through the skin or cause dermal irritation and burns. Many of the poisons discussed have important industrial uses and may even be capable of causing mass-casualty disasters (e.g., factory event or during a train derailment). However, on a day-to-day basis, as a prehospital clinician you are most likely to encounter these toxins in a patient's home or workplace.

Ethylene Glycol

Ethylene glycol, one of the toxic alcohols, is found in automotive antifreeze, brake fluid, and deicers due to its ability to prevent both overheating and freezing of substances. Reportedly, its sweet taste increases the chance of large accidental ingestions by children and pets, but it is thought that roughly 70% of cases of ethylene glycol poisoning occur in adults. Often, adult patients have a history of alcohol use disorder and have not been able to obtain their normal ethanol source and thus resort to ethylene glycol ingestion as a substitute.

Pathophysiology

Ethylene glycol is metabolized into glycolic acid and oxalic acid by the enzyme alcohol dehydrogenase in the liver. These two metabolites cause most of the significant toxicity, acidosis, and kidney damage associated with ethylene glycol ingestion. The oxalic acid binds calcium in the body to form calcium oxalate crystals in the kidneys, resulting in renal failure. This process causes hypocalcemia, which increases the risk of cardiac dysrhythmias. The crystal deposition can cause severe joint pain, peripheral nerve dysfunction, and cardiomyopathy. Glycolic acid is the primary cause of acidosis and is also nephrotoxic, though the mechanism of injury is not understood.

Signs and Symptoms

Ethylene glycol toxicity typically occurs in the following three stages:

- *Stage 1: Neurologic (1 to 12 hours after ingestion).* Characterized by CNS effects, including signs of intoxication such as slurred speech, ataxia, sleepiness, nausea and vomiting, convulsions, hallucinations, stupor, and coma.
- *Stage 2: Cardiopulmonary (12 to 36 hours after ingestion).* Characterized by cardiopulmonary effects, which may include tachypnea secondary to metabolic acidosis, cyanosis, pulmonary edema, or cardiac arrest.
- *Stage 3: Renal (24 to 72 hours after ingestion).* Affects the renal system and may include flank pain, oliguria, crystalluria, proteinuria, anuria, hematuria, or uremia.

Some patients do not go through all stages but may exhibit life-threatening problems early due to their medical history and amount ingested. Life-threatening signs and symptoms include intoxication, headache, CNS depression, respiratory difficulty, metabolic acidosis, hypocalcemia, cardiovascular collapse, renal, seizures, and coma.

Differential Diagnosis

Patients with ethylene glycol ingestion may initially have an unremarkable physical examination until enough toxic metabolites build up to cause signs and symptoms. Differential diagnosis may also include ethanol or other toxic alcohol intoxication (methanol, diethylene glycol, isopropyl alcohol), hypoglycemia, infection, trauma, and electrolyte imbalance.

Treatment

Supportive care, antidote administration, and hemodialysis are the core treatments for ethylene glycol poisoning. Supportive care focuses on airway and hemodynamic management. Administer either ethanol or fomepizole as an antidote to inhibit further toxic metabolite production by competing for binding sites on the alcohol dehydrogenase enzyme molecule, which prefers ethanol and fomepizole over ethylene glycol. Ironically, patients who coingest ethanol are partially protected from the toxic effects of ethylene glycol until the ethanol is metabolized. Cofactor therapy consisting of pyridoxine (vitamin B_6) and thiamine (vitamin B_1) will boost ethylene glycol metabolism down a different pathway, particularly in patients with a history of alcohol use disorder, as these vitamins are classically lacking in their diet. Overall, however, hemodialysis is the definitive treatment for ethylene glycol poisoning to remove any remaining ethylene glycol and the toxic metabolites while also correcting the acidosis.

Prehospital Setting

In addition to basic treatment, obtain a detailed patient history, especially regarding the time of ingestion and possible coingestions. Establish IV access for rehydration and for antidote therapy when needed. Administer sodium bicarbonate for metabolic acidosis and diazePAM for seizures as necessary. Transport the patient rapidly to a hospital for hemodialysis.

In-Hospital Setting

Outside of supportive management, the hospital will typically administer fomepizole as the antidote. When ethanol or fomepizole is used, ethylene glycol metabolism is blocked and delayed, allowing for it to be excreted by the kidneys before it can be metabolized into toxic metabolites.

Lab work may include an ethanol level and a serum osmolality, which allows calculation of the osmolal gap; an elevated osmolal gap suggests toxic alcohol ingestion. Few hospital labs can provide ethylene glycol levels, so treatment often begins based on the history. Check serum calcium levels and venous blood gas analysis to guide management.

Hypocalcemia may be present in severe poisoning and requires calcium replenishment. Sodium bicarbonate administration is indicated for metabolic acidosis, along with hemodialysis, which offers definitive treatment by removing toxic metabolites from the blood.

Methanol

Methanol (methyl alcohol or wood alcohol), a common household solvent, is a component of windshield-washer fluid, paint, gasoline treatments, and canned tabletop fuels such as Sterno. It is also extensively used in industry as a solvent and reagent. Methanol may be intentionally ingested as an ethanol substitute, although most poisonings appear to be accidental or suicidal. Methanol is very volatile, so inadvertent inhalation is also possible and may cause aspiration pneumonitis. Methanol is absorbed through the skin, unlike many other toxic alcohols, though absorption is relatively low.

Pathophysiology

Methanol itself is not toxic, but its metabolites, formaldehyde and formic acid, are very toxic. Formic acid may cause irreversible blindness through retinal injury, lactate-associated metabolic acidosis (by inhibiting ATP production in the electron transport chain), and neurologic and cardiovascular toxicity. Symptom onset is usually delayed 12 to 24 hours until the toxic metabolites have accumulated.

Signs and Symptoms

Methanol initially causes inebriation, but to a lesser degree than the other alcohols. Early signs and symptoms mimic ethanol intoxication, including slurred speech, ataxia, drowsiness, and nausea and vomiting. More severe toxicity manifests as nausea and vomiting, abdominal pain, respiratory difficulty, headache, vertigo, ataxia, sedation, seizures, and coma. Vision complaints such as blurred vision and visual haziness are an initial hallmark of methanol poisoning. The initial onset of symptoms can be rapid, occurring in as little as 30 minutes, or delayed up to 24 hours, depending on the dose and route of entry. Mortality is associated with severe acidosis and cerebral edema.

Differential Diagnosis

Perform a thorough history and physical exam to determine the etiology. The differential diagnosis includes electrolyte imbalance, ethanol or other toxic alcohol ingestion, sedative-hypnotic ingestion, hypoglycemia, and infection.

Treatment

As with other drug intoxications, check a serum glucose level. Consider naloxone if the patient exhibits respiratory depression, which may be due to concurrent opioid ingestion, though respiratory depression will not improve if due only to toxic alcohol ingestion.

Prehospital Setting

Treatment consists of maintaining the patient's airway, breathing, and circulation. Airway management is important due to altered mental status along with possible respiratory depression. If intubation occurs, attempt to hyperventilate initially to compensate for likely metabolic acidosis. Identification of the offending substance, including documentation of ingredients or taking a picture of the product, if available, can help guide resuscitative and treatment efforts.

In-Hospital Setting

Hospital treatment consists of supportive care, antidote (fomepizole) administration to prevent toxic metabolite production, and hemodialysis as indicated. Supportive care should focus on maintaining an airway and hemodynamic stability. Administer cofactor therapy with thiamine to facilitate formic acid elimination. Decontamination is not helpful with gastric lavage or activated charcoal. Hemodialysis may be indicated in severe exposures if the patient complains of visual symptoms, severe acidosis is present, or serum methanol levels are high.

Lab studies are indicated by the findings. In severe methanol intoxication, obtain a serum alcohol level, electrolytes, venous blood gas, lactic acid, and serum bicarbonate level. The serum methanol level can be measured directly in some labs, or it can be estimated by calculating the osmolal gap and the metabolic acidosis.

Isopropyl Alcohol

Isopropyl alcohol (isopropanol/rubbing alcohol) is another of the toxic alcohols, though it is less toxic than either methanol or ethylene glycol. It is commonly found in hand sanitizer, perfumes, paint thinners, mouthwash, and other household supplies. Isopropyl alcohol is often abused as an alternative to ethanol. In high doses, it can cause hemorrhagic gastritis, vomiting, and hypotension.

Pathophysiology

Isopropanol is quickly absorbed in the stomach and metabolized into acetone, which is not particularly toxic. Notably, isopropyl alcohol is twice as strong a CNS depressant as ethyl alcohol and is known for the phrase, "twice as drunk, twice as long." Isopropyl alcohol may also induce hypotension due to vasodilation, though this is easily managed with IV fluids and possible vasopressor support.

Signs and Symptoms

Signs and symptoms of isopropyl toxicity include confusion, lethargy, CNS depression, respiratory depression, ketonemia, ketonuria, mild hypothermia, hypotension, and coma. As a result of acetone production, you may notice a fruity breath odor like that of a person with DKA. Unlike other toxic alcohols, isopropyl alcohol does not cause acidosis.

Differential Diagnosis

A thorough physical exam and patient history help determine the etiology of the toxicity. Differential diagnosis includes hypoglycemia, ethanol or other toxic alcohol intoxication, infection, and DKA.

Treatment

Perform a serum glucose test to rule out alternative etiologies of altered mental status. Consider naloxone if the patient exhibits respiratory depression and you suspect opioids, though note that naloxone will not change respiratory status if it is depressed only due to isopropyl alcohol. Because of the low toxicity of the isopropyl metabolites, fomepizole therapy is not indicated.

Prehospital Setting

In the field, treatment is mainly supportive. Maintain airway, breathing, and circulation, and establish IV access for fluid resuscitation and medication administration.

In-Hospital Setting

Hospital treatment is similar to prehospital treatment, which emphasizes supportive care through fluid resuscitation and aspiration prevention. Proton pump inhibitors or H2 blockers may help with hemorrhagic gastritis.

In severe intoxication, the lab workup may include blood gas analysis, serum electrolytes, and ethanol level primarily to assess for other toxic alcohols. Notably, kidney function may appear impaired as acetone falsely elevates the creatinine level.

Carbon Monoxide

In the United States, carbon monoxide (CO), a colorless/odorless gas produced from incomplete combustion of organic fuel, is a leading cause of morbidity and mortality from poisoning. Sources include household furnaces, space heaters, generators, gas stoves, gas and charcoal grills, motor vehicles, and smoke from house fires. In addition, methylene chloride, a chemical used as a paint stripper, degreaser, and industrial solvent, is metabolized to CO in the liver if ingested. Ingestion or significant inhalation exposure to methylene chloride can therefore cause delayed CO toxicity.

Pathophysiology

Carbon monoxide induces toxicity in many ways. Most commonly, CO preferentially binds the oxygen sites on hemoglobin with a greater affinity than oxygen. The resulting conformational change in the hemoglobin molecule prevents oxygen release to the tissues/cells despite normal serum PaO_2. CO also binds the mitochondrial cytochrome oxidase and impairs energy production by oxidative phosphorylation. The result is hypoxemia and acidosis, similar to the effects of cyanide. CO also binds to cardiac myoglobin and decreases oxygen extraction in heart muscle, thus contributing to cardiac ischemia. Finally, CO toxicity induces free-radical formation, inflammatory mediators, and delayed lipid peroxidation, eventually inducing cellular apoptosis (programmed cell death).

Signs and Symptoms

Symptoms of CO toxicity range from mild to fatal, depending on the concentration and the duration of exposure. Patients often describe fatigue, headache, myalgia, nausea, and vomiting, similar to a flulike illness. Severe toxicity can cause chest pain, shortness of breath, syncope, ataxia, seizure, and coma. In high concentrations, CO is considered a knockdown agent, meaning it causes rapid toxicity and loss of consciousness. In addition to primary cellular toxicity, the combined toxic effects of CO can induce myocardial ischemia, decreased contractility, vasodilation, and hypotension.

The vital signs of a patient with CO toxicity may be normal or grossly abnormal. Pulse oximetry is typically falsely normal as the oximeter cannot differentiate between carboxyhemoglobin and oxyhemoglobin (see Chapter 3, *Respiratory Disorders*). Cherry-red skin, a classic but uncommon late examination finding in patients with light skin tones, is due to the presence of oxygenated venous blood because of the combined inability of hemoglobin to unload oxygen and of tissue to extract it. Pulmonary examination may reveal pulmonary edema caused by either cardiogenic failure or primary pulmonary toxicity. The abdominal exam is generally unremarkable except for nausea and vomiting.

Neurologically, mild gait and balance abnormalities indicate significant exposure, whereas altered mental status and seizure coincide with severe toxicity. The patient may have focal neurologic deficits attributable to CO-induced stroke. In contrast to focal deficits caused by localized tissue hypoxia, these sequelae often involve memory, personality, and behavior. Symptoms may not develop for several weeks after recovery from the actual intoxication. Patients who have lost consciousness or had periods of hypotension are at risk for such delayed adverse effects, but it is difficult to predict their occurrence or severity.

Differential Diagnosis

Mild CO toxicity is probably underrecognized because its symptoms are generally mild and resemble flulike illness. The diagnosis may be further delayed because unintentional CO exposures tend to occur in cold-weather months when furnaces are in use and the incidence of viral illness increases.

Diagnosis of CO toxicity depends heavily on gathering accurate information from the scene. Multiple patients in the same setting with similar symptoms may suggest CO intoxication. The patient(s) may have been in an enclosed space such as a garage, with a motor running from a space heater, power generator, combustion engine, or other appliance. Household poisoning from a faulty furnace can provoke symptoms in several family members at once. Another clue might be the resolution of symptoms when the patient leaves the exposure source and the return of symptoms on reentering. Animals are often affected by CO poisoning earlier and more severely than humans exposed to the same source. Most fire departments are equipped with CO meters, which can detect elevated levels of the dangerous gas at the scene, thereby accelerating diagnosis and treatment. Some EMS agencies now also have access to CO-oximetry, a device that allows for measurement of a patient's CO level like pulse oximetry for oxygen. These methods of identifying CO in the environment or in a patient are less effective than the small and relatively inexpensive devices that many EMS agencies carry in their "first due" bags. These devices sound an alarm when the bag enters an environment with high CO, and they have been reported to be the first indicator of both a toxic environment and a valuable method of identifying patients with vague symptoms as a CO poisoning.

In patients with direct CO exposure, carboxyhemoglobin is measured only once, because the level cannot increase after the patient is removed from the source of CO. Patients with suspected exposure to methylene chloride, however, require prolonged observation and repeated testing to ensure that toxicity has peaked, because the carboxyhemoglobin level rises as the body metabolizes methylene chloride over at least 8 to 12 hours.

Patients may develop other problems to consider on your differential, including lactic acidosis, myocardial ischemia, cerebral ischemia, pulmonary edema, cyanide toxicity, electrolyte disturbance, and thermal burns.

Treatment

Prehospital Setting

The most important treatment for the patient and clinician is immediate removal from the CO source. Even a brief exposure can be toxic if the gas is sufficiently concentrated. After moving the patient to a safe location, place the patient on high-flow oxygen delivered through a nonrebreathing mask. Increasing the fraction of inspired oxygen (FiO_2) displaces CO from hemoglobin and reduces the half-life of CO on room air from about 6 hours to 3, and from about 3 hours to 90 minutes on 100% FiO_2. Hyperbaric oxygen can reduce the half-life to about 23 minutes.

If endotracheal intubation is required, maintain the patient on 100% FiO_2. Continuous positive airway pressure (CPAP) may also benefit the patient. Treat cardiac dysrhythmias as usual after oxygen administration. Hypotension often responds to IV fluids and vasopressors when needed.

It is unclear if hyperbaric oxygen therapy definitively benefits patients after CO exposure (**Tip Box 14-2**).

TIP BOX 14-2

Treatment of CO Exposure with Hyperbaric Therapy

The treatment of CO exposure with hyperbaric therapy is controversial. Consensus is lacking on the best approach after removing the patient from the environment and placing them on high-concentration oxygen. Regionalization of emergency health care systems may best coordinate and standardize the care of these patients in your area.

Most hospitals do not have hyperbaric chambers available, so a regional plan should include hyperbaric sites, available physicians, and necessary resources. An emergency physician can discuss with the hyperbaricist to determine if hyperbaric therapy and subsequent transfer are indicated.

Notify the fire department or local hazardous material responders to identify, isolate, evacuate, and ventilate structures, especially those with multiple occupants.

In-Hospital Setting

In addition to the physical examination, supplemental laboratory and radiographic data are used to evaluate patients with CO toxicity. Obtain and analyze a venous blood gas sample on a CO-oximetry device to determine the carboxyhemoglobin level. An elevated carboxyhemoglobin level aids in diagnosis, but the specific level does not predict toxicity or outcome. For example, a critical patient who has received prolonged oxygen supplementation prior to lab analysis may have normal CO levels due to treatment but still have underlying pathology, whereas a patient with only mild symptoms may have a significantly elevated level. Clinical signs and symptoms may be more reliable.

In the emergency department, high-flow oxygen or CPAP/bilevel positive airway pressure (BPAP) is continued to hasten the dissociation of CO from hemoglobin along with hemodynamic management.

Hyperbaric oxygen therapy remains controversial. It is unclear whether there are true benefits associated with this therapy. Hyperbaric oxygen chambers are either monoplace or multiplace, in reference to the number of patients each can accommodate. A monoplace chamber is roughly the size of a casket and can accommodate only one person at a time. A multiplace chamber is a small room in which several patients can be treated at once. Oxygen is pumped into the room at increasing pressure. Hyperbaric oxygen further decreases the half-life of CO to roughly 25 minutes. It is worth noting that barotrauma may occur in hyperbaric management due to high pressure, leading to possible sinus pain and tympanic membrane injury or rupture.

Specific criteria for determining the need for hyperbaric oxygen have been poorly defined. Currently, severe, persistent symptoms, including altered mental status, coma, seizure, focal neurologic deficits, hypotension, chest pain, myocardial infarction, and syncope, are accepted indications for hyperbaric oxygen therapy. Those with milder symptoms should receive high-flow oxygen or CPAP/BPAP with 100% FiO_2 until symptoms resolve.

In treating CO exposure, pregnant patients represent a special patient population. Fetal hemoglobin binds CO with greater affinity than maternal hemoglobin, leading to a high carboxyhemoglobin concentration in the fetus, which is compounded by decreased oxygen delivery. Maternal carboxyhemoglobin levels do not reflect fetal levels. Severe fetal toxicity, long-term neurologic deficits, and fetal demise have been reported with maternal exposure. Children born to patients with mild CO toxicity have done well.

Hyperbaric oxygen therapy presents a theoretical threat to the fetus, but the risk has not been substantiated. Pregnant patients with CO toxicity should undergo hyperbaric oxygen therapy if significant symptoms develop. As with nonpregnant patients, the specific carboxyhemoglobin level at which therapy should be initiated is not known, but 20% has been suggested.

Cyanide

Cyanide is a toxic compound rooted in chemical warfare, first employed by Napoleon III and subsequently in both World Wars. It has also gained notoriety for its role in mass casualties such as the Jonestown, Guyana, mass suicide in the 1970s.

Most cyanide exposures are unintentional, primarily through chemical reactions in laboratory work, as well as exposure through structural fires and smoke inhalation from combustion of synthetic polyesters, rubber, wool, and silk. Cyanide toxicity may also occur in the hospital setting with nitroprusside, a medication that lowers blood pressure but also partially degrades into cyanide.

Pathophysiology

Cyanide causes toxicity primarily by inhibiting the electron transport chain, thus disrupting ATP production, the primary energy source of every cell. The result is inadequate energy production and profound lactic acidosis. Secondarily, cyanide is directly neurotoxic via excessive NMDA receptor activation, leading to increased intracellular calcium levels and induction of cell death.

Signs and Symptoms

There is no sign or symptom unique to cyanide poisoning, though rapid (seconds to minutes following exposure) deterioration of high oxygen–utilizing organ systems (e.g., cardiovascular and neurologic) suggests cyanide toxicity. From a cardiovascular standpoint, bradycardia and hypertension may be seen early with quick progression to hypotension and reflex tachycardia. In patients with lighter skin tones, cherry-red skin color may occur due to venous blood that is rich in oxygen because it could not be extracted due to electron transport chain blockade. For those who survive acute toxicity, delayed neurologic symptoms similar to those of Parkinson disease may develop over time.

Differential Diagnosis

Consider exposure to other toxic compounds, particularly CO and thermal burns if the exposure is due to a structural fire, a common source for both cyanide and CO. Sequelae of cyanide exposure such as cardiovascular collapse, neurologic dysfunction, and respiratory failure may also suggest other etiologies leading to cardiac/cerebral ischemia, metabolic derangement, and hypoglycemia.

Treatment

Like many other toxins, supportive care is paramount, including airway assessment and cardiopulmonary support. Antidote administration as early as possible is vital as well. Historically, nitrites and thiosulfate were the main treatment, but now hydroxocobalamin is preferred. Research has shown that hydroxocobalamin and thiosulfate combined may provide greater benefit than either alone. Cobalt moieties within hydroxocobalamin bind cyanide to form cyanocobalamin, or active vitamin B_{12}. Cyanocobalamin is then excreted by the kidneys. Administration of hydroxocobalamin is associated with deep red to purple staining of body excretions (urine) and secretions and interferes with some colorimetric laboratory studies, including chemistries, for several days. Amyl nitrite ampules for inhalation (formerly included in cyanide antidote kits) are no longer available.

Prehospital Setting

Patient and personal safety take precedence. If the patient is coming from a structural fire, work on extraction from this immediate danger before providing further medical care. Decontamination and proper PPE are essential, particularly if the cyanide exposure is due to a nonfire source, such as laboratory exposure. Once in a safe place, quickly assess and intervene for airway patency, breathing support, and cardiovascular support. If available in your agency, and if suspicion for cyanide toxicity is high, administer whichever antidote is available. Otherwise, continue supportive measures, including oxygen supplementation at 100% FiO_2 en route to the hospital.

In-Hospital Setting

Continue supportive measures in the hospital. If high suspicion for cyanide poisoning is present, administer either hydroxocobalamin or thiosulfate. Due to the rapid deterioration potential in this patient population, lab work and imaging are not indicated to guide management but may be obtained during empiric resuscitation. These include chest x-ray, CBC, electrolyte levels, liver function tests, ECG, and cardiac enzymes. Note that a markedly elevated lactic acid (> 8 mmol/L) is highly suggestive of cyanide toxicity.

Hydrogen Sulfide

Hydrogen sulfide is a toxic gas that is a serious, but rare, cause of toxicity. This gas is commonly produced by bacteria as a by-product of protein decomposition, as well as a by-product in paper mills, refineries, and asphalt. It has a characteristic odor of rotten eggs. Hydrogen sulfide can be found in various industries, including petroleum and mining, and it also can accumulate in sewers and in manure pits on farms.

Pathophysiology

Hydrogen sulfide is typically absorbed through inhalation and may induce chemical irritation of mucous membranes, including the mouth, nares, and eyes. Mechanistically, hydrogen sulfide acts like cyanide toxicity and inhibits the electron transport chain. Unlike cyanide, however, hydrogen sulfide induces reactive oxygen species that cause oxidative damage to cells/tissues and also inhibits glycolysis—another pathway cells use to produce energy. Notably, prolonged exposure to hydrogen sulfide paralyzes the olfactory nerve, thus giving the false impression that the gas has dissipated and is no longer a threat. This may lead to further exposure.

Signs and Symptoms

Prolonged exposure and high inhaled doses may induce rapid neurologic and cardiopulmonary decompensation, leading to cardiac/respiratory arrest. Typically, patients who are removed rapidly and early from the source of hydrogen sulfide rapidly improve with likely full recovery. Unfortunately, delayed neurologic deficits, including memory loss, behavioral changes, muscle rigidity, and ataxia, may occur some time after exposure due to progressive neurologic injury.

Differential Diagnosis

Differential diagnosis is driven by known environmental risk factors and the patient's personal history. Other toxic inhalation gases must be considered. Evaluate for cardiovascular and respiratory failure as well as for easily reversible causes, such as dehydration and hypoglycemia.

Treatment

Treatment is mainly supportive, including oxygen supplementation, airway protection, and ventilatory support with CPAP/BPAP or direct mechanical ventilation, depending on the patient's mental status and respiratory drive. Administer IV fluid resuscitation with possible vasopressors as needed for hemodynamic support. There is no ideal antidote. Sodium nitrite may help by creating methemoglobinemia but must be administered as soon as possible with close monitoring for subsequent hemodynamic compromise. Notably, check methemoglobin levels following sodium nitrite administration. Additional antidotes may include hydroxocobalamin and cobinamide.

Prehospital Setting

As with cyanide, patient and personal safety are priority. Only those in proper respiratory PPE (self-contained breathing apparatus [SCBA]) should be permitted to enter the exposure site to immediately remove the patient and minimize further hydrogen sulfide absorption. Once safe to do so, apply oxygen at 100% FiO_2 and implement standard ACLS evaluation/management as indicated. Sodium nitrite or hydroxocobalamin may be considered according to local protocol, if available.

In-Hospital Setting

Supportive care continues in the hospital along with antidote administration: sodium nitrite, hydroxocobalamin, and cobinamide. Monitor hemodynamics closely. Support ventilation with high positive end-expiratory pressure (PEEP), particularly if there is evidence of pneumonitis or acute lung injury. Lab work consists of venous blood gas analysis, electrolytes, cardiac enzymes, liver and renal function tests, and lactic acid. Though controversial, hyperbaric oxygen may benefit this patient population as well.

Corrosives

Corrosives are a broad category of chemicals that corrode metal and destroy tissue on contact. Several federal agencies, including the Department of Transportation (DOT) and the Environmental Protection Agency (EPA), define precise parameters for corrosive solutions. The corrosivity of a solution—that is, its ability to oxidize and chemically disintegrate materials—is determined partly by its pH. The standard pH scale runs from an acidic low of 0 to a basic/alkaline high of 14, with both extremes being corrosive. The scale is logarithmic, meaning that a difference in 1 on the scale correlates with a 10 times difference in strength (e.g., a pH of 3 is 10 times more acidic than a pH of 4). A neutral or normal pH is 7.0. The DOT defines a strong acid as a solution with a pH less than 2 and a strong base with a pH greater than 12.5. Even acids and bases that do not reach these extremes in pH can be harmful depending on duration and location.

Acids and bases may cause serious chemical reactions when mixed together, typically generating heat along with toxic gases. For example, mixing household bleach (hypochlorite) with an ammonia-based cleaner generates chloramine gas. Examples of acids and bases are given in Table 14-15.

Table 14-15 Selected Acids and Bases

Acids	Alkalis (Bases)
▪ Battery acid ▪ Drain cleaners ▪ Hydrochloric acid ▪ Hydrofluoric acid ▪ Sulfuric acid ▪ Nitric acid ▪ Phosphoric acid ▪ Acetic acid ▪ Citric acid ▪ Formic acid ▪ Trichloroacetic acid ▪ Phenol	▪ Drain cleaners ▪ Refrigerants ▪ Fertilizers ▪ Anhydrous ammonia ▪ Lye ▪ Sodium hydroxide ▪ Bleach ▪ Sodium hypochlorite ▪ Lime ▪ Calcium oxide ▪ Sodium carbonate ▪ Lithium hydride

Acids and alkaline solutions are found commonly in household chemicals; we use them to open clogged drains, treat swimming pools, polish metal, and clean everything from toilet bowls to wheel rims. Acids are also found in the foods we eat. Vinegar, for instance, is composed of about 5% to 10% acetic acid, and many soft drinks contain phosphoric acid.

In industry, acids and alkaline solutions are used as chemical reagents, catalysts, and industrial cleaning agents. Ammonia is a widely used and available corrosive and flammable chemical. It is used in agriculture as a fertilizer and in industry as a refrigerant (in the form of a liquefied gas) and chemical reagent. In addition to these legitimate uses, ammonia is a primary ingredient in methamphetamine production. Several people have died of chemical burns sustained when this flammable gas ignited while they were manufacturing ("cooking") methamphetamine.

Pathophysiology

The pathophysiology of various acid and base exposures varies widely. First, acid burns and alkali burns are different. Acids produce necrosis by denaturing proteins, forming an eschar that limits penetration of the acid—a process called coagulation necrosis. Bases (often referred to as alkalis or caustics), in contrast, produce liquefaction necrosis (**Figure 14-7**). (Hydrofluoric acid, which tends to produce liquefaction necrosis like an alkali, is an exception to this rule.) Liquefaction necrosis causes a more penetrating injury in which cell membranes break down and dissolve, essentially forming soap. Consequently, a hallmark of caustic exposure is that the skin feels slick or slimy. This process, called saponification, results in a deeper burn that is more difficult to decontaminate. Pain is often delayed in these exposures.

Second, the severity of the burn depends on several variables, including the pH, physical form (solid, liquid, or gas), and concentration of the corrosive as well as the

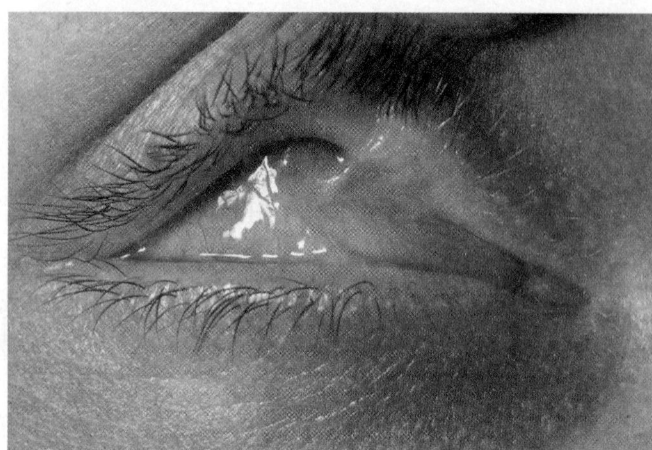

Figure 14-7 Liquefaction necrosis due to hydrofluoric acid exposure.

surface area involved and the contact time. Ingestion of solid alkali pellets such as lye causes severe GI burns because the pellets remain in prolonged contact with the esophagus and stomach. Full-thickness or circumferential esophageal burns can be complicated by strictures (narrowing scar tissue) that form as the burns heal.

Signs and Symptoms

Hydrofluoric acid, or hydrogen fluoride, is dangerous because it is highly corrosive while causing deep tissue penetration and inducing acute systemic toxicity even though it is a weak acid. The fluoride ion is the most electronegative ion and therefore binds and sequesters calcium and magnesium in the body. A white or yellowish-white precipitate of calcium fluoride salt may form beneath the skin in patients with hydrofluoric acid burns. Severe exposures can cause systemic hypocalcemia and hypomagnesemia. Industrial strength hydrofluoric acid is 35% and will cause immediate, direct burns and tissue damage upon contact. Disruption of cellular membranes induced by hydrofluoric acid also causes hyperkalemia as intracellular potassium is released. Cardiac dysrhythmias attributed to either hyperkalemia and/or hypocalcemia are the likely causes of most deaths not directly attributable to caustic injury. Other acids and bases may cause many differing symptoms depending on several variables (e.g., pH, contact area, duration of contact), including dermatitis, skin/mucosal burns, respiratory distress, and dehydration.

Complications

Evaluate hemodynamic and fluid status as severe burns can cause dehydration from insensible fluid loss associated with loss of barrier protection. If ingested, GI strictures and irritation are possible and may warrant endoscopy for evaluation once the patient is stable. Pneumonitis and cardiovascular symptoms may occur if the solution is inhaled along with special exposures such as hydrofluoric acid described previously.

Treatment

Prehospital Setting

If there is skin contact, copiously irrigate the site with soap and water, normal saline, or lactated Ringer's (whichever you have available). The goal is to wash as much of the offending substance off as possible. Do not try to neutralize the substance (e.g., apply a basic solution if the patient was exposed to an acid, or vice versa) because an exothermic reaction may occur. Simple decontamination with water is safe because a relatively small quantity of acid is being washed away by a large quantity of water. The heat generated by the chemical reaction is absorbed by the cool water. Take care not to induce hypothermia when decontaminating patients for more than a few minutes.

Carry out decontamination procedures in an area with good ventilation and adequate space. The amount of time to irrigate depends on the corrosive, its concentration, and the size of the body surface area affected. For ocular decontamination, there are two typical approaches: (1) irrigate the eyes for 15 minutes with water or normal saline, or (2) extend irrigation time to 30 to 60 minutes with a Morgan irrigation lens or IV tubing and topical anesthetic if available. Check the initial pH of the cornea using litmus paper if available and monitor every 10 to 20 minutes for pH correction. Irrigate until pH is neutral; if you are unable to test the pH, err on the side of safety and continue to irrigate until at the hospital. Inadequate irrigation may cause irreversible damage leading to blindness.

Flush the skin with water for at least 5 minutes, though flushing/irrigation will typically require longer periods of time. Flushing can continue during transport, as long as contaminated water is isolated in a reservoir such as an emesis basin. Test the area with litmus paper (pH paper) to determine whether decontamination is complete.

Do not attempt GI decontamination following presumed caustic ingestion given the risk of further GI injury or aspiration. The poison control center or medical control may advise you to dilute the acid by giving the patient milk or water to drink following a minor ingestion.

If decontamination is not rapidly completed, the acid produces intense pain at the site of contact. This may become necrotic and form an eschar if not adequately irrigated in an appropriate amount of time. GI damage from acid ingestion may include burns of the mouth, esophagus, and stomach; with time, the acid may even be absorbed by the bloodstream, presenting as acidosis.

Hydrofluoric acid burns require special consideration. Fluoride ions can be bound by either calcium or magnesium. Therefore, any hydrofluoric acid burns should be treated with calcium gluconate or calcium chloride and magnesium to replenish body stores and to prevent cardiac dysrhythmias. The antidote for hydrofluoric acid skin burns is thorough decontamination with water, followed by application of topical calcium gluconate gel. Because of the penetrating nature of fluoride burns, apply calcium gluconate to the burn site repeatedly and continuously even after completing initial decontamination and treatment. Deeper burns may require subcutaneous injections of calcium gluconate. Cover burns and wounds with dry, sterile dressings.

In the case of alkali (base) burns, copiously and continuously flush the wounds en route to the emergency department. Alkali exposures burn longer and deeper, causing greater tissue damage.

In-Hospital Setting

Lab workups may be necessary following corrosive exposures. The extent of the workup depends on the type of corrosive, strength of the corrosive, the surface area of the burn, and the route of exposure. Localized burns do not typically require lab workups. Severe burns, however, warrant a CBC, blood glucose level, electrolyte studies, creatinine, serum urea nitrogen, creatine kinase, a coagulation profile, and a urinalysis. Hydrofluoric acid burns require calcium, magnesium, and potassium levels, along with an ECG, to identify any systemic effects, in addition to broader lab workups that may be indicated by the severity of the exposure.

Thoroughly decontaminate any corrosive exposure area. In addition, because many corrosives are volatile, you may need to secure the airway. Endotracheal intubation may be indicated for ingestion or facial burns. Corrosive burns affecting a large body surface area require fluid therapy analogous to fluid resuscitation given after thermal burns. As with most skin injuries, infection can complicate long-term recovery.

Nitrites and Sulfa Drugs That Cause Methemoglobinemia

Compounds such as nitrites and nitrates, which can oxidize the iron in hemoglobin, cause **methemoglobinemia**. Many chemicals and medications can cause methemoglobinemia, some of which are listed in Table 14-16.

Overuse of certain medications such as nitroprusside and benzocaine sprays (commonly used for oral ulcers or teething) can cause methemoglobinemia. In rural areas, biologic processes such as fermentation after silos are filled with grain can create nitrites. Peak toxicity occurs about a week after filling. Agricultural groundwater and well water contamination with fertilizers such as ammonium nitrate can cause methemoglobinemia and cyanosis in infants, known as "blue baby syndrome."

Table 14-16 Selected Chemicals That Cause Methemoglobinemia

- Aniline dyes
- Aromatic amines
- Arsine
- Chlorates
- Chlorobenzene
- Chromates
- Combustion products
- Dimethyl toluidine
- Naphthalene
- Nitric acid
- Nitric oxides
- Nitrites (such as butyl nitrite and isobutyl nitrite)
- Nitroaniline
- Nitrobenzene
- Nitrofurans
- Nitrophenol
- Nitrosobenzene
- Nitrous oxides
- Resorcinol
- Silver nitrate
- Trinitrotoluene

Pathophysiology

The pathophysiology of methemoglobinemia can be inferred from its antidote, methylene blue, which was first used by Dr. Madison Cawein in the Kentucky Appalachian Mountains in the early 1960s. Oxygen and other oxidizers naturally convert a small percentage of hemoglobin to methemoglobin on a continuous basis via oxidation of iron in oxyhemoglobin to methemoglobin. NADH methemoglobin reductase is an enzyme that can correct this oxidation by converting ferric (Fe^{3+}) methemoglobin back to ferrous (Fe^{2+}) hemoglobin. The "Kentucky blue" people, as they are known, have a mutation in the enzyme NADH methemoglobin reductase. Affected individuals have a blue skin tone that makes them appear cyanotic (**Figure 14-8**). This coloring is not caused by oxygen-deprivation cyanosis, but rather by methemoglobin, which is a dark bluish-brown color. Cawein empirically administered methylene blue to these patients, correctly surmising that it would eliminate their blue pallor by acting as an electron donor (reducing agent) to convert methemoglobin back to hemoglobin. The symptoms associated with methemoglobinemia are due to inadequate oxygen delivery to peripheral tissues. The classic presentation is a pulse oximetry reading of about 85% despite adequate oxygen supplementation.

Signs and Symptoms

Patients with methemoglobinemia due to nitrate and nitrite poisoning have altered levels of consciousness, including anxiety, confusion, and stupor. Methemoglobinemia causes a slate-gray cyanosis. Nausea and vomiting, dizziness, and headache are common. Severe signs and symptoms may include cerebral ischemia,

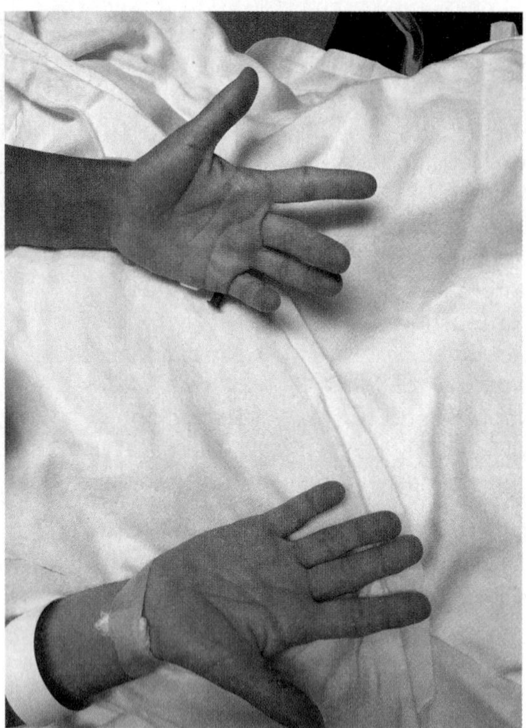

Figure 14-8 Methemoglobinemia.

hypotension, and respiratory distress, which can lead to cardiovascular collapse and asphyxiation.

Differential Diagnosis

Recognizing methemoglobinemia can be challenging because the patient may have only mild complaints. Pulse oximetry is inaccurate with methemoglobinemia because the methemoglobin interferes with measurement of oxyhemoglobin. Typically, pulse oximetry will give a reading in the high 80s that is unresponsive to additional oxygen supplementation. Special oximetry devices are available that can evaluate for methemoglobinemia. The differential diagnosis must include any cause for clinical hypoxia. A thorough history and physical assessment assist in discovering the correct etiology.

Methemoglobinemia can be diagnosed quickly in the field with a blood-drop test. Place a drop of blood on a 4 × 4-inch gauze pad. If it is chocolate brown and does not turn red in a few minutes with exposure to atmospheric oxygen, you can suspect methemoglobinemia with confidence because carboxyhemoglobin turns red when it oxidizes, whereas methemoglobin does not.

Treatment

As previously mentioned, the antidote to nitrate and nitrite poisoning is methylene blue, which assists with conversion of methemoglobin back to oxyhemoglobin. Paradoxically, at high concentrations, methylene blue acts as an oxidizing agent and may actually cause methemoglobinemia and even hemolysis.

Prehospital Setting

Provide supportive care, including maintenance of airway, breathing, and circulation. Administer supplemental oxygen. Ensure that the patient has been removed from the offending environment and thoroughly decontaminated. Decontamination is also important to prevent cross contamination.

In-Hospital Setting

Treatment is based on symptom severity. External decontamination is important to prevent continued intoxication and avoid cross contamination of health care personnel and of the emergency department environment. Obtain a methemoglobin level.

Mild exposures resolve on their own, whereas more severe exposures require intervention with supportive care and antidote methylene blue therapy. Supplemental oxygen is crucial to ensure that the remaining hemoglobin becomes fully saturated with oxygen. Patients in whom methylene blue is contraindicated may benefit from hyperbaric oxygen therapy or exchange transfusion.

Environmental Toxins: Poisoning by Envenomation

Environmental toxicology studies the effects of chemicals in the environment. A wide variety of environmental toxins, such as animal venom and microbial and plant toxins, can have adverse effects on humans. Many of the cardiovascular and neurologic effects of natural toxins are treated in ways similar to those used to treat other toxic exposures, as outlined in the preceding sections. However, several specific toxic mechanisms and clinical manifestations require directed therapy.

In the United States, you may treat patients for envenomation by *Latrodectus* (black widow spider), *Loxosceles* (brown recluse spider), or Buthidae (scorpions). Although envenomation by any of these arthropods can be painful, death is rare. The linchpins of treatment are supportive care and symptomatic management with opioids and anxiolytics. Table 14-17 summarizes toxicity, mechanism of action, and recommended treatment for each type of arthropod envenomation.

About 5,000 snakebites occur each year in the United States, with only one to three deaths. Venomous snakes can be found throughout the continental United States

Table 14-17 Arthropod Toxicity

Arthropod	Toxin	Toxic Mechanism	Clinical Manifestations	Treatment
Latrodectus mactans (black widow)	Alpha-latrotoxin	Presynaptic calcium channel opening with release of multiple vasoactive and myoactive neurotransmitters	Nausea, vomiting, sweating at bite site, tachycardia, hypertension, muscle cramping	DiazePAM, fentaNYL Consider antivenom for severe toxicity.
Loxosceles reclusa (brown recluse)	Sphingomyelinase-D Hyaluronidase	Sphingomyelinase-D: local tissue destruction, intravascular clotting Hyaluronidase: promotes tissue penetration	Local: tissue necrosis and ulcer formation Systemic: loxoscelism, including fever, vomiting, rhabdomyolysis, disseminated intravascular coagulation, hemolysis	Local wound care, tetanus prophylaxis, and analgesia Supportive care for systemic toxicity
Centruroides exilicauda (bark scorpion)	Neurotoxins I–IV	Sodium channel opening with repeated depolarization and neurotransmitter release	Local paresthesias, tachycardia, hypertension, salivation, diaphoresis, muscle fasciculations, opsoclonus (roving eye movements)	Tetanus prophylaxis, wound care, anxiolysis, analgesia Severe toxicity may be treated with antivenom.

and Alaska. The two families of venomous snakes are as follows:

1. The Crotalidae (pit vipers), a family that comprises rattlesnakes (including the eastern and western diamondback, pygmy, and massasauga varieties), cottonmouths (water moccasins), and copperheads
2. The Elapidae (coral snakes)

Snake venom toxicity and mode of action vary between the families.

Many marine creatures deliver venom via bites or stings, producing intense pain at the site of envenomation. Some of these organisms—jellyfish, fire coral, and sea anemones—inject toxins with stinging cells called nematocysts. Other organisms, such as sea urchins and stingrays, have spines that inject venom deeper into the tissue, causing trauma as well as envenomation.

Recall from the discussion of the AMLS Assessment Pathway earlier in the chapter that scene safety is always of foremost importance. Many venomous animals can envenomate again, even after death. Identification of venomous animals can be extremely helpful; however, you should never pursue or handle the live animal. A photograph or detailed description will suffice.

Black Widow Spider

The black widow spider lives in all parts of the continental United States. It is usually found outdoors in woodpiles, brush, sheds, or garages, and may hitchhike into the home on outdoor-stored items such as firewood or Christmas trees.

Identification

The female black widow is recognizable by its bulbous, shiny black abdomen and red hourglass marking on the ventral surface (**Figure 14-9**). The spider is usually an inch or less in length. Its venom is a potent neurotoxin. The male black widow is brown, about half the size of the female, and nonvenomous.

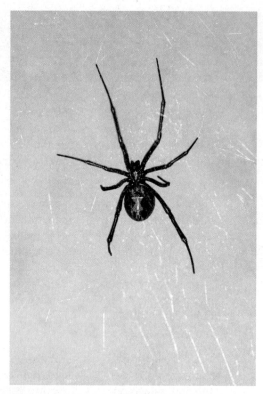

Figure 14-9 Female black widow spider with red hourglass marking on underside of abdomen.

Signs and Symptoms

Signs and symptoms of black widow envenomation include muscle spasms; nontender abdominal rigidity; and immediate severe, localized pain, redness, and swelling at the site. The patient may describe the bite as a bee sting–like sensation. You might observe two small fang marks spaced 1 mm apart. Systemic effects of envenomation may include nausea and vomiting, diaphoresis (sweating) at the bite site, muscle spasms, severe pain, or a decreased level of consciousness.

Treatment

Prehospital treatment is mainly supportive. Administer analgesics and antiemetics for pain and nausea. Treat muscle spasms with benzodiazepines such as diazePAM, LORazepam, or midazolam. Monitor and treat hypertension as needed. Antivenom is available for black widow envenomation, making identification of the spider and rapid transport to the facility important.

Brown Recluse Spider

The brown recluse spider lives in dark, dry locations, including inside houses, in relatively warm climates. In the United States, the recluse is found in Hawaii, the South, the Midwest, and the Southwest. Most envenomations occur in states in the south-central region of the country.

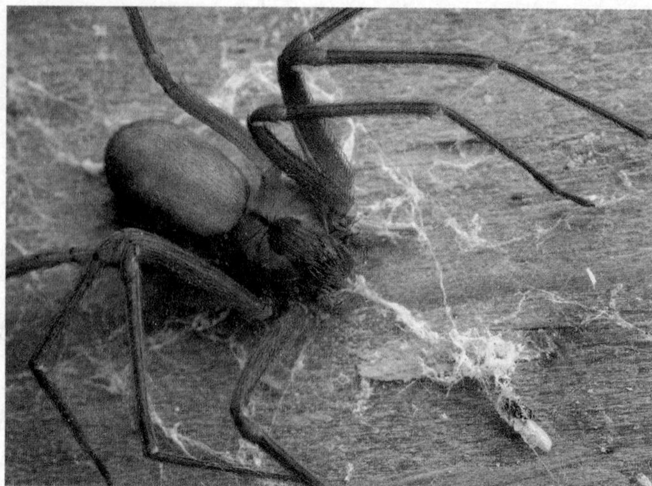

Figure 14-10 Brown recluse spider. Note the dark, violin-shaped marking on the spider's back.

Identification

The recluse is tan to brown, with a distinctive violin-shaped marking on its back (it is also known as the "violin spider" or the "fiddle-back spider"; **Figure 14-10**). Its body can be up to three-fourths of an inch long. Another identifying feature is that it has six eyes, rather than the usual eight. The eyes are arranged in a semicircle in pairs of three.

Signs and Symptoms

The venom of the brown recluse is a cocktail of at least 11 peptides that possess a variety of cytotoxic properties. The necrotic venom produces a classic bull's-eye lesion at the injection site. Many envenomations occur at night while the patient is asleep. The bite is painless and initially begins as a small blister (papule), sometimes surrounded by a white halo (**Figure 14-11**). Over the next 24 hours, localized pain, redness, and swelling develop. During the next few days or weeks, tissue necrosis develops at the site, and the redness and swelling begin to spread. The necrosis makes the wound slow to heal, and it may be visible months after the bite (**Figure 14-12**).

Although local effects are most common, systemic symptoms of brown recluse envenomation include malaise, chills, fever, nausea and vomiting, and joint pain. Life-threatening symptoms may include bleeding disorders such as disseminated intravascular coagulation and hemolytic anemia. Of note, necrotic wounds of other etiologies may often be falsely attributed to spider

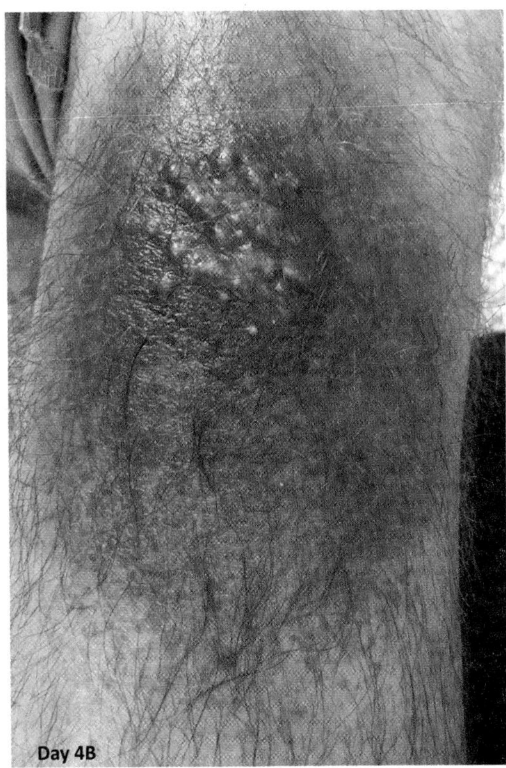

Figure 14-11 Brown recluse spider bite. A severe reaction in which infarction, bleeding, and blistering have occurred.

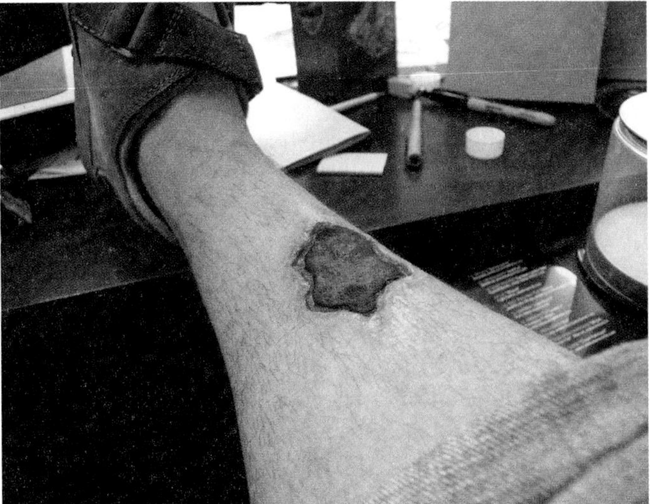

Figure 14-12 Necrotic ulceration from a brown recluse spider bite.

bites. Maintain a broad differential (sepsis, necrotizing soft-tissue infection, abscess, etc.) for systemically sick patients with necrotizing wounds.

Treatment

Prehospital care should focus on airway management and pain control. Treatment is supportive. Clean and dress the wound, apply a cold compress to the envenomation site, and transport the patient for medical evaluation.

FentaNYL is the opioid of choice to treat envenomation because it does not produce the histamine release associated with other opioids. Specific antidotes to brown recluse envenomation have been investigated, but because of serious potential adverse effects and lack of effectiveness, their use is not recommended.

Scorpions

In 2020, 11,393 scorpion stings were reported in the United States, with no fatalities. More than 600 scorpion species are found in the United States, but only the bark or sculptured scorpion of the desert Southwest is dangerous to humans. Scorpions are nocturnal and hide under objects and buildings during the day. They may enter buildings, especially at night.

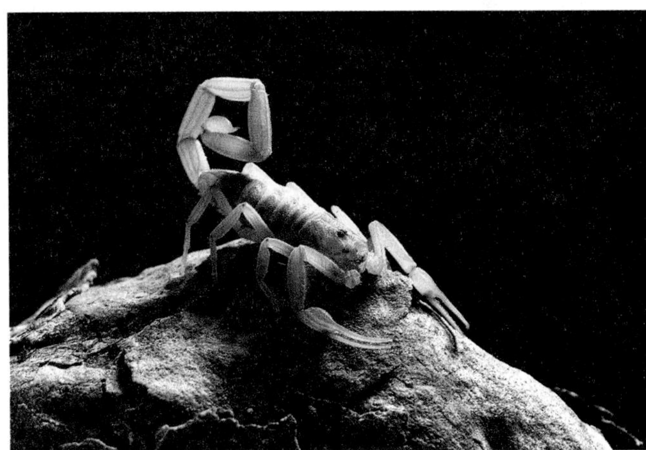

Figure 14-13 Arizona bark scorpion (*Centruroides exilicauda*).

Identification

Scorpions are yellowish-brown, may be striped, and are about 1 to 3 inches long (**Figure 14-13**). The scorpion injects venom stored in a bulb at the base of a stinger on the end of its tail. It usually injects only a small amount of poison. The sculptured scorpion is active from April to August and hibernates during the winter.

Signs and Symptoms

Systemic effects are usually only seen in small children (< 20 kg [44 lb]) or debilitated adults and primarily cause neuromuscular dysfunction. Symptoms can include slurred speech, restlessness, salivation, abdominal cramping, nausea and vomiting, rotatory nystagmus, muscle fasciculations (twitching), and seizures. Seizures are rare, and the much more common muscle fasciculations may easily be mistaken for seizures; if the patient appears to be having a generalized tonic-clonic seizure but is awake, then seizure is highly unlikely. Symptoms typically peak within 5 hours of envenomation. If redness and swelling are present at the injection site, a bark scorpion is probably not responsible for the sting because its venom does not induce localized inflammation. The venom of the bark scorpion is a neurotoxin that initially produces a burning or tingling sensation, followed by numbness. The toxin is a mixture of proteins and polypeptides that affect voltage-dependent ion channels, especially the sodium channels involved in nerve signaling. A secondary effect of envenomation is CNS stimulation through sympathetic neurons.

Treatment

Begin treatment by managing airway, breathing, and circulation and by calming the patient. Offer supportive care for respiratory depression. Clean the wound, and apply a cold compress (not ice). The technique of applying a lymphatic tourniquet (a wide band with moderate tightness, not to be confused with arterial tourniquet) is controversial. Tourniquet application is not recommended for any envenomations due to difficulty of proper application and monitoring, as well as a lack of supportive evidence.

Administer NSAIDs for local pain. Avoid giving opioid analgesics if the patient is experiencing respiratory symptoms, as this may exacerbate them. Provide transport to the hospital. Antivenom is available for scorpion stings in endemic locations.

Megalopyge opercularis—the Asp or Puss Caterpillar

Megalopyge opercularis, the "asp" or "puss" caterpillar, is the larva of the southern flannel moth and is the most toxic caterpillar in North America. It is most commonly found in Texas but is also seen from New Jersey to Florida. Exposures peak in June–July and again in September–October annually. Occasional multiple exposures can occur when larvae fall from trees onto children. Ocular and oral exposures present the most concerning problems. This 2-cm long, teardrop-shaped, furry caterpillar (**Figure 14-14**) has urticating hairs that break off and release venom into the skin, rapidly causing intense throbbing, burning pain, and erythema. Hemorrhagic vesicles may last up to 5 days. Reported systemic symptoms include nausea, vomiting, and numbness. Treatment consists of adhesive tape to remove spines/hairs from the skin, soap and water to remove the venom, oral antihistamines to relieve itching, and occasionally stronger pain medication or corticosteroids for intense inflammation.

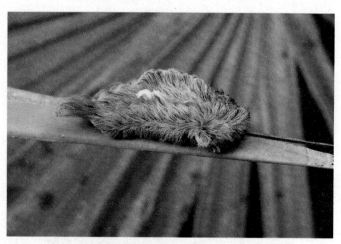

Figure 14-14 A puss caterpillar.

Crotalids (Pit Vipers)

In the United States, nearly all snake envenomations can be attributed to the Crotalidae family, the pit vipers. Crotalids are native to every state in the United States except Maine and Hawaii. In 2020, 4,670 known pit viper envenomations were reported to U.S. poison centers, with three deaths reported, all from rattlesnakes.

Identification

Pit vipers are named for the distinctive pits that form grooves in the maxillary bone on each side of their triangular head between the nares and eyes. They have vertical elliptical pupils and long, hinged fangs (**Figure 14-15**).

Signs and Symptoms

Signs and symptoms of crotalid envenomation include distinctive fang marks at the injection site, accompanied by redness, pain, swelling, and oozing that may precede compartment syndrome (an unusual finding). Systemic effects can include the following:

- Thirst
- Sweating
- Chills
- Weakness
- Dizziness
- Tachycardia
- Metallic taste in the mouth
- Nausea and vomiting
- Diarrhea
- Hypotension
- Clotting defects

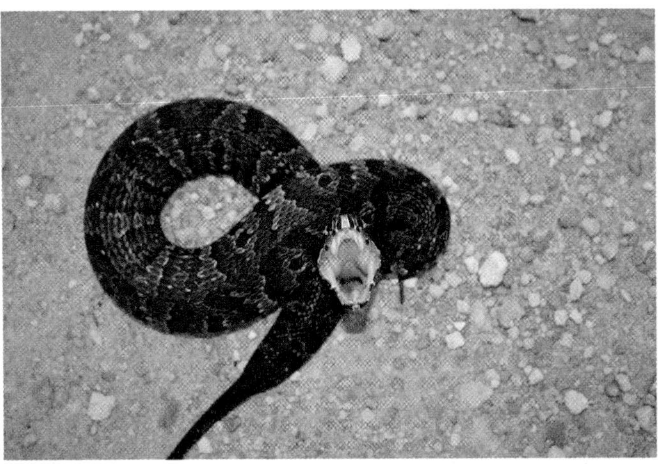

A

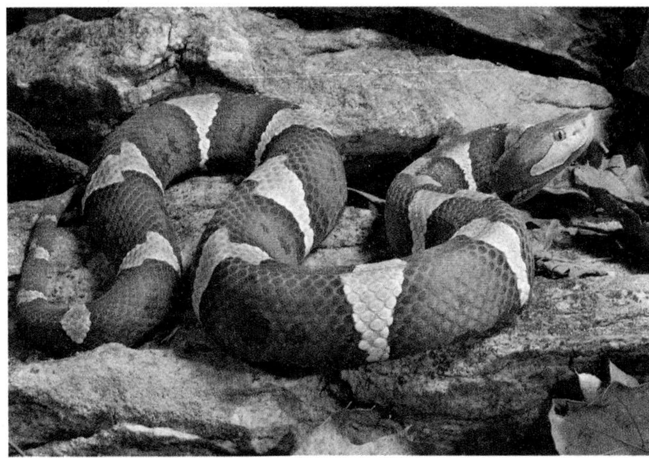

B

Figure 14-15 **A.** Water moccasin (cottonmouth) snake. **B.** Southern copperhead (*Agkistrodon contortrix contortrix*) has markings that make it almost invisible when lying in leaf litter.

- Respiratory distress
- Numbness and tingling around the head (with some species)

Despite coagulation abnormalities, significant bleeding complications of envenomation are rarely reported, though certainly possible. The primary morbidity is associated with local tissue injury. Neurotoxicity, such as paresthesias and weakness, is associated with only select species of crotalids, primarily the Mojave rattlesnake (*Crotalus scutulatus*) in the United States. Crotalid envenomation is associated with injury and significant morbidity, but fatalities are rarely reported. Pit viper venom consists of multiple peptides and enzymes, the aggregate effect of which primarily leads to tissue and muscle injury, as well as consumption and depletion of clotting factors, including platelets and fibrinogen. Although disseminated intravascular coagulopathy has been reported with severe envenomation, coagulopathy, thrombocytopenia, and hypofibrinogenemia develop in most patients without the microangiopathic clotting and associated tissue injury seen in disseminated intravascular coagulopathy. Intravascular envenomation can lead to disseminated intravascular coagulopathy, hypotension, and death. Approximately 25% of bites are considered dry, meaning that little or no venom is delivered with the bite.

Treatment

Treatment consists of supporting airway, breathing, and circulation; removing rings or any constricting jewelry; and elevating the affected limb (after arrival to the health care facility) to ameliorate the degree of local tissue injury. Administer fentaNYL for pain.

Immobilize the limb with a splint, but do not suction, incise, or apply cold packs to the wound. Snakebite suction kits are not effective and should not be used. Do not attempt to constrict the affected area with a tourniquet. The primary morbidity associated with crotalid envenomation is local tissue injury and the potential for compartment syndrome, whereas systemic toxicity is relatively minor by comparison. Therefore, the goal of prehospital care is to immobilize the affected extremity to prevent systemic spread. Avoid patient exertion and keep the patient calm to keep the heart rate down.

Antivenom is available for crotalid envenomation, so rapid transport to an appropriate medical facility is critical. Two varieties of antivenom are currently available in the United States: Crofab and Anavip. Although there are molecular and manufacturing differences between the two, either will suffice if indicated. Antivenom should be administered at a health care facility in consultation with a medical toxicologist. Indications for antivenom administration include rapidly progressive edema, neurotoxicity, clinically significant coagulopathy, compartment syndrome, or risk of airway obstruction. Observe the patient closely for a possible allergic reaction to the antivenom, although it rarely occurs.

Tissue injury and limb dysfunction due to lymphedema may take weeks or months to resolve, and physical therapy may be necessary. In rare cases, surgical intervention and fasciotomy may also be necessary to treat compartment syndrome or other complications. However, the primary treatment for compartment syndrome is more antivenom.

Patient destination decisions vary throughout the United States regarding what type of facility and what type of physicians should care for snakebite patients. Regional protocols may dictate where you transport. An envenomation is typically not a surgical disease and is managed with observation and coagulopathy prevention or therapy. A physician knowledgeable in coagulation management (e.g., an emergency physician) is sufficient. Occasionally, a compartment syndrome may develop, and appropriate consultation should be available. It is preferred to coordinate with a receiving facility and ensure that they have antivenom available or can be obtained rapidly. This does not necessarily need to be a trauma center.

Elapids

In the United States, snakes of the elapid genus *Micrurus*, the coral snakes, are found in the Southeast (eastern variety) and Southwest (Arizona variety). Seventy-six coral snake envenomations were reported to U.S. poison centers in 2020 with no deaths. Of note, each year dozens of exotic snakebites are reported in the United States. Many of these snakes are also elapids, although not native to the United States.

Identification

Coral snakes are smaller than pit vipers and have round pupils, a narrow head, small fixed fangs, and no pits on the head (**Figure 14-16**). They can be identified by their distinctive alternating horizontal bands of black, pale yellow or white, and deep orange or red. Some nonvenomous snakes (such as the king snake) mimic this color pattern, but imperfectly. The old saying, "Red on yellow, kill a fellow; red on black, venom lack," can distinguish between the coral snake and its imposters. However, the rhyme applies only to coral snakes native to the United States.

Signs and Symptoms

Coral snake envenomation is uncommon because of the snake's docile nature; its short, fixed teeth; and its small size. Severe envenomations, however, can cause skeletal muscle paralysis and difficulty breathing. Signs and symptoms include fang marks, swelling, redness, and localized numbness at the injection site. Systemic effects, some of which may be delayed for 12 to 24 hours, include the following:

- Weakness
- Drowsiness
- Slurred speech or salivation
- Ataxia
- Paralysis of the tongue and larynx
- Drooping eyelids
- Dilated pupils
- Abdominal pain
- Nausea and vomiting
- Seizures
- Respiratory distress
- Hypotension

The venom of a coral snake contains a mixture of hydrolytic toxins and a neurotoxin that blocks acetylcholine receptor sites. It has more significant neurologic effects than pit viper venom and may induce paralysis and respiratory failure, but only 40% of bites cause envenomation.

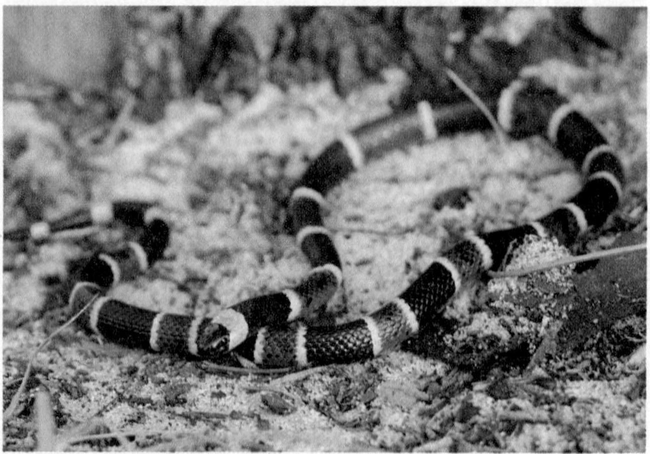

Figure 14-16 Texas coral snake (*Micrurus tener tener*) and the eastern coral snake (*M. fulvius*) have a potent neurotoxic venom, but are secretive, and bites are uncommon.

Treatment

Initial management of elapid envenomation consists primarily of supportive care. If respiratory symptoms are noted, be prepared to intubate the patient. As with crotalids, lymphatic tourniquets are not recommended. Decontaminate the wound with water or normal saline, keep the affected extremity below the heart, and encourage the patient to remain quiet and still. Immobilize the limb with a splint and start an IV line with a volume-expanding crystalloid fluid. Do not incise or apply cold packs to the wound.

No U.S. Food and Drug Administration–approved antivenom is currently available. Small supplies of expired antivenom exist and are tested annually for effectiveness. In eastern coral snake–endemic regions (Texas, Florida), the antivenom is available, so rapid transport to an appropriate medical facility is critical. If the patient is not transported to a hospital for evaluation, this should be considered a high-risk refusal, as elapid envenomation may be asymptomatic for 12 to 24 hours. All coral snake bites should prompt at least 24 hours of observation for any sign of respiratory compromise. Treat with antivenom promptly if respiratory distress develops.

Jellyfish

Many jellyfish stings cause only minor local dermal irritation and pain, but some species can produce more severe symptoms. The Portuguese man o' war can produce intense pain, welts, and muscle cramping, and the box jellyfish (*Chironex fleckeri*) can produce systemic toxicity (**Figure 14-17**). Jellyfish have long tentacles equipped with nematocysts that discharge and deposit venom on contact with skin. Drowning deaths have been reported when victims incapacitated by severe pain have been unable to swim to shore.

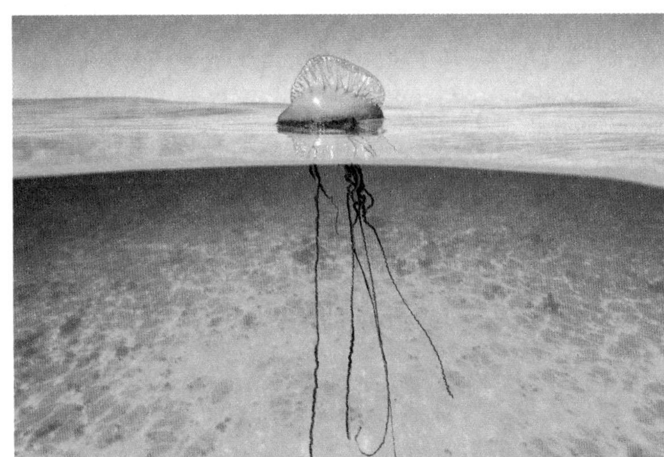

A

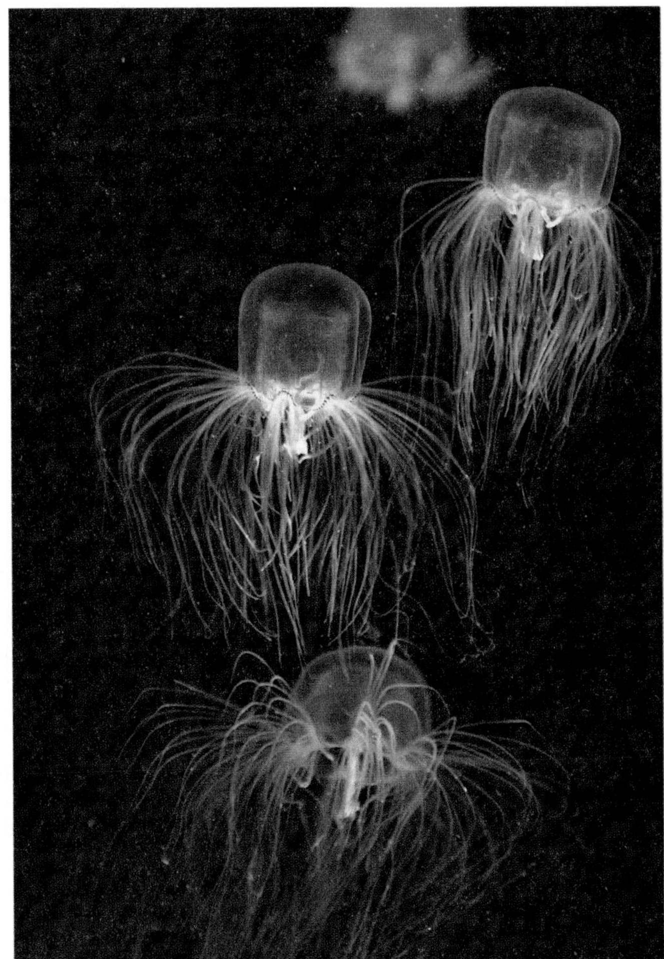

B

Figure 14-17 A. Atlantic Portuguese man o' war. **B.** Box jellyfish swimming just beneath the water surface.

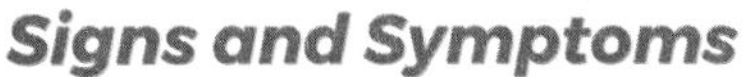

Signs and Symptoms

Jellyfish envenomation can cause the following signs and symptoms:

- Intense localized pain
- Swelling and skin discoloration along the line of tentacle contact (classically a whiplike rash; **Figure 14-18**)
- Nausea and vomiting
- Respiratory difficulty
- Cardiovascular toxicity that infrequently results in cardiac dysrhythmia and death

Treatment

The primary recommendations for treating jellyfish stings are to administer opioids and antihistamines, apply salt water, and place the affected area in warm (43°C to 45°C [110°F to 113°F]) water. Carefully remove nematocysts with a gloved hand and forceps or by scraping with a straight-edged tool (e.g., credit card) or a knife. Researchers have studied various methods of removing nematocysts, including flushing the area with water, vinegar, urine, or ethanol and applying commercially available products such as StingEze. Do not use fresh water, because the difference in osmolarity (compared with salt water) causes embedded nematocysts to fire. Vinegar is beneficial in some species, but intensifies symptoms in others. Optimal treatment depends on geographic location. In the United States, where *Physalia physalis*, or the Portuguese man-o-war, is of greatest concern, use sea water (not vinegar). In the Indo-Pacific region, where

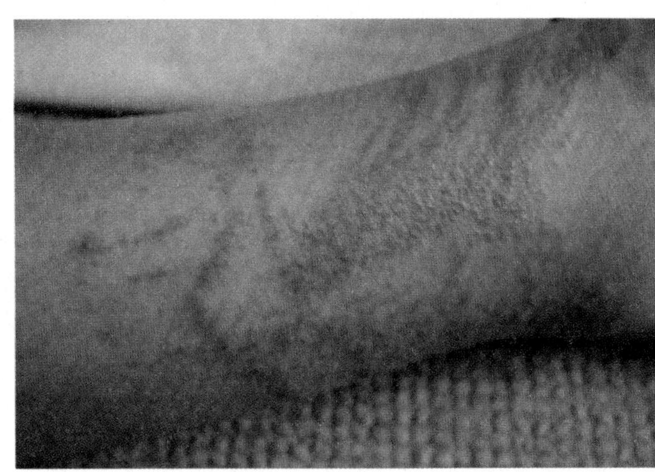

Figure 14-18 Whiplike pattern typical of a jellyfish sting.

Chironex fleckeri and *Carukia barnesi* are of concern, apply vinegar. Antivenom is of uncertain benefit and, in any case, is available only for box jellyfish stings and only in Australia and New Zealand.

Spinous Sea Creatures

Many species of fish and echinoderms have venomous spines. Venom from such spinous sea animals produces similar symptoms of varying severity, but the treatment is standard.

A stingray tail is armed with a serrated spine within an integumentary sheath that not only delivers venom but can also deliver significant traumatic injuries (**Figure 14-19**). The tail reflexively whips dorsally and may penetrate deeply into tissue, causing intrathoracic and intra-abdominal injuries that have sometimes been fatal to divers (e.g., Steve Irwin, the "Crocodile Hunter").

Sea urchins and other echinoderms have spines of varying lengths that typically envenomate humans when stepped on. Fish of the Scorpionidae family have venomous spines as well. This family includes the scorpion fish, the lionfish, and the stonefish, which is responsible for the most severe toxicity (**Figure 14-20**).

Signs and Symptoms

Toxicity from spinous marine animals causes severe local irritation and pain that may radiate proximally. Systemic symptoms can include nausea, vomiting, and cardiovascular instability. Envenomations are occasionally fatal.

Treatment

All venom from spinous creatures is heat labile, which means that heat will neutralize it. Prolonged immersion in hot water is associated with improvement in toxicity. The water temperature and the duration of immersion should be limited only by the patient's tolerance. Surgical intervention may be required to repair traumatic damage after stingray impalement.

The spines and stingers of all these fish and rays are brittle, often breaking off during exposure and attempted removal. Plain radiography is generally suggested to ensure that all fragments have been completely removed. Treat lacerations from spines. Update tetanus prophylaxis and consider giving antibiotic therapy covering normal skin flora and selected marine bacteria (e.g., *Vibrio parahaemolyticus*). Antivenom therapy is available and recommended for only a few species, including the stonefish, because of the potency of its venom.

Biting Sea Creatures

Sea snakes, cone snails, and the blue-ring octopus are all capable of delivering venom through bites/stings. Sea snake venom contains several toxins that primarily produce myotoxicity and neurotoxicity. Severe rhabdomyolysis and paralysis may occur.

Treatment

Supportive care and antivenom administration are the primary therapies recommended for marine envenomation. The following are specific recommendations:

- Blue-ring octopus venom consists of tetrodotoxin, a peripheral nervous system sodium channel blocker that causes paresthesia, paralysis, and respiratory depression in severe toxicity. Treatment is supportive.

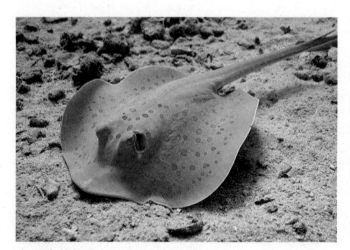

Figure 14-19 Blue-spotted stingray.

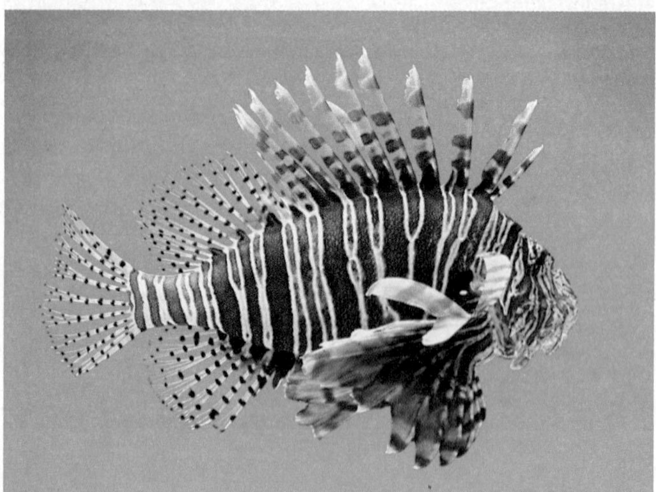

Figure 14-20 Adult lionfish.

Table 14-18 Mechanisms of Marine Foodborne Intoxication

Toxin	Source	Mechanism	Description	Clinical Manifestations	Treatment
Brevetoxin	Shellfish	Neuromuscular sodium channel opening	Neurotoxic shellfish poisoning	GI upset, paresthesia, hot/cold reversal	Supportive
Ciguatoxin	Reef fish (e.g., amberjack, barracuda, grouper, snapper)	Neuromuscular sodium channel opening	Seafood poisoning from ingestion of fish that ingested other fish that were toxic (dinoflagellates)	Paresthesia, GI upset, hot/cold reversal, bradycardia, hypotension	Supportive cyclic antidepressants for prolonged neuropathy
Saxitoxin	Shellfish	Neuromuscular sodium channel blockade	Paralytic shellfish poisoning	Numbness, paresthesia, muscle weakness, paralysis, respiratory failure	Supportive
Tetrodotoxin	Puffer fish (fugu), blowfish	Neuromuscular sodium channel blockade	Neurotoxin that blocks nerve cell action potential	GI upset, paresthesia, numbness, ascending paralysis, respiratory failure	Supportive
Domoic acid	Mussels	Glutamate and kainic acid analogs	Amnesic shellfish poisoning	GI upset, memory loss, coma, seizures	Supportive
Histidine	Tuna, mackerel, skipjack	Histamine production due to improper cooling	Scombroid fish poisoning	Upper body erythema, pruritus, bronchospasm, angioedema	Antihistamines

GI, Gastrointestinal.

- Cone snail bites may cause severe local pain and systemic sequelae of muscle weakness, coma, and cardiovascular collapse. Again, supportive therapy is indicated.

Poisonings Related to Seafood Consumption

A number of fish may cause systemic toxicity in a patient when ingested. Concern for suspected ingestions should be prompted when faced with these symptoms in the appropriate clinical setting. Table 14-18 summarizes these marine foodborne toxicities.

Toxic Plants and Mushrooms

Most plants and mushrooms are nontoxic or only slightly toxic, but plant ingestion can cause GI, cardiovascular, and neurologic toxicity through various mechanisms. Of the thousands of exposures annually, fatalities blamed on plants or mushrooms are rare. Most plant poisonings are accidental and involve household plants or ornamentals ingested by children. The categories of plant poisonings are GI irritants, dermatitis inducers, and oxalate-containing plant ingestions.

In any toxic plant or mushroom ingestion, gather a comprehensive patient history and collect a sample of the ingested material for later identification or laboratory analysis. Poison control centers and wilderness medicine resources can help you identify specific species and gauge their level of toxicity. It is not possible to become familiar with all the different poisonous plants and mushrooms in North America or with the mosaic of signs and symptoms they cause, but it is helpful to know how to approach a patient suspected of having ingested a toxic plant or mushroom. Generally, supportive care represents the backbone of therapy following exposure to toxic plants. Antidotes are available for certain plant toxins.

Plant Toxicity

Toxic plant exposure may be a result of touching, ingestion, or inhalation. The most dangerous exposures are often caused by smoking or by drinking tea made from a toxic plant.

The most common form of plant toxicity is local inflammation. Depending on the mechanism of exposure, this will most likely present as dermal, mucosal, or GI irritation. Early decontamination will increase patient comfort and prevent further exposure to the patient or responders.

Cardiac glycoside plants contain naturally occurring toxins similar to digoxin (see section on cardioactive agents). Plants containing cardiac glycosides, such as the lily of the valley, are popular as ornamental flowers and sometimes accidentally ingested, especially by children. The digoxin-like property of these plants increases the force of myocardial contraction and decreases the conduction rate of the AV node. Toxicity after ingestion of these plants is similar to toxicity after acute digoxin ingestion. The incidence of plant-induced cardiac glycoside toxicity is low, with only 1% of plant exposures attributable to cardiac glycoside plants. Mortality from plant cardiac glycoside toxicity is rare, and the rate is much lower than that associated with pharmaceutical digitalis toxicity. Other cardiotoxic plants include aconite (or monkshood), which contains a toxic alkaloid that may cause ventricular dysrhythmia.

Plants such as jimson weed and nightshade (*Atropa belladonna*) have anticholinergic toxicity. Hemlock and tobacco may cause nicotinic toxicity, causing muscle fasciculations and/or weakness, seizures, tachycardia, hypertension, and altered mental status; they may also induce the muscarinic SLUDGE symptoms. Many stone fruits (such as peaches, cherries, and almonds) contain amygdalin (like cyanide) in their seeds or pits. See previous sections in this chapter for more information on anticholinergic, cholinergic, and cyanide toxicities.

Identification

Following are examples of common plants that contain digoxin-like glycoside toxins (**Figure 14-21**):

- Foxglove (*Digitalis purpurea*)
- Lily of the valley (*Convallaria majalis*)
- Oleander (*Nerium oleander*)
- Red squill (*Urginea maritima*)
- Yellow oleander (*Thevetia peruviana*)

Signs and Symptoms

Irritating chemicals in many plants may produce redness or irritation at the site of contact, so begin by examining the patient's oropharynx for redness, irritation, swelling, or blistering. Excessive salivation, lacrimation, and diaphoresis may also be present. Abdominal effects of toxicity may include nausea and vomiting, cramps, and diarrhea. Severe exposures may diminish the patient's level of consciousness or induce a coma.

Acute toxicity from plants containing cardiac glycosides often initially presents with nonspecific GI symptoms. It may also induce hyperkalemia and neurologic symptoms such as altered mental status and weakness. Chronic toxicity likewise manifests with GI symptoms but can also cause weight loss, diarrhea, anorexia, hypokalemia, and hypomagnesemia. In both acute and chronic exposures, the patient usually reports a variety of cardiac symptoms, including palpitations, light-headedness, dizziness, shortness of breath, and chest pressure. Almost any type of dysrhythmia other than a rapidly conducted atrial dysrhythmia may occur and can rapidly evolve into a life-threatening ventricular tachycardia.

Differential Diagnosis

Remember that toxic plants will present with a wide variety of symptoms according to their underlying mechanisms. Maintain a wide differential when the history points to a plant exposure.

Diagnosis of plant toxicity depends on gathering accurate information from the scene and the patient. Ask whether the exposure was accidental or intentional and whether other people were also exposed. The poisoning may represent a suicide attempt, which may make the patient history unreliable. Examination of emesis may reveal plant material. The presence of cardiac glycoside plants in the environment should arouse suspicion if you detect cardiac dysrhythmia during the physical exam.

Treatment

The general steps in treating any plant toxicity include providing supportive care, minimizing further toxin absorption, neutralizing absorbed toxin using an antidote,

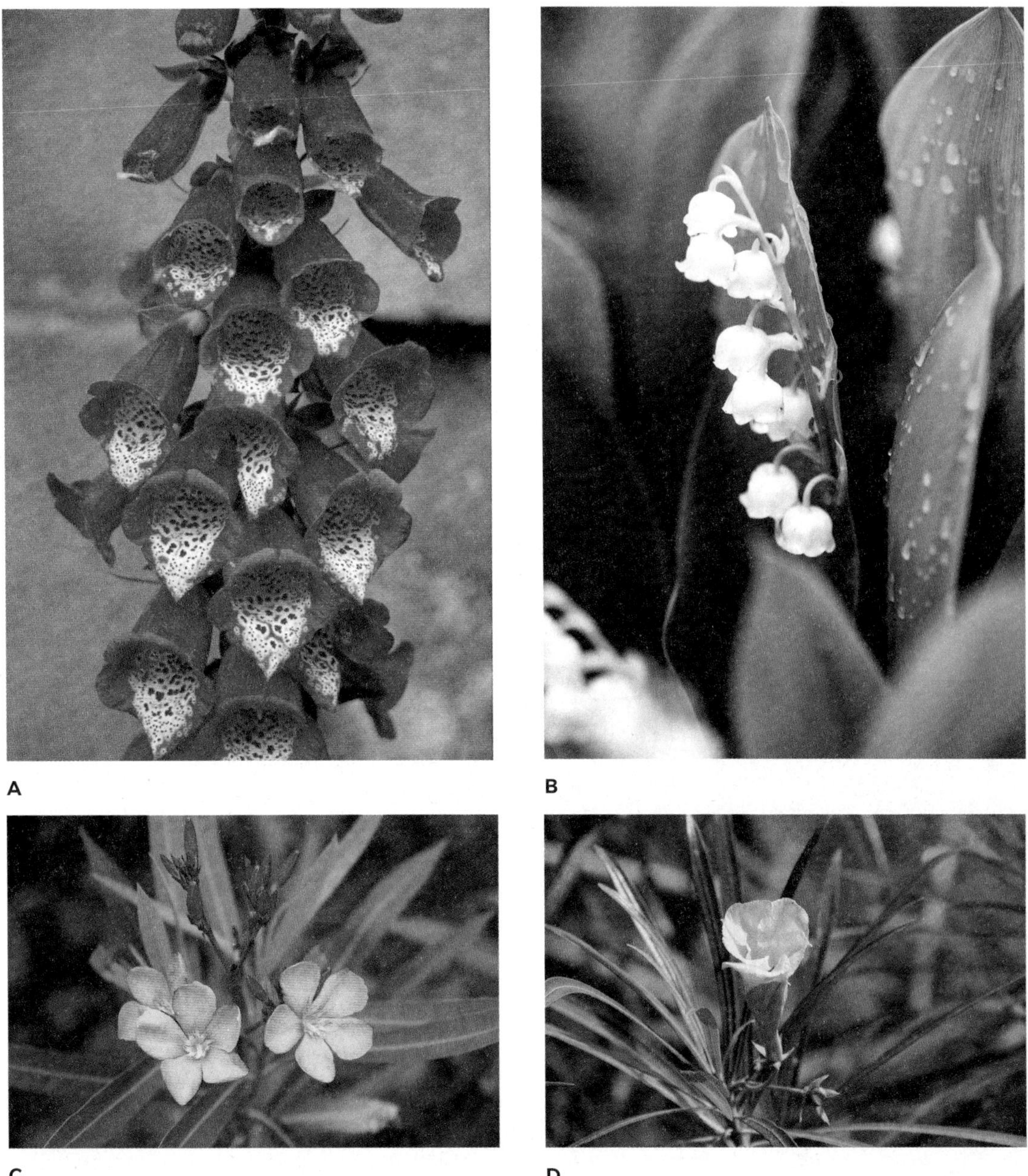

Figure 14-21 **A.** *Digitalis purpurea* (foxglove). **B.** Lily of the valley (*Convallaria majalis*). **C.** *Nerium oleander* (common oleander) plants have white or pink flowers and long, narrow seed pods. **D.** *Thevetia peruviana* (yellow oleander) has yellow flowers with smooth seed pods known as "lucky nuts," which are composed of green flesh surrounding a hard brown seed.

and treating any complications. Perform early decontamination, including consideration of GI decontamination in appropriate patients. Appropriate protocols for support of airway, breathing, and circulation should be followed.

Specific treatments are available for plants that cause cardiac glycoside, anticholinergic, and cyanide toxicities. Management of cardiac glycosides in the prehospital setting consists primarily of supportive care and transportation to the hospital for further evaluation and testing. Digoxin-specific Fab fragments may be given for hyperkalemia or hemodynamic instability. Physostigmine should be given to patients with anticholinergic toxicity (e.g., from Jimson weed or diphenhydrAMINE) with altered mental status. Cyanide toxicity (stone fruits) may be treated with cyanide antidote kits. Administer atropine to patients with bradycardia.

Mushroom Poisoning

Mushroom poisoning can be either accidental or intentional. Children sometimes ingest unknown mushrooms, and adults who forage for mushrooms for food can make mistakes and pick poisonous mushrooms. Hallucinogenic mushrooms may be ingested accidentally or intentionally; the age group most often affected seems to be children and young adults between the ages of 6 and 19 years. The cyclopeptide group of mushrooms, which includes the *Amanita* and *Galerina* genera, contains potent hepatotoxins (liver toxins) and accounts for most lethal exposures (**Figure 14-22**). General supportive care provides the most good until the patient can be evaluated in the emergency department. Many mushroom toxicities present with early symptoms. However, if a patient develops symptoms after 6 hours have passed, this is highly concerning for severe disease. A thorough history may be required to connect mushroom ingestion to late-presenting symptoms.

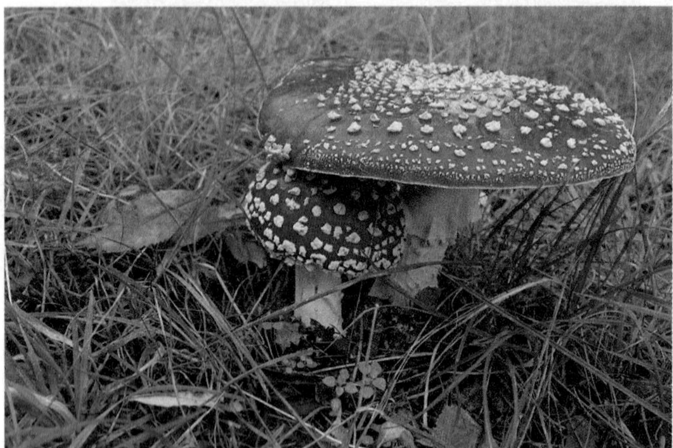

Figure 14-22 *Amanita muscaria* mushroom.

Putting It All Together

When you are a first responder for a patient exposed to a toxin, the initial scene and patient assessment challenges can be daunting. Maintain a heightened level of awareness for situations and patients that may present safety issues. Your AMLS training and skills can then help you organize a methodical health care plan. First you must know the extent of the threat of the toxic exposure to yourself and your patient, and then you must be able to implement appropriate safety precautions in addition to treating your patient's medical emergency.

Become familiar with local, regional, state, and federal agencies that can offer support in these situations. If mutual aid is required, those agencies should be contacted immediately for activation. As always, the AMLS Assessment Pathway provides the appropriate approach to evaluating the patient's presenting signs and symptoms, determining a working diagnosis, and arriving at an effective treatment plan. In toxicologic emergencies in particular, the patient's historical information can provide key clues to medical management that will stabilize the patient and improve outcomes.

SCENARIO SOLUTION

- Differential diagnoses may include sympathomimetic intoxication (cocaine, amphetamine, ePHEDrine, phencyclidine), stroke, autonomic hyperreflexia, or alcohol withdrawal.
- To narrow your differential diagnosis, complete a more thorough history of the patient's past and present illness. Question his roommate about the use of alcohol or other drugs. Perform a physical examination that includes vital sign assessment, stroke scale, pupil assessment, evaluation of heart and breath sounds, ECG monitoring and a 12-lead ECG, pulse oximetry, capnography, and blood glucose analysis. If you suspect autonomic hyperreflexia, look for a trigger such as a full bladder that could be the source of the problem.
- The patient has signs that indicate an exaggerated sympathetic response. Administer oxygen if indicated. Establish vascular access. Continue to monitor the ECG. Further treatment will depend on the rest of your assessment findings. If you suspect sympathomimetic overdose or alcohol withdrawal, treat with a benzodiazepine and IV fluid administration. If the patient has signs of stroke, transport him to the closest appropriate center. If the patient's exam points to autonomic hyperreflexia, transport if the source of the problem is not immediately resolved.

SUMMARY

- Ensure safety before entering any scene that may be contaminated, and consider airborne toxins that could be dangerous.
- Obtain a thorough history, including available drugs/toxins, time of ingestion, and dose. Ask bystanders and witnesses for additional information.
- Maintain supportive care for comatose patients, including airway management and administration of glucose, thiamine, and small doses of naloxone if necessary.
- Obtain an accurate core temperature, and institute temperature normalization strategies if necessary.
- Gauge perfusion status by monitoring mental status, urine output, blood pressure, capillary refill time, and acid–base status. Initiate invasive monitoring as time allows.
- Contact a poison control center early in the encounter to aid appropriate diagnosis and treatment of any toxicologic disorder if allowed by protocol.
- Performing a thorough assessment and obtaining a complete history can help eliminate secondary exposure by identifying contamination early.
- Presentation of signs and symptoms of exposure varies with different contaminants, on the basis of volatility, duration, and route of exposure.

Key Terms

anticholinergic The effects of substances that block the effect of acetylcholine. These can be used to treat conditions such as urinary incontinence. Anticholinergic symptoms include flushed skin, dry mount/eyes/skin, dilated pupils, delirium/confusion, fever, and urinary retention.

benzodiazepines A class of drugs that has a depressant effect on the central nervous system, which can be used in treatment of anxiety, panic disorders, seizures, and as a muscle relaxant, among other conditions.

cholinergic The effect of substances that lead to acetylcholine acting as a neurotransmitter. These effects include cramps, lacrimation, diarrhea, salivation, weakness, and muscle fasciculations.

delirium An acute mental disorder characterized by confusion, disorientation, restlessness, clouding of consciousness, incoherence, fear, anxiety, excitement, and often illusions.

gastrointestinal decontamination Any attempt to limit absorption or hasten elimination of a toxin from a patient's gastrointestinal tract. Examples include activated charcoal, gastric lavage, and whole-bowel irrigation. Although these methods do have a small role in toxicology, their use is not routinely recommended and should be discussed with a poison control center or medical toxicologist.

huffing The act of pouring an inhalant onto a cloth or into a bag and inhaling the substance, usually to alter one's mental status.

intoxication The state of being poisoned by a drug or other toxic substance; the state of being inebriated because of excessive alcohol consumption.

methemoglobinemia The presence of methemoglobin in the blood, which prevents the ability of hemoglobin to carry and transport oxygen to the tissues. Hemoglobin is converted to methemoglobin by nitrogen oxides and sulfa drugs.

packers Persons who ingest a large quantity of well-packed drugs for smuggling. These carefully prepared packages are less likely to rupture than those ingested by stuffers, but toxicity can be severe if they do because of the large amount of drug present.

stuffers Persons who hastily ingest small packets of poorly packaged drugs to evade law enforcement and to avoid drug confiscation. The dose is much lower than that seen with packers, but the likelihood of toxicity is much greater because the packages, meant for distribution, are likely to open in the patient's stomach or bowel.

toxidrome A specific syndrome-like group of symptoms associated with exposure to a given poison.

Bibliography

Acetadote [package insert]. Cumberland Pharmaceuticals, Inc., March 2004.

Afp. 'Crocodile Hunter' Steve Irwin stabbed hundreds of times by stingray, cameraman reveals. *The Telegraph*. March 10, 2014. https://www.telegraph.co.uk/news/worldnews/australiaandthepacific/australia/10687502/Crocodile-Hunter-Steve-Irwin-stabbed-hundreds-of-times-by-stingray-cameraman-reveals.html

American Academy of Clinical Toxicology & European Association of Poisons Centres and Clinical Toxicologists. Position paper: single-dose activated charcoal. *Clin Toxicol*. 2005;43(2):61–87.

Auerbach P. *Wilderness Medicine*. 7th ed. Elsevier; 2017.

Bailey B. Glucagon in beta blocker and calcium channel blocker overdoses: a systematic review. *J Toxicol Clin Toxicol*. 2003;41: 595–602.

Benson BE, Hoppu K, Troutman WG, et al. Position paper update: gastric lavage for gastrointestinal decontamination. *Clin Toxicol*. 2013;51(3):140–146.

Bar-Oz B, Levichek Z, Koren G. Medications that can be fatal for a toddler with one tablet or teaspoonful: a 2004 update. *Pediatr Drugs*. 2004;6(2):123–126.

Bilici R. Synthetic cannabinoids. *North Clin Istanbul*. 2014; 1(2):121–126. PMID: 28058316.

Brent J, Burkhart K, Dargan P, et al. *Critical Care Toxicology: Diagnosis and Management of the Critically Poisoned Patient*. Springer; 2017.

Budisavljevic MN, Stewart L, Sahn SA, et al. Hyponatremia associated with 3,4-methylenedioxy-methyamphetamine ("ecstasy") abuse. *Am J Med Sci*. 2003;326:89–93.

Bush DM, Woodwell D. *Update: Drug-Related Emergency Department Visits Involving Synthetic Cannabinoids*. The CBHSQ Report. October 16, 2014. Substance Abuse and Mental Health Services Administration, Center for Behavioral Health Statistics and Quality. This report was previously published as: *The DAWN Report: Update: Drug-Related Emergency Department Visits Involving Synthetic Cannabinoids*. October 16, 2014. Substance Abuse and Mental Health Services Administration, Center for Behavioral Health Statistics and Quality.

Caravati EM. Hallucinogenic drugs. In Dart RC, ed. *Medical Toxicology*, 3rd ed. Lippincott; 2004:1103–1111.

Cater RE. The use of sodium and potassium to reduce toxicity and toxic side effects from lithium. *Med Hypotheses*. 1986;20:359–383.

Centers for Disease Control and Prevention. *2018 Annual Surveillance Report of Drug-Related Risks and Outcomes—United States*. Surveillance Special Report. Centers for Disease Control and Prevention, U.S. Department of Health and Human Services. August 31, 2018. https://www.cdc.gov/drugover dose/pdf/pubs/2018-cdc-drug-surveillance-report.pdf

Centers for Disease Control and Prevention. U.S. overdose deaths in 2021 increased half as much as in 2020—but are still up 15%. May 11, 2022. https://www.cdc.gov/nchs/pressroom/nchs_press_releases/2022/202205.htm

Centers for Disease Control and Prevention. *Web-based Injury Statistics Query and Reporting System (WISQARS)*. 2021. http://www.cdc.gov/injury/wisqars/fatal.html

Chance BC, Erecinska M, Wagner M. Mitochondrial responses to carbon monoxide. *Ann NY Acad Sci*. 1970;174:193–203.

Chandler DB, Norton RL, Kauffman J. Lead poisoning associated with intravenous methamphetamine use—Oregon, 1988. *MMWR Morb Mortal Wkly Rep*. 1989;38:830–831.

Chyka PA, Seger D. Position statement: single-dose activated charcoal. *J Toxicol Clin Toxicol*. 1997;35:721–741.

Clark RF, Wethern-Kestner S, Vance MV, Gerkin R. Clinical presentation and treatment of black widow spider envenomation: a review of 163 cases. *Ann Emerg Med*. 1992;21(7):782–787.

Coupey SM. Barbiturates. *Pediatr Rev*. 1997;18:260–264.

Crane EH. *Highlights of the 2011 Drug Abuse Warning Network (DAWN) Findings on Drug-Related Emergency Department Visits*. The CBHSQ Report. February 22, 2013. Center for Behavioral Health Statistics and Quality, Substance Abuse and Mental Health Services Administration, Rockville, MD. Substance Abuse and Mental Health Services Administration, Center for Behavioral Health Statistics and Quality. June 19, 2014. *The DAWN Report: Emergency Department Visits Involving Methamphetamine: 2007 to 2011*. Rockville, MD.

Currance PL, Clements B, Bronstein AC. *Emergency Care for Hazardous Materials Exposure*. 3rd ed. Mosby; 2005.

Eddleston M, Ariaratnam CA, Meyer WP, et al. Multiple-dose activated charcoal in acute self-poisoning: a randomized controlled trial. *Lancet*. 2008;371:579–587.

Eddleston M, Eyer P, Worek F, et al. Pralidoxime in acute organophosphorus insecticide poisoning—a randomised controlled trial. *PLoS Med*. 2009;6(6):e1000104.

Emerson TS, Cisek JE. Methcathinone ("cat"): a Russian designer amphetamine infiltrates the rural Midwest. *Ann Emerg Med*. 1993;22:1897–1903.

Forrester MB. *Megalopyge opercularis* caterpillar stings reported to Texas poison centers. *Wilderness Environ Med*. 2018;29(2): 215–220.

Frierson J, Bailly D, Shultz T, et al. Refractory cardiogenic shock and complete heart block after unsuspected verapamil—SR and atenolol overdose. *Clin Cardiol*. 1991;14:933–935.

Garnier R, Guerault E, Muzard D, et al. Acute zolpidem poisoning—analysis of 344 cases. *J Toxicol Clin Toxicol*. 1994;32:391–404.

Graham SR, Day RO, Lee R, et al. Overdose with chloral hydrate: a pharmacological and therapeutic review. *Med J Aust*. 1988;149:686–688.

Gummin DD, Mowry JB, Beuhler MC, et al. 2020 annual report of the American Association of Poison Control Centers' National Poison Data System (NPDS): 38th annual report. *Clin Toxicol (Phila)*. 2021;59(12):1282–1501.

Hariman RJ, Mangiardi LM, McAllister RG, et al. Reversal of the cardiovascular effects of verapamil by calcium and sodium: differences between electrophysiologic and hemodynamic responses. *Circulation*. 1979;59:797–804.

Heard KJ. Acetylcysteine for acetaminophen poisoning. *N Engl J Med*. 2008;359(3):285–292.

Hedegaard H, Miniño AM, Warner M. *Drug overdose deaths in the United States, 1999–2017*. NCHS Data Brief, no 329. 2018. National Center for Health Statistics.

Hendren WC, Schreiber RS, Garretson LK. Extracorporeal bypass for the treatment of verapamil poisoning. *Ann Emerg Med.* 1989;18:984–987.

Hesse B, Pedersen JT. Hypoglycaemia after propranolol in children. *Acta Med Scand.* 1973;193:551–552.

Hoegholm A, Clementson P. Hypertonic sodium chloride in severe antidepressant overdosage. *J Toxicol Clin Toxicol.* 1991;29: 297–298.

Horowitz AL, Kaplan R, Sarpel G. Carbon monoxide toxicity: MR imaging in the brain. *Radiology.* 1987;162:787–788.

Kattimani S, Bharadwaj B. Clinical management of alcohol withdrawal: a systematic review. *Ind Psychiatry J.* 2013; 22(2):100–108.

Kerns W II, Schroeder D, Williams C, et al. Insulin improves survival in a canine model of acute beta blocker toxicity. *Ann Emerg Med.* 1997;29:748–757.

Kitchens CS, Van Mierop LHS. Envenomation by the eastern coral snake (*Micrurus fulvius fulvius*). *J Am Med Assoc.* 1987;258:1615–1618.

Kline JA, Tomaszewski CA, Schroeder JD, et al. Insulin is a superior antidote for cardiovascular toxicity induced by verapamil in the anesthetized canine. *J Pharm Exp Ther.* 1993;267:744–750.

Koren G, Nachmani A. Drugs that can kill a toddler with one tablet or teaspoonful: a 2018 updated list. *Clin Drug Investig.* 2019;39:217.

Kunkel DB, Curry SC, Vance MV, et al. Reptile envenomations. *J Toxicol Clin Toxicol.* 1983–1984;21:503–526.

Lange RA, Cigarroa RG, Yancy CW, et al. Potentiation of cocaine-induced coronary vasoconstriction by beta-adrenergic blockade. *Ann Intern Med.* 1990;112:897–903.

Lee WM. Acetaminophen (APAP) hepatotoxicity—Isn't it time for APAP to go away? *J Hepatol.* 2017;67:1324–1331.

Lefebvre KA, Robertson A. Domoic acid and human exposure risks: a review. *Toxicon.* 2010;56(2):218–230.

Leonard LG, Scheulen JJ, Munster AM. Chemical burns: effect of prompt first aid. *J Trauma.* 1982;22:420–423.

Long H, Nelson LS, Hoffman RS. A rapid qualitative test for suspected ethylene glycol poisoning. *Acad Emerg Med.* 2008;15: 688–690.

Love JN, Sachdeva DK, Curtis LA, et al. A potential role for glucagon in the treatment of drug-induced symptomatic bradycardia. *Chest.* 1998;114:323–326.

McCarron MM, Schulze BW, Thompson GA, et al. Acute phencyclidine intoxication. Clinical patterns, complications, and treatment. *Ann Emerg Med.* 1981;10:290–297.

Miura T, Mitomo M, Kawai R, et al. CT of the brain in acute carbon monoxide intoxication: characteristic features and prognosis. *AJNR Am J Neuroradiol.* 1985;6:739–742.

Moss MJ, Warrick BJ, Nelson LS, et al. ACMT and AACT position statement: preventing occupational fentanyl and fentanyl analog exposure to emergency responders. *Clin Toxicol (Phila).* 2018;56(4):297–300.

National Association of Emergency Medical Technicians. *PHTLS: Prehospital Trauma Life Support.* 10th ed. Public Safety Group; 2023.

National Institute on Drug Abuse. Benzodiazepines and opioids. https://nida.nih.gov/research-topics/opioids/benzodiazepines-opioids. Updated November 7, 2022.

National Institute on Drug Abuse. "Flakka" (alpha PVP). https://nida.nih.gov/research-topics/commonly-used-drugs-charts#bath-salts. Updated September 19, 2023.

National Institute on Drug Abuse. Synthetic cannabinoids (K2/spice). DrugFacts. https://nida.nih.gov/publications/drugfacts/synthetic-cannabinoids-k2spice. Updated June 2020.

National Institute on Drug Abuse; National Institutes of Health; U.S. Department of Health and Human Services. *Monitoring the Future: 2018 Survey Results: Teen Drug Use.* https://nida.nih.gov/research-topics/monitoring-the-future/survey-results-2021-infographic

Nelson L, Howland MA, Lewin NA, et al. *Goldfrank's Toxicologic Emergencies.* 11th ed. McGraw-Hill Education; 2019.

Olson KR, Anderson IB, Benowitz NL, et al. *Poisoning & Drug Overdose.* 7th ed. McGraw Hill Education; 2017.

Ostapowicz G, Fontana RJ, Schiodt FV, et al. Results of a prospective study of acute liver failure at 17 tertiary care centers in the United States. *Ann Intern Med.* 2002;137:947–954.

Pena BM, Krauss B. Adverse events of procedural sedation and analgesia in a pediatric emergency department. *Ann Emerg Med.* 1999;34:483–491.

Pentel PR, Benowitz NL. Tricyclic antidepressant poisoning—management of arrhythmias. *Med Toxicol.* 1986;1:101–121.

Prescott LF. Paracetamol overdosage: pharmacological considerations and clinical management. *Drugs.* 1983;25:290–314.

Raphael JC, Elkharrat D, Jars-Guincestre MC, et al. Trial of normobaric and hyperbaric oxygen for acute carbon monoxide intoxication. *Lancet.* 1989;2(8660):414–419.

Roth BA, Vinson DR, Kim S. Carisoprodol-induced myoclonic encephalopathy. *J Toxicol Clin Toxicol.* 1998;36:609–612.

Seger DL. Flumazenil—treatment or toxin? *J Toxicol Clin Toxicol.* 2004;42:209–216.

Signs and symptoms of various concentrations of carboxyhemoglobin levels. *UpToDate.* https://www.uptodate.com/contents/image?imageKey=SURG%2F106164

St. Onge M, Anseeuw K, Cantrell FL, et al. Experts consensus recommendations for the management of calcium channel blocker poisoning in adults. *Crit Care Med.* 2017;45(3): e306–315.

St. Onge M, Dubé PA, Gosselin S, et al. Treatment for calcium channel blocker poisoning: a systematic review. *Clin Toxicol.* 2014;52(9):926–944.

Suchard JR, LoVecchio F. Envenomations by rattlesnakes thought to be dead. *N Engl J Med.* 1999;340:1930.

Tracy DK, Wood DM, Baumeister D. Novel psychoactive substances: types, mechanisms of action, and effects. *BMJ.* 2017; 356:i6848.

Traylor J, Singhal M. Ciguatera toxicity. *StatPearls.* https://www.ncbi.nlm.nih.gov/books/NBK482511/. Updated February 7, 2023.

Van Hoesen KB, Camporesi EM, Moon RE, et al. Should hyperbaric oxygen be used to treat the pregnant patient for acute carbon monoxide poisoning? A case report and literature review. *J Am Med Assoc.* 1989;261:1039–1043.

Wason S, Lacouture PG, Lovejoy FH. Single high-dose pyridoxine treatment for isoniazid overdose. *J Am Med Assoc.* 1981; 246:1102–1104.

Weaver LK, Hopkins RO, Chan KJ, et al. Hyperbaric oxygen for acute carbon monoxide poisoning. *N Engl J Med.* 2002; 347:1057–1067.

Wiley CC, Wiley JF II. Pediatric benzodiazepine ingestion resulting in hospitalization. *J Toxicol Clin Toxicol*. 1998;36:227–231.

Woodward C, Pourmand A, Mazer-Amirshahi M. High dose insulin therapy, an evidence based approach to beta blocker /calcium channel blocker toxicity. *DARU J Pharm Sci*. 2014; 22:36.

Yildiz S, Aktas S, Cimsit M, et al. Seizure incidence in 80,000 patient treatments with hyperbaric oxygen. *Aviat Space Environ Med*. 2004;75:992–994.

Zakharov S, Vaneckova M, Seidl Z, et al. Successful use of hydroxocobalamin and sodium thiosulfate in acute cyanide poisoning: a case report with follow-up. *Basic Clin Pharmacol Toxicol*. 2015;117:209–212.

Glossary

absorption How the body takes in a specific drug.

acidosis An abnormal increase in the hydrogen ion concentration in the blood resulting from an accumulation of an acid or the loss of a base; indicated by a blood pH below the normal range.

acute coronary syndrome (ACS) An umbrella term that refers to a group of conditions caused by myocardial ischemia (insufficient blood supply to the heart muscle that results from coronary artery disease), including unstable angina, ST-segment elevation myocardial infarction (STEMI), and non–ST-segment elevation myocardial infarction (NSTEMI).

acute lung injury/acute respiratory distress syndrome (ALI/ARDS) Syndrome that typically occurs in ill patients, characterized by alveolar and pulmonary capillary breakdown leading to edema and alveolar collapse; this leads to severe hypoxemia and difficult ventilation.

acute mountain sickness (AMS) Illness from exposure to a high-altitude environment that presents with a variety of mild to moderate symptoms, including headache, weakness, fatigue, and body aches.

acute myocardial infarction (AMI) Commonly known as a "heart attack"; occurs when the blood supply to part of the heart is interrupted, causing heart cells to die. This is most commonly due to blockage of a coronary artery following the rupture of plaque within the wall of an artery. The resulting ischemia and decreased supply of oxygen, if left untreated, can cause damage and/or death of heart muscle tissue.

adaptive immune response The body's secondary response to infection. It has memory. It uses T cells (helper and killer) and B cells and their antibodies and the classic pathway of the complement cascade to accelerate or potentiate (slow) the response to infection.

Addison disease An endocrine disease caused by a deficiency of corticosteroid hormones produced by the adrenal cortex. The disease is characterized by nausea, vomiting, abdominal pain, and tanning of the skin.

adrenal crisis An endocrine emergency caused by a deficiency of corticosteroid hormones produced by the adrenal cortex. The disease is characterized by nausea, vomiting, abdominal pain, hypotension, hyperkalemia, and hyponatremia.

Advanced Medical Life Support (AMLS) Assessment Pathway A dependable framework to support the reduction of morbidity and mortality by using an assessment-based approach to determine a differential diagnosis and effectively manage a broad range of medical emergencies.

aerobic metabolism The normal metabolism that utilizes oxygen.

afterload In the intact heart, the pressure against which the ventricle ejects blood. It is impacted by the transmural pressure, peripheral vascular resistance, and the physical characteristics and volume of blood in the arterial system.

altered mental status Any decrease in normal level of wakefulness, change in mentation, or behavior that is not normal for a particular patient.

anaerobic metabolism The metabolism that takes place in the absence of oxygen; the principal by-product is lactic acid.

angioedema A vascular reaction that may have an allergic, hereditary, drug-induced, or other non-allergic cause and may result in profound swelling of the face, upper airway, and other regions of the body.

anosognosia Lack of insight caused by a neurologic condition such as a psychiatric disorder.

antibodies Immunoglobulins produced by lymphocytes in response to bacteria, viruses, or other antigenic substances.

antibodies Proteins produced by plasma cells/B cells in response to a specific antigen. Also known as immunoglobulins, they are the key component of the adaptive immune response.

anticholinergic The effects of substances that block the effect of acetylcholine. These can be used to treat conditions such as urinary incontinence. Anticholinergic symptoms include flushed skin, dry mouth/eyes/skin, dilated pupils, delirium/confusion, fever, and urinary retention.

antiemetics Substances that prevent or alleviate nausea and vomiting.

antigen A substance, usually a protein, that the body recognizes as foreign and that can evoke an immune response.

apneustic center A portion of the pons that assists in creating longer, slower respirations.

apoptosis Programmed cell death. Cytokines signal an infected or damaged host cell to die, preventing further escalation of infection to additional host cells.

assessment-based patient management Utilizing the patient's cardinal presentation; historical, diagnostic, and physical exam findings; and one's own critical-thinking skills as a health care professional to diagnose and treat a patient.

assisted reproductive technology (ART) Fertility treatments that help women become pregnant.

ataxia Loss of coordination of muscle control, which can lead to gait disturbance or extremity clumsiness. May be due to many causes, including peripheral nerve, spinal cord, or brain dysfunction, often of the cerebellum, which controls coordination.

atelectasis The collapse of the alveolar air spaces of the lungs.

B cells Lymphocytes that mature in the bone marrow and play an important role in the adaptive immune response. Also known as plasma cells, they produce antibodies (IgA, IgE, IgG, and IgM) that play a role in the body's immune response.

barotrauma Injury resulting from severe changes in barometric pressure, typically from rapid ascent after diving.

basophils Cells containing secretory granules that release histamine and heparin. They play a key role in the innate immune response.

benzodiazepines A class of drugs that has a depressant effect on the central nervous system, which can be used in treatment of anxiety, panic disorders, seizures, and as a muscle relaxant, among other conditions.

bias A tendency, preference, or inclination (either known or unknown) toward or against something or someone that prevents objectivity.

bipolar disorder A disorder with discrete episodes of both decreased mood (depressive episodes) and elevated mood (manic or hypomanic episodes).

blood pressure The tension exerted by blood on the arterial walls. Blood pressure is calculated using the following equation: Blood pressure = Flow × Resistance.

bloodborne pathogens (BBP) Pathogenic microorganisms that are transmitted via human blood and cause disease in humans; examples include hepatitis B virus and human immunodeficiency virus.

blood-brain barrier A filtering mechanism of the capillaries that carry blood to the brain and spinal cord tissue, blocking the passage of certain substances.

Boyle's law At a constant temperature, the volume of a gas is inversely proportional to its pressure (if you double the pressure of gas, you halve its volume; written as PV = K, where P = pressure, V = volume, and K = a constant).

capillary refill Time for tissues to reperfuse after compression (e.g., nail beds, fingers, toes).

carboxyhemoglobin Hemoglobin bound to carbon monoxide.

cardiac cycle A complete cardiac movement or heartbeat. The period from the beginning of one heartbeat to the beginning of the next; from diastole through systole.

cardiac output The effective volume of blood expelled by either ventricle of the heart per unit of time (usually volume per minute). It is equal to the stroke volume multiplied by the heart rate.

cardiac output The volume of blood pumped by the heart over time. Cardiac output is often recorded in liters per minute. It can be calculated as the heart rate times the stroke volume (the volume of blood pumped in a single cardiac contraction).

cardiac tamponade Also known as "pericardial tamponade"; an emergent condition in which fluid accumulates in the pericardium (the sac that surrounds the heart) and restricts the amount of blood that can reenter the heart. If the amount of fluid increases slowly (such as in hypothyroidism), the pericardial sac can expand to contain a liter or more of fluid prior to tamponade occurring. If the fluid increases rapidly (as may occur after trauma or myocardial rupture), as little as 100 mL can cause tamponade.

cardinal presentation The patient's primary presenting sign or symptom from the clinician's perspective; often this is similar to the patient's chief complaint, but it may be an objective finding such as unconsciousness or choking.

cerebral perfusion pressure (CPP) Represents the pressure gradient driving cerebral blood flow (CBF) and therefore oxygen and metabolite delivery; it is the difference between the mean arterial pressure (MAP) and the intracranial pressure (ICP). CPP = MAP − ICP.

cerebrospinal fluid (CSF) A transparent, slightly yellowish fluid in the subarachnoid space around the brain and spinal cord.

chemokines A subclass of cytokines (signaling proteins) released by cells that cause the attraction of other cells to the area (i.e., chemotaxis).

chemoreceptors Chemical receptors that sense changes in the composition of blood and body fluids. The primary chemical changes registered by chemoreceptors are those involving levels of hydrogen (H^+), carbon dioxide (CO_2), and oxygen (O_2).

cholinergic The effect of substances that lead to acetylcholine acting as a neurotransmitter. These effects include cramps, lacrimation, diarrhea, salivation, weakness, and muscle fasciculations.

clinical decision making The ability to integrate assessment findings and test data with experience and evidence-based guidelines to make decisions regarding the most appropriate treatment.

clinical reasoning The combination of good judgment with clinical experience to make accurate diagnoses and initiate proper treatment. This process assumes the clinician has a strong foundation of clinical knowledge.

coagulation cascade Causes clot formation and regulation after exposure to tissue damage. It can be triggered by the extrinsic or intrinsic pathway and by platelet or cell damage.

cognitive bias A systematic error in thinking that impacts how one interprets information from the environment and distorts judgment in favor of or against certain ideas, actions, or people.

communicable diseases Any disease transmitted from one person or animal to another either directly, by contact with excreta or other discharges from the body; or indirectly, by means of substances or inanimate objects such as contaminated drinking glasses, toys, or water, or by vectors such as flies, mosquitoes, ticks, or other insects.

complement cascade Complement can be triggered to be activated indirectly by exposure to a pathogen in the innate immune response, causing opsonization of the invading microbe, sending additional signals in the area to cause inflammation and phagocytosis. It can also be triggered directly by exposure to specific antibodies to the invading pathogen. This leads to formation of the membrane attack complex under the classic complement cascade in the adaptive immunity response.

complement Inactive proteins produced by the liver that play a key role in the innate and adaptive immune responses.

contaminated A condition of being soiled, stained, touched, or otherwise exposed to harmful agents, making an object potentially unsafe for use as intended or without barrier techniques; for example, entry of infectious or toxic materials into a previously clean or sterile environment.

culture of safety An organizational culture in which leaders, directors, and staff emphasize safety over opposing goals.

Cushing triad Hypertension; bradycardia; and rapid, deep, or irregular respirations.

cytokines Signaling proteins released by cells that initiate further response by the surrounding cells.

decision-making capacity The ability to understand choices, the risks and rewards of choices, and alternatives available so as to make an informed decision for oneself.

decompression sickness A broad range of signs and symptoms caused by nitrogen bubbles in blood and tissues coming out of solution on ascent.

decontamination The process of removing foreign material such as blood, body fluids, or radioactivity; it does not eliminate microorganisms, but is a necessary step preceding disinfection or sterilization.

delirium An acute mental disorder characterized by confusion, disorientation, restlessness, clouding of consciousness, incoherence, fear, anxiety, excitement, and often illusions.

dendritic cells Act as a messenger between the innate immune response and the adaptive immune response. They present pieces of the invading microbe, known as antigens, along their cell surface.

diabetic ketoacidosis (DKA) An acute endocrine emergency caused by a lack of insulin. The condition is characterized by an elevated blood glucose level, ketone production, metabolic acidosis, dehydration, nausea, vomiting, abdominal pain, and tachypnea.

differential diagnoses The possible causes of the patient's clinical condition.

distribution The distribution of a medication throughout the body (between the plasma and the other body components).

drowning The process of experiencing respiratory impairment from submersion or immersion in liquid.

dysarthria Garbled speech (but of one's intended words) due to cranial nerve motor dysfunction (distinguish from expressive and receptive aphasia).

elimination The process by which a drug is excreted from the body. In humans, this is typically via the kidneys or the liver. Physiologic effects on these organs can affect how fast or how much of a medication is removed from the body.

embolus A particle that travels in the circulatory system and obstructs blood flow when it becomes lodged in a smaller artery. A blood clot is the most common type of embolus, but fat (after long bone fracture), atherosclerotic, and air (diving) emboli can also occur.

endemic A disease that is present in the community at a given baseline level over time, such as herpes or chickenpox.

end-tidal carbon dioxide ($ETCO_2$) The CO_2 level in the expired air at the end of expiration.

eosinophils Cells containing secretory granules that release histamine and cytokines. They play a key role in parasitic infections and allergic reactions.

epidemic A disease that affects a significantly large number of people at the same time and spreads rapidly through a demographic segment of the human population.

epidemiology The study of the determinants of disease events in populations.

exercise-associated hyponatremia A condition due to prolonged exertion in a hot environment coupled with excessive hypotonic fluid intake that leads to nausea; vomiting; and, in severe cases, mental status changes and seizures (also known as exertional hyponatremia).

exposure incidents Being in the presence of or subjected to a force or influence (e.g., viral exposure, heat exposure).

expressive aphasia Inability to speak intended words due to dysfunction of the cerebral speech center (Broca's area) in the left frontal lobe (distinguish from dysarthria).

fomite An inanimate object that can become contaminated with an infectious pathogen and spread disease.

frostbite Localized damage to tissues resulting from prolonged exposure to extreme cold.

frostnip Early frostbite, characterized by numbness and pallor without significant tissue damage.

gas exchange The process in which oxygen in the alveoli is taken up by circulating blood cells and carbon dioxide from the bloodstream is released to air in the alveoli.

gastrointestinal (GI) Pertaining to the organs of the gastrointestinal tract. The GI tract links the organs involved in consumption, processing, and elimination of nutrients. Components include the mouth, pharynx, esophagus, stomach, small and large intestines, and rectum/anus.

gastrointestinal decontamination Any attempt to limit absorption or hasten elimination of a toxin from a patient's gastrointestinal tract. Examples include activated charcoal, gastric lavage, and whole-bowel irrigation. Although these methods do have a small role in toxicology, their use is not routinely recommended and should be discussed with a poison control center or medical toxicologist.

gastroparesis A medical condition characterized by paresis (partial paralysis) of the stomach, resulting in food remaining in the stomach for an abnormally long time.

gender expression The way a person communicates gender identity to the outside world.

gender identity The personal sense of one's own gender.

gender The internal sense of how someone identifies in relation to the socially constructed roles and characteristics of men and women, rather than biological characteristics.

granulocytes A type of a white blood cell with secretory granules in its cytoplasm; that is, a neutrophil, basophil, or eosinophil.

heat illness A spectrum of illnesses related to excessive heat exposure or heat generation, ranging from rash and cramps to heat exhaustion and heatstroke.

hematemesis Vomiting of bright red blood, indicating upper gastrointestinal bleeding.

hematochezia Passage of red blood through the rectum.

hemiparesis Unilateral mild to moderate weakness, usually occurring on the opposite side of the body from the stroke (distinguish from hemiplegia).

hemiplegia Paralysis or severe weakness on one side of the body (distinguish from hemiparesis).

hemorrhagic stroke Damage to the brain from bleeding in the brain tissue (intracerebral), most commonly related to hypertension, or into the subarachnoid space, often due to rupture of an aneurysm or arteriovenous malformation.

high-altitude cerebral edema (HACE) Brain swelling and dysfunction associated with exposure to high altitudes.

high-altitude pulmonary edema (HAPE) A noncardiogenic form of pulmonary edema (fluid accumulation in the lungs) that occurs in high altitudes.

history of present illness (HPI) Information about the patient's chief complaint and related symptoms. The primary elements of the HPI can be obtained by using the OPQRST and SAMPLER mnemonics. It is the most important element of patient assessment.

hospital-acquired infection/ health care–associated infection (HAI) An infection acquired from exposure to an infectious agent at a health care facility, defined as at least 72 hours after hospitalization.

huffing The act of pouring an inhalant onto a cloth or into a bag and inhaling the substance, usually to alter one's mental status.

human trafficking Using force, fraud, or coercion to obtain some type of forced labor or commercial sex act (sexual slavery).

hypercapnia An abnormally elevated carbon dioxide level in the blood, caused by hypoventilation or lung disease. It may also be caused by exposure to environments containing abnormally high concentrations of carbon dioxide, or by rebreathing exhaled carbon dioxide. Usually defined as a carbon dioxide level > 45 mm Hg. This term is interchangeable with hypercarbia.

hyperosmolar hyperglycemic syndrome (HHS) An endocrine emergency characterized by a high plasma glucose concentration, absent ketone production, and increased serum osmolality (> 315 mOsm/kg). The syndrome causes severe dehydration, nausea, vomiting, abdominal pain, and tachypnea.

hyperthermia Unusually elevated body temperature above 38.5°C (101.3°F).

hypobaric hypoxia Low oxygen content caused by low atmospheric pressure.

hypoglycemia A plasma glucose concentration of > 70 mg/dL. This condition is often associated with signs and symptoms such as sweating, cold skin, tachycardia, and altered mental status.

hypothermia Core body temperature below 35°C (95°F); at lower temperatures, it may induce cardiac arrhythmia and precipitate a decline in mental status.

hypovolemia Abnormally decreased volume of circulating blood in the body, due to loss of either blood or plasma.

ideal body weight (IBW) A measure used for medication dosing. IBW (kg) = 50 (males) or 45.5 (females) + 2.3 kg × each inch over 5 feet.

immune system Protects the body from invading pathogens; includes the spleen, thymus, bone marrow, lymphatic system, T cells, and B cells.

indications Conditions or circumstances for which a medication is administered.

infectious diseases Diseases caused by another living organism or virus, which may or may not be transmissible to another person.

innate immune response The body's initial response to a foreign microbe. It has no memory and is nonspecific. The type of response incorporates the alternative complement pathway, natural killer cells, granulocytes, monocytes, and mast cells.

intervention Action taken to improve something, such as administering medication for a medical issue.

intimate partner violence (IPV) Violence by a spouse or partner (current or former) in an intimate domestic relationship against the other spouse or partner.

intoxication The state of being poisoned by a drug or other toxic substance; the state of being inebriated because of excessive alcohol consumption.

intracranial pressure (ICP) A measure of the hydrostatic pressure of the intracranial CSF fluid. Swelling (cerebral edema), increased volume of CSF (hydrocephalus), tumor, and intracranial hemorrhage can increase the ICP. If ICP is increased significantly, perfusion to the brain can be impaired and brain structures can herniate, causing severe neurologic impairment and death.

intussusception Prolapse of one segment of the bowel into the lumen of adjacent bowel. This kind of intestinal obstruction may involve segments of the small intestine, colon, or terminal ileum and cecum.

ischemia Insufficient oxygen and nutrient delivery to an organ or tissue caused by decreased blood flow, severe anemia or hypoxia, or an increased metabolic demand, which leads to damage or dysfunction of the tissue.

ischemic stroke A stroke that occurs when a thrombus or embolus obstructs a blood vessel, diminishing blood flow to and causing injury to the affected area of the brain.

Korsakoff syndrome Chronic and irreversible condition involving cognitive dysfunction, especially memory loss, due to prolonged thiamine deficiency.

Ludwig angina A deep-space infection of the floor of the mouth and anterior neck just below the mandible.

lymphocytes White blood cells that are part of the immune system; they are differentiated as B cells and T cells.

macrophages Monocytes capable of engulfing an invading pathogen or infected host cell.

mean arterial pressure (MAP) The average pressure in a patient's arteries during one cardiac cycle, an indicator of perfusion to vital organs; to calculate MAP: SBP + (2 × DBP) / 3

medication concentration The amount of a drug in the body related to the concentration of the drug measured in a biologic fluid (blood).

melena Abnormal black, tarry stool that has a distinctive odor and contains digested blood; results from an upper gastrointestinal source of bleeding.

menarche Onset of menstruation and fertility.

menopause End of menstruation and fertility.

metabolism The process by which a drug is broken down (degraded) into inactive components or to active metabolites causing an effect on the body.

metabolites Breakdown products of a drug, Inactive metabolites no longer exert a pharmacologic effect; active metabolites continue to exert a metabolic effect (which may be the same or different from the parent drug's effect).

methemoglobinemia The presence of methemoglobin in the blood, which prevents the ability of hemoglobin to carry and transport oxygen to the tissues. Hemoglobin is converted to methemoglobin by nitrogen oxides and sulfa drugs.

monocytes White blood cells that can differentiate into macrophages or dendritic cells. They play a key role in the innate immune response.

myxedema coma Severe hypothyroidism associated with cold intolerance, weight gain, weakness, and declining mental status.

necrosis Unregulated cell death caused by factors external to the cell, such as bacterial toxins or injury.

neurotransmitters Chemical substances that are released at the end of a nerve fiber by the arrival of a nerve impulse (action potential) and, by diffusing across the synapse or junction, cause the transfer of the impulse to another nerve fiber, a muscle fiber, or some other structure.

neutrophils Cells containing secretory granules and comprising greater than 50% granulocytes. They play a key role in the innate immune response by enveloping invading pathogens and releasing enzymes and cytokines to destroy the invading microbe and alert the host immune response.

nitrogen narcosis A state resembling alcohol intoxication produced by nitrogen gas dissolved in the blood at high ambient pressure.

noninvasive positive-pressure ventilation (NIPPV) A procedure in which positive pressure is provided through the upper airway by some type of mask or other noninvasive device.

non–ST-elevation myocardial infarction (NSTEMI) A type of myocardial infarction that is not associated with ST-segment elevation on electrocardiogram (ECG) recordings. It is diagnosed on the basis of laboratory tests for elevated cardiac enzymes.

normalization of deviance Occurs when an improper practice or standard gradually becomes tolerable and accepted, resulting in repeated deviant behavior (without disastrous results) that then becomes the procedural norm.

nosocomial infection See hospital-acquired infection/health care–associated infection (HAI).

ophthalmoplegia Abnormal function of the eye muscles.

opsonization The act of marking a foreign microbe or antigen for phagocytosis or a dead cell for recycling. Surfactant in the lung can cover invading microbes and mark them for phagocytosis as part of the innate immune response. Complement proteins can also cover or mark an invading microbe or antigen as part of the innate immune response. Antibodies can identify and mark an invading microbe as part of the adaptive immune response.

packers Persons who ingest a large quantity of well-packed drugs for smuggling. These carefully prepared packages are less likely to rupture than those ingested by stuffers, but toxicity can be severe if they do because of the large amount of drug present.

pandemic A disease occurring throughout the population of a large part of the world.

parenteral Pertaining to treatment other than through the digestive system.

pattern recognition A process of recognizing and classifying data based on past knowledge and experience.

perfusion The delivery of oxygenated blood to body tissues.

pericarditis A condition in which the tissue surrounding the heart (pericardium) becomes inflamed. It can be caused by several factors, but is often related to a viral infection.

peritonsillar abscess An abscess in the submucosal space adjacent to the tonsils. This abscess and its accompanying inflammation can cause the uvula to deviate to the opposing side.

personality disorders A group of mental disorders that cause an inflexible and unhealthy way of thinking, behaving, and functioning that impacts daily life and relationships.

phagocytes Cells that can engulf a foreign cell or an infected host cell. Include macrophages and neutrophils.

pharmacodynamics The effect that a drug exerts on the body. It is based on where and which receptors, enzymes, or other proteins a drug binds to in the body.

pharmacokinetics The absorption, distribution, metabolism, and excretion of medications.

pharmacokinetics What the body does to a drug; how the drug is absorbed, metabolized, and excreted.

pharmacology The study of interactions between substances and living organisms.

pleurae Thin membranes that surround and protect the lungs (visceral) and line the chest cavity (parietal).

pneumotaxic center Located in the pons, this center generally controls the rate and pattern of respiration.

polymerase chain reaction (PCR) A laboratory method used to replicate DNA that is leveraged to test for the presence of genetic material from organisms, including viruses.

preload The volume of blood in the ventricle at the end of diastole. It reflects venous return and the stress or stretch on the ventricular wall. Also called end-diastolic volume.

primary survey The process of initially assessing the airway, breathing, circulation, and disability status to identify and manage life-threatening conditions and establish priorities for further assessment, treatment, and transport.

proprioception Sensory function that provides the awareness of the location of one's own body parts relative to the rest of the body.

pulmonary embolism (PE) The sudden blockage of a pulmonary artery by a blood clot, often originating from a deep vein in the legs or pelvis, that embolizes and travels to the lung. Symptoms include tachycardia, hypoxia, and hypotension.

pulse pressure The difference between the systolic and diastolic blood pressures.

pulse pressure The difference between the systolic and diastolic blood pressures; normal pulse pressure is 30 to 40 mm Hg.

pulsus paradoxus An exaggeration of the normal inspiratory decrease in systolic blood pressure, defined by an inspiratory fall of systolic blood pressure of > 10 mm Hg.

receptors Chemical structures that receive or interact with a drug or hormone and transduce signals, which may be integrated into a biologic system. Receptors typically relay, amplify, or integrate a chemical or electrical signal.

referred pain Pain felt at a site different from that of an injured or diseased organ or body part.

reflective listening A communication technique in which you listen to a speaker, and then repeat back what you heard to confirm the speaker was understood.

respiration (1) Physiologically, the transfer of oxygen from the environment to the cells of the body and the reciprocal transfer of carbon dioxide from the body to the environment. (2) Biochemically, the generation of energy through the oxidation of nutrients.

respiratory failure A disorder in which the lungs become unable to perform their basic task of gas exchange—that is, the transfer of oxygen from inhaled air into the blood and the transfer of carbon dioxide from the blood into exhaled air.

retrovirus Any of a family of ribonucleic acid (RNA) viruses containing reverse transcriptase, an enzyme, in the virion; examples include human immunodeficiency virus (HIV1, HIV2) and human T-cell lymphotropic virus.

schizophrenia A mental disorder that causes a breakdown between thoughts, emotions, and behavior that leads to faulty perceptions, loss of reality, inappropriate behavior, and difficulty with daily functioning and relationships.

secondary survey An in-depth systematic head-to-toe physical examination, including vital signs.

seizure An episode of abnormal neuronal activity in the cerebral cortex that can cause loss of or alteration in consciousness, convulsions or tremors, incontinence, behavior changes, subjective changes in perception (taste, smell, fears), and other symptoms.

sepsis The body's response to potentially life-threatening infection.

septic abortion A severe infection of the uterus associated with an induced or spontaneous abortion.

sex The biological characteristics a person was born with or assigned at birth, such as anatomy and physiology with reproductive organs, chromosomes, and hormones.

sexual assault Nonconsensual sexual contact.

sexually transmitted infections (STIs) Infections transmitted through sexual contact.

shock index (SI) A measure of hemodynamic status particularly useful in patients with compensated shock. It is calculated by dividing the heart rate by the systolic blood pressure, with a normal range of 0.5 to 0.7. Increasing values, particularly > 0.9, indicate worsening hemodynamic status.

shock A condition of profound hemodynamic and metabolic disturbance characterized by failure of the circulatory system to maintain adequate perfusion to vital organs. It may result from inadequate blood volume, cardiac function, or vasomotor tone or from obstruction to blood flow.

side effects Unexpected or untoward effects caused by a drug that occur in addition to the desired therapeutic effect of a medication.

signs Objective evidence that a health care professional observes, feels, sees, hears, touches, or smells.

social determinants of health Nonclinical factors that impact a person's health outcomes, including income, education, age, health literacy, racism, environment, housing, and social mobility, as well as access to health care, transportation, safe food and water.

somatic (parietal) pain Generally well-localized pain caused by an irritation of the nerve fibers in the parietal peritoneum or other tissues (e.g., musculoskeletal system). Physical findings include sharp, discrete, localized pain accompanied by tenderness to palpation, guarding of the affected area, and rebound tenderness.

stable angina Symptoms of chest pain, shortness of breath, or other equivalent symptoms that occur predictably with exertion, then resolve with rest, suggesting the presence of a fixed coronary lesion that prevents adequate perfusion with increased demand.

standard precautions Guidelines recommended by the Centers for Disease Control and Prevention for reducing the risk of transmission of bloodborne and other pathogens in hospitals. Standard precautions apply to (1) blood; (2) all body fluids, secretions, and excretions except sweat, regardless of whether or not they contain blood; (3) nonintact skin; and (4) mucous membranes.

ST-elevation myocardial infarction (STEMI) A type of acute myocardial infarction associated with ST-elevation in a vascular distribution on 12-lead electrocardiogram (ECG) recordings. These attacks carry a substantial risk of death and disability and call for a quick response by a system geared toward reperfusion therapy.

stigma Viewing someone in a negative way due to a characteristic, trait, or condition the person has.

stroke center Hospital or receiving facility that is designated as an appropriate facility with appropriate resources to receive, assess, and treat patients with suspected stroke. Regional authorities that designate stroke centers often use outside accrediting organizations to ensure that the center meets standards for preparedness and care.

stroke volume The amount of blood ejected by the ventricle during each heartbeat.

stroke A brain injury that occurs when blood flow to a part of the brain is obstructed or interrupted or when nontraumatic bleeding in the brain damages brain cells from increased pressure. (See ischemic stroke and hemorrhagic stroke.)

stuffers Persons who hastily ingest small packets of poorly packaged drugs to evade law enforcement and to avoid drug confiscation. The dose is much lower than that seen with packers, but the likelihood of toxicity is much greater because the packages, meant for distribution, are likely to open in the patient's stomach or bowel.

symptoms Subjective perceptions by patients indicating what they feel, such as nausea, or have experienced, such as a sensation of seeing flashing lights.

T cells Lymphocytes that mature in the thymus and play an important role in escalating the adaptive immune response. There are two types: helper and cytotoxic/killer.

tension pneumothorax A life-threatening condition that results from progressive worsening of a simple pneumothorax (an accumulation of air under pressure in the pleural space). It can lead to progressive restriction of venous return, which leads to decreased preload, then systemic hypotension.

therapeutic communication A communication process in which the health care clinician uses effective communication skills to obtain information about the patient's condition, including the use of the four Es: engagement, empathy, education, and enlistment.

thermoregulation The process by which the body compensates for environmental extremes.

thoracentesis A procedure to remove fluid or air from the pleural space.

thoracic duct Located in the left upper thorax; the largest lymph vessel in the body. It returns the excess fluid that is not collected by the veins from the lower extremities and abdomen to the venae cavae.

thoracostomy A procedure in which an opening is made through the skin into the pleural cavity; a tube is often placed through the opening to facilitate drainage of air, blood, or other fluid.

thrombus A blood clot that forms in a blood vessel and causes obstruction where it forms.

thyroid storm An endocrine emergency characterized by hyperfunction of the thyroid gland. This disorder is associated with fever, tachycardia, nervousness, altered mental status, and hemodynamic instability.

thyrotoxicosis A condition of elevated thyroid hormone levels, which often leads to signs and symptoms of tachycardia, tremor, weight loss, and high-output heart failure.

toxidrome A specific syndrome-like group of symptoms associated with exposure to a given poison.

transgender Persons whose gender identity or gender expression does not conform to that typically associated with the sex to which they were assigned at birth.

transient ischemic attack (TIA) Sometimes referred to as a "mini stroke," TIA is a condition of low or interrupted blood flow to a part of the brain, causing transient ischemia and strokelike symptoms that resolve within 24 hours. A TIA is considered a warning sign of an impending stroke.

trauma-informed care Clinical approach acknowledging that a patient's previous experiences affect their responses to subsequent health care issues and encounters.

ultrasound Also called sonography or diagnostic medical sonography; an imaging method that uses high-frequency sound waves to produce precise images of structures within the body.

unstable angina Angina of increased frequency, severity, or occurring with less intensive exertion than the baseline. It suggests the narrowing of a static lesion, causing further limitations of coronary blood flow with increased demand.

virulence The power of a microorganism to produce disease.

visceral pain Poorly localized pain that occurs when the walls of the hollow organs are stretched, thereby activating the stretch receptors. This kind of pain is characterized by a deep, persistent ache ranging from mild to intolerable and commonly described as cramping, burning, and gnawing.

viscus (pl. viscera) An organ enclosed within a body cavity. Typically used to refer to hollow organs such as esophagus, stomach, and intestines.

volvulus A condition in which a segment of the gastrointestinal tract twists on itself, causing a closed loop bowel obstruction. Often the feeding blood vessels also become twisted, blocking the flow of blood and leading to ischemia and eventually infarction of the involved loop of bowel. This most commonly occurs in the cecum and sigmoid regions of the large intestine but may involve the stomach and small intestine.

Wernicke encephalopathy A disorder caused by deficiency of thiamine (vitamin B1) and characterized by a triad of symptoms: acute confusion, ataxia, and ophthalmoplegia.

working diagnosis The presumed cause of the patient's condition, arrived at by evaluating all assessment information thus far obtained while conducting further diagnostic testing to definitively diagnose the illness.

Index

Note: Page numbers followed by "*f*" and "*t*" refer to figures and tables, respectively.

A

C

F

J

K

L

M

N

P

Q

R

S

T

W

Z